MOSBY'S
TEXTBOOK FOR

LONG-TERM CARE ASSISTANTS

THIRD EDITION

With 792 Illustrations

MOSBY'S

TEXTBOOK FOR

LONG-TERM CARE ASSISTANTS

THIRD EDITION

Sheila A. Sorrentino, RN, PhD
Curriculum and Health Care Consultant
Normal, Illinois

Bernie Gorek, RNC, GNP, MA
Director of Residential Care and Services,
Bonell Good Samaritan Center
Greeley, Colorado

Mosby

St. Louis Baltimore Boston Carlsbad Chicago Minneapolis New York Philadelphia Portland
London Milan Sydney Tokyo Toronto

Mosby
Dedicated to Publishing Excellence

Editor-in-Chief: Sally Schrefer
Senior Editor: Susan R. Epstein
Associate Developmental Editor: Maria Broeker
Project Manager: John Rogers
Project Specialists: Kathleen L. Teal and Betty Hazelwood
Designer: Kathi Gosche
Manufacturing Manager: Linda Ierardi

Third Edition

Composition by Graphic World, Inc.
Printing by Von Hoffman Press

Mosby, Inc.
11830 Westline Industrial Drive
St. Louis, Missouri 63146

International Standard Book Number 0-323-00709-0

99 00 01 02 03 / 9 8 7 6 5 4 3 2 1

Dedication

To the Sorrentino girl cousins—family and friends:

Mary Beth

Linda

Sandra

Judy (in memorium)

Sharyn

Mary Lou

Janice

Regina

Sheila A. Sorrentino

To my loving husband, Tom, who offers emotional and technical support

To my beautiful daughter, Stacy, who is always there for me

To my awesome son, Thane, who helps me see the lighter side of life

Bernie Gorek

Reviewers

Marie Bailey, RN
Home Care Nurse
Personal Home Care
New Baltimore, Michigan

Patrick Debold, MSE
Vice President of Education
ConCorde Career Colleges
Kansas City, Missouri

Adrienne Garbarino, RN, ADN
Inservice Coordinator
Lapeer County Medical Care Facility
Lapeer, Michigan

Jana Gilbertson, RN, CDONA
Group Clinical Services Manager
Beverly Health Care
Louisville, Kentucky

Diann Muzyka, RN, BSN, MSN
Instructor/Coordinator, Patient Care Skills
Columbus State Community College
Columbus, Ohio

Virginia Pettyjohn, RN, ADN, BSN
Instructor, Assistant to the Health Coordinator
Indian Hills Community College
Ottumwa, Iowa

Acknowledgments

Textbooks are written and published by the combined efforts of many people. The planning, manuscript development and review, design, and production processes involve the insights, talents, and contributions of many individuals. We are especially grateful to:

The very special residents and staff of Bonell Good Samaritan Center in Greeley, Colorado, for providing inspiration and advice for this book and for their cooperation during our photography session.

Art Hess, Administrator of Bonell Good Samaritan Center in Greeley, Colorado, for providing inspiration and advice.

Tess Masters, nursing assistant instructor at the community CNA training center in Greeley, Colorado, for providing valuable input and sharing ideas.

Carol Miller, Employment Specialist at OSF St. Joseph Medical Center in Bloomington, Illinois, for providing resources and information.

Sandra Sorrentino Bookhout for helping us prepare for art and photography.

Cherie Whyms and the staff and residents at Pleasant Living Rehabilitation and Skilled Nursing Center in Edgewater, Maryland, for their cooperation and assistance during a photography session.

Rick Brady of Riva, Maryland, our photographer and friend.

The artists at Graphic World, Inc. in St. Louis, Missouri, for their talented work.

Our families, friends, and the Mosby staff who provided family photographs for the chapter opening design: Joan Baltusis, Graquel Hutchinson, Kathy Teal, Elizabeth Gorek, Wendy McCarville, Gail Brower, Denise Fundanish, Carol Chiarello, Rosemary Stendeback, Billi Carcheri, Martha Fluke, Kristin Geen, Yvette Webber-Davis, Jan Waters, Jay Walton, Traci Goldstein, Toni Linstedt, Oliver Tillman, Karen Breeden, Ross and Dale Sorrentino, Anthony and Frances Sorrentino, and Margaret Askew.

Marie Bailey, Patrick Debold, Adrienne Garbarino, Jana Gilbertson, Diann Muzyka, and Virginia Pettyjohn for reviewing the manuscript and for their candor and suggestions. They have contributed to the thoroughness and accuracy of this book.

The people at Mosby, especially Suzi Epstein, Maria Broeker, Graquel Hutchinson and the members of John Roger's production team—Betty Hazelwood, Kathy Teal, and Kathi Gosche. Suzi gave us valuable insights, guidance, and support. Maria and Graquel handled numerous details and manuscript needs. Betty Hazelwood was again amazing as a copy editor. Her attention to detail enhanced the quality of this book. Kathy Teal again produced an excellent page layout making the proofreading and production process easy and pleasant. And Kathi Gosche's book and cover design is uniquely creative and colorful.

To all those who contributed to this effort in any way, we are sincerely grateful.

Sheila A. Sorrentino
Bernie Gorek

Preface to the Instructor

Mosby's Textbook for Long-Term Care Assistants is intended to prepare students to function in the traditional nursing assistant role in nursing centers. We believe that an ethical and legal imperative exists to provide such individuals with the necessary education and training for safe, effective, and sensitive functioning. Focusing on nursing assistant skills and functions, safety, and the psychosocial approach to resident care, the book emphasizes the needs of older persons and other persons requiring long-term care. Sensitivity to the resident as a person with dignity and value is central to the essence of this book. We believe that students must appreciate the resident as a person with a past, a present, and a future. In every chapter, caring, understanding, resident rights, and respect for residents as individuals with dignity and value are important attitudes conveyed to the student.

Also critical to safe and effective functioning is the need to understand the legalities of the role and delegation principles. Because nursing centers vary in their use of nursing assistants, the responsibilities and limitations of nursing assistants are emphasized throughout the book and specifically in Chapter 2, which focuses on the ethical and legal aspects of the role. The nursing assistant role also is predicated on a positive work ethic. This concept also is integrated throughout the book, with specific workplace behaviors addressed in Chapter 3.

These concepts and principles—safety, sensitivity to the resident as a person, ethical and legal aspects, and work ethics—serve as the guiding framework for this book. Additional organizational strategies and values include:

- The need for nursing assistants to be aware of and understand their work environment and the individuals in that environment.
- Respect for the resident as a physical, social, psychological, and spiritual being with basic needs and protected rights.
- Recognizing the role of cultural heritage in health and illness practices.
- An understanding of body structure and function for the safe and competent performance of psychomotor skills.
- That learning proceeds from the simple to the complex. Concepts and procedures integral to other activities and functions (safety, body mechanics, medical asepsis) are presented early as those are skills basic to the nursing assistant role. More complex content and skills follow.
- That the nursing process is the basis for planning and delivering nursing care and that nursing assistants must follow the resident's care plan.

Content Issues

Various factors were considered in deciding content issues: minimum standards of the Omnibus Budget Reconciliation Act of 1987; various state curricula and training requirements; practice trends relating to restraints, subacute care, and advanced roles for assistive personnel; the changing clientele in nursing centers resulting from managed care; the special needs of residents with dementia; cultural influences; work settings; and the need for a positive work ethic. These issues were accommodated through additional content and with special features and design elements. New content includes:

- Delegation principles
- Workplace violence
- Child abuse and domestic abuse
- Work ethics **(new chapter)**
- Communication techniques
- Dealing with the angry person
- Nursing process (including nursing diagnoses)
- Dealing with conflict
- Fall prevention (risk factors, safety measures, use of bed rails)
- Restraints (complications, alternatives, safety guidelines, safety measures)
- Handling hazardous substances
- Risk management
- Personal safety practices
- Surgical asepsis (including principles and practices and donning and removing sterile gloves)
- Leg and foot ulcers
- Wound care
- Comfort **(new chapter)**
- Oxygen needs **(new chapter)**
- Mental health problems
- Development disabilities **(new chapter)**

Features and Design

In addition, considerable attention was given to making the text readable and user friendly. Therefore several design elements were retained and new ones added (see Student Preface, p. xiii).

- Chapter opening photos show progression through the life span. They are intended to sensitize the student to the journey of life from infancy through old age and from the past into the present and the future. We want the student to understand that the resident is not just an older person with illness and disabilities. Rather, the resident is someone with a rich, colorful, historical, and emotional past who has contributed in countless ways to the world we share today. We want the student to treat the resident's past, present, and future with dignity and respect.
- Key terms with definitions appear at the beginning of each chapter and are in bold print throughout the text. The definitions also are presented in the text.
- Boxes are used to list principles, rules, signs and symptoms, and other information. The boxes present an efficient way for instructors to highlight content and provide useful study guides for students. Bullets are used for each item in a list rather than numbers.
- Icons in section headings alert the reader to an associated procedure. Procedure boxes contain the same icon. ***(New!)***
- Procedure boxes are divided into Pre-Procedure, Procedure, and Post-Procedure steps. Labeling and color gradients also differentiate the sections. ***(New!)***
- A *Quality of Life* section in the procedure boxes reminds the student to knock before entering the room, address the person by name, and introduce one's self by name and title. ***(New!)***
- The skills included in the National Nurse Aide Assessment Program (NNAAP™) Skills Examination are designated in the title bar of the procedure boxes. ***(New!)***
- *Subacute Care* boxes alert the student to special information and insights about subacute care. Whereas other books dedicate a chapter to subacute care, we feel that there are no nursing skills or knowledge unique to subacute care. Compartmentalizing subacute care with a dedicated chapter would compromise our organizational approach using basic nursing concepts. Therefore subacute care is integrated throughout the text and is designated by a special design element. ***(New!)***
- *Residents With Dementia* boxes focus on special information and insights about caring for persons with dementia. ***(New!)***
- *Caring About Culture* boxes are intended to help the student learn to appreciate the importance of cultural diversity and how culture influences health and illness practices. ***(New!)***
- Because the requirements of the Omnibus Budget Reconciliation Act of 1987 (OBRA) markedly influence the care given in nursing centers, OBRA requirements are once again integrated throughout the text. In this edition, all references to OBRA are highlighted by a special screen and with a vertical OBRA label in the margin. ***(New!)***
- A *Quality of Life* section at the end of each chapter bridges the focus of the chapter with how to protect the person's quality of life when giving care.
- Review questions are found at the end of each chapter. They are followed by the page number where the answers are listed.

We hope that this book will serve you and your students well. Our intent is to provide you and your students with the information needed to teach and learn safe and effective care during this time of dynamic change in health care.

Sheila A. Sorrentino, RN, BSN, MA, MSN, PhD
Bernie Gorek, RNC, GNP, MA

Preface to the Student

This book was designed for you. It was designed to help you learn. The book is a useful resource as you gain experience and expand your knowledge.

This preface gives some study guidelines and helps you use this book. When you are given a reading assignment, do you read from the first page to the last page without stopping? How much do you remember? You will learn more if you use a study system. A useful study system has these steps:

- Survey or preview
- Question
- Read and record
- Recite and review

Survey or Preview

Before you start a reading assignment, preview or survey the assignment. This gives you an idea of what the assignment covers. It also helps you recall what you already know about the subject. Carefully look over the assignment. Preview the chapter title, headings, subheadings, and terms or ideas in bold print or italics. Also survey the objectives, key terms, first paragraph, boxes and the summary and review questions at the end of the chapter. Previewing takes only a few minutes. Remember, previewing helps you become familiar with the material.

Question

After previewing, you need to form questions to answer while you read. Questions should relate to what might be asked on a test or how the information applies to giving care. Use the title, headings, and subheadings to form questions. Avoid questions that have one-word answers. Questions that begin with what, how, or why are helpful. While reading, you may find that a question does not help you study. If so, just change the question. Remember, questioning sets a purpose for reading. So changing a question only makes this step more useful.

Read and Record

Reading is the next step. Reading is more productive after determining what you already know and what you need to learn. Read to find answers to your questions. The purpose of reading is to:

- Gain new information
- Connect the new information to what you know already

Break the assignment into smaller parts. Then answer your questions as you read each part. Also, mark important information. The information can be marked by underlining, highlighting, or making notes. Underlining and highlighting remind you what you need to learn. You need to go back and review the marked parts later. Making notes results in more immediate learning. When making notes, you write down important information in the margins or in a notebook. Use words and summary statements that will jog your memory about the material.

After reading the assignment, you need to remember the information. To remember the material, you must work with the information. This step involves organizing information into a study guide. Study guides have many forms. Diagrams or charts help show relationships or steps in a process. Much of the information in this text is organized in this manner to help you learn. Note taking in outline format also is very useful. The following is a sample outline.

1. Main heading
   a. Second level
   b. Second level
      i. Third level
      ii. Third level
2. Main heading

Recite and Review

Finally, recite and review. Use your notes and the study guides. Answer the questions you formed earlier. Also answer any other questions that came up during the reading and the review questions at the end of the chapter. Answer all questions out loud (recite).

Reviewing is more about *when* to study rather than *what* to study. You already determined what to study during the preview, question, and reading steps. The best times to review the material are right after the first study session, one week later, and regularly before a test or midterm or final examination.

We want you to enjoy learning. We also want you to enjoy your work. You and your work are important. You and the care you give may be bright spots in a person's day. This book was designed also to help you study. Special design features are described on the next pages.

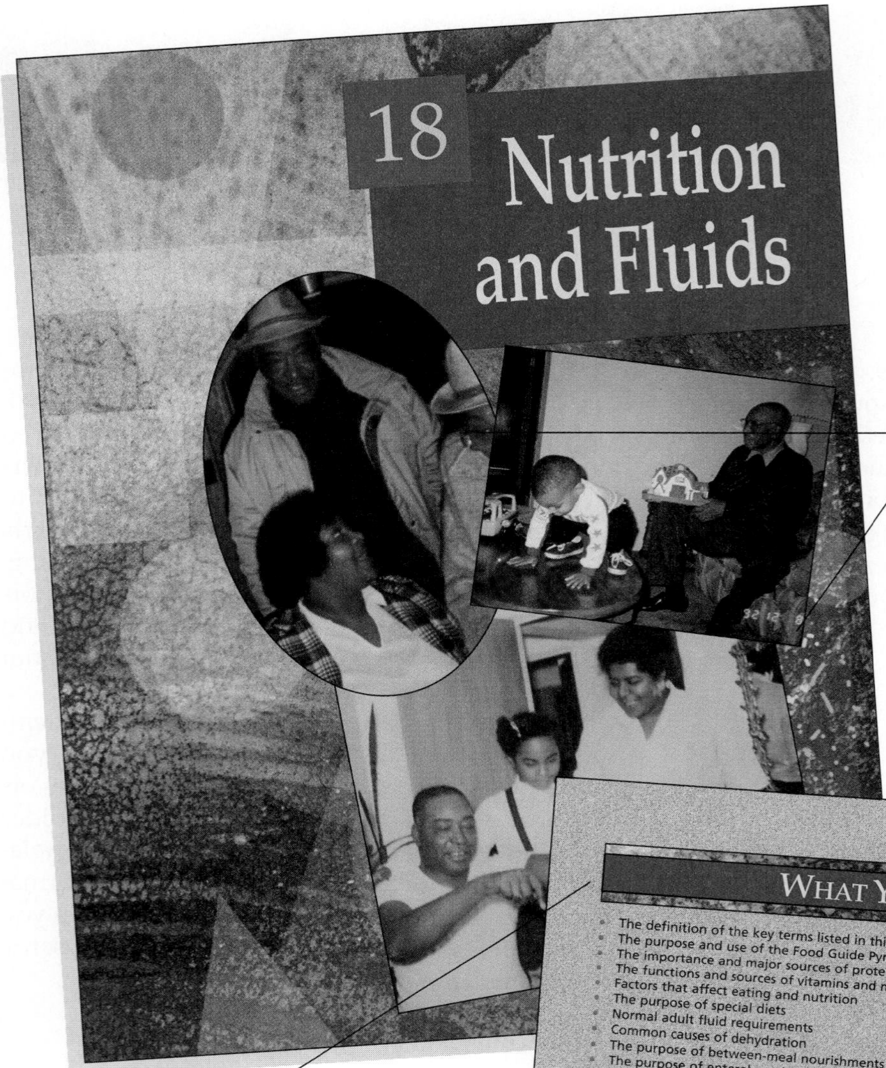

Chapter opening photos show the journey of life from infancy through old age and from the past into the present and the future. We want you to understand that the resident is not just an older person with illness and disabilities. Rather, the resident is someone with a rich, colorful, historical, and emotional past who has contributed in countless ways to the world we share today.

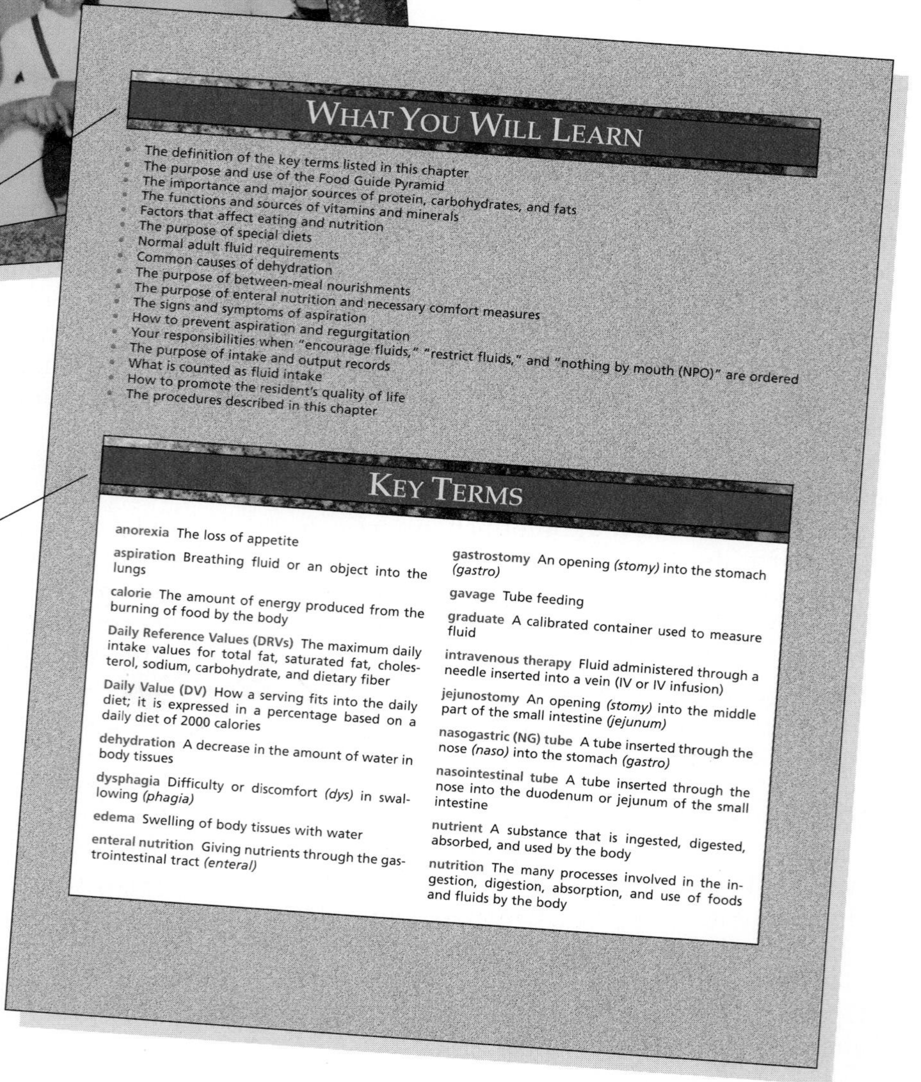

What You Will Learn

- The definition of the key terms listed in this chapter
- The purpose and use of the Food Guide Pyramid
- The importance and major sources of protein, carbohydrates, and fats
- The functions and sources of vitamins and minerals
- Factors that affect eating and nutrition
- The purpose of special diets
- Normal adult fluid requirements
- Common causes of dehydration
- The purpose of between-meal nourishments
- The purpose of enteral nutrition and necessary comfort measures
- The signs and symptoms of aspiration
- How to prevent aspiration and regurgitation
- Your responsibilities when "encourage fluids," "restrict fluids," and "nothing by mouth (NPO)" are ordered
- The purpose of intake and output records
- What is counted as fluid intake
- How to promote the resident's quality of life
- The procedures described in this chapter

Key Terms

anorexia The loss of appetite

aspiration Breathing fluid or an object into the lungs

calorie The amount of energy produced from the burning of food by the body

Daily Reference Values (DRVs) The maximum daily intake values for total fat, saturated fat, cholesterol, sodium, carbohydrate, and dietary fiber

Daily Value (DV) How a serving fits into the daily diet; it is expressed in a percentage based on a daily diet of 2000 calories

dehydration A decrease in the amount of water in body tissues

dysphagia Difficulty or discomfort *(dys)* in swallowing *(phagia)*

edema Swelling of body tissues with water

enteral nutrition Giving nutrients through the gastrointestinal tract *(enteral)*

gastrostomy An opening *(stomy)* into the stomach *(gastro)*

gavage Tube feeding

graduate A calibrated container used to measure fluid

intravenous therapy Fluid administered through a needle inserted into a vein (IV or IV infusion)

jejunostomy An opening *(stomy)* into the middle part of the small intestine *(jejunum)*

nasogastric (NG) tube A tube inserted through the nose *(naso)* into the stomach *(gastro)*

nasointestinal tube A tube inserted through the nose into the duodenum or jejunum of the small intestine

nutrient A substance that is ingested, digested, absorbed, and used by the body

nutrition The many processes involved in the ingestion, digestion, absorption, and use of foods and fluids by the body

What You Will Learn tells what is presented in the chapter.

Key Terms are the important words and phrases in the chapter. Definitions are given for each term. The key terms introduce you to the chapter content. They are also useful study guides.

Residents With Dementia boxes alert you to the special considerations that are necessary when caring for persons with dementia.

Boxes and tables contain important rules, principles, guidelines, signs and symptoms, and other information in a list format. They identify important information and are useful study guides for reviewing.

OBRA content is screened and has a vertical label to alert you to requirements of the Omnibus Budget Reconciliation Act of 1987.

302 Mosby's Textbook for Long-Term Care Assistants

RESIDENTS WITH DEMENTIA

Some residents are confused and may resist care at times. They may move quickly and without warning. Or they may pull away from you during care. Some residents try to hit or kick caregivers. These unexpected movements can cause skin tears. When giving care to a resident who resists care, ask the nurse for help. Never force care on a resident. See Chapter 27 for approaches to use when caring for residents who are confused and resist care. Always follow the care plan.

BOX 14-2 MEASURES TO PREVENT SKIN TEARS

- Follow the care plan for moving, dressing, and bathing residents.
- Keep residents' skin well lubricated. Follow the care plan.
- Offer fluids to keep residents hydrated. Follow the care plan.
- Dress and undress residents carefully.
- Dress residents in soft clothing with long sleeves and legs, such as sweat suits.
- Keep your fingernails short and smoothly filed.
- Keep residents' fingernails and toenails short and smoothly filed. If you are not allowed to trim toenails, report long and rough toenails to the nurse.
- Do not wear rings with large stones.
- Follow the safety rules in Chapter 10 when lifting and transferring residents to and from beds and wheelchairs.
- Be patient and stay calm when caring for confused or agitated residents or those who resist care.
- Pad bed rails and wheelchair arms and foot pedals. Follow the care plan.

lower legs are common sites for skin tears. Many residents have very thin and fragile skin. Even a small amount of pressure can cause a skin tear.

Causes

Skin tears are caused by shearing (see Chapter 10), pulling, or direct pressure on the skin. For example, a skin tear can occur by bumping a hand, arm, or leg on a bed rail, wheelchair foot pedal, or other hard surface. A caregiver can cause a skin tear by holding on to a resident's arm or leg too tightly when moving the person. Buttons or zippers pulled across fragile skin can also cause a skin tear. Skin tears are painful. They provide a portal of entry for microbes. You must notify the nurse immediately if you cause or find a skin tear on a resident. (*See Residents With Dementia.*)

Residents at Risk

Residents at risk for skins tears are those who:

- Require moderate to complete help in moving
- Have poor nutrition
- Have poor hydration
- Have altered mental awareness
- Are very thin

Prevention

You can help prev...

... residents ... Box 14-2

...kin tear ... Elastic ...e heal- ... when ... injury. ...pecific

PRESSURE ULCERS

A **pressure ulcer (decubitus ulcer, bed sore, pressure sore)** is any injury caused by unrelieved pressure. It usually occurs over a bony prominence. Prominence means to stick out. Therefore a bony prominence is an area where the bone sticks out or projects out from the flat surface of the body. The shoulder blades, elbows, hip bones, sacrum, knees, ankle bones, heels, and toes are bony prominences (see Figure 14-1).

Causes

Pressure, friction, and shearing are common causes of skin breakdown and pressure ulcers. Other factors include breaks in the skin, poor circulation to an area, moisture, dry skin, and irritation by urine and feces.

Pressure occurs when the skin over a bony prominence is squeezed between hard surfaces. The bone itself is one hard surface. The other is usually the mattress or chair seat. The squeezing or pressure prevents blood flow to the skin and underlying tissues. Lack of

12 Mosby's Textbook for Long-Term Care Assistants

THE OMNIBUS BUDGET RECONCILIATION ACT OF 1987

OBRA In 1987 the U.S. Congress passed the **Omnibus Budget Reconciliation Act (OBRA).** OBRA is a federal law concerned with the quality of life, health, and safety of residents. Nursing centers must provide care in a manner and in a setting that maintains or improves each resident's quality of life, health, and safety. Training and competency evaluation of nursing assistants are also OBRA requirements (see Chapter 2). Many other requirements must be met as well.

Resident Rights

Nursing center residents have certain rights under federal and state laws. Residents have rights as citizens of the United States. They also have rights relating to their everyday lives and care in a nursing center. Nursing centers must protect and promote resident rights. Residents must be able to exercise their rights without interference from the center. Some residents are incompetent (not able) and cannot exercise their rights. Legal guardians exercise rights for them.

Nursing centers must inform residents of their rights. They must be informed orally and in writing. Such information is given before or during admission to the center. It must be given in the language used and understood by the resident.

Privacy and confidentiality. Residents have the right to personal privacy. The resident's body must not be exposed unnecessarily. Only those workers directly involved in care, treatments, or examinations should be present. The resident must give consent for others to be present. For example, a student may want to observe a procedure or treatment. The resident's consent is necessary for the student to be an observer. OBRA A resident also has the right to use the bathroom in private. Privacy must be maintained for personal care activities as well.

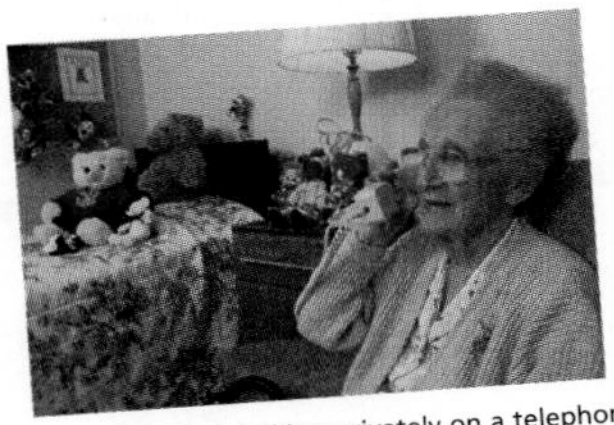

Fig. 1-4 A resident talking privately on a telephone.

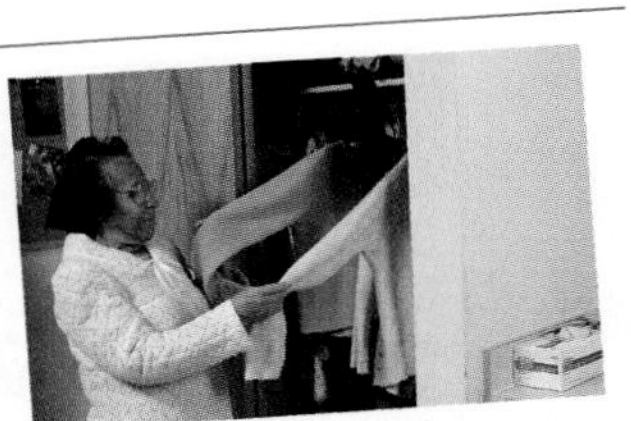

Fig. 1-5 A resident choosing what clothing to wear.

Residents also have the right to visit with others in private. They have the right to visit in an area where they cannot be seen or heard by others. The center must try to provide private space when it is requested. Offices, chapels, dining rooms, meeting rooms, and conference rooms can be used if available. OBRA

The right to visit in private also involves telephone conversations (Fig. 1-4). In addition, residents have the right to send and receive mail without interference by others. Mail sent and received by the resident must not be opened by others without the resident's permission.

Information about the resident's care, treatment, and condition must be kept confidential. Medical and financial records also are confidential. The resident must give consent for them to be released to other centers or individuals. Consent is not needed for the release of medical records when the resident is being transferred to another center. Records also can be released without the resident's consent when they are required by law or for insurance purposes.

Throughout this textbook you will be reminded to keep information about the person confidential. Providing for privacy and keeping medical and personal information confidential show respect for the person. They also protect the person's dignity. The right to privacy and confidentiality are discussed in Chapter 2.

Personal choice. OBRA requires that residents be free to choose their own doctors. They also have the right to participate in planning their own care and treatment. This means that residents have the right to choose activities, schedules, and care based on their personal preferences. For example, residents have the right to choose when to get up and go to bed, what to wear, how to spend their time, and what to eat (Fig. 1-5). They also can choose companions and visitors inside and outside of the center. OBRA

Personal choice is important for quality of life, dignity, and self-respect. You will be reminded throughout this book to allow the person's preferences whenever it is safely possible.

Bolded type is used to highlight the key terms in the text. You again see the key term and read its definition. This helps reinforce your learning.

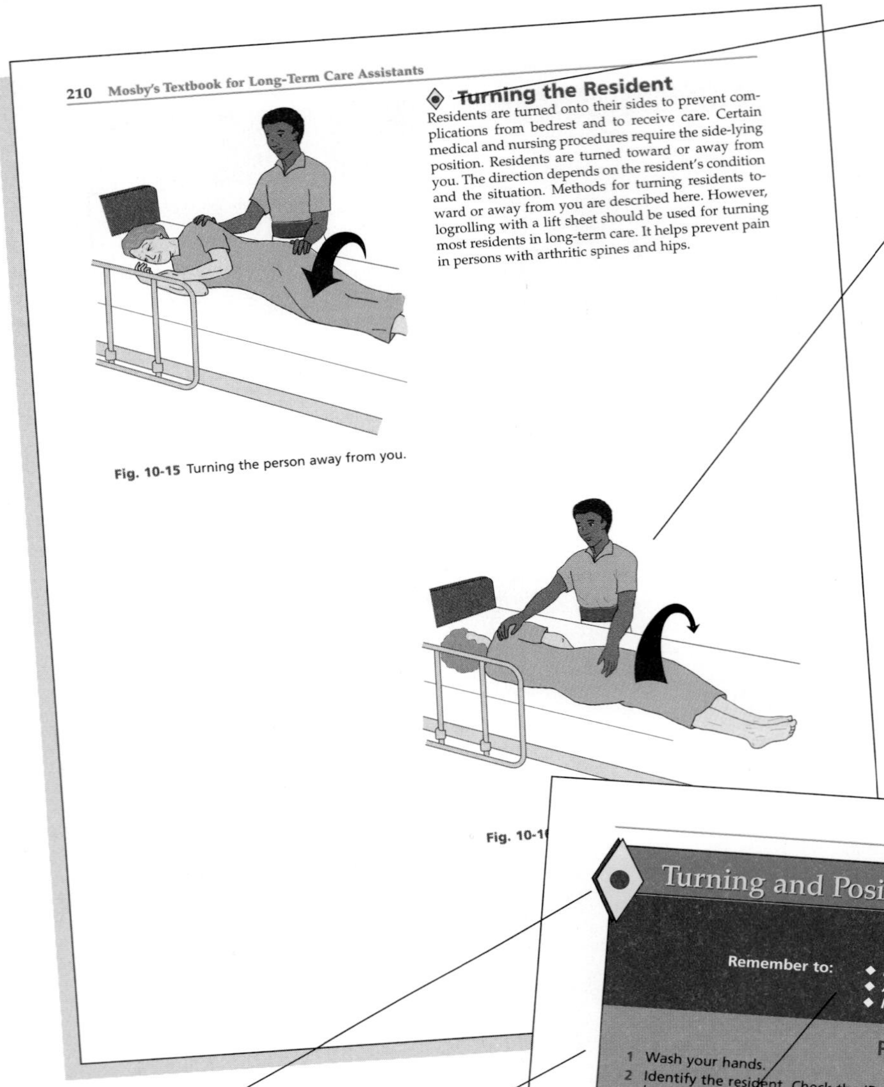

210 Mosby's Textbook for Long-Term Care Assistants

◈ Turning the Resident

Residents are turned onto their sides to prevent complications from bedrest and to receive care. Certain medical and nursing procedures require the side-lying position. Residents are turned toward or away from you. The direction depends on the resident's condition and the situation. Methods for turning residents toward or away from you are described here. However, logrolling with a lift sheet should be used for turning most residents in long-term care. It helps prevent pain in persons with arthritic spines and hips.

Fig. 10-15 Turning the person away from you.

Fig. 10-1

Icons in the headings alert you to an associated procedure. Procedure boxes contain the same icon.

Color illustrations and photographs visually present a key idea, concept, or procedure step. They help you apply and remember the written material.

NNAAP™ in the procedure title bar alerts you to those skills that are part of the National Nurse Aide Assessment Program (NNAAP™). **(NOTE: All states do not participate in NNAAP. Ask your instructor for a list of the skills tested in your state.)**

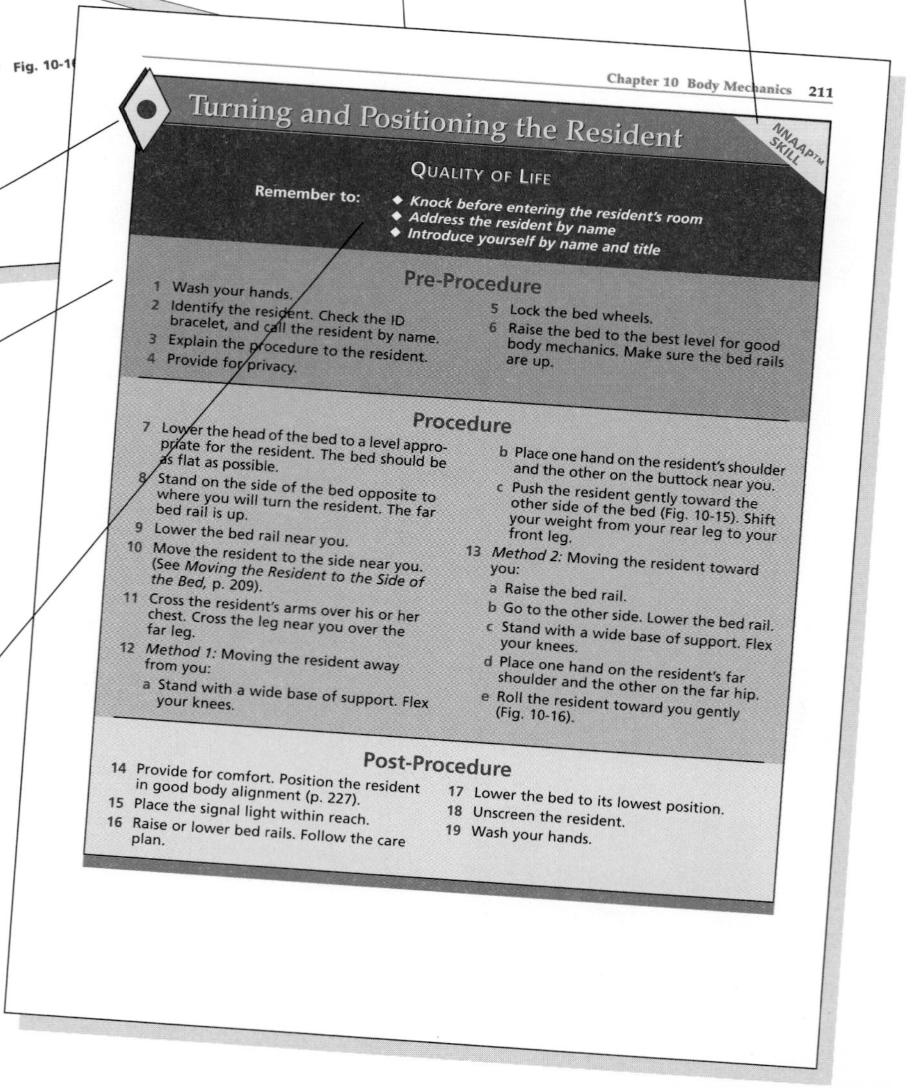

Chapter 10 Body Mechanics 211

Turning and Positioning the Resident

NNAAP™ SKILL

QUALITY OF LIFE

Remember to:
- Knock before entering the resident's room
- Address the resident by name
- Introduce yourself by name and title

Pre-Procedure

1 Wash your hands.
2 Identify the resident. Check the ID bracelet, and call the resident by name.
3 Explain the procedure to the resident.
4 Provide for privacy.
5 Lock the bed wheels.
6 Raise the bed to the best level for good body mechanics. Make sure the bed rails are up.

Procedure

7 Lower the head of the bed to a level appropriate for the resident. The bed should be as flat as possible.
8 Stand on the side of the bed opposite to where you will turn the resident. The far bed rail is up.
9 Lower the bed rail near you.
10 Move the resident to the side near you. (See *Moving the Resident to the Side of the Bed*, p. 209).
11 Cross the resident's arms over his or her chest. Cross the leg near you over the far leg.
12 *Method 1:* Moving the resident away from you:
  a Stand with a wide base of support. Flex your knees.
  b Place one hand on the resident's shoulder and the other on the buttock near you.
  c Push the resident gently toward the other side of the bed (Fig. 10-15). Shift your weight from your rear leg to your front leg.
13 *Method 2:* Moving the resident toward you:
  a Raise the bed rail.
  b Go to the other side. Lower the bed rail.
  c Stand with a wide base of support. Flex your knees.
  d Place one hand on the resident's far shoulder and the other on the far hip.
  e Roll the resident toward you gently (Fig. 10-16).

Post-Procedure

14 Provide for comfort. Position the resident in good body alignment (p. 227).
15 Place the signal light within reach.
16 Raise or lower bed rails. Follow the care plan.
17 Lower the bed to its lowest position.
18 Unscreen the resident.
19 Wash your hands.

Procedure icon

Procedures are written in a step-by-step format. They are divided into Pre-Procedure, Procedure, and Post-Procedure sections for easy studying.

Quality of Life in the procedure boxes reminds you to knock before entering the room, to call the resident by name, and to introduce yourself by name and title. These simple courtesies show respect for the resident as a person.

Caring About Culture boxes contain information to help you learn about the various practices of other cultures.

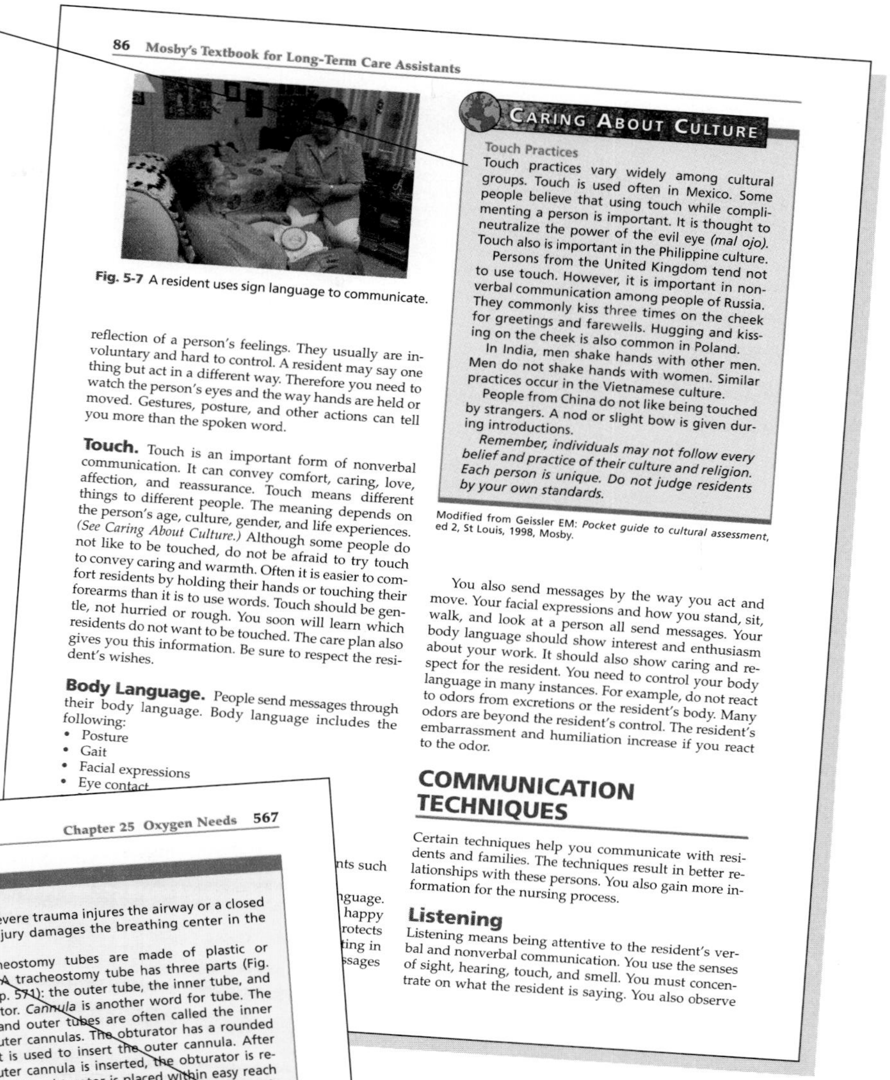
86 Mosby's Textbook for Long-Term Care Assistants

Fig. 5-7 A resident uses sign language to communicate.

reflection of a person's feelings. They usually are involuntary and hard to control. A resident may say one thing but act in a different way. Therefore you need to watch the person's eyes and the way hands are held or moved. Gestures, posture, and other actions can tell you more than the spoken word.

Touch. Touch is an important form of nonverbal communication. It can convey comfort, caring, love, affection, and reassurance. Touch means different things to different people. The meaning depends on the person's age, culture, gender, and life experiences. *(See Caring About Culture.)* Although some people do not like to be touched, do not be afraid to try touch to convey caring and warmth. Often it is easier to comfort residents by holding their hands or touching their forearms than it is to use words. Touch should be gentle, not hurried or rough. You soon will learn which residents do not want to be touched. The care plan also gives you this information. Be sure to respect the resident's wishes.

Body Language. People send messages through their body language. Body language includes the following:
- Posture
- Gait
- Facial expressions
- Eye contact

CARING ABOUT CULTURE

Touch Practices

Touch practices vary widely among cultural groups. Touch is used often in Mexico. Some people believe that using touch while complimenting a person is important. It is thought to neutralize the power of the evil eye *(mal ojo)*. Touch also is important in the Philippine culture.

Persons from the United Kingdom tend not to use touch. However, it is important in nonverbal communication among people of Russia. They commonly kiss three times on the cheek for greetings and farewells. Hugging and kissing on the cheek is also common in Poland.

In India, men shake hands with other men. Men do not shake hands with women. Similar practices occur in the Vietnamese culture.

People from China do not like being touched by strangers. A nod or slight bow is given during introductions.

Remember, individuals may not follow every belief and practice of their culture and religion. Each person is unique. Do not judge residents by your own standards.

Modified from Geissler EM: *Pocket guide to cultural assessment*, ed 2, St Louis, 1998, Mosby.

You also send messages by the way you act and move. Your facial expressions and how you stand, sit, walk, and look at a person all send messages. Your body language should show interest and enthusiasm about your work. It should also show caring and respect for the resident. You need to control your body language in many instances. For example, do not react to odors from excretions or the resident's body. Many odors are beyond the resident's control. The resident's embarrassment and humiliation increase if you react to the odor.

COMMUNICATION TECHNIQUES

Certain techniques help you communicate with residents and families. The techniques result in better relationships with these persons. You also gain more information for the nursing process.

Listening

Listening means being attentive to the resident's verbal and nonverbal communication. You use the senses of sight, hearing, touch, and smell. You must concentrate on what the resident is saying. You also observe

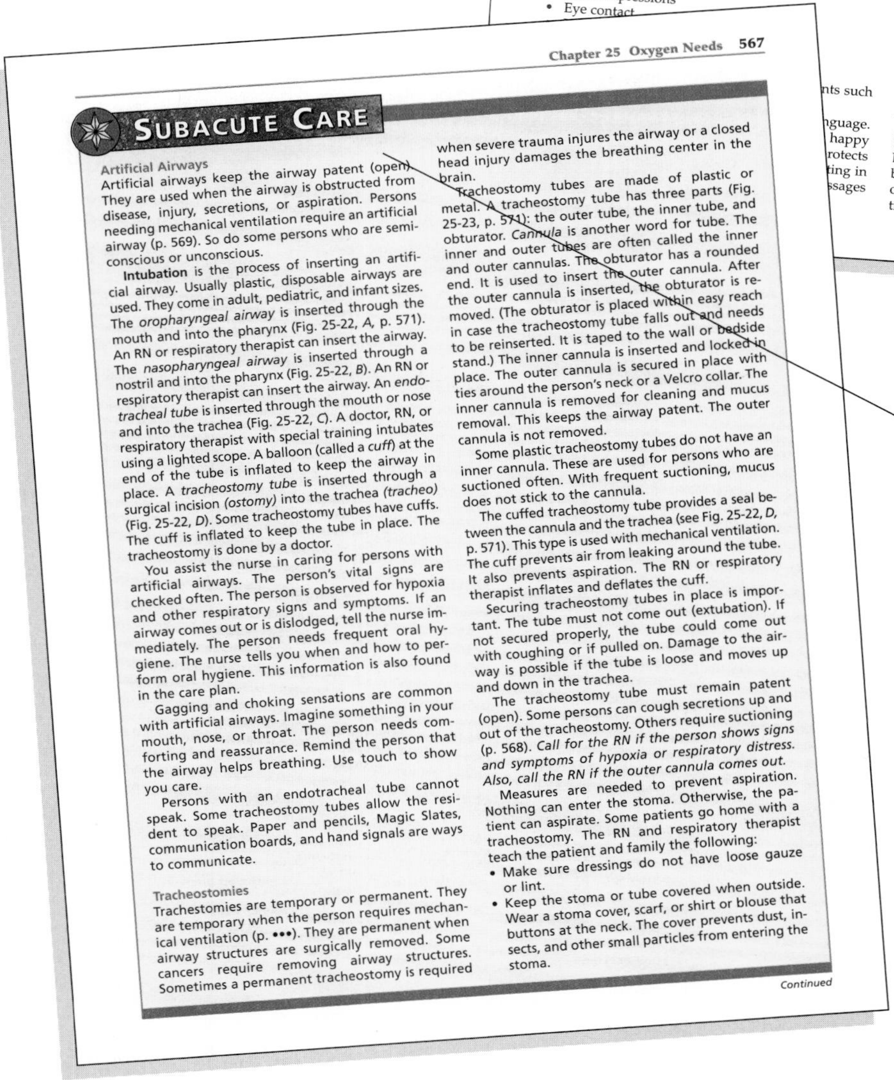
Chapter 25 Oxygen Needs 567

SUBACUTE CARE

Artificial Airways

Artificial airways keep the airway patent (open). They are used when the airway is obstructed from disease, injury, secretions, or aspiration. Persons needing mechanical ventilation require an artificial airway (p. 569). So do some persons who are semiconscious or unconscious.

Intubation is the process of inserting an artificial airway. Usually plastic, disposable airways are used. They come in adult, pediatric, and infant sizes. The *oropharyngeal airway* is inserted through the mouth and into the pharynx (Fig. 25-22, *A*, p. 571). An RN or respiratory therapist can insert the airway. The *nasopharyngeal airway* is inserted through a nostril and into the pharynx (Fig. 25-22, *B*). An RN or respiratory therapist can insert the airway. An *endotracheal tube* is inserted through the mouth or nose and into the trachea (Fig. 25-22, *C*). A doctor, RN, or respiratory therapist with special training intubates using a lighted scope. A balloon (called a *cuff*) at the end of the tube is inflated to keep the airway in place. A *tracheostomy tube* is inserted through a surgical incision *(ostomy)* into the trachea *(tracheo)* (Fig. 25-22, *D*). Some tracheostomy tubes have cuffs. The cuff is inflated to keep the tube in place. The tracheostomy is done by a doctor.

You assist the nurse in caring for persons with artificial airways. The person's vital signs are checked often. The person is observed for hypoxia and other respiratory signs and symptoms. If an airway comes out or is dislodged, tell the nurse immediately. The person needs frequent oral hygiene. The nurse tells you when and how to perform oral hygiene. This information is also found in the care plan.

Gagging and choking sensations are common with artificial airways. Imagine something in your mouth, nose, or throat. The person needs comforting and reassurance. Remind the person that the airway helps breathing. Use touch to show you care.

Persons with an endotracheal tube cannot speak. Some tracheostomy tubes allow the resident to speak. Paper and pencils, Magic Slates, communication boards, and hand signals are ways to communicate.

Tracheostomies

Trachestomies are temporary or permanent. They are temporary when the person requires mechanical ventilation (p. •••). They are permanent when airway structures are surgically removed. Some cancers require removing airway structures. Sometimes a permanent tracheostomy is required when severe trauma injures the airway or a closed head injury damages the breathing center in the brain.

Tracheostomy tubes are made of plastic or metal. A tracheostomy tube has three parts (Fig. 25-23, p. 571): the outer tube, the inner tube, and obturator. *Cannula* is another word for tube. The inner and outer tubes are often called the inner and outer cannulas. The obturator has a rounded end. It is used to insert the outer cannula. After the outer cannula is inserted, the obturator is removed. (The obturator is placed within easy reach in case the tracheostomy tube falls out and needs to be reinserted. It is taped to the wall or bedside stand.) The inner cannula is inserted and locked in place. The outer cannula is secured in place with ties around the person's neck or a Velcro collar. The inner cannula is removed for cleaning and mucus removal. This keeps the airway patent. The outer cannula is not removed.

Some plastic tracheostomy tubes do not have an inner cannula. These are used for persons who are suctioned often. With frequent suctioning, mucus does not stick to the cannula.

The cuffed tracheostomy tube provides a seal between the cannula and the trachea (see Fig. 25-22, *D*, p. 571). This type is used with mechanical ventilation. The cuff prevents air from leaking around the tube. It also prevents aspiration. The RN or respiratory therapist inflates and deflates the cuff.

Securing tracheostomy tubes in place is important. The tube must not come out (extubation). If not secured properly, the tube could come out with coughing or if pulled on. Damage to the airway is possible if the tube is loose and moves up and down in the trachea.

The tracheostomy tube must remain patent (open). Some persons can cough secretions up and out of the tracheostomy. Others require suctioning (p. 568). *Call for the RN if the person shows signs and symptoms of hypoxia or respiratory distress. Also, call the RN if the outer cannula comes out.*

Measures are needed to prevent aspiration. Nothing can enter the stoma. Otherwise, the patient can aspirate. Some patients go home with a tracheostomy. The RN and respiratory therapist teach the patient and family the following:
- Make sure dressings do not have loose gauze or lint.
- Keep the stoma or tube covered when outside. Wear a stoma cover, scarf, or shirt or blouse that buttons at the neck. The cover prevents dust, insects, and other small particles from entering the stoma.

Continued

Subacute Care boxes contain information about the special needs and nursing care required by persons in subacute care units.

Quality of Life box at the end of each chapter bridges the focus of the chapter with how to protect the resident's rights and enhance the person's quality of life when giving care.

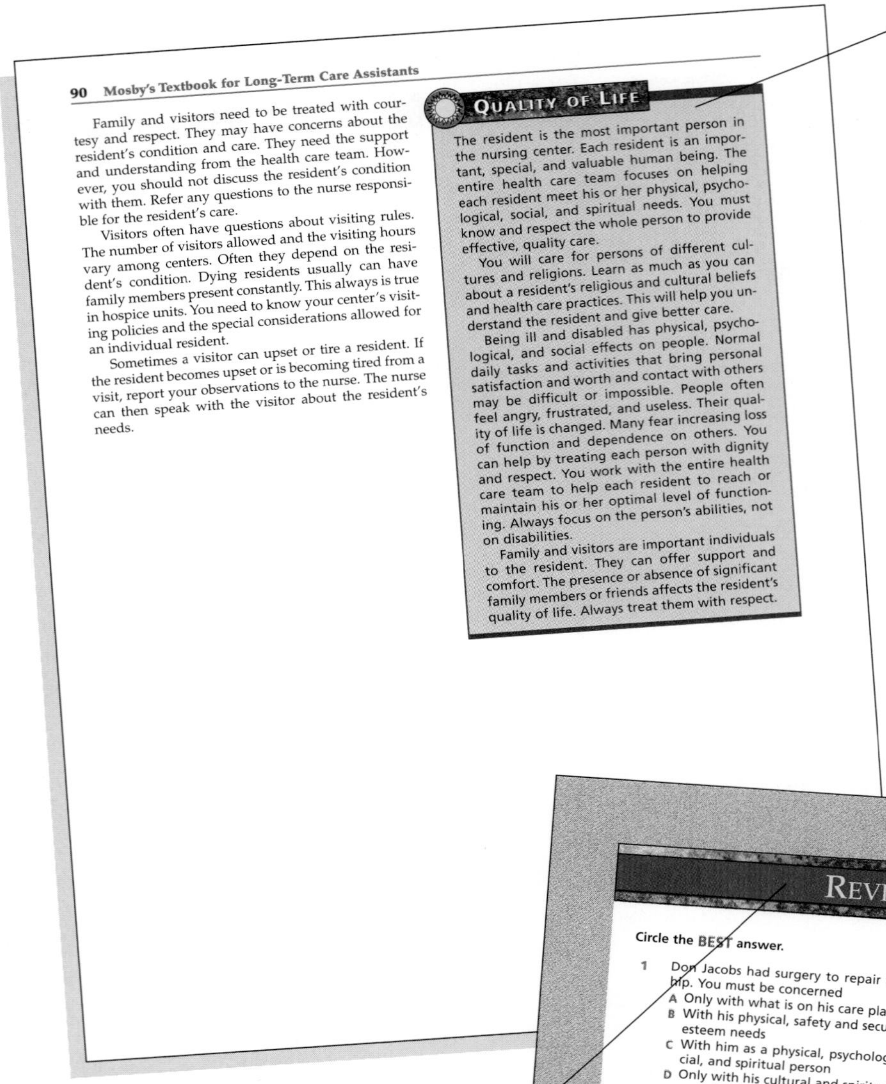

90 Mosby's Textbook for Long-Term Care Assistants

Family and visitors need to be treated with courtesy and respect. They may have concerns about the resident's condition and care. They need the support and understanding from the health care team. However, you should not discuss the resident's condition with them. Refer any questions to the nurse responsible for the resident's care.

Visitors often have questions about visiting rules. The number of visitors allowed and the visiting hours vary among centers. Often they depend on the resident's condition. Dying residents usually can have family members present constantly. This always is true in hospice units. You need to know your center's visiting policies and the special considerations allowed for an individual resident.

Sometimes a visitor can upset or tire a resident. If the resident becomes upset or is becoming tired from a visit, report your observations to the nurse. The nurse can then speak with the visitor about the resident's needs.

QUALITY OF LIFE

The resident is the most important person in the nursing center. Each resident is an important, special, and valuable human being. The entire health care team focuses on helping each resident meet his or her physical, psychological, social, and spiritual needs. You must know and respect the whole person to provide effective, quality care.

You will care for persons of different cultures and religions. Learn as much as you can about a resident's religious and cultural beliefs and health care practices. This will help you understand the resident and give better care.

Being ill and disabled has physical, psychological, and social effects on people. Normal daily tasks and activities that bring personal satisfaction and worth and contact with others may be difficult or impossible. People often feel angry, frustrated, and useless. Their quality of life is changed. Many fear increasing loss of function and dependence on others. You can help by treating each person with dignity and respect. You work with the entire health care team to help each resident to reach or maintain his or her optimal level of functioning. Always focus on the person's abilities, not on disabilities.

Family and visitors are important individuals to the resident. They can offer support and comfort. The presence or absence of significant family members or friends affects the resident's quality of life. Always treat them with respect.

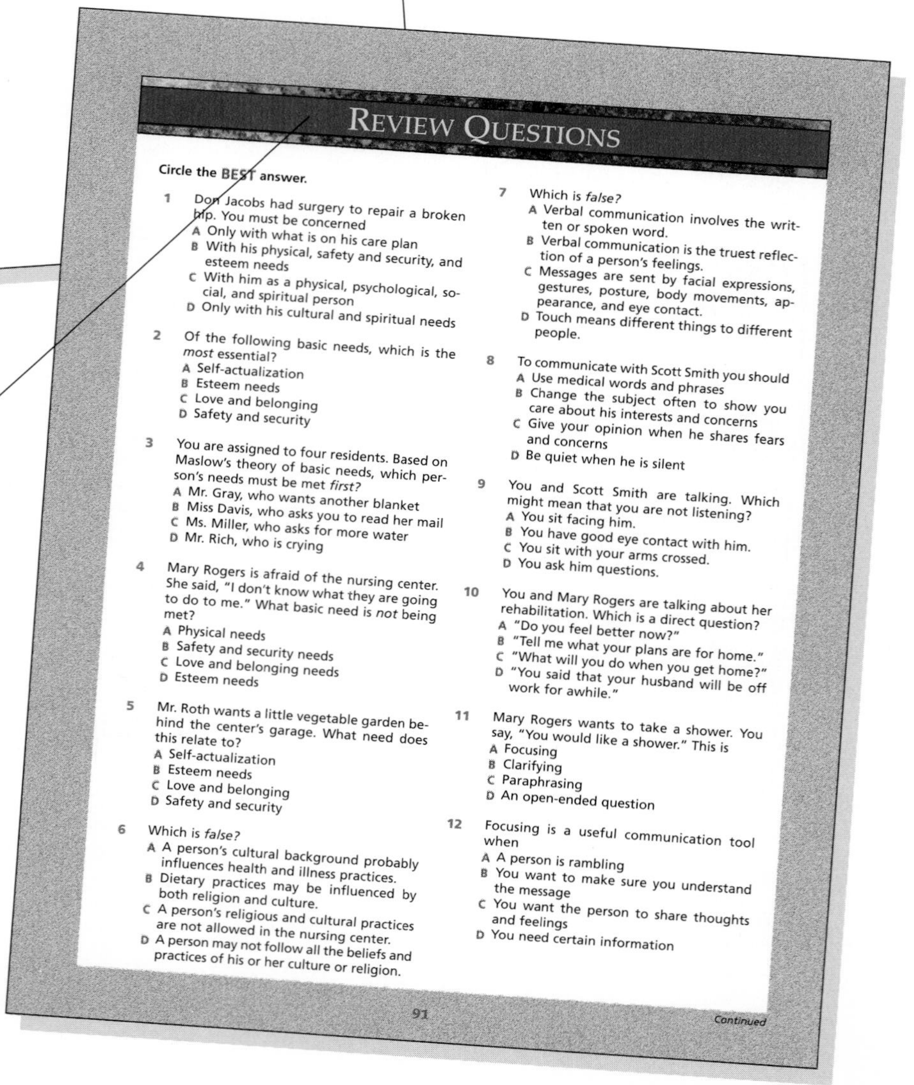

REVIEW QUESTIONS

Circle the BEST answer.

1 Don Jacobs had surgery to repair a broken hip. You must be concerned
A Only with what is on his care plan
B With his physical, safety and security, and esteem needs
C With him as a physical, psychological, social, and spiritual person
D Only with his cultural and spiritual needs

2 Of the following basic needs, which is the *most* essential?
A Self-actualization
B Esteem needs
C Love and belonging
D Safety and security

3 You are assigned to four residents. Based on Maslow's theory of basic needs, which person's needs must be met *first?*
A Mr. Gray, who wants another blanket
B Miss Davis, who asks you to read her mail
C Ms. Miller, who asks for more water
D Mr. Rich, who is crying

4 Mary Rogers is afraid of the nursing center. She said, "I don't know what they are going to do to me." What basic need is *not* being met?
A Physical needs
B Safety and security needs
C Love and belonging needs
D Esteem needs

5 Mr. Roth wants a little vegetable garden behind the center's garage. What need does this relate to?
A Self-actualization
B Esteem needs
C Love and belonging
D Safety and security

6 Which is *false?*
A A person's cultural background probably influences health and illness practices.
B Dietary practices may be influenced by both religion and culture.
C A person's religious and cultural practices are not allowed in the nursing center.
D A person may not follow all the beliefs and practices of his or her culture or religion.

7 Which is *false?*
A Verbal communication involves the written or spoken word.
B Verbal communication is the truest reflection of a person's feelings.
C Messages are sent by facial expressions, gestures, posture, body movements, appearance, and eye contact.
D Touch means different things to different people.

8 To communicate with Scott Smith you should
A Use medical words and phrases
B Change the subject often to show you care about his interests and concerns
C Give your opinion when he shares fears and concerns
D Be quiet when he is silent

9 You and Scott Smith are talking. Which might mean that you are not listening?
A You sit facing him.
B You have good eye contact with him.
C You sit with your arms crossed.
D You ask him questions.

10 You and Mary Rogers are talking about her rehabilitation. Which is a direct question?
A "Do you feel better now?"
B "Tell me what your plans are for home."
C "What will you do when you get home?"
D "You said that your husband will be off work for awhile."

11 Mary Rogers wants to take a shower. You say, "You would like a shower." This is
A Focusing
B Clarifying
C Paraphrasing
D An open-ended question

12 Focusing is a useful communication tool when
A A person is rambling
B You want to make sure you understand the message
C You want the person to share thoughts and feelings
D You need certain information

91 Continued

Review Questions are a useful study guide. They help you to review what you have learned. They can be used also when studying for a test or the compentency evaluation. Answers are given at the back of the book beginning on p. 695.

Contents

1 Introduction to Long-Term Care

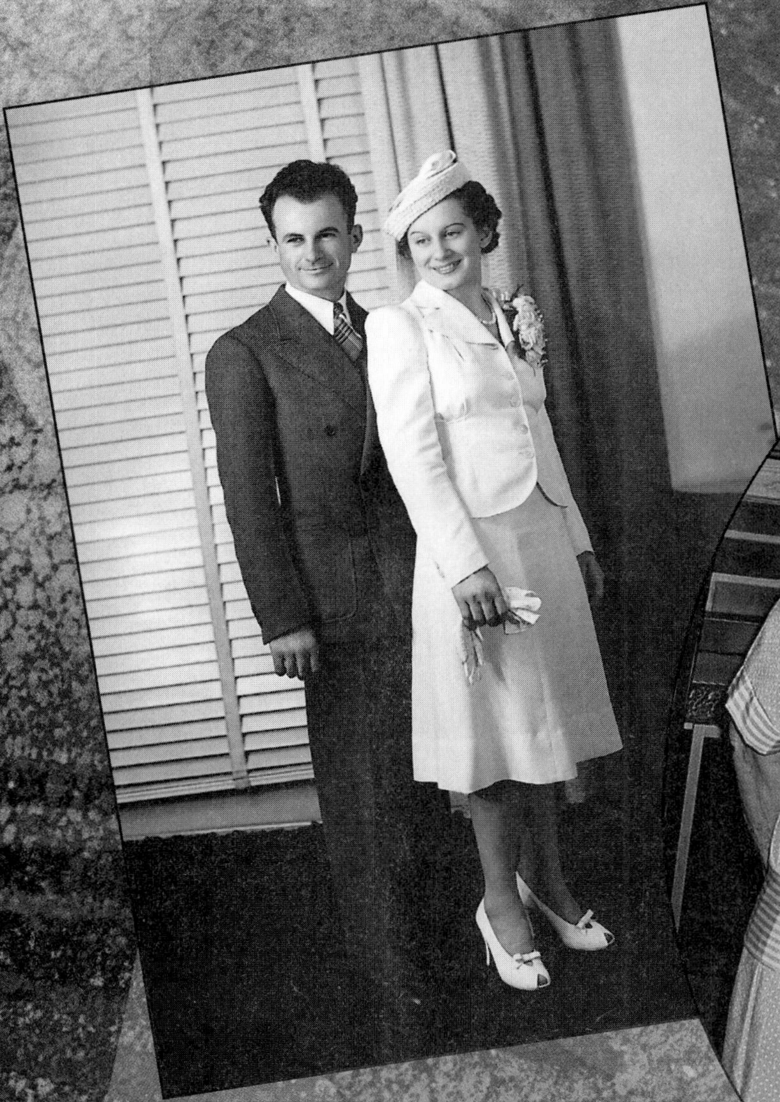

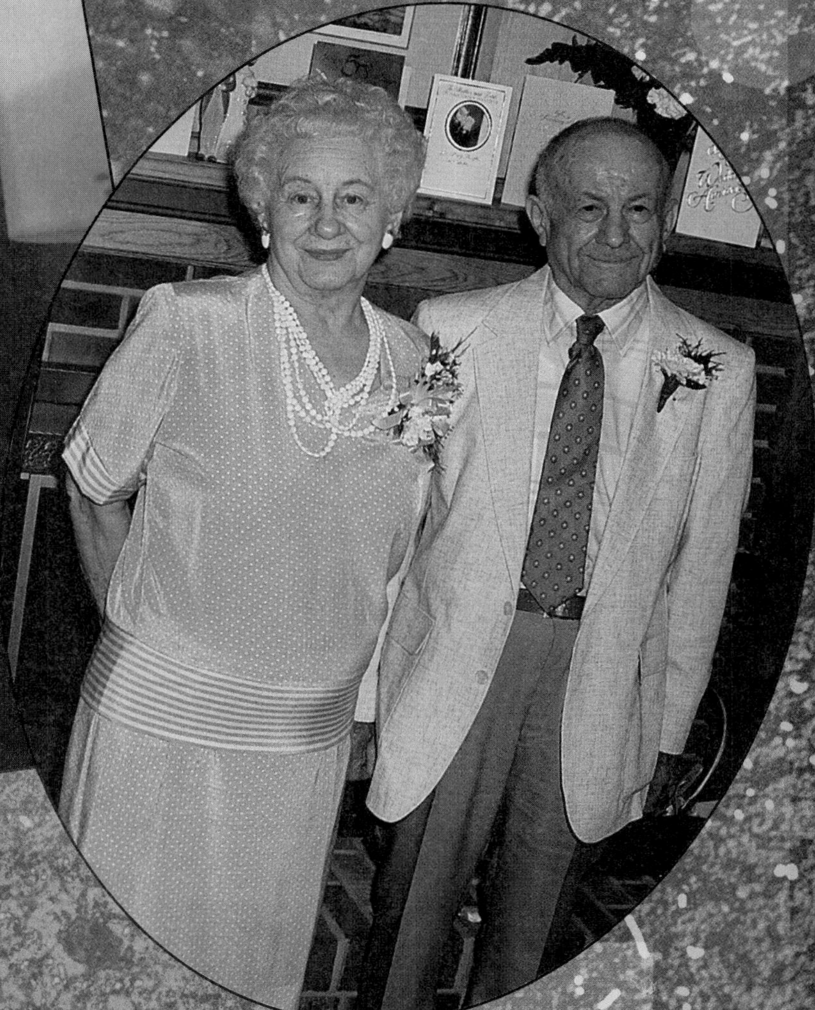

What You Will Learn

- The definition of the key terms listed in this chapter
- The types, purposes, and organization of long-term care centers
- The differences between RNs, LPNs/LVNs, and nursing assistants
- Three programs that pay for health care
- How diagnosis-related groups (DRGs) affect Medicare and Medicaid payments
- The requirements of the Omnibus Budget Reconciliation Act of 1987
- The purpose of the Joint Commission on Accreditation of Healthcare Organizations

Key Terms

acute illness A sudden illness from which the person is expected to recover

Alzheimer's disease A disease that affects brain tissue; persons suffer increasing memory loss and confusion until they cannot meet their simplest personal needs

assisted living facility A board and care facility or residential care facility

board and care facility A facility that provides custodial care to a few independent residents, often in a home setting; no licensed nurse is required; also called an *assisted living facility or residential care facility*

case management A method of organizing nursing care; a case manager (an RN) coordinates resident care from admission through discharge and into the home setting

chronic illness An illness, slow or gradual in onset, for which there is no known cure; the illness can be controlled and complications prevented

deconditioning The process of becoming weak from illness or lack of exercise; the loss of muscle strength as a result of inactivity

functional nursing A method of organizing nursing care; nursing staff perform specific tasks for all assigned residents

group insurance plan An insurance plan bought by a group for individuals

hospice A health care facility or program for persons dying from a terminal illness

interdisciplinary health care team A variety of health workers who work together to provide health care for residents

licensed practical nurse (LPN) An individual who has completed a 1-year nursing program and who has passed the licensing examination for practical nurses; called *licensed vocational nurse (LVN)* in some states

Medicaid A health insurance program sponsored by state and federal governments

Medicare A health insurance plan administered by the Social Security Administration of the federal government

nurse practitioner (NP) A registered nurse with advanced training in physical examination and assessment; some states allow NPs to diagnose and prescribe under a doctor's supervision

nursing assistant An individual who gives basic nursing care under the supervision of an RN or an LPN/LVN; also called *nurse's aide, nursing attendant,* and *health care assistant*

nursing center A facility that provides health care services to residents who require regular or continuous care; licensed nursing staff is required; commonly called a *nursing home* or *nursing facility*

nursing facility (NF) Nursing center or nursing home

nursing home Nursing facility or nursing center

nursing team The individuals involved in providing nursing care: RNs, LPNs/LVNs, and nursing assistants

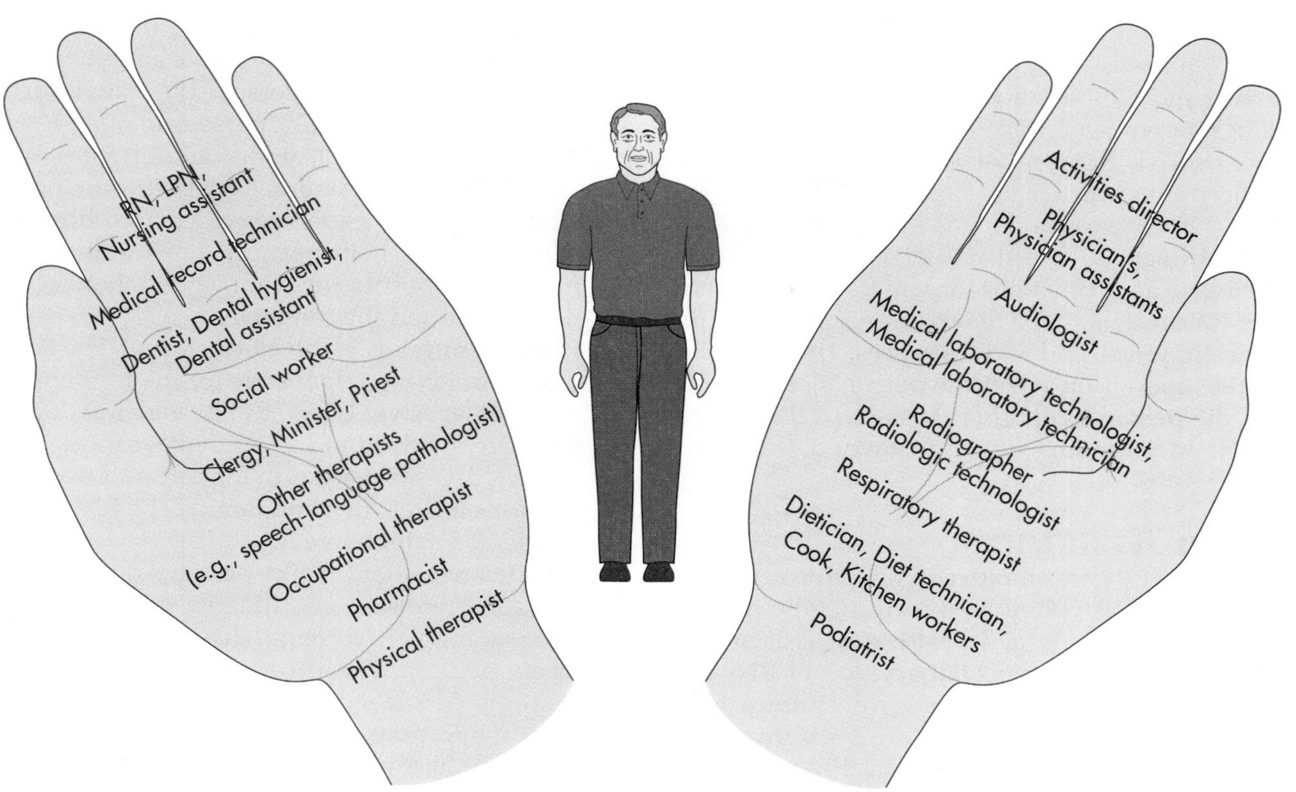

Fig. 1-3 Members of the interdisciplinary health care team, with the resident as the focus of care.

Registered Nurses

A **registered nurse (RN)** studies for 2 years at a community college, 2 or 3 years in a hospital-based diploma program, or 4 years at a college or university. Nursing and the biological, social, and physical sciences are studied. The graduate nurse takes a licensing examination offered by a state board of nursing. The examination must be passed for the nurse to become *registered* and receive a license to practice. RNs must be licensed by the state in which they practice.

RNs assess, make nursing diagnoses, plan, implement, and evaluate nursing care (see Chapter 4). An RN identifies a person's nursing problems and develops a care plan. The RN is responsible for making sure that the nursing team follows the care plan. The RN also delegates nursing care to LPNs/LVNs and nursing assistants. The RN then evaluates the effect of the care plan and nursing care on the resident. The resident is helped to become independent and is taught ways to stay or become healthy. Family teaching also is provided.

The RN is responsible for carrying out the doctor's orders. The RN may carry out the orders or delegate them to LPNs/LVNs or nursing assistants. RNs do not diagnose diseases or illnesses or prescribe treatments or medications. However, RNs can study to become clinical nurse specialists or nurse practitioners. These RNs are involved in diagnosing and prescribing within the limits of their state laws.

RNs work as staff nurses, charge nurses, nurse managers, supervisors, directors of nursing, and instructors. Their job opportunities depend on their education, professional abilities, and experience.

Nurse Practitioners

A **nurse practitioner (NP)** is an RN who has had additional education in physical examination and assessment. Some states require a nurse practitioner to be certified by the state board of nursing. Nurse practitioners may specialize in many areas. Most NPs who work in nursing centers are either family nurse practitioners (FNPs) or gerontological nurse practitioners (GNPs). GNPs specialize in the care of older persons. NPs work for doctors or under the direction of the center's medical director. The NP assists the nursing staff in assessing residents. The NP may be permitted to write orders for medications and treatments for uncomplicated illnesses or other problems.

Licensed Practical Nurses and Licensed Vocational Nurses

A **licensed practical nurse (LPN)** completes 1 year of study in a hospital-based nursing program, community college, vocational school, or technical school. Some programs are 18 months long. Some public high schools offer 2-year programs. Students study nursing, body structure and function, basic psychology, arithmetic, and communication skills. Graduates take a licensing examination for practical nursing. When the test is passed, the individual receives a license to practice and the title of *licensed practical nurse*. The title *licensed vocational nurse (LVN)* is used in some states. Like RNs, practical or vocational nurses must have a license to practice nursing.

LPNs/LVNs work under the supervision of RNs, licensed physicians, and licensed dentists. Their responsibilities and functions are more limited than those of RNs. LPNs/LVNs have less education in the biological, physical, and social sciences. They function with little supervision when the person's care is simple and the person's condition is stable. LPNs/LVNs assist RNs in providing nursing care and with complex procedures.

Nursing Assistants

Nursing assistants are employed in nursing centers to assist nurses in providing care to residents. Nurse's aide, nursing attendant, and health care assistant are other titles. Under the direct supervision of RNs and LPNs/LVNs, nursing assistants give simple, basic nursing care. Nursing assistants are very important members of the interdisciplinary health care team. They provide much of the care to residents.

OBRA

The Omnibus Budget Reconciliation Act (OBRA) of 1987 requires that nursing assistants have formal training and pass a competency evaluation. Nursing assistant courses are offered by community colleges, technical schools, and high school vocational programs. Others are offered by nursing education departments in nursing centers and hospitals. Before OBRA, some nursing assistants received on-the-job training instead of a formal course. (Nursing assistant training and competency evaluation are discussed in Chapter 2.)

You may wish to continue your education to become an RN or LPN/LVN. Community colleges and 4-year colleges and universities in your area can help you select the best program to meet your needs, abilities, and financial situation.

NURSING CARE PATTERNS

Safe and effective nursing care is provided in different ways. The nursing care pattern depends on how many persons need care, the available staff, and the cost.

- **Functional nursing** focuses on tasks and jobs. Each nursing team member has specific functions or tasks to do. For example, one RN gives all medications. Another RN changes all dressings and gives all treatments. LPNs/LVNs give baths, take vital signs, and weigh everyone. Nursing assistants make beds, serve meal trays, and feed patients.
- **Team nursing** involves a team of nursing staff led by an RN. The RN determines the amount and kind of care needed by each person. The team leader delegates the care of specific persons to other RNs and to LPNs/LVNs. The team leader delegates nursing tasks, procedures, and activities to nursing assistants. The team leader delegates according to the resident's needs and team member abilities. Team members report to the team leader about observations made and the care given.
- **Primary nursing** involves total care. The primary nurse (an RN) is responsible for the resident's total care. Other RNs, LPNs/LVNs, and nursing assistants are involved in the resident's care as needed. The RN gives bedside nursing care and teaches and counsels the resident and family. The RN also plans the person's discharge.
- **Case management** is like primary nursing. A case manager (an RN) coordinates the person's care from admission through discharge and into the home setting. The case manager communicates with the person's doctor and the health care team. Communication also occurs with the insurance company and with community agencies involved in the resident's care. The case manager makes sure that the resident's care is well planned. The case manager also helps all team members to work together. *(See Subacute Care, p. 11.)*

PAYING FOR HEALTH CARE

Health care is costly. Even after the person leaves the hospital or long-term care center, bills often continue for doctor visits, medicines, medical supplies, and home care. Most people cannot afford large medical bills. Some avoid medical care because they cannot pay. Others pay doctor bills even if it means going without food or medicine. Worry, fear, and emotional upset occur about paying for health care. If the person has insurance, part of or all health care costs are covered. Rarely is the total cost of long-term care covered.

Health care is a major focus in today's society. The goals are to provide health care access to everyone and to reduce the high cost of care. Government leaders have proposed many changes. Efforts to reduce health care costs include managed care and prospective payment systems. More changes are likely. Before managed care and prospective payment are presented, a general discussion of insurance programs is necessary.

- **Private insurance plans** are bought by individuals, and **group insurance plans** are bought by a group for individuals. These plans rarely pay for long-term care. If long-term care is covered, there usually are strict limits regarding eligibility for coverage, amount paid, and length of stay. Long-term

SUBACUTE CARE

Case management is often used in subacute care.

care insurance also can be purchased. However, there are limits on coverage. Policies should be reviewed before purchase.

- **Medicare** is a health insurance plan administered by the Social Security Administration of the federal government. Benefits are for persons 65 years of age and older. Younger, disabled people also may be covered. Monthly premiums are paid by those insured. Medicare has two parts. Part A pays for some hospital costs during a specified time period (see diagnosis-related groups in the next section). Long-term care and home care costs are included if certain regulations are met. Part B pays for some medical expenses, such as doctor visits, diagnostic tests, and treatments. Part B may cover such things as physical therapy, language therapy, and hospital equipment for home use if ordered by a doctor. Medicare benefits and regulations are complex and change often. Your local Social Security office can provide information and answer questions.
- **Medicaid** is a health insurance program sponsored by the state and federal governments. Benefits, regulations, and eligibility requirements vary from state to state. Persons younger than 65 may qualify. Blind and disabled persons and low-income families usually are eligible. Medicaid usually pays for hospital services, doctors' fees, x-ray and laboratory tests, home care, family planning, dental and eye care, immunizations, and rehabilitation. There is no insurance premium. However, the amount paid for each covered service is limited.

Prospective Payment Systems

Prospective payment systems limit the amounts paid by insurance companies, Medicare, and Medicaid. Prospective relates to *before* care. The amount paid for services is determined before the person receives care.

Diagnosis-related groups (DRGs) help reduce Medicare and Medicaid costs. Under the DRG system, Medicare and Medicaid payments are determined *before* the person receives hospital care.

Each DRG has specific diagnoses. Length of stay and treatment costs are determined for each diagnosis. The hospital is paid the predetermined amount for persons covered by Medicare and Medicaid. If the hospital's treatment costs are less than the DRG amount, the hospital keeps the extra money. If costs are greater, the hospital takes the loss.

BOX 1-1 TYPES OF MANAGED CARE

Health maintenance organization (HMO) provides health care services for a prepaid fee. For the fee, persons receive needed services offered by the organization. Some need only an annual physical examination but others require hospital care. Whatever services are used, the cost is covered by the prepaid fee. HMOs emphasize preventing disease and maintaining health. Keeping someone healthy costs far less than treating illness.

Preferred provider organization (PPO) is a group of doctors and hospitals that provides health care at reduced rates. Usually the arrangement is made between the PPO and an employer or an insurance company. Employees or those insured are given reduced rates for the services used. The person can choose any doctor or hospital in the PPO.

Managed Care

Managed care deals with the delivery and payment of health care. Insurance companies contract with doctors and hospitals for reduced rates or discounts. The insured person uses those doctors and agencies providing the lower rates. If others are used, the care may be covered only in part or not at all. The person pays for costs not covered by insurance.

Managed care limits the person's choice of where to go for health care. It also places limits on which doctors provide the care. Health maintenance organizations and preferred provider organizations (Box 1-1) are common managed care arrangements. Managed care generally involves private and group insurance plans. However, many states require managed care for Medicaid and Medicare participants.

Managed care as preapproval for services. Many insurance companies must approve the need for health care services. If the need is approved, the insurance company pays for the services. If preapproval or precertification is not obtained, the person pays for the health care. This preapproval process and the monitoring of care is also called *managed care*. It reduces unneeded medical and surgical services and procedures. The insurance company decides what to pay. With HMO or PPO contracts, the insurance company may decide where the person goes for the services.

Insurance companies have RNs who handle the preapproval process. The process varies depending on the insurance plan.

THE OMNIBUS BUDGET RECONCILIATION ACT OF 1987

In 1987 the U.S. Congress passed the **Omnibus Budget Reconciliation Act (OBRA).** OBRA is a federal law concerned with the quality of life, health, and safety of residents. Nursing centers must provide care in a manner and in a setting that maintains or improves each resident's quality of life, health, and safety. Training and competency evaluation of nursing assistants are also OBRA requirements (see Chapter 2). Many other requirements must be met as well.

Resident Rights

Nursing center residents have certain rights under federal and state laws. Residents have rights as citizens of the United States. They also have rights relating to their everyday lives and care in a nursing center. Nursing centers must protect and promote resident rights. Residents must be able to exercise their rights without interference from the center. Some residents are incompetent (not able) and cannot exercise their rights. Legal guardians exercise rights for them.

Nursing centers must inform residents of their rights. They must be informed orally and in writing. Such information is given before or during admission to the center. It must be given in the language used and understood by the resident.

Privacy and confidentiality. Residents have the right to personal privacy. The resident's body must not be exposed unnecessarily. Only those workers directly involved in care, treatments, or examinations should be present. The resident must give consent for others to be present. For example, a student may want to observe a procedure or treatment. The resident's consent is necessary for the student to be an observer. A resident also has the right to use the bathroom in private. Privacy must be maintained for personal care activities as well.

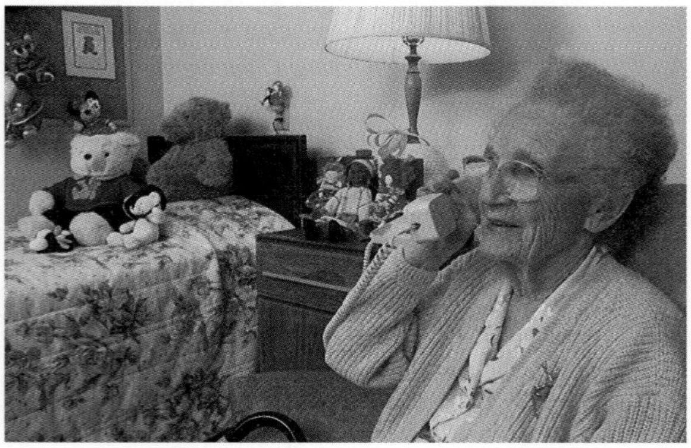

Fig. 1-4 A resident talking privately on a telephone.

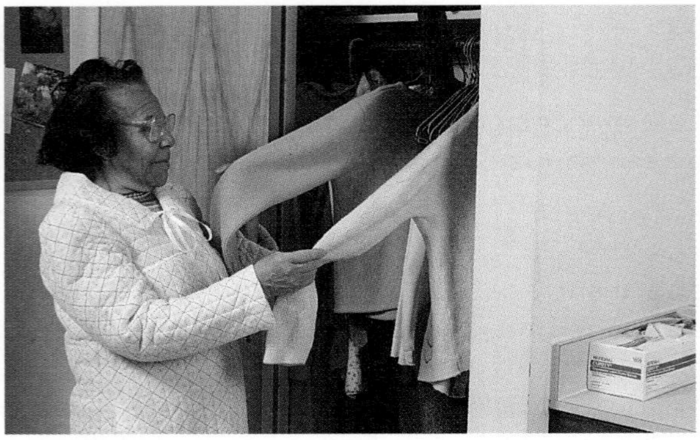

Fig. 1-5 A resident choosing what clothing to wear.

Residents also have the right to visit with others in private. They have the right to visit in an area where they cannot be seen or heard by others. The center must try to provide private space when it is requested. Offices, chapels, dining rooms, meeting rooms, and conference rooms can be used if available.

The right to visit in private also involves telephone conversations (Fig. 1-4). In addition, residents have the right to send and receive mail without interference by others. Mail sent and received by the resident must not be opened by others without the resident's permission.

Information about the resident's care, treatment, and condition must be kept confidential. Medical and financial records also are confidential. The resident must give consent for them to be released to other centers or individuals. Consent is not needed for the release of medical records when the resident is being transferred to another center. Records also can be released without the resident's consent when they are required by law or for insurance purposes.

Throughout this textbook you will be reminded to keep information about the person confidential. Providing for privacy and keeping medical and personal information confidential show respect for the person. They also protect the person's dignity. The right to privacy and confidentiality are discussed in Chapter 2.

Personal choice. OBRA requires that residents be free to choose their own doctors. They also have the right to participate in planning their own care and treatment. This means that residents have the right to choose activities, schedules, and care based on their personal preferences. For example, residents have the right to choose when to get up and go to bed, what to wear, how to spend their time, and what to eat (Fig. 1-5). They also can choose companions and visitors inside and outside of the center.

Personal choice is important for quality of life, dignity, and self-respect. You will be reminded throughout this book to allow the person's preferences whenever it is safely possible.

Disputes and grievances. Residents have the right to voice concerns, questions, and complaints about care or treatment. The dispute or grievance may involve another resident. It may be about treatment or care that was not given. The center must promptly try to correct the situation. The resident must not be punished in any way for voicing the dispute or grievance.

Participation in resident and family groups. Residents have the right to participate in resident and family groups. This means that residents have the right to form groups. In addition, a resident's family has the right to meet with the families of other residents. These groups can discuss concerns and suggest ways to improve quality of life in the center. They also can plan activities for residents and families. The group can provide support and reassurance for group members. Residents also have the right to participate in social, religious, and community activities. They have the right to assistance in getting to and from activities of their choice.

Care and security of personal possessions. Residents have the right to keep and use personal possessions. Available space and the health and safety of other residents can affect the type and amount of personal possessions allowed. A person's property must be treated with care and respect. Although the items may not have value to you, they are important to the resident. They also relate to personal choice, dignity, and quality of life.

The center must take reasonable measures to protect the person's property. Items should be labeled with the resident's name. The center must investigate reports of lost, stolen, or damaged items. Police assistance sometimes is necessary. The resident and family probably will be advised not to keep jewelry and other expensive items in the center.

You must protect yourself and the center from being accused of stealing a resident's property. Do not go through a resident's closet, drawers, purse, or other space without the person's knowledge and consent. Have another worker with you and the resident or legal guardian present if it is necessary to inspect closets and drawers. The worker serves as a witness to your activities.

Freedom from abuse, mistreatment, and neglect. OBRA states that residents have the right to be free from verbal, sexual, physical, or mental abuse (see Chapter 2).

Residents also have the right to be free from involuntary seclusion. Involuntary seclusion is separating the resident from others against his or her will. It also can mean keeping the person confined to a certain area or away from his or her room without consent. If the person is incompetent, involuntary seclusion occurs against the legal guardian's consent.

No one can abuse, neglect, or mistreat the resident. This includes center staff members, volunteers, staff members from other agencies or groups, other residents, family, visitors, and legal guardians. Nursing centers must have policies and procedures for investigating suspected or reported cases of resident abuse. Also, nursing centers cannot employ persons who have been convicted of abusing, neglecting, or mistreating individuals (see Chapter 2).

Freedom from restraint. Residents have the right not to have body movements restricted. Restraints and certain drugs can restrict body movements. Some drugs can restrain the person because they affect mood, behavior, and mental function. Sometimes residents need to be restrained to protect them from harming themselves or others. A doctor's order is necessary for restraints to be used. Restraints cannot be used for the convenience of the staff. Restraints are discussed in Chapter 8.

Quality of life. OBRA requires that nursing centers care for residents in a manner that promotes dignity, self-esteem, and physical, psychological, and emotional well-being. Protecting the rights of residents is one way to promote quality of life. Personal choice, privacy, participating in group activities, having personal property, and freedom from restraint show respect for the person.

The resident should be spoken to in a polite and courteous manner (see Chapter 5). Giving good, honest, and thoughtful care will enhance the resident's quality of life.

Activities. Activities are important to a resident's quality of life. OBRA requires that nursing centers provide activity programs that meet the interests and physical, mental, psychosocial, and spiritual needs of each resident (Fig. 1-6, p. 14). Such activities must allow personal choice and promote physical, intellectual, social, spiritual, and emotional well-being. Many centers provide religious services for spiritual health. You will be responsible for assisting residents to and from activity programs. You also may be assigned to help residents with activities.

Environment. The center's environment must promote quality of life. The environment must be clean, safe, and as homelike as possible. Letting the resident have personal possessions enhances quality of life. It allows personal choice and promotes a homelike setting. The safe environment is discussed in Chapter 8. The furniture and equipment in a resident's room are discussed in Chapter 11. Information relating to temperature and sound levels also is presented.

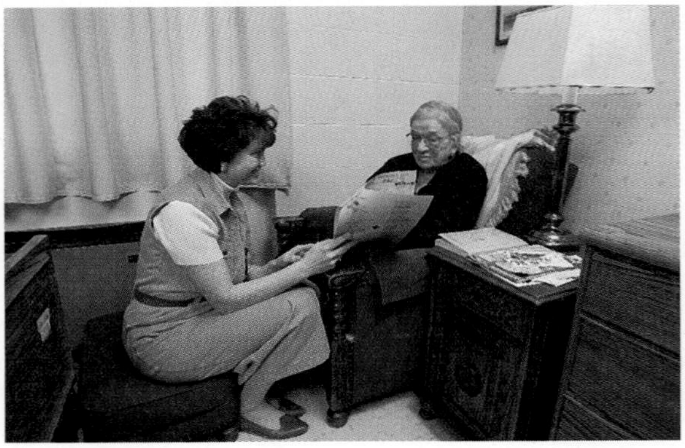

Fig. 1-6 An activities director and resident discuss the schedule of activities at the center.

THE JOINT COMMISSION ON ACCREDITATION OF HEALTHCARE ORGANIZATIONS

The Joint Commission on Accreditation of Healthcare Organizations (JCAHO) develops standards and practices for hospitals, nursing centers, and home health care agencies. JCAHO improves the quality of care to the public through voluntary accreditation. Accreditation is an approval process. To become accredited, the facility must meet certain standards of care.

Some centers choose to become accredited by JCAHO. JCAHO accreditation is another way for a center to show that it provides quality care. Centers may get JCAHO accreditation for long-term, dementia, and subacute care. Centers pay an application fee and are surveyed. JCAHO accreditation is not required. *(See Subacute Care, p. 14.)*

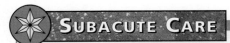

SUBACUTE CARE

A center with a subacute unit may need JCAHO accreditation before insurance companies will pay for care.

QUALITY OF LIFE

The focus of care in all nursing centers is always the resident. All residents are helped to become or remain as independent as possible. Helping residents reach and maintain their highest level of functioning helps promote their quality of life.

Nursing centers have an interdisciplinary health care team. Team members work together to provide quality resident care.

In 1987 the U.S. Congress passed the Omnibus Budget Reconciliation Act (OBRA). OBRA is a federal law concerned with quality of life, health, and safety of residents. All care provided in nursing centers must maintain or improve each resident's quality of life. The information and procedures in this book help you provide the best possible care. Everything you do as a nursing assistant must maintain and improve each resident's quality of life, health, and safety. If you remember this, your job will be rewarding and enjoyable.

REVIEW QUESTIONS

Circle the BEST answer.

1 Helping persons return to their highest physical and psychological functioning is known as
- A Detection and treatment of disease
- B Promotion of health
- C Rehabilitation
- D Disease prevention

2 Rehabilitation starts when
- A The person is ready to be discharged from the center
- B The person is admitted to the center
- C The doctor writes the order
- D The interdisciplinary health care team feels that the resident is ready

3 The person who controls policy in a nursing center is
- A The director of nurses
- B The administrator
- C The owner
- D The interdisciplinary health care team

4 A health care program for dying residents is called
- A A hospice
- B A board and care facility
- C An intermediate care facility
- D A hospital

5 The nursing team includes all of the following *except*
- A Registered nurses
- B Doctors
- C Nursing assistants
- D LPNs/LVNs

6 The person responsible for the entire nursing staff and the activities involved in providing safe nursing care is the
- A RN
- B Doctor
- C Director of nursing
- D Owner

7 These statements are about nursing assistants. Which is *false?*
- A They assist nurses in giving care
- B OBRA requires that they complete a training program
- C They can be supervisors
- D They are supervised by RNs and LPNs/LVNs

8 Nursing tasks are delegated according to the resident's needs and a staff member's abilities. This nursing care pattern is called
- A Team nursing
- B Functional nursing
- C Case management
- D Managed care

9 Which statement is *false?*
- A Medicare is for persons 65 years of age and older and for some disabled persons.
- B DRGs affect Medicare and Medicaid payments.
- C Most insurance programs pay all costs of long-term care.
- D Persons younger than 65 years may be eligible for Medicaid.

Circle T if the statement is true or F if the statement is false.

10 T F You have the right to open a resident's mail.

11 T F The resident has the right to decide what he or she will wear.

12 T F You can search the resident's closets and drawers to look for lost items.

13 T F Residents can offer suggestions to improve the center.

14 T F Residents can be restrained to prevent them from leaving the center.

15 T F Residents must be free from abuse, neglect, and mistreatment.

16 T F Allowing personal choice is important for the resident's quality of life.

17 T F Participation in activities is important for the resident's quality of life.

18 T F Nursing centers must be JCAHO accredited.

Answers to these questions are on p. 695.

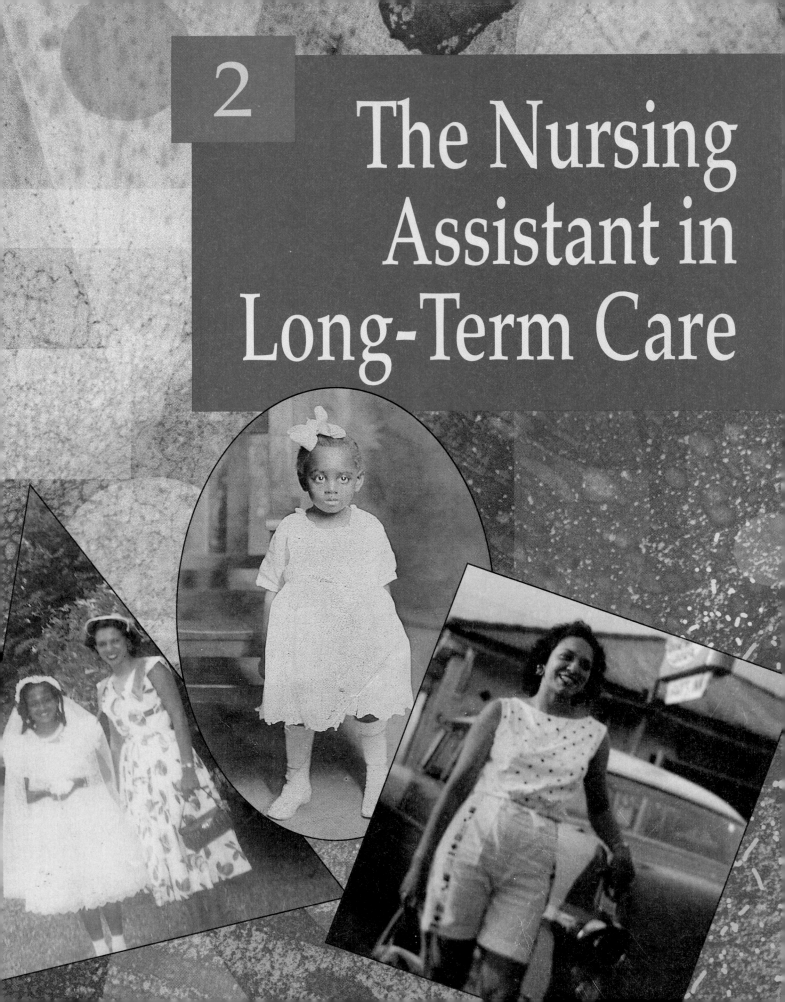

2 The Nursing Assistant in Long-Term Care

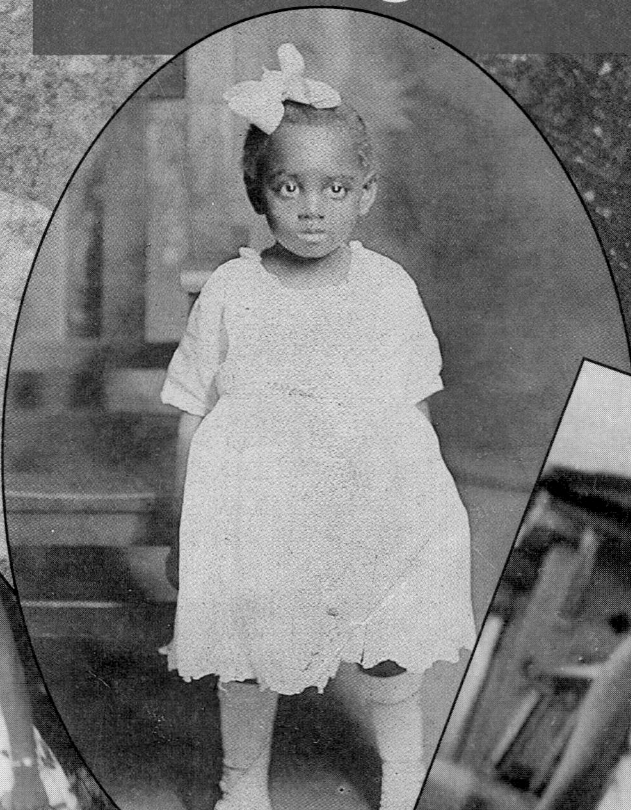

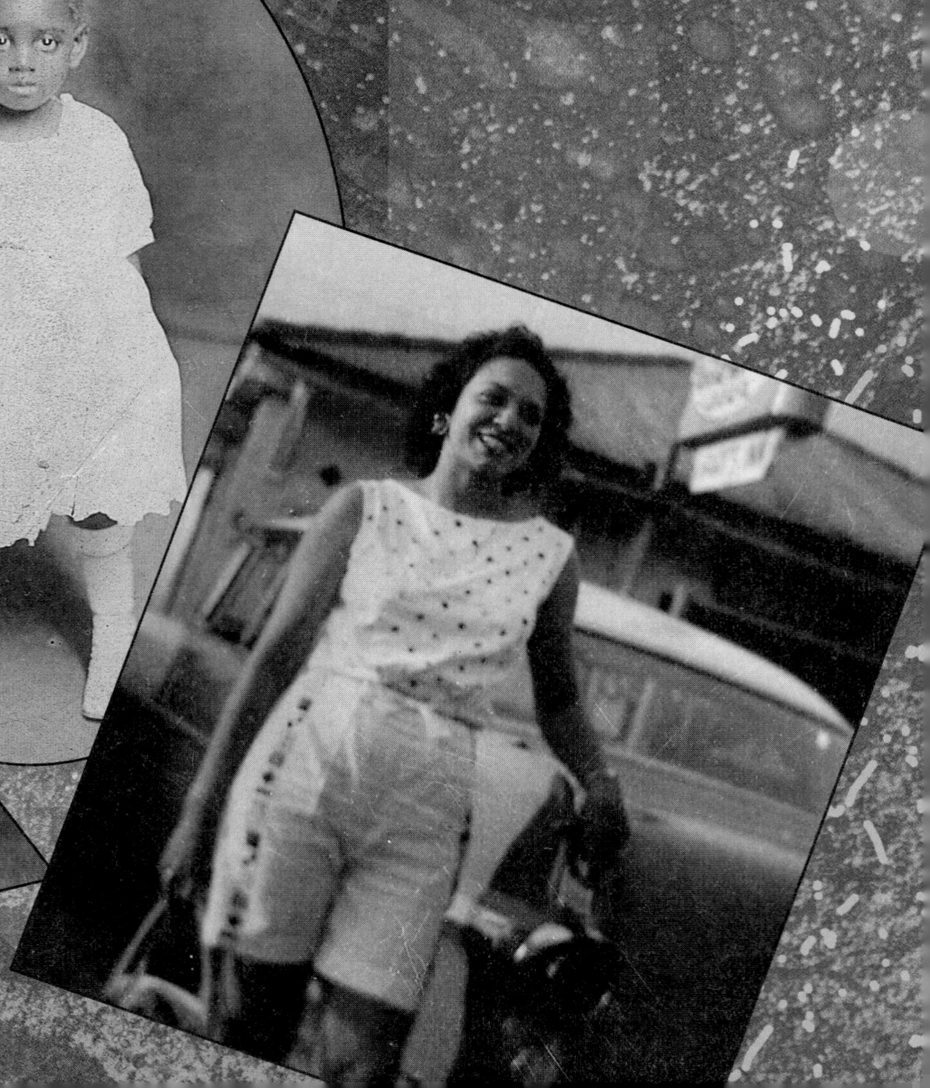

What You Will Learn

- The definition of the key terms listed in this chapter
- The history and current trends affecting nursing assistants
- How nurse practice acts affect nursing assistants
- The information contained in the nursing assistant registry and other OBRA requirements
- The functions, roles, responsibilities, and role limits of nursing assistants
- Why a job description is important
- The educational requirements for nursing assistants
- The delegation process and the "five rights of delegation"
- How you will use the "five rights of delegation"
- Your responsibilities when accepting or refusing a delegated task
- How to prevent negligent acts
- Examples of false imprisonment, defamation, assault, battery, and fraud
- How to protect the right to privacy
- The purpose of informed consent
- The elements of child, elderly, and domestic abuse
- Your role in relation to wills

Key Terms

accountable Being responsible for one's actions and the actions of others who perform delegated tasks; answering questions about and explaining one's actions and the actions of others

assault Intentionally attempting or threatening to touch a person's body without the person's consent

battery Unauthorized touching of a person's body without the person's consent

civil law Laws concerned with relationships between people; private law

crime An act that violates a criminal law

criminal law Laws concerned with offenses against the public and society in general; public law

defamation Injuring a person's name and reputation by making false statements to a third person

delegate Authorizing another person to perform a task

ethics Knowledge of what is right conduct and wrong conduct

false imprisonment Unlawful restraint or restriction of a person's movement

fraud Saying or doing something to trick, fool, or deceive another person

invasion of privacy Violating a person's right not to have his or her name, photograph, or private affairs exposed or made public without giving consent

job description listing of the responsibilities and functions the agency expects you to perform

law A rule of conduct made by a government body

libel Defamation through written statements

malpractice Negligence by a professional person

negligence An unintentional wrong in which a person fails to act in a reasonable and careful manner and causes harm to a person or to the person's property

preceptor A staff member who guides

responsibility The duty or obligation to perform some act or function

Continued

KEY TERMS—cont'd

slander Defamation through oral statements

task A function, procedure, activity, or work that does not require an RN's professional knowledge or judgment

tort A wrong committed against a person or the person's property

will A legal statement of how a person wishes to have property distributed after death

Federal and state laws and agency policies combine to define the roles and functions of each health team member. All health care personnel must protect residents from harm. To protect residents from harm, you must understand your roles and responsibilities. You need to know what you can and cannot do, what is right conduct and wrong conduct, and your legal limits. Supervised by RNs and LPNs/LVNs, you perform selected nursing tasks. Laws, job descriptions, and residents' condition influence how you function. So does the amount of supervision you need.

Protecting residents from harm also involves a complex set of rules and standards of conduct. These rules and standards form the legal and ethical aspects of care.

HISTORY AND CURRENT TRENDS

Nursing practice has a long history involving nursing assistants. For decades they assisted nurses in giving resident care. Commonly called *nurse's aides* or *nursing assistants*, they gave basic bedside nursing care. Bathing and feeding residents were common tasks. So were making beds, repositioning residents, and assisting with elimination. Their work was similar in hospitals and nursing homes throughout the United States. Until the 1980s, no training or experience was required. Nurses gave on-the-job training. Some hospitals, nursing homes, and schools offered nursing assistant courses.

Before the 1980s, team nursing was a common nursing care pattern. Team members included RNs, LPNs/LVNs, and nursing assistants. An RN was the team leader. The RN made team member assignments according to each resident's needs and condition. The education and experiences of each staff member also influenced assignments. Team members communicated with the team leader about resident care and observations.

Primary nursing became popular in hospitals in the 1980s. RNs planned and gave resident care. With this nursing care pattern, hospitals eliminated many LPN/LVN and nursing assistant positions. Often only RNs were hired to give resident care.

Meanwhile, nursing homes continued to rely on nursing assistants for resident care. To improve the quality of life of nursing home residents, the U.S. Congress passed the Omnibus Budget Reconciliation Act of 1987 (OBRA). The law sets minimum training and competency evaluation requirements for nursing assistants working in nursing homes. This law requires each state to set rules for nursing assistant training and evaluation. A state's requirements must be met before a person can work as a nursing assistant in a nursing home in that state. OBRA

Home care also increased during the 1980s. Prospective payment systems greatly affected this trend. Prospective payment systems limit how much insurance companies, Medicare, and Medicaid pay for health care (see Chapter 1). To reduce health care costs, hospital lengths of stay also are shortened. There-fore patients are discharged earlier than in the past. These persons are often still quite ill. Often skilled nursing care in a long-term care center or home care is required.

FEDERAL AND STATE LAWS

The U.S. Congress makes federal law. A federal law applies to all 50 states. Individual state legislatures make state law. A state law applies in that specific state. You must know the federal and state laws that affect your work.

Nurse Practice Acts

Each state has a nurse practice act. Intended to protect the public's welfare and safety, the law regulates nursing practice in that state. Definitions are given for RNs and LPNs/LVNs. Their scope of practice and education and licensing requirements are described. The law protects the public from persons practicing nursing without a license. That is, it prevents persons who do not meet the state's education and licensing requirements from performing nursing functions.

The law allows for revoking or suspending a nurse's license to practice. The reasons for such action include:

- Being convicted of a crime in any state
- Selling or distributing drugs
- Using the resident's drugs for oneself
- Placing residents in danger from the excessive use of alcohol or drugs
- Demonstrating grossly negligent nursing practice
- Being convicted of abusing or neglecting children or older persons

- Violating the act and its rules and regulations
- Demonstrating incompetent behaviors
- Aiding or assisting another person to violate the act and its rules and regulations
- Making medical diagnoses or prescribing medicines and treatments

A state's nurse practice act is used to determine the nursing tasks that nursing assistants can perform. Legal and advisory opinions about nursing assistants are based on the act. So are any state laws that regulate nursing assistant roles and functions. If you perform a task beyond the legal limits of your role, you could be practicing nursing without a license. This creates serious legal problems for you and the nurse supervising your work.

The Omnibus Budget Reconciliation Act of 1987

In 1987 the U.S. Congress passed the Omnibus Budget Reconciliation Act (OBRA). It is a federal law and applies to all 50 states. The law addresses training for nursing assistants working in long-term care. It requires each state to have a nursing assistant training and competency evaluation program. Nursing assistants working in nursing centers and hospital long-term care units must meet federal and state training and competency requirements.

State requirements vary. However, OBRA requires at least 75 hours of instruction. Sixteen of those hours involve supervised practical training. Such training occurs in a laboratory or clinical setting. The student actually performs nursing care and procedures on another person. A nurse supervises this practical training (clinical practicum or clinical experience).

The training program includes the knowledge and skills needed by nursing assistants to give basic nursing care. Areas of study include:

- Communication
- Infection control
- Safety and emergency procedures
- Resident rights
- Basic nursing skills
- Personal care skills
- Feeding techniques
- Elimination procedures
- Skin care
- Transferring, positioning, and turning techniques
- Dressing
- Ambulating residents
- Range-of-motion exercises
- Signs and symptoms of common diseases
- How to care for cognitively impaired residents (those who have problems with thinking and memory)

Competency Evaluation

The competency evaluation program includes a written test and a skills test (see Appendix, p. 722). The written test involves multiple-choice questions. Each question has 4 possible answers. Only 1 answer is correct. The number of questions varies from state to state. The skills evaluation involves the demonstration of nursing skills. You will have to perform certain skills learned in your training program.

The written and skills competency evaluations are done after you complete your training program. Your instructor or supervisor can help you find where to take the tests and how to complete the required application form. There is a fee for the competency evaluation. This fee must be sent with your application. If you are employed by a nursing center, the employer must pay this fee. You will be notified about the location and time of the tests after your application has been processed.

Your training program will prepare you for the competency evaluation. If the first attempt was unsuccessful, you can retest. OBRA allows three attempts to complete the evaluation successfully.

Nursing Assistant Registry

OBRA requires each state to have a nursing assistant registry. The registry is an official record or listing of persons who have successfully completed a nursing assistant training and competency evaluation program. The registry contains the following information about each nursing assistant:

- Full name, including maiden name and any married names
- Last known home address
- Social Security number
- Date of birth
- Last known employer, date hired, and date employment was terminated
- Date the competency evaluation was passed
- Information about findings of abuse, neglect, or dishonest use of property. This includes the nature of the offense and evidence supporting the finding. If a hearing was held, the date and its outcome are included. The person has the right to include a statement disputing the finding. All information remains in the registry for at least 5 years.

Any nursing center or agency can access registry information. The nursing assistant also receives a copy of all information in her or his registry file. The copy is provided when the entry is first included in the registry and when information is changed or added. The nursing assistant can correct inaccurate information.

Other OBRA Requirements

OBRA also requires retraining and a new competency evaluation program for nursing assistants who have not worked for 2 consecutive years (24 months). For example, you completed a training and competency evaluation. After working as a nursing assistant, you quit your job. You were either not working or you worked in some other field for 2 or more years. Now you want to work as a nursing assistant again. OBRA requires that you take another training and competency evaluation program. This is to ensure that your knowledge and skills are current for safe care. It does not matter how long you worked as a nursing assistant, but how long you did not work.

OBRA

Regular in-service education and performance reviews are other OBRA requirements. Nursing centers must provide 12 hours of in-service training per year to nursing assistants. A nursing assistant's work also will be evaluated regularly. These are ways to help ensure that nursing assistants have the knowledge and skills to give safe, effective care.

THE ROLE OF A NURSING ASSISTANT

OBRA

Nurse practice acts, OBRA, state laws, and legal and advisory opinions give direction to what nursing assistants can do. To protect residents from harm, you must understand what you can do, what you cannot do, and the legal limits of your role. In some states this is called *scope of practice.*

Nursing assistants function under the supervision of RNs and, in some states, LPNs/LVNs. You assist nurses in giving care. You also perform nursing procedures and tasks involved in the resident's care. Often you function without a nurse in the room. At other times you help nurses give bedside nursing care. The following rules should help you understand your role:

- You are an assistant to the nurse.
- A nurse assigns and supervises your work.
- You report any changes in a resident's physical or mental status to the nurse.
- You do not make decisions about what should or should not be done for a resident.
- If you do not understand directions or instructions, ask the nurse for clarification before going to the resident.
- Perform no function or task that you have not been prepared to do or that you do not feel comfortable performing without the supervision of a nurse.

Generally, you assist nurses in meeting the hygiene, safety, nutrition, exercise, elimination, and oxygen needs of residents. Related functions include lifting and moving residents, observing them, and helping promote physical comfort.

FUNCTIONS AND RESPONSIBILITIES

The functions and responsibilities of a nursing assistant vary among nursing centers. **Responsibility** is a duty or obligation to perform some act or function and to be able to answer for one's actions. Nursing assistants perform the procedures in this book. Some procedures are more advanced than others.

You will perform functions and procedures relating to the personal hygiene, safety, comfort, nutrition, exercise, and elimination needs of residents. You also will perform related functions such as lifting and moving residents, making observations, and collecting specimens. Because you provide care over many months, you will play an important role in the residents' psychological comfort. In addition, you may assist with the admission and discharge of residents and measure temperatures, pulses, respirations, and blood pressures.

Your training may prepare you to perform certain procedures. Your employer may not allow nursing assistants to perform some procedures. Other centers may ask you to perform procedures that you did not learn.

There are certain functions, procedures, and tasks that you should never perform. State laws and rules limit nursing assistant functions. It is extremely important that you understand what you cannot do as a nursing assistant. Box 2-1 describes the limits of the nursing assistant role. Job descriptions for nursing assistants reflect those laws and rules.

Job Description

The **job description** lists the responsibilities and functions the agency expects you to perform (Box 2-2, pp. 22-23). It also identifies the educational requirements for nursing assistants. These requirements are based on state laws or recommendations that limit what nursing assistants can do.

Always request a written job description when you apply for a job. Ask questions about the job description during your job interview. Before accepting a job, tell the employer about functions you do not know how to do. Also advise the employer of functions you are opposed to doing for moral or religious reasons. Have a clear understanding of what is expected of you before taking a job. Do not take a job that requires you to:

- Act beyond the legal limits of your role
- Function beyond your educational limits
- Perform acts that are against your moral or religious principles

No one can force you to perform a function, task, or procedure that is beyond the legal limits of nursing assistants. Jobs may be threatened for refusing to follow an RN's orders. Often staff obey out of fear. That is why you must understand the roles and responsibilities of nursing assistants. You also need to know the functions you can safely perform, the things you should never do, and your job description. Under-

Box 2-1 Limits of the Nursing Assistant Role

- **Never give medications.** This includes medication given orally, rectally, by injection, by application to the skin, or directly into the bloodstream through an intravenous line. There have been times when a nurse has brought a medication to a resident's room while the resident was in the bathroom or busy with some other activity. The nurse then instructed the nursing assistant to give the medication to the resident later. In this (and other similar situations) you should respectfully, but firmly, refuse to follow the nurse's direction. If you give a medication, you are performing a function and a responsibility beyond the scope of nursing assistants.
- **Never insert tubes or objects into a resident's body openings or remove them from the body.** You must not insert tubes into the resident's bladder, esophagus, trachea, nose, ears, bloodstream, or body openings that have been surgically created. Exceptions to the rule are those procedures in this textbook that you will study and practice with your instructor's supervision.
- **Never take verbal or telephone orders from doctors.** You might answer the telephone or be near a doctor who wants to give you an order. You should politely give your name and title, ask the doctor to wait, and promptly find a nurse to speak with the doctor.
- **Never perform procedures that require sterile technique.** With sterile technique, all objects that will be in contact with the resident's body are free of all microorganisms. Sterile technique and procedures require skills, knowledge, and judgment beyond the training you will receive. You can assist a nurse during a sterile procedure. However, you must never perform the procedure yourself.
- **Never tell the resident or family the resident's diagnosis or medical or surgical treatment plans.** The doctor is responsible for informing the resident and family about the diagnosis and treatment. Nurses may provide further explanations about what the doctor has already told the resident and family if they seem confused.
- **Never diagnose or prescribe treatments or medications for residents.** Only doctors can diagnose and prescribe.
- **Never supervise other nursing assistants.** Nurses are responsible for supervising nursing assistants. You will not be trained to supervise the work of others. Supervising other nursing assistants can have serious legal consequences.
- **Never just ignore an order or request to do something that you cannot do or that is beyond your scope of practice as a nursing assistant.** Promptly explain to the nurse why you cannot carry out the order or request. The nurse assumes you are doing what you were told unless you explain otherwise. Resident care cannot be neglected.

standing the ethical and legal aspects of your role is equally important (pp. 26-31).

Center Policies and Procedures

When employed, you will complete the center's orientation program. Center policies and procedures are explained and your skills checked. That is, the center has you perform nursing procedures and tasks to make sure you can do them safely and correctly. Also, you are shown how to use the center's supplies and equipment.

Some centers have preceptor programs. A **preceptor** is a staff member who guides. In a preceptor program, a staff nurse or nursing assistant helps you become familiar with the center layout so you can find what you need (Fig. 2-1). The preceptor may introduce

Text continued on p. 24

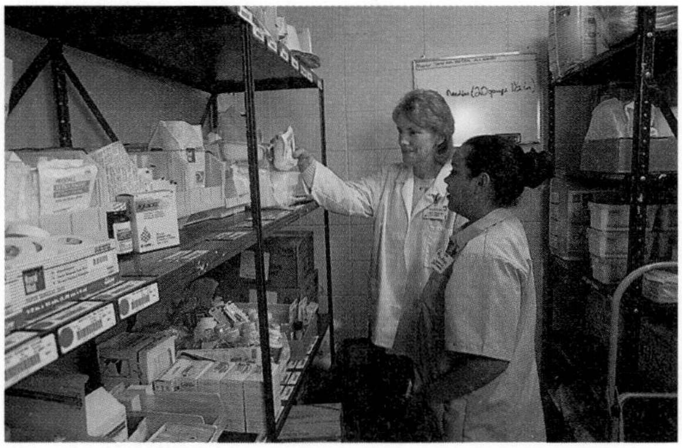

Fig. 2-1 A nurse preceptor shows a new nursing assistant where to find supplies.

Box 2-2 Job Description for Nursing Assistants

Nursing Assistant

Employee Name: ____________________

The Evangelical Lutheran Good Samaritan Society Job Description

Supervised by: ____________________

Job Summary

Primary Purpose of Job
To provide care to assigned residents in a caring, safe, and efficient manner

Essential Job Functions
Responsible to perform the following according to Good Samaritan mission, facility standards, procedures, and individualized resident care plans:

Resident care

1. Dressing/undressing	Helps residents with dressing and undressing and maintaining proper clothing.
2. Grooming	Assists residents in maintaining proper and clean appearance.
3. Bathing	Assists residents with bathing and maintaining cleanliness of all body areas.
4. Toileting/elimination	Helps residents with toileting needs.
5. Nutrition	Helps residents with meals and in meeting dietary needs.
6. Movement	Assists residents in transferring, repositioning, and walking.
7. Psychosocial care	Accommodates residents' needs through responding appropriately to residents' verbal/nonverbal expressions of needs.
8. Spiritual care	Assures residents' spiritual needs are met by willing employees (self or others).

Resident rights

1. Property	Safeguards residents' property.
2. Living areas	Keeps residents' living areas pleasant and orderly.
3. Dignity/privacy/confidentiality	Maintains residents' self-esteem, privacy, and confidentiality of personal information.
4. Independence/choice	Provides residents with opportunities for independence and choice consistent with their care plans.
5. Advocacy	Assures residents rights are protected and that all residents, families, and significant others are made aware of resident rights.

Communication

1. Monitor/document	Measures body functions and documents care provided to residents.
2. Resident status	Receives and shares information; observes and reports residents' conditions to appropriate staff.
3. Cooperation	Works with team members and other staff members in a helpful, respectful, and courteous manner.
4. Socialization	Assists residents in meeting their social needs through interaction with staff, family, and other residents.
5. Customer service	Responds appropriately to residents' requests for help and maintains positive relationships with residents' friends and family members; responds promptly to residents' call lights.

Modified from The Evangelical Lutheran Good Samaritan Society, Sioux Falls, S.D.

CONT'D
BOX 2-2

JOB DESCRIPTION FOR NURSING ASSISTANTS

Safety	Maintains safe work practices and follows facility safety procedures.
Infection control	Follows facility infection control procedures.
Other basic responsibilities	
1. Attendance	Arrives on time for work and is ready to perform assigned tasks.
2. Personal hygiene/ appearance	Meets facility hygiene and appearance standards.
3. Time management	Prioritizes and completes work assignments within reasonable and agreed-upon timeframes.
4. Conduct/policies/ procedures	Follows facility conduct standards and policies and procedures, performing all work alcohol and drug free.
5. In-service training/ meetings	Meets requirements for in-service training and meeting attendance per facility policy and state and federal requirements.
6. Continuous quality improvement	Actively participates and works to identify and improve quality and work outcomes individually and as part of a team.
7. Technology skills	Seeks to learn and utilize appropriate equipment and trends in technology.
8. Professional certification/ licensure/standards	Maintains required certification/qualifications and associated standards.
Other	Performs other related duties as assigned.

Minimum Hiring Requirements

Following are the minimum requirements to be hired into this job:

1. Knowledge	Basic ability to communicate and comprehend; ability to measure and comprehend certain quantities. (A high school education or higher educaton is <u>not</u> required to be hired into this job.)
2. Prior experience	Prior work experience may not be required to be hired into this job.
3. Basic abilities	Ability to meet the physical and mental abilities of the job as outlined in Physical and Mental Abilities Profile. (Reasonable accommodation for qualified disabilities will be considered by the employer on an individual basis as provided under the Americans with Disabilities Act.)
4. Special abilities/training	Ability to meet conditions of employment applicable to the facility. Completion of an accredited nursing assistant training program or ability to satisfactorily complete an accredited training program approved by the facility and the state in which the facility is located.

Acknowledgment

I have read and understand the essential job functions and the physical and mental abilities required for this job. My questions have been addressed, and by signing this page I acknowledge receipt of a copy of this job description.

Signature of Employee ______________________________ Date ____________ you to residents and other staff. Preceptors also help you organize your work and feel comfortable as part of the nursing team. A nursing assistant preceptor is not your supervisor. Only RNs and LPNs/LVNs can supervise. Depending on the center, the preceptor program can last from 2 to 4 weeks. It is designed to help you succeed in your new role and to ensure quality and safe resident care.

DELEGATION

Nurse practice acts give RNs and LPNs/LVNs certain responsibilities and the authority to perform nursing tasks. **Responsibility** is the duty or obligation to perform some act or function. For example, RNs are responsible for supervising LPNs/LVNs and nursing assistants. Only RNs can carry out this responsibility.

In nursing, a **task** is a function, procedure, activity, or work that does not require an RN's professional knowledge or judgment. **Delegate** means to authorize another person to perform a task. The person must be competent to perform the task in a given situation. For example, you know how to give a complete bed bath. However, Mr. Jones was just admitted to the subacute unit from the hospital. Mr. Jones has multiple injuries from an auto accident. He has neck injuries and is at risk for paralysis. His left leg is fractured in three places, and he has a full leg cast. He has two IVs, a retention catheter, a nasogastric tube, and a tracheostomy. In this situation, giving a bed bath to Mr. Jones is complicated. The RN gives the bath and asks you to assist.

Who Can Delegate

Nurse practice acts allow RNs to delegate tasks to LPNs/LVNs and nursing assistants. Some states allow LPNs/LVNs to delegate tasks to nursing assistants. RNs and LPNs/LVNs can delegate tasks only within their scope of practice.

When making delegation decisions, nurses must protect the resident's health and safety. The delegating nurse remains accountable for the delegated task. To be **accountable** means to be responsible for one's actions and the actions of others who perform delegated tasks. It also involves answering questions about and explaining one's actions and the actions of others.

The delegating nurse must make sure that the task was completed safely and correctly. If the RN delegates, the RN is responsible for the delegated task. If the LPN/LVN delegates, the LPN/LVN is responsible for the delegated task. Remember, the RN is also responsible for supervising the practice of LPNs/LVNs. Therefore the RN also is accountable for the tasks that LPNs/LVNs delegate to nursing assistants. The RN is accountable for all resident care.

Nursing assistants cannot delegate. You cannot delegate any task to other nursing assistants. You can ask another nursing assistant to help you. However you cannot ask or tell another person to do your work.

Some states allow LPNs/LVNs to have supervisory roles in long-term care settings. The LPN/LVN delegates tasks to nursing assistants. The LPN/LVN follows the delegation process and the "five rights of delegation."

Delegation Process

Delegated tasks must be within the legal limits of what nursing assistants can do. Before delegating tasks to you, the nurse must know:

- What tasks your state allows nursing assistants to perform
- The tasks included in your job description
- What you were taught in your training program
- What skills you learned and how they were evaluated
- About your work experiences

The nurse uses this information to make delegation decisions. The nurse is likely to discuss this information with you. This is so the nurse can get to know you, your abilities, and your concerns. Whenever your work with a new nurse, you should meet to discuss your training and work experience. You may be a new employee or new to the nursing unit. Or the nurse may be someone new. In any case, it is wise for the nurse to get to know you and for you to get to know the nurse.

Center policies, guidelines, and the job description for nursing assistants state what tasks nurses can delegate to you. These documents must be consistent with state laws, rules, and legal opinions about the roles and functions of nursing assistants. However, even if a task is in your job description, a nurse does not have to delegate it to you. The nurse must consider the circumstances when delegating.

The nurse makes delegation decisions after considering the questions in Box 2-3. The resident's needs, the task, and the person performing the task must fit. The nurse can decide to delegate the task to you. Or the nurse can decide not to delegate the task. If the resident's needs and the task require the knowledge, judgment, and skill of an RN, the RN completes the task. You may be asked to assist.

You must not be offended or get angry if you are not allowed to perform a task that is part of your job description and that is usually delegated to you. The nurse makes a decision that is best for the resident at the time. That decision is also best for you at that time. You do not want to perform a task that requires an RN's judgment and critical thinking skills. For example, you may routinely care for Mrs. Mills. You take her vital signs and assist her with bathing, dressing, and grooming. You also assist her with ambulation

Box 2-3 Factors Affecting Delegation Decisions

- What is the resident's condition? Is it stable or likely to change?
- What are the resident's basic needs at this time?
- What is the resident's mental function at this time?
- What are the resident's emotional and spiritual needs at this time?
- Can the resident assist with his or her care? Does the resident depend on others for care?
- Is the task something the nurse can delegate?
- For this resident, does the task require the knowledge, judgment, and skill of an RN or LPN/LVN?
- How often will the nurse have to assess the resident?
- Can the task harm the resident? If yes, how?
- What effect will the task have on the resident?
- Is it safe for the resident if the task is delegated to you?
- Do you have the training and experience to perform the task, given the resident's current status? Is your training documented? How were your training and skills evaluated?
- How often have you performed the task?
- What other tasks were delegated to you?
- Do you have the time to perform the task safely?
- Is a nurse available to supervise you?
- How much supervision will you need?
- Will you need more directions as you perform the task?
- Is a nurse available to help or take over if the resident's condition changes or problems arise?

twice each day. Mrs. Mills becomes ill. She has an elevated temperature, is weak, and is not eating well. The RN wants to observe and evaluate the change in her condition. The RN delegates the care to another nurse. Although you can provide routine care for Mrs. Mills, at this time she needs the nurse's judgment and knowledge.

The person's circumstances are central factors in making delegation decisions. Delegation decisions should always result in the best care for the resident. A nurse places a resident's health and safety at risk with poor delegation decisions. Also, the nurse may face serious legal problems. If you perform a task that places the resident at risk, you also can face serious legal problems.

The five rights of delegation. The following five rights of delegation summarize the delegation process. These are based on guidelines developed by the National Council of State Boards of Nursing:

- *The right task*—Can the task be delegated? Does the nurse practice act allow the RN or LPN/LVN to delegate the task? Is the task in the job description for nursing assistants?
- *The right circumstances*—What are the resident's physical, mental, emotional, and spiritual needs at this time?
- *The right person*—Do you have the training and experience to safely perform the task for this resident?
- *The right directions and communication*—The nurse must give clear directions. The nurse tells you what to do, when to do it, what observations to make, and when to report back. The nurse allows questions and helps you set priorities.
- *The right supervision*—The nurse guides, directs, and evaluates the care you give. The nurse demonstrates tasks as necessary and is available to answer questions. The less experience you have performing a task, the more supervision you need. Complex tasks require greater supervision than basic tasks. Also, the resident's circumstances affect how much supervision you need. The nurse assesses how the task affected the resident and how well you performed the task. To help you learn and give better care, the nurse tells you what you did well and what you can do to improve your work.

Your Role in Delegation

You must remember that you perform delegated tasks for or on a person. You must perform the task safely to protect the person from harm.

You have two choices when a nurse delegates a task to you. You either agree or refuse to do the task. You should use the "five rights of delegation" to make your choice. Before accepting a delegated task, you need to answer the questions in Box 2-4 on p. 26.

Accepting a task. When you agree to perform a task, you are responsible for your own actions. Remember, what you do or fail to do can bring harm to the resident. You must complete the task safely. You must ask for help when you are unsure or have questions about a task. You must communicate with the nurse by reporting what you did and your observations.

Box 2-4 The Five Rights of Delegation for Nursing Assistants

The Right Task
- Does your state allow nursing assistants to perform the task?
- Were you trained to do the task?
- Do you have experience performing the task?
- Is the task in your job description?

The Right Circumstances
- Do you have experience performing the task, given the resident's condition and needs?
- Do you understand the purpose of the task for the resident?
- Can you perform the task safely under the current circumstances?
- Do you have the equipment and supplies to safely complete the task?
- Do you know how to use the equipment and supplies?

The Right Person
- Are you comfortable performing the task?
- Do you have concerns about performing the task?

The Right Directions and Communication
- Did the nurse give clear directions and instructions?
- Did you review the task with the nurse?
- Do you understand what the nurse expects?

The Right Supervision
- Is a nurse available to answer questions?
- Is a nurse available if the resident's condition changes or if problems occur?

Modified from the National Council of State Boards of Nursing Inc., Chicago, Ill.

Refusing a task. You have the right to say "no." Sometimes refusing to follow the nurse's directions is your right and duty. You should refuse to perform a task when:
- The task is beyond the legal limits of your role.
- The task is not in your job description.
- You were not prepared to perform the task safely.
- The task could harm the resident.
- The resident's condition has changed.
- You do not know how to use the supplies or equipment.
- The nurses's directions are unethical, illegal, or against center policies.
- The nurse's directions are unclear or incomplete.
- A nurse is not available for supervision.

Protect residents and yourself by using common sense. Ask yourself if what you are doing is safe for the person.

As explained in Box 2-1, you must never ignore an order or request to do something. You must communicate your concerns to the nurse. If the task is within the legal limits of your role and in your job description, the nurse can help you feel more comfortable with the tasks. The nurse can answer your questions, demonstrate the task, and show you how to use supplies and equipment. The nurse can help you as needed, observe you performing the task, and check on you often. The nurse also can arrange for needed training.

With good communication, you and the nurse should be able to work out any problems. If not, try talking to the nurse or supervisor. When work problems continue, talk to someone whom you trust and can confide in. For example, your instructor or another professional can help you sort out work problems.

You must not refuse a delegated task simply because you do not like or want to do the task. You must have sound reasons for your refusal. Otherwise, you could place the resident at risk for harm. You also risk losing your job.

ETHICAL ASPECTS

Ethics is concerned with what is right conduct and wrong conduct. It involves morals and making choices or judgments about what should or should not be done. An ethical person behaves and acts in the right way and does not bring harm to the person.

Ethical behavior also involves not being prejudiced or biased. A person who is prejudiced or biased makes judgments and has opinions before knowing the facts. Judgments and opinions usually are based a person's own values and standards. Such values are derived from the person's culture, religion, education, and life experiences. The resident's situation may be very different from your own. For example:
- Children decide that their elderly mother needs nursing home care after leaving the hospital. In your culture, children take care of elderly parents at home.

- A resident has multiple tattoos and body piercings. You do not believe in tattooing or body piercing.
- An 80-year-old man has a living will that says he should not be resuscitated. You believe that everything possible should be done to save life.

You must not judge the person by your own values or standards. You must not avoid persons whose standards and values are different from your own.

Ethical dilemmas involve making choices. You must decide what is the right thing to do. For example:

- A co-worker was late for work 3 days this week. You find her in an empty room drinking from a thermos. You also smell alcohol on her breath. She asks you not to tell anyone.
- An older resident has bruises all over her body. She told the RN that they are from a fall. Later she tells you that her son is very mean to her. She asks you not to tell anyone.

Professional groups have codes of ethics. The code involves rules, or standards of conduct, for group members to follow. The American Nurses Association (ANA) has a code of ethics for RNs. The National Federation of Licensed Practical Nurses (NFLPN) has one for LPNs/LVNs. No formal code of ethics exists for nursing assistants. However, the rules of conduct in Box 2-5 can guide your thinking and behavior. JCAHO requires centers to have a code of ethics to guide the care given. See Chapter 3 for ethical behavior in the workplace.

Box 2-5 Rules of Conduct for Nursing Assistants

- Respect each person as an individual.
- Perform no act that is not within the legal limits of your role.
- Perform no act for which you have not been adequately prepared.
- Take no drug without the prescription and supervision of a doctor.
- Carry out the directions and instructions of the nurse to your best possible ability.
- Complete each task safely.
- Be loyal to your employer and co-workers.
- Act as a responsible citizen at all times.
- Recognize the limits of your role and knowledge.
- Keep resident information confidential.
- Consider the resident 's needs to be more important than your own.

LEGAL ASPECTS

Whereas ethics is concerned with what you *should* or *should not do*, laws tell you what you *can* and *cannot do*. A **law** is a rule of conduct made by a government body such as the U.S. Congress or a state legislature. Laws protect the public welfare and are enforced by the government.

Criminal laws are concerned with offenses against the public and against society in general. A violation of a criminal law is called a **crime**. A person found guilty of a crime is fined or sent to prison. Murder, robbery, rape, and kidnapping are examples of crimes.

Civil laws deal with the relationships between people. Examples of civil laws are those that involve contracts and nursing practice. A person found guilty of breaking a civil law usually has to pay a sum of money to the injured person.

Torts

Tort comes from a French word meaning *wrong*. Torts are part of civil law. A **tort** is committed by an individual against another person or the person's property. Torts may be intentional or unintentional.

Unintentional torts. **Negligence** is an unintentional wrong. The person did not mean or intend to cause harm. The negligent person failed to act in a reasonable and careful manner and thereby caused harm to the person or property of another. The person at fault failed to do what a reasonable and careful person would have done. Or the individual did what a reasonable and careful person would not have done. The negligent individual may have to pay damages (a sum of money) to the injured person.

Malpractice is negligence by professionals. A person has professional status because of training, education, and the service provided. Nurses, doctors, dentists, lawyers, and pharmacists are examples of professional people.

You are legally responsible (liable) for your own actions. What you do or do not do can lead to a lawsuit if harm results to the person or property of another. A nurse may direct you to do something beyond the legal limits of your role. Or you may be asked to do something beyond your education. Giving medications is an example. You may be told not to worry, that the nurse will be responsible if anything happens. The nurse is liable as your supervisor. However, you are not relieved of personal liability. You are responsible for your own actions. Remember, sometimes refusing to follow the RN's directions is your right and duty (p. 26).

Intentional torts. Intentional torts are acts meant to be harmful. Defamation (libel and slander), assault and battery, false imprisonment, invasion of privacy, and fraud are intentional torts.

Defamation is injuring the name and reputation of a person by making false statements to a third person. **Libel** is making false statements in print, writing, or through pictures or drawings. **Slander** is making false statements orally. Protect yourself from defamation by never making false statements about a resident, a co-worker, or any other person. Examples of defamation include:

- Implying or suggesting that a person has a sexually transmitted disease
- Saying that a resident is insane or mentally ill
- Implying or suggesting that a person is corrupt or dishonest

Assault and battery may result in both civil and criminal charges. **Assault** is intentionally attempting or threatening to touch a person's body without the person's consent. The person fears bodily harm. Threatening to "tie down" an uncooperative resident is an example of assault. **Battery** is the actual touching of a person's body without the person's consent. Consent is the important factor in assault and battery. The person must consent to any procedure, treatment, or other act that involves touching the body. The person has the right to withdraw consent at any time.

Consent is more than a person's verbal okay or signature on a form. For consent to be valid, it must be informed consent. Protect yourself from assault and battery by explaining to the person what is to be done and get the person's consent. Consent may be verbal ("yes" or "okay") or a gesture (a nod, turning over for a back rub, or holding out an arm for a blood pressure measurement).

False imprisonment is the unlawful restraint or restriction of a person's freedom of movement. Threat of restraint or actual physical restraint is false imprisonment. Preventing a person from leaving the agency also is false imprisonment.

Every person has the right not to have his or her name, photograph, or private affairs exposed or made public without having given consent. Violating this right is an **invasion of privacy.** You must treat residents with respect and ensure their privacy. Only staff involved in the residents care should see, handle, or examine the person's body. The precautions listed in Box 2-6 help ensure the right to privacy.

Fraud is saying or doing something to trick, fool, or deceive another person. The act is fraud if it does or could cause harm to a person or the person's property. Telling a resident or family that you are an RN is fraud. So is giving incomplete or inaccurate information on a job application.

Informed Consent

Informed consent recognizes a person's right to decide what will be done to his or her body and who can touch his or her body. Consent is informed when the

Box 2-6 Protecting the Resident's Right to Privacy

- Keep all resident information confidential.
- Make sure the resident is covered when being moved in corridors.
- Screen the resident as in Figure 2-2, and close the door when giving care. Also close drapes and window shades.
- Expose only the body part involved in a treatment or procedure (Fig. 2-3).
- Do not discuss the resident or the resident's treatment with anyone except the nurse supervising your work. "Shop talk" is a common cause of invasion of privacy.
- Ask visitors to leave the room when care is given.
- Do not open the resident's mail.
- Allow the resident to visit with others and to use the telephone in private.

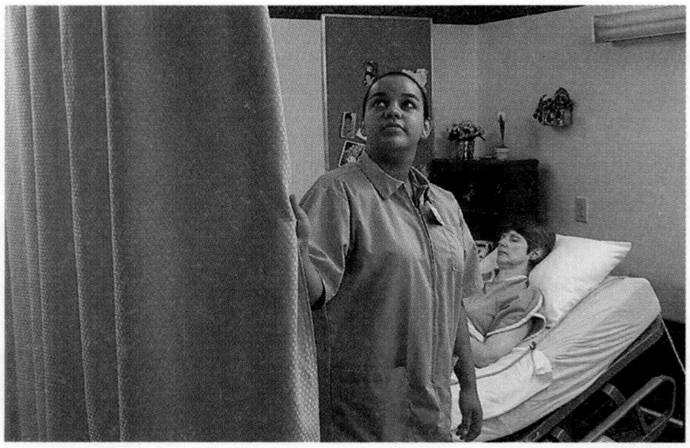

Fig. 2-2 The nursing assistant pulls the curtain around the bed to provide for the resident's privacy.

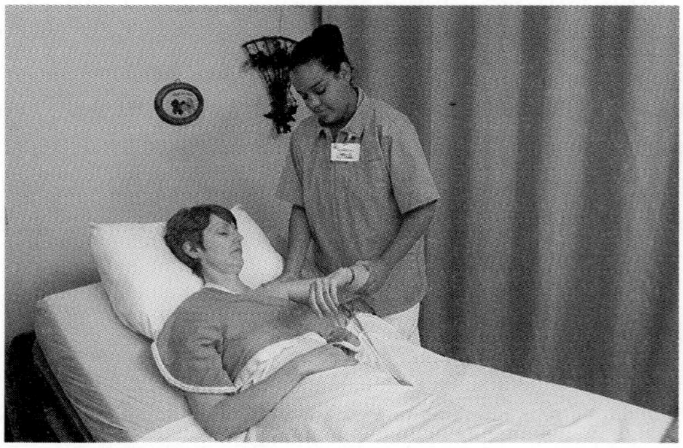

Fig. 2-3 Only the body part involved in the procedure is exposed.

person clearly understands the reason for a treatment, what will be done, how it will be done, who will do it, and the expected outcomes. The person also must understand other treatment options and the effects of not having the treatment. The doctor is responsible for informing the person about all aspects of treatment.

Often consent is needed for persons under legal age (usually 18 years of age). A parent or legal guardian gives consent. Mentally incompetent persons also cannot give legal consent. Persons who are unconscious, sedated, or confused are not mentally competent to give legal consent. Persons with certain mental health disorders are also incompetent to give consent. Consent is given by a responsible party—a husband, wife, son, daughter, or a legal representative. As with consent given by the resident, consent by a responsible party must be informed consent.

Consent is given when the person enters the nursing center. A form is signed giving general consent to treatment. Special consent forms are required before residents are admitted to secured Alzheimer's units. Certain procedures performed by the doctor may also require special consents. The doctor is responsible for informing the person about all aspects of the procedure. The RN may be given this responsibility. You are never responsible for obtaining written consent.

Wills

A **will** is a legal statement of how a person wishes to have property distributed after death. There is no ethical or legal reason why you cannot witness the signing of a will if you are asked to do so. You also may refuse to witness the signing of a will without fear of legal liability. A resident or family member may ask you to help prepare a will. You should politely refuse. Explain that you do not have the necessary knowledge or legal ability to prepare a will. Ask a nurse to speak to the resident or family member about contacting a lawyer.

Do not witness a resident's will if you are named in the will. To do so would prevent you from receiving that which had been left to you. As a witness, you may have to testify that the resident was of sound mind when the will was signed. You also should be prepared to testify that the resident stated that the document being signed was his or her last will.

Be sure to tell your supervisor that you were asked to witness a resident's will. Many centers have policies that do not allow employees to witness wills. You must know your center's policy before you agree to witness the signing of a will. If you have questions, ask your supervisor.

REPORTING ABUSE

Abuse is more evident in today's society. Abuse has one or more of the following elements:

- Willful causing of injury
- Unreasonable confinement
- Intimidation (to make afraid with threats of force or violence)
- Punishment
- Deprivation of goods or services needed for physical, mental, or psychosocial well-being

With abuse, one or more of these elements result in physical harm, pain, or mental anguish. Protection against abuse extends to persons in a coma. With child and elderly abuse, the abuser is usually a family member or a caregiver. All states require the reporting of child abuse and elderly abuse. In domestic abuse (domestic violence), the abuser is a partner. The victim is responsible for reporting the abuse and filing criminal charges.

It is important that all members of the health care team understand how abuse is defined. It is also important that you know your role in reporting suspected abuse.

Elderly Abuse

There are different forms of elderly abuse:

- *Physical abuse* involves hitting, slapping, kicking, pinching, and beating. It also includes corporal punishment—punishment inflicted directly on the body, such as beatings, lashings, or whippings. Neglect is also physical abuse. It involves depriving the person of needed medical services or treatment. Neglect is also failure to provide food, clothing, hygiene, and other basic needs. In nursing centers, neglect includes but is not limited to leaving persons lying or sitting in urine or feces, isolating persons in their rooms or other areas, and failing to answer call bells.
- *Verbal abuse* is the use of oral or written words or statements that speak badly of, sneer at, criticize, or condemn the person. Verbal abuse includes unkind gestures.
- *Involuntary seclusion* is confining the person to a specific area. Elderly people have been locked in closets, basements, attics, and other spaces.
- *Financial abuse* is when the elderly person's money is used by another person.
- *Mental abuse* includes humiliation, harassment, and threats of being punished or deprived of needs such as food, clothing, care, a home, or a place to sleep.
- *Sexual abuse* is when the person is harassed about sex or is attacked sexually. The person may be forced to perform sexual acts out of fear of punishment or physical harm.

There are many signs of elderly abuse. The abused person may show only some of the signs listed in Box 2-7 on p. 30.

OBRA

OBRA and state laws require the reporting of elderly abuse. If abuse is suspected, it must be reported. Where and how to report suspected abuse vary in each

Box 2-7 Signs of Elderly Abuse

- Living conditions are unsafe, unclean, or inadequate.
- Personal hygiene is lacking. The resident is unclean, and clothes are dirty.
- Weight loss—the person shows signs of poor nutrition and inadequate fluid intake.
- Frequent injuries—circumstances behind the injuries are strange or seem impossible.
- Old and new bruises are seen.
- The resident seems very quiet or withdrawn.
- The resident seems fearful, anxious, or agitated.
- The resident does not seem to want to talk or answer questions.
- The resident is restrained or locked in a certain area for long periods of time. Toilet facilities, food and water, and other necessary items cannot be reached.
- Private conversations are not allowed. The caregiver is present during all conversations.
- The resident seems anxious to please the caregiver.
- Medications are not taken properly. Medications are not purchased, or too much or too little medication is taken.
- Visits to the emergency room may be frequent.
- The resident may go from one doctor to another. Some people do not have a doctor.

state. You may suspect that a resident is being abused. If so, discuss the situation and your observations with the nurse. Give as much information as possible. The nurse then contacts the appropriate members of the health team. Community agencies that investigate elderly abuse also are contacted. They act immediately if there is a life-threatening situation. Sometimes the help of police or the courts is necessary. Nursing centers must have and follow procedures for investigating all cases of suspected abuse.

Helping abused elderly persons is not always easy or possible. The abuse may never be reported or recognized. Sometimes the investigating agency may be unable to gain access to the person. Sometimes elderly persons are abused by their children. A victim may want to protect the child. Some victims are embarrassed or believe the abuse is deserved. A victim may be afraid of what will happen. He or she may think that the present situation is better than no care at all. Some people fear not being believed if they report the abuse themselves.

Child Abuse

If you work in a long-term care center that cares for children, you must have knowledge about child abuse. Child abuse occurs at every social level. It occurs in low- , middle- , and high-income families. The abuser may have little education or be highly educated. The abuser is usually a household member (parent, a parent's partner, brother or sister, nanny) or someone known to the family. Risk factors for child abuse include the following:

- Stress
- Family crisis (divorce, unemployment, relocation, poverty, crowded living conditions)
- Drug or alcohol abuse
- Abuser history of being abused as a child
- Discipline beliefs that include physical punishment
- Lack of emotional attachment to the child
- A child with birth defects or chronic illness
- A child with a personality or behaviors that the abuser considers "different" or unacceptable
- Unrealistic expectations for the child's behavior or performance
- Families that move frequently and do not have family or friends nearby

Types of child abuse. Abuse differs from neglect. *Physical neglect* involves depriving the child of food, clothing, shelter, and medical care. *Emotional neglect* involves not meeting the child's need for affection and attention.

Physical abuse is intentionally injuring the child. Death can occur from physical abuse. Sexual abuse is using, persuading, or forcing a child to engage in sexual conduct. It may take several forms:

- Rape—forced sexual intercourse without the person's consent
- Molestation—sexual advances toward a child. Molesting includes kissing, touching, or fondling sexual areas. The abuser may kiss, touch, or fondle the child. Or the child is forced to kiss, touch, or fondle the abuser.
- Incest—sexual activity between family members. The abuser may be a stepparent, brother or sister, stepbrother or stepsister, aunt or uncle, cousin, or grandparent.
- Child pornography—photographing or videotaping a child involved in sexual acts.
- Child prostitution—forcing a child to engage in sexual activity for money. Usually the child is forced to have many sexual partners.

Box 2-8 lists the signs of physical and sexual abuse. Behaviors of the child and parents may arouse suspicion that something is wrong. The child may be quiet and withdrawn and fear adults. Sometimes children are afraid to go home. Sudden behavior changes are common in sexual abuse. Bed-wetting, thumb-

Box 2-8 Signs and Symptoms of Child Abuse

Physical Abuse
- Bruises on the face (lips, mouth, cheeks), back, buttocks, abdomen, chest, and inner thighs
- Welts on the face (lips, mouth, cheeks), back, buttocks, abdomen, chest, and inner thighs
  - The shape of the object causing the welt may be evident. The shape may be of a belt, belt buckle, wooden spoon, chain, clothes hanger, rope, or other object.
- Burns and scalds on the feet, hands, back, or buttocks
  - Intentional burns leave a pattern from the item causing the burn: cigarette, iron, curling iron, ropes, stove burner, and radiator.
  - In scalds, the area immersed in the hot liquid is clearly marked. For example, with a scald to the hand, the hand looks like a glove. A scald to a foot looks like a sock.
- Fractures of the nose, skull, arms, or legs
- Bite marks

Sexual Abuse
- Bleeding, cuts, and bruises of the genitalia, anus, or mouth
- Stains or blood on underclothing
- Painful urination
- Vaginal discharge
- Genital odor
- Difficulty walking or sitting
- Pregnancy

sucking, loss of appetite, poor grades, and running away from home are some examples.

Parents give different stories about what happened. Injuries are blamed on play accidents or other children. Frequent emergency room visits are common.

Child abuse is a complex syndrome. Many more behaviors, signs, and symptoms are present than discussed here. Health care professionals must be alert for signs and symptoms of child abuse. State laws require that suspected child abuse be reported. However, it is important not to falsely accuse someone. If you suspect child abuse, share your concerns with the nurse. As with elderly abuse, give as much information as you can. The nurse will contact appropriate members of the health team and child protection agencies.

Domestic Abuse

Domestic abuse occurs in relationships. One partner has power and control over the other. Such power and control occur through abuse. Fear and harm occur. Types of abuse include physical, sexual, verbal, economic, or social. Usually more that one type of abuse is present in the relationship:

- *Physical abuse* is unwanted punching, slapping, biting, pulling hair, or kicking. Other forms of violence include burns and the use of weapons. Physical injuries occur. Death is a constant threat.
- *Sexual abuse* is unwanted sexual contact.
- *Verbal abuse* involves unkind and hurtful remarks. The remarks leave the person feeling unwhole, unattractive, and with little value.
- *Economic abuse* involves controlling money. Having or not having a job, pay checks, money gifts from family and friends, and money for household expenses (food, clothing) are controlled by the abuser.
- *Social abuse* is controlling friendships and other relationships. The abuser controls phone calls, use of the car, leaving the home, and visits with family and friends.

Nursing center residents can be victims of domestic abuse. For example, a husband or wife can slap a resident during a visit. Or a spouse may use the resident's money for his or her own benefit. Like child and elderly abuse, domestic abuse is complex. The victim often hides the abuse and protects the abusive partner. However, unlike child and elderly abuse, many state laws do not require that health professionals report suspected domestic abuse. However, health professionals have an ethical responsibility to provide emotional support and to give information about safety and community resources. If you suspect that a person is a victim of domestic abuse, share your concerns with the RN. The RN will gather additional information as necessary to help the person.

Quality of Life

Residents have the right to a comfortable and safe environment. Residents always are protected from harm. To protect residents from harm, you must understand your roles and responsibilities. What you do and how you do it affect the residents' quality of life.

OBRA was passed by the U.S. Congress in 1987 to improve the quality of life of nursing home residents. The law requires training and competency evaluation programs for nursing assistants working in long-term care. These programs provide nursing assistants with the knowledge and skills needed to give basic nursing care. You must always practice within the legal limits of your role. Doing so protects residents from harm and promotes their quality of life.

REVIEW QUESTIONS

Circle T if the statement is true or F if the statement is false.

1 T F You must perform all tasks and procedures as directed by the nurse.

2 T F You make decisions about what should be done for residents.

3 T F All health care facilities let nursing assistants perform the same procedures and tasks.

4 T F You should have a written job description before employment.

5 T F You should never give a resident medication unless told to do so by an RN.

6 T F You can take verbal or telephone orders from doctors.

7 T F You must respect the values, beliefs, and feelings of residents.

8 T F You should take drugs only under the advice and supervision of a doctor.

9 T F Alcohol must never be consumed on duty.

10 T F OBRA requires a training program and a competency evaluation for nursing assistants.

11 T F The nursing assistant registry is private and confidential.

12 T F OBRA requires retraining if you have not worked for 2 consecutive years.

13 T F Laws are ethical standards of right conduct and wrong conduct.

14 T F You are always responsible for your own actions.

15 T F Assault is attempting or threatening to touch another person without that person's consent.

16 T F False imprisonment is the illegal restraint of another person's movement.

17 T F A resident has the right to have information about treatment and care kept private and confidential.

18 T F You cannot witness the signing of a will.

19 T F Mr. Hart has the right to decide what will be done to his body.

20 T F A health care worker is guilty of negligence. The person can be sent to prison.

21 T F You are responsible for obtaining the person's informed consent in writing.

22 T F State laws require the reporting of child, elderly, and domestic abuse.

23 T F Domestic abuse always involves violence.

Circle the BEST answer.

24 Nursing practice is regulated by
- A The Omnibus Budget Reconciliation Act of 1987
- B Medicare and Medicaid
- C Nurse practice acts
- D All of the above

25 What state law affects what nursing assistants can do?
- A The state's nurse practice act
- B The Omnibus Budget Reconciliation Act of 1987
- C Medicare
- D Medicaid

26 You perform a nursing task not allowed by your state. Which is *true?*
- A If an RN delegated the task, there is no legal problem.
- B You could be found guilty of practice nursing without a license.
- C Performing the task is allowed if it is in your job description.
- D If you complete the task safely, there is no legal problem.

REVIEW QUESTIONS—cont'd

27 These statements are about delegation. Which is *false?*
- **A** RNs can delegate their responsibilities to you.
- **B** A delegated task must be safe for the resident.
- **C** The delegated task must be in your job description.
- **D** The delegating nurse is responsible for the safe completion of the task.

28 A task is in your job description. Which is *false?*
- **A** The nurse must always delegate the task to you.
- **B** The nurse delegates the task to you if the resident's circumstances are right.
- **C** The nurse must make sure you have the necessary education and training.
- **D** You must have clear directions before you perform the task.

29 A nurse delegates a task to you. You must
- **A** Complete the task
- **B** Decide if you can accept the task or if you must say "no"
- **C** Delegate the task to someone else if you are too busy to complete the task
- **D** Ignore the request if you do not know how to perform the task

30 You are responsible for
- **A** Completing tasks safely
- **B** Delegation
- **C** The "five rights of delegation"
- **D** Delegating tasks to nursing assistants

31 You can refuse to perform a task for the following reasons except
- **A** The task is beyond the legal limits of your role
- **B** The task is not in your job description
- **C** You do not like the task
- **D** A nurse is not available to supervise you

32 You decide to refuse to perform a task. Your first action is to
- **A** Delegate the task to another nursing assistant
- **B** Communicate your concerns to the nurse
- **C** Ignore the request
- **D** Talk to the nurse's supervisor

33 The doctor orders several laboratory tests for a resident. The resident wants to know why. Who is responsible for telling the resident?
- **A** The doctor
- **B** You
- **C** The RN
- **D** Any health team member

34 Which is not a crime?
- **A** Negligence
- **B** Murder
- **C** Robbery
- **D** Rape

35 A resident's photograph is made public without his consent. This is
- **A** Battery
- **B** Fraud
- **C** Invasion of privacy
- **D** Malpractice

36 A resident asks if you are a nurse. You answer "yes." This is
- **A** Negligence
- **B** Fraud
- **C** Libel
- **D** Slander

37 Which is not a sign of elderly abuse?
- **A** Stiff joints and joint pain
- **B** Old and new bruises
- **C** Poor personal hygiene
- **D** Frequent injuries

38 You suspect a resident has been abused. What should you do?
- **A** Tell the family.
- **B** Call a state agency.
- **C** Tell the nurse.
- **D** Ask the resident if he or she has been abused.

Answers to these questions are on p. 695.

3 Work Ethics

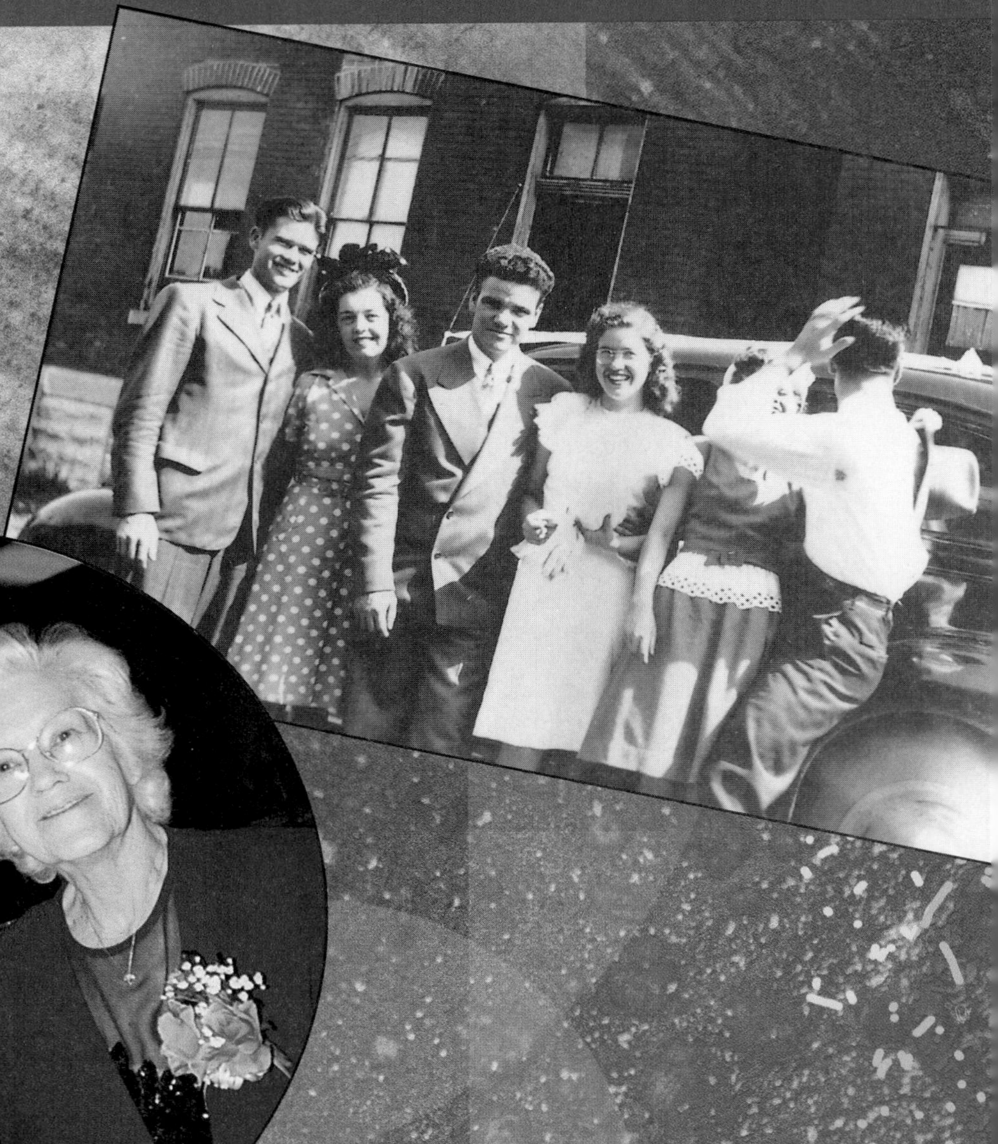

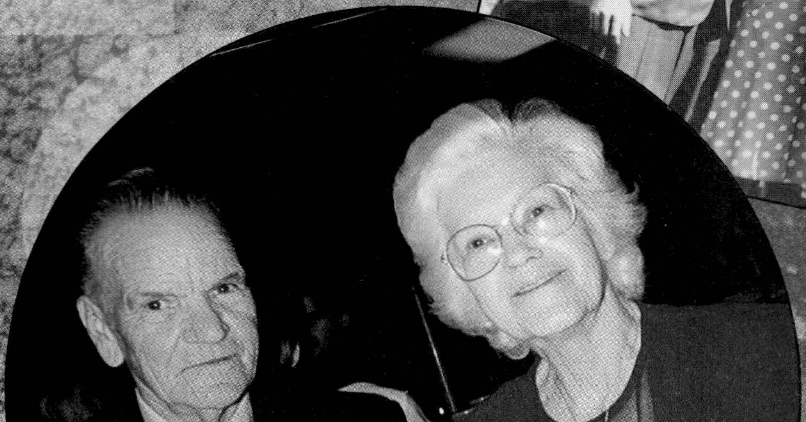

What You Will Learn

- The definition of the key terms listed in this chapter
- The practices for professional appearance
- The qualities and characteristics of a successful nursing assistant
- Good health and personal hygiene practices
- What you should do to get a job
- How to prepare for work by planning for childcare and transportation
- Ethical behavior on the job
- What is meant by harassment and sexual harassment
- How to resign from a job
- The common reasons for losing a job

Key Terms

confidentiality Trusting others with personal and private information

courtesy A polite, considerate, or helpful comment or act

gossip Spreading rumors or talking about the private matters of others

harassment Troubling, tormenting, offending, or worrying a person by one's behavior or comments

work ethics Behavior in the workplace

As explained in Chapter 2, ethics deals with right conduct and wrong conduct. It involves making choices and judgments about what or what not to do. An ethical person does the right thing. In the workplace, certain behaviors (conduct), choices, and judgments are expected. Therefore **work ethics** deals with behavior in the workplace. Your conduct reflects your choices and judgments. Your appearance, what you say, how you behave, and how you treat and work with others are all part of work ethics. To get and keep a job you must conduct yourself in the right way.

PERSONAL HEALTH, HYGIENE, AND APPEARANCE

The health team sets an example for others. Residents, families, and visitors expect the team to look and act healthy. For example, a person has reason to question health team members who smoke, especially when the person is told to stop smoking. You are a member of the health team. Therefore your personal health, appearance, and hygiene deserve careful attention.

Your Health

Residents and employers trust you. They believe you will give careful and effective care. To fulfill this trust you must be physically and mentally healthy. Otherwise you cannot function at your best. Your job as a nursing assistant requires physical stamina and a positive outlook.

- *Diet*—Good nutrition involves eating a balanced diet from the Food Guide Pyramid (see Chapter 18). Start your day with a good breakfast. To maintain your weight, the number of calories taken in must equal your energy needs. To lose weight, caloric intake must be less than energy needs. Limit your intake of foods from the fats, oils, and sweets groups. Avoid salty foods and crash diets.
- *Sleep and rest*—Adequate sleep and rest are needed to stay healthy and to do your job well. Most adults need about 7 hours of sleep daily. Fatigue, lack of energy, and irritability mean you need more rest and sleep.
- *Body mechanics*—You will bend, carry heavy objects, and lift, move, and turn residents. These activities place stress and strain on your body. You need to use your muscles effectively (see Chapter 10).

- *Exercise*—Exercise is needed for muscle tone, circulation, and weight control. Walking, running, swimming, and biking are good forms of exercise. You will feel better physically and mentally with regular exercise. Consult your doctor before starting a vigorous exercise program.
- *Your eyes*—Your eyes deserve special care and respect. Good vision is needed in your work. You will read instructions and measure blood pressures and temperatures. These involve fine measurements. Inaccurate readings can place residents in danger. Have your eyes examined, and wear glasses or contact lenses as prescribed. Make sure you have enough light when reading or doing fine work.
- *Smoking*—Smoking causes lung cancer, lung diseases, and many heart and circulatory disorders. Cigarette smoke can offend others. Smoke odors stay on a person's breath, hands, clothing, and hair. Therefore handwashing and good personal hygiene are essential. Many centers do not allow employees to smoke in the buildings.
- *Drugs*—Some drugs affect thinking, feeling, behavior, and functioning. They affect a person's ability to work effectively. A person who works under the influence of drugs places residents in danger. Take only those drugs that are prescribed by a doctor and only in the way prescribed.
- *Alcohol*—Alcohol is a drug that depresses the brain. It affects thinking, balance, coordination, and mental alertness. Never report to work under the influence of alcohol or drink alcohol while working. Doing so puts residents, co-workers, and you own safety at risk.

Your Hygiene

You must pay careful attention to your personal cleanliness. Prevent offensive body odors by bathing daily and using a deodorant or antiperspirant. Brush your teeth after meals and use a mouthwash regularly to prevent breath odors. Shampoo often, and style hair in an attractive and simple way. Keep fingernails clean, short, and neatly shaped. Clothing must be clean and wrinkle free.

Special hygiene measures are necessary during menstrual periods. Change tampons or sanitary napkins often, especially if flow is heavy. Wash your genital area with soap and water at least twice a day. Handwashing is necessary after going to the bathroom, changing tampons or sanitary napkins, and washing the genital area.

Foot care prevents odors and infection. Your feet should be bathed daily and dried thoroughly between the toes. Cut toenails straight across after bathing or soaking them in water.

Your Appearance

Good health and personal hygiene practices help you look and feel well. Box 3-1 describes practices and suggestions to help you look neat, clean, and professional (Fig. 3-1).

GETTING A JOB

You may know where you want to work. If not, there are some simple ways to find out about job openings. One place is the classified ad sections of newspapers. The local state employment service is also a source. You may hear about jobs from people you know. You can also directly contact the facilities where you would like to work. Phone book yellow pages list health care facilities.

The nursing center for your student clinical experience is another place to look. The staff always look at students as future employees. They watch how students treat residents and co-workers. They look for the qualities and characteristics described in Box 3-2 on p. 38. So you are really being considered for a job while still a student. This is one more reason to always display good work ethics. If that nursing center is not hiring, the staff may know of places looking for nursing assistants.

What Employers Look For

Before applying for a job or interviewing, think about what employers want in those they hire. If you had your own business, whom would you want to hire? Answering that question helps you better understand the employer's point of view.

Employers want employees who:

- Are well groomed
- Are dependable and on time for work
- Have the skills and training needed to do the job
- Are motivated and eager to learn
- Have the values and attitudes that fit with the center

Caring about others is a common trait of health team members. Nursing assistants must care enough to want to make the life of a person happier, easier, or less painful. Good work ethics involves certain traits, attitudes, and manners. These qualities and characteristics are described in Box 3-2 on p. 38. They are necessary for you to function effectively in your role (Fig. 3-2, p. 38).

Respecting residents' property also is important. Nursing assistants handle valuables and personal property on a daily basis. You must handle residents' personal property carefully and prevent damage.

Applicants who look good communicate many things to the employer. You have only one chance to make a good first impression. A well-groomed person

Box 3-1 Practices for a Professional Appearance

- Uniforms fit well and are modest in length and style.
- Uniforms are clean, pressed, and mended. Wear a clean uniform daily.
- Wear your name badge or photo ID at all times when on duty.
- Underclothes are clean and fit properly. They are changed daily and are an appropriate color. Colored undergarments can be seen through white and light colored uniforms.
- Jewelry is not worn. Most centers let employees wear wedding rings; some allow engagement rings. Large rings and bracelets can scratch residents. Confused or combative persons can easily pull off necklaces, brace-lets, and earrings.
- Stockings and socks are clean, well fitting, and changed daily.
- Shoes are comfortable, give needed support, and fit properly. Clean and polish shoes often. Wash laces and replace them as necessary. Open-toe shoes and sandals should not be worn.
- Fingernails are clean, short, and neatly shaped.
- Nail polish is not worn. Chipped nail polish provides a place for microorganisms to grow and multiply.
- Hairstyles are simple and attractive. Hair is off your collar and away from you face. Use simple pins, combs, barrettes, and bands to keep long hair up and in place.
- Makeup is modest in amount and moderate in color. Avoid a painted and severe appearance.
- Perfume, cologne, and after-shave lotions are not worn. They may offend and nauseate residents.

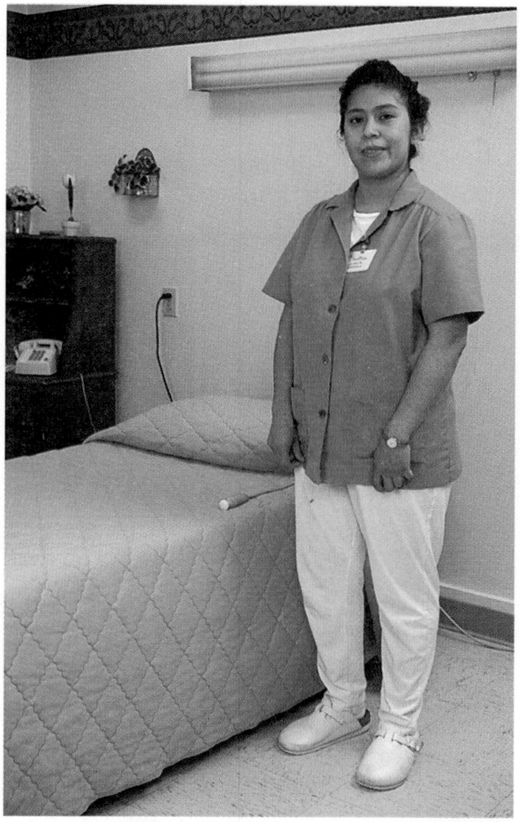

Fig. 3-1 The nursing assistant is well groomed. Her uniform and shoes are clean. Her hair has a simple style and is out of her face and off of her collar. No jewelry is worn.

Box 3-2 Qualities and Characteristics for Good Work Ethics

Dependability	Report to work on time and when scheduled. Perform delegated tasks and keep obligations and promises.
Consideration	Respect the person's physical and emotional feelings. Be gentle and kind toward residents, families, and co-workers.
Cheerfulness	Greet and talk to people in a pleasant manner. Do not be moody, bad tempered, or unhappy while at work.
Empathy	Look at things from the person's point of view—put yourself in the person's position. Always ask yourself how you would feel if you had the person's problem?
Trustworthiness	Residents and staff members have confidence in you. They believe you will keep resident information confidential. They trust you not to gossip about residents, co-workers, doctors, or the health team.
Respectfulness	Residents have rights, values, beliefs, and feelings. If they differ from yours, do not criticize or condemn the person. Treat the person with respect and dignity at all times. Also show respect for supervisors and co-workers.
Courtesy	Be polite and courteous to residents, families, visitors, and co-workers. Address people by title and name ("Mr. Tyler," "Ms. Crane," "Dr. Gilson"). Other courtesies include explaining to the person what you are going to do, saying "please" and "thank you," and not interrupting others unnecessarily.
Conscientiousness	Be careful, alert, and exact in following instructions. Give thorough care with knowledge and skill. Always give your best possible effort.
Honesty	Truthfully and accurately report the amount and kind of care given, your observations, and any errors.
Cooperation	Willingly help and work with others. Also take that "extra step" during busy and stressful times.
Enthusiasm	Be eager, interested, and excited about your work. What you are doing is important.
Self-awareness	Know your own feelings, strengths, and weaknesses. You need to understand yourself before you can understand your residents.

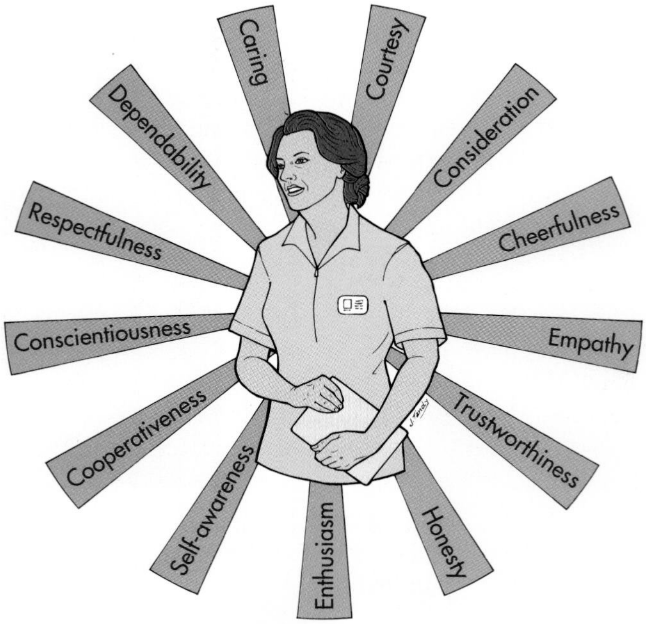

Fig. 3-2 Good work ethics involve these qualities and characteristics.

is likely to get the job over someone who is sloppy, has wrinkled or dirty clothes, and has body or breath odors. Proper dress for an interview is discussed later in this section.

The importance of being dependable is discussed on p. 45. Health care facilities provide services to people. Staff must be at work on time and when scheduled. Undependable people cause everyone problems. Other staff take on extra work. Fewer people give care. Quality of care can easily suffer. Supervisors spend time trying to find out if the person is coming to work. They also have to find someone else to cover for the absent employee. If you had your own business, you would want people to be at work when expected. Otherwise your business would be less efficient and productive.

Employers need to know that you can perform required job skills. The employer requests proof of the required training. OBRA requires that long-term centers hire nursing assistants who have completed a state-approved training and competency evaluation program. The employer requests proof of training and also checks your record in the state nursing assistant registry. Some states require centers to do criminal background checks on all applicants before a job offer is made.

OBRA

Job Applications

The employer asks you to complete a job application (Fig. 3-3, pp. 40-42). You get the application from the personnel office or human resources office. You may be asked to complete the application in that office. Some employers have you take the application home and return it by mail or in person. Make sure you are well groomed and behave pleasantly when seeking or returning a job application. It may be your first chance to make a good impression.

Refer to the guidelines in Box 3-3 when completing a job application. How you fill it out may mean the difference between getting or not getting the job. The application may also be your first chance to impress the employer. A neat, legible, and complete application gives a better image than one that is sloppy or incomplete. Remember, employers use applications to screen out unqualified applicants.

The Job Interview

A job interview is the employer's chance to get to know and evaluate you. It also lets you find out more about the center. Remember, employers hire well-groomed, dependable, and skilled people.

The interview may be when you complete the job application. Some employers review the application first to see if you are qualified. Box 3-4 on p. 43 lists common interview questions. Prepare your answers to these questions before the interview. Also prepare a typed list of your skills to give to the interviewer.

Text continued on p. 43

Box 3-3 Guidelines for Completing a Job Application

- Read the directions first, and then follow them. The directions may ask you to use black ink and to print. Following directions is important on the job. Employers look at job applications to see if you can follow directions.
- Write neatly. Your writing must be legible. A messy application gives a bad image. Legible writing lets the employer have the correct information. You will not be contacted if the employer cannot read your telephone number. You may miss getting the job.
- Complete the entire application. If something does not apply to you, write "N/A" for nonapplicable or draw a line through the space. This tells the employer that you read the section and that you did not skip the item on purpose.
- Report any felony convictions as directed. Write "no" or "none" if you were arrested but not convicted. Some states require criminal background checks.
- Provide information about employment gaps. If you did not work for a time, the employer wonders why. Provide this information to give the employer a good impression about your honesty. Reasons include going to school, staying home to raise children, caring for an ill family member, or your own illness.
- Tell why you left a job, if asked. Be brief but honest. People leave a job for one that pays better or career advancement. Other reasons include those given above for employment gaps. If you were fired from a job, give an honest but positive response.
- Provide references as requested. Be prepared to give the names, titles, addresses, and telephone numbers of at least three references. You should have this information written down before completing an application. (Always ask references if an employer can contact them). You may get the job faster or over another applicant if the employer can quickly check references. If they are missing or incomplete, the employer waits for all of the information. This wastes your time and the employer's time. Also, the employer wonders if you are hiding something with incomplete reference information.
- Be honest in all your responses. Lying on an application is fraud. It is grounds for being fired.

OSF HEALTHCARE — A commitment to life.

APPLICATION FOR EMPLOYMENT

OSF St. Francis Hospital
3401 Ludington Street, Escanaba, MI 49829

OSF Saint Joseph Hospital
1005 Julien Street, Belvidere, IL 61008

OSF Saint Anthony Medical Center
5666 E State Street, Rockford, IL 61108

OSF Saint James Hospital
610 E Water Street, Pontiac, IL 61764

OSF St. Joseph Medical Center
2200 E Washington Street, Bloomington, IL 61701

OSF Saint Francis Medical Center
530 NE Glen Oak Avenue, Peoria, IL 61637

OSF St. Mary Medical Center
3333 N Seminary, Galesburg, IL 61401

OSF St. Francis Continuation Care and Nursing Home Center
210 S Fifth Street, Burlington, IA 52601

OSF St. Anthony's Continuing Care Center
767 30th Street, Rock Island, IL 61201

OSF HEALTHPLANS, INC.
300 SW Jefferson Street, Peoria, IL 61602

OSF SAINT FRANCIS, INC.
4541 N Prospect, Peoria, IL 61614

OSF HEALTHCARE SYSTEM
800 NE Glen Oak Avenue, Peoria, IL 61603

NAME — LAST — FIRST — MIDDLE INITIAL — POSITION DESIRED — DATE

OSF HealthCare is an equal opportunity employer and does not discriminate because of age, sex, race, creed, color, religion, national origin, marital status, disability, or other protected status.

PLEASE PRINT

LAST NAME	FIRST NAME	MIDDLE INITIAL	SOCIAL SECURITY NO.
STREET ADDRESS, CITY, STATE, ZIP			HOME PHONE ( ) / ALTERNATE PHONE ( )
POSITION(S) DESIRED	DATE AVAILABLE		PAYRATE DESIRED
HAVE YOU EVER APPLIED AT OSF HEALTHCARE BEFORE? ☐ YES ☐ NO	WHEN?	WHERE?	WHAT POSITION?
WERE YOU EVER EMPLOYED BY OSF HEALTHCARE BEFORE? ☐ YES ☐ NO	IF YES, WHEN? UNDER WHAT LAST NAME?	WHAT FACILITY?	WHAT CAPACITY?
IF UNDER AGE 18, GIVE BIRTHDATE.	ARE YOU A U.S. CITIZEN OR AN ALIEN LEGALLY AUTHORIZED TO WORK IN THE U.S.A.? ☐ YES ☐ NO		
DO YOU HAVE ANY RELATIVES WORKING AT THIS FACILITY? ☐ YES ☐ NO	IF YES, PLEASE LIST NAMES AND RELATIONSHIP		

Have you ever pled guilty to or been convicted of any criminal offense (other than minor traffic violations)? ❑ *Yes* ❑ *No*
If "yes," please explain. Note: A criminal conviction is not an automatic bar to employment.

EMPLOYMENT DATA

WHAT SHIFT(S) ARE YOU WILLING TO WORK? 1ST 2ND 3RD OTHER: ______	CIRCLE DAYS YOU CAN WORK MON. TUES. WED. THURS. FRI. SAT. SUN. / ARE YOU WILLING TO WORK OT IF REQUIRED? ☐ YES ☐ NO	ARE YOU WILLING TO WORK WEEKENDS? ☐ YES ☐ NO HOLIDAYS? ☐ YES ☐ NO	STATUS DESIRED ☐ FULL-TIME ☐ PART-TIME ☐ PRN ☐ TEMPORARY
WHAT PROMPTED YOUR APPLICATION? (PLEASE BE SPECIFIC) ☐ EMPLOYEE REFERRAL ______ ☐ NEWSPAPER ______ ☐ OWN ACCORD ______ ☐ JOB LINE ______ ☐ OTHER ______			IF APPLYING FOR PART-TIME, HOW MANY HOURS PER WEEK ARE YOU ABLE TO WORK? ______

Form No. Z8020 (Rev. 10/96) *MFI*

Fig. 3-3 A sample job application. *(Courtesy OSF Healthcare System, Peoria, Ill.)*

EDUCATION

	NAME & ADDRESS OF SCHOOL	COURSE OF STUDY	CIRCLE LAST YEAR COMPLETED	DID YOU GRADUATE	LIST DEGREE OR DIPLOMA
HIGH SCHOOL			1 2 3 4	☐ YES ☐ NO	
COLLEGE			1 2 3 4	☐ YES ☐ NO	
POST GRADUATE			1 2 3 4	☐ YES ☐ NO	
OTHER					

IF NOW ATTENDING SCHOOL, PLEASE GIVE ANTICIPATED GRADUATION DATE.

EMPLOYMENT HISTORY

PRESENT OR MOST RECENT EMPLOYER

NAME OF EMPLOYER	STREET ADDRESS, CITY, STATE, ZIP	PHONE NUMBER ( )
YOUR LAST NAME AT THAT TIME?	JOB TITLE	DATE OF EMPLOYMENT FROM: TO:
REASON FOR LEAVING?	SUPERVISOR'S NAME	ENDING SALARY
CONTACT FOR REFERENCE? IF NO, WHY? ☐ YES ☐ NO	DUTIES, SKILLS, EQUIPMENT USED:	

PREVIOUS EMPLOYERS LIST MOST RECENT FIRST

NAME OF EMPLOYER	STREET ADDRESS, CITY, STATE, ZIP	PHONE NUMBER ( )
YOUR LAST NAME AT THAT TIME?	JOB TITLE	DATE OF EMPLOYMENT FROM: TO:
REASON FOR LEAVING?	SUPERVISOR'S NAME	ENDING SALARY
CONTACT FOR REFERENCE? IF NO, WHY? ☐ YES ☐ NO	DUTIES, SKILLS, EQUIPMENT USED:	
NAME OF EMPLOYER	STREET ADDRESS, CITY, STATE, ZIP	PHONE NUMBER ( )
YOUR LAST NAME AT THAT TIME?	JOB TITLE	DATE OF EMPLOYMENT FROM: TO:
REASON FOR LEAVING?	SUPERVISOR'S NAME	ENDING SALARY
CONTACT FOR REFERENCE? IF NO, WHY? ☐ YES ☐ NO	DUTIES, SKILLS, EQUIPMENT USED:	
NAME OF EMPLOYER	STREET ADDRESS, CITY, STATE, ZIP	PHONE NUMBER
YOUR LAST NAME AT THAT TIME?	JOB TITLE	DATE OF EMPLOYMENT FROM: TO:
REASON FOR LEAVING?	SUPERVISOR'S NAME	ENDING SALARY
CONTACT FOR REFERENCE? IF NO, WHY? ☐ YES ☐ NO	DUTIES, SKILLS, EQUIPMENT USED:	

I HEREBY GIVE PERMISSION TO OSF HEALTHCARE TO CONTACT THE EMPLOYERS LISTED ABOVE TO OBTAIN ANY INFORMATION DEEMED RELEVANT. I COMPLETELY RELEASE OSF HEALTHCARE AND THE PROVIDERS OF THE INFORMATION FROM ANY AND ALL LIABILITY ARISING OUT OF INQUIRIES MADE OR INFORMATION PROVIDED RELATIVE TO MY APPLICATION FOR EMPLOYMENT EVEN IF SUCH INFORMATION IS NEGATIVE AND/OR ADVERSELY AFFECTS MY APPLICATION FOR EMPLOYMENT.

DATE ______________________ APPLICANT SIGNATURE ______________________

Fig. 3-3, cont'd A sample job application.

PROFESSIONAL LICENSES, REGISTRATIONS, AND/OR CERTIFICATIONS

ARE YOU CURRENTLY: ☐ REGISTERED ☐ LICENSED ☐ CERTIFIED

TYPE	STATE ISSUED	DATE	NO.
TYPE	STATE ISSUED	DATE	NO.
TYPE	STATE ISSUED	DATE	NO.

HAVE YOU EVER HAD YOUR LICENSES, REGISTRATION OR CERTIFICATION REVOKED, SUSPENDED OR PUT ON PROBATION? ❑ YES ❑ NO
IF YES, PLEASE EXPLAIN.

IF THE JOB YOU ARE APPLYING FOR REQUIRES THE DRIVING OF A MOTOR VEHICLE WHILE ON DUTY, PLEASE PROVIDE THE FOLLOWING INFORMATION:

DRIVER'S LICENSE NO. ______________________ STATE ______________

ADDITIONAL SKILLS

PLEASE CHECK ANY SKILLS BELOW IN WHICH YOU ARE PROFICIENT:

- ❑ TYPING ________ WPM
- ❑ SHORTHAND OR SPEEDWRITING
- ❑ MACHINE TRANSCRIPTION
- ❑ MEDICAL TERMINOLOGY
- ❑ FOREIGN LANGUAGE ______________
- ❑ OTHER: ______________

COMPUTER SKILLS: (SPECIFY SOFTWARE)

- ❑ WINDOWS
- ❑ WORD PROCESSING
- ❑ SPREADSHEET
- ❑ DATABASES
- ❑ GRAPHICS
- ❑ ALPHANUMERIC DATA ENTRY _____ SPH

PLEASE NOTE ANY ADDITIONAL SKILLS, EXPERIENCE, OR TRAINING THAT YOU FEEL IS IMPORTANT. PLEASE INCLUDE EQUIPMENT OR COMPUTER SOFTWARE USED.

I UNDERSTAND THAT IF I MAKE ANY FALSE STATEMENTS, MISREPRESENTATIONS, OR OMISSIONS ON THIS APPLICATION OR DURING THE HIRING PROCESS, I MAY BE REFUSED EMPLOYMENT OR, IF EMPLOYED, I MAY BE TERMINATED, REGARDLESS OF WHEN DISCOVERED. IN CONSIDERATION OF MY EMPLOYMENT, I AGREE TO CONFORM TO THE RULES, REGULATIONS AND PHILOSOPHY AND VALUES OF OSF HEALTHCARE. I UNDERSTAND THIS APPLICATION IS NOT INTENDED TO BE A CONTRACT OF EMPLOYMENT. I UNDERSTAND THAT MY EMPLOYMENT CAN BE TERMINATED AT ANY TIME AND FOR ANY REASON, AT THE OPTION OF EITHER OSF HEALTHCARE OR MYSELF. I UNDERSTAND THAT NO ONE OTHER THAN AN ADMINISTRATOR HAS ANY AUTHORITY TO ENTER INTO ANY AGREEMENT FOR EMPLOYMENT FOR ANY SPECIFIED PERIOD OF TIME OR TO MAKE ANY AGREEMENT CONTRARY TO THE FOREGOING AND THAT ANY SUCH AGREEMENT MUST BE IN WRITING, SIGNED BY AN ADMINISTRATOR, AND NOTARIZED. I ALSO UNDERSTAND THAT I WILL BE REQUIRED TO COMPLETE A MEDICAL EXAMINATION WHICH MAY INCLUDE A DRUG SCREEN AND A CRIMINAL BACKGROUND CHECK BEFORE BEGINNING EMPLOYMENT. I UNDERSTAND THIS APPLICATION AND ANY INFORMATION IN IT MAY BE SHARED WITH ANY OSF HEALTHCARE ENTITY.

APPLICANT SIGNATURE ______________________ DATE ______________

Fig. 3-3, cont'd A sample job application. *(Courtesy OSF Healthcare System, Peoria, Ill.)*

Box 3-4 Common Interview Questions

- Tell me about yourself.
- Please tell me about your career goals.
- What are you doing currently to achieve these goals?
- Describe what you consider to be professional behavior.
- Tell me about your last job.
- What did you like the most about your last job? What did you like the least?
- Why did you leave your last job?
- What would your supervisor and co-workers tell me about your dependability? Your skills? Your ability to adapt?
- Of all your functions, which presented the most difficulty for you?
- How did you handle this difficulty?
- How do you set priorities?
- In what ways have your past experiences prepared you for this position?
- If there is one thing that you could change about your last job, what would it be?
- How do you handle problems with residents and co-workers?
- Why do you want to work here?
- Why should this center hire you?

Your appearance is important. You must make a good impression. You need to be neat, clean, and well groomed (Fig. 3-4). Your dress is also important. Box 3-5 gives guidelines on how to dress for an interview.

You must be on time. It shows you are dependable. If you have not been to the center or do not know where it is, a dry run may be useful. Go to the center some day before your interview. Note how long it takes to get there and where to park. Also ask where to find the personnel office. A dry run gives you an idea of the time it takes to get from your home to the personnel office.

When you arrive for the interview, give the receptionist your name and your purpose for being there. Also give the interviewer's name. Then take a seat in the waiting area. Sit quietly in a professional manner. Do not smoke or chew gum. Use the time to review your answers to the common interview questions. Remember, waiting may be part of the interview. You need to wait patiently. The interviewer may ask the receptionist about you—how you presented yourself when you arrived and what you did while waiting. You must be polite and friendly at all times. Remember to smile.

Box 3-5 Grooming and Dressing for an Interview

- Take a bath, brush your teeth, and wash your hair.
- Use a deodorant or antiperspirant.
- Make sure your hands and fingernails are clean.
- Apply makeup in a simple, attractive manner.
- Style your hair so that it is neat and attractive. You may want to wear it as you would for work.
- Do not wear jeans, shorts, tank tops, halter tops, or other casual clothing.
- Wear a simple dress, skirt (or slacks) and blouse (sweater), or suit (women). Men should wear a suit or dark slacks, shirt and tie, and a jacket. A long-sleeved white or light blue shirt is best.
- Make sure clothing is pressed and in good repair. Sew on loose buttons, and mend garments as needed.
- Wear socks (men and women) or hose (women). Hose should be free of runs and snags.
- Make sure shoes are polished and in good repair.
- Avoid heavy perfumes, colognes, and aftershaves. A lightly scented fragrance is acceptable.
- Wear only simple jewelry that complements your clothes.
- Stop in the restroom when you arrive at the interview location. Check to make sure that your hair, makeup, and clothes are in place.

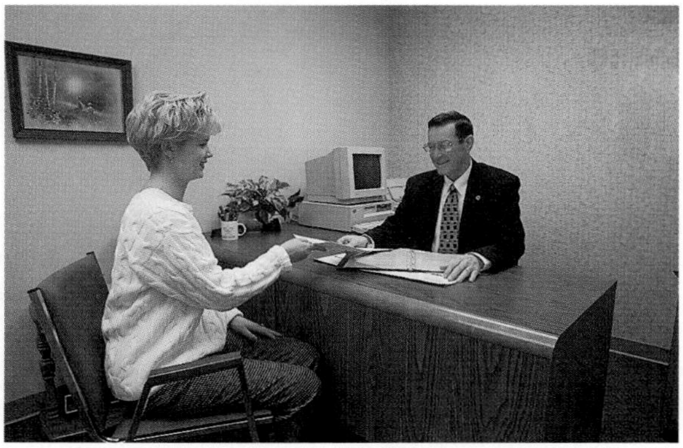

Fig. 3-4 Simple slacks and sweater are worn for a job interview. Note that the applicant sits with her back straight and legs together.

Greet the interviewer in a polite, courteous manner. A firm handshake is correct for both men and women. Address the interviewer as Mr., Mrs., Ms., Miss, or Dr. Then remain standing until asked to take a seat. When sitting, use good posture and sit in a professional manner (see Fig. 3-4). If the interviewer offers you a beverage, it is correct to accept. Remember to thank the person.

Good eye contact with the interviewer is important. Look directly at the interviewer when answering or asking questions. Poor eye contact can communicate negative information. This negative information includes being shy, insecure, or dishonest or lacking interest. Also watch your body language (see Chapter 5). Body language relates to facial expressions, gestures, postures, and body movements. What you say is important. However, how you use and move your body also communicates a great deal. Avoid distracting habits such as biting your nails, playing with jewelry or clothing, crossing your arms, and swinging your legs back and forth. Keep your mind on the interview. Do not touch or read things on the interviewer's desk.

The interview lasts 15 to 45 minutes. Answer honestly and to the best of your ability. Speak clearly and with confidence. Avoid short answers and long answers. "Yes" and "no" answers give little information. You generally want to give a brief explanation of "yes" and "no" responses.

The interviewer is likely to ask about your skills. Give him or her your skill list. The employer may ask about a skill not on your list. Explain that you are willing to learn the skill if your state allows nursing assistants to perform the task.

Whenever you look for employment, you want to find the right job for you. A right match is important. You do not want a job that is not right for you. Nor does the employer want to hire someone who will not be happy in the job or at the center. At the end of the interview you will have the chance to ask questions. Asking questions shows your interest in the job. Box 3-6 lists some questions to ask during your interview. The interviewer's answer will help you decide if the job is right for you.

You should also review the job description with the interviewer. If you have any questions, ask them at this time. Also advise the interviewer of any functions you cannot perform because of training, legal, ethical, or religious reasons. An honest talk with the interviewer prevents problems later.

Also ask questions about starting salary, work hours, the attendance policy, your job description, uniform and dress code requirements, and the center's new employee orientation program. Remember to ask about benefits such as health and disability insurance, vacation, and continuing education.

Box 3-6 Questions to Ask the Interviewer

- Which of my job functions do you think are the most important?
- What employee qualities and characteristics are most important to you?
- What nursing care pattern is used here? (See Chapter 1.)
- Who will I be working with?
- When are performance evaluations done? Who does them? How are they done?
- What performance factors are evaluated?
- How does my supervisor handle problems?
- What are the most common reasons that nursing assistants quit their job here?
- What are the most common reasons that nursing assistants lose their job here?
- How do you see my job in the next year? In the next 5 years?
- What is the greatest reward from my job?
- What is the greatest challenge of my job?
- What do you enjoy the most about nursing assistants who work here?
- Why should I work here rather than in another center?
- Why are you interested in hiring me?
- May I have a tour of the center and the unit I will be working on? Will you introduce me to my supervisor and co-workers?

The interviewer signals when the interview is over. You will be thanked for coming for the interview. You may be offered a job at this time. Or the interviewer tells you when to expect a call. Follow-up is acceptable. Ask the interviewer when you can check on your application. Before leaving, thank the interviewer and tell the person that you look forward to hearing from him or her.

A written thank-you note is advised. Write this the day of or the day after the interview. Your writing must be neat and legible. Use a computer or typewriter if your writing is hard to read. The thank-you note should include:

- The date
- The interviewer's formal name using Mr., Mrs., Ms., Miss, or Dr.
- A statement thanking the person for the interview
- Comments about the interview, the center, and your eagerness to hear about the job
- Your signature using your first and last names

Accepting a Job

Accept the job that is best for you. You can apply at several places and have many interviews. Take time to think about any offers before accepting one. If you have more questions about the center, ask them before accepting the job. Discussing the offer with a relative, friend, co-worker, or your instructor may help you with your decision.

When you accept a job, agree on a starting date and time. Find out where to report on your first day. Ask for the employee handbook and other center information. Read all materials before you start working.

PREPARING FOR WORK

Having a job is a privilege. It is not a right or something due to you. You earned the job by getting the necessary education and training. You succeeded in a job interview. Now you must function well and work well with others to keep your job.

You must work when scheduled. This means getting to work on time and staying through the entire shift. Absences and tardiness (being late) are among the most common reasons for losing a job. Childcare and transportation issues often interfere with getting to work and getting to work on time. You need to plan in advance for childcare and transportation. Do not wait until it is time to leave for work.

Childcare

Someone needs to care for your children when you leave for work, while you are at work, and before you get home from work. Also plan for the following emergencies:

- Your childcare provider is ill or unable to care for your children that day.
- A child becomes ill while you are at work.
- You will be late getting home from work.

Transportation

Plan for how you get to and from work. If you drive your own car, keep the car in good working order. Keep plenty of gas in the car, or leave early enough to get gas.

Car pooling is another option. Every member of the car pool has responsibilities to each other. If the driver is late leaving or picking one person up, everyone is late for work. If one person is not ready when the driver arrives, everyone in the car pool is late for work. Car pool with persons you trust to be ready and on time. When you drive, make sure you leave and pick others up on time. When a passenger, be ready when the driver arrives.

Public transportation (buses and trains) is common in large cities. Know your bus or train schedule. Know what other bus or train you can take if delays occur. Always make sure you have enough money for your fares to and from work.

ON THE JOB

You will have contact with residents, visitors, and co-workers. How you look, how you behave, and what you say affect everyone in the center. Working when scheduled, being cheerful and friendly, performing delegated tasks, helping others, and being kind in what you do and say are part of good work ethics. OSF Saint Francis Medical Center's (Peoria, Ill.) *Employee Handbook* says it best:

> You are what people see when they arrive here; yours are they eyes they look into when they're frightened and lonely. Yours are the voices people hear when they ride the elevators, when they try to sleep, and when they try to forget their problems. You are what they hear on their way to appointments which could affect their destinies, and what they hear after they leave those appointments. Yours are the comments people hear when you think they can't.
>
> Yours is the intelligence and caring that people hope they'll find here. If you're noisy, so is the medical center. If you're rude, so is the medical center. And if you're wonderful, so is the medical center.

Remember, you are an important member of the health care team. How well you work with others and how you feel about your job will affect the quality of care you give to residents.

Attendance

You must report to work when scheduled and on time. The entire unit is affected when just one person is late (p. 39). You must call your supervisor if you will be late or cannot go to work. Attendance policies are explained in your employee handbook. You must follow these policies. Poor attendance can cause you to lose your job.

Being on time does not mean arriving at the center when your shift begins. It means being ready to work when your shift starts. Remember, you need to store your coat, purse, backpack, and other personal items. You might need to use the restroom when you arrive at the center. Plan to arrive on your nursing unit a few minutes early. This gives you time to greet others and settle yourself.

Attendance is more than getting to work when scheduled and on time. You must stay the entire shift. Preparing for childcare emergencies is important. Watching the clock as the shift ends gives a bad image. Working overtime is sometimes necessary. You need to prepare to stay longer if necessary. You should report off duty to the nurse in charge before you leave.

Your Attitude

You need to show a positive attitude about your job. Show that you are happy to be at the center and that you enjoy your work. Listen to others, and be willing to learn. Stay busy, and use your time well. You must demonstrate the qualities and characteristics described in Box 3-2. The work you do is important. Nurses, residents, and families rely on you to give good care. They also expect you to be pleasant and respectful. You need to believe that you and your work are valuable to the center.

Always think before you speak. The following statements signal a negative attitude:

- "I can't. I'm too busy."
- "I didn't do it."
- "It's not my fault."
- "Don't blame me."
- "It's not my turn. I did it yesterday."
- "Nobody told me."
- "I can't come to work today. I have a headache."
- "That's not my job."
- "You didn't tell me that you needed it right away."
- "I work harder than anyone else."
- "No one appreciates what I do."

Gossip

To **gossip** means to spread rumors or talk about the private matters of others. Gossiping is unprofessional. It can hurt others. The following guidelines will help you avoid being a part of gossip:

- Remove yourself from a group or situation where gossip is occurring.
- Do not make or repeat any comment that can hurt a resident, family member, co-worker, or the center.
- Do not make or repeat any comment that you do not know to be true. Remember, making or writing false statements about another person is defamation (see Chapter 2).
- Do not talk about residents, visitors, family members, co-workers, or the center at home or in social settings.

Confidentiality

Resident information is private and personal. **Confidentiality** means to trust others with personal and private information. Resident information is shared only among health team members involved in the person's care. Privacy and confidentiality are resident rights (see Chapter 1). Center and co-worker information also is confidential.

Avoid talking about residents, the center, or co-workers where others are present. Share information only with the nurse supervising your work. Avoid talking about residents, the center, or co-workers in hallways, elevators, dining areas, or outside the center. Others not involved in the situation may overhear you. Residents and visitors are very alert to what is said. Other residents or visitors can overhear you and think you are talking about them or their loved one. Misinformation and the wrong impressions are given about the resident's condition. You can easily upset the resident or family. Therefore you must be very careful about what you say, how you say it, when you say it, and where you say it.

Avoid eavesdropping. To eavesdrop means to listen in or overhear the conversations of others. When you eavesdrop, you invade another person's privacy.

Intercom systems require special considerations (see Chapter 4). Some centers have intercom systems to allow communication between the bedside and the nurses' station. Residents use the intercom to signal when they need help. A staff member at the nurses' station answers the intercom. The nursing team also uses the intercom to communicate with other team members. Be careful what you say over the intercom. It is like a loudspeaker. Others nearby can hear what you are saying.

Personal Hygiene and Appearance

How you look affects the way people think about you and the center. If staff are clean and neat, people think the center is clean and neat. They think the center is unclean if staff are messy and unkempt.

Attire that is accepted in home and social settings is often unacceptable in the work setting. You cannot wear jeans, halter tops, tank tops, or short skirts. Clothing must not be sexual in nature. That is, females cannot show cleavage, the tops of breasts, or the upper thigh. Males must avoid tight pants and exposing their chest. Only the top shirt button can be open.

Follow these guidelines for good personal hygiene and appearance in the work setting:

- Practice personal hygiene (p. 35).
- Follow the guidelines for professional appearance listed in Box 3-1.
- Follow the center's dress code.
- Tend to grooming needs in private. Use the restroom to brush hair, freshen make-up, apply lipstick, or floss or brush your teeth.
- Do not chew gum or tobacco or smoke while on duty.
- Cover tattoos. They may offend residents, visitors, and co-workers.
- Do not wear jewelry in pierced eyebrows, nose, lips, or tongue while on duty.

Speech and language. Your speech and language must be professional. Accepted speech and language in home and social settings may be unacceptable at work. The words you use when talking to family and friends may offend residents, visitors, and co-workers. Remember the following:

- Do not swear or use foul, vulgar, or abusive language.
- Do not use slang.
- Control the volume and tone of your voice. Speak softly and gently.
- Speak clearly. Persons with hearing problems may have difficulty hearing you (see Chapter 26).
- Do not shout or yell.
- Do not fight or argue with residents, families, or co-workers.

Courtesies

A **courtesy** is a polite, considerate, or helpful comment or act. Courtesies are easy. They require little time or energy. And they mean so much to people. Even the smallest act of kindness can brighten someone's day.

- Address others by Miss, Mrs. Ms. Mr., or Dr. Call a person by first name only if he or she asks you to do so.
- Say "please." Begin or end each request with "please."
- Say "thank you" when someone does something for you.
- Apologize to others. Say "I'm sorry" when your make a mistake or hurt someone. Even little things—like bumping into someone in the hallway—require an apology.
- Be thoughtful of others. Compliment others as appropriate. Wish others a happy birthday, a happy day or weekend off, or a happy holiday.
- Wish residents and families well when they leave the center. "Stay well" or "stay healthy" is a good phrase to use.
- Hold doors open for others. If you are at the door first, open the door and let others pass through. In business, men and women hold doors open for each other.
- Hold elevator doors open for others coming down the hallway.
- Help others willingly when asked.
- Praise others. If you see a co-worker do or say something that impresses you, tell that person. Also tell your co-workers.
- Do not take credit for another person's deed. Give the person credit for the action.

Personal Matters

You are employed to do a job. Personal matters cannot interfere with the job. Otherwise resident care is neglected. You could lose your job for tending to personal matters while at work. Practice the following to keep personal matters separate from the workplace:

- Make personal phone calls only during breaks and lunch. Use a public pay phone.
- Do not let family and friends visit you on the unit. If they must see you, arrange for them to meet you for lunch.
- Arrange personal appointments (doctor, dentist, lawyer, beauty, and others) for times when you are not scheduled to work.
- Do not use center computers, printers, fax machines, or photocopiers for your personal use.
- Do not take center supplies (pens, paper, and others) for your personal use.
- Do not discuss personal problems at work.
- Control your emotions. If you need to cry or express anger, do so in a private place. Get yourself together quickly and return to your work.
- Avoid borrowing money from or lending money to co-workers. This includes lunch money and bus or train fares. Borrowing and lending can lead to problems with co-workers.
- Do not engage in fund-raising activities at work. Do not sell your child's candy or raffle tickets to co-workers.
- Do not carry personal pagers or cellular phones while at work.

Meals and Breaks

Everyone has a meal time and two breaks during an 8-hour shift. The meal time is usually 30 minutes long. Breaks are usually for 15 minutes. Meals and breaks are scheduled so that some staff are always on the unit. Staff remaining on the unit cover for the staff at meal or on break.

Staff members have responsibilities to each other. Leave for and return from your meal or break on time. That way other staff can have their meals or break. Do not take longer than you are allowed. Also, remember to tell the nurse when you leave and return to the unit.

Job Safety

Safety involves protecting residents, visitors, co-workers, and yourself from harm. Every employee is responsible for job safety. Negligent behavior affects the safety of others (see Chapter 2). Safety practices are presented throughout this book. The following guidelines are important no matter what you are doing:

- Understand the roles, functions, and responsibilities in your job description.
- Be familiar with the contents and policies in personnel and procedure manuals.
- Know the difference between right and wrong.
- Know what you can and cannot do.
- Develop the desired qualities and characteristics of nursing assistants.
- Follow the nurse's directions and instructions.

- Question unclear instructions and things you do not understand.
- Help others willingly when asked.
- Follow center rules and regulations.
- Ask for any training that you might need.
- Accurately report measurements, observations, the care given, resident complaints, and any errors.
- Accept responsibility for your actions. Admit when you are wrong or make mistakes. Do not blame others. Do not make excuses for your actions.

Planning and Organizing Your Work

Working well with others includes working in an organized and efficient way. You will give nursing care to residents. You also will perform routine tasks on the nursing unit. Some assignments must be completed by a certain time. Other tasks or functions are to be done by the end of the shift. You must plan and organize your work to give safe, thorough care and to make good use of your time. The guidelines in Box 3-7 will help you to plan and organize your work.

Box 3-7 Planning and Organizing Your Work

- Discuss priorities with the nurse.
- Know the routine of your shift and nursing unit.
- List care or procedures that are on a schedule. Some persons are turned or offered the bedpan every 2 hours.
- Estimate how much time is needed for each person, procedure, and task.
- Identify which tasks and procedures can be done while residents are eating, visiting, or involved in activities or therapies.
- Plan care around meal times, visiting hours, recreational activities, social activities, and therapies.
- Identify situations in which you will need help from a co-worker. Ask a co-worker to help you, and give the approximate time when you will need help.
- Schedule any equipment or rooms if necessary. Some centers have only one shower or bathtub to a nursing unit. You will need to schedule the room for resident use.
- Review the procedures to be performed and gather needed supplies beforehand.
- Do not waste time. Stay focused on your work.
- Do not leave a messy work area. Make sure resident rooms are neat and orderly. Also clean utility areas.
- Be a self-starter. That is, have initiative. Ask others if they need help, follow unit routines, stock supply areas, and clean utility rooms. Stay busy.

HARASSMENT

Harassment means troubling, tormenting, offending, or worrying a person by one's behavior or comments. Harassment can be sexual. Or it can involve one's age, race, ethnic background, religion, or disability. What you say and do must be respectful of others. You must not offend others by your gestures, remarks, or use of touch. Nor can you offend others with jokes or pictures. Harassment is not legal in the workplace.

Sexual Harassment

Sexual harassment involves unwanted sexual behaviors by another. The behavior may be a sexual advance or request for a sexual favor. It can be in the form of a comment or touch. The behavior interferes with the person's work and comfort. In extreme cases, the person's job may be threatened if sexual favors are not granted.

Victims of sexual harassment may be men or women. Men harass women or men. Women harass men or women. If you feel that you are being harassed, you must report the situation to your supervisor and the human resource officer.

You must be careful about what you say or do. Even innocent remarks and behaviors can be viewed as harassment. Employee orientation programs include information about harassment. If you are not sure about your own or another person's remarks or behaviors, discuss the situation with your supervisor. You cannot be too careful.

RESIGNING FROM A JOB

A new job closer to home, with better pay, or with new opportunities may prompt you to leave your current job. Going to school, childcare responsibilities, and illness are other reasons. Whatever the reason, you need to inform your employer. Give a written notice. Prepare a letter of resignation, or complete a form in the human resources office. Giving 2 weeks' notice is a good practice. It is never good practice to leave a job without notice. Doing so can have a negative impact on resident care. Include the following in your written notice:

- Your reason for leaving
- The last date you will work
- Comments thanking the employer for the opportunity to work in the center

An exit interview is common practice. You and the employer talk before you leave the center. Usually the employer asks what you liked about the center and your job. Often employees are asked how the center can improve.

LOSING A JOB

Remember, a job is a privilege. You must perform your job well and protect residents from harm. Not being awarded a pay raise or losing your job results from poor performance. Failure to follow a center policy is often grounds for termination. So is failure to get along with others. Box 3-8 lists the many reasons why you can lose your job. Protect your job by performing to the best of your ability. Always practice good work ethics.

QUALITY OF LIFE

Your job as a nursing assistant is important. Residents, families, and visitors believe that you will give safe and effective care. Residents and employers trust that you will work your assigned schedule, arrive at work on time, stay for your entire shift, and complete your assignments. They also expect you to be well groomed, pleasant, and courteous. Your work ethics have an impact on the resident's quality of life. Good work ethics help residents to feel safe, secure, loved, and cared for. If you care enough to want to make the lives of residents happier, easier, and less painful, you will practice good work ethics.

BOX 3-8 COMMON REASONS FOR LOSING A JOB

- Poor attendance—not showing up for work or excessive tardiness (being late)
- Abandonment—leaving the job during your shift without permission from the nurse
- Falsifying a record—application or resident record
- Violent behavior in the workplace
- Possessing weapons in the work setting—guns, knives, explosives, or other dangerous items
- Possessing, using, or distributing alcohol in the work setting
- Possessing, using, or distributing drugs in the work setting (this excludes taking drugs ordered by a doctor)
- Taking a resident's drug for your own use or giving it to others
- Harassment—see p. 48
- Using offensive speech and language
- Stealing the center's or a resident's property
- Destroying the center's or a resident's property
- Showing disrespect to residents, visitors, coworkers, or supervisors
- Abusing or neglecting a resident
- Invading a person's privacy
- Failing to maintain resident, center, or coworker confidentiality (includes access to computer information)
- Using the employer's supplies and equipment for your own use
- Defamation—see Gossiping and p. 28 in Chapter 2
- Abusing lunch and break periods
- Sleeping on the job
- Violating center dress code
- Violating any center policy
- Failing to follow center procedures for providing resident care
- Tending to personal matters while on duty

Review Questions

Circle T if the statement is true or F if the statement is false.

1 T F Uncorrected eye problems can affect the resident's safety.

2 T F Childcare and transportation issues require planning before going to work.

3 T F Being on time for work means arriving at your center when your shift begins.

4 T F Failure to maintain confidentiality is grounds for losing your job.

5 T F You must be careful what you say over the intercom system.

6 T F You do not follow the center's dress code. You can lose your job.

7 T F You can use the center's computer for your personal use.

8 T F You should carry a personal pager so family members can reach you.

9 T F You should be familiar with center policy and procedure manuals.

10 T F Harassment is legal in the workplace.

Circle the BEST answer.

11 To perform your job well you need the following *except*
A Adequate sleep and rest
B Regular exercise
C Drugs and alcohol
D Good nutrition

12 Good personal hygiene for work involves the following *except*
A Bathing daily
B Using a deodorant or antiperspirant
C Brushing teeth after meals
D Keeping fingernails long and polished

13 You are getting ready for work. You should do the following *except*
A Press and mend your uniform
B Wear your name badge or photo ID
C Wear jewelry
D Style your hair so it is up and off the collar

14 Linda Ames applied for a job at West Bay Nursing Center. When should she ask questions about the job description?
A After she completes the application
B Before she completes the application
C When her interview is scheduled
D During the interview

15 Lying on an employment application is
A Negligence
B Fraud
C Libel
D Slander

16 When completing a job application you should do the following *except*
A Write neatly and clearly
B Provide references
C Give information about employment gaps
D Leave spaces blank that do not apply to you

17 Which of these qualities and characteristics do employers look for?
A Cooperation
B Courtesy
C Dependability
D All of the above

18 Empathy is
A Feeling sorry for residents
B Seeing things from the other person's point of view
C Being polite to others
D All of the above

19 What should you wear to a job interview?
A A uniform
B Party clothes
C A simple dress or suit
D What is most comfortable

20 Which behavior is inappropriate during a job interview?
- A Good eye contact with the interviewer
- B Shaking hands with the interviewer
- C Asking the interviewer questions
- D Crossing your arms and legs

21 Which response to an interview question is *best?*
- A "Yes" or "no"
- B Long answers
- C Brief explanations
- D Short answers

22 Which statement reflects a positive work attitude?
- A "It's not my fault."
- B "Please show me how this works."
- C "That's not my job."
- D "I did it yesterday. It's her turn."

23 A co-worker tells you that a doctor and nurse are dating. This is
- A Gossip
- B Eavesdropping
- C Confidential information
- D Sexual harassment

24 Which is professional speech and language?
- A Speaking clearly
- B Using vulgar and abusive words
- C Shouting
- D Arguing

25 Which is not a courteous act?
- A Saying "please" and "thank you"
- B Expecting others to open doors for you
- C Saying "I'm sorry"
- D Complimenting others

26 You are on your break. Which is *false?*
- A You can make personal phone calls.
- B Family members can meet you for lunch.
- C You can take a few extra minutes if necessary.
- D The nurse needs to know that you are off the unit.

27 You are organizing your work. You should do the following *except*
- A Discuss priorities with the nurse
- B Ask others if they need help
- C Stay busy
- D Plan care so that you can watch the resident's TV

28 A letter of resignation should include the following *except*
- A Your reason for leaving
- B The last day you will work
- C A thank-you to the employer
- D What problems you had during your work

Answers to these questions are on p. 695.

4 Communicating With the Health Team

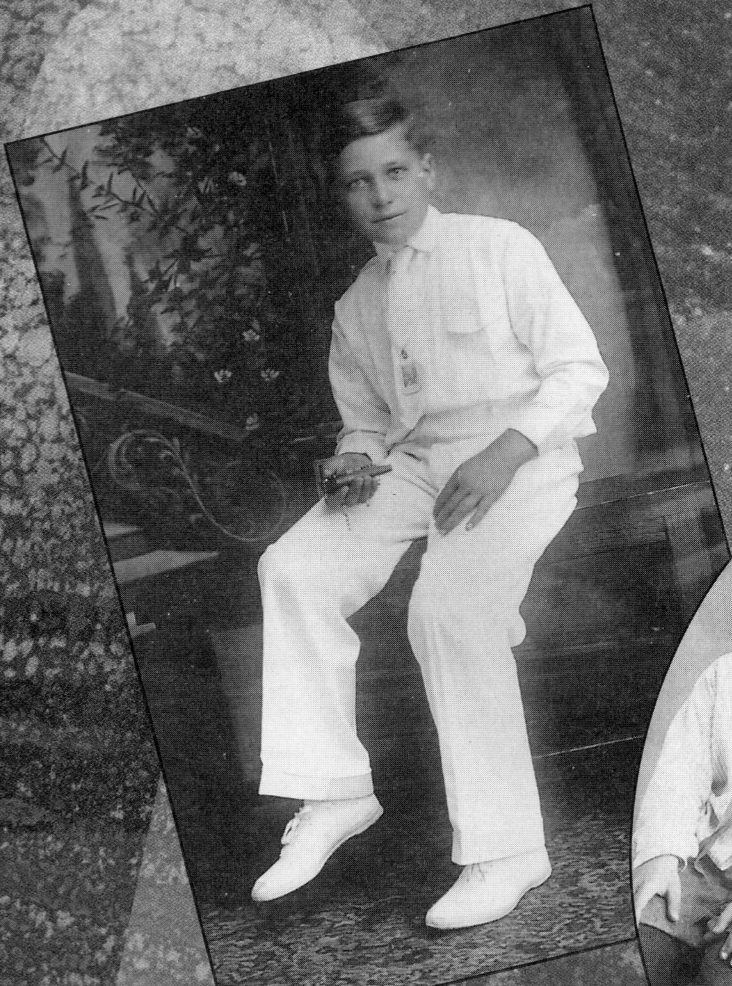

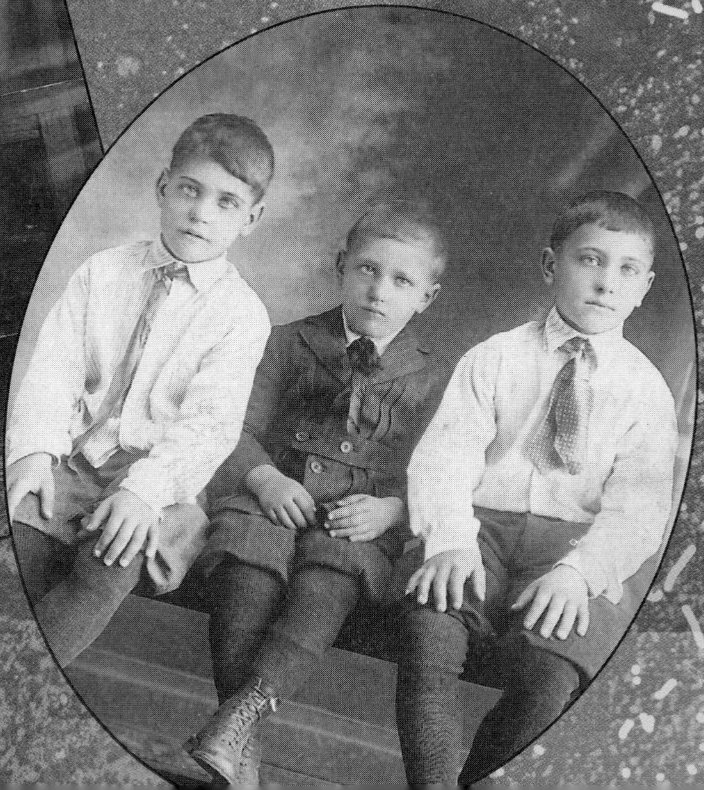

What You Will Learn

- The definition of the key terms listed in this chapter
- Why health team members need to communicate
- The rules for effective communication
- The purpose, parts, and information found in the medical record
- The legal and ethical aspects of medical records
- The purpose of the Kardex
- Your role in the nursing process
- Information to collect about a resident using sight, hearing, touch, and smell
- The information to include when reporting to the nurse
- The basic rules for recording
- How to use the 24-hour clock
- Medical terminology and abbreviations
- How computers are used in health care
- How to protect the resident's right to privacy when using computers
- The rules for answering the telephone
- How to deal with conflict

Key Terms

abbreviation A shortened form of a word or phrase

assessment Collecting information about the resident

chart Another term for the medical record

charting Recording

communication The exchange of information; a message sent is received and interpreted by the intended person

comprehensive care plan A written guide giving direction about the nursing care a resident should receive

conflict A clash between opposing interests and ideas

evaluation Measuring if the goals in the planning step of the nursing process were met

goal That which is desired in or by the resident as a result of nursing care

implementation Performing or carrying out nursing measures in the care plan

interdisciplinary progress note A written description of the care given and the resident's response and progress

Kardex A type of card file that summarizes information found in the medical record—medications, treatments, diagnosis, routine care measures, special equipment used, and special needs

medical diagnosis The identification of a disease or condition by a doctor

medical record A written account of a resident's illness and response to the treatment and care given by the health team; chart

nursing diagnosis A statement describing a health problem that can be treated by nursing measures

nursing intervention An action or measure taken by the nursing team to help the resident reach a goal

nursing process The method used by RNs to plan and deliver nursing care; its five steps are assessment, nursing diagnosis, planning, implementation, and evaluation

objective data Information that can be seen, heard, felt, or smelled by another person; signs

observation Using the senses of sight, hearing, touch, and smell to collect information about a resident

prefix A word element placed at the beginning of a word to change the meaning of the word

recording Writing or charting resident care and observations

Continued

KEY TERMS—cont'd

reporting A verbal account of resident care and observations

root A word element containing the basic meaning of the word

signs Objective data

subjective data That which is reported by a person and cannot be observed by using the senses; symptoms

suffix A word element placed at the end of a root to change the meaning of the word

symptoms Subjective data

triggers Clues for the resident assessment protocols

word element A part of a word

Health team members must communicate with one another to provide coordinated and effective resident care. They share information about what was done and what needs to be done for the resident. Information about the resident's response to treatment is also shared.

Consider this example of communication by the health care team. The doctor ordered a blood test for Mrs. Carter. Food affects the test results. Mrs. Carter cannot have breakfast until a laboratory technician takes a blood sample. The nurse asks the dietary department not to send Mrs. Carter's breakfast until notified. She explains to Mrs. Carter why breakfast will be delayed. The nurse also tells you about the breakfast delay. The laboratory technician draws the blood sample and tells the nurse that the resident may have breakfast. The nurse orders the meal. A dietary worker brings the tray to the nursing station. You are asked to serve Mrs. Carter's tray. When she finishes eating, you remove the tray and observe what she ate. You report your observations to the nurse. The nurse records your observations in Mrs. Carter's record. Because the team members communicated with one another and the resident, Mrs. Carter's care was coordinated and effective. She understood that she was not neglected or forgotten.

OBRA

You will communicate with the health care team (called the *interdisciplinary health care team* by OBRA). However, you will have more direct and frequent communication with the nursing team. You need to understand the basic elements and rules of communication. Then you can learn ways to communicate resident information to the health care team. (Communication with residents and families is discussed in Chapter 5.)

COMMUNICATION

Communication is the exchange of information—a message sent is received and interpreted by the intended person. For communication to be effective, words must have the same meaning for the sender and the receiver of the message. The words "small," "moderate," and "large" often are used in health care. However, the words mean different things to different people. Is small the size of a dime or the size of a half-dollar? In health care, different meanings can cause serious problems. Try to avoid words with more than one meaning.

Using words familiar to people you communicate with is important. You will learn medical terminology as you study and gain experience as a nursing assistant. If someone uses an unfamiliar term, ask for an explanation. If you do not understand the message sent to you, communication does not occur. Likewise, do not use terms unfamiliar to residents.

Try to be brief and concise when communicating. Do not add unrelated or unnecessary information. Stay on the subject, avoid wandering in thought, and do not get wordy. Being brief and concise reduces the chance of omitting important details.

Give information in a logical and orderly manner. Organize your thoughts so you can present them logically and in the right order. Think about what happened step-by-step. Give the information to the nurse in that way.

Present facts, and be specific. The receiver should have a clear picture of what you are communicating. Asking for clarification or for more information should not be necessary. Telling the nurse that a resident's temperature is 100.2° F is more specific and factual than saying the "temperature is up."

THE MEDICAL RECORD

The resident's **medical record (chart)** is a written account of the resident's condition and response to care and treatment. It provides a way for the health care team to communicate information about the resident.

The record is permanent and can be used many years later if a resident's health history is needed. The record is a legal document. It can be used in court as evidence of the resident's problems, treatment, and care.

The record has many forms organized into sections for easy use. Chart organization may vary among nursing centers. Each page is stamped with the person's name, room number, and other identifying information. This helps prevent errors and improper placement of records. The record includes the resident's:

- Admission sheet
- History
- Physical examination results
- Doctor's orders
- Doctor's progress notes
- Interdisciplinary progress notes
- Graphic sheet
- Laboratory results
- X-ray examination reports
- IV therapy record
- Respiratory therapy record
- Consultation report
- Assessments from nursing, social services, dietary services, and recreational therapy
- Special consents

Health team members record information on forms for their department and service. Other health team members read the information to find the care provided and the resident's response.

Members of the health care team record data on the progress notes and on forms for their department or service. The information is then available to other health care team members who need to know what care has been given and the resident's response (Fig. 4-1).

Nursing centers have policies about the contents of resident records and about who may see them. There are policies about how often to make recordings and who records information on the specific forms. There also are policies about acceptable abbreviations, correcting errors, the color of ink to use, and how to sign entries. You need to know your center's policies.

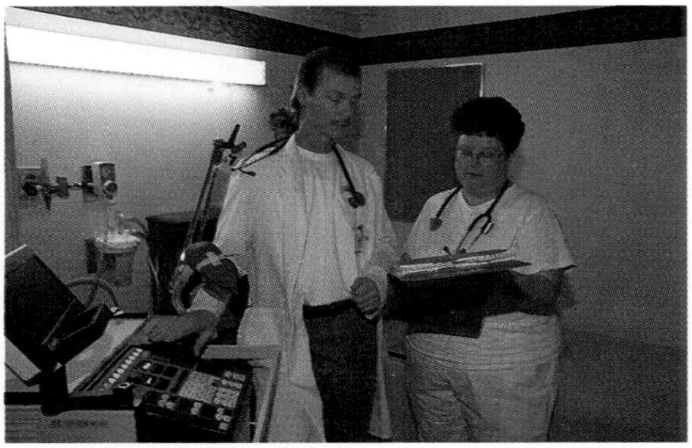

Fig. 4-1 The nurse and respiratory therapist review a resident's chart.

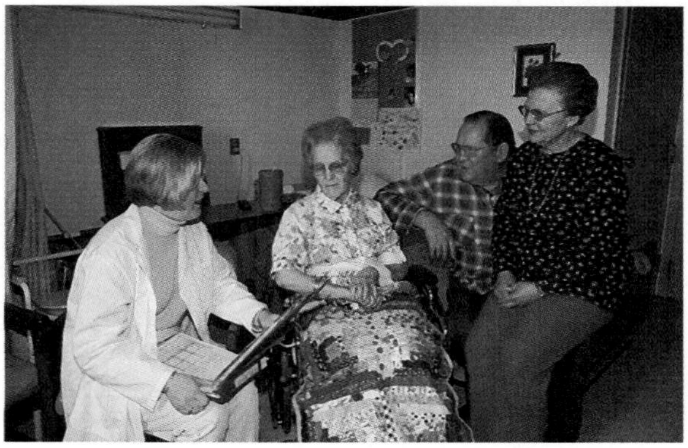

Fig. 4-2 A nurse, resident, and family members review the chart together.

Some centers do not let nursing assistants write in the chart. They believe this is the nurse's responsibility. Others allow and rely on nursing assistants to record observations and care.

Usually all professional health care workers involved in a resident's care have access to the chart. Those not directly involved in the resident's care are not allowed to review the record. Cooks, laundry and housekeeping staff members, and office clerks have no need to see resident records. Some centers do not let nursing assistants read charts. The nurse shares necessary resident information with them.

Remember that you have an ethical and a legal responsibility to keep resident information confidential. Only health team members involved in the resident's care need to read the chart. You may have a friend or relative in the center. If you are not involved in that resident's care, you have no right to review that resident's chart. To review the chart is an invasion of privacy.

Many centers let residents see their records if they ask to do so. In some states it is their legal right. You should know your employer's policy about residents or their guardians seeing a resident's chart. If a resident or guardian asks you for the chart, report the request to your supervisor. The nurse is responsible for dealing with the request (Fig. 4-2).

The following parts of the medical record relate to your work as a nursing assistant.

The Admission Sheet

The admission sheet is completed when the person is admitted to the center. It contains identifying information about the resident: legal name, birth date, age, gender (male or female), current address, marital status, and Medicare or Social Security number. The name of the resident's responsible party or guardian

Date	Time	Nursing Margin	Other Depts Margin

Name ______________________ Birthdate ____________

Admission Date ______________________ Medical Rec. # ____________

Physician ______________________

GSS #239

INTER-DISCIPLINARY PROGRESS NOTES

Rev. 2-1-81

Fig. 4-3 Interdisciplinary progress note. *(Courtesy Evangelical Lutheran Good Samaritan Society, Sioux Falls, South Dakota.)*

also is included. Other information includes known allergies, diagnosis, date and time of admission, religion, church, and the doctor's name. Advance directives (the resident's wishes about resuscitation and life support measures—see Chapter 32) also may be found here. An identification (ID) number is given to each resident and included on the admission sheet.

You might use the admission sheet to learn background information about a resident. You also might use it to fill out other forms that require some of the same information. In that way the resident or guardian does not have to answer the same questions several times.

Interdisciplinary Progress Notes

The **interdisciplinary progress note** is a written description of the care given and the resident's response (Fig. 4-3). These notes include the signs and symptoms the nurse observes about the resident. Nurses use the progress notes to record information about special treatments and medications that are given. Resident teaching and counseling, procedures performed by the doctor, and visits by other health care team members are recorded in the interdisciplinary progress notes.

OBRA

Nurses in long-term care do not chart daily in the progress notes unless there was a change in the resident's condition, an unusual event, or a problem. However, OBRA requires that summaries of care be written at least quarterly (every 3 months). These summaries reflect the resident's progress toward the goals established in the resident care plan and the resident's response to care. Some centers require more frequent summaries. *(See Subacute Care, pp. 58-61.)*

Activities-of-Daily-Living Flow Sheet

The activities-of-daily-living (ADL) flow sheet (Fig. 4-4, pp. 58-61) is used to record a resident's ability to perform ADL. This flow sheet may contain information about hygiene, food and fluids, bowel and bladder elimination, rest and sleep, activities, and social interactions.

Other Types of Flow Sheets

Other flow sheets are used to record any series of measurements or observations made at frequent intervals. For example, a resident's pulse, respirations, and blood pressure may need to be measured every 15 minutes. Or a resident with a heart condition may be weighed daily (Fig. 4-5, p. 62). These measurements are recorded on flow sheets designed for this purpose. The intake and output record is another type of flow sheet (see Chapter 18).

> **SUBACUTE CARE**
>
> In subacute care units, charting may be required every shift.

THE KARDEX

Some centers use the Kardex system. The **Kardex** is a type of card file that summarizes the resident's care plan, current diagnosis, routine care measures, special equipment used, and any special needs (Fig. 4-6, p. 63). There is a card for each resident. It contains some of the information found in the resident's record. The Kardex card is a quick and easy source of resident information.

NURSING PROCESS

Nurses must communicate with each other about the resident's strengths, problems, needs, and care. Information is communicated through the nursing process. The **nursing process** is the method used by nurses to plan and deliver nursing care. It has five steps: assessment, nursing diagnosis, planning, implementation, and evaluation. The purpose of the nursing process is to meet the resident's nursing needs. It requires good communication between the resident and the nursing team.

Each step is important. If done in order with good communication, the nursing process helps residents reach desired goals. Nursing care is organized and has purpose. All members of the nursing team do the same things for the resident and have the same goals. The resident feels safe and secure with consistent care.

The nursing process is ongoing. That is, it constantly changes as new information is gathered and as the resident's needs change. You will see the continuous nature of the nursing process as each step is explained.

Assessment

Assessment involves collecting information about the resident. Nurses gather information from many sources. A nursing history is taken to find out about current and past health problems. The family's health history also is important. Many diseases are genetic. That is, the risk for certain diseases is inherited from parents. For example, if a mother had breast cancer, her daughters are at risk. The nurse reviews information collected by the doctor. If available, past medical records are reviewed. The nurse also reviews laboratory and other test reports.

Text continued on p. 62

WC#_______ Walker#_______ 199__ JAN FEB MAR APR MAY JUN JUL AUG SEP OCT NOV DEC

DATE	ORDER/INSTRUCTION	TIME	1	2	3	4	5	6	7	8	9	10	11	12	13	14	15	16	17	18	19	20	21	22	23	24	25	26	27	28	29	30	31
	Bath & Shampoos every____ & ____on____shift Tub, Shower, Bedbath	11-7																															
		7-3																															
		3-11																															
	Oral Care Own/Dentures/None I = Independent A = Assist SU = Setup	11-7																															
		7-3																															
		3-11																															
	Dressing I = Independent A = Assist SU = Setup T = Total Care	11-7																															
		7-3																															
		3-11																															
	Grooming: Washing, Face, Hands, Combing Hair I = Independent A = Assist SU = Setup T = Total Care	11-7																															
		7-3																															
		3-11																															
	Trim nails weekly	11-7																															
		7-3																															
		3-11																															
	Lotion arms and legs twice daily	11-7																															
		7-3																															
		3-11																															
	Shave men daily	11-7																															
		7-3																															
		3-11																															
	Initials	11-7																															
		7-3																															
		3-11																															

INITIALS	SIGNATURE	INITIALS	SIGNATURE	INITIALS	SIGNATURE

PATIENT STICKER DIAGNOSIS ALLERGIES SPECIAL INSTRUCTIONS:

(revised 2/97)

Fig. 4-4 Activities of daily living flow sheet. *(Courtesy Evangelical Lutheran Good Samaritan Society, Sioux Falls, South Dakota.)*

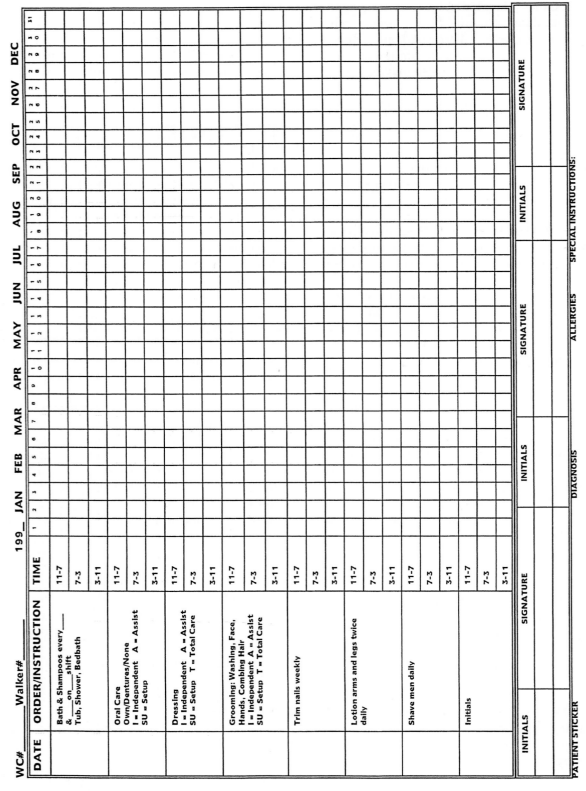

WC#_______ Walker#_______ 199_ JAN FEB MAR APR MAY JUN JUL AUG SEP OCT NOV DEC

DATE	ORDER/INSTRUCTION	TIME	1	2	3	4	5	6	7	8	9	10	11	12	13	14	15	16	17	18	19	20	21	22	23	24	25	26	27	28	29	30	31
	Bowel Movements L = Large M = Medium S = Small I = Incontinent	11-7																															
		7-3																															
		3-11																															
	Weight Bearing Status TT = Toe Touch AT = As tol P = Partial F = Full NWB = Not wt bearing	11-7																															
		7-3																															
		3-11																															
	Transfer Status ML = Medilift SBA = Stand By Assist; Assist of 1 or 2	11-7																															
		7-3																															
		3-11																															
	Activity A = Ambulate GC = Gerichair T = Turn every 2 hrs W/C = Wheelchair	11-7																															
		7-3																															
		3-11																															
	Safety LT = Lap Tray SR = Siderails BA = Bed Alarm SB = Seat Belt	11-7																															
		7-3																															
		3-11																															
	Feeding Status I = Independen S = Set up/cue F = Staff feed SP = Swallow Precautions; TL = Thickened Liquids	Breakfast																															
		Lunch																															
		Supper																															
	Amount of Food Taken in %	Breakfast																															
		Lunch																															
		Supper																															
	Initials	11-7																															
		7-3																															
		3-11																															

INITIALS	SIGNATURE	INITIALS	SIGNATURE	INITIALS	SIGNATURE

PATIENT STICKER DIAGNOSIS ALLERGIES SPECIAL INSTRUCTIONS:

Fig. 4-4, cont'd For legend see opposite page.

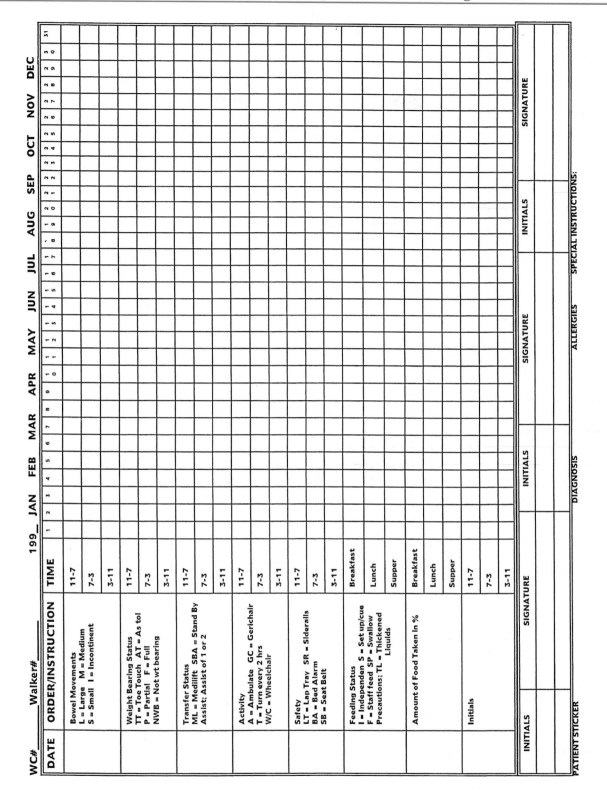

WC#_____ Walker#_____ 199__ JAN FEB MAR APR MAY JUN JUL AUG SEP OCT NOV DEC

DATE	ORDER/INSTRUCTION	TIME	1	2	3	4	5	6	7	8	9	10	11	12	13	14	15	16	17	18	19	20	21	22	23	24	25	26	27	28	29	30	31
	Amount of Snacks Taken in %	AM																															
		PM																															
		HS																															
	Vital Signs Every _____	11-7																															
		7-3																															
		3-11																															
	Weight Every _____																																
	Intake and Output	11-7																															
		7-3																															
		3-11																															
	Initials	11-7																															
		7-3																															
		3-11																															

INITIALS	SIGNATURE	INITIALS	SIGNATURE	INITIALS	SIGNATURE

PATIENT STICKER DIAGNOSIS ALLERGIES SPECIAL INSTRUCTIONS:

Fig. 4-4, cont'd Activities of daily living flow sheet. *(Courtesy Evangelical Lutheran Good Samaritan Society, Sioux Falls, South Dakota.)*

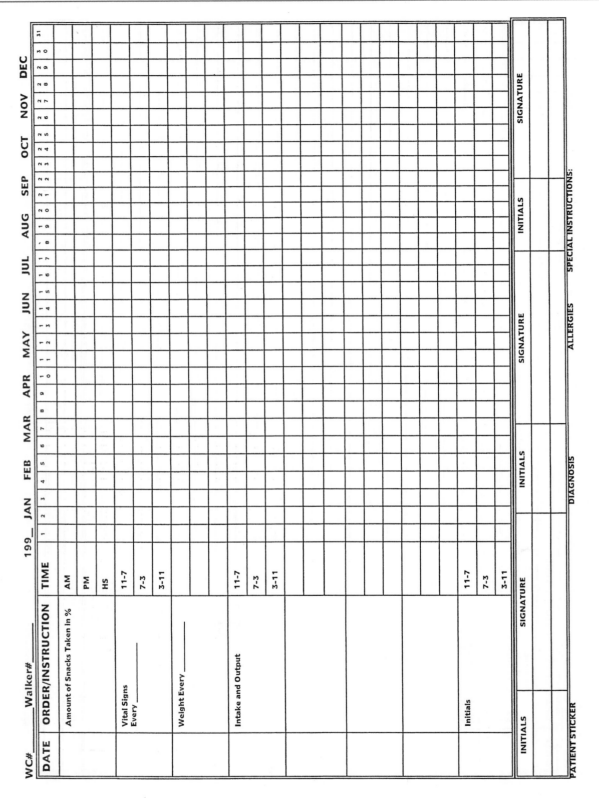

WC#_______Walker#_______ 199_ JAN FEB MAR APR MAY JUN JUL AUG SEP OCT NOV DEC

DATE	ORDER/INSTRUCTION	TIME	1	2	3	4	5	6	7	8	9	10	11	12	13	14	15	16	17	18	19	20	21	22	23	24	25	26	27	28	29	30	31
	Initials	11-7																															
		7-3																															
		3-11																															

INITIALS	SIGNATURE	INITIALS	SIGNATURE	INITIALS	SIGNATURE

PATIENT STICKER DIAGNOSIS ALLERGIES SPECIAL INSTRUCTIONS:

(revised 2/97 c:\wpdocs\starcare\rescar3.frm

Fig. 4-4, cont'd For legend see opposite page.

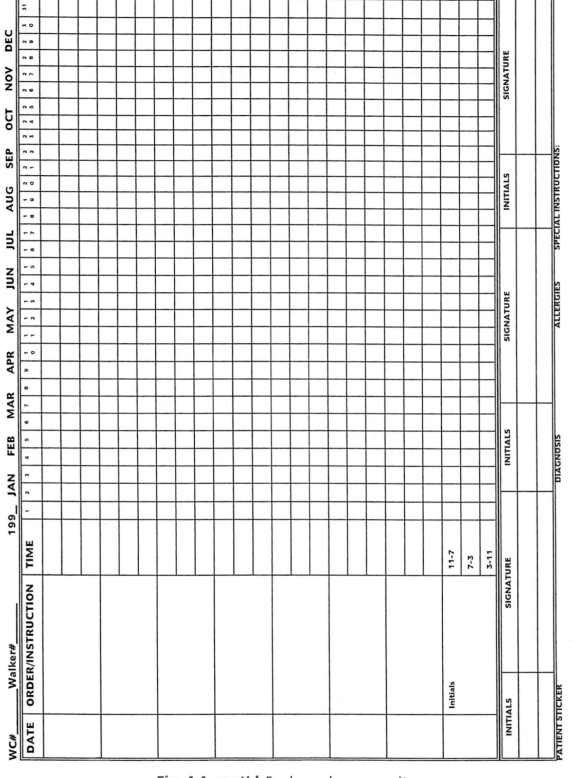

Date	Time	Weight	T	P	R	BP				Signatures

Name ______________________ Birthdate ______________

Admission Date ______________________ Medical Rec. # ______________

Physician ______________________

©1980 The Ev. Lutheran Good Samaritan Society

GSS #243

VITAL SIGNS RECORD

Rev. 2-12-82

Fig. 4-5 Vital signs and daily-weight flow sheet. *(Courtesy Evangelical Lutheran Good Samaritan Society, Sioux Falls, South Dakota.)*

An RN performs a physical assessment. Information is collected about each body system. The RN also assesses the resident's mental status. Information is gathered by observing the resident. You play an important role in the assessment step. You make many observations as you give care and talk to residents.

Observation is using the senses of sight, hearing, touch, and smell to collect information. You see the way the resident lies, sits, or walks. You see flushed or pale skin and reddened or swollen body areas. You listen to the resident breathe, talk, and cough. You use a stethoscope to listen to the heartbeat and to measure blood pres-

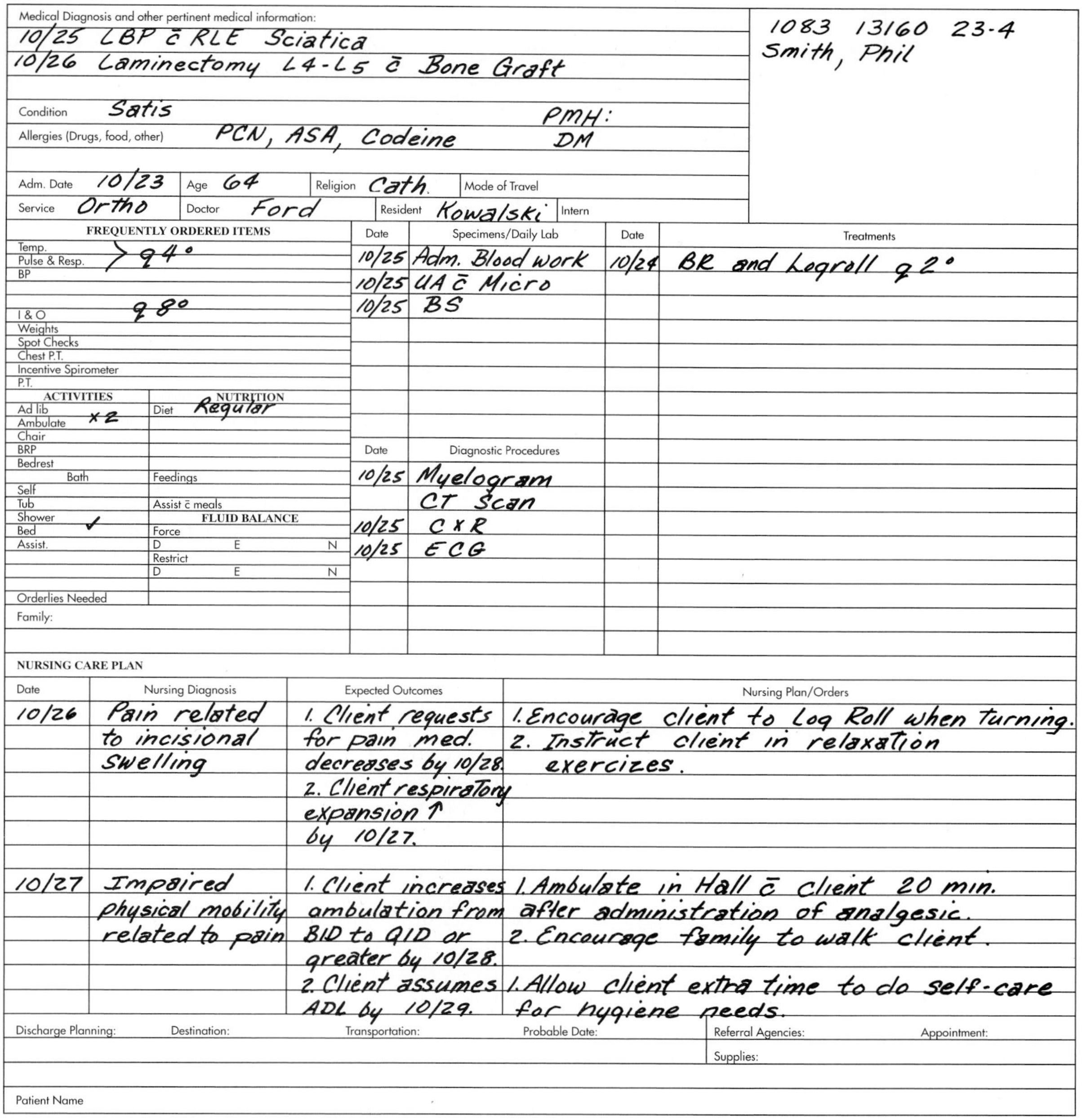

Medical Diagnosis and other pertinent medical information:
10/25 LBP c̄ RLE Sciatica
10/26 Laminectomy L4-L5 c̄ Bone Graft

1083 13160 23-4
Smith, Phil

Condition: Satis
PMH: DM
Allergies (Drugs, food, other): PCN, ASA, Codeine

Adm. Date: 10/23 | Age: 64 | Religion: Cath. | Mode of Travel:
Service: Ortho | Doctor: Ford | Resident: Kowalski | Intern:

FREQUENTLY ORDERED ITEMS
Temp. / Pulse & Resp. / BP: q4°
I & O: q8°
Weights
Spot Checks
Chest P.T.
Incentive Spirometer
P.T.

ACTIVITIES: Ad lib; Ambulate x2; Chair; BRP; Bedrest
NUTRITION: Diet Regular; Feedings; Assist c̄ meals
Bath: Self; Tub; Shower ✓; Bed; Assist.
FLUID BALANCE: Force D E N; Restrict D E N
Orderlies Needed
Family:

Date	Specimens/Daily Lab
10/25	Adm. Blood work
10/25	UA c̄ Micro
10/25	BS

Date	Treatments
10/24	BR and Logroll q2°

Date	Diagnostic Procedures
10/25	Myelogram
	CT Scan
10/25	CXR
10/25	ECG

NURSING CARE PLAN

Date	Nursing Diagnosis	Expected Outcomes	Nursing Plan/Orders
10/26	Pain related to incisional swelling	1. Client requests for pain med. decreases by 10/28. 2. Client respiratory expansion ↑ by 10/27.	1. Encourage client to Log Roll when turning. 2. Instruct client in relaxation exercizes.
10/27	Impaired physical mobility related to pain	1. Client increases ambulation from BID to QID or greater by 10/28.	1. Ambulate in Hall c̄ client 20 min. after administration of analgesic. 2. Encourage family to walk client.
		2. Client assumes ADL by 10/29.	1. Allow client extra time to do self-care for hygiene needs.

Discharge Planning: | Destination: | Transportation: | Probable Date: | Referral Agencies: | Appointment: | Supplies:
Patient Name

Fig. 4-6 A sample Kardex. *(From Potter PA, Perry AG:* Fundamentals of nursing: concepts, process, and practice, *ed 4, St Louis, 1997, Mosby.)*

sure. When touching the resident, you collect information about skin temperature and feel if the skin is moist or dry. You also use touch to take the resident's pulse. Smell is used to detect body, wound, and breath odors and unusual odors from urine and bowel movements.

Information observed about a resident is called objective data. **Objective data (signs)** are seen, heard, felt, or smelled. You can feel a pulse, and you can see urine. However, you cannot feel or see the resident's pain, fear, or nausea. **Subjective data (symptoms)** are things a resident tells you that you cannot observe through your senses.

Box 4-1 on pp. 64-65 lists the basic observations you need to make and report to the nurse. Make notes of your observations. They help when you report to the nurse. They also help when recording observations. Carry a note pad and pen in your pocket to note observations as you make them.

The assessment step never ends. The nursing team collects new information with every resident contact. New observations are made, and residents share more information. Families often add more information.

Box 4-1 Basic Patient Observations

Ability to Respond
- Is the person easy or difficult to arouse?
- Is the person able to give his or her name, the time, and location when asked?
- Does the person identify others accurately?
- Does the person answer questions correctly?
- Does the person speak clearly?
- Are instructions followed correctly?
- Is the person calm, restless, or excited?
- Is the person conversing, quiet, or talking a lot?

Movement
- Can the person squeeze your fingers with each hand?
- Can the person move arms and legs?
- Are the person's movements shaky or jerky?
- Does the person complain of stiff or painful joints?

Pain or Discomfort
- Where is the pain located? (Ask the person to point to the pain.)
- Does the pain go anywhere else?
- When did the pain begin?
- What was the person doing when the pain began?
- How long does the pain last?
- How does the person describe the pain?
  - Sharp
  - Severe
  - Knifelike
  - Dull
  - Burning
  - Aching
  - Comes and goes
  - Depends on position
- Was medication given?
- Did medication help relieve the pain? Is pain still present?
- Is the person able to sleep and rest?
- What is the position of comfort?

Skin
- Is the skin pale or flushed?
- Is the skin cool, warm, or hot?
- Is the skin moist or dry?
- What color are the lips and nails?
- Are sores or reddened areas present?
- Are bruises present? Where are they located?
- Does the person complain of itching?

Eyes, Ears, Nose, and Mouth
- Is there drainage from the eyes?
- Are the eyelids closed?
- Are the eyes reddened?
- Does the person complain of spots, flashes, or blurring?
- Is the person sensitive to bright lights?
- Is there drainage from the ears?
- Can the person hear? Is repeating necessary? Are questions answered appropriately?
- Is there drainage from the nose?
- Can the person breathe through the nose?
- Is there breath odor?
- Does the person complain of a bad taste in the mouth?
- Does the person complain of painful gums or teeth?

Respirations
- Do both sides of the person's chest rise and fall with respirations?
- Is breathing noisy?
- Does the person complain of difficulty breathing?
- What is the amount and color of sputum?
- What is the frequency of the person's cough? Is it dry or productive?

Bowels and Bladder
- Is the abdomen firm or soft?
- Does the person complain of gas?
- What is the amount, color, and consistency of bowel movements?
- What is the frequency of bowel movements?
- Does the person have pain or difficulty urinating?
- What is the amount of urine?
- Does urine have a foul smell?
- Is the person able to control the passage of urine?
- What is the frequency of urination?

CONT'D
BOX 4-1 BASIC PATIENT OBSERVATIONS

Appetite
- Does the person like the diet?
- How much of the food on the tray is eaten?
- What are the person's food preferences?
- How much liquid was taken?
- What are the person's liquid preferences?
- How often does the person drink liquids?
- Is the person experiencing nausea?
- What is the amount and color of material vomited?
- Does the person have hiccups?
- Is the person belching?

Activities of Daily Living
- Can the person perform personal care without help?
  - Bathing?
  - Brushing teeth?
  - Combing and brushing hair?
  - Shaving?
- Does the person use the toilet, commode, bedpan, or urinal?
- Is the person able to feed self?
- Is the person able to walk?
- What amount and kind of assistance is needed?

OBRA

OBRA requires the use of the minimum data set (MDS) for residents of long-term care centers (see Appendix A, p. 712.) The MDS is an assessment and screening tool. The form is completed when the resident is admitted to the center. It provides extensive information about the resident. Examples include the resident's memory, communication, hearing and vision, physical function, and activities. A nurse completes the MDS. The nurse uses your observations in completing the MDS. The RN responsible for resident care has the final responsibility for information on the MDS. The MDS is updated to include new information before each care conference. A new MDS is completed once a year and whenever a change occurs in the resident's health status. An RN must sign the MDS. The RN's signature means that the MDS is complete and accurate.

Nursing Diagnosis

The RN uses information from the assessment to make a nursing diagnosis. A **nursing diagnosis** is a statement describing a health problem that can be treated by nursing measures. The health problem may exist or may develop. Nursing diagnoses and medical diagnoses are different. A **medical diagnosis** is the identification of a disease or condition by a doctor. Medical diagnoses include cancer, pneumonia, chicken pox, stroke, heart attack, infection, AIDS, and diabetes. Medications, therapies, and surgery are ordered by doctors to cure or heal.

A resident may have many nursing diagnoses. Remember that nursing deals with the total person. Therefore nursing diagnoses involve the physical, emotional, social, and spiritual needs of residents. Nursing diagnoses may change or new ones may be added as the RN gains more information about the resident through assessment. Box 4-2 on pp. 66-67 lists the nursing diagnoses approved by the North American Nursing Diagnosis Association (NANDA).

Planning

Priorities and goals are set during planning. Measures or actions to help the resident meet the goals are chosen. The resident, family, and other members of the health care team help the nurse plan. JACHO requires nursing assistant involvement in planning care.

Priorities relate to what is most important for the resident. Maslow's theory of basic needs is useful for setting priorities (Chapter 5). Maslow describes the needs that all humans have. The needs are arranged in order of importance. Some needs are required for life and survival, such as oxygen, water, and food. The needs necessary for life and survival must be met before all other needs. They have priority and must be met first.

Goals are then set. A **goal** is that which is desired in or by a resident as a result of nursing care. Goals are aimed at the resident's highest level of well-being and functioning: physical, emotional, social, spiritual. Goals promote health and prevent health problems. They also promote the person's rehabilitation.

Nursing interventions are chosen after goals are set. An intervention is an action or measure. A **nursing intervention** is an action or measure taken by the nursing team to help the resident reach a goal. In this book, nursing intervention, nursing action, and nursing measure mean the same thing. A nursing intervention does not need a doctor's order. However, some nursing measures come from a doctor's order. For example, a doctor orders that Mrs. Lange walk 50 yards two times a day. The nurse includes this order in the care plan.

Box 4-2 Nursing Diagnoses Approved by the North American Nursing Diagnosis Association (NANDA)

- Activity Intolerance
- Activity Intolerance, Risk for
- Adaptive Capacity: Intracranial, Decreased
- Adjustment, Impaired
- Airway Clearance, Ineffective
- Anxiety
- Aspiration, Risk for
- Bathing/Hygiene Self Care Deficit
- Body Image Disturbance
- Body Temperature, Risk for Altered
- Breastfeeding, Effective
- Breastfeeding, Ineffective
- Breastfeeding, Interrupted
- Breathing Pattern, Ineffective
- Cardiac Output, Decreased
- Caregiver Role Strain
- Caregiver Role Strain, Risk for
- Communication, Impaired Verbal
- Community Coping, Ineffective
- Community Coping, Potential for Enhanced
- Confusion, Acute
- Confusion, Chronic
- Constipation
- Constipation, Colonic
- Constipation, Perceived
- Coping, Defensive
- Decisional Conflict (Specify)
- Denial, Ineffective
- Diarrhea
- Disuse Syndrome, Risk for
- Diversional Activity Deficit
- Dressing/Grooming Self Care Deficit
- Dysreflexia
- Energy Field Disturbance
- Environmental Interpretation Syndrome, Impaired
- Family Coping: Ineffective, Compromised
- Family Coping: Ineffective, Disabling
- Family Coping: Potential for Growth
- Family Processes, Altered: Alcoholism
- Family Processes, Altered
- Fatigue
- Fear
- Feeding Self-Care Deficit
- Fluid Volume Deficit
- Fluid Volume, Risk for Deficit
- Fluid Volume Excess
- Gas Exchange, Impaired
- Grieving, Anticipatory
- Grieving, Dysfunctional
- Growth and Development, Altered
- Health Maintenance, Altered
- Health-Seeking Behaviors (Specify)
- Home Maintenance Management, Impaired
- Hopelessness
- Hyperthermia
- Hypothermia
- Incontinence, Bowel
- Incontinence, Functional
- Incontinence, Reflex
- Incontinence, Stress
- Incontinence, Total
- Incontinence, Urge
- Individual Coping, Ineffective
- Infant Behavior, Disorganized
- Infant Behavior, Risk for Disorganized
- Infant Feeding Pattern, Ineffective
- Injury, Risk for
- Infection, Risk for
- Knowledge Deficit (Specify)
- Loneliness, Risk for
- Management of Therapeutic Regimen, Ineffective: Community
- Management of Therapeutic Regimen, Ineffective: Families
- Management of Therapeutic Regimen, Ineffective: Individual
- Management of Therapeutic Regimen, Ineffective: Individuals
- Management of Therapeutic Regimen, Noncompliance (Specify)
- Memory, Impaired
- Neglect, Unilateral
- Neurovascular Dysfunction, Risk for Peripheral
- Nutrition, Altered: Less Than Body Requirements
- Nutrition, Altered: More Than Body Requirements
- Nutrition, Altered: Potential for More Than Body Requirements
- Oral Mucous Membrane: Altered
- Pain
- Pain, Chronic

(From North American Nursing Diagnosis Association: *NANDA nursing diagnoses: Definitions and classification 1999-2000*, Philadelphia, 1999, The Association.)

Box 4-2 Nursing Diagnoses Approved by the North American Nursing Diagnosis Association (NANDA) CONT'D

- Parent/Infant/Child Attachment, Risk for Altered
- Parental Role Conflict
- Parenting, Altered
- Parenting, Risk for Altered
- Perioperative Positioning Injury, Risk for
- Personal Identify Disturbance
- Physical Mobility, Impaired
- Poisoning, Risk for
- Post-Trauma Response
- Powerlessness
- Protection, Altered
- Rape-Trauma Syndrome
- Rape-Trauma Syndrome: Compound Reaction
- Rape-Trauma Syndrome: Silent Reaction
- Relocation Stress Syndrome
- Role Performance, Altered
- Self-Esteem, Chronic Low
- Self-Esteem Disturbance
- Self-Esteem, Situational Low
- Self-Mutilation, Risk for
- Sensory/Perceptual Alterations (Specify visual, auditory, kinesthetic, gustatory, tactile, olfactory)
- Sexual Dysfunction
- Sexuality Patterns, Altered
- Skin Integrity, Impaired
- Skin Integrity, Risk for Impaired
- Sleep Pattern Disturbance
- Social Interaction, Impaired
- Social Isolation
- Spiritual Distress
- Spiritual Well-Being, Potential for Enhanced
- Suffocation, Risk for
- Swallowing, Impaired
- Thermoregulation, Ineffective
- Thought Process, Altered
- Tissue Integrity, Impaired
- Tissue Perfusion, Altered: (Specify renal, cerebral, cardiopulmonary, gastrointestinal, or peripheral)
- Toileting Self-Care Deficit
- Trauma, Risk for
- Urinary Elimination, Altered
- Urinary Retention
- Ventilation, Inability to Maintain Spontaneous
- Ventilatory Weaning Response, Dysfunctional (DVWR)
- Violence, Risk for Self-Directed or Directed at Others

OBRA requires regular interdisciplinary care planning (IDCP) conferences for each resident. It is attended by members of the interdisciplinary health care team involved in the resident's care.

OBRA

The **comprehensive care plan** is a written guide about the care a resident should receive. The health care team develops the comprehensive care plan. The care plan includes the nursing diagnoses and goals. It consists of resident problems; goals for care, and actions to take to help the resident solve problems.

The problems identified on the MDS give **triggers** (clues) for the resident assessment protocols (RAPs) (see Appendix A, p. 712). RAPs are guidelines that help the health care team develop the resident's care plan. For example, Mr. Smith is deconditioned. Deconditioning is the process of becoming weak from illness or lack of exercise. The MDS shows that Mr. Smith cannot do his activities of daily living (ADL). This triggers the RAPs, which provide guidelines for actions to solve the problem. The goal is for Mr. Smith to be independent in all ADL. Health care team members from three disciplines (occupational therapy, physical therapy, and nursing) work to solve one problem. The actions to help Mr. Smith reach the goal are as follows:

- Occupational therapy to work with Mr. Smith on ADL (activities of daily living) daily
- Physical therapy to work with Mr. Smith on strengthening exercises daily
- Nursing staff member to walk Mr. Smith 20 feet twice daily

The care plan must also identify the resident's strengths. For example, Mrs. Jones may be able to walk without help. This is a strength, which increases her independence. It is important that the care team help Mrs. Jones continue to walk on her own.

A comprehensive care plan is developed for each resident. Care plan suggestions are welcomed from all health care team members, including nursing assistants. You should use the care plan as a guide to provide individualized resident care.

Care plan forms vary in each center. Often the care plan is included in the resident's record or in a Kardex (see Fig. 4-6). The plan must be carried out. The health care team revises the care plan if the resident's needs change.

Implementation

Implementation means to perform or carry out. The **implementation** step is performing or carrying out nursing measures in the care plan. Care is given in this step.

Nursing measures range from simple to complex. Nurses delegate measures that are within your legal limits and job description. Nurses often ask you to assist with complex measures.

You report the care given to the nurse. Some centers allow you to record care. Reporting and recording are done *after* giving care, not before. Also remember to report or record your observations. Observing is part of assessment. New observations may change the nursing diagnoses, causing changes in the nursing care plan. You need to know about any changes in the nursing care plan so that you can give the correct care.

Evaluation

Evaluation means to measure. The **evaluation** step involves measuring if the goals in the planning step were met. The nurse evaluates the progress made. Goals may be met totally, in part, or not at all. Information from assessment is used for evaluation. Changes in nursing diagnoses, goals, and the care plan may result from evaluation.

The nursing process never ends. Nurses constantly collect information about the resident. As the resident's needs change, the nursing process changes. Nursing diagnoses, goals, and the care plan may change. You play an important part in the nursing process. You make and report observations. The RN uses the information for nursing diagnoses, goals, and the care plan. You may help develop the care plan. In the implementation step, you perform nursing actions and measures written in the care plan. Your observations are used for the evaluation step.

RESIDENT CARE CONFERENCES

OBRA requires two types of resident care conferences. One is the interdisciplinary care planning (IDCP) conference, and the other is a problem-focused conference.

The IDCP conference is held regularly to review and update resident care plans or to develop care plans for new residents. This conference includes the RN in charge of the resident's care, the doctor, and health team members from other disciplines. Such disciplines include dietary, recreation, rehabilitation therapies, and social work. The resident and a family member also are included. OBRA

Problem-focused conferences are held when there is a single problem affecting a resident's care. Only health care team members directly involved in the problem attend. The resident or the resident's family may be asked to attend.

The resident has the right to participate in his or her care planning. OBRA requires that the resident be included in this process. The resident may refuse actions suggested by the health care team. OBRA

Nursing assistants often are included in both types of conferences. They are encouraged to share their suggestions and observations.

REPORTING AND RECORDING OBSERVATIONS

Reporting and recording promote communication among health team members. Both are accounts of what was done for and observed about the resident. **Reporting** is the verbal account of care and observations. **Recording** or **charting** is the written account of observations and care.

Reporting

You report resident care and observations to the nurse. Reports must be prompt, thorough, and accurate. Always tell the nurse the resident's name, room and bed number, and the time your observations were made or the care given. Report only those things that you observed or did yourself. Give reports as the resident's condition requires or as often as requested by the nurse. Immediately report any changes from normal or changes in the resident's condition. Use your written notes to give a specific, concise, and descriptive report (Fig. 4-7).

The nurse gives a report at the end of the shift to the nursing team of the oncoming shift (called the *end-of-shift report*). Information is shared about the resident care given and the care that must be given. Information about the resident's condition also is included. Some centers have all nursing team members hear the end-of-shift report as they come on duty. Others have nursing assistants perform routine tasks while RNs and LPNs/LVNs hear the report.

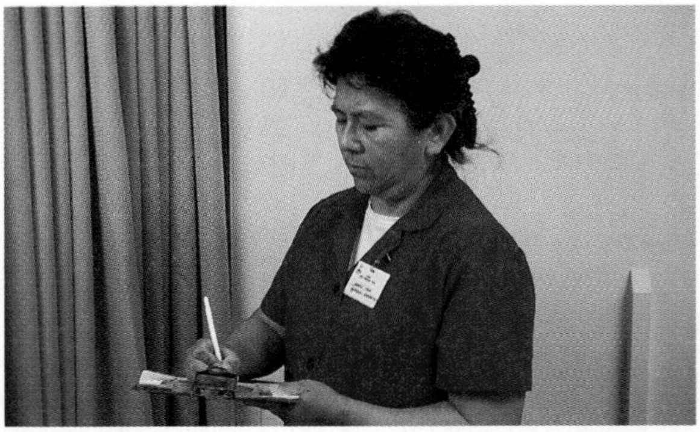

Fig. 4-7 Nursing assistant uses notes when reporting.

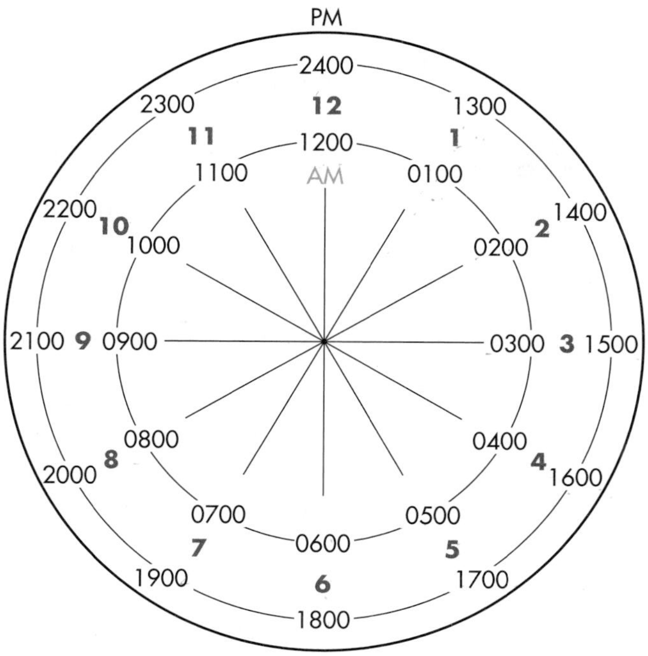

Fig. 4-8 The 24-hour clock.

Recording

When recording on the resident's chart, you must communicate clearly and thoroughly. You must follow the rules in Box 4-3. Anyone who reads your charting should know:

- What you observed
- What you did
- The resident's response

Recording time. The 24-hour clock (military time or international time) has four digits (Fig. 4-8). The first two digits are for the hour: 0100=1:00 AM; 1300=1:00 PM. The last two digits are for minutes: 0110=1:10 AM. The AM and PM abbreviations are not used.

As Box 4-4 on p. 70 shows, the hour is the same for morning times, but AM is not used. For PM times, add 12 to the clock time. If it is 2:00 PM, add 12 and 2 for 1400. For 8:35 PM, add 12 and 835 for 2035.

Box 4-3 Rules for Recording

- Always use ink.
- Include the date and the time whenever a recording is made. Use conventional time (AM or PM) or 24-hour clock time according to center policy.
- Make sure writing is legible and neat.
- Use only center approved abbreviations (p. 70).
- Use correct spelling, grammar, and punctuation.
- Never erase or use correction fluid if you make an error. Cross out the incorrect part, write "error" or "mistaken entry" over it, and rewrite the part. Follow center policy for correcting errors.
- Sign all entries with your name and title as required by center policy.
- Do not skip lines. Draw a line through the blank space of a partially completed line or to the end of a page. This prevents others from recording in a space with your signature.
- Make sure each form is stamped with the person's name and other identifying information.
- Record only what you observed and did yourself.
- Never chart a procedure or treatment until after its completion.
- Be accurate, concise, and factual. Do not record judgments or interpretations.
- Record in a logical and sequential manner.
- Be descriptive. Avoid terms with more than one meaning.
- Use the person's exact words whenever possible. Use quotation marks to show that the statement is a direct quote.
- Chart any changes from normal or changes in the person's condition. Also chart that you informed the nurse and the time you made the report.
- Do not omit information.
- Record safety measures such as raising bed rails, assisting a person when up, or reminding someone not to get out of bed. This will help protect you if the person falls.

MEDICAL TERMINOLOGY AND ABBREVIATIONS

Medical terminology and abbreviations are used to communicate in health care. They are presented throughout this book. If someone uses a word or phrase that you do not understand, ask a nurse to explain its meaning. Otherwise, communication is not effective. You may also want to buy a medical dictionary so you can learn new words.

Like all words, medical terms are made up of parts, or **word elements**. These elements are combined in various ways to form medical terms. A term is translated by separating the word into its elements. Important word elements are prefixes, roots, and suffixes.

BOX 4-4 24-HOUR CLOCK

Conventional Time	24-Hour Clock
1:00 AM	0100
2:00 AM	0200
3:00 AM	0300
4:00 AM	0400
5:00 AM	0500
6:00 AM	0600
7:00 AM	0700
8:00 AM	0800
9:00 AM	0900
10:00 AM	1000
11:00 AM	1100
12:00 noon	1200
1:00 PM	1300
2:00 PM	1400
3:00 PM	1500
4:00 PM	1600
5:00 PM	1700
6:00 PM	1800
7:00 PM	1900
8:00 PM	2000
9:00 PM	2100
10:00 PM	2200
11:00 PM	2300
12:00 midnight	2400 or 0000

Prefixes, Roots, and Suffixes

A **prefix** is a word element placed at the beginning of a word. A prefix changes the meaning of the word. The prefix *olig* (scant, small amount) is placed before the word *uria* (urine) to make *oliguria.* It means a scant amount of urine. Prefixes are always combined with other word elements. They are never used alone. Most prefixes are Greek or Latin. Box 4-5 on pp. 71-72 lists commonly used prefixes.

The **root** is a word element that contains the basic meaning of the word. It is combined with another root, with prefixes, and with suffixes to form a medical term. Roots are mainly from Greek and Latin. A vowel (an *o* or an *i*) is added when two roots are combined or when a suffix is added to a root. The vowel makes pronunciation easier. See Box 4-5 for most common roots.

A **suffix** is a word element placed at the end of a root to change the meaning of the word. Suffixes are not used alone. Like prefixes and roots, they are from Greek and Latin. When translating medical terms, begin with the suffix. For example, *nephritis* means inflammation of the kidney. It was formed by combining *nephro* (kidney) and *itis* (inflammation). See Box 4-5 for common suffixes.

Medical terms are formed by combining word elements. The important things to remember are that prefixes always come before roots and suffixes always come after roots. A root can be combined with prefixes, roots, or suffixes. The prefix *dys* (difficult) is combined with the root *pnea* (breathing). This forms the term *dyspnea,* meaning difficulty in breathing.

Roots can be combined with suffixes. The root *mast* (breast) combined with the suffix *ectomy* (excision or removal) forms the term *mastectomy.* It means the removal of a breast.

Combining a prefix, root, and suffix is another way to form medical terms. *Endocarditis* consists of the prefix *endo* (inner), the root *card* (heart), and the suffix *itis* (inflammation). Endocarditis means inflammation of the inner part of the heart.

Abdominal Regions

The abdomen is divided into regions (Fig. 4-9, p. 73) to help describe the location of body structures, pain, or discomfort. The regions are the:

- Right upper quadrant (RUQ)
- Left upper quadrant (LUQ)
- Right lower quadrant (RLQ)
- Left lower quadrant (LLQ)

Directional Terms

Certain terms describe the position of one body part in relation to another. These terms give the direction of the body part when a person is standing and facing forward. The following directional terms come from some of the prefixes listed in this chapter:

- *Anterior (ventral)*—located at or toward the front of the body or body part
- *Distal*—the part farthest from the center or from the point of attachment
- *Lateral*—relating to or located at the side of the body or body part
- *Medial*—relating to or located at or near the middle or midline of the body or body part
- *Posterior (dorsal)*—located at or toward the back of the body or body part
- *Proximal*—the part nearest to the center or to the point of origin

Abbreviations

Abbreviations are shortened forms of words or phrases. They save time and space in written communication. Each center has a list of accepted abbreviations. Obtain the list when you are hired, and use only the abbreviations accepted by the center. If you are unsure whether an abbreviation is acceptable, write the term out in full to communicate accurately.

Common abbreviations are listed on the inside of the back cover for easy reference.

Box 4-5 MEDICAL TERMINOLOGY

Prefixes

prefix	**meaning**
a-, an-	without, not, lack of
ab-	away from
ad-	to, toward, near
ante-	before, forward, in front of
anti-	against
auto-	self
bi-	double, two, twice
brady-	slow
circum-	around
contra-	against, opposite
de-	down, from
dia-	across, through, apart
dis-	apart, free from
dys-	bad, difficult, abnormal
ecto-	outer, outside
en-	in, into, within
endo-	inner, inside
epi-	over, on, upon
eryth-	red
eu-	normal, good, well, healthy
ex-	out, out of, from, away from
hemi-	half
hyper-	excessive, too much, high
hypo-	under, decreased, less than normal
in-	in, into, within, not
infra-	within
inter-	between
intro-	into, within
leuk-	white
macro-	large
mal-	bad, illness, disease
meg-	large
micro-	small
mono-	one, single
neo-	new
non-	not
olig-	small, scant
para-	beside, beyond, after
per-	by, through
peri-	around
poly-	many, much
post-	after, behind
pre-	before, in front of, prior to
pro-	before, in front of
re-	again, backward
retro-	backward, behind
semi-	half
sub-	under, beneath
super-	above, over, excess
supra-	above, over
tachy-	fast, rapid
trans-	across
uni-	one

Roots

root (combining vowel)	**meaning**
abdomin (o)	abdomen
aden (o)	gland
adren (o)	adrenal gland
angi (o)	vessel
arterio	artery
arthr (o)	joint
broncho	bronchus, bronchi
card, cardi (o)	heart
cephal (o)	head
chole, chol(o)	bile
chondr (o)	cartilage
colo	colon, large intestine
cost (o)	rib
crani (o)	skull
cyan (o)	blue
cyst (o)	bladder, cyst
cyt (o)	cell
dent (o)	tooth
derma	skin
duoden (o)	duodenum
encephal (o)	brain
enter (o)	intestines
fibr (o)	fiber, fibrous
gastr (o)	stomach
gloss (o)	tongue
gluc (o)	sweetness, glucose
glyc (o)	sugar
gyn, gyne, gyneco	woman
hem, hema, hemo, hemat (o)	blood
hepat (o)	liver
hydr (o)	water
hyster (o)	uterus
ile (o), ili (o)	ileum
laparo	abdomen, loin, or flank
laryng (o)	larynx
lith (o)	stone
mamm (o)	breast, mammary gland
mast (o)	mammary gland, breast
meno	menstruation
my (o)	muscle
myel (o)	spinal cord, bone marrow
necro	death
nephr (o)	kidney
neur (o)	nerve
ocul (o)	eye
oophor (o)	ovary
ophthalm (o)	eye
orth (o)	straight, normal, correct
oste (o)	bone
ot (o)	ear
ped (o)	child, foot

Continued

BOX 4-5—CONT'D MEDICAL TERMINOLOGY

Roots—cont'd

root (combining vowel)	meaning
pharyng (o)	pharynx
phleb (o)	vein
pnea	breathing, respiration
pneum (o)	lung, air, gas
proct (o)	rectum
psych (o)	mind
pulmo	lung
py (o)	pus
rect (o)	rectum
rhin (o)	nose
salping (o)	eustachian tube, uterine tube
splen (o)	spleen
sten (o)	narrow, constriction
stern (o)	sternum
stomat (o)	mouth
therm (o)	heat
thoraco	chest
thromb (o)	clot, thrombus
thyr (o)	thyroid
toxic (o)	poison, poisonous
toxo	poison
trache (o)	trachea
urethr (o)	urethra
urin (o)	urine
uro	urine, urinary tract, urination
uter (o)	uterus
vas (o)	blood vessel, vas deferens
ven (o)	vein
vertebr (o)	spine, vertebrae

Suffixes

suffix	meaning
-algia	pain
-asis	condition, usually abnormal
-cele	hernia, herniation, pouching
-centesis	puncture and aspiration of
-cyte	cell

Suffixes—cont'd

suffix	meaning
-ectasis	dilation, stretching
-ectomy	excision, removal of
-emia	blood condition
-genesis	development, production, creation
-genic	producing, causing
-gram	record
-graph	a diagram, a recording instrument
-graphy	making a recording
-iasis	condition of
-ism	a condition
-itis	inflammation
-logy	the study of
-lysis	destruction of, decomposition
-megaly	enlargement
-meter	measuring instrument
-metry	measurement
-oma	tumor
-osis	condition
-pathy	disease
-penia	lack, deficiency
-phagia	to eat or consume; swallowing
-phasia	speaking
-phobia	an exaggerated fear
-plasty	surgical repair or reshaping
-plegia	paralysis
-ptosis	falling, sagging, drooping, down
-rrhage, -rrhagia	excessive flow
-rrhaphy	stitching, suturing
-rrhea	profuse flow, discharge
-scope	examination instrument
-scopy	examination using a scope
-stasis	maintenance, maintaining a constant level
-stomy, -ostomy	creation of an opening
-tomy, -otomy	incision, cutting into
-uria	condition of the urine

COMPUTERS IN HEALTH CARE

The use of computers is common in health care. Information systems collect, send, record, and store information. The information is retrieved when needed. Resident records and care plans are kept on computers in more and more nursing centers. Instead of recording on the resident's chart, it is easier, faster, and more efficient to enter information into a computer (Fig. 4-10).

Computers also are used to monitor certain measurements such as blood pressures, temperatures, and heart rates. The computer recognizes normal and abnormal measurements. When the abnormal is sensed, an alarm alerts the nursing staff. Computerized moni-

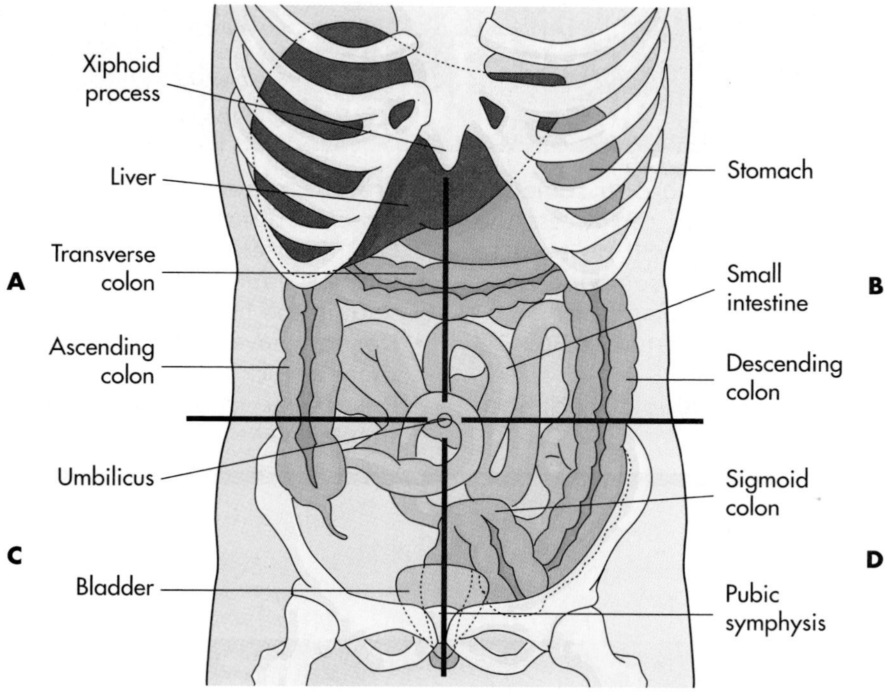

Fig. 4-9 The four regions of the abdomen. **A,** Right upper quadrant. **B,** Left upper quadrant. **C,** Right lower quadrant. **D,** Left upper quadrant.

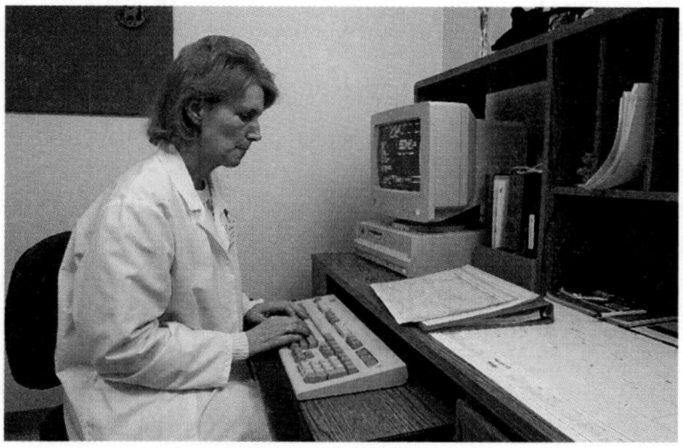

Fig. 4-10 Nurse enters information into the computer.

toring is common in hospitals. It may be used also in skilled nursing units.

Computers save time. The quality and safety of resident care are increased. Less information is omitted from the residents' records, and fewer errors are made in recording. Records are more complete, and personnel are more efficient.

Computers are easy to use, and vast amounts of information are stored in them. Therefore the resident's right to privacy must be protected. Only certain individuals may use the computer. They have their personal codes (passwords) that are used to access the computer. Nursing assistants usually are not allowed to use the computer. If allowed access, you must follow the ethical and legal considerations related to privacy, confidentiality, and defamation. Rules to protect privacy when using a computer are found in Box 4-6 on p. 74.

Learning to use a computer is easy and fun. If you have the opportunity to use the computer where you work, you should do so. If you know how to use computers, you have an additional skill that makes you more employable.

TELEPHONE COMMUNICATIONS

In some centers clerical staff members answer the telephones on the nursing units. Others do not have a clerical staff on the nursing units. In any case, there are times when you must answer the telephone. Good telephone communication skills are essential. The caller cannot see you. Therefore, how you speak and sound are important. Your tone of voice, how clearly you speak, and your attitude give much information. You must speak as professionally on the telephone as you would speak to the person face-to-face.

Most centers have policies about answering the telephone. Know your center's policy. The guidelines in Box 4-7 on p. 74 can help you be professional and courteous.

Box 4-6 Rules to Protect Privacy When Using the Computer

- Do not tell anyone your password. If someone has your password, that person can access the computer under your name. It will be hard to prove that entries were made by someone else.
- Change your password on a regular basis.
- Follow the rules for recording listed in Box 4-3 (p. 69).
- Enter information carefully. Double-check your entries.
- Prevent others from seeing what is on the screen. Do not leave the computer unattended. Log off after making an entry.
- Position equipment so that the screen cannot be seen in the hallway.
- Do not leave printouts where others can read them or pick them up.
- Destroy or shred any computer-printed worksheets.

Box 4-7 Guidelines for Answering Telephones

- Answer the call after the first ring if possible. Business manners call for the phone to be answered by the fourth ring.
- Do not answer the phone in a rushed or hasty manner.
- Give a courteous greeting, identify the area, and give your name and title. For example: "Good morning. Three center. Jeff North, nursing assistant."
- Write the following information when taking a message: the caller's name and telephone number (include area code and extension number), the date and time, and the message.
- Repeat the message and telephone number back to the caller.
- Ask the caller to "Please hold" if necessary. However, find out who is calling first, and then ask if the caller can hold. Do not put callers with an emergency on hold.
- Do not lay the phone down or cover the receiver with your hand when not speaking to the caller. The caller may overhear confidential conversations.
- Return to a caller on hold within 30 seconds. Ask if the caller can wait longer or if the call can be returned.
- Do not give confidential information to any caller. Remember, information about residents and employees is confidential. Refer such calls to an RN.
- Transfer the call if appropriate. Tell the caller that you are going to transfer the call. Give the name of the department if appropriate. Give the caller the phone number in case the call gets disconnected or the line is busy.
- End the conversation politely. Thank the person for calling and say good-bye.
- Give the message to the appropriate person.

DEALING WITH CONFLICT

People bring their own values, attitudes, opinions, experiences, and expectations to the work setting. Differences often lead to conflict. **Conflict** is described as a clash between opposing interests and ideas. Disagreements, misunderstandings, arguments, and unrest occur.

Conflicts arise over issues or events. Work schedules, absences, and the amount and quality of work performed are examples. The problems must be worked out. Otherwise, unkind words or actions may occur. The work environment becomes unpleasant, and resident care is affected.

Communication and good work ethics are essential for preventing and resolving conflicts. Identify and solve problems before they become major issues. The following guidelines can help you deal with conflict:

- Ask your supervisor for some time to talk privately. Explain the situation, and ask for advice in solving the problem. Give facts and specific examples.
- Approach the person with whom you have a conflict. Ask to talk privately. Be polite and professional in your approach.
- Agree on a time and place to talk.
- Talk in a private setting. Others should not be able to see or hear you and your co-worker.
- Explain the problem and what is bothering you. Give facts and specific behaviors.
- Listen to the person's response. Do not interrupt the person.
- Identify ways to solve the problem. Offer your own thoughts, and ask for the co-worker's ideas.
- Schedule a date and time to review the situation.
- Thank the person for meeting with you.
- Implement the solutions.
- Review the situation as scheduled.

QUALITY OF LIFE

Communication among health care team members is essential for effective and coordinated resident care. Communication that is factual, concise, and understandable and presented in a logical manner helps the health care team provide a high quality of care to residents. Information that is false or incomplete can cause a resident harm.

Remember that resident information is personal and confidential. You must always protect the resident's right to privacy. Confidential information is shared only with the health care team members involved in a resident's care. It is never shared with the resident's family or friends without the resident's permission.

The resident has the right to participate in his or her care planning. OBRA requires that the resident be included in this process. The resident may refuse actions suggested by the health care team. Involving the resident in the care planning process helps the health care team meet the resident's needs more effectively. You are an important member of the team. Sharing your observations and suggestions can help the team provide more effective care.

REVIEW QUESTIONS

Circle T if the statement is true or F if the statement is false.

1 T F The health team communicates to provide effective and coordinated resident care.

2 T F Mrs. Reece was discharged from St. Jude's Nursing Center. Her chart is destroyed to protect her right to privacy.

3 T F The medical record is not used in a lawsuit because of the right to privacy.

4 T F Nursing assistants generally have access to all medical records in the center.

5 T F Information is collected about a person using the senses.

6 T F Subjective data are signs noted when observing a person.

7 T F The comprehensive care plan lists the medications and treatments ordered by the doctor.

8 T F Nursing assistants are not involved in the interdisciplinary care conference.

9 T F Never give confidential information to anyone over the telephone.

Circle the BEST answer.

10 When communicating, you should do the following *except*
A Use terms that have more than one meaning
B Be brief and concise
C Present information logically and in sequence
D Give facts and be specific

11 These statements are about medical records. Which is *false?*
A The record is used to communicate information about the resident.
B The record is a written account of the resident's illness and response to treatment.
C The record is a written account of care given by the health team.
D Anyone working in the center can read the medical record.

12 A person is weighed daily. The measurement is recorded on the
A Admission sheet
B Graphic sheet
C Flow sheet
D Nurses' notes

13 Where does the RN describe the nursing care given?
A Nursing care plan
B Interdisciplinary progress notes
C Graphic sheet
D Kardex

14 Measures in the comprehensive care plan are carried out. What step of the nursing process is this?
A Nursing diagnosis
B Planning
C Implementation
D Evaluation

15 Which statement is *true?*
A The nursing process is done without the resident's involvement.
B Nursing assistants are responsible for the nursing process.
C The nursing process is used to communicate the resident's care.
D All of the above

REVIEW QUESTIONS—cont'd

16 The comprehensive care plan
- A Is written by the doctor
- B Consists of actions the health care team takes to help a resident
- C Is the same for all residents
- D Is also called the Kardex

17 When recording information, you should do the following, *except*
- A Use ink
- B Include the date and time
- C Erase if you make an error
- D Sign all entries with your name and title

18 These statements are about recording. Which is *false?*
- A Use the person's exact words when possible.
- B Record only what you observed and did yourself.
- C Do not skip lines.
- D To save time, chart a procedure before it is completed.

19 In the evening you note that the clock says 9:26. In 24-hour clock time you record this as
- A 9:26 PM
- B 926
- C 0926
- D 2126

20 You are learning medical terminology. You know that a suffix is
- A Placed at the beginning of the word
- B Placed after a root
- C A shortened form of a word or phrase
- D Describes the body's position

21 These statements are about computers in health care. Which is *false?*
- A Computers are used to collect, send, record, and store information.
- B The resident's privacy must be protected.
- C All employees have the same password.
- D Computers link one department to another.

22 You answer a resident's phone in the center. How should you answer?
- A "Good morning. Mrs. Park's room."
- B "Good morning. Third floor."
- C "Hello."
- D "Good morning. Mrs. Reece's room. Jill Brown, nursing assistant, speaking."

23 A co-worker is often late for work. You have extra work in her absence. In resolving the conflict you should do the following *except*
- A Explain the problem to your supervisor
- B Discuss the matter during the end-of-shift report
- C Give facts and specific instances
- D Suggest ideas to solve the problem

Answers to these questions are on pp. 695-696.

5 Communicating With the Resident

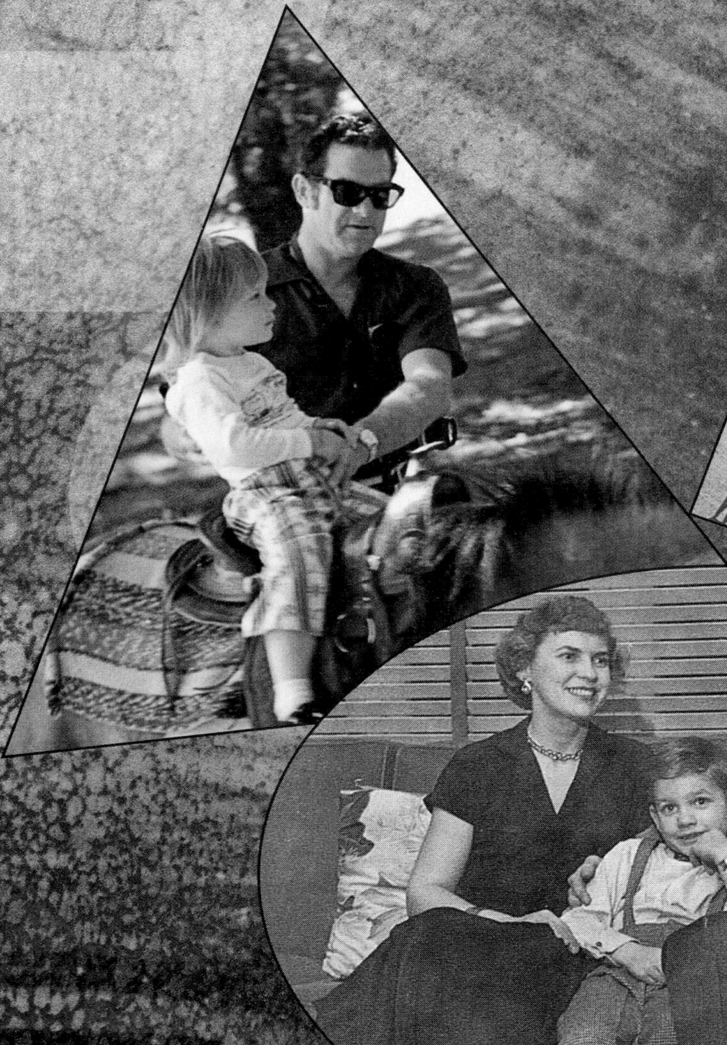

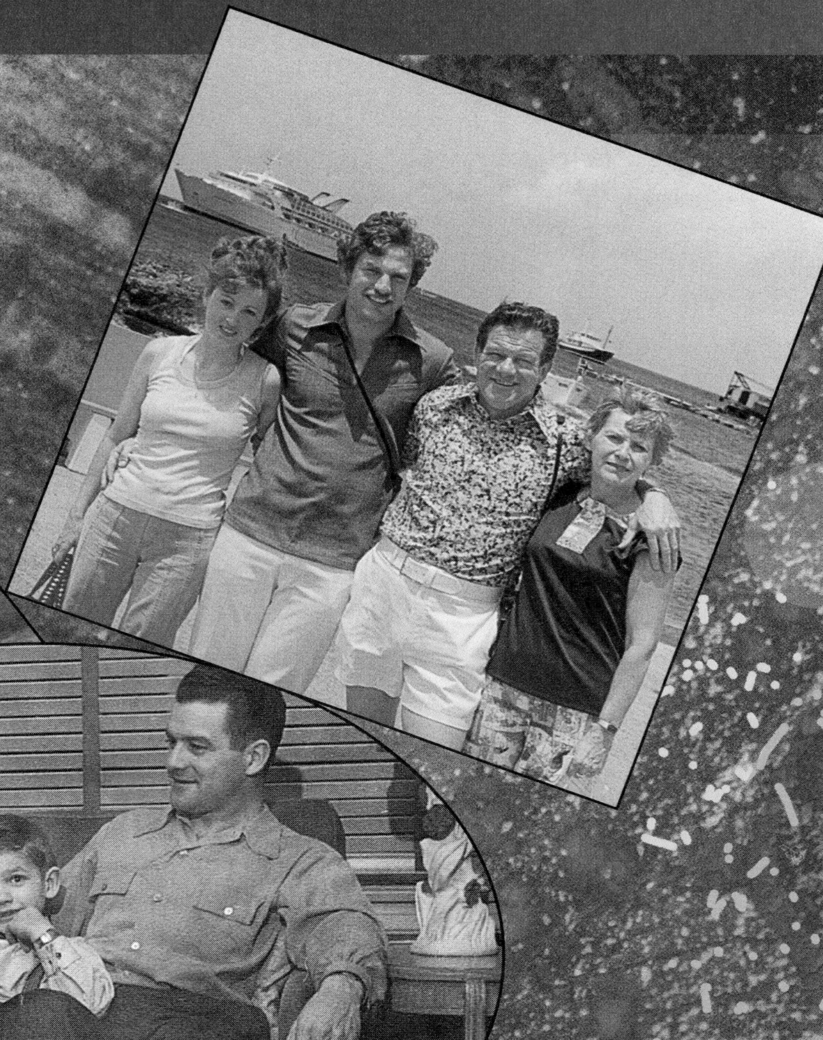

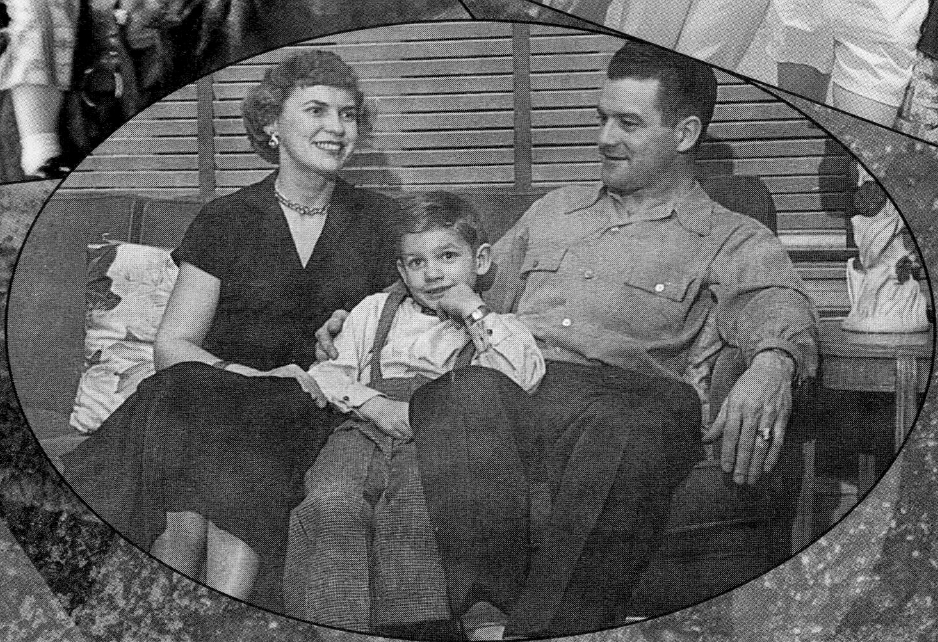

What You Will Learn

- The definition of the key terms listed in this chapter
- The parts that make up the whole person
- The basic needs for life identified by Abraham Maslow
- How culture and religion influence health and illness
- The psychological and social effects of illness
- The types of residents cared for in nursing centers
- How to promote a resident's quality of life
- The elements needed for effective communication
- How verbal and nonverbal communication are used
- The techniques and barriers to effective communication
- How to deal with the angry person
- Why family and visitors are important to residents
- The courtesies given to residents and visitors

Key Terms

body language Facial expressions, gestures, posture, and body movements that send messages to others

comatose The inability to respond to verbal stimuli

culture The values, beliefs, habits, likes, dislikes, customs, and characteristics of a group of people that are passed from one generation to the next

need That which is necessary or desirable for maintaining life and mental well-being

nonverbal communication Communication that does not involve words

optimal level of function A person's highest potential for mental and physical performance

paraphrasing Restating the person's message in your own words

religion Spiritual beliefs, needs, and practices

self-actualization Experiencing one's potential

self-esteem Thinking well of oneself, seeing oneself as useful, and being well thought of by others

verbal communication Communication that uses the written or spoken word

The resident is the most important person in the nursing center. Age, religion, nationality, education, occupation, and life-style are some factors that make each resident unique. Each resident is an important, special, valuable human being. The resident must be treated as a person who thinks, acts, feels, and makes decisions.

You will care for many residents; most of them are elderly. Keep in mind that each resident is a unique person. You need to understand the fears, needs, and rights of that person. Also, you need to understand the losses that the person may have suffered. This is especially true of older residents. Many have lost homes, family members, friends, and body functions. They also may have lost their roles in families or communities. This chapter helps you understand and communicate with the residents you will serve, help, and care for.

THE RESIDENT AS A PERSON

Too often a resident is referred to as a room number, such as "12A needs a pain pill," rather than "Mrs. Brown in 12A needs a pain pill." This strips the person of his or her identity and reduces the individual to a thing. Residents often are denied the dignity and respect of being called by their titles, such as Mrs. Jones, Mr. Smith, or Miss Turner. Instead, they are called Jane, Tom, or Mary. Some have been called Grandma, Papa, or sweetheart. Never call residents by their first name or any other name unless asked by the person to do so. Residents are not things, your relatives, or children. They are complex, adult human beings. To give effective care, you must be aware of the whole person.

The whole person has physical, social, psychological, and spiritual parts. These parts are woven together and cannot be separated (Fig. 5-1). Each part relates to and depends on the others. As a social being, a person speaks and communicates with others. Physically, the brain, mouth, tongue, lips, and throat structures must function for speech. Communication is also psychological. It involves the thinking and reasoning abilities of the mind. To consider only the physical part is to ignore the resident's ability to think, make decisions, and interact with others. You also ignore the fact that the resident is a living person with a life history of experiences, joys, sorrows, and needs.

Health care workers must be aware of the whole person. Disability and physical illness affect the person socially, psychologically, and spiritually. For example, Mr. Lund had a stroke. He can no longer care for his physical needs without help. He had to give up his home. Relationships with his wife and children are changed. He is angry with God for letting this happen to him. The health care team must plan his care to help him deal with all of these problems. You must know and respect the whole person to provide effective, quality care.

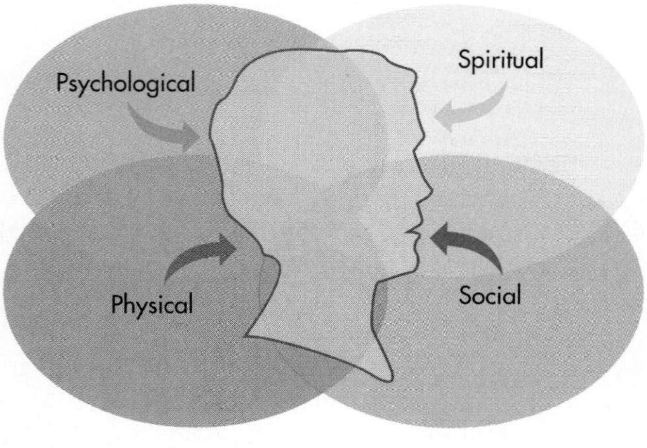

Fig. 5-1 A person is a physical, psychological, social, and spiritual being. The parts overlap and cannot be separated.

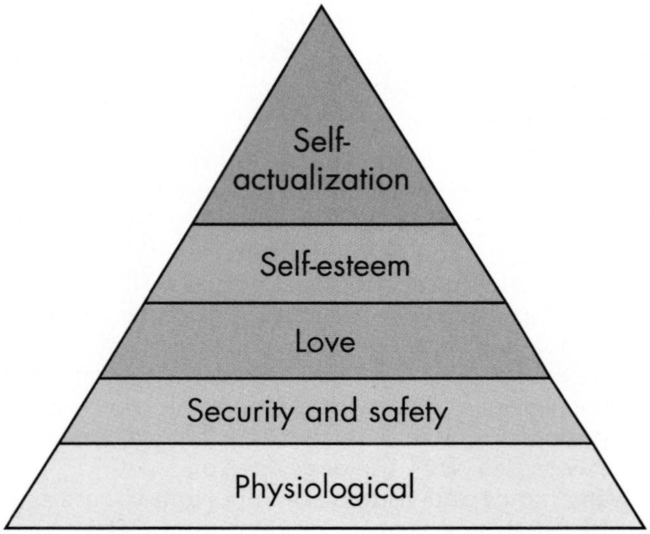

Fig. 5-2 Basic needs for life as described by Maslow. These needs—from the lowest to the highest level—are physiological needs, the need for safety and security, the need for love and belonging, the need for self-esteem, and the need for self-actualization.

NEEDS

A **need** is that which is necessary or desirable for maintaining life and mental well-being. According to Abraham Maslow, a famous psychologist, certain basic needs must be met if a person is to survive and function. These needs are arranged in order of importance. Lower-level needs must be met before higher-level needs. These basic needs, from the lowest level to the highest, are physiological or physical needs, the need for safety and security, the need for love and belonging, self-esteem needs, and the need for self-actualization (Fig. 5-2). People normally meet their own needs. When they cannot, it is usually because of disease, illness, injury, or advanced age. Those who are ill or injured usually seek help from doctors, nurses, and other health care providers.

Physiological Needs

Oxygen, food, water, elimination, rest, and shelter are required for life. These needs are the most important for survival. They must be met before higher-level needs. A person dies within minutes without oxygen. Without food or water, a person feels weak and ill within a few hours. The kidneys and intestines must function normally. Otherwise poisonous wastes build up in the blood. If the problem is not corrected, the person dies. Without enough rest and sleep, a person becomes exhausted.

You will assist other health care team members in helping residents meet their physical needs. You need to develop a true appreciation of these physical needs. Most people take them for granted until a problem develops. How do you feel when you have difficulty breathing or feel as if you are choking? How do you react when you are thirsty, hungry, or do not get enough sleep?

The Need for Safety and Security

Safety and security needs relate to protection from harm, danger, and fear. Many people are afraid of nursing centers. Some procedures involve strange equipment and cause pain or discomfort. People feel safer and more secure if they understand the procedure. They should know why and how a procedure is to be done. The person also needs to know who will do it and what sensations or feelings to expect.

Many persons feel a loss of security and safety when admitted to a nursing center. They are not in the familiar, secure setting of their home. They are in a strange place, with strange routines and with strangers to care for them. Often they become frightened and confused. Treat them with kindness, understanding, and patience to help them feel secure. Show them their new surroundings, listen to their concerns, and explain all routines and procedures. You may have to repeat explanations and directions many times for several days or weeks until the resident feels safe and unafraid. Be patient.

The Need for Love and Belonging

The need for love and belonging relates to love, closeness, affection, belonging, and meaningful relationships with others. There are cases where people slowly became weaker and unable to care for themselves, or have died, because of lack of love and belonging. This is particularly true of older persons who have outlived families and friends. Family, friends, and the health care team can meet love and belonging needs. Remember that the center becomes the new home for many persons. It is important that you help the resident feel loved and accepted. Remind the resident that you are there to provide care for him or her.

The Need for Self-Esteem

Esteem means the worth, value, or opinion one has of a person. **Self-esteem** needs relate to thinking well of oneself, seeing oneself as useful, and being well thought of by others. Nursing center residents often lack self-esteem because they are older, disabled, or chronically ill. An older man once built his own home, worked a farm, and supported and raised a family. Now he cannot dress or feed himself because of painful arthritis. How might he feel about himself? A woman has lost her hair because of cancer treatments. She may feel unattractive and less than whole. Persons with slow, crippling diseases or those who have lost a limb also may feel less than whole. You must treat residents with respect. Although it takes more time, encourage residents to do as much for themselves as possible. This helps increase self-esteem.

The Need for Self-Actualization

Self-actualization means experiencing one's potential. It involves learning, understanding, and creating to the limit of a person's capacity. This is the highest-level need. Rarely, if ever, is it totally met. Most people constantly try to learn and understand more. The need for self-actualization can be postponed, and life will continue.

CULTURE AND RELIGION

Culture is defined as the values, beliefs, habits, likes, dislikes, customs, and characteristics of a group of people that are passed from one generation to the next. The resident's culture influences health beliefs and practices. Culture also influences the resident's behavior in a nursing center.

You will care for persons of different cultures. People in the United States come from various cultures, races, and nationalities. Therefore you may care for residents from cultures that differ from your own. They may have family practices, food preferences, hygiene habits, and clothing styles that are different from yours. The resident also may speak and understand a foreign language. Some cultural groups have beliefs about the causes and cures of illnesses. *(See Caring About Culture [Health Care Beliefs], p. 82.)* They may perform certain rituals aimed at ridding the body of disease. *(See Caring About Culture [Sick Care Practices], p. 82.)* They may also have beliefs and rituals about death and dying (see Chapter 32). Learn as much as you can about a resident's cultural beliefs and health care practices. This will help you provide care that meets the resident's needs.

Religion relates to spiritual beliefs, needs, and practices. Like culture, a person's religion influences health and illness practices. Religions may have beliefs and practices about diet, healing, days of worship, birth, and death.

Most Americans are Jewish, Protestant, or Roman Catholic. There also are many Moslems, Buddhists, and Hindus. Many residents find religion to be a source of comfort and strength during illness. They may want to pray and observe certain religious practices. If religious services are held in your center, assist

CARING ABOUT CULTURE

Health Care Beliefs

Some cultures believe that health involves a balance between hot and cold. In Mexico and the Dominican Republic, hot and cold imbalances are thought to cause disease. "Hot" conditions include fever, infections, diarrhea, constipation, and ulcers. "Cold" conditions include cancer, earaches, menstrual periods, headaches, colds, and paralysis.

In Vietnam, foods and medicine are given to restore the hot-cold balance. Hot foods and medicines are given for "cold" illnesses; cold foods and medicines are given for "hot" illnesses.

Remember, individuals may not follow every belief and practice of their culture and religion. Each person is unique. Do not judge residents by your own standards.

Modified from Giger JN, Davidhizar RE: *Transcultural nursing: Assessment and intervention*, ed 2, St Louis, 1995, Mosby.

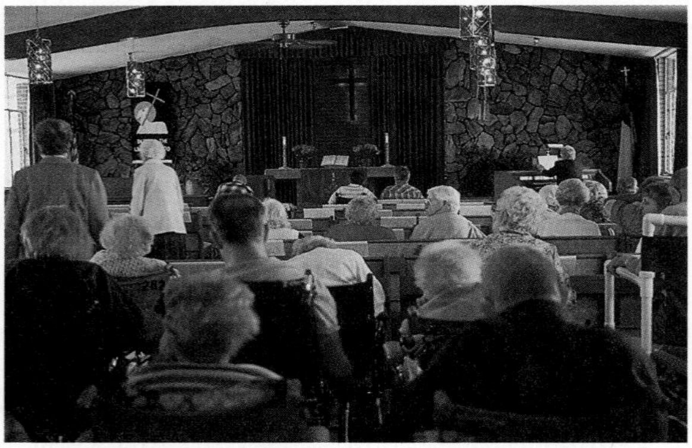

Fig. 5-3 Residents attend a religious service at a nursing center.

residents to attend the services if they wish (Fig. 5-3). A resident may want to leave the center to attend services or have a visit from a spiritual leader or adviser. You need to report the request to the nurse. A resident may want the pastor to visit in the room. If so, make sure the room is neat and orderly and that there is a chair for the cleric to use. Be sure the resident and pastor have privacy during the visit.

The nursing process reflects the person's culture and religion. The health care team and the resident plan measures that include the person's cultural and religious practices.

You need to respect and accept the resident's culture and religion. When you meet people from other cultures or religions, take time to learn about their beliefs and practices. This helps you understand the resident and give better care.

Individuals may not follow all the beliefs and practices of their culture or religion. Some people may not practice a religion. Remember that each person is unique. Avoid judging residents by your standards.

CARING ABOUT CULTURE

Sick Care Practices

Folk practices are common in the Vietnamese culture. Such practices include *cao gio,* rubbing the skin with a coin. This is done to treat the common cold. Skin pinching *(bat gio)* is used for headaches and sore throats. Herbal teas and soups are common remedies for many different signs and symptoms.

Russian folk practices also include herbs. Herbs are taken in drinks or in enemas. For headaches, an ointment is placed behind the ears and temples. It is also at the back of the neck. There are different treatments for backache. One involves making a dough of dark rye flour and honey. The dough is placed on the spinal column.

Folk healers are seen in Mexico and among some Mexican Americans. Folk healers include a family member skilled in healing practices passed down from one generation to another. Folk healers are sometimes sought outside the family. A *jerbero* uses herbs and spices to prevent or cure disease. A *curandero* (*curandera* if female) deals with serious physical and mental illnesses. Witches use magic. A male witch is called a *brujos*; a female witch is called a *brujas.*

Remember, individuals may not follow every belief and practice of their culture and religion. Each person is unique. Do not judge residents by your own standards.

Modified from Giger JN, Davidhizar RE: *Transcultural nursing: Assessment and intervention*, ed 2, St Louis, 1995, Mosby.

EFFECTS OF ILLNESS AND DISABILITY ON THE RESIDENT

People are not sick and disabled because they want to be. Being ill and injured has physical, psychological, and social effects on people. Normal activities—such as work, driving a car, preparing meals, doing yard work, or taking part in hobbies—may be difficult or impossible. These daily activities bring personal satisfaction, worth, and contact with others. People often feel angry, frustrated, and useless when unable to perform them. These feelings may become even greater if others must perform routine functions for them. Some residents also feel alone and isolated if they have outlived friends and family. They may direct anger at you. Try to remember that they are angry at the situation and not at you personally. If you do not know how to respond to a resident's anger, ask the nurse for help (p. 88).

Chronically ill and disabled residents may have many fears and anxieties about living in a nursing center. They may feel lonely and believe families and friends have abandoned them. They may fear being dependent on strangers. Many may fear increasing loss of function. Some will express their fears. Others will not or cannot. You will work closely with these residents. You can anticipate these concerns and help the resident feel safe, secure, and loved. You can take an extra minute to "visit," to quietly hold a hand, or to give a hug.

Show your willingness to take care of their personal needs. Respond promptly, and treat each person with respect and dignity. You may not be able to prevent increasing loss of function. You can, however, help the resident maintain his or her **optimal level of functioning.** This refers to a person's highest potential for mental and physical performance. Encourage the person to be as independent as possible. Always focus on the person's abilities, not on the disabilities.

Hospital patients often are treated as sick, dependent people. Encouraging this "sick role" in a nursing center reduces the resident's quality of life. Your job, and that of all health care workers, is to improve the resident's quality of life. You can do this by helping each person regain or maintain as much physical and mental function as possible.

RESIDENTS YOU WILL CARE FOR

You will care for different types of residents. Most are older. Some are mentally alert and oriented but have chronic illnesses or disabilities that keep them from living alone or with family (Fig. 5-4). Others are too confused and disoriented to care for themselves. Still others are recovering from fractures, acute illnesses, or surgery. You may care for terminally ill residents (residents who are dying). These residents need special care to maintain comfort and make their last days as peaceful as possible.

Alert, and Oriented Residents

Many residents are alert and oriented. They know who they are, where they are, the year, and the time of day.

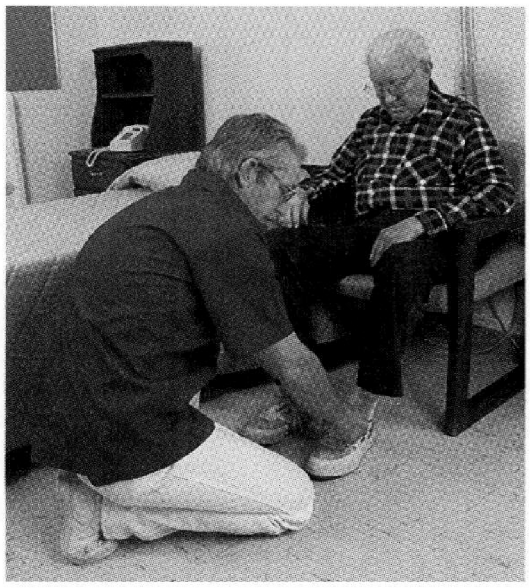

Fig. 5-4 This older man requires the services of a long-term care center.

These residents have physical problems that require care in a nursing center. Some are paralyzed from a stroke, injury, or birth defect. Others have a disabling disease such as arthritis or multiple sclerosis. Still others suffer from chronic heart, liver, kidney, or respiratory disease. The amount of care required depends on the degree of disability. Because these residents are alert and oriented, they may have problems adjusting to a nursing center. You need to help these residents accept the nursing center as home.

Confused and Disoriented Residents

Many residents are mildly to severely confused and disoriented. Some simply have trouble remembering where the dining room is or the month and year. Others are more confused and disoriented—for example, thinking they are in another city waiting for a train. The most severely disoriented persons do not even know who they are. Sometimes the confusion and disorientation are temporary. This is especially true for newly admitted residents. For other residents, such as those with Alzheimer's disease, the confusion and disorientation are permanent and become worse. Chapter 27 discusses how to work with all types of confused residents.

Complete Care Residents

You will take care of very physically disabled residents who are also confused and disoriented. These residents require total assistance with all activities of daily living (ADL). They cannot meet any of their own needs. Nor can they tell you what they need or want. The health care team must take special care to keep these residents clean, safe, and comfortable. You must remember that these residents have the right to be treated with respect and compassion. Touch, massage, and music may provide comfort and decrease loneliness.

Short-Term Residents

Some residents stay in a center for a short time. Short-term residents are called *patients* in some centers because they do not plan to make the center their home. *(See Subacute Care.)* The goal is to help these residents increase their strength and mobility so they can return home or to their former living situation. Some residents are so ill that they need skilled care. They may need IV therapy, tube feedings, special wound care, intense rehabilitation, or other treatments. Others may need special therapy programs: physical, occupational, speech and language, respiratory, or special restorative nursing care. You will assist other health care workers in helping these residents return to their optimal level of functioning.

Some people are cared for at home and are admitted to nursing centers for short stays. This is *respite care.* The caregiver has time to take a vacation, take care of business, or simply to rest. Respite care may last from a few days to several weeks.

SUBACUTE CARE

Persons requiring subacute care may be younger than most other residents. They may be recovering from fractures, acute illness, or surgery.

Terminally Ill Residents

Terminally ill residents are dying. They may have advanced cancer or liver, kidney, respiratory, or heart disease. Some may have AIDS. Some are alert and oriented; others are comatose. **Comatose** residents cannot respond to verbal stimuli but may still feel pain. They may show pain by grimacing or groaning. Some residents have a great deal of pain and need frequent care to maintain comfort. Pain medication can help. You should promptly report any sign of discomfort to the nurse. Pain medication is important, but so is the care you give. Turning and positioning, gentle back rubs, touch, and holding a hand are very effective in promoting comfort and peace. Many centers work closely with hospice programs to provide quality care to dying residents (see Chapter 1).

COMMUNICATING WITH THE RESIDENT

Remember, communication involves sending and receiving messages. You communicate with residents every time you give care. You give information to the resident, and the resident gives information to you. Your body sends messages all the time—at the bedside, in the hallway, at the nurses' station, in the dining room, and everywhere else. Residents and families are aware of what you say. They also are aware of what you do. Good work ethics and understanding the person are necessary for good communication. What you say and do also are important.

Effective Communication

Several elements are necessary for effective communication between you and the resident. You must:

- Understand and respect the resident as a person.
- View the person as more than a disease or an illness. The person is a physical, psychological, social, and spiritual human being.
- Appreciate the person's problems and frustrations from being sick.
- Recognize and respect the person's rights.
- Accept and respect the person's religion and culture.

The communication rules discussed in Chapter 4 apply when you communicate with residents. Remember to:

- Use words that have the same meaning to both you and the person.
- Avoid medical terminology and other words that are unfamiliar to the person.
- Communicate in a logical and orderly manner. Do not wander in thought.
- Give specific and factual information.
- Be brief and concise.
- Give the resident time to process (understand) the information that you give.
- Ask questions to be sure you were understood. Repeat information as often as necessary. Repeat exactly what you said so the person does not have to process a new message. This is especially important for residents with hearing problems.
- Be patient. Residents with memory problems may ask the same question several times a day. Do not remind them that you are repeating information. Accept their memory loss as you would any other disability.

You will use both verbal and nonverbal communication when relating to your residents. Knowing how to use both methods will help you communicate effectively.

VERBAL AND NONVERBAL COMMUNICATION

Communication is what you say and do. You communicate verbally and nonverbally with residents. You must use both methods effectively.

A B C D

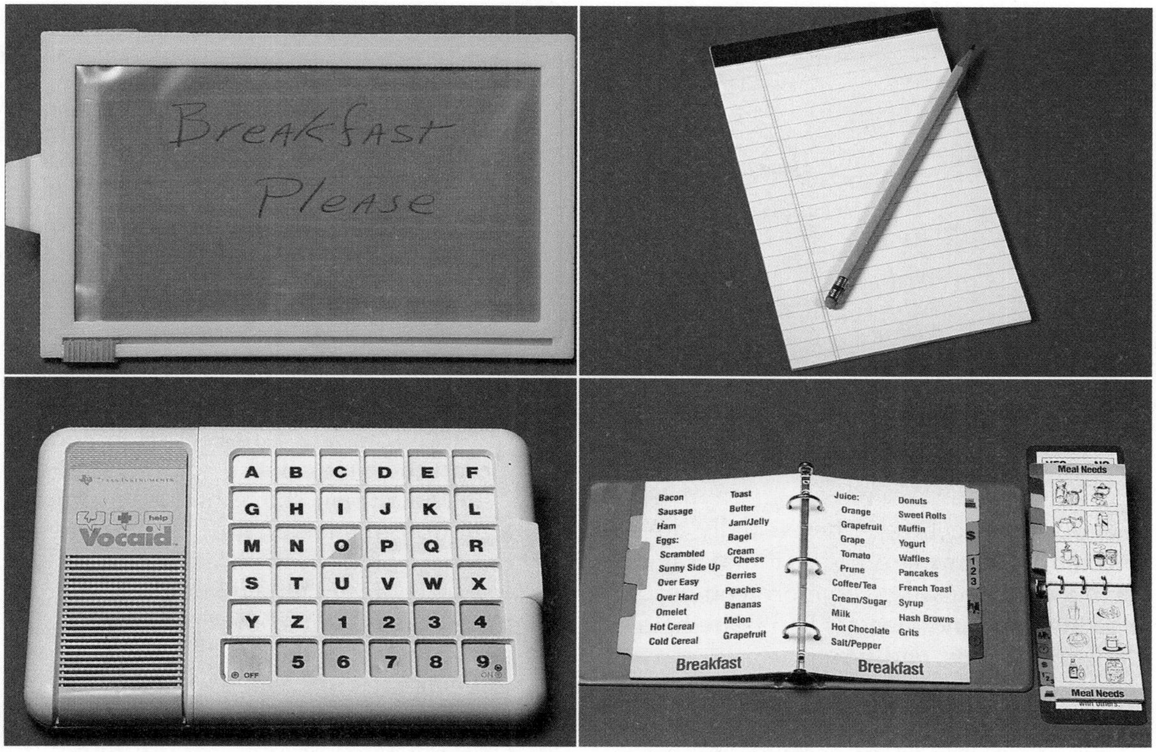

Fig. 5-5 **A,** Magic Slate. **B,** Paper and pencil. **C,** Electronic talking aid. **D,** Communication and picture binders.

Verbal Communication

Words are used in **verbal communication.** The words are spoken or written. Verbal communication is used to talk with residents, to find out how they are feeling, and to share information with them.

Written communication is used when a resident cannot speak or hear but can read. Magic Slates, paper and pencil, communication boards, or electronic talking aids (Fig. 5-5) are used. If a resident cannot speak or read, you need to provide a way for the resident to communicate needs. The nurse tells you how to communicate with the resident. If the resident can hear but cannot speak or read, ask questions that are answered yes or no with nods, blinks, or other gestures. A picture board may be helpful (Fig. 5-6). You will write messages to communicate with residents who are deaf or who have severe hearing problems. When writing messages for those with poor vision, use a black felt pen on white paper. Print the message in large letters. Persons who are deaf may use sign language and written messages to communicate (Fig. 5-7 on p. 86).

Your communication with residents should be kind, courteous, and friendly. This may be hard when residents are not courteous in return. Remember that residents who are the hardest to deal with probably need your kindness the most.

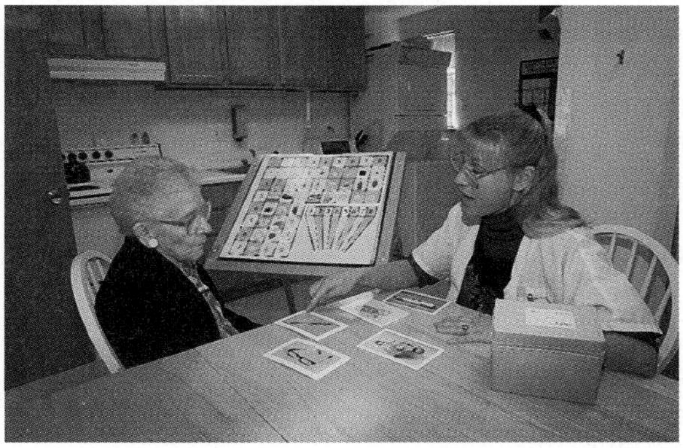

Fig. 5-6 A picture board is used to communicate with the resident.

Nonverbal Communication

Nonverbal communication (body language) does not rely on words. Gestures, facial expressions, posture, body movements, touch, and smell are examples of how messages are sent and received without the use of words. Nonverbal messages are considered a truer

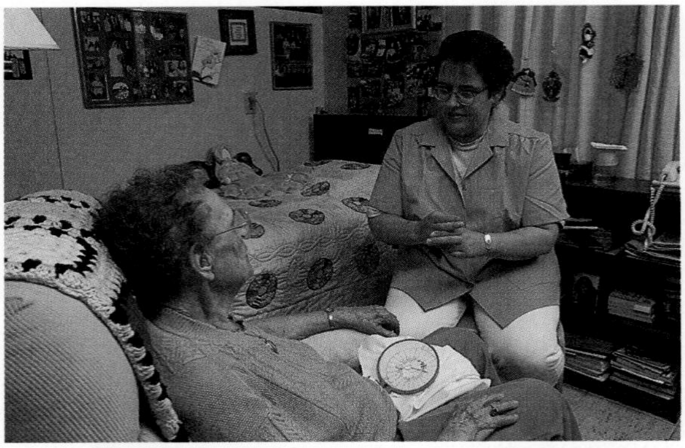

Fig. 5-7 A resident uses sign language to communicate.

reflection of a person's feelings. They usually are involuntary and hard to control. A resident may say one thing but act in a different way. Therefore you need to watch the person's eyes and the way hands are held or moved. Gestures, posture, and other actions can tell you more than the spoken word.

Touch. Touch is an important form of nonverbal communication. It can convey comfort, caring, love, affection, and reassurance. Touch means different things to different people. The meaning depends on the person's age, culture, gender, and life experiences. *(See Caring About Culture.)* Although some people do not like to be touched, do not be afraid to try touch to convey caring and warmth. Often it is easier to comfort residents by holding their hands or touching their forearms than it is to use words. Touch should be gentle, not hurried or rough. You soon will learn which residents do not want to be touched. The care plan also gives you this information. Be sure to respect the resident's wishes.

Body Language. People send messages through their body language. Body language includes the following:

- Posture
- Gait
- Facial expressions
- Eye contact
- Hand movements
- Gestures
- Body movements
- Appearance (dress, hygiene, and adornments such as jewelry, perfume, and cosmetics)

Residents send messages with their body language. Slumped posture may mean the person is not happy or feeling well. A resident may deny pain but protects the affected body part by standing, lying, or sitting in a certain way. Residents send many other messages with body language.

CARING ABOUT CULTURE

Touch Practices

Touch practices vary widely among cultural groups. Touch is used often in Mexico. Some people believe that using touch while complimenting a person is important. It is thought to neutralize the power of the evil eye *(mal ojo).* Touch also is important in the Philippine culture.

Persons from the United Kingdom tend not to use touch. However, it is important in nonverbal communication among people of Russia. They commonly kiss three times on the cheek for greetings and farewells. Hugging and kissing on the cheek is also common in Poland.

In India, men shake hands with other men. Men do not shake hands with women. Similar practices occur in the Vietnamese culture.

People from China do not like being touched by strangers. A nod or slight bow is given during introductions.

Remember, individuals may not follow every belief and practice of their culture and religion. Each person is unique. Do not judge residents by your own standards.

Modified from Geissler EM: *Pocket guide to cultural assessment*, ed 2, St Louis, 1998, Mosby.

You also send messages by the way you act and move. Your facial expressions and how you stand, sit, walk, and look at a person all send messages. Your body language should show interest and enthusiasm about your work. It should also show caring and respect for the resident. You need to control your body language in many instances. For example, do not react to odors from excretions or the resident's body. Many odors are beyond the resident's control. The resident's embarrassment and humiliation increase if you react to the odor.

COMMUNICATION TECHNIQUES

Certain techniques help you communicate with residents and families. The techniques result in better relationships with these persons. You also gain more information for the nursing process.

Listening

Listening means being attentive to the resident's verbal and nonverbal communication. You use the senses of sight, hearing, touch, and smell. You must concentrate on what the resident is saying. You also observe

Caring About Culture

Eye Contact Practices
Direct eye contact is practiced among the people of Poland and Russia. However, direct eye contact is rude in Mexican and Vietnamese cultures. In the United Kingdom, staring is a part of good listening.

Blinking also has meaning. In the Vietnamese culture, blinking means that a message is received. It indicates understanding in the United Kingdom.

Remember, individuals may not follow every belief and practice of their culture and religion. Each person is unique. Do not judge residents by your own standards.

Modified from Geissler EM: *Pocket guide to cultural assessment*, ed 2, St Louis, 1998, Mosby.

nonverbal clues. The resident's nonverbal communication can support what the resident says. Or it can show other feelings. For example, Mr. Hart says, "I want to go to a nursing home. That way my daughter won't have to stay home to care for me." However, you see tears in his eyes and he looks away from you. His verbal says happy, but his nonverbal shows sadness.

Listening requires that you care and have interest. The following guidelines are important:

- Face the resident.
- Have good eye contact with the resident. *(See Caring About Culture.)*
- Lean toward the resident (Fig. 5-8). Do not sit back with your arms crossed.
- Respond to the resident. Nod your head. Say "uh huh," "mmm," and "I see." Repeat what the resident says, and ask questions.
- Avoid the barriers to effective communication (p. 88).

Paraphrasing

Paraphrasing is restating a person's message in your own words. You use fewer words than the person did to send the message. Paraphrasing serves three purposes:

- It shows you are listening.
- It lets the person see if you understand the message sent.
- It promotes further communication.

The person usually responds to your statement. For example:

Resident: My wife was crying after she spoke with the doctor. I don't know what he said to her.
You: You don't know why your wife was crying.
Resident: He must have told her that I have a tumor.

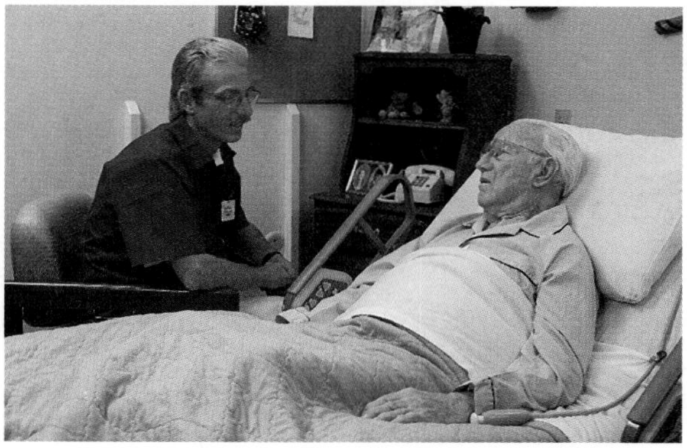

Fig. 5-8 The nursing assistant shows he is listening by facing the resident, having good eye contact, and leaning toward the resident.

Direct Questions

Direct questions focus on specific information. You ask the person something you need to know. Some direct questions have "yes" or "no" answers. Others require the person to give more information. For example:

You: Mr. Hart, do you want to shave this morning?
Resident: Yes.
You: Mr. Hart, when would you like to shave and have your bath?
Resident: Could we start in about 15 minutes? I'd like to call my son first.
You: Yes, we can start in 15 minutes. Did you have a bowel movement today, Mr. Hart?
Resident: No.
You: You said you didn't eat well this morning. Can you tell me what you ate?
Resident: I only had toast and coffee. I just don't feel like eating this morning.

Open-Ended Questions

Open-ended questions lead or invite the person to share thoughts, feelings, or ideas. The person chooses what to talk about. Answers require more than a "yes" or "no." However, the person controls what is talked about and the information given. Consider these examples:

- "What do you like about living with your daughter?"
- "Tell me about your grandson."
- "What was your wife like?"
- "What do you like about being retired?"

The person chooses how to answer the question. Responses to open-ended questions generally are longer and give more information than direct questions.

Clarifying

Clarifying lets you make sure that you understand the message. You can ask the person to repeat the

message, say you do not understand, or restate the message. For example:
- "Could you say that again?"
- "I'm sorry, Mr. Hart. I don't understand what you mean.
- "Are you saying that you want to go home?"

Focusing
Focusing is dealing with a specific topic. It is useful when a person rambles or wanders in thought. For example, Mr. Hart talks at length about his favorite foods and places to eat. You need to know why he did not eat breakfast. You focus the conversation on breakfast by saying: "Let's talk about today's breakfast. You said you didn't feel like eating."

Silence
Silence is a very powerful way to communicate. Sometimes, especially during sad times, you do not need to say anything. Just being there shows you care. At other times, silence gives you or the resident time to think, organize thoughts, or choose words. Silence is useful when making difficult decisions. It is also useful when the resident is upset and needs time to regain control. Silence on your part shows caring and respect for the resident's situation and feelings.

Sometimes pauses or long silences are uncomfortable. Do not think you need to talk when the resident is silent. The resident may need silence. Dealing with silence gets easier as you gain experience in you role.

Barriers to Effective Communication
Communication may fail for many reasons. You and the resident must use and understand the same language. Otherwise, messages sent will not be accurately interpreted. Communication barriers prevent sending and receiving messages effectively. Communication fails. The following are communication barriers:
- *Using unfamiliar language.* You and the resident must use and understand the same language. If not, messages are not accurately interpreted.
- *Changing the subject.* Either you or the resident changes the subject when the topic is uncomfortable. Avoid changing the subject whenever possible.
- *Giving your opinion.* This tells the resident that you are judging his or her values, behavior, or feelings. Let others express their feelings and concerns without adding your opinion, making a judgment, or jumping to conclusions.
- *Talking a lot when others are silent.* Excessive talking is usually the result of nervousness and discomfort with silence. Silences have meaning. They convey acceptance, rejection, fear, or the need for quiet and time to think.
- *Failing to listen.* Communication is blocked if you fail to listen with interest and sincerity. Do not pretend to listen. This causes inappropriate responses and conveys a lack of interest and caring. You can miss important complaints of pain, discomfort, or other abnormal sensations that must be reported to the nurse.
- *Giving pat answers.* "Don't worry," "Everything will be okay," and "Your doctor knows best" block communication. These make residents feel that you are ridiculing their concerns, feelings, and fears. They think you do not care about what they think or feel.
- *Illness.* Some central nervous system disorders affect speech and body movements. The person may be unable to speak. Disorders that affect movement interfere with nonverbal communication.

THE ANGRY PERSON
Anger is a common emotion seen in residents and families. The many causes of anger include fear, pain, and death and dying. Loss of body function and losing control of one's health and life also cause anger. So do long waits for treatment or to see the doctor.

Anger also is a symptom of diseases that affect thinking and behavior. Residents who abuse alcohol and drugs are likely to show anger. Residents with dementia may also strike out in anger. Some people are generally angry. Few things please or make them happy.

Anger is communicated verbally and nonverbally. Verbal outbursts, shouting, raised voices, and rapid speech are common. The resident tells you what to do or threatens you or the center. Some people are silent when angry. Others are uncooperative and may refuse to answer questions. Nonverbal signs of anger include rapid movements, pacing, clenched fists, and a reddened face. Glaring and getting close to you when speaking are other signs. Violent behaviors can occur.

Good communication is important to prevent and deal with anger. Follow the guidelines in Box 5-1.

BOX 5-1 DEALING WITH THE ANGRY PERSON

- Recognize frustrating and frightening situations. Put yourself in the person's situation. How would you feel? How would you want to be treated?
- Treat the person with dignity and respect.
- Answer the person's questions clearly and thoroughly. Ask the nurse to answer questions you cannot answer.
- Keep the person informed. Tell the person what you are going to do and when.
- Do not keep the person waiting for long periods. Answer call bells promptly. If you tell the person that you will do something for him or her, do it promptly.
- Explain the reason for long waits. Ask if there is something you can get or do for the person to increase his or her comfort.
- Stay calm and professional if the person directs anger and hostility toward you. Often the person is not angry at you, but at another person or situation.
- Do not argue with the person.
- Listen and use silence. The person may feel better if able to express angry feelings.
- Protect yourself from violent behaviors (see Chapter 8).
- Report the person's behavior to the nurse. Discuss how you should deal with the person.

CARING ABOUT CULTURE

Family Roles in Sick Care

In Vietnam, all family members are involved in the person's care. A similar practice is common in Russia and in China. Family members bathe, feed, and comfort the person. However, women in Mexico cannot give care at home if it involves touching the genitals of adult men.

Remember, individuals may not follow every belief and practice of their culture and religion. Each person is unique. Do not judge residents by your own standards.

Modified from Geissler EM: *Pocket guide to cultural assessment*, ed 2, St Louis, 1998, Mosby.

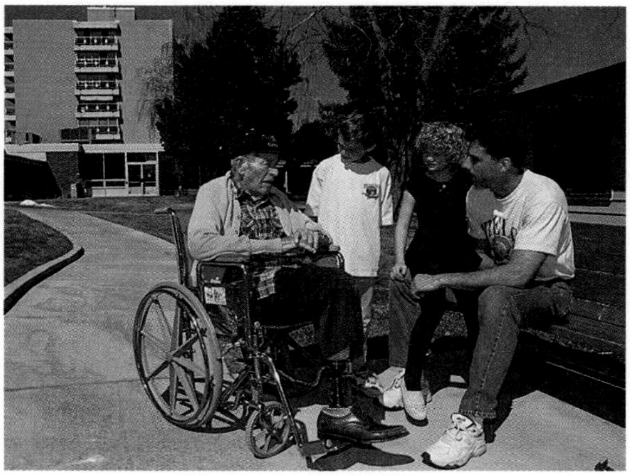

Fig. 5-9 A resident visits with his family.

THE RESIDENT'S FAMILY AND FRIENDS

Family and friends can help meet the resident's needs for safety and security, love and belonging, and esteem. They can offer support and comfort and lessen feelings of loneliness. Some also help with the resident's care. *(See Caring About Culture.)* This helps both the family and the resident. The family knows they are doing something to help the resident, and the resident's physical and emotional needs are met. The presence or absence of significant family members or friends affects the resident's quality of life.

The resident has the right to visit with family and friends in private and without unnecessary interruptions (Fig. 5-9). Sometimes care must be given while visitors are present. Remember the resident's right to privacy. The resident's body should not be exposed in the presence of visitors. Politely ask visitors to leave the room, and show them a comfortable place to wait. Promptly tell visitors when they can return. If a spouse or close family member wants to help you and the resident gives consent, allow that person to stay.

Family and visitors need to be treated with courtesy and respect. They may have concerns about the resident's condition and care. They need the support and understanding from the health care team. However, you should not discuss the resident's condition with them. Refer any questions to the nurse responsible for the resident's care.

Visitors often have questions about visiting rules. The number of visitors allowed and the visiting hours vary among centers. Often they depend on the resident's condition. Dying residents usually can have family members present constantly. This always is true in hospice units. You need to know your center's visiting policies and the special considerations allowed for an individual resident.

Sometimes a visitor can upset or tire a resident. If the resident becomes upset or is becoming tired from a visit, report your observations to the nurse. The nurse can then speak with the visitor about the resident's needs.

Quality of Life

The resident is the most important person in the nursing center. Each resident is an important, special, and valuable human being. The entire health care team focuses on helping each resident meet his or her physical, psychological, social, and spiritual needs. You must know and respect the whole person to provide effective, quality care.

You will care for persons of different cultures and religions. Learn as much as you can about a resident's religious and cultural beliefs and health care practices. This will help you understand the resident and give better care.

Being ill and disabled has physical, psychological, and social effects on people. Normal daily tasks and activities that bring personal satisfaction and worth and contact with others may be difficult or impossible. People often feel angry, frustrated, and useless. Their quality of life is changed. Many fear increasing loss of function and dependence on others. You can help by treating each person with dignity and respect. You work with the entire health care team to help each resident to reach or maintain his or her optimal level of functioning. Always focus on the person's abilities, not on disabilities.

Family and visitors are important individuals to the resident. They can offer support and comfort. The presence or absence of significant family members or friends affects the resident's quality of life. Always treat them with respect.

REVIEW QUESTIONS

Circle the BEST answer.

1 Don Jacobs had surgery to repair a broken hip. You must be concerned
- A Only with what is on his care plan
- B With his physical, safety and security, and esteem needs
- C With him as a physical, psychological, social, and spiritual person
- D Only with his cultural and spiritual needs

2 Of the following basic needs, which is the *most* essential?
- A Self-actualization
- B Esteem needs
- C Love and belonging
- D Safety and security

3 You are assigned to four residents. Based on Maslow's theory of basic needs, which person's needs must be met *first?*
- A Mr. Gray, who wants another blanket
- B Miss Davis, who asks you to read her mail
- C Ms. Miller, who asks for more water
- D Mr. Rich, who is crying

4 Mary Rogers is afraid of the nursing center. She said, "I don't know what they are going to do to me." What basic need is *not* being met?
- A Physical needs
- B Safety and security needs
- C Love and belonging needs
- D Esteem needs

5 Mr. Roth wants a little vegetable garden behind the center's garage. What need does this relate to?
- A Self-actualization
- B Esteem needs
- C Love and belonging
- D Safety and security

6 Which is *false?*
- A A person's cultural background probably influences health and illness practices.
- B Dietary practices may be influenced by both religion and culture.
- C A person's religious and cultural practices are not allowed in the nursing center.
- D A person may not follow all the beliefs and practices of his or her culture or religion.

7 Which is *false?*
- A Verbal communication involves the written or spoken word.
- B Verbal communication is the truest reflection of a person's feelings.
- C Messages are sent by facial expressions, gestures, posture, body movements, appearance, and eye contact.
- D Touch means different things to different people.

8 To communicate with Scott Smith you should
- A Use medical words and phrases
- B Change the subject often to show you care about his interests and concerns
- C Give your opinion when he shares fears and concerns
- D Be quiet when he is silent

9 You and Scott Smith are talking. Which might mean that you are not listening?
- A You sit facing him.
- B You have good eye contact with him.
- C You sit with your arms crossed.
- D You ask him questions.

10 You and Mary Rogers are talking about her rehabilitation. Which is a direct question?
- A "Do you feel better now?"
- B "Tell me what your plans are for home."
- C "What will you do when you get home?"
- D "You said that your husband will be off work for awhile."

11 Mary Rogers wants to take a shower. You say, "You would like a shower." This is
- A Focusing
- B Clarifying
- C Paraphrasing
- D An open-ended question

12 Focusing is a useful communication tool when
- A A person is rambling
- B You want to make sure you understand the message
- C You want the person to share thoughts and feelings
- D You need certain information

Continued

13 Which is *not* a barrier to communication?
A Using silence
B Giving your opinions
C Changing the subject
D Illness

14 A resident is angry. Which is *false?*
A Listening and use of silence are important.
B You can tell the resident to calm down, and everything will be fine.
C You should report the resident's behavior to the nurse.
D You should treat the resident with dignity and respect.

Answers to these questions are on p. 696.

6 Body Structure and Function

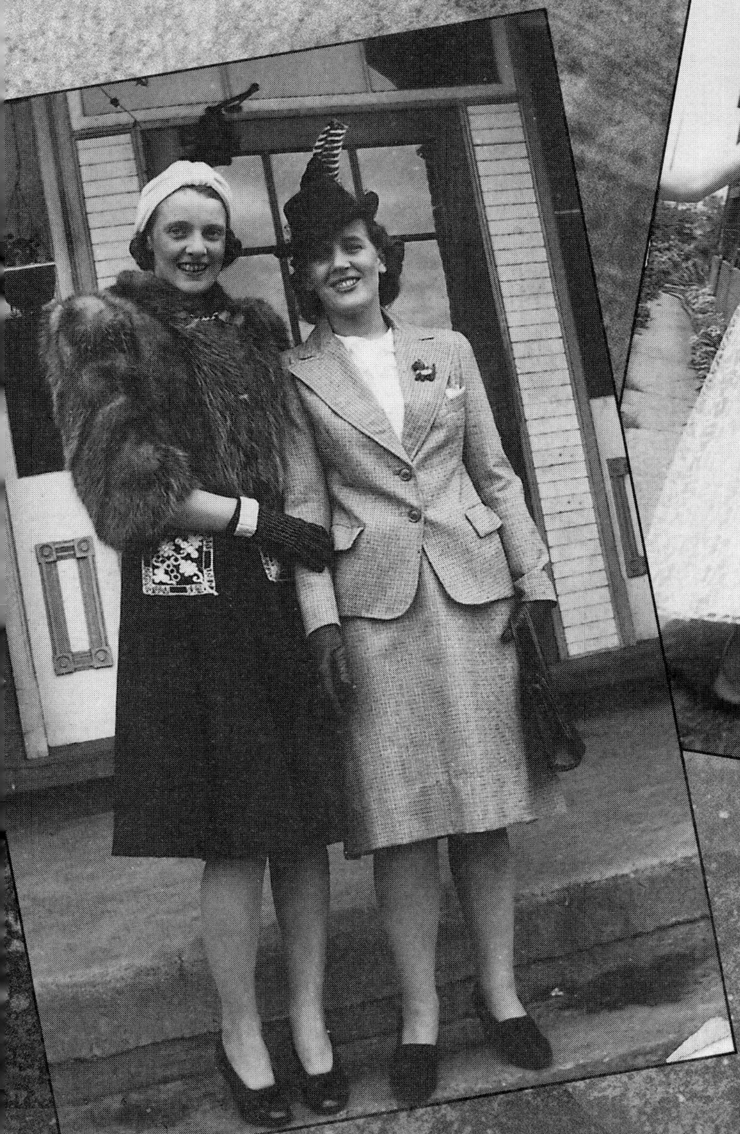

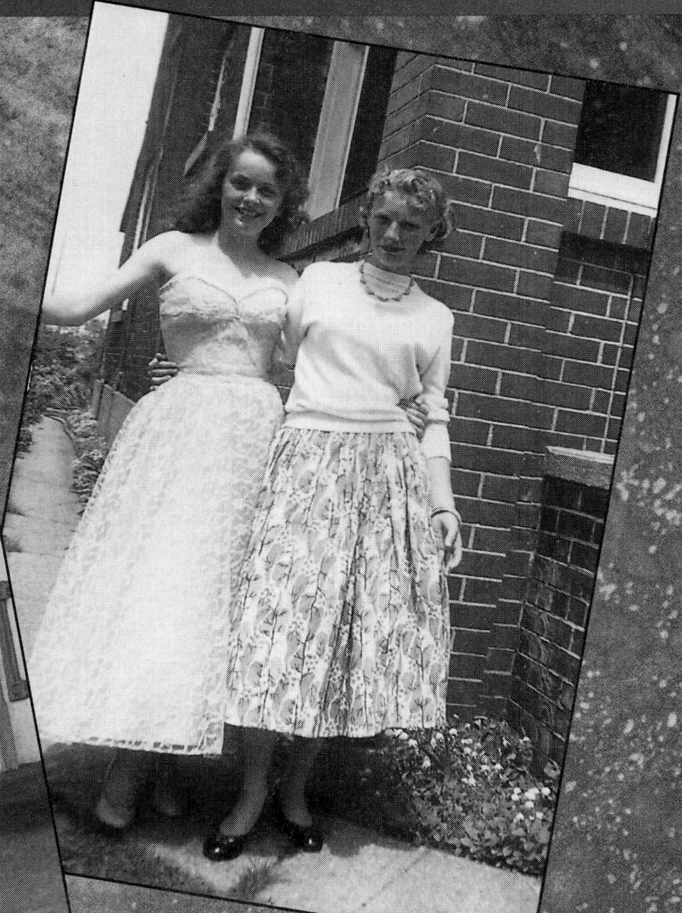

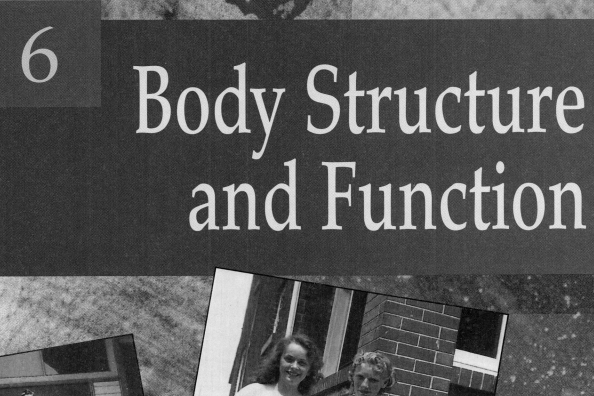

WHAT YOU WILL LEARN

- The definition of the key terms listed in this chapter
- The basic structures of the cell and how cells divide
- The four types of tissue
- The structures of each body system
- The functions of each body system

KEY TERMS

artery A blood vessel that carries blood away from the heart

capillary A tiny blood vessel; food, oxygen, and other substances pass from the capillaries to the cells

cell The basic unit of body structure

digestion The process of physically and chemically breaking down food so that it can be absorbed for use by the cells

hemoglobin The substance in red blood cells that carries oxygen and gives blood its color

hormone A chemical substance secreted by the glands into the bloodstream

immunity Protection against a disease or infection; the person will not get or be affected by the disease

menstruation The process in which the lining of the uterus breaks up and is discharged from the body through the vagina

metabolism The burning of food for heat and energy by the cells

organ Groups of tissues with the same function

peristalsis Involuntary muscle contractions in the digestive system that move food through the alimentary canal

system Organs that work together to perform special functions

tissue A group of cells with similar functions

vein A blood vessel that carries blood back to the heart

NOTE: Students are responsible for only those terms mentioned in the text. Additional terms used in labeling figures throughout this chapter are for illustrative purposes only.

You will help residents meet their basic needs. Their bodies cannot work at peak efficiency because of illness, disease, injury, or advanced age. As a result, residents often need medical and nursing care. You will be directed to provide care and perform procedures to promote physical and emotional comfort, physical and spiritual healing, and a return to the highest possible level of functioning. A basic knowledge of the body's normal structure and function will help you understand certain signs, symptoms, and behaviors, reasons for care, and purposes of procedures. This knowledge should result in safer, more efficient resident care. The changes in body structure and function that occur with aging are discussed in Chapter 7.

CELLS, TISSUES, AND ORGANS

The basic unit of body structure is the **cell**. Each cell has the same basic structure. However, the function, size, and shape of cells may be different. Cells are so small that a microscope is needed to see them. Cells need food, water, and oxygen to live and perform their functions.

The cell and its basic structures are shown in Figure 6-1. The *cell membrane* is the outer covering that encloses the cell and helps it hold its shape. The *nucleus* is the control center of the cell; it directs the cell's activities. The nucleus is in the center of the cell. The *cytoplasm* is the portion of the cell that surrounds

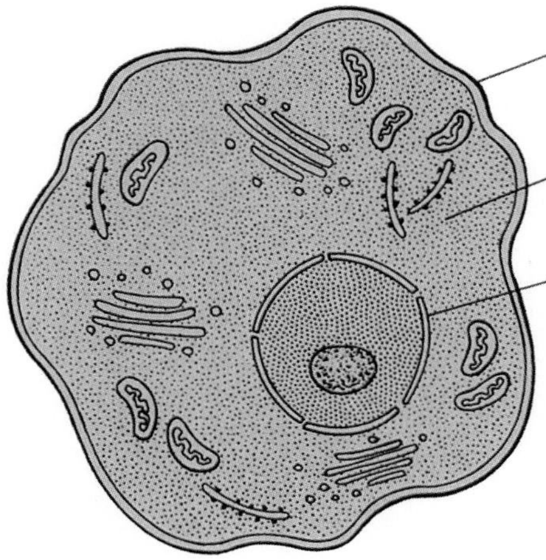

Fig. 6-1 Parts of a cell.

the nucleus. Cytoplasm contains many smaller structures that perform cell functions. The *protoplasm,* which means "living substance," refers to all of the structures, substances, and water within the cell. Protoplasm is a semiliquid substance much like egg white.

Chromosomes are threadlike structures within the nucleus. Each cell has 46 chromosomes. Chromosomes contain *genes.* Genes control the physical and chemical traits inherited by children from their parents. Inherited traits include height, eye color, and skin color.

Besides controlling cell activities, the nucleus is responsible for cell reproduction. Cells reproduce by dividing in half. The process of cell division is called *mitosis.* Cell division is needed for growth and repair of body tissues. During mitosis, the 46 chromosomes arrange themselves in 23 pairs. As the cell divides, the 23 pairs of chromosomes are pulled in half. The two new cells are identical, and each contains 46 chromosomes (Fig. 6-2).

The cells are the body's building blocks. Groups of cells with similar functions combine to form **tissues.** The body has four basic types of tissue:

- *Epithelial tissue* covers internal and external body surfaces. Tissue that lines the nose, mouth, respiratory tract, stomach, and intestines is epithelial tissue. So are the skin, hair, nails, and glands.
- *Connective tissue* anchors, connects, and supports other body tissues. Connective tissue is found in every part of the body. Bones, tendons, ligaments, and cartilage are connective tissue. Blood is a form of connective tissue.
- *Muscle tissue* allows the body to move by stretching and contracting. There are three types of muscle tissue (p. 98).
- *Nerve tissue* receives and carries impulses to the brain and back to body parts.

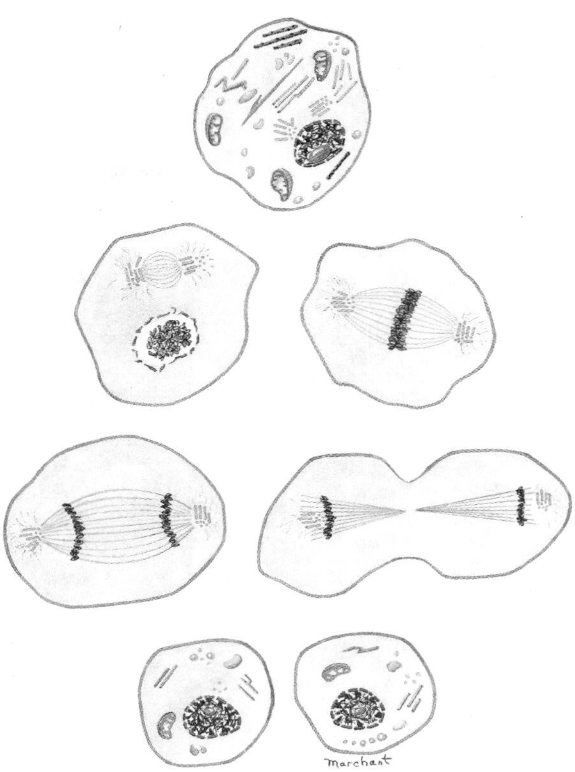

Fig. 6-2 Cell division.

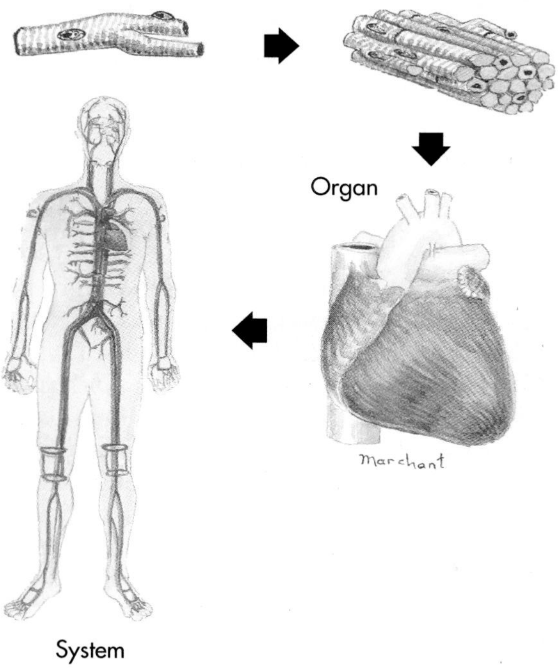

Fig. 6-3 Organization of the body.

Groups of tissues form **organs.** An organ performs one or more functions. Examples of organs are the heart, brain, liver, lungs, and kidneys. **Systems** are formed by organs that work together to perform special functions (Fig. 6-3).

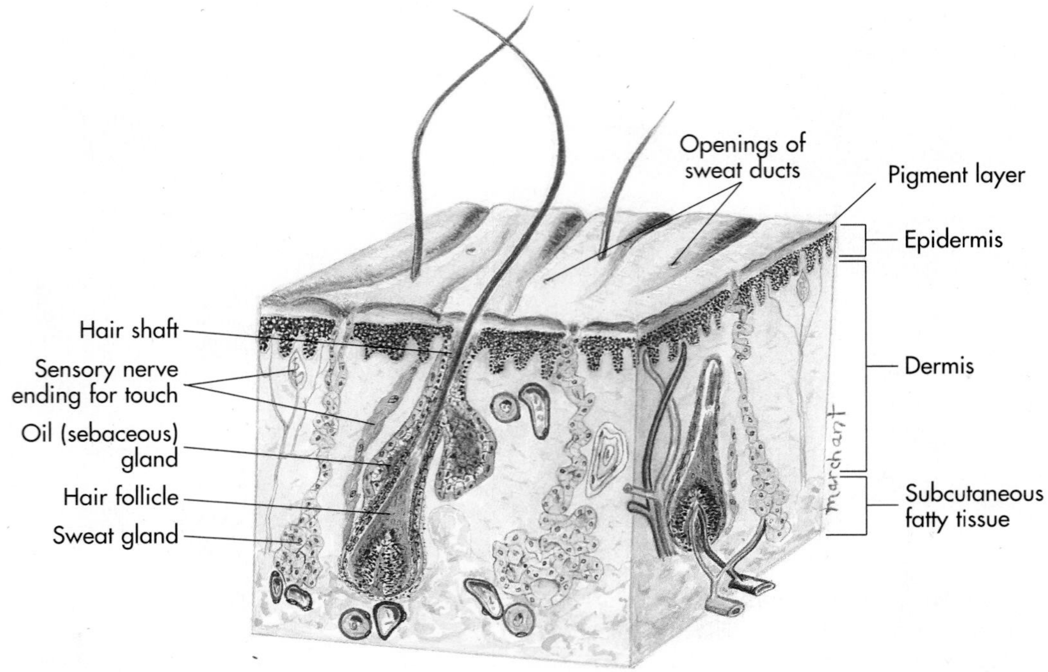

Fig. 6-4 Layers of the skin.

THE INTEGUMENTARY SYSTEM

The *integumentary system,* or skin, is the largest system of the body. *Integument* means covering. The skin is the body's natural covering. Skin is made up of epithelial, connective, and nerve tissue, as well as oil and sweat glands. There are two skin layers: the epidermis and the dermis (Fig. 6-4). The *epidermis* is the outer layer; it contains living cells and dead cells. The dead cells were once deeper in the epidermis and were pushed upward as other cells divided. Dead cells constantly flake off and are replaced by living cells. Living cells also die and flake off. Living cells of the epidermis contain *pigment.* Pigment gives skin its color. The epidermis has no blood vessels and few nerve endings. The *dermis* is the inner layer of the skin and is made up of connective tissue. Blood vessels, nerves, sweat glands, oil glands, and hair roots are found in the dermis.

Oil glands, sweat glands, hair, and *nails* are skin appendages. The entire body, except the palms of the hands and soles of the feet, is covered with hair. Hair in the nose, eyes, and ears protects these organs from dust, insects, and other foreign objects. Nails protect the tips of fingers and toes. Nails help fingers pick up and handle small objects. Sweat glands help the body regulate temperature. Sweat consists of water, salt, and a small amount of wastes. Sweat is secreted through pores in the skin. The body is cooled as sweat evaporates. Oil glands lie near hair shafts. They secrete an oily substance into the space near the hair shaft. Oil travels to the skin surface, helping to keep the hair and skin soft and shiny.

The skin has many important functions. It is the protective covering of the body. Bacteria and other substances are prevented from entering the body. The skin prevents excessive amounts of water from leaving the body and protects organs from injury. Nerve endings in the skin sense both pleasant and unpleasant stimulation. There are nerve endings over the entire body. The body is protected because cold, pain, touch, and pressure are sensed. The skin helps regulate body temperature. Blood vessels dilate (widen) when temperature outside the body is high. More blood is brought to the body surface for cooling during evaporation. When blood vessels constrict (narrow), the body retains heat because less blood reaches the skin.

THE MUSCULOSKELETAL SYSTEM

The musculoskeletal system provides the framework for the body and allows the body to move. This system also protects and gives the body shape. Besides bones and muscles, the system has ligaments, tendons, and cartilage.

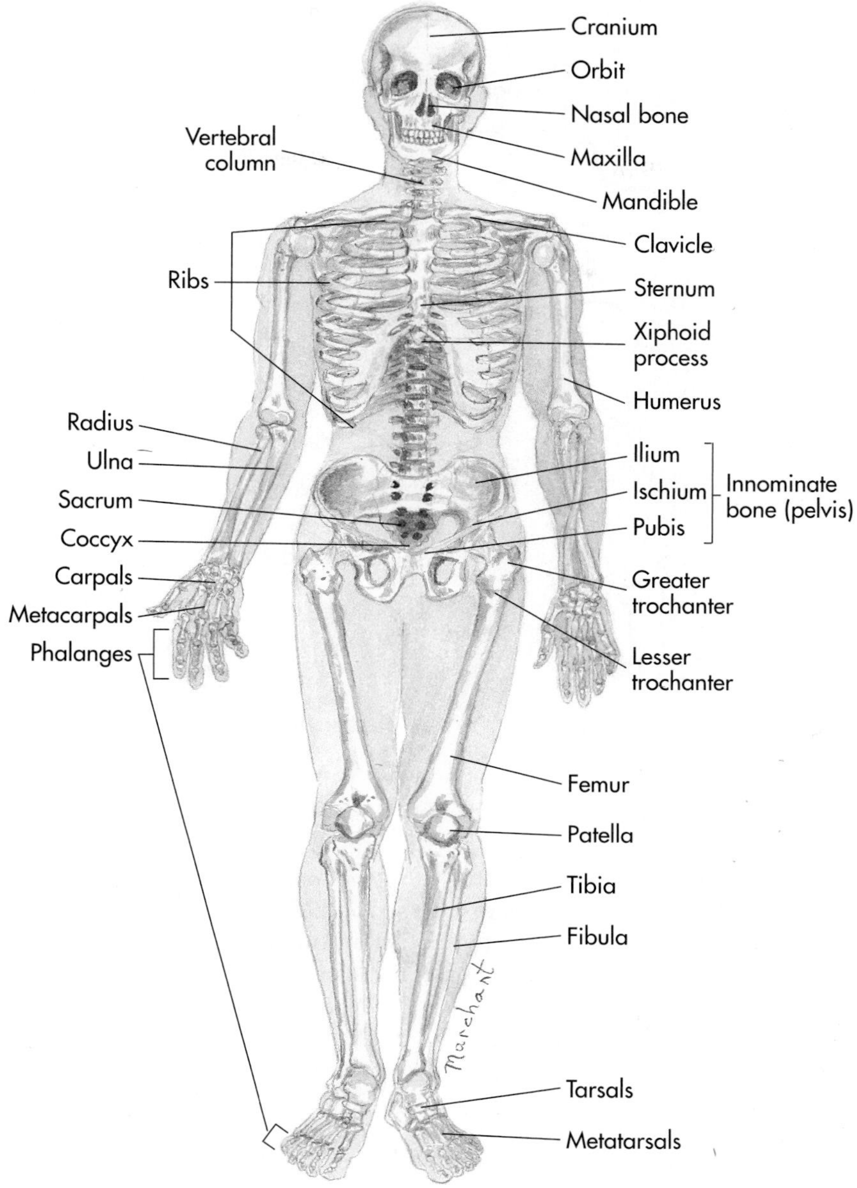

Fig. 6-5 Bones of the body.

Bones

The human body has 206 bones (Fig. 6-5). There are four types of bones:

- *Long bones* bear the weight of the body. Leg bones are long bones.
- *Short bones* allow skill and ease in movement. Bones in the wrists, fingers, ankles, and toes are short bones.
- *Flat bones* protect the organs. Such bones include the ribs, skull, pelvic bones, and shoulder blades.
- *Irregular bones* are the vertebrae in the spinal column. They allow various degrees of movement and flexibility.

Bones are hard, rigid structures that are made up of living cells. They are covered by a membrane called *periosteum.* Periosteum contains blood vessels that supply bone cells with oxygen and food. Inside the hollow centers of the bones is a substance called *bone marrow.* Blood cells are manufactured in the bone marrow.

Joints

A *joint* is the point at which two or more bones meet. Joints allow movement (see Chapter 19). *Cartilage* is the connective tissue at the end of long bones. Cartilage cushions the joint so that bone ends do not rub together. The *synovial membrane* lines the joints. The

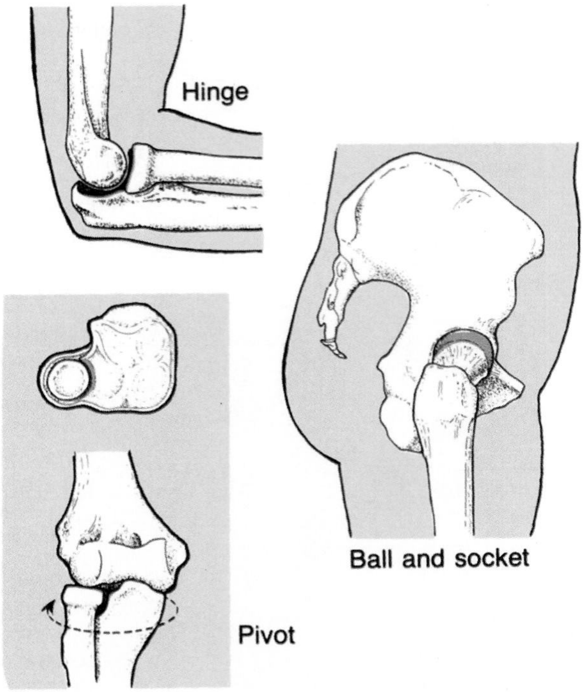

Fig. 6-6 Types of joints. *(Modified from Austrin M, Austrin H:* Learning medical terminology: a worktext, *ed 8, St Louis, 1995, Mosby.)*

membrane secretes *synovial fluid.* Synovial fluid acts as a lubricant so the joint can move smoothly. Bones are held together at the joint by strong bands of connective tissue called *ligaments.*

There are three types of joints (Fig. 6-6):

- *Ball-and-socket joint* allows movement in all directions. It is made up of the rounded end of one bone and the hollow end of another bone. The rounded end of one fits into the hollow end of the other. The joints of the hips and shoulders are ball-and-socket joints.
- *Hinge joint* allows movement in one direction. The elbow is a hinge joint.
- *Pivot joint* allows turning from side to side. The skull is connected to the spine by a pivot joint.

Muscles

There are more than 500 muscles in the human body (Figs. 6-7 and 6-8). Some are voluntary, and others are involuntary. *Voluntary muscles* can be consciously controlled. Muscles attached to bones *(skeletal muscles)* are voluntary. Arm muscles do not work unless you move your arm; likewise for leg muscles. Skeletal muscles are *striated;* that is, they look striped or streaked. *Involuntary muscles* work automatically and cannot be consciously controlled. Involuntary muscles control the action of the stomach, intestines, blood vessels, and other body organs. Involuntary muscles are also called *smooth muscles.* They look smooth, not streaked or striped. *Cardiac muscle* is in the heart. Although it is an involuntary muscle, it appears striated like skeletal muscle.

Muscles perform three important body functions:

- Movement of body parts
- Maintenance of posture
- Production of body heat

Strong, tough connective tissues called *tendons* connect muscles to bones. When muscles contract (shorten), tendons at each end of the muscle cause the bone to move. The body has many tendons; the Achilles tendon is shown in Figure 6-8. Some muscles constantly contract to maintain the body's posture. When muscles contract, they burn food for energy, resulting in the production of heat. The greater the muscular activity, the greater the amount of heat produced in the body. Shivering is a way the body produces heat when exposed to cold. The shivering sensation is from rapid, general muscle contractions.

THE NERVOUS SYSTEM

The nervous system controls, directs, and coordinates body functions. The two main divisions of the nervous system are the *central nervous system (CNS)* and the *peripheral nervous system (PNS).* The central nervous

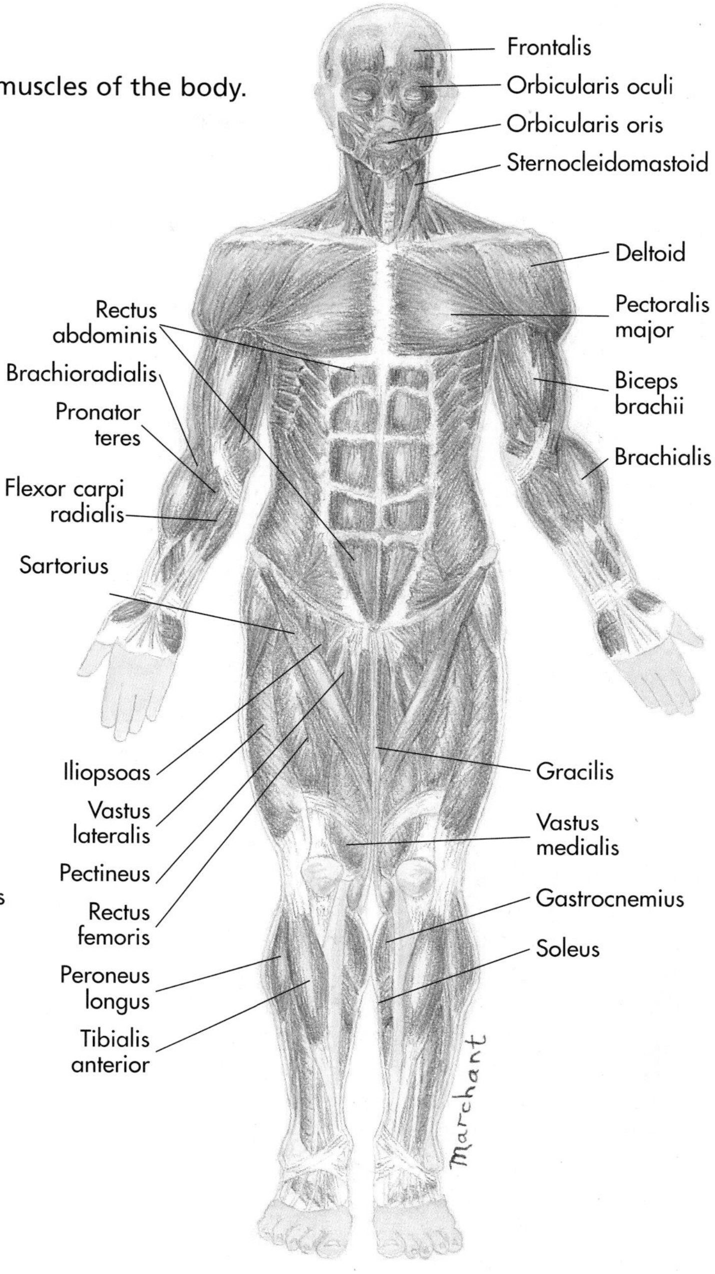

Fig. 6-7 Anterior view of the muscles of the body.

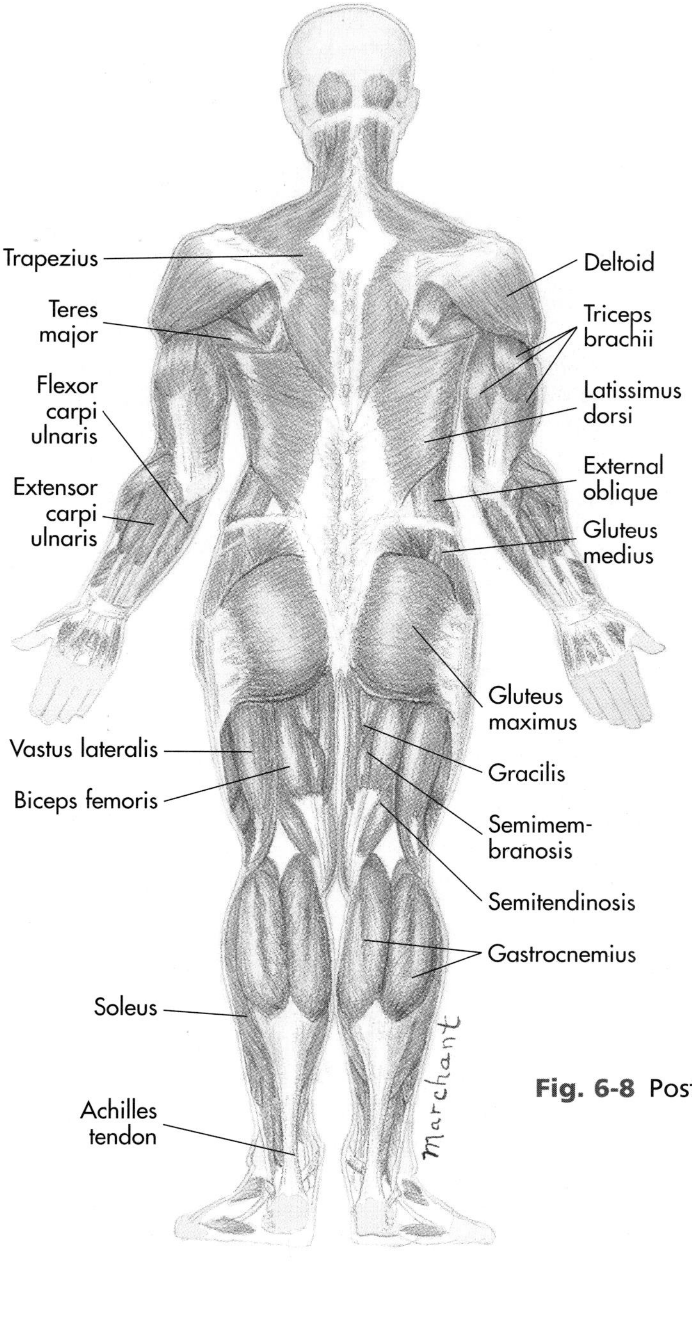

Fig. 6-8 Posterior view of the muscles of the body.

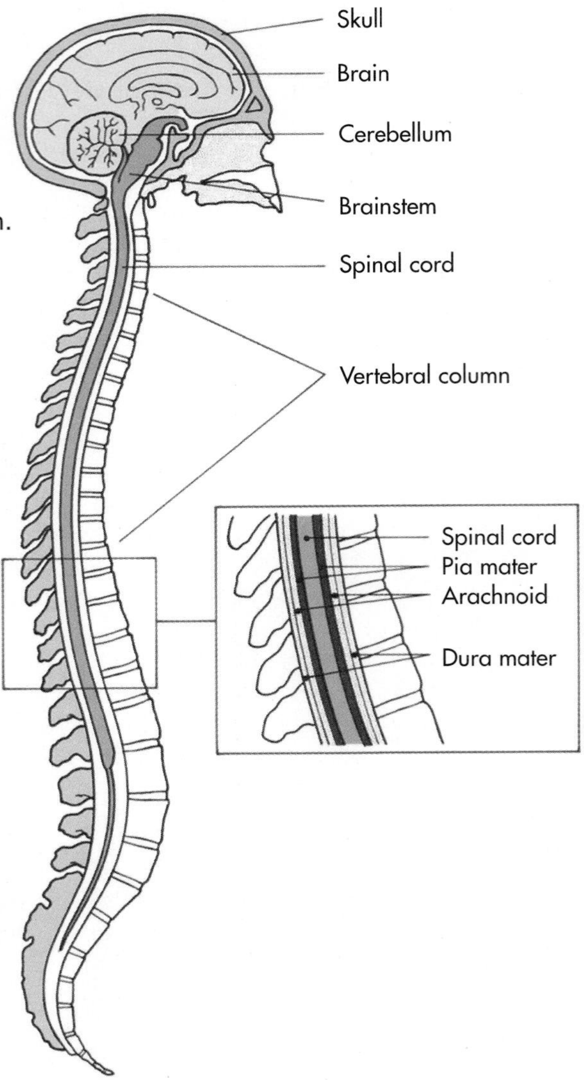

Fig. 6-9 Central nervous system.

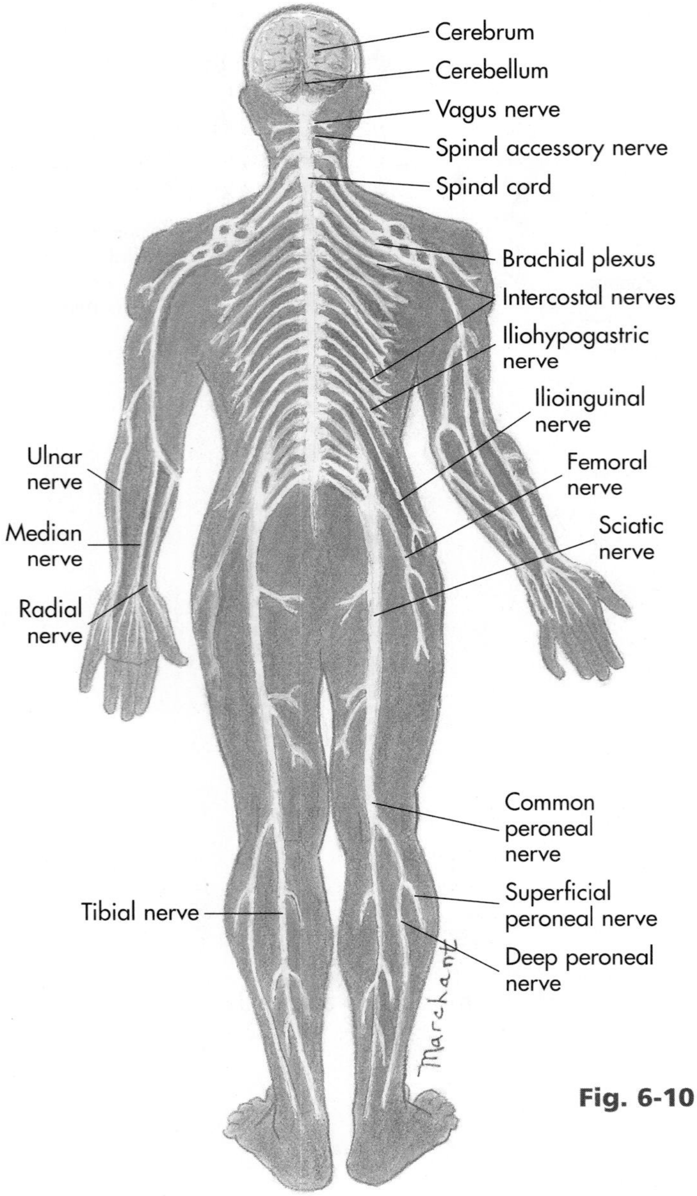

Fig. 6-10 Peripheral nervous system.

system consists of the *brain and spinal cord* (Fig. 6-9). The peripheral nervous system involves the nerves throughout the body (Fig. 6-10). Nerves carry messages or impulses to and from the brain. Nerves are connected to the spinal cord. The nerve cell, called a *neuron,* is the basic unit of the nervous system. Threadlike projections from the cytoplasm of the neuron are called nerve fibers. The nerve fibers that bring impulses to the cell are called *dendrites.* The fibers that carry impulses away from the neurons are called *axons.* A neuron usually has only one axon. Dendrites may be short or as long as 3 feet.

Receptors, or *end-organs,* are found inside and outside of the body. Each receptor is attached to a neuron by a dendrite. A stimulus is received by the receptor and travels to the brain. Such stimuli include heat, cold, touch, smell, hearing, vision, balance, hunger, and thirst. If the body or body part must respond to the stimulus, the brain sends an impulse through the neurons to the proper muscles and glands.

Nerves are easily damaged and take a long time to heal. Some nerve fibers have a protective covering called a *myelin sheath.* The myelin sheath also insulates the nerve fiber. Nerve fibers covered with myelin can conduct impulses faster than those fibers without the protective covering.

The Central Nervous System

The central nervous system consists of the brain and spinal cord. The brain is covered by the skull. The three main parts of the brain are the *cerebrum,* the *cerebellum,* and the *brainstem* (Fig. 6-11).

The cerebrum is the largest part of the brain. It is the center of thought and intelligence. The cerebrum is divided into two halves called the right and left *hemispheres.* The right hemisphere controls movement and activities on the body's left side. The left hemisphere controls the right side. The outside of the cerebrum is called the *cerebral cortex.* The cerebral cortex controls the highest functions of the brain. These include reasoning, memory, consciousness, speech, voluntary muscle movement, vision, hearing, sensation, and other activities.

The cerebellum regulates and coordinates body movements. The smooth movements of voluntary muscles and balance are possible because of control by the cerebellum. Injury to the cerebellum results in jerky movements, loss of coordination, and muscle weakness.

The brainstem connects the cerebrum to the spinal cord. Important structures within the brainstem are the *midbrain, pons,* and *medulla.* The midbrain and pons relay messages between the medulla and the cerebrum.

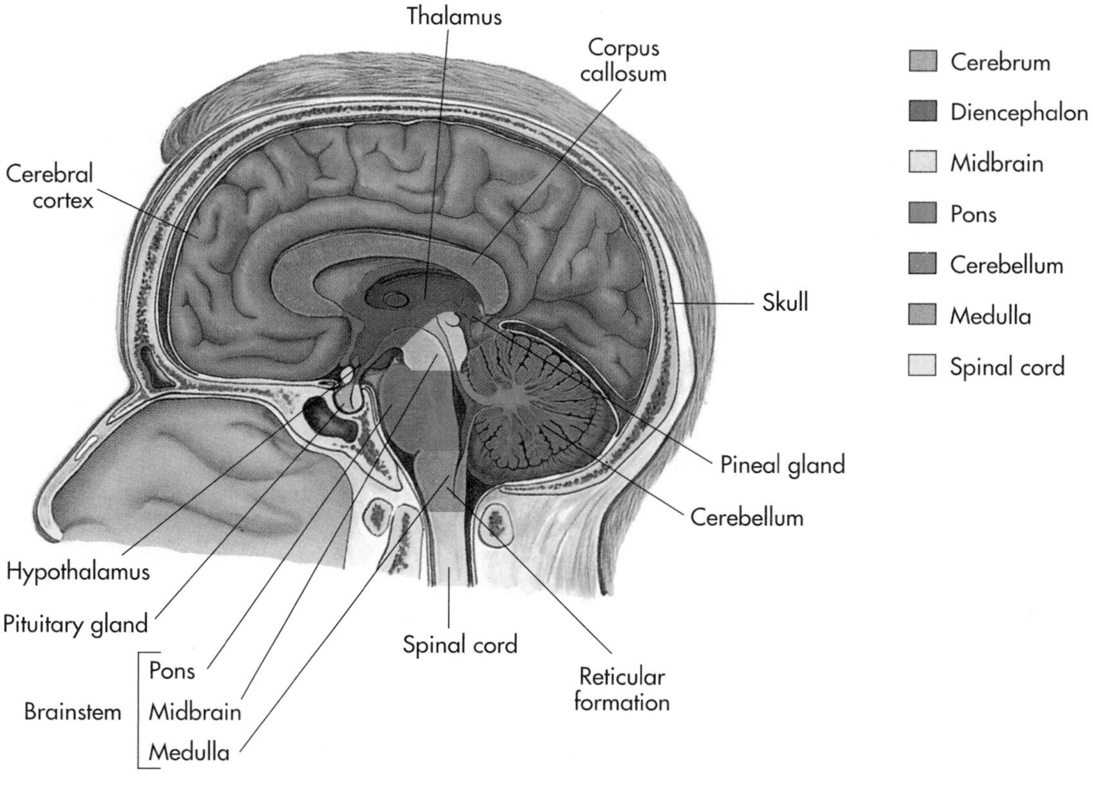

Fig. 6-11 The brain. *(From Thibodeau GA, Patton KT:* The human body in health & disease, *ed 2, St Louis, 1997, Mosby.)*

The medulla is directly below the pons. Heart rate, breathing, blood vessel size, swallowing, coughing, and vomiting are some functions controlled by the medulla. The brain is connected to the spinal cord at the lower end of the medulla.

The spinal cord lies within the spinal column. The cord is about 18 inches long. Pathways that conduct messages to and from the brain are contained within the cord.

The brain and spinal cord are covered and protected by three layers of connective tissue called *meninges.* The outer layer lies next to the skull. It is a tough covering called the *dura mater.* The middle layer is called the *arachnoid.* The inner layer is the *pia mater.* The space between the middle and inner layers is the *arachnoid space.* The space is filled with fluid called *cerebrospinal fluid.* It circulates around the brain and spinal cord. Cerebrospinal fluid protects the central nervous system. It cushions shocks that could easily injure structures of the brain and spinal cord.

The Peripheral Nervous System

The peripheral nervous system has 12 pairs of *cranial nerves* and 31 pairs of *spinal nerves.* Cranial nerves conduct impulses between the brain and the head, neck, chest, and abdomen. They conduct impulses for smell, vision, hearing, pain, touch, temperature, pressure, and voluntary and involuntary muscle control. Spinal nerves carry impulses from the skin, extremities, and the internal body structures not supplied by cranial nerves.

Some peripheral nerves with special functions form the *autonomic nervous system.* This system controls involuntary muscles and certain body functions. The functions include the heartbeat, blood pressure, intestinal contractions, and glandular secretions. These functions occur automatically. The autonomic nervous system is divided into the *sympathetic nervous system* and the *parasympathetic nervous system.* These divisions balance one another. The sympathetic nervous system tends to speed up functions. The parasympathetic nervous system slows them down. When you are angry, frightened, excited, or exercising, the sympathetic nervous system is stimulated. The parasympathetic system is activated when you relax or when the sympathetic system is under stimulation for too long.

The Sense Organs

The five major senses are sight, hearing, taste, smell, and touch. Receptors for taste are in the tongue and are called *taste buds.* Receptors for smell are in the nose. Touch receptors are found in the dermis, especially in the toes and fingertips.

The eye. Receptors for vision are in the eyes. The eye is a delicate organ that can be easily injured. Bones of the skull, eyelids and eyelashes, and tears protect the eyes from injury. Eye structures are shown in Figure 6-12. The eye has three layers:

- The *sclera,* the white of the eye, is the outer layer. It is made of tough connective tissue.
- The *choroid* is the second layer. Blood vessels, the *ciliary muscle,* and the *iris* make up the choroid. The iris gives the eye its color. The opening in the middle of the iris is the *pupil.* Pupil size varies with the amount of light entering the eye. The pupil constricts (narrows) in bright light and dilates (widens) in dim or dark places.
- The *retina* is the inner layer of the eye. Receptors for vision and the nerve fibers of the optic nerve are contained in the retina.

Light enters the eye through the *cornea.* The cornea is the transparent part of the outer layer that lies over the eye. Light rays pass to the *lens,* which lies behind the pupil. The light is then reflected to the retina and carried to the brain by the optic nerve.

The *aqueous chamber* separates the cornea from the lens. The chamber is filled with a fluid called *aqueous humor.* The fluid helps the cornea keep its shape and position. The *vitreous body* is behind the lens. The vitreous body is a gelatin-like substance that supports the retina and maintains the eye's shape.

The ear. The ear is a sense organ that functions in hearing and balance. It is divided into the *external ear, middle ear,* and *inner ear.* Ear structures are shown in Figure 6-13.

The external ear (outer part) is called the *pinna* or *auricle.* Sound waves are guided through the external ear into the *auditory canal.* Glands in the auditory canal secrete a waxy substance called *cerumen.* The auditory canal extends about 1 inch to the *eardrum.* The eardrum *(tympanic membrane)* separates the external ear and middle ear.

The middle ear is a small space that contains the eustachian tube and three small bones called *ossicles.* The eustachian tube connects the middle ear and the throat. Air enters the eustachian tube so that there is equal pressure on both sides of the eardrum. The ossicles amplify sound received from the eardrum and transmit the sound to the inner ear. The three ossicles are:

- The *malleus,* which looks like a hammer
- The *incus,* which resembles an anvil
- The *stapes,* which is shaped like a stirrup

The inner ear consists of the *semicircular canals* and the *cochlea.* The cochlea, which looks like a snail shell, contains fluid. The fluid carries sound waves received from the middle ear to the *auditory nerve.* The auditory nerve then carries the message to the brain.

The three semicircular canals are involved with balance. They sense the head's position and changes in position and send messages to the brain.

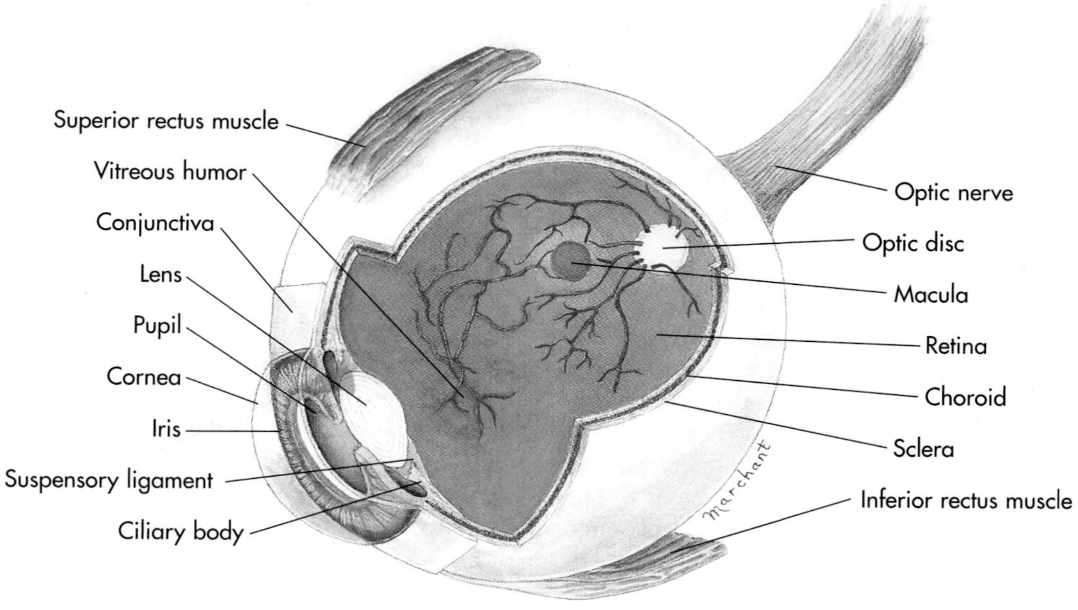

Fig. 6-12 The eye.

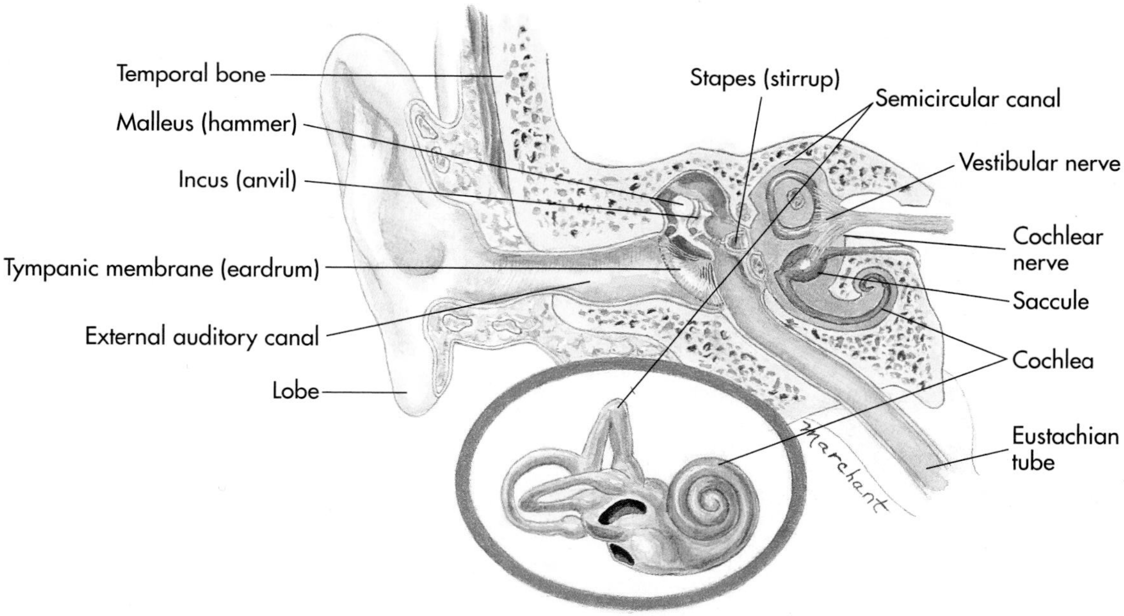

Fig. 6-13 The ear.

THE CIRCULATORY SYSTEM

The circulatory system is made up of the blood, heart, and blood vessels. The heart pumps blood through the blood vessels. The circulatory system has many important functions. Blood carries food, oxygen, and other substances to the cells. Blood also removes waste products from cells. Regulation of body temperature is aided by the blood and blood vessels. Heat from muscle activity is carried by the blood to other body parts. Blood vessels in the skin dilate if the body needs to be cooled. They constrict if heat should be kept in the body. The circulatory system also produces and carries cells that defend the body from disease-causing microorganisms.

The Blood

The blood consists of blood cells and a liquid called *plasma*. Plasma is mostly water. It carries blood cells to other body cells. Plasma also carries other substances needed by cells for proper functioning. Food (proteins, fats, and carbohydrates), hormones (p. 111), chemicals, and waste products are among the many substances carried in the plasma.

Red blood cells are called *erythrocytes*. They give the blood its red color because of a substance in the cell called **hemoglobin.** As red blood cells circulate through the lungs, hemoglobin picks up oxygen. The hemoglobin carries oxygen to the cells. When the blood is bright red, hemoglobin in the red blood cells is saturated (filled) with oxygen. As blood circulates through the body, oxygen is given to the cells. The cells release carbon dioxide (a waste product), which is picked up by the hemoglobin. Red blood cells saturated with carbon dioxide make the blood look dark red.

There are about 25 trillion (25,000,000,000,000) red blood cells in the body. About 4 to 5 million cells are in a cubic millimeter of blood (the size of a tiny drop). These cells live for 3 or 4 months. They are destroyed by the liver and spleen as they wear out. Bone marrow produces new red blood cells. About 1 million new red blood cells are produced every second.

White blood cells, called *leukocytes*, are colorless. They protect the body against infection. There are 5,000 to 10,000 white blood cells in a cubic millimeter of blood. At the first sign of infection, white blood cells rush to the site of the infection and begin to multiply rapidly. The number of white blood cells increases when there is an infection in the body. White blood cells are also produced by the bone marrow. They live about 9 days.

Platelets (thrombocytes) are necessary for the clotting of blood. They also are produced by the bone marrow. There are about 200,000 to 400,000 platelets in a cubic millimeter of blood. A platelet lives about 4 days.

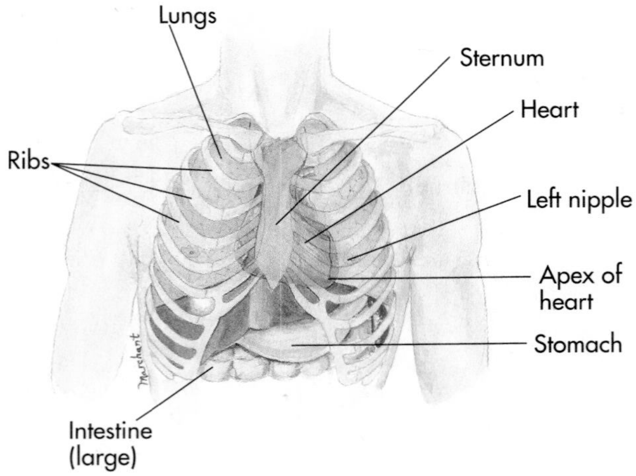

Fig. 6-14 Location of the heart in the chest cavity.

The Heart

The heart is a muscle. It pumps blood through the blood vessels to the tissues and cells. The heart lies in the middle to lower part of the chest cavity toward the left side (Fig. 6-14). The heart is hollow and has three layers (Fig. 6-15):

- The *pericardium* is the outer layer. It is a thin sac covering the heart.
- The *myocardium* is the second layer. This layer is the thick, muscular portion of the heart.
- The *endocardium* is the inner layer. The endocardium is the membrane lining the inner surface of the heart.

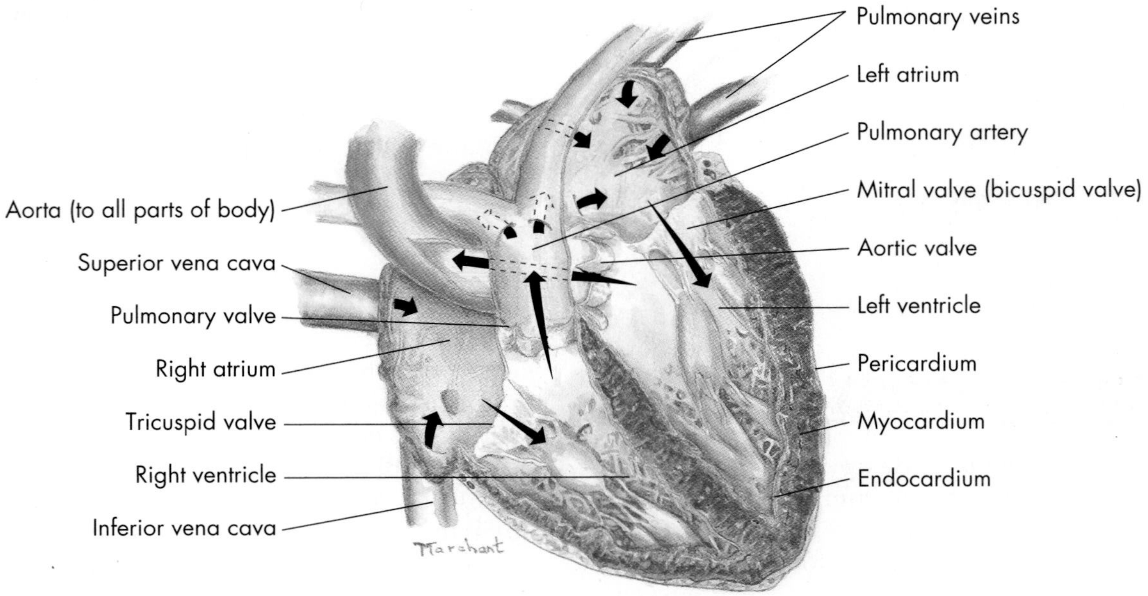

Fig. 6-15 Structures of the heart.

The heart has four chambers (see Fig. 6-15). Upper chambers receive blood and are called the *atria.* The *right atrium* receives blood from body tissues. The *left atrium* receives blood from the lungs. Lower chambers are called *ventricles.* Ventricles pump blood. The *right ventricle* pumps blood to the lungs for oxygen. The *left ventricle* pumps blood to all parts of the body.

Valves are located between the atria and ventricles. The valves allow blood to flow in one direction. They prevent blood from flowing back into the atria from the ventricles. The *tricuspid valve* is between the right atrium and right ventricle. The *mitral valve (bicuspid valve)* is between the left atrium and left ventricle.

There are two phases of heart action. During *diastole,* the resting phase, heart chambers fill with blood. During *systole,* the working phase, the heart contracts. Blood is pumped through the blood vessels when the heart contracts.

The Blood Vessels

Blood flows to body tissues and cells through the blood vessels. There are three groups of blood vessels: arteries, capillaries, and veins. **Arteries** carry blood away from the heart. Arterial blood is rich in oxygen. The *aorta* is the largest artery. The aorta receives blood directly from the left ventricle. The aorta branches into other arteries that carry blood to all parts of the body (Fig. 6-16). These arteries branch into smaller parts within the tissues. The smallest branch of an artery is an *arteriole.* Arterioles connect with blood vessels called **capillaries.** Capillaries are very tiny vessels. Food, oxygen, and other substances pass from capillaries into the cells. Waste products, including carbon dioxide, are picked up from cells by the capillaries. Waste products are carried back to the heart by the veins.

Veins return blood to the heart. They are connected to the capillaries by *venules.* Venules are small veins. Venules begin branching together to form veins. The many branches of veins also branch together as they near the heart to form two main veins (see Fig. 6-16). The two main veins are the *inferior vena cava* and the *superior vena cava.* Both empty into the right atrium. The inferior vena cava carries blood from the legs and trunk. The superior vena cava carries blood from the head and arms. Venous blood is dark red because it contains little oxygen and a lot of carbon dioxide.

Blood flow through the circulatory system is diagramed in Figure 6-15 and can be summarized as follows:

1 Venous blood, poor in oxygen, empties into the right atrium.
2 Blood flows through the tricuspid valve into the right ventricle.
3 The right ventricle pumps blood into the lungs to pick up oxygen.
4 Oxygen-rich blood from the lungs enters the left atrium.
5 Blood from the left atrium passes through the mitral valve into the left ventricle.
6 The left ventricle pumps the blood to the aorta, which branches off to form other arteries.
7 The arterial blood is carried to the tissues by arterioles and to the cells by capillaries.
8 The cells and capillaries exchange oxygen and nutrients for carbon dioxide and waste products.
9 Capillaries connect with venules. Venules carry blood that contains carbon dioxide and waste products.
10 The venules form veins.
11 Veins return blood to the heart.

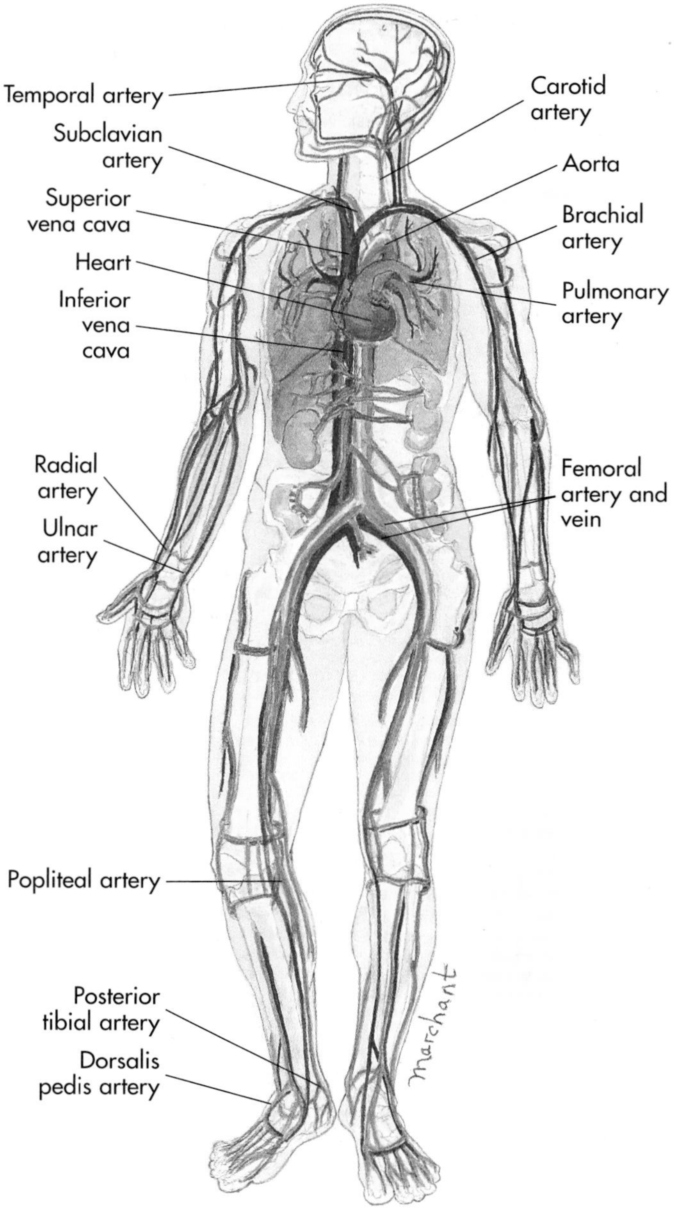

Fig. 6-16 Arterial and venous systems.

THE RESPIRATORY SYSTEM

Oxygen is needed for survival. Every cell needs oxygen. Air contains about 20% oxygen—enough to meet body needs under normal conditions. The respiratory system brings oxygen into the lungs and eliminates carbon dioxide. The process of supplying the cells with oxygen and removing carbon dioxide from them is called *respiration*. Respiration involves *inhalation* (breathing in) and *exhalation* (breathing out). The terms *inspiration* (breathing in) and *expiration* (breathing out) also are used. The respiratory system is shown in Figure 6-17.

Air enters the body through the *nose*. The air then passes into the *pharynx* (throat), a tube-shaped passageway for both air and food. Air passes from the pharynx into the *larynx* (the voice box). A piece of cartilage called the *epiglottis* acts like a lid over the larynx. The epiglottis prevents food from entering the airway during swallowing. During inhalation the epiglottis lifts up to let air pass over the larynx. Air passes from the larynx into the *trachea* (the windpipe). The trachea divides at its lower end into the *right bronchus* and *left bronchus*. Each bronchus enters a lung. Upon entering the lungs, the bronchi further divide several times into smaller branches called *bronchioles*. Eventually the bronchioles subdivide and end in tiny one-celled air sacs called *alveoli*. Alveoli look like small clusters of grapes. They are supplied by capillaries. Oxygen and carbon dioxide are exchanged between the alveoli and capillaries. Blood in the capillaries picks up oxygen from the alveoli. Then the blood is returned to the left side of the heart and pumped to the rest of the body. Alveoli pick up carbon dioxide from the capillaries for exhalation.

The lungs are spongy tissues filled with alveoli, blood vessels, and nerves. Each lung is divided into lobes. The right lung has three lobes; the left lung has two. The lungs are separated from the abdominal cavity by a muscle called the *diaphragm*. Each lung is covered by a two-layered sac called the *pleura*. One layer is attached to the lung and the other to the chest wall. The pleura secretes a very thin fluid that fills the space between the layers. The fluid prevents the layers from rubbing together during inhalation and exhalation. A bony framework consisting of the ribs, sternum, and vertebrae protects the lungs.

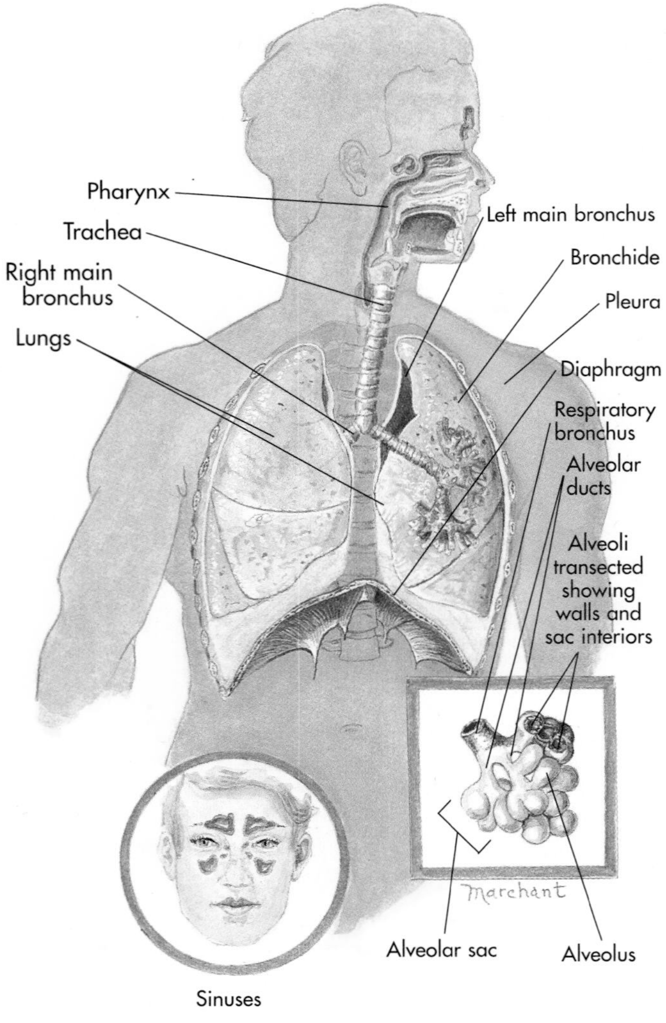

Fig. 6-17 Respiratory system.

THE DIGESTIVE SYSTEM

The digestive system breaks down food physically and chemically so it can be absorbed for use by the cells. This process is called **digestion.** The digestive system is also called the *gastrointestinal system (GI system)*. The system also eliminates solid wastes from the body. The digestive system consists of the *alimentary canal (GI tract)* and the accessory organs of digestion (Fig. 6-18). The alimentary canal is a long tube extending from the mouth to the anus. Its major parts are the mouth, pharynx, esophagus, stomach, small intestine, and large intestine. The accessory organs of digestion are the teeth, tongue, salivary glands, liver, gallbladder, and pancreas.

Digestion begins in the *mouth*. The mouth is also called the *oral cavity*. The oral cavity receives food and prepares it for digestion. Using chewing motions, the *teeth* cut, chop, and grind food into smaller particles for digestion and swallowing. The *tongue* aids in chewing and swallowing. *Taste buds* on the tongue's surface contain nerve endings. Taste buds allow sweet, sour, bitter, and salty tastes to be sensed. *Salivary glands* in the mouth secrete saliva. Saliva moistens food particles for easier swallowing and begins to digest food. During swallowing, the tongue pushes food into the pharynx.

The *pharynx* (throat) is a muscular tube. The act of swallowing is continued as the pharynx contracts. Con-

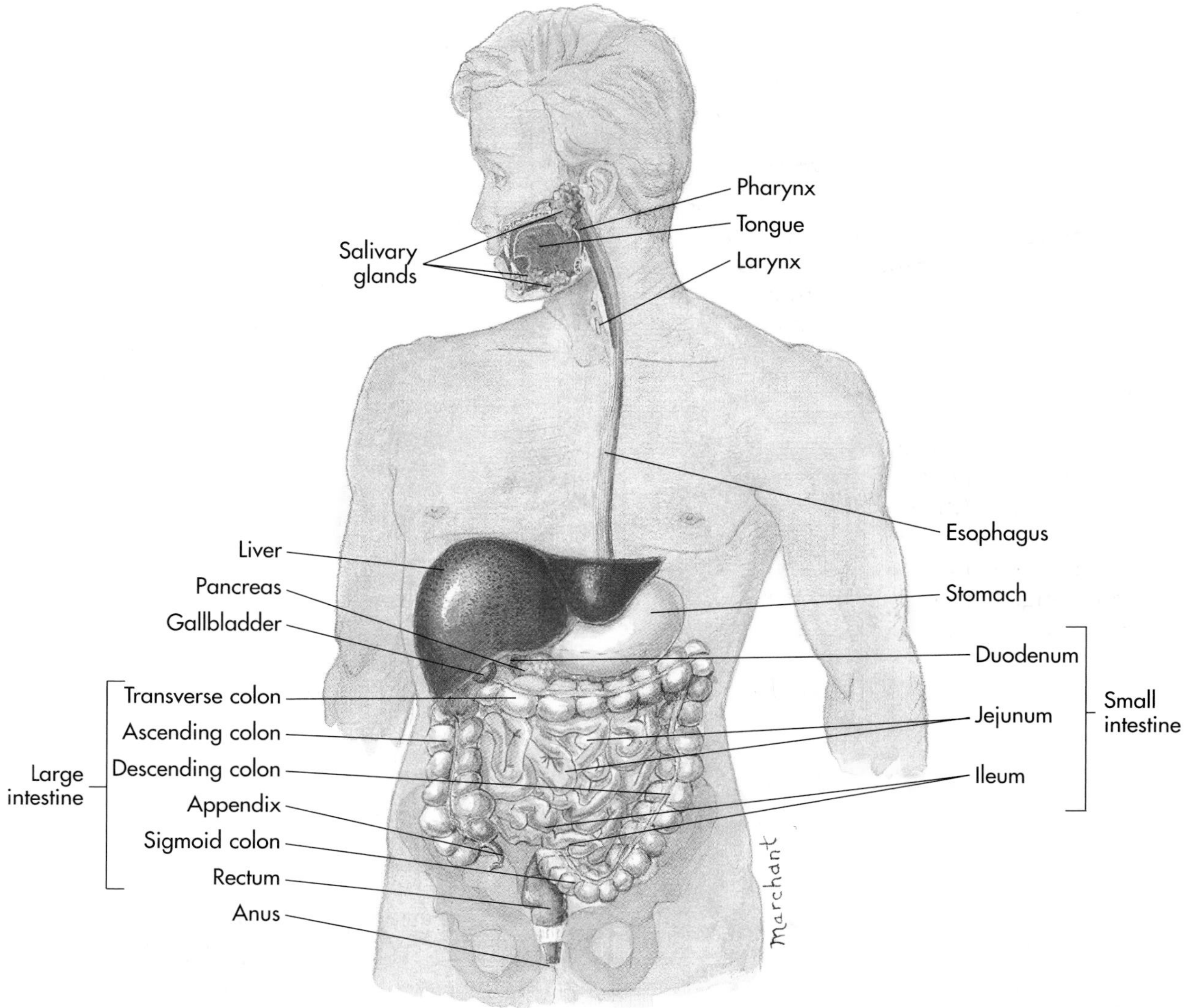

Fig. 6-18 Digestive system.

traction of the pharynx pushes food into the *esophagus.* The esophagus is a muscular tube about 10 inches long. It extends from the pharynx to the stomach. Involuntary muscle contractions called **peristalsis** move food down the esophagus into the stomach.

The *stomach* is a muscular, pouch-like sac in the upper left portion of the abdominal cavity. Strong stomach muscles stir and churn food to break it up into even smaller particles. The stomach is lined with a mucous membrane containing glands that secrete *gastric juices.* Food is mixed and churned with the gastric juices to form a semiliquid substance called *chyme.* Through peristalsis, the chyme is pushed from the stomach into the small intestine.

The *small intestine* is about 20 feet long and has three parts. The first part is the duodenum. In the *duodenum,* more digestive juices are added to the chyme. One is called *bile.* Bile is a greenish liquid produced by the *liver* and stored in the *gallbladder.* Juices from the *pancreas* and small intestine also are added to the chyme. The digestive juices chemically break down food so that it can be absorbed.

Peristalsis moves the chyme through the two remaining portions of the small intestine: the *jejunum* and the *ileum.* Tiny projections called *villi* line the small intestine. Villi absorb the digested food into the capillaries. Most of the absorption of food takes place in the jejunum and ileum.

Some chyme remains undigested. The undigested chyme passes from the small intestine into the *large intestine (large bowel* or *colon).* The colon absorbs most of the water from the chyme. The remaining semisolid material is called *feces.* Feces consist of a small amount of water, solid wastes, and some mucus and germs. These are the waste products of digestion. Feces pass through the colon into the *rectum* by peristalsis. Feces pass out of the body through the anus.

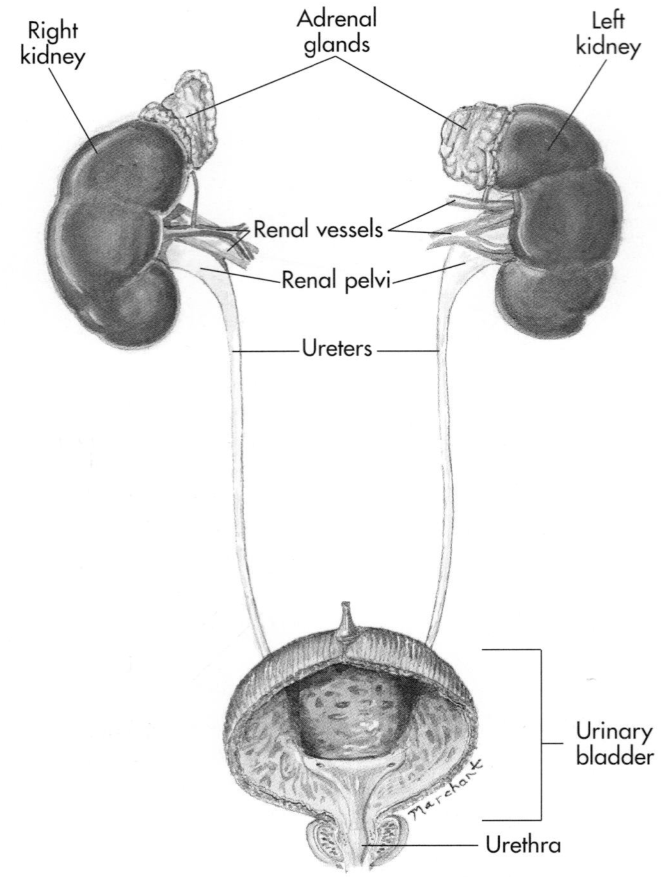

Fig. 6-19 Urinary system.

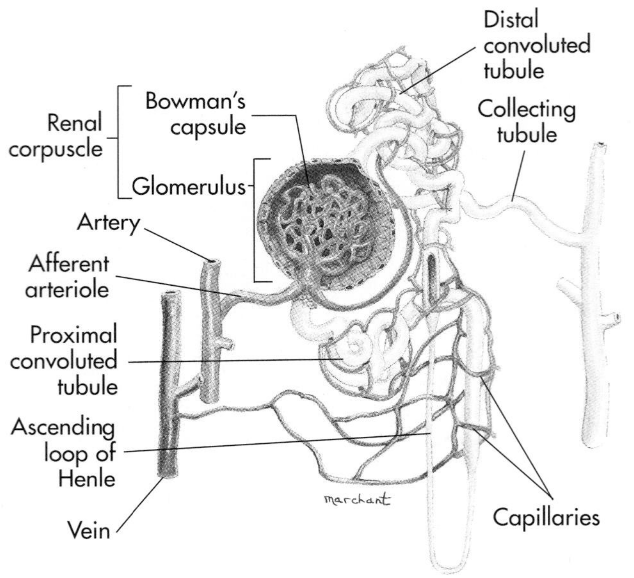

Fig. 6-20 A nephron.

THE URINARY SYSTEM

Wastes are removed from the body through the respiratory system, the digestive system, and the skin. The digestive system rids the body of solid wastes. The lungs rid the body of carbon dioxide. Water and other substances are contained in sweat. There are other waste products in the blood as a result of body cells burning food for energy. The functions of the urinary system are to remove waste products from the blood and to maintain water balance within the body. The structures of the urinary system are shown in Figure 6-19.

The *kidneys* are two bean-shaped organs in the upper abdomen. They lie against the muscles of the back on each side of the spine. They are protected by the lower edge of the rib cage.

Each kidney has over a million tiny *nephrons* (Fig. 6-20). The nephron is the basic working unit of the kidney. Each nephron has a *convoluted tubule,* which is a tiny coiled tubule. Each convoluted tubule has a *Bowman's capsule* at one end. The capsule partially surrounds a cluster of capillaries called a *glomerulus.* Blood passes through the glomerulus and is filtered by the capillaries. The fluid portion of the blood is squeezed into the Bowman's capsule. The fluid then passes into the tubule. Most of the water and other necessary substances are reabsorbed by the blood and recirculated in the body. The rest of the fluid and the waste products form *urine* in the tubule. Urine flows through the tubule to a *collecting tubule.* All of the collecting tubules within the millions of nephrons drain into the *renal pelvis* within the kidney.

A tube, called the *ureter,* is attached to the renal pelvis of the kidney. Each ureter is about 10 to 12 inches long. The ureters carry urine from the kidneys to the *bladder.* The bladder is a hollow, muscular sac situated toward the front in the lower part of the abdominal cavity. Urine is stored in the bladder until the desire to urinate is felt. The need to urinate usually occurs when there is about half a pint (250 ml) of urine in the bladder. Urine passes from the bladder through the urethra. The opening at the end of the urethra is the *meatus.* Urine passes from the body through the meatus. Urine is a clear, yellowish fluid.

THE REPRODUCTIVE SYSTEM

Human reproduction results from the union of a female sex cell and a male sex cell. Structures of the male reproductive system and female reproductive system are different. The differences allow for the process of reproduction.

The Male Reproductive System

The structures of the male reproductive system are shown in Figure 6-21. The *testes (testicles)* are the male sex glands. Sex glands are also called *gonads.* The two testes are oval or almond-shaped glands. Male sex cells are produced in the testes. Male sex cells are

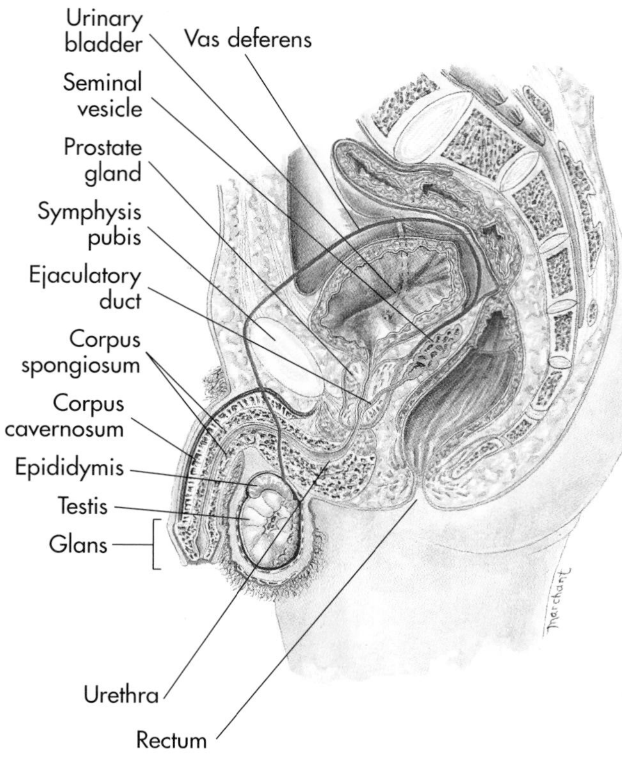

Fig. 6-21 Male reproductive system.

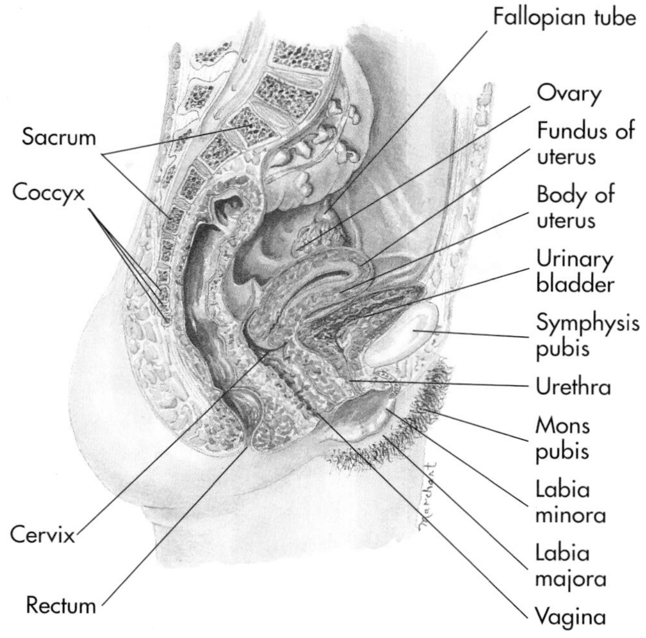

Fig. 6-22 Female reproductive system.

called *sperm cells. Testosterone,* the male hormone, also is produced in the testes. This hormone is needed for the functioning of the reproductive organs and for the development of the male's secondary sex characteristics. Male secondary sex characteristics include facial hair; pubic and axillary hair; hair on the arms, chest, and legs; deepening of the voice; and increase in neck and shoulder sizes. The testes are suspended between the thighs in a sac called the *scrotum.* The scrotum is made of skin and muscle.

Sperm travel from the testis to the *epididymis.* The epididymis is a coiled tube on top and to the side of the testis. From the epididymis, sperm travel through a tube called the *vas deferens.* Eventually each vas deferens joins a *seminal vesicle.* The two seminal vesicles store sperm and produce *semen.* Semen is a fluid that carries sperm from the male reproductive tract. The ducts of the seminal vesicles unite to form the *ejaculatory duct.* The ejaculatory duct passes through the prostate gland.

The *prostate gland,* shaped like a doughnut, lies just below the bladder. The gland secretes fluid into the semen. As the ejaculatory ducts leave the prostate, they join the *urethra,* which also runs through the prostate. The urethra is the outlet for both urine and semen. The urethra is contained within the penis.

The *penis* is outside of the body and has *erectile* tissue. When a man becomes sexually excited, blood fills the erectile tissue. This causes the penis to become enlarged, hard, and erect. The erect penis can enter the vagina of the female reproductive tract. The semen, which contains sperm, is then released into the female vagina.

The Female Reproductive System

The structures of the female reproductive system are shown in Figure 6-22. The female gonads are two almond-shaped glands called *ovaries.* There is an ovary on each side of the uterus in the abdominal cavity. The ovaries contain ova, or eggs. Ova are the female sex cells. One ovum (egg) is released monthly during the woman's reproductive years. Release of an ovum from an ovary is called *ovulation.* The ovaries also secrete the female hormones *estrogen* and *progesterone.* These hormones are needed for the functioning of the reproductive system and the development of secondary sex characteristics in the female. These include increase in breast size, pubic and axillary hair, slight deepening of the voice, and widening and rounding of the hips.

When an ovum is released from an ovary, it travels through a *fallopian tube.* There are two fallopian tubes—one on each side. The tubes are attached at one end to the uterus. The ovum travels through the fallopian tube to the *uterus.* The uterus is a hollow, muscular organ shaped like a pear. The uterus is in the center of the pelvic cavity behind the bladder and in front of the rectum. The main part of the uterus is the *fundus.* The neck or narrow section of the uterus is the *cervix.* Tissue lining the uterus is called the *endometrium.* There are

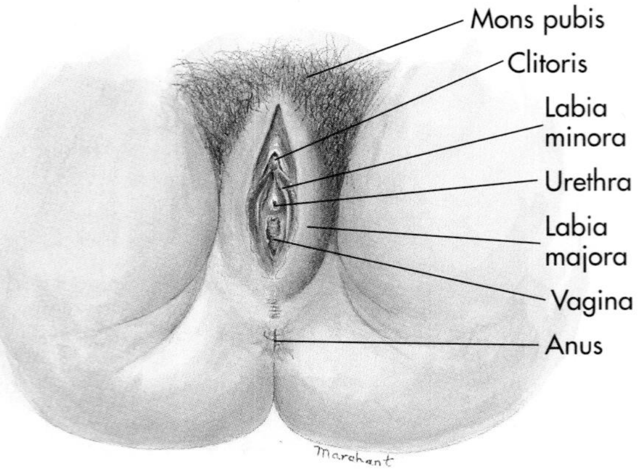

Fig. 6-23 External female genitalia.

many blood vessels in the *endometrium.* If sex cells from the male and female unite into one cell, that cell implants into the endometrium, where it grows into a baby. The uterus serves as a place for the unborn baby to grow and receive nourishment.

The cervix of the uterus projects into a muscular canal called the *vagina.* The vagina opens to the outside of the body and is located just behind the urethra. The vagina receives the penis during sexual intercourse and serves as part of the birth canal. Glands in the vaginal wall keep it moistened with secretions. In young girls, the external vaginal opening is partially closed by a membrane called the *hymen*. The hymen ruptures when the female has intercourse for the first time.

The external genitalia of the female are referred to as the *vulva* (Fig. 6-23). The *mons pubis* is a rounded, fatty pad over a bone called the *symphysis pubis.* The mons pubis is covered with hair in the adult female. The *labia majora* and *labia minora* are two folds of tissue on each side of the vaginal opening. The *clitoris* is a small organ composed of erectile tissue. The clitoris becomes hard when sexually stimulated.

The *mammary glands (breasts)* are considered organs of reproduction because they secrete milk after childbirth. The glands are located on the outside of the chest. They are made up of glandular tissue and fat (Fig. 6-24). The milk drains into ducts that open onto the nipple.

Menstruation. The endometrium is rich in blood to nourish the cell that grows into an unborn baby *(fetus).* If pregnancy does not occur, the endometrium breaks up and is discharged through the vagina to the outside of the body. This process is called **menstruation.** Menstruation occurs about every 28 days. Therefore it is also called the *menstrual cycle.*

The first day of the cycle begins with menstruation. Blood flows from the uterus through the vaginal opening. Menstrual flow usually lasts 3 to 7 days. Ovulation occurs during the next phase of the cycle. An ovum matures in an ovary and is released. Ovulation usually occurs on or about day 14 of the cycle. Meanwhile, estrogen and progesterone (the female hormones) are secreted by the ovaries. These hormones cause the endometrium to thicken for possible pregnancy. If pregnancy does not occur, the hormones decrease in amount. Blood supply to the endometrium decreases because of the decrease in hormones. The endometrium breaks up and is discharged through the vagina. Another menstrual cycle begins.

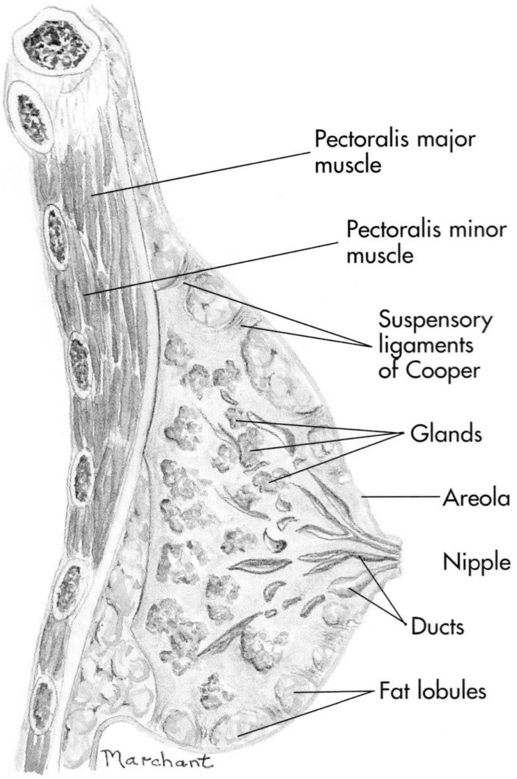

Fig. 6-24 The female breast.

Fertilization. For reproduction to occur, a male sex cell (sperm) must unite with a female sex cell (ovum). The uniting of the sperm and ovum into one cell is called *fertilization.* A sperm has 23 chromosomes, and an ovum has 23 chromosomes. When the two cells unite, the fertilized cell has 46 chromosomes.

During intercourse, millions of sperm are deposited in the vagina. Sperm travel up the cervix, through the uterus, and into the fallopian tubes. If a sperm and an ovum unite in a fallopian tube, fertilization occurs and results in pregnancy. The fertilized cell travels down the fallopian tube to the uterus. After a short time, the fertilized cell implants in the thick endometrium and grows during pregnancy.

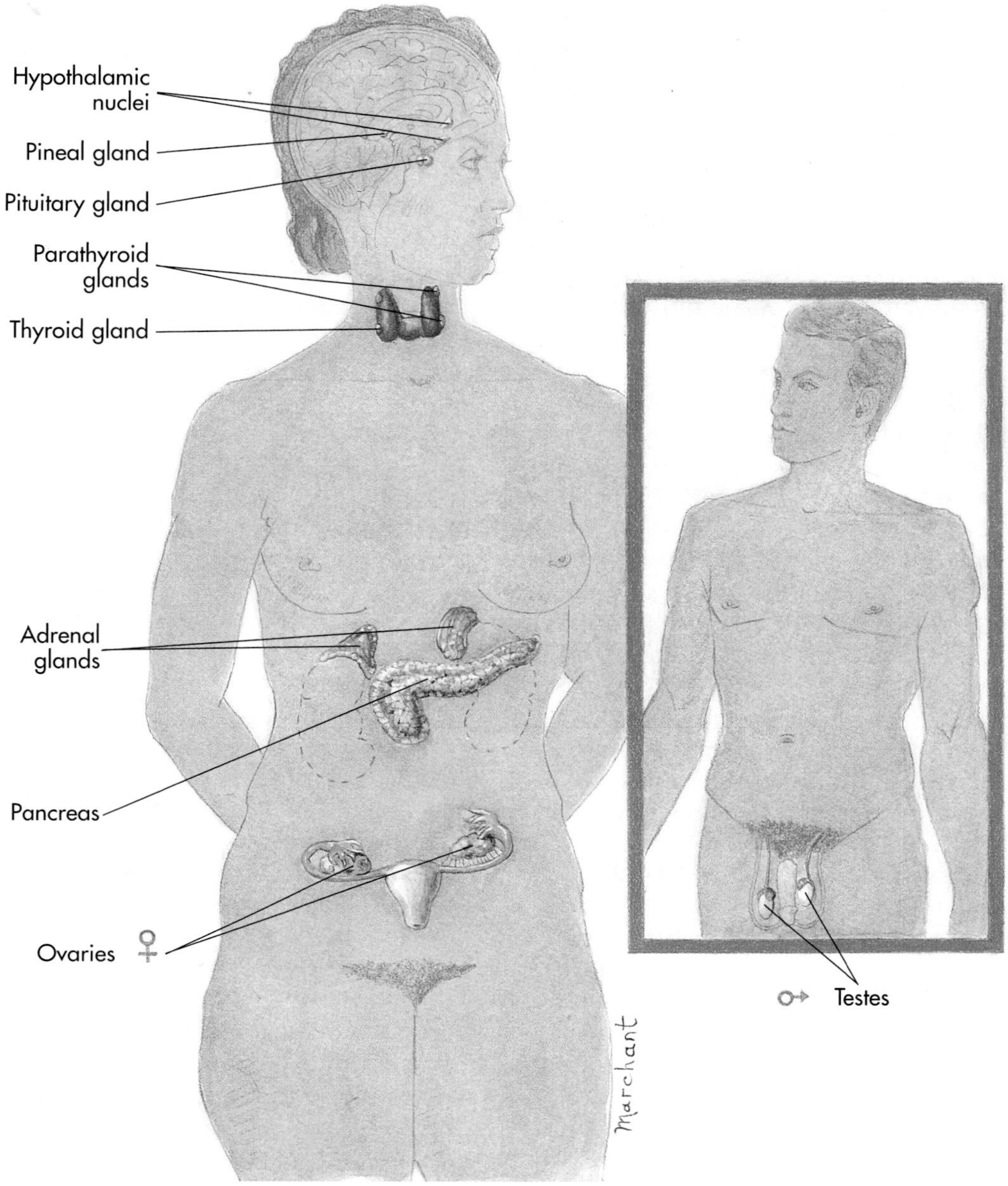

Fig. 6-25 Endocrine system.

THE ENDOCRINE SYSTEM

The endocrine system is made up of glands called the *endocrine glands* (Fig. 6-25). The endocrine glands secrete chemical substances called **hormones** into the bloodstream. Hormones regulate the activities of other organs and glands in the body.

The *pituitary gland* is called the *master gland.* About the size of a cherry, it is at the base of the brain behind the eyes. The pituitary gland is divided into the anterior pituitary lobe and the posterior pituitary lobe. The *anterior pituitary lobe* secretes important hormones. *Growth hormone* is needed for the growth of muscles, bones, and other organs. Adequate amounts of growth hormone are needed throughout life to maintain normal-size bones and muscles. Growth is stunted if a baby is born with deficient amounts of the growth hormone. Too much of the hormone causes excessive growth.

Thyroid-stimulating hormone (TSH) also is secreted by the anterior pituitary lobe. The thyroid gland requires thyroid-stimulating hormone for proper function. *Adrenocorticotropic hormone (ACTH)* is another hormone secreted by the anterior lobe. This hormone stimulates the adrenal gland. The anterior lobe also secretes hormones that regulate the growth, development, and function of the male and female reproductive systems.

The *posterior pituitary lobe* secretes *antidiuretic hormone (ADH)* and *oxytocin.* Antidiuretic hormone prevents the kidneys from excreting excessive amounts of water. Oxytocin causes the uterine muscles to contract during childbirth.

The *thyroid gland,* shaped like a butterfly, is in the neck in front of the larynx. *Thyroid hormone (TH)* is secreted by the thyroid gland. *Thyroxine* is another term for thyroid hormone. Thyroid hormone regulates **metabolism.** Metabolism is the burning of food for heat and energy by the cells. Too little thyroid hormone results in slowed body processes, slowed movements, and weight gain. Too much of the hormone causes increased metabolism, excess energy, and weight loss. If a baby is born with deficient amounts of thyroid hormone, physical and mental growth will be stunted.

The *parathyroid glands* secrete *parathormone.* There are four parathyroid glands. Two are located on each side of the thyroid gland. Parathormone regulates the body's use of calcium. Calcium is needed for the proper function of nerves and muscles. Insufficient amounts of calcium cause *tetany.* Tetany is a state of severe muscle contraction and spasm. If untreated, tetany can cause death.

There are two *adrenal glands.* An adrenal gland is on the top of each kidney. The adrenal gland has two parts: the *adrenal medulla* and the *adrenal cortex.* The adrenal medulla secretes *epinephrine* and *norepinephrine.* These hormones stimulate the body to quickly produce energy during emergencies. Heart rate, blood pressure, muscle power, and energy all increase. The adrenal cortex secretes three groups of hormones that are essential for life. The *glucocorticoids* regulate metabolism of carbohydrates. They also control the body's response to stress and inflammation. The *mineralocorticoids* regulate the amount of salt and water that is absorbed and lost by the kidneys. The adrenal cortex also secretes small amounts of male and female sex hormones.

The pancreas secretes *insulin.* Insulin regulates the amount of sugar in the blood available for use by the cells. Insulin is needed for sugar to enter the cells. If there is too little insulin, sugar cannot enter the cells. If sugar cannot enter the cells, excess amounts of sugar build up in the blood. This condition is called *diabetes mellitus.*

The *gonads* are the glands of human reproduction. Male sex glands (testes) secrete *testosterone.* Female sex glands (ovaries) secrete *estrogen* and *progesterone.*

THE IMMUNE SYSTEM

The immune system protects the body from disease and infection. Abnormal body cells can grow into tumors. Sometimes the body produces substances that cause the body to attack itself. Microorganisms (bacteria, viruses, and other germs) in the environment can lead to an infection. The immune system defends against threats inside and outside the body.

The immune system provides the body with immunity. **Immunity** means that a person has protection against a disease or infection. The person will not get or be affected by the disease. *Specific immunity* is the body's reaction to a specific threat. *Nonspecific immunity* is the body's reaction to anything it does not recognize as a normal body substance.

Special cells and substances produce immunity:

- *Antibodies*—normal body substances that recognize abnormal or unwanted substances. They attack and destroy such substances.
- *Antigens*—abnormal or unwanted substances. An antigen causes the body to produce antibodies. The antibodies attack and destroy the antigens.
- *Phagocytes*—types of white blood cells that digest and destroy microorganisms and other unwanted substances.
- *Lymphocytes*—types of white blood cells that produce antibodies. Lymphocyte production increases as the body responds to an infection.
- *B lymphocytes (B cells)*—cause the production of antibodies that circulate in the plasma. The antibodies react to specific antigens.
- *T lymphocytes (T cells)*—destroy invading cells. *Killer T cells* produce poisonous substances near the invading cells. Some T cells attract other cells; these other cells destroy the invaders.

When the body senses an antigen (an unwanted substance), the immune system is activated. Phagocyte and lymphocyte production increases. Phagocytes destroy invaders through digestion. The lymphocytes produce antibodies that attack and destroy the unwanted substances.

QUALITY OF LIFE

The human body is made up of several systems. Each system has its own structures and functions. The body systems are related to and depend on each other for proper functioning and survival. Injury or disease of one part of the system affects the entire system and the whole body.

Basic knowledge of the body's normal structure and function should result in safer, more efficient resident care. The knowledge you receive in this chapter will help you better understand the reasons for the care you give. Always treat the resident's body with dignity and respect.

REVIEW QUESTIONS

Circle the BEST answer.

1 The basic unit of body structure is the
A Cell
B Neuron
C Nephron
D Ovum

2 The outer layer of the skin is called the
A Dermis
B Epidermis
C Integument
D Myelin

3 Which is not a function of the skin?
A Providing the protective covering for the body
B Regulating body temperature
C Sensing cold, pain, touch, and pressure
D Providing the shape and framework for the body

4 Which part allows movement?
A Bone marrow and periosteum
B Synovial membrane
C Joints
D Ligaments

5 Skeletal muscles
A Are under involuntary control
B Appear smooth
C Are under voluntary control
D Appear striped and smooth

6 The highest functions of the brain take place in the
A Cerebral cortex
B Medulla
C Brainstem
D Spinal nerves

7 Besides hearing, the ear is involved with
A Regulating body movements
B Balance
C Smoothness of body movements
D Controlling involuntary muscles

8 The liquid part of the blood is the
A Hemoglobin
B Red blood cell
C Plasma
D Alveolus

9 Which part of the heart pumps blood to the body?
A Right atrium
B Right ventricle
C Left atrium
D Left ventricle

10 Which carry blood away from the heart?
A Capillaries
B Veins
C Venules
D Arteries

11 Oxygen and carbon dioxide are exchanged
A In the bronchi
B Between the alveoli and capillaries
C Between the lungs and the pleura
D In the trachea

12 The process of digestion begins in the
A Mouth
B Stomach
C Small intestine
D Colon

13 Most food absorption takes place in the
A Stomach
B Small intestine
C Colon
D Large intestine

14 Urine is formed by the
A Jejunum
B Kidneys
C Bladder
D Liver

15 Urine passes from the body through
A The ureters
B The urethra
C The anus
D Nephrons

16 The male sex gland is called the
A Penis
B Semen
C Testis
D Scrotum

Continued

17 The male sex cell is the
A Semen
B Ovum
C Gonad
D Sperm

18 The female sex gland is the
A Ovary
B Fallopian tube
C Uterus
D Vagina

19 The discharge of the lining of the uterus is called
A The endometrium
B Ovulation
C Fertilization
D Menstruation

20 The endocrine glands secrete substances called
A Hormones
B Mucus
C Semen
D Insulin

21 The immune system protects the body from
A Low blood sugar
B Disease and infection
C Falling and loss of balance
D Stunted growth and loss of fluid

Answers to these questions are on p. 696.

7 The Older Person

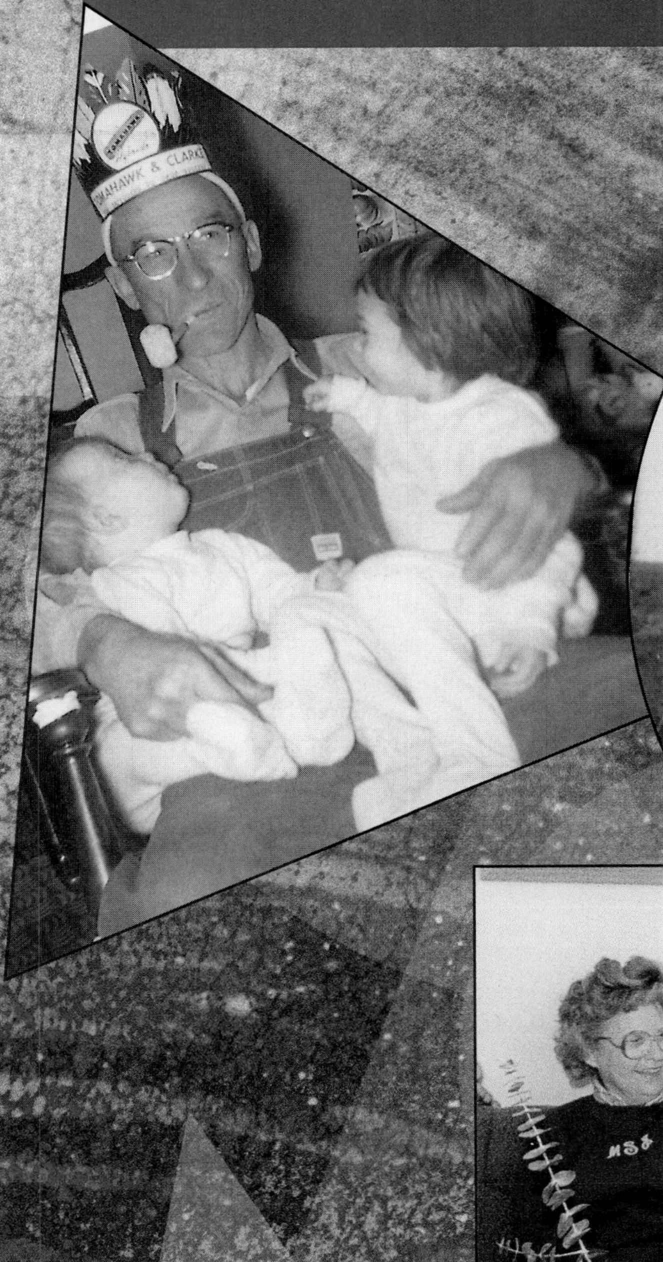

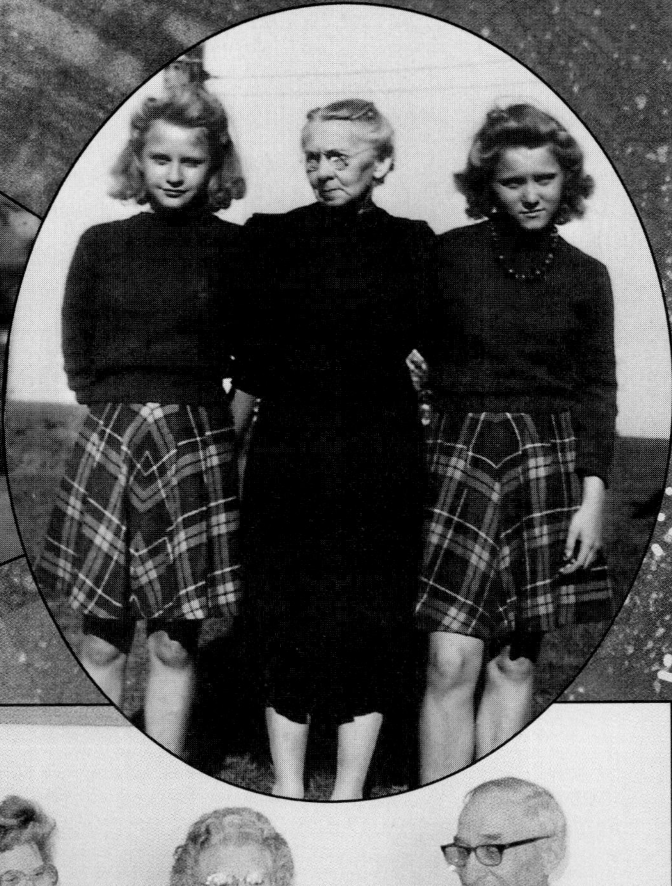

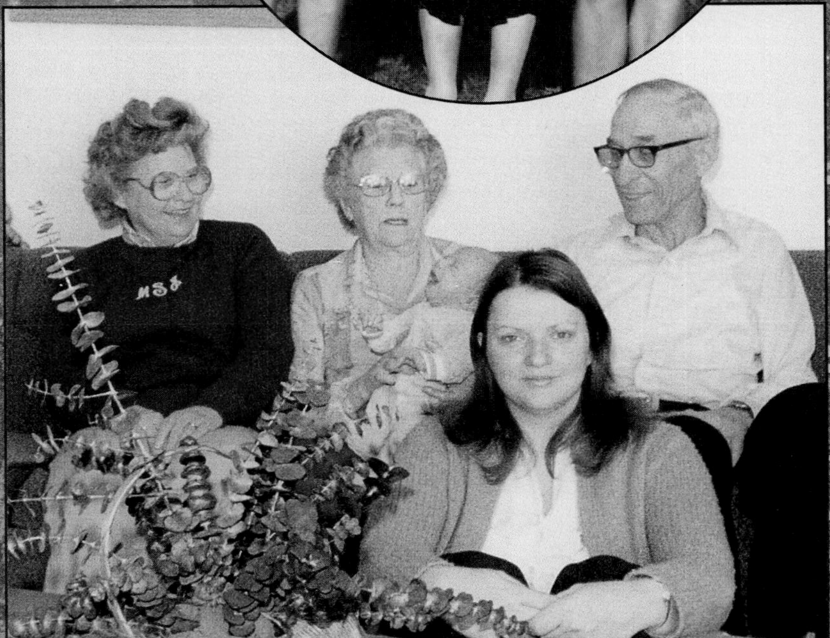

What You Will Learn

- The definition of the key terms listed in this chapter
- The effects of retirement
- Common changes in social relationships of older persons
- How the death of a spouse affects the survivor
- Changes in body systems as a result of aging
- Housing alternatives for older persons
- Why nursing center residents may avoid social relationships
- How to promote the resident's quality of life

Key Terms

dysphagia Difficulty *(dys)* swallowing *(phagia)*

dyspnea Difficult, labored, or painful *(dys)* breathing *(pnea)*

geriatrics The care of aging people

gerontology The study of the aging process

menopause The cessation of the menstrual cycle

old Those persons between the ages of 65 and 85

old-old Those persons over the age of 85

presbyopia Age-related *(presby)* farsightedness (*opia* means eye)

young-old Those persons between the ages of 55 and 65

The number of older persons is increasing every day. People are living longer and are healthier than before. Most people can expect to live into their 70s. Many live into their 80s and 90s. More and more people are living past 100.

But what is old? There are different age ranges for the young-old, the old, and the old-old. The **young-old** are between the ages of 55 and 65. The **old** are between the ages of 65 and 85. The **old-old** are people over age 85. However, these age categories are not magical. Individuals age at different rates. Many individuals are healthy, active, and alert well into their 90s.

Gerontology is the study of the aging process. **Geriatrics** is the care of the aged. Aging is a normal part of the life cycle. It is not a disease. Normal changes occur in body structure and function throughout the life span. However, certain physical changes increase the risk for illness, chronic disease, and disability. Most changes occur gradually. How and why these changes occur are not clearly understood. Most people adapt very well to these changes and lead happy, meaningful lives. Many continue to live in their own home. Fewer than 10% of older persons live in a nursing center .

PSYCHOLOGICAL AND SOCIAL EFFECTS OF AGING

Aging is a complex process. Physical changes occur in all body systems. Graying hair, wrinkles, and slower movements are physical reminders of growing old. These physical changes can affect self-esteem; they can threaten self-image, feelings of self-worth, and independence. All are important to a fulfilling and happy life.

Social roles change as people age. An older parent may depend on an adult child for care. Retirees must develop a new role to replace the work role. Many older persons must adjust to the death of a spouse, relatives, and friends. The person is also faced with his or her own death.

Growing old is a difficult process socially, psychologically, and physically. Each person copes with age-related changes differently. Some factors that affect how a person copes with changes are:

- Health status
- Life experiences
- Financial resources
- Education
- Social support systems

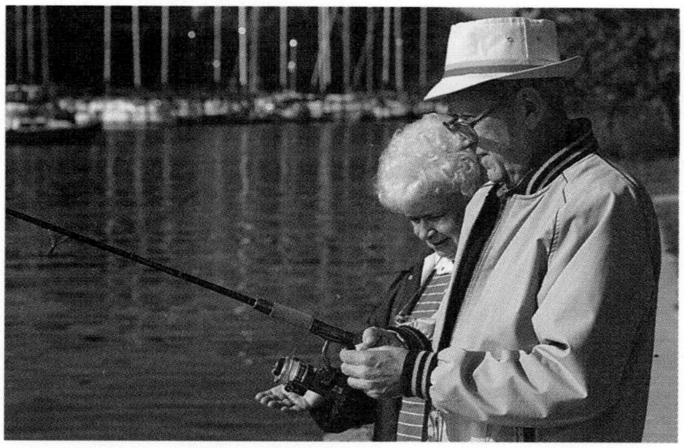

Fig. 7-1 A retired couple enjoying fishing together.

Retirement

People commonly retire at the age of 65. Some retire earlier. Others work until the age of 70 or longer. Retirement is a reward for a lifetime of hard work. The person has earned the right not to work and can now relax and enjoy life (Fig. 7-1). Travel, leisure, and doing whatever one wants are retirement "benefits." Many people enjoy retirement. Others are not as lucky. Some must retire because of chronic disease or disability. Poor health and medical bills can make retirement very difficult.

Work has social and psychological effects. Work helps meet the basic needs of love, belonging, and esteem. Work brings personal satisfaction and usefulness. Friendships develop and co-workers share day-to-day events. Leisure activities, recreation, and companionship often involve co-workers. Some people need work for psychological and social fulfillment. Retirement can be hard for them. Some retired people have part-time jobs or do volunteer work (Fig. 7-2). Such activities promote feelings of usefulness and well-being.

Retirement usually means reduced income. For some people, the monthly Social Security check is the only income. Retirement and aging do not mean fewer expenses. There still may be rent or house payments. Food, clothing, taxes, and gas, electricity, and water bills are other expenses. Car expenses, home repairs, medicine, and health care are other costs. So are entertainment and gifts for children and grandchildren. Retirement can cause severe money problems. Some people plan for retirement with savings, investments, retirement plans, and insurance.

Social Relationships

Social relationships change throughout life. (*See Caring About Culture.*) Children grow up and move away. They have their own family. Many live far away from older parents. Older family members and friends die,

A

B

Fig. 7-2 A, This retired woman does volunteer work at a nursing center. **B,** This retired woman is a foster grandmother.

> **CARING ABOUT CULTURE**
>
> **Communicating in a Foreign Language**
>
> Some older persons speak and understand a foreign language. Communication occurs with family and friends who speak the same language. They also share cultural values and practices. These relatives and friends may move away or die. The person may not have anyone to talk with and may not be understood by others. Greater loneliness and isolation for the foreign-speaking person may result.

move away, or become disabled. These changes can cause feelings of loneliness and isolation. Separation from children and the lack of companionship with people their own age are common causes of loneliness in older persons.

Many older people adjust to these changes. Hobbies, church and community activities, and new friends help prevent loneliness. Some communities and organizations sponsor bus trips to ball games, shopping, plays, and concerts. Being a grandparent

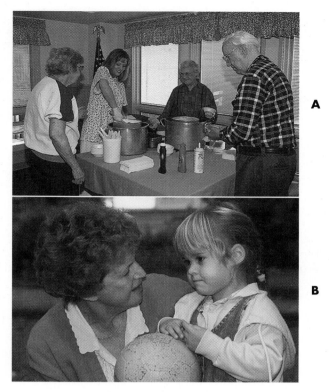

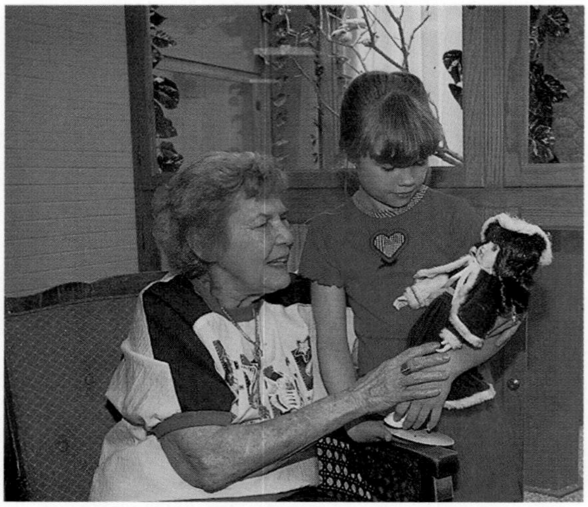

Fig. 7-3 An older woman plays with her grandchild.

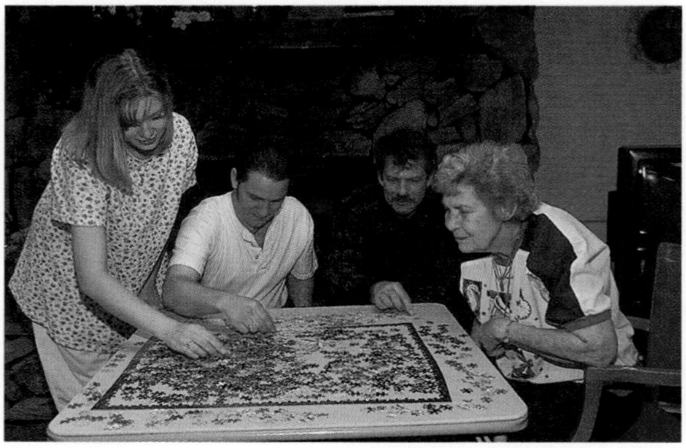

Fig. 7-4 This older woman is included in family activities.

can bring great love and enjoyment (Fig. 7-3). Being included in family activities helps prevent loneliness. It also allows the older person to feel useful and wanted (Fig. 7-4).

Some children care for their older parents. This is a social change for the parent and child. Parents and children change roles. Instead of the parent caring for the child, the child cares for the parent. This role change makes some older persons feel more secure. Others feel unwanted, in the way, and useless. Some feel a loss of dignity and self-respect. Tensions may develop among the child, parent, and other household members. Lack of privacy, disagreements, and criticisms about housekeeping, child rearing, cooking, and friends are common causes of tension.

Death of a Partner

As couples grow older, the chances increase that one partner will die. Women usually live longer than men. Therefore becoming a widow is a reality for many women.

A person may try to prepare psychologically for the death of a life partner. When death does occur, however, the loss is devastating. No amount of preparation is ever enough for the emptiness and changes that result. The person loses a lover, friend, companion, and confidant. The survivor's grief can be very great. Serious physical and mental health problems can result. Some lose the will to live or attempt suicide.

PHYSICAL EFFECTS OF AGING

Certain physical changes are a normal part of aging. The changes occur in everyone (Table 7-1). The changes are gradual and may go unnoticed as the person adjusts to them. Some people age faster than others. The rate and degree of change vary with each person. Body processes slow down. Energy level and body efficiency decline.

Illness, injury, or disability does not always accompany normal aging. Quality of life does not have to decline. The changes in body processes take place over many years. This lets the person adjust to such things as reduced activity and mobility.

The Integumentary System

The skin loses its elasticity and fatty tissue layer. As a result, the skin thins and sags. Folds, lines, and wrinkles appear. Oil gland and sweat gland secretions decrease. Dry skin develops. The skin is fragile and easily injured. Skin breakdown and pressure ulcers are dangers.

Loss of the skin's fatty layer makes the person more sensitive to cold. Sweaters, lap blankets, socks, and extra blankets often are needed for warmth. Older persons need protection from drafts and extreme cold. Often thermostat settings are higher than normal.

Dry skin is easily damaged and causes itching. A tub bath, shower, or bed bath twice a week usually is enough for cleanliness. Partial baths are taken at other times. Only mild soaps are used. Some nursing centers use soap substitutes. Soaps may be used to clean only the underarms, perineum, and under female breasts. Often soap is not used on the arms, legs, back, chest, and abdomen. Lotions, oils, and creams can prevent drying and itching. Deodorants usually are not needed because of decreased sweat gland secretion. Personal hygiene and skin care are discussed in Chapters 13 and 14.

Nails become thick and tough. Feet usually have poor circulation. A nick or cut can lead to a serious infection. Sometimes amputation is necessary to fight the infection (see Chapter 26). Nail and foot care are described in Chapter 14.

Table 7-1 Physical Changes During the Aging Process

System	Changes
Integumentary	Skin becomes less elastic Fatty tissue layer is lost Skin thins and sags Skin is fragile and easily injured Folds, lines, and wrinkles appear Decreased secretion of oil and sweat glands Dry skin develops Itching Increased sensitivity to cold Nails become thick and tough Whitening or graying hair Loss or thinning of hair
Musculoskeletal	Muscles atrophy and strength decreases Bone mass decreases Bone strength decreases Bone becomes brittle; can break easily Vertebrae shorten Joints become stiff and painful Hip and knee joints become flexed Gradual loss of height Loss of strength Decreased mobility
Nervous	Reduction in nerve cells Slower nerve conduction Reflexes slow Slower response to stimuli Reduced blood flow to the brain Progressive loss of brain cells Shorter memory Forgetfulness Confusion Dizziness Changes in sleep patterns Reduced sensitivity to touch and pain Decreased senses of smell and taste Eyelids thin and wrinkle Less tear secretion
Nervous—cont'd	Pupils less responsive to light Decreased vision at night or in dark rooms Difficulty seeing green and blue colors Poor vision Changes in auditory nerve Eardrums atrophy High-pitched sounds not heard Wax secretion decreases Hearing loss
Circulatory	Heart pumps with less force Arteries narrow and are less elastic Less blood flows through narrowed arteries Weakened heart has to work harder to pump blood through narrowed vessels
Respiratory	Respiratory muscles weaken Lung tissue becomes less elastic Difficulty breathing (dyspnea) Decreased strength for coughing
Digestive	Decreased saliva production Difficulty swallowing (dysphagia) Decreased appetite Decreased secretion of digestive juices Difficulty digesting fried and fatty foods Indigestion Loss of teeth Decreased peristalsis, causing flatulence and constipation
Urinary	Kidney function decreases Blood flow to the kidneys is reduced Kidneys atrophy Urine becomes concentrated

Continued

CONT'D TABLE 7-1 PHYSICAL CHANGES DURING THE AGING PROCESS

System	Changes	System	Changes
Urinary—cont'd	Bladder muscles weaken Urinary incontinence may occur	Reproductive *Female*—cont'd	Loss of fat and elastic tissue in external genitalia Breasts are less firm
Reproductive *Female*	Cessation of menstrual activity Decreased estrogen production Ovaries and uterus decrease in size Vaginal walls are thinner, dryer, and less elastic	*Male*	Testosterone level decreases Force of ejaculation decreases Sperm count is reduced Testes are smaller Prostate gland is enlarged Erection develops more slowly

Older persons may complain of cold feet. Socks help. Hot water bottles and heating pads are not used. The risk of burns is very great. Fragile skin, poor circulation, and decreased sensitivity to heat and cold increase the risk of burns.

The risk of skin cancer increases with age. Prolonged sun exposure is a known cause. Other skin growths are common in older persons. They include seborrheic keratosis and senile keratosis. *Seborrheic keratosis* is a wart-type lesion of the skin. The lesion looks like a greasy, yellow or brown wart. (Seborrheic comes from the Latin word *sebum,* meaning sweat; *kerat* means horny; *osis* means condition of.) *Senile keratosis* is a raised, thickened area that is brown or gray. (*Senile* comes from the Latin word for old.) The areas become scaly. These lesions can become malignant (cancerous) if untreated (see Chapter 26). Skin disorders increase with age but rarely cause death if treated early.

White or gray hair is common. Men lose a lot of hair. Hair thins on both men and women. Thinning occurs on the head, in the pubic area, and under the arms. Hair tends to be drier. This is from decreased scalp oil production. Brushing helps stimulate circulation and oil production. Shampooing frequency depends on personal choice. Usually it decreases with age. Shampooing should be done as often as necessary to maintain hygiene and comfort. Women and men may wear wigs because of thinning hair. Some color their hair to cover graying.

The Musculoskeletal System

Muscles atrophy (shrink) and decrease in strength. Bone mass decreases. Minerals, especially calcium, are lost from the bones. Bones decrease in strength, become brittle, and break easily. These changes are severe in some older persons. For them, simply turning in bed can cause fractures (broken bones). Vertebrae shorten. Joints become stiff and painful. Hip and knee joints become slightly flexed (bent). These changes result in gradual loss of height, loss of strength, and decreased mobility.

Older persons need to be as active as possible. Activity, exercise, and diet help prevent bone loss and muscle strength. Walking is one of the best exercises. Exercise groups and range-of-motion exercises are helpful. The diet should be high in protein, calcium, and vitamins. Remember, bones can break easily. You must protect the person from injury and prevent falls (see Chapter 8). Turn and move the person gently and carefully. A resident may need help and support getting out of bed and in walking.

The Nervous System

Nerve cells are lost. Nerve conduction is slower. Reflexes are slower. Therefore responses to stimuli are slower. For example, an older person who slips is more likely to fall than is a younger person. The message telling the brain the person has slipped travels slowly. The message from the brain needed to prevent the fall also travels slowly. Thus the persons falls.

Blood flow to the brain is reduced. This may cause dizziness, increasing the risk for falls. Measures to prevent falls are practiced (see Chapter 8). Residents are reminded to get up slowly from the bed or chair to prevent dizziness (see Chapter 19).

A progressive loss of brain cells occurs. Reduced blood flow and loss of brain cells affect personality and mental function. Memory is shorter, and forgetfulness increases. The ability to respond slows. Confusion, dizziness, and fatigue may occur. Older people often remember events in the distant past better than those in the recent past. Many older persons stay mentally active and involved in current events. They show fewer personality and mental changes. (See Chapter 27 for the care of persons with confusion and dementia).

Changes in sleep patterns occur. The older persons tend to have more difficulty falling asleep, wake often during the night, and have less deep sleep. They may rest or nap more during the day to prevent fatigue.

The senses. Aging affects touch, smell, taste, sight, and hearing. Touch and sensitivity to pain are reduced. So is the ability to feel heat and cold. These changes increase the older person's risk for injury. Injuries and diseases that normally cause much pain may go unnoticed. The person may feel only minor discomfort. Therefore older residents are protected from injury. Safety measures are practiced when heat and cold are applied (see Chapter 24). The skin is carefully inspected for signs of breakdown. Good skin care and the measures to prevent pressure ulcers are practiced (see Chapter 14).

Smell and taste are important when eating. These senses dull and cause a decrease in appetite. The number of taste buds decreases with aging. The tongue senses only sweet, salty, bitter, and sour. Sweet and salty tastes are lost first. That is why older residents often complain that food has no taste. This is also why they often ask for more salt or sugar on their food.

The eye. Many changes occur in the eye. Eyelids thin and wrinkle. Tear secretion is less. Therefore eye irritation easily occurs from such things as dust and air pollutants. The pupil becomes smaller and less responsive to light. This causes decreased vision at night or in dark rooms. It takes longer for the eye to adjust to changes in the amount of light. The person has problems seeing when going from a dark room into a brighter room or from a brighter room into a darker one. The ability to see clearly is reduced. This creates the need for eyeglasses. The lens of the eye (see Fig. 6-12, p. 103) yellows. Therefore green and blue colors are harder to see.

Older persons become more and more farsighted. Age-related farsightedness is called **presbyopia.** (*Presby* relates to aging or being old; *opia* comes from the Latin word for eye). The lens becomes more rigid with age. It is harder for the eye to shift from far vision to near vision and from near vision to far vision. These changes increase the risk of falls and other accidents, especially where lighting is poor and on stairs. Always make sure that residents wear their eyeglasses. Their rooms need to be well lit. Nightlights help them see when they are up during the night.

The ear. Changes occur in the auditory nerve. Eardrums atrophy (shrink). The ability to hear high-pitched sounds decreases or is lost. Severe hearing loss occurs if these changes progress. A hearing aid may be needed for the affected ear. Hearing aids must be clean and correctly placed in the ear. Wax secretion decreases. Wax becomes harder and thicker with age. This wax is easily impacted (wedged in the ear) and can increase hearing loss. A doctor or nurse removes the wax.

The Circulatory System

The heart muscle becomes less efficient. Blood is pumped through the body with less force. The person may not have problems when resting. Activity, exercise, excitement, and illness increase the body's need for oxygen and nutrients. If damaged or severely weakened, the heart may be unable to meet these needs.

Arteries narrow and loose their elasticity. Less blood flows through them. Poor circulation occurs in many body parts. A weakened heart must work harder to pump blood through narrowed vessels.

Exercise helps maintain health and well-being. Walking is good exercise for the healthy older adult. Many older persons exercise daily. They walk, jog, golf, bicycle, hike, ski, play tennis, swim, or play other sports. Nursing center residents are kept as active as possible.

Although many older adults are quite active, others are less fortunate. Sometimes cardiovascular changes are severe. Affected persons need rest periods during the day. Daily activities are planned to avoid overexertion. Such persons should not walk long distances, climb many stairs, or carry heavy objects. Personal care items, television, telephone, and other needed items should be nearby. A moderate amount of daily exercise helps to stimulate circulation. Exercise also helps prevent thrombi (blood clots) in leg veins. Active or passive range-of-motion exercises are needed by persons confined to bed (see Chapter 19). Doctors may order certain exercises and activity limits.

The Respiratory System

Respiratory muscles weaken, and lung tissue becomes less elastic. Lung changes may not be obvious at rest. However, difficult, labored, or painful breathing **(dyspnea)** may occur with activity. (*Dys* means difficult; *pnea* means breathing). The person may not have enough strength to cough and clear the upper airway of secretions. Respiratory infections and diseases may develop. These can severely threaten the older person's life.

Measures are necessary to promote normal breathing. Heavy bed linens should not cover the chest. They can prevent normal chest expansion. Turning, repositioning, and deep breathing help prevent respiratory complications from bedrest. Breathing usually is easier in the semi-Fowler's position (see Chapter 10). The person should be as active as possible.

The Digestive System

Many changes occur in the digestive system. Salivary glands produce less saliva. This can cause difficulty in swallowing **(dysphagia).** (*Dys* means difficult; *phagia* means swallowing.) Dulled senses of taste and smell cause a decrease in appetite. Secretion of digestive juices decreases. As a result, fried and fatty foods are hard to digest and may cause indigestion. Loss of teeth and ill-fitting dentures make chewing difficult. This results in digestion problems. Hard to chew foods are avoided—usually high-protein foods such as meat. High-protein foods are needed for a balanced diet. Grinding or chopping meat makes it easier to chew and swallow. Decreased peristalsis results in slower emptying of the stomach and colon. Flatulence and constipation are common from decreased peristalsis (see Chapter 17).

Dry, fried, and fatty foods should be avoided. This helps lessen difficulty in swallowing and indigestion. Good oral hygiene and denture care improve the ability to taste. Some persons do not have natural teeth or dentures. Their food is pureed or ground. Often high-fiber foods are avoided even though they help prevent constipation. High-fiber foods are hard to chew and can irritate the intestines. They include apricots, celery, and fruits and vegetables with skins and seeds. Foods providing soft bulk often are ordered for persons with chewing difficulties or constipation. These foods include whole-grain cereals and cooked fruits and vegetables.

Aging requires certain dietary changes. Older people need fewer calories than younger people do. Energy and activity levels are lower. More fluids are needed to aid chewing, swallowing, and digestion. The person needs foods that prevent constipation and musculoskeletal changes. High-protein foods are needed for tissue growth and repair. However, the diets of some older persons lack protein. High-protein foods generally are expensive.

The Urinary System

Kidney function decreases with age The kidneys atrophy (shrink). Blood flow to the kidneys is reduced. Removal of body wastes is less efficient. Urine is more concentrated. The risk of urinary tract infection increases. The ureters, bladder, and urethra lose tone and elasticity. The bladder stores less urine. This causes more frequent urination. Many older persons have to urinate several times during the night. Urinary incontinence may occur (see Chapter 16). In men, the prostate gland enlarges. This puts pressure on the urethra. Difficulty passing urine and more frequent urination occur.

Adequate fluids are necessary. Too little fluid can damage the kidneys and cause urinary tract infections. Intake should include water, fruit juices, milk, and gelatin. The person should have a choice in the type of fluids served. Make sure water is available to all residents who are permitted to have water. Remind them to drink, and offer fluids often to those who need help. Most fluids should be ingested before 5:00 PM (1700). This reduces the need to urinate during the night. Bladder training programs may be necessary for those with urinary incontinence. Indwelling catheters sometimes are needed. Urinary elimination is discussed in Chapter 16.

The Reproductive System

Aging causes changes in the reproductive system of both women and men. However, sexual activity need not decrease. It is an important and enjoyable part of the lives of many older people (see Chapter 30).

Female. The ovaries produce less estrogen and progesterone. This results in changes in the menstrual cycle and a woman's ability to reproduce. These changes usually begin around age 40. **Menopause** (the cessation of the menstrual cycle) is completed by the mid-50s for most women. The ovaries and uterus decrease in size. There is loss of subcutaneous fat and elastic tissue in the external genitalia. They also shrink in size. The vaginal walls become thinner, dryer, and less elastic. This can lead to itching and painful intercourse. Lubricants and estrogen replacement creams may be helpful. Decreased muscle tone and elasticity cause breasts to be less firm and to sag.

Male. In men, fewer healthy sperm are produced. The force of ejaculation is decreased. Testosterone levels decrease somewhat. The testes become less firm and smaller. The prostate gland often enlarges. The enlarged prostate gland may compress the urethra and cause difficulty urinating. In severe cases, it prevents the flow of urine and surgery is needed. Erection develops more slowly. The ability to regain erection after completion of intercourse is reduced.

HOUSING OPTIONS

A house is more than a place to live. For most people, a house has family memories and is a link to neighbors and the community. It is a source of pride and self-esteem. Aging can bring a need to change living arrangements.

Most older persons live in their own homes. Some choose to give up their homes; others are forced to. Reduced income, taxes, home repairs, and the inability to do yard work are influencing factors. Some older people retire to warmer climates. Others do not want a large home when children are gone. Some cannot care for themselves.

Living with Family

Sometimes older brothers, sisters, and cousins live together. They provide companionship for each other. They also can share living expenses. They can care for each other during illness or disability. One may have the caregiver role if the other is ill or disabled.

Some older persons live with their adult children. (*See Caring About Culture*) The elderly parent (or parents) moves in with the child, or the child moves into the parent's home. The elderly parent may be healthy, may need some supervision, or may be ill or disabled. Some adult children are caregivers for ill or disabled parents. Often children care for parents to avoid nursing home care. They try the caregiver role first. A nursing center is an option if they cannot give needed care.

Living with an adult child is a social change. The parent, adult child, and the child's family all need to adjust. Sleeping arrangements may change if there is no spare bedroom. The parent may need a hospital bed. It may need to go in a living room, dining room, or bedroom.

The adult child's family still needs time alone. Other brothers and sisters may help give care. Respite care (see Chapter 1) is an option for weekends and vacations. Home care agencies can provide nurses or home health care aides. Many community and church groups have volunteers who help give care.

Adult day-care centers. Many adult children need to work even though the elderly parent cannot be left alone. Adult day-care centers provide meals, supervision, and activities for older persons. Some provide transportation to and from the center.

Caring About Culture

Parents Living With Children

Cultural attitudes toward older adults vary. Generally, whites expect older parents to care for themselves and not depend on adult children for care. Other cultures have higher levels of respect for aging adults than do whites. Such cultural groups include blacks, Asians, Hispanics, and Native Americans. In Asian cultures, it is common for the oldest son to assume responsibility for aging parents. Aging Hispanics commonly are invited to live with a family member.

Modified from Lueckenotte AG: *Gerontologic nursing*, St Louis, 1996, Mosby.

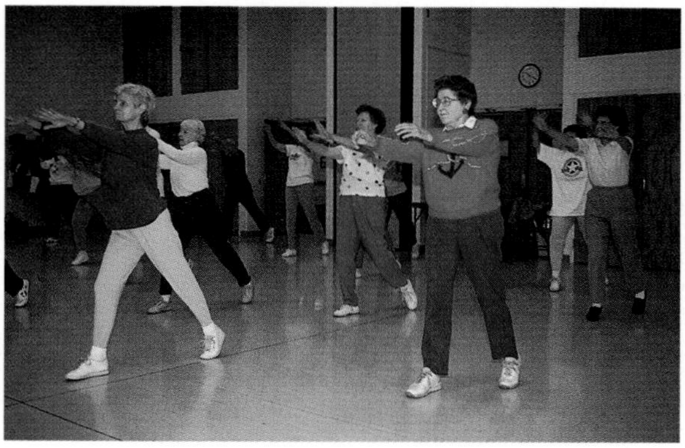

Fig. 7-5 An adult day-care center.

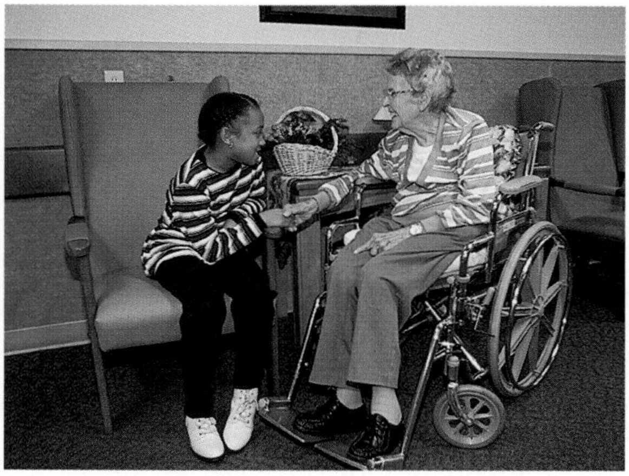

Fig. 7-6 An older adult and young child interact together.

Requirements vary. Some require that the person be able to walk, using a cane or walker if needed. Others allow wheelchairs. Most require that the person be capable of some self-care activities.

Many activities are available at the center. Examples include cards, board games, movies, crafts, dancing, walks, exercise groups, and lectures (Fig. 7-5). Some provide bowling and swimming opportunities. All activities are supervised. Needed assistance is given.

Some areas have intergenerational day-care centers. Children and older persons are in the same center (Fig. 7-6). Both groups benefit. The elders and children work together on some activities. They eat together and play together. Young children bring out much joy and caring in older persons, whether healthy, ill, or disabled. The children give older persons purpose, love, and affection. In turn, children learn about aging. They also receive love and affection from older persons.

Small rural communities may not have access to adult day-care programs. Home care services may also be limited in some areas.

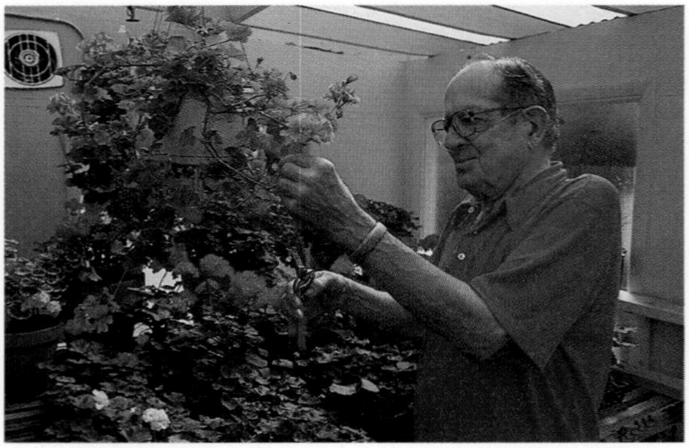

Fig. 7-7 This man enjoys gardening.

Apartments

Apartments have some advantages for older persons. The owner is responsible for maintenance, yard work, snow removal, and major appliances. Older persons are still independent. They can keep personal belongings. However, rent and utility bills are costly expenses. Many older persons enjoy gardening and yard work (Fig. 7-7). Apartment living usually does not provide those opportunities.

Residential Hotels

Some cities have residential hotels. Private rooms or efficiency apartments are rented. Food services may include a dining room, cafeteria, or room service. Some provide recreational activities and emergency medical services. Most hotels are close to shopping areas, churches, and other civic services. The disadvantages of residential hotels and apartments are similar disadvantages.

Senior Citizen Housing/ Congregate Housing

In many areas, state and federal funds were used to build housing for senior citizens. Older people can live independently in an apartment near others of the same age. Buildings have wheelchair access, handrails, elevators, and other safety measures. Some apartments are furnished. Appliances are placed to meet the special needs of older persons.

Many services are available. A dining area and a nurse or doctor on call are common. A daily telephone call is made to check on each tenant. Transportation usually is available to church, the doctor, or shopping areas. Tenants pay monthly rent. If government funds are involved, rent usually is less than that for a regular apartment.

Personal Care Boarding Homes

Personal care boarding homes provide lodging, meals, laundry, supervision, and some help with personal needs. Residents have their own room but not an apartment. They share common areas and eat meals together. Homes vary in size. Some have 4 residents. Others have 30 or more residents. The care provided and government regulation vary from state to state. Residents pay monthly rent. Some board-and-care homes also receive government funds.

Adult foster care. These board-and-care homes provide assistance for as many as four functionally disabled adults. Care is given in the provider's own home. Developmentally disabled persons (see Chapter 28) and mentally ill persons (see Chapter 26) are served. So are frail, older persons.

Services include lodging, meals, laundry, and help with shopping and transportation. Caregivers also make sure that residents get needed medical attention. Adult foster homes provide a family-like setting. They serve both private pay and state-funded residents. They are usually licensed by the state.

Nursing Centers

Nursing centers are housing options for older persons who cannot care for themselves (see Chapter 1). Nursing centers offer different levels of care. Assisted-living centers provide merely room, food, and laundry services. Others centers provide nursing, rehabilitation, dietary, recreational, social, and religious services.

Some people stay in nursing centers for the rest of their life. Others stay until they can return home. The nursing center is the person's temporary or permanent home. The surroundings are made as homelike as possible (Fig. 7-8).

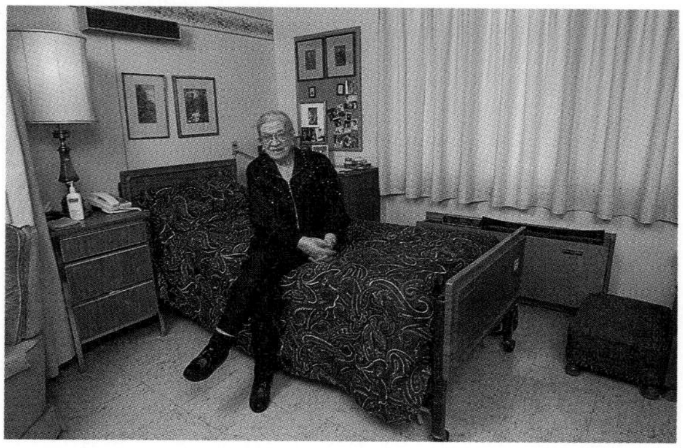

Fig. 7-8 The atmosphere of a nursing center is as homelike as possible.

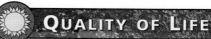

Nursing centers are designed to meet the special needs of older and disabled persons. Physical changes of aging and the safety needs of older persons are considered in the center's design and construction. The following features are desirable in a nursing center:

- Elevators or a one-level building
- Spacious and uncluttered areas
- Handrails along hallways
- Adequate lighting without shadows or glares
- Carpeted or not heavily waxed floors
- Pleasant landscaping
- Variations in the use of color
- Acoustics for noise control
- Ventilation for control of odors
- Smoke detectors and a sprinkling system
- Emergency exits
- Windows with a pleasant view of the outdoors

Many centers have independent living units. These are small apartments. They are occupied by older persons living alone or by older couples. Tenants take care of themselves and take their own medicine. Food services are available. Help is nearby if needed. Little supervision or assistance is needed.

Many hospitals have long-term care units. They are for persons who still need skilled care but not at the level once required. Some eventually go home. Others transfer to nursing centers.

OBRA

Most nursing centers receive Medicare or Medicaid funds. Such centers must meet OBRA requirements (see Chapters 1 and 2). OBRA protects the resident's rights and sets standards to promote quality of life. Funding is lost if requirements are not met. Unannounced surveys are conducted to determine if nursing centers are meeting OBRA requirements.

Quality of Life

Moving to a nursing center can renew feelings of loneliness and isolation. Making new friends helps residents adjust to the center and improves their quality of life. Most residents develop new social relationships at the center. Others avoid social contacts. Some people are quiet, private persons. You need to respect their wishes for privacy. Some residents cannot visit with friends or get to activities without assistance. Offer to take them to visit in a friend's room or to a special activity. Those trying to cope with many losses may find it hard to talk to others. Encourage the person to talk about the losses. He or she may find that other residents have similar losses.

Urinary frequency or incontinence may cause older persons to avoid social activities. They are taken to the bathroom before the event or visit or given incontinent briefs (see Chapter 16). People usually need to feel good about their appearance before feeling comfortable with others. Help residents with grooming (shaving, make-up, hair). Help them to dress in clothes of their choosing. Make sure that dentures, eyeglasses, and hearing aids are in place.

Review Questions

Circle the BEST answer.

1 People between the ages of 65 and 85 are
A Young-old
B Old
C Old-old
D Elderly

2 The study of the aging process is called
A Geriatrics
B Dysphagia
C Gerontology
D Dyspnea

3 Retirement usually results in
A Lower income
B Physical changes from aging
C Less free time
D Financial security

4 Which does *not* cause loneliness in older persons?
A Children have moved away
B Difficulty communicating with others
C Relatives and friends have died or moved
D Contact with family and friends

5 When older persons live with their children, they often feel
A Independent
B Wanted and a part of things
C Useless
D Dignified

6 Death of a partner results in the loss of a
A Friend
B Companion
C Lover
D All of the above

7 Skin changes occur during aging. Care should include all of the following *except*
A Providing lap robes for warmth
B Applying lotion
C Using soap daily
D Providing good skin care

8 An older person has cold feet. You should
A Provide socks
B Apply a hot water bottle
C Soak the feet in hot water
D Apply a heating pad

9 Changes occur in the musculoskeletal system. Which is *false?*
A Bones become brittle and can break easily.
B Bedrest is needed because of loss of strength.
C Joints become stiff and painful.
D Range-of-motion exercises slow the rate of musculoskeletal changes.

10 Changes occur in the nervous system. Which is *true?*
A More sleep is needed than when younger.
B Recent events are remembered better than past events.
C Sensitivity to pain is reduced.
D Confusion occurs in every older person.

11 Changes occur in the eye. Which is *false?*
A Night vision is decreased.
B Blue and green colors are the easiest colors to see.
C Eyelids thin and wrinkle.
D The eye is easily irritated by dust.

12 Common causes of hearing loss in older persons include the following *except*
A Changes in the auditory nerve
B Atrophy of the eardrums
C Impacted ear wax
D Ear infections

13 Arteries narrow and lose their elasticity. These changes result in
A A slower heart rate
B Lower blood pressure
C Less blood in the body
D Poor circulation to many parts of the body

14 An older person has cardiovascular changes. Care should include the following *except*
- A Placing personal items in a convenient location
- B A moderate amount of daily exercise
- C Planning activities to avoid exertion
- D Walking long distances

15 Respiratory changes occur with aging. Which is *false?*
- A Heavy bed linens prevent normal chest expansion.
- B Frequent turning and repositioning are necessary for the person on bedrest.
- C The side-lying position is the best for breathing.
- D The person should be as active as possible.

16 Older persons should avoid dry foods because of
- A Decrease in saliva
- B Loss of teeth or ill-fitting dentures
- C Decreased amount of digestive juices
- D Decreased peristalsis

17 Changes occur in the digestive system. The older person should avoid the following *except*
- A Fruits and vegetables with skin and seeds
- B Dry and fatty foods
- C Raw apricots and celery
- D Protein foods

18 Changes occur in the urinary system. Which is *true?*
- A Kidneys increase in size.
- B Fluids are important for kidney function.
- C The bladder becomes larger.
- D There is increased blood flow to the kidneys.

19 The doctor has ordered an increased fluid intake for an older resident. You should
- A Give most of the fluid before noon
- B Give most of the fluid before 1700
- C Offer only water
- D Start a bladder training program

20 Which housing option does *not* allow older persons to live independently?
- A Apartments
- B Residential hotels
- C Senior citizen housing
- D A nursing center

21 Changes occur in the female reproductive system. Which is *true?*
- A Vaginal walls become thinner and dryer.
- B Estrogen levels increase.
- C Ovaries increase in size.
- D The ability to reproduce continues.

22 Changes occur in the male reproductive system. Which is *false?*
- A Testosterone levels decrease.
- B The testes are smaller.
- C Erection develops more slowly.
- D The prostate gland decreases in size.

Answers to these questions are on p. 696.

8 Safety

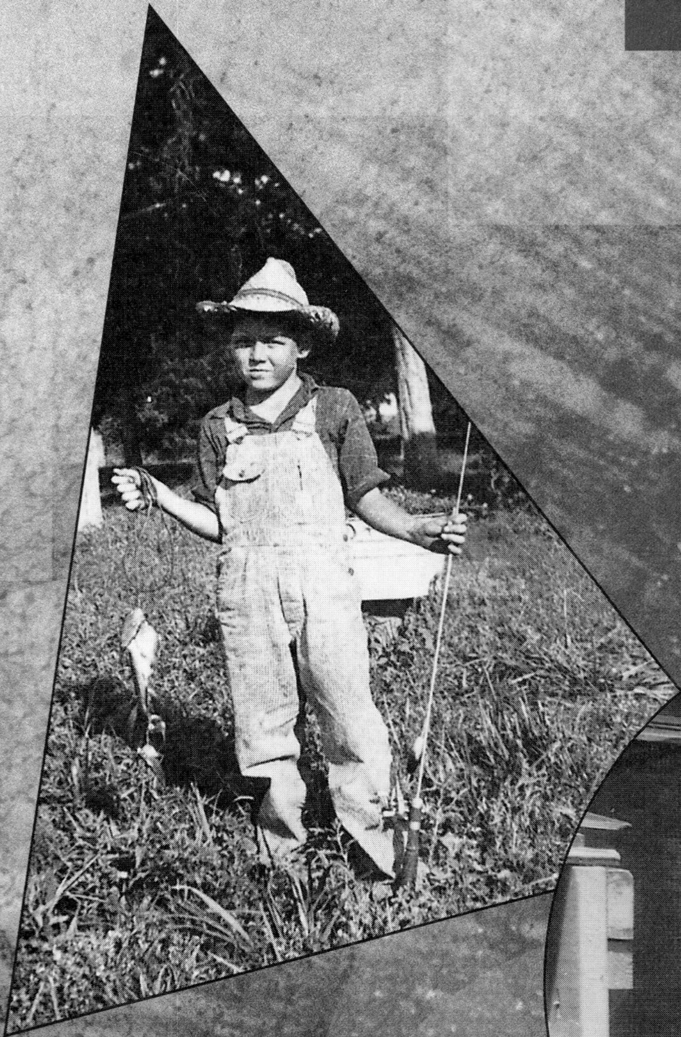

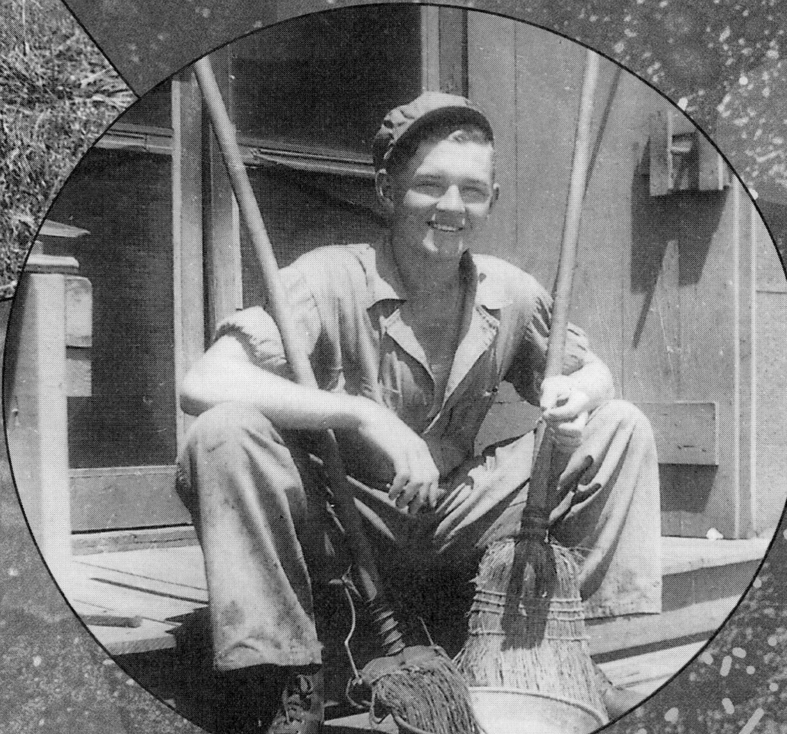

What You Will Learn

- The definition of the key terms listed in this chapter
- Why some persons are at risk for accidents
- Common safety hazards in nursing centers
- The safety measures for preventing falls, burns, poisoning, and suffocation
- Why residents are identified before receiving care and how to accurately identify them
- How to prevent equipment accidents
- The purpose and complications of restraints and how to use them safely
- Restraint alternatives
- How to handle hazardous substances
- The safety measures related to fire prevention and the use of oxygen
- What to do if there is a fire
- Examples of natural and man-made disasters
- How to report accidents and errors
- How to protect yourself from workplace violence
- Your role in risk management
- The procedures described in this chapter

Key Terms

active physical restraint A restraint attached to the person's body and to a stationary (nonmovable) object; movement and access to one's body are restricted

coma A state of being unaware of one's surroundings and being unable to react or respond to people, places, or things

dementia A set of chronic signs and symptoms in which a person loses memory and the ability to think and reason

disaster A sudden catastrophic event in which many people are injured and killed and property is destroyed

ground That which carries leaking electricity to the earth and away from an electrical appliance

hazardous substance Any chemical that presents a physical hazard or a health hazard in the workplace

hemiplegia Paralysis on one side of the body

paraplegia Paralysis from the waist down

passive physical restraint A restraint near but not directly attached to the person's body; it does not totally restrict freedom of movement and allows access to certain body parts

quadriplegia Paralysis from the neck down

restraint Any item, object, device, garment, material, or chemical that restricts a person's freedom of movement or access to one's body

suffocation When breathing stops from the lack of oxygen

Safety is a basic need of everyone. Awareness of safety needs is very important in nursing centers. Nursing center residents are at great risk for falls. For many, the fall results in serious injury. People tend to fall when ill or physically impaired. Some accidents and injuries cause death. Therefore the health care team must know and address the safety risks faced by residents.

You and the entire health care team are responsible for resident safety. Accidents are prevented by focusing on the environment, proper equipment, movement training, personal safety, and medication management. You must practice ordinary and sometimes extraordinary precautions to keep residents safe. The goal is to minimize the resident's risk of accidents and injuries without limiting mobility and independence. However, you must not interfere with the resident's rights as outlined by OBRA (see Chapter 1).

OBRA

OBRA and JCAHO standards require that nursing centers follow safety policies and procedures. These are designed to keep residents, visitors, and staff safe. You play a key role in resident safety. The procedures in this book will help you provide safe care.

THE SAFE ENVIRONMENT

Every staff member is responsible for providing a safe environment. A safe environment is one in which a resident has a very low risk of illness or injury. The person feels safe and secure, both physically and mentally. The risk of infection, falls, burns, poisoning, or other injuries is low. Temperature and noise are at comfortable levels. Smells are pleasant. There is enough lighting and room to move about safely. The person is not afraid and has few worries and concerns.

ACCIDENT RISK FACTORS

Some residents cannot protect themselves. Age, impaired vision or hearing, reduced awareness, and limited mobility are some factors. To provide for safety, you need to know the factors that increase a resident's risk of accidents.

Age

Most residents are elderly. They are at risk for accidents because of changes in their bodies from aging and chronic illness. They have decreased strength and move slowly. Some are unsteady. If balance is affected, they may fall easily. These changes prevent quick and sudden movements to avoid dangers. Other factors make older persons prone to accidents and injuries. These include decreased sensitivity to heat and cold, poor vision, hearing problems, and a dulled sense of smell.

RESIDENTS WITH DEMENTIA

Some persons suffer from dementia. **Dementia** is a set of chronic signs and symptoms in which a person loses memory and the ability to think and reason (see Chapter 27). It is caused by diseases and injuries. Persons with dementia are confused and disoriented and have a reduced awareness of their surroundings. Persons with dementia, especially those who are older, are very prone to accidents and injury. They are dangerous to themselves because of poor judgment. They no longer know what is safe and what is dangerous. They may access closets, cupboards, or other unsafe and unlocked areas. They may eat or drink cleaning chemicals, medicines, or other poisons. They depend on the health care team for all their safety needs.

Awareness of Surroundings

People need to know their surroundings to protect themselves from injury. Some residents are totally unaware of their surroundings. These residents are unconscious or in a coma. **Coma** is defined as a state of being completely unaware of one's surroundings and unable to react or respond. It is caused by illness or injury. A person in a coma cannot react or respond to people, places, or things. This person must rely on you and others for protection. *(See Residents With Dementia.)*

Agitated and Aggressive Behavior

Some residents have agitated and aggressive behaviors. Causes include confusion, pain, decreased awareness of surroundings, and fear of what may happen. These residents are at risk for accidents. They also may put other residents at risk. The health care team must provide a safe environment for these residents (see Chapter 27). Planning is done during a resident care conference.

Impaired Vision

Persons with poor vision have difficulty seeing objects. They are in danger of falling or tripping over equipment, furniture, or electrical cords. They also may have problems reading container labels. They may think that perfume, aftershave lotion, hand lotion, or cleaning agents are substances to eat and drink.

Impaired Hearing

Residents with impaired hearing may have problems hearing warning signals or fire alarms. They may not hear approaching meal carts, medicine carts, or residents in wheelchairs. All staff must make sure that hearing-impaired persons are out of the way when moving carts, wheelchairs, or other equipment through hallways.

Smell and Touch

Illness and aging affect the senses of smell and touch. When smell is reduced, a person may not detect smoke or gas fumes. When touch is reduced, burns are a risk. The person has difficulty sensing the difference between heat and cold. Some residents have a decreased pain sense. They can injure themselves without knowing it. For example, a resident with new shoes develops a blister without feeling it. If the person has poor circulation to the legs and feet, the blister can become a more serious wound.

Impaired Mobility

Some residents have disabling diseases or injuries that make it impossible to move out of danger. Some persons with arthritis cannot walk or propel wheelchairs. Some residents are paralyzed. **Paraplegia** is paralysis from the waist down. **Quadriplegia** is paralysis from the neck down. Persons with **hemiplegia** are paralyzed on one side of the body. These people may be unable to sense pain, heat, or cold. They may be aware of their surroundings and danger but cannot physically move to safety. Part of your job is to keep them safe.

Medications

Drugs can affect people in many ways. This is especially true of older persons. Side effects include loss of balance, reduced awareness, confusion, disorientation, drowsiness, and lack of coordination. These changes may cause the resident to be fearful and uncooperative. Report any changes in a resident's behavior to the nurse. Also report any resident complaint to the nurse.

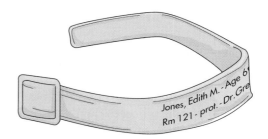

Fig. 8-1 Resident identification bracelet.

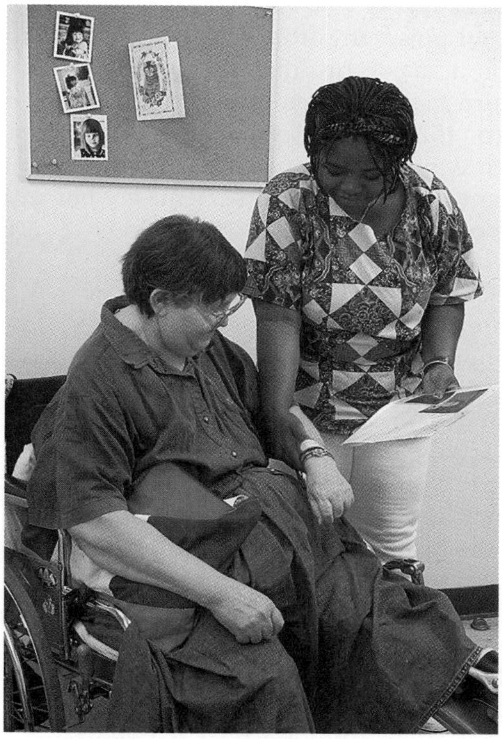

Fig. 8-2 The resident's ID bracelet is compared with the assignment sheet to accurately identify the resident.

SAFETY IN THE NURSING CENTER

Providing a safe setting for residents is the responsibility of the entire health care team. You must properly identify residents so that they receive the right care and treatment. You must be alert to safety hazards that can cause poisoning, burns, suffocation, infection, and falls. If you cannot correct a safety hazard, promptly tell the nurse.

Identifying Residents

You will care for several residents. Each has different treatments, therapies, and activity limits. You must protect residents from infections, falls, and equipment-related accidents. Safety also involves giving the right care to the right person. A resident's life and health are threatened if the wrong care is given.

Most residents receive identification (ID) bracelets when admitted to the center. The resident's name, room and bed number, age, religion, doctor, center name, and other identifying information are shown on the bracelet (Fig. 8-1).

The ID bracelet is used to identify the resident before giving care (Fig. 8-2). Also call the resident by name while checking the ID bracelet. Calling the resident by name is a courtesy that is given as the person is being touched and before providing care. However, calling the resident by name is not a reliable way to identify the resident. Confused, disoriented, drowsy, or hearing-impaired residents may respond to any name.

Residents who are alert and oriented may choose not to wear an ID bracelet. The resident's refusal to wear an ID bracelet is noted on the care plan. Follow center policy and the resident's care plan to accurately identify the resident.

Some nursing centers have identification systems that use photographs. The resident's photograph is taken at admission. The photograph is placed in his or her medical record for identification purposes. If your center uses such a system, you must learn to use it safely.

Preventing Poisoning

Accidental poisoning from poor vision or mental confusion is a major health hazard in nursing centers. Make sure that residents cannot reach hazardous materials (p. 152). Follow center policy and procedures for storing personal care items (mouthwash, lotion, deodorant, and others). These items are harmful when swallowed.

Preventing Burns

Burns are a leading cause of death, especially among children and older persons. Smoking, spilled hot liquids, electrical appliances, and very hot bath water are common causes of burns in nursing centers.

The following safety measures can prevent burns:

- Be sure residents smoke only in smoking areas.
- Do not leave smoking materials at the bedside unless the resident can be trusted to smoke alone and only in smoking areas. Check the resident's care plan.
- Supervise the smoking of residents who cannot protect themselves.
- Do not allow smoking in bed.
- Do not allow smoking near oxygen tanks or concentrators (p. 153).
- Check equipment for frayed cords and proper operation (p. 157).
- Do not use resident-owned electrical items until they are safety checked. This is done by the maintenance department.
- Do not allow space heaters in resident rooms or recreational areas.
- Do not allow residents to sleep with heating pads.
- Do not use electric blankets.
- Check the temperature of the bath water before assisting the resident into the tub (Fig. 8-3).

A

B

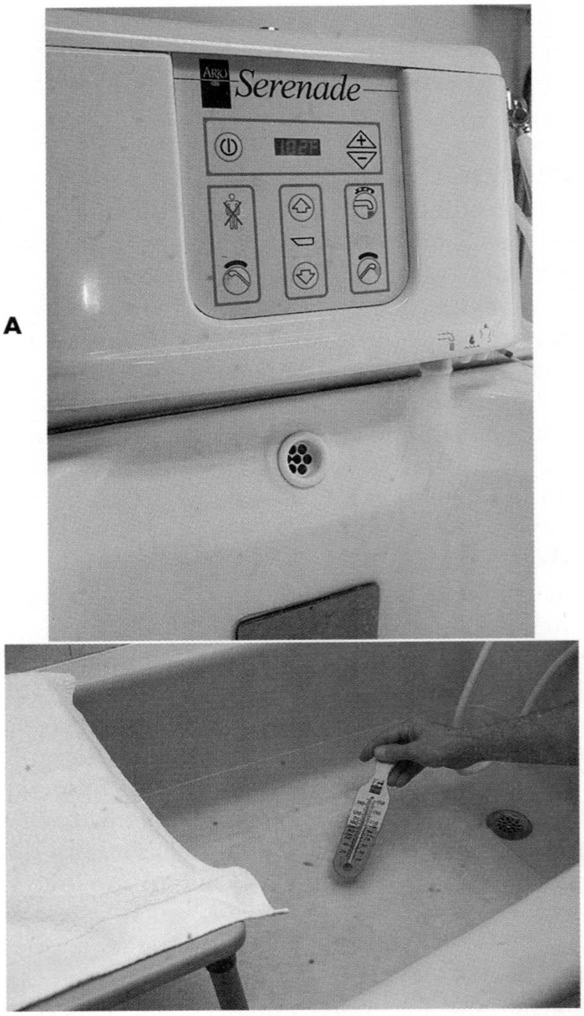

Fig. 8-3 **A,** This digital display shows bath water temperature. **B,** The nursing assistant use a bath thermometer to check bath water temperature.

Preventing Suffocation

Suffocation is the termination of breathing that results from lack of oxygen. Death occurs if the person does not start breathing again. Common causes include choking on an object, drowning, inhaling gas or smoke, strangulation, and electrical shock. Carbon monoxide poisoning results from a lack of oxygen. The person breathes in air filled with carbon monoxide rather than oxygen. Faulty exhaust systems on cars and damaged furnaces are common causes of carbon monoxide poisoning. The following safety measures can help prevent suffocation:

- Cut food into small, bite-size pieces for residents who cannot do so themselves.
- Be sure dentures are in place.
- Make sure the resident can properly chew and swallow the food served.
- Report loose teeth or dentures to the nurse.
- Check the resident's care plan for swallowing problems before giving between-meal snacks or beverages. Some residents ask for items that they cannot swallow.
- Tell the nurse immediately if a resident is having difficulty swallowing.

- Do not give oral foods and fluids to residents with feeding tubes (see Chapter 18).
- Never leave a resident unattended in the bathtub.
- Move all residents from the area if you smell gas or smoke.
- Position residents in bed properly (see Chapter 10).
- Use restraints properly (p. 138).
- Make sure that all electrical cords and appliances are in good repair (p. 137).

Preventing Infection

The spread of infection is a major hazard in health care facilities. Infections are caused by microorganisms that easily spread from one person to another. The older, chronically ill, and disabled persons are at risk for infections. Infections increase their health problems. Good handwashing helps prevent the spread of infection. Chapter 9 describes how to prevent infections.

Preventing Falls

Falls are the most common accidents in nursing centers. The risk of falling increases with age. Most falls are in persons between the ages of 65 and 85. A history of falls increases a person's risk of falling.

Most falls occur in the evening, between 1800 (6:00 PM) and 2100 (9:00 PM). Falls also are more likely during shift changes. Shift changes occur between 0600 (6:00 AM) and 0800 (8:00 AM) and between 1400 (2:00 PM) and 1600 (4:00 PM).

Besides the accident risk factors (p. 130), residents have other problems that increase their risk of falling (Box 8-1). Therefore nursing centers have fall prevention programs. Box 8-2 on p. 134 lists safety measures that help prevent falls. These are part of the center's fall prevention program and the resident's care plan. The care plan also lists measures for the resident's specific risk factors.

Some falls will occur in nursing centers. The health care team must work with the resident and family to decrease the risk of falls without decreasing quality of life. The health care team must make sure the resident's environment is safe. Besides the measures listed in Box 8-2, some common sense measures can greatly reduce the number of falls in nursing centers:

- Keep resident rooms free of clutter.
- Let residents use only wheelchairs, walkers, and canes that work properly. The device must properly fit the individual resident.
- Keep residents properly positioned in beds, chairs, and wheelchairs.
- Use the correct equipment and procedures to move and transfer residents from beds and chairs. Follow the person's care plan.
- Use special cushions to prevent falls (Fig. 8-6 on p. 135). Follow the person's care plan.
- Pay attention to bed and chair alarms. They alert staff when a resident is getting up from a bed or chair. Some alarms are secured to the bed or chair with a cord attached to the resident. The alarm sounds when the cord is pulled. Other alarms are weight sensitive. They sound when the resident's weight is shifted (see Fig. 8-4).
- Check the resident often. Careful and frequent observation by the nursing staff is very important.
- Keep residents involved in meaningful activities.
- Use bed rails and other safety devices as directed. Follow the person's care plan.

Text continued on p. 136

Box 8-1 Factors Increasing the Risk of Falling

- A history of falls
- Weakness
- Slow reaction time
- Poor vision
- Confusion
- Disorientation
- Decreased mobility
- Foot problems
- Shoes that fit poorly
- Elimination needs
- Urinary incontinence
- Dizziness and lightheadedness
- Dizziness on standing
- Joint pain and stiffness
- Muscle weakness
- Low blood pressure
- Balance problems
- Medication side effects
  - Low blood pressure when standing or sitting
  - Drowsiness
  - Fainting
  - Dizziness
  - Poor muscle coordination
  - Unsteadiness
  - Frequent urination
  - Confusion and disorientation
  - Visual impairment
- Excessive alcohol use
- Depression
- Strange surroundings
- Poor judgment
- Memory problems
- Care equipment (e.g., IV poles, drainage tubes and bags)
- Improper use of wheelchairs, walkers, canes, and crutches

Box 8-2 Safety Measures to Prevent Falls

- Good lighting is provided in rooms, hallways, and bathrooms.
- Light switches (including those in bathrooms) are within reach and easy to find.
- Night-lights are placed in bedrooms, hallways, and bathrooms.
- Handrails are on both sides of stairs and hallways. They also are in bathrooms.
- Safety rails and grab bars are in showers and tubs and by the toilet.
- Scatter, area, and throw rugs are not used.
- Floor coverings are one color. Bold designs can cause dizziness in older persons.
- Floors have nonglare, nonslip surfaces.
- Nonskid wax is used on hardwood, tiled, or linoleum floors.
- Floors and stairs are uncluttered. They are free of electrical cords and other items that can cause tripping.
- Floors are free of spills and excess furniture.
- Electric and extension cords are out of the way.
- Furniture is arranged for easy movement.
- Rearranging furniture is avoided.
- Chairs have armrests that give support when sitting and standing.
- A telephone and lamp are at the bedside.
- Tubs and showers have nonslip surfaces or nonslip bath mats.
- Nonskid shoes and slippers are worn. Long shoelaces are avoided.
- Clothing fits properly. Clothing is not loose and does not drag on the floor. Belts are tied or secured in place.
- Fluid needs are met.
- Glasses and hearing aids are worn as needed. Reading glasses are not worn when the resident is up and about.
- The resident is taught how to use the signal light (see Chapter 11).
- The signal light is always within the resident's reach.
- The resident is asked to call for assistance when help is needed to get out of bed or a chair or to walk.
- Signal lights are answered promptly. The resident may need immediate assistance or may not wait for help.
- Frequent checks are made on residents with poor judgment or memory.
- Residents at risk for falling are in rooms close to the nurses' station.
- Companionship is provided. Arrangements are made for sitters, companions, or volunteers to be with the person at risk for falling.
- Electronic warning devices are used. Weight-sensitive alarms for beds and chairs sense when the person tries to get up (Fig. 8-4).
- Explanations are given when medical devices are used and treatments are performed.
- Pillows or wedge pads or seats keep the resident correctly positioned (see Chapter 10).
- Nonslip strips are on the floor next to the bed and in the bathroom.
- The resident is assisted to the bathroom as soon as requested. Or the bedpan, urinal, or commode is provided.
- The resident is assisted to the bathroom, or the bedpan, urinal, or commode is offered at regular times.
- The bedpan, urinal, or commode is kept within easy reach of residents able to use the device without assistance.
- A warm drink, soft lights, or a back massage is used to calm the agitated resident.
- Barriers are used to prevent wandering (Fig. 8-5).
- The bed is in the lowest horizontal position except when giving bedside nursing care. The distance from the bed to the floor is reduced if the resident falls or gets out of bed.
- A mattress or special mat is placed on the floor beside a resident's bed. This reduces the chance of injury if the resident falls or gets out of bed.
- Bed rails are used properly when ordered. They are in the up position when the bed is raised.
- Crutches, canes, and walkers have nonskid tips.
- Wheelchair brakes are in working order.
- Wheels of beds, wheelchairs, and stretchers are locked when transferring residents.
- Caution is used when turning corners, entering corridor intersections, and going through doors. You could injure a resident coming from the other direction.
- A safety check is made of the room after visitors leave. They may have lowered a bed rail, removed the signal light, moved a walker out of reach, or brought an item that could present dangers to the resident.

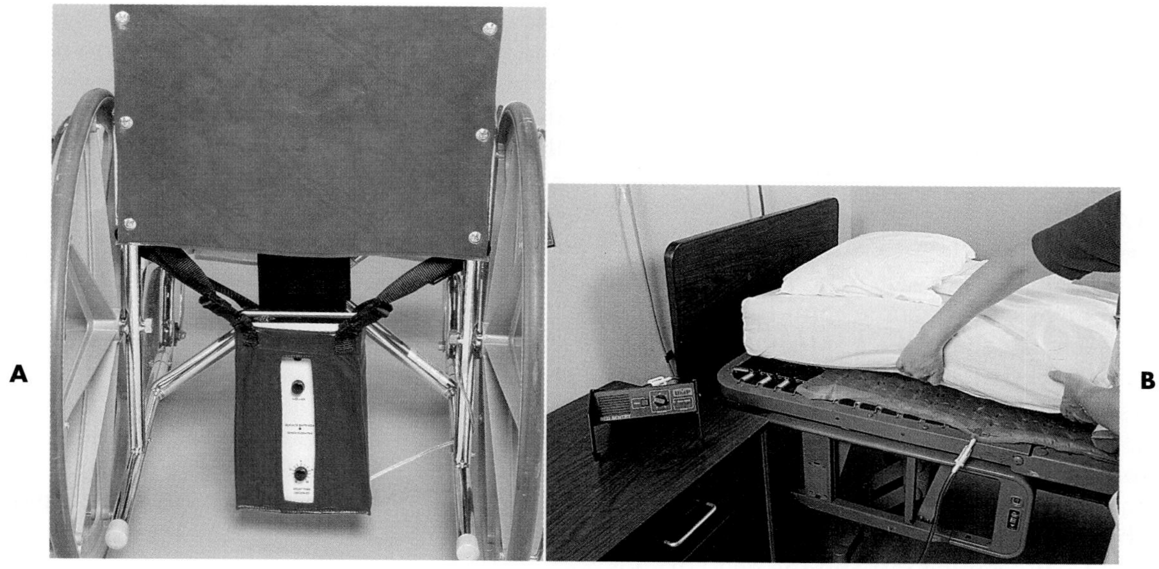

Fig. 8-4 Weight-sensitive alarm. *(**A**, Courtesy J.T. Posey Co., Arcadia, Calif.)*

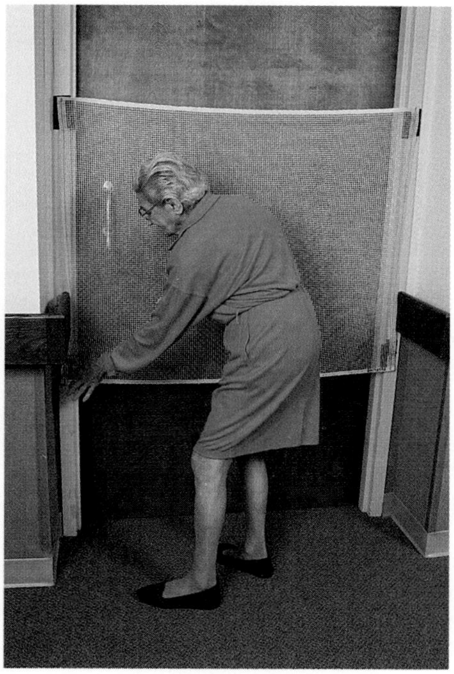

Fig. 8-5 Barriers prevent wandering.

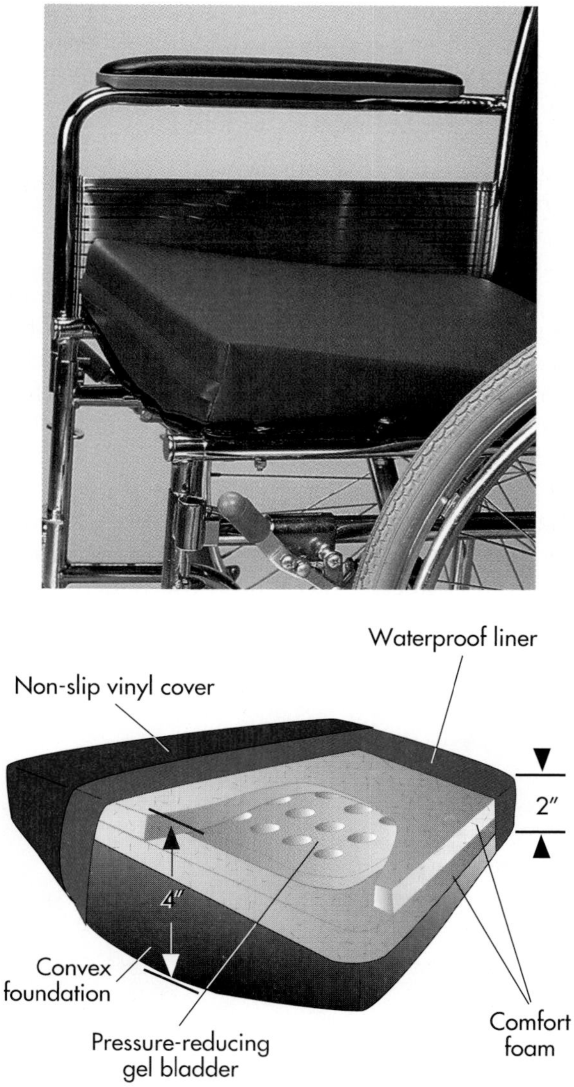

Fig. 8-6 Special cushions prevent falls. *(Courtesy J.T. Posey Co., Arcadia, Calif.)*

Bed rails. Bed rails (side rails) on hospital beds are raised and lowered. They lock in place with levers, latches, or buttons. Bed rails are half, three quarters, or the full length of the bed (Fig. 8-7). Sometimes two rails are placed on each side when half-length rails are used. One is for the upper part of the bed and the other for the lower part.

The nurse tells you when to raise bed rails. They are usually necessary for persons who are unconscious or sedated with medication. Some confused or disoriented residents require them. If a resident requires bed rails, keep the rails up at all times except when giving bedside nursing care.

Bed rails are hazards for residents trying to get out of bed without help. A resident can get caught or entangled in the rail. They also can get caught or entangled in bed rail gaps. Gaps occur between half-length rails and between the rail and the head or foot of the bed. These hazards are great risks for confused, disoriented, and restrained residents (p. 138).

Bed rails prevent residents from getting out of bed. Therefore they are considered restraints under the Omnibus Budget Reconciliation Act of 1987 (OBRA). Using bed rails as a restraint is not allowed unless they are necessary to treat a resident's medical symptoms. Bed rails may be used to increase a resident's mobility. Some residents feel safer with bed rails up. Others use them for changing positions in bed. Under OBRA, the resident or the resident's legal representative must give consent for raised bed rails (p. 140). The need for bed rails must be carefully documented in the resident's record and on the care plan. This law applies to nursing centers and hospital long-term care units.

The Joint Commission on Accreditation of Healthcare Organizations (JCAHO) also has standards for bed rail use in nursing centers. Bed rails are allowed when the resident's clinical condition requires them. The use of bed rails must be in the resident's best interest.

The procedures in this book include using bed rails. This helps you to remember their importance and how to use them correctly. You will know which residents use bed rails from change of shift report, the care plan, and your assignment sheet. If a resident uses his or her rights under OBRA not to have bed rails, they are not used. You can then omit the steps asking you to lower the bed rails at the beginning of the procedure and to raise the bed rails at the end of the procedure. *However, whenever the bed is raised to give care or perform a procedure, the bed rails must be raised to prevent the person from falling. Always explain to the person why bed rails are used.*

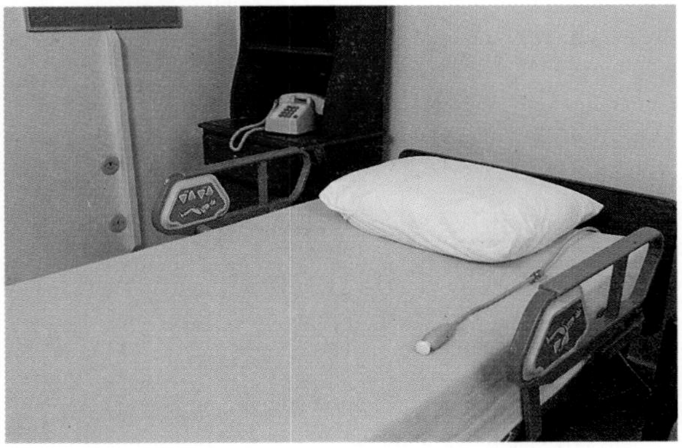

Fig. 8-7 Bed rails.

Hand rails and grab bars. Hand rails are in hallways, stairways, and bathrooms (Fig. 8-8). They provide support for residents who are weak or unsteady when walking. They also provide support for sitting down on or getting up from a toilet. Grab bars are along bathtubs for use in getting in and out of the tub.

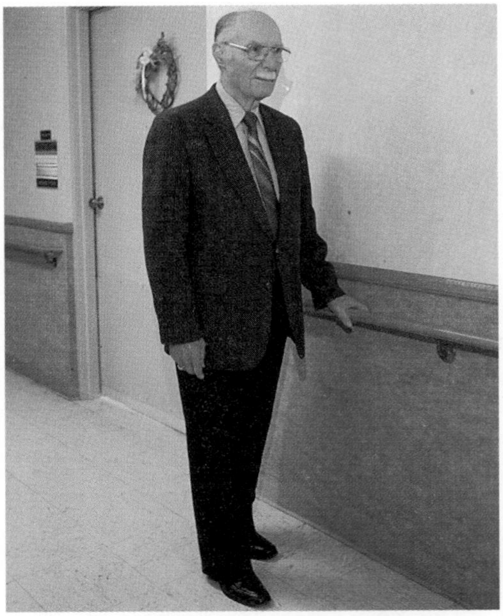

Fig. 8-8 Handrails provide support when walking.

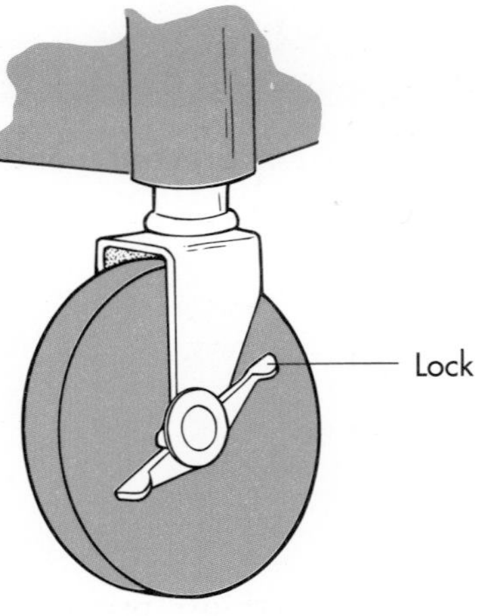

Fig. 8-9 Lock on a bed wheel.

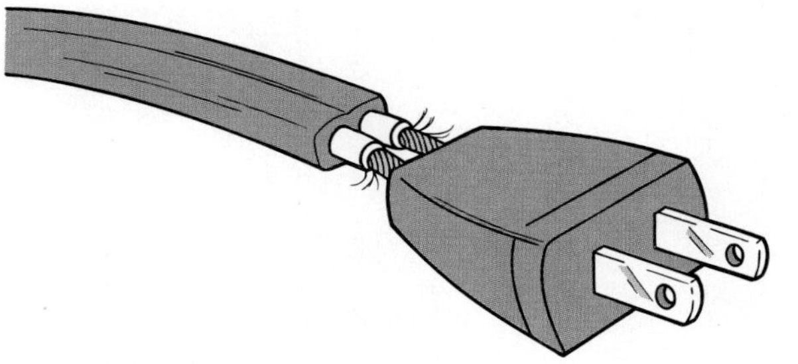

Fig. 8-10 Frayed electrical cord.

Wheel locks. Bed legs have wheels or casters. A caster is a small wheel that lets the bed move easily. Each wheel or caster has a lock to prevent the bed from moving (Fig. 8-9). Lock bed wheels when giving bedside care. Also lock them when you transfer a resident to and from the bed. Wheelchair and stretcher wheels also are locked during transfers. You or the resident can be injured if the bed, wheelchair, or stretcher moves.

Preventing Equipment Accidents

All equipment is unsafe if broken, not used correctly, or not functioning properly. Inspect all equipment before use. Check glass and plastic items for cracks, chips, and sharp or rough edges. All these can cause cuts, stabs, or scratches. Follow the Bloodborne Pathogen Standard (see Chapter 9). Do not use or give damaged equipment to residents.

Electrical equipment must function properly and be in good repair. Frayed cords (Fig. 8-10) and overloaded electrical outlets (Fig. 8-11) can cause electrical shocks. Such shocks can cause death and fires. Frayed cords and broken equipment must be repaired by a trained person.

Three-pronged plugs (Fig. 8-12) are used on all electrical equipment. Two prongs carry electrical current. The third prong is the ground. A **ground** carries leaking electricity to the earth and away from the item. If a ground is not used, leaking electricity can be conducted to a person and cause electrical shocks and possible death. Immediately report any shock received while using a piece of equipment. Send the item for repair immediately.

Warning signs of a faulty electrical item include:

- Shocks
- Loss of power or a power outage
- Dimming or flickering lights
- Sparks
- Sizzling or buzzing sounds
- Burning odor
- Loose plugs

Practice these safety measures when using equipment:

- Follow center policies and procedures.
- Read all caution and warning labels.

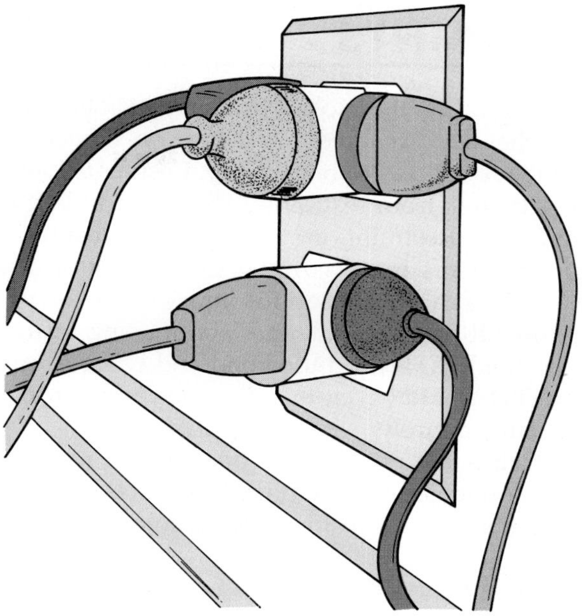

Fig. 8-11 Overloaded electrical outlet.

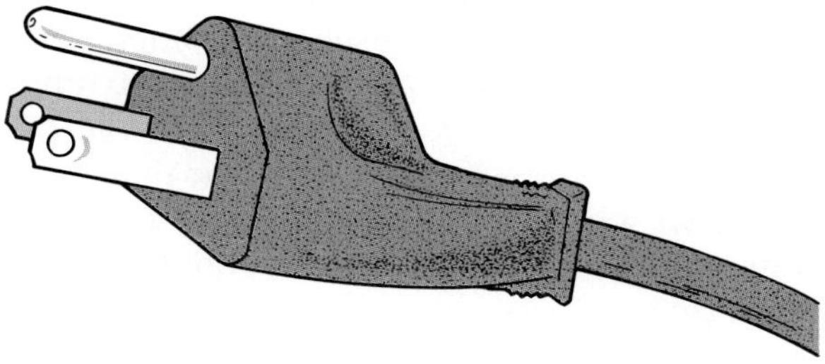

Fig. 8-12 A three-pronged plug.

- Do not use unfamiliar equipment. Ask for needed training. Also ask the nurse to supervise you the first time you use the item.
- Use equipment only for its intended purpose.
- Make sure the item works before you begin.
- Make sure you have all needed equipment. For example, if you need to plug in an item, an outlet must be available.
- Place a "do not use" sticker on broken equipment. Complete a repair request form, and explain the problem.
- Notify the nurse about broken equipment.
- Do not try to repair broken equipment yourself.

An incident report (p. 161) is completed if a resident, visitor, or staff member has an equipment-related accident. The Safe Medical Devices Act requires that nursing centers report equipment-related illnesses, injuries, and deaths.

RESTRAINTS

A **restraint** is any item, object, device, garment, material, or chemical that restricts a person's freedom of movement or access to one's body. Residents have the right to be free from restraints. This is a resident right under OBRA. Restraints are used only as a last resort to protect residents from harming themselves or others.

Restraints can cause serious injury and even death. Therefore OBRA has guidelines about using restraints. So does the JCAHO and the Food and Drug Administration (FDA). However, this does not prevent the use of restraints entirely.

Restraints are not used to discipline a resident or for staff convenience. Discipline is any action that punishes or penalizes a resident. Convenience is any action that:

- Controls the resident's behavior
- Requires less effort by the center
- Is not in the resident's best interests

According to OBRA, restraints are used only when necessary to treat a resident's medical symptoms. Restraints may be necessary to ensure the physical safety of the resident or other persons. That is, residents are protected from harming themselves or others. Certain behaviors can be harmful to the resident or to others in the area. They include:

- Getting out of bed or a chair or wheelchair or off of a stretcher when help is needed
- Crawling over bed rails or the foot of the bed
- Interfering with treatment (pulling out tubes, removing dressings, or disconnecting equipment)
- Wandering in or away from the center
- Behaving in an agitated or combative way toward staff, family, or other persons

Restraints were once used to prevent falls. However, research shows that restraints cause falls. Falls occur when residents try to get free of the restraints. More serious injuries occur from falls in restrained persons than in nonrestrained persons.

Restraints were commonly used for persons who were confused, showed poor judgment, or had behavior problems. Older persons were restrained more often than younger persons. *Now, OBRA requires that all other alternatives must be tried before using restraints.*

Physical and Chemical Restraints

OBRA's legal definition of *physical restraints* includes the following key points:

- May be any manual method, physical or mechanical device, material, or equipment
- Is attached to or next to the person's body
- Cannot be easily removed by the person
- Restricts freedom of movement or access to one's body

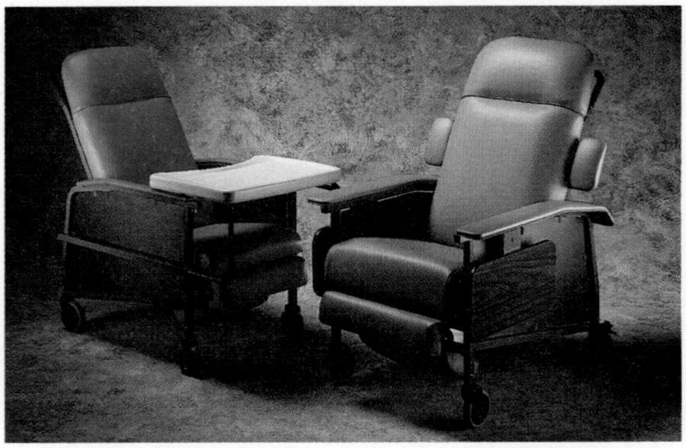

Fig. 8-13 The geriatric chair is a physical restraint. (Courtesy Invacare Corp., Elyria, Ohio.)

A restraint confines the person to a bed or chair or prevents movement of a body part. Restraints are applied to the chest, waist, elbows, wrists, hands, or legs. According to OBRA, certain furniture or barriers also prevent free movement. Geriatric chairs (Geri-chairs) or chairs with attached trays are examples (Fig. 8-13). Such chairs are often used for residents who need support to sit up. Placing any chair so close to a wall that the resident cannot move is another form of restraint. Bed rails are also restraints. So are sheets tucked in so tightly that they restrict movement.

Chemical restraints are drugs used to prevent a certain behavior or movement. OBRA defines chemical restraints as drugs used for discipline or staff convenience and not required for medical treatment. OBRA does not allow the use of chemical restraints. However, drugs may be used to help confused or disoriented residents. These residents may become anxious, agitated, or aggressive. The doctor may order medication to control these behaviors. The goal is to control the behavior without making the resident sleepy and unable to function at his or her highest level. Residents whose behavior cannot be controlled usually are transferred to a facility that can meet their special needs. The safety of all residents must be considered.

Complications of Restraint Use

Box 8-3 lists the many complications from restraint use. Injuries occur as the resident tries to get free of the restraint. Cuts, bruises, and fractures are common injuries. Injuries also occur from using the wrong restraint, applying it wrong, or keeping it on too long. *The most serious risk from restraints is death from strangulation.* There are also mental effects. Being restrained affects a person's dignity and self-esteem. Depression, anger, and agitation are common in restrained persons. So are embarrassment, humiliation, and mistrust.

Restraints are medical devices. The Safe Medical Device Act applies if a restraint causes illness, injury, or death.

Box 8-3 Risks of Restraint Use

- Agitation
- Anal incontinence (see Chapter 17)
- Anger
- Bruises
- Cuts
- Dehydration
- Depression
- Embarrassment
- Fractures
- Humiliation
- Mistrust
- Nerve injuries
- Nosocomial infection (see Chapter 9)
- Pneumonia
- Pressure ulcers (see Chapter 14)
- Strangulation
- Urinary incontinence (see Chapter 16)
- Urinary tract infection

Restraint Alternatives

OBRA OBRA, JCAHO, and the FDA do not forbid the use of restraints. Restraints are allowed only after trying all other alternatives. Box 8-4 lists restraint alternatives. The health care team selects alternatives for the resident's nursing care plan.

Safety Guidelines

If a restraint is used, the least restrictive method is used. Remember the following about using restraints:

- OBRA *Restraints are used to protect the resident. OBRA does not allow the use of restraints for staff convenience.* Restraining a resident is thought to be easier for the staff than properly supervising and observing the resident. Actually, a restrained resident requires more staff time for care, supervision, and observation. A restraint is used only when it is the best safety precaution for the resident. It is not used to punish uncooperative residents.
- OBRA *Restraints require a doctor's order.* OBRA, JCAHO, state laws, and FDA warnings protect persons from unnecessary restraint. Centers must have policies and procedures about restraint use. If a resident needs restraining for medical reasons, a written doctor's order is required. The doctor gives the reason for the restraint, what to use, and how long to use the restraint. This information is on the resident's care plan and your assignment sheet. You need to know the laws and policies about using restraints where you work.

Box 8-4 Alternatives to Restraints

- Diversion activities: television, videos, music, games, books, relaxation tapes, and so on
- Pillows and positioning aids
- Keeping the signal light within reach
- Meeting food, fluid, and elimination needs
- Visits by family, friends, and volunteers
- Arranging for companions and sitters
- Spending time with the resident
- Reminiscing with the resident
- A calm, quiet environment
- Allowing wandering in a safe area
- Exercise programs
- Outdoor time
- Jobs or tasks the resident consents to
- Electronic warning devices on beds and doors
- Measures to prevent falls (see Box 8-2)
- Reclining chairs
- Frequent observation
- Moving the resident closer to the nurses' station
- Explaining all procedures and care measures
- Frequent explanations about required medical equipment or devices
- Orienting confused individuals to person, time, and place; providing calendars and clocks
- Good lighting
- Consistent staff assignments
- Promoting uninterrupted sleep

- *OBRA requires using the least restrictive method.* An **active physical restraint** attaches to the person's body and to a stationary (nonmovable) object. It restricts the person's movement or body access. Vest, leg, arm, wrist, hand, and some belt restraints are active physical restraints. A **passive physical restraint** is near but not directly attached to the person's body. It does not totally restrict freedom of movement and allows access to certain body parts. Passive physical restraints are the least restrictive. OBRA
- *Restraints are used only after trying other methods to protect the resident.* Some people can harm themselves or others. The care plan must include measures to protect the resident and to prevent the resident from harming others. Restraints lessen the resident's dignity. They are allowed only after other measures fail to provide needed protection (see Box 8-4). Many fall prevention measures are restraint alternatives (see Box 8-2).

- *Unnecessary restraint is false imprisonment (see Chapter 2).* If told to apply a restraint, you must clearly understand the need. If not, politely ask about its use. If you apply a restraint unnecessarily, you could face false imprisonment charges.
- *OBRA requires informed consent for restraint use.* The resident must understand the reason for the restraint. The resident is told how the restraint will help the planned medical treatment. The resident is told also about risks of restraint use. If the resident cannot give informed consent, the resident's legal representative is given the information. Either the resident or legal representative must give consent. Restraints cannot be used without consent. The doctor or nurse provides the necessary information and obtains informed consent.
- *The manufacturer's instructions are followed.* The manufacturer gives specific instructions about applying and securing the restraint. Failure to follow the instructions could affect the resident's safety. You could be negligent for improperly applying or securing a restraint.
- *The restrained resident's basic needs are met by the health care team.* The restraint must be snug and firm, but not tight. Tight restraints interfere with circulation and breathing. The resident must be comfortable and able to move the restrained part to a limited and safe extent. OBRA requires checking the resident at least every 15 minutes. Meet food, fluid, comfort, safety, exercise, and elimination needs.
- *Restraints are applied with enough help to protect the resident and staff from injury.* Residents in immediate danger of harming themselves or others are restrained quickly. Combative and agitated people can hurt themselves and the staff when restraints are applied. Enough staff members are needed to complete the task safely and efficiently.
- *Restraints can increase a resident's confusion and agitation.* Whether confused or alert, people are aware of restricted body movements. They may try to get out of the restraint or struggle or pull at it. Many restrained residents beg anyone who passes by to set them free or to help release them. These behaviors are often viewed as signs of confusion. Confusion increases in some persons because they do not understand what is happening to them. Restrained residents need repeated explanations and reassurance. Spending time with them has a calming effect.
- *OBRA requires that the resident's quality of life be protected.* Restraints are used for as short a time as possible. The resident's care plan must show how restraint use is slowly reduced. The goal is to meet the resident's needs using as little restraint as possible. Besides meeting physical needs, you must meet the resident's psychosocial needs. These needs are met by visiting with the resident and explaining the purpose of the restraints.

Restraints are dangerous. Injuries and deaths have occurred from improper restraint use and poor resident observation. *The resident is observed at least every 15 minutes or more often as required by the care plan.* Complications from restraints are prevented, such as interferences with breathing and circulation. Practice the safety measures in Box 8-5 when caring for a restrained person.

Reporting and Recording

Information about restraints is recorded in the resident's medical record. You might apply restraints or care for a restrained resident. To meet OBRA requirements, report the following to the nurse:

- The type of restraint applied
- The reason for the application
- Safety measures taken (e.g., bed rails padded and up)
- The time you applied the restraint
- The time you removed the restraint
- The care given when the restraint was removed
- The color and condition of the resident's skin
- The pulse felt in the restrained extremity
- Complaints of a tight restraint, difficulty breathing, and pain, numbness, or tingling in the restrained part

Text continued on p. 144

Box 8-5 Safety Measures for Using Restraints

- Use the restraint specified by the health care team and the care plan. The least restrictive device is used.
- Apply a restraint only after receiving instruction about its proper use. Demonstrate proper application to the nurse before using it on any resident.
- Use the correct size as instructed by the nurse. Small restraints are tight. They cause discomfort, agitation, restricted breathing, or reduced circulation. Strangulation is a risk from big or loose restraints.
- Use only restraints that have manufacturer's instructions. Read the manufacturer's warning labels. Note the front and back of the restraint.
- Follow the manufacturer's instructions. Some restraints are safe for bed, chair, and wheelchair use. Others are used only with certain equipment.
- Do not use sheets, towels, tape, rope, straps, bandages, or other items to restrain a resident.
- Use intact restraints. Look for tears, frayed edges, missing loops or straps, or other damage.
- Do not use restraints to position a resident on a toilet.
- Follow center policies and procedures when applying restraints.
- Position the resident in good body alignment before applying the restraint (see Chapter 10).
- Pad bony areas and skin to prevent pressure and injury from the restraint.
- Secure the restraint. It should be snug but allow some movement of the restrained part. If the restraint is applied to the chest, make sure that the resident can breathe easily. A flat hand should slide between the restraint and the resident's body (Fig. 8-14, p. 142).
- Criss-cross vest restraints in front (Fig. 8-15, p. 142). Do not criss-cross restraints in the back unless part of the manufacturer's instructions. Criss-crossing vests in the back can cause death from strangulation.
- Tie restraints according to center policy. The policy should follow the manufacturer's instructions. The knot must be easily released in an emergency. Quick-release knots often are used (Fig. 8-16, p. 143). Some restraints have quick-release buckles.
- Secure straps out of the resident's reach.
- Secure the restraint to the movable part of the bed frame or to the bed springs (see Fig. 8-16, p. 143). Never secure restraints to the bed rails. The resident can reach bed rails to release knots or buckles. Also, injury to the resident is likely when raising or lowering bed rails. For chairs, secure straps to the wheelchair or the chair frame (Fig. 8-17, p. 143).
- Pad the bed rails as in Figure 8-18 on p. 143. Padded bed rails prevent the resident from getting caught (entrapment) between the rails (Fig. 8-19, p. 143). Entrapment can occur between:
  - The bars of a bed rail
  - The space between half-length (split) bed rails
  - The bed rail and mattress
  - The headboard or footboard, bed rail, and mattress
- Keep full bed rails up when using a vest or belt restraint if required by the manufacturer's instructions and center policy. If the bed rails are not up, the resident could fall off the bed and strangle on the restraint. Remember to pad bed rails following the manufacturer's instructions and center policy.
- Position the resident in a chair so the hips are well to the back of the chair. If using a belt restraint, apply it at a 45-degree angle over the hips (Fig. 8-20, p. 144).
- Do not use back cushions when a resident is restrained in a chair. If the cushion moves out of place, slack occurs in the straps. Strangulation could result if the resident slides forward or down from the extra slack (Fig. 8-21, p. 144).
- Check the resident's circulation every 15 minutes if wrist or leg restraints are applied. You should feel a pulse at a pulse site below the restraint. Fingers or toes should be warm and pink. Notify the nurse immediately if:
  - You cannot feel a pulse
  - Fingers or toes are cold, pale, or blue in color
  - The resident complains of pain, numbness, or tingling in the restrained part
  - The skin is red or damaged
- Check the resident every 15 minutes for safety and comfort. Also check the position of the restraint, especially in the front and back.
- Keep scissors in your pocket. In an emergency, cutting the tie may be faster than untying the knot. Never leave scissors at the bedside or where the resident can reach them.

Continued

CONT'D BOX 8-5 SAFETY MEASURES FOR USING RESTRAINTS

- Remove the restraint and reposition the resident every 2 hours. Give skin care and perform range-of-motion exercises at this time.
- Meet the resident's basic needs. The resident must have food and fluids. Offer water often to prevent dehydration. Help the resident meet elimination needs at least every 2 hours. Injuries often occur when restrained residents try to go to the bathroom.
- Make sure the signal light is always within the resident's reach.
- Report to the nurse every time the restraint is released. Report your observations made and the care given. Follow center policy for recording.

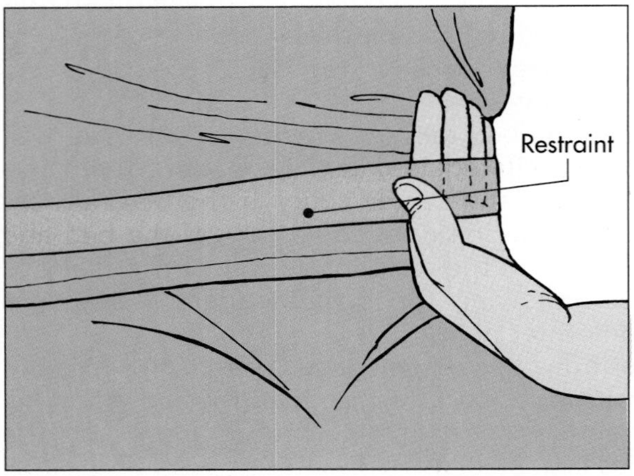

Fig. 8-14 A flat hand should slide between the restraint and the person.

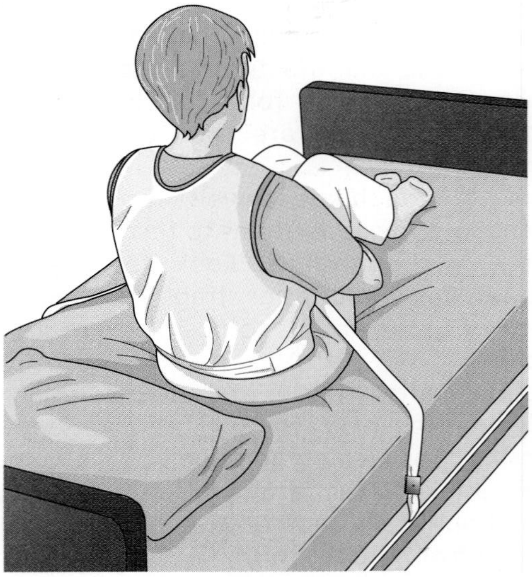

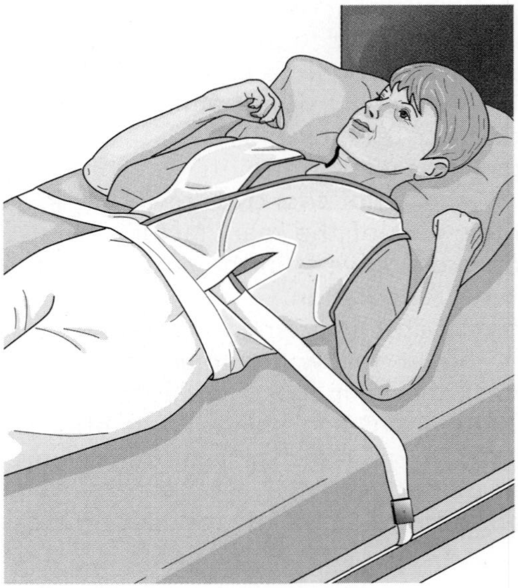

Fig. 8-15 Vest restraint criss-crosses in front.

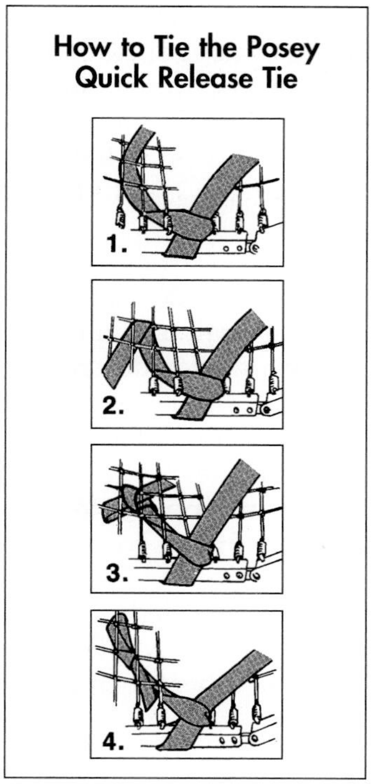

Fig. 8-16 The Posey quick-release tie. *(Courtesy J.T. Posey Co., Arcadia, Calif.)*

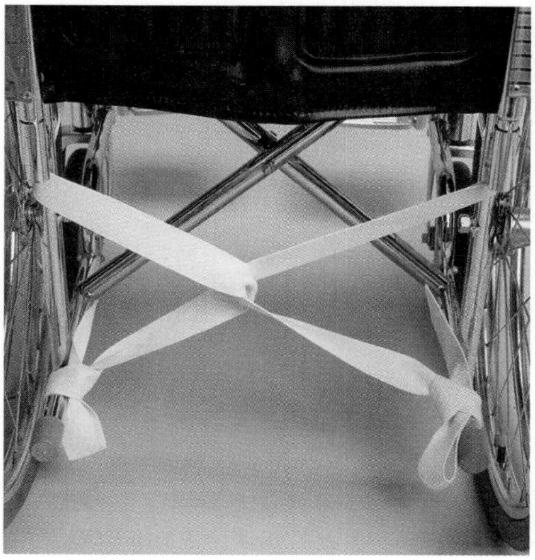

Fig. 8-17 The restraint straps are secured to the wheelchair frame using a quick-release tie. *(Courtesy J.T. Posey Co., Arcadia, Calif.)*

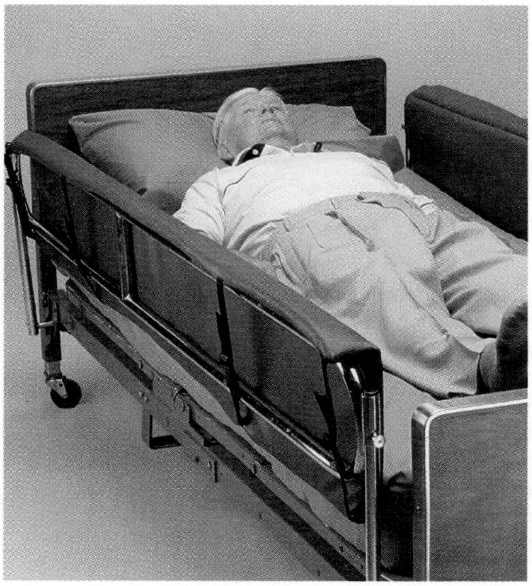

Fig. 8-18 Padded bed rails. *(Courtesy J.T. Posey Co., Arcadia, Calif.)*

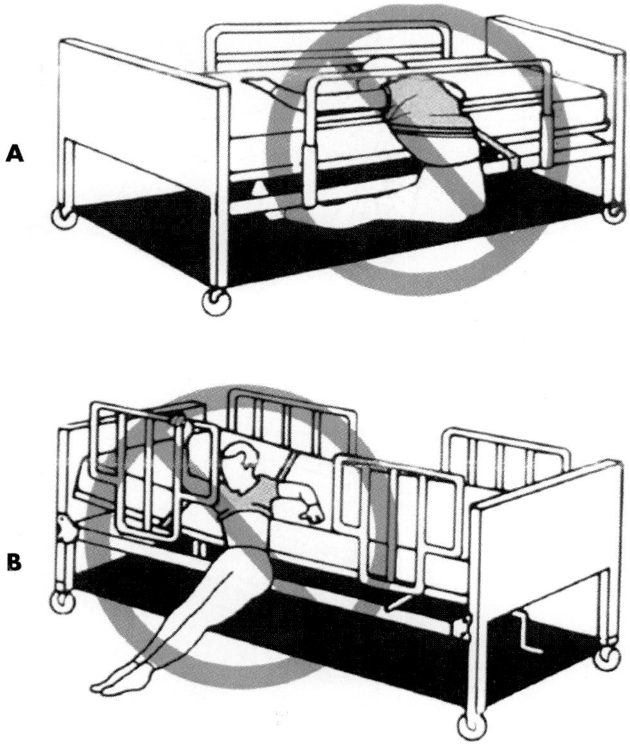

Fig. 8-19 A, The person is caught in the bed rail. **B,** Half-length bed rails are dangerous for the restrained person. *(Courtesy J.T. Posey Co., Arcadia, Calif.)*

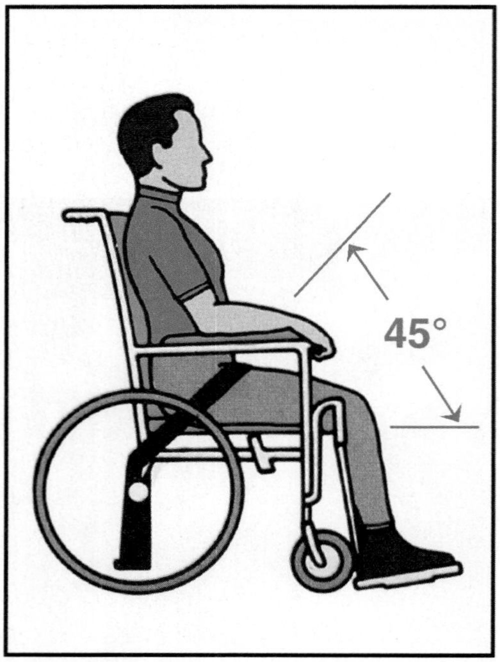

Fig. 8-20 The safety belt is at a 45-degree angle over the person's hips. *(Courtesy J.T. Posey Co., Arcadia, Calif.)*

Types of Restraints

Restraints are made of cloth or leather. Cloth restraints (soft restraints) are belts, straps, and vests. They are applied to the wrists, ankles, hands, waist, and chest. Leather restraints are applied to the wrists and ankles. They are used in extreme cases of resident agitation and combativeness.

◈ Wrist restraints and ankle restraints. These restraints limit the movement of arms and legs. They are often described by their application points:

- *2-point restraints* are applied to two extremities. The wrists are common sites.
- *3-point restraints* are applied to three extremities. They are usually applied to both wrists and one ankle.
- *4-point restraints* are applied to all four extremities. They are applied to both wrists and both ankles.

The nurse tells you where to apply the restraints.

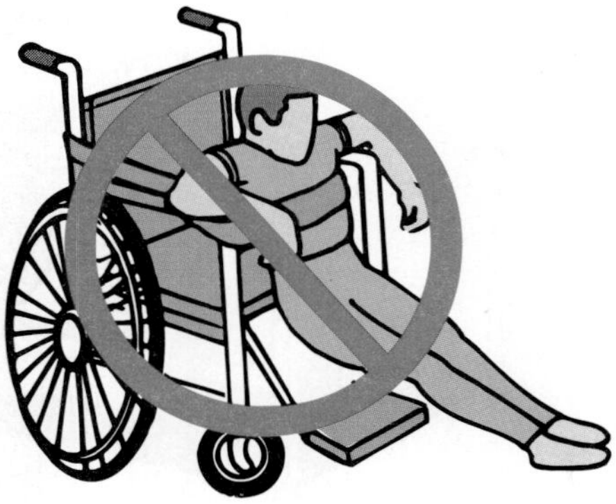

Straps to prevent sliding should always be over the thighs—NOT around the waist or chest. Straps should be at a 45° angle and secured to the chair under the seat, not behind the back. They should be snug but comfortable and not restrict breathing. If a belt or vest is too loose or applied around the waist, the person may slide partially off the seat—resulting in the possible suffocation and death.

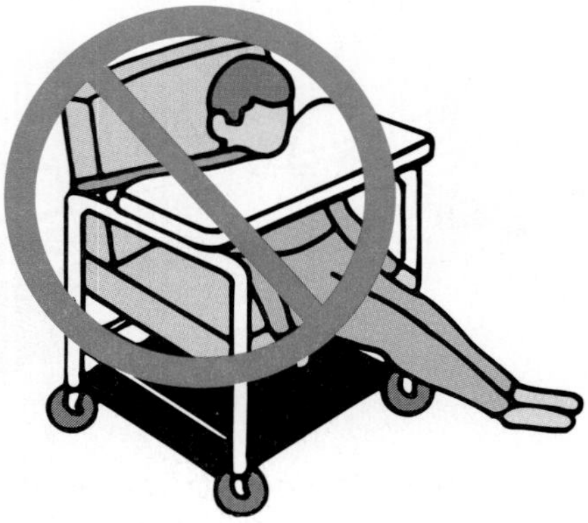

Tray tables (with or without a belt or vest) pose potential danger if the person should slide partly under the table and become caught. This could result in suffocation and death. Make sure the person's hips are positioned at the back of the chair—this may necessitate the use of an anti-slide material (Posey Grip), a pommel cushion, or a restrictive device if the person shows any tendency to slide forward.

Fig. 8-21 Strangulation could result if the person slides forward or down because of the extra slack in the restraint. *(Courtesy J.T. Posey Co., Arcadia, Calif.)*

Applying Wrist and Ankle Restraints

Quality of Life

Remember to:
- ***Knock before entering the resident's room***
- ***Address the resident by name***
- ***Introduce yourself by name and title***

Pre-Procedure

1 Get the number of restraints you need.
2 Wash your hands.
3 Identify the resident. Check the ID bracelet against the assignment sheet.
4 Explain the procedure to the resident.
5 Provide for privacy.

Procedure

6 Make sure the resident is comfortable and in good body alignment (Chapter 10).
7 Apply the restraint following the manufacturer's instructions. Place the soft part toward the skin (Fig. 8-22).
8 Secure the restraint so it is snug but not tight. Make sure that you can slide two fingers under the restraint (Fig. 8-23).
9 Tie the ends to the movable part of the bed frame or to the bed springs. Use an agency-approved knot.
10 Repeat steps 7, 8, and 9 for a 2-point, 3-point, or 4-point application.

Post-Procedure

11 Place the signal light within the resident's reach.
12 Unscreen the resident.
13 Wash your hands.
14 Check the resident and the restraints at least every 15 minutes. Check the pulse, color, and temperature of the restrained parts. Report your observations to the nurse.
15 Do the following at least every 2 hours:
- Remove the restraints.
- Reposition the resident.
- Meet the resident's food, fluids, and elimination needs.
- Give skin care.
- Perform range-of-motion exercises or ambulate the resident. Follow the care plan.
- Reapply the restraints.

16 Report and record your observations and the care given.

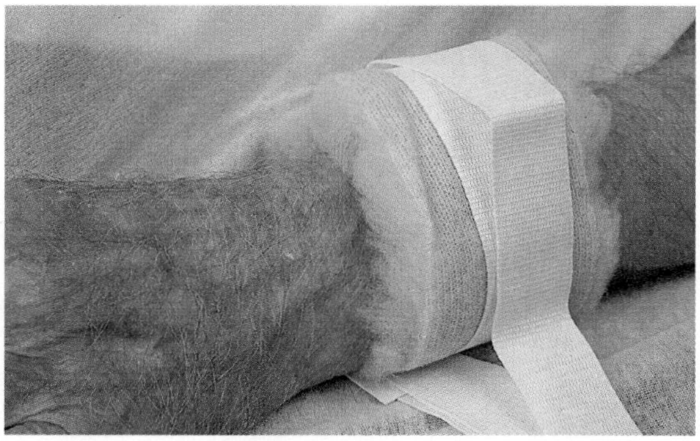

Fig. 8-22 The soft part of the restraint is toward the skin.

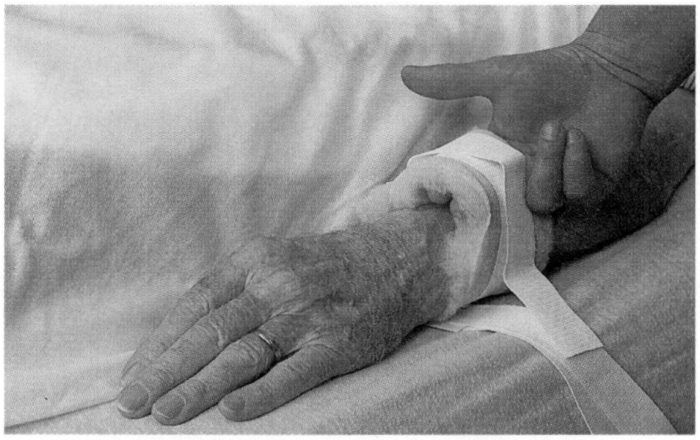

Fig. 8-23 Two fingers should fit between the restraint and the wrist.

Mitt restraints. Hands are placed in mitt restraints. They prevent finger use but do not prevent hand, wrist, or arm movements. Mitt restraints are thumbless and prevent the resident from scratching, pulling out tubes, or removing dressings. The resident holds a hand roll to keep the fingers in a normal position. Hand rolls are not needed with padded mitts (Fig. 8-24).

Applying Mitt Restraints

Quality of Life

Remember to:
- *Knock before entering the resident's room*
- *Address the resident by name*
- *Introduce yourself by name and title*

Pre-Procedure

1 Collect the following equipment:
- Two mitt restraints
- Two washcloths or two commercial hand rolls if the mitts are not padded
- Tape if washcloths are used

2 Make the hand rolls as in Figure 8-25, or use commercial ones.

3 Wash your hands.

4 Identify the resident. Check the ID bracelet against the assignment sheet.

5 Explain the procedure to the resident.

6 Provide for privacy.

Procedure

7 Make sure the resident's hands are clean and dry.

8 Give the resident a hand roll to hold if a padded mitt is not used.

9 Apply the mitt restraint (Fig. 8-26). Follow the manufacturer's instructions.

10 Tie the ends to the movable part of the bed frame or to the bed springs. Use a center-approved knot.

11 Repeat steps 8, 9, and 10 for the other hand.

Post-Procedure

12 Place the signal light within the resident's reach.

13 Unscreen the resident.

14 Wash your hands.

15 Check the resident and the restraints at least every 15 minutes.

16 Do the following at least every 2 hours:
- Remove the restraints.
- Reposition the resident.
- Meet the resident's needs for food, fluids, and elimination.
- Give skin care.
- Perform range-of-motion exercises, or ambulate the resident. Follow the care plan.
- Reapply the restraints.

17 Report and record your observations and the care given.

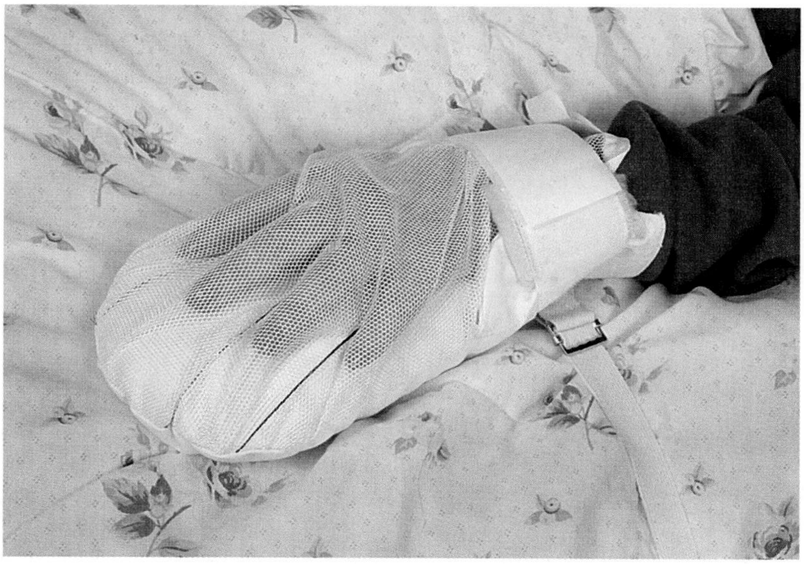

Fig. 8-24 Padded mitt restraint.

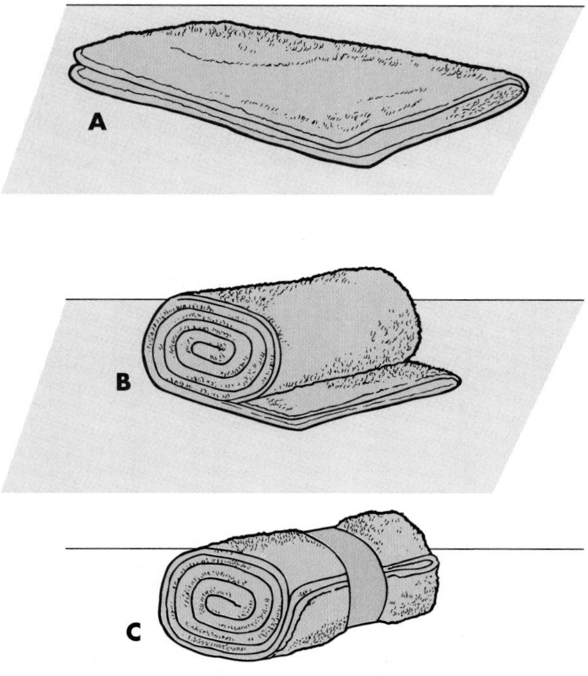

Fig. 8-25 Make a hand roll from a washcloth. **A,** Fold the washcloth in half. **B,** Roll up the washcloth. **C,** Tape the rolled washcloth.

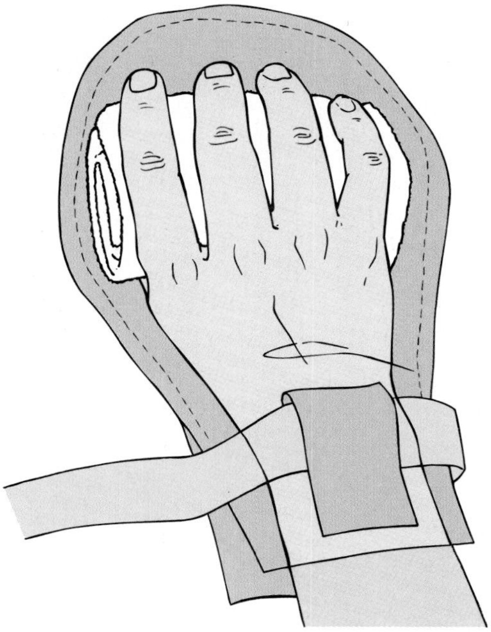

Fig. 8-26 Mitt restraint. The person is holding a hand roll.

◈ **Vest restraints.** Vest restraints are applied to the chest. The resident cannot get out of bed or out of a chair. The resident's arms are put through the sleeves so the vest crosses in front (see Fig. 8-15). *Vest restraints always cross in the front*. The vest must *never* cross in the back. If it crosses in the back, there is only a small neck opening at the front. Strangulation can occur from the small neck opening if the resident slides down in the bed or chair. The restraint is always applied over a gown, pajamas, or clothes.

Vest restraints carry great risks to the resident's life. Death can occur from strangulation. If the resident becomes caught in the restraint, it can become so tight that the resident's chest cannot expand to inhale air. The resident quickly suffocates and dies. Correct application of a restraint is always important. In the case of vest restraints it is critical. Therefore you are advised to only assist the nurse in its application. It is best that the nurse assume full responsibility for the application of a vest restraint.

Applying a Vest Restraint

QUALITY OF LIFE

Remember to:

- ◆ ***Knock before entering the resident's room***
- ◆ ***Address the resident by name***
- ◆ ***Introduce yourself by name and title***

Pre-Procedure

1 Collect the following:
- Vest restraint (the nurse tells you the size)
- Pads for the bed rails

2 Get assistance if needed.

3 Wash your hands.

4 Identify the resident. Check the ID bracelet against the assignment sheet.

5 Explain the procedure to the resident.

6 Provide for privacy.

Procedure

7 Put the pads on the bed rails if the resident is in bed.

8 Assist the resident to a sitting position.

9 Apply the restraint with your free hand. Follow the manufacturer's instructions. Remember, the vest crosses in front.

10 Make sure the vest is free of wrinkles in the front and back.

11 Help the resident lie down if he or she is in bed.

12 Bring the ties through the slots.

13 Make sure the resident is comfortable and in good body alignment (see Chapter 10).

14 Secure the straps to the movable part of the bed frame, the bedsprings, or to the chair or wheelchair. Use a center-approved knot.

15 Slide a flat hand under the restraint (see Fig. 8-14). Adjust the straps as needed so the restraint is snug but not tight.

Post-Procedure

16 Place the signal light within the resident's reach.

17 Raise the bed rails.

18 Unscreen the resident.

19 Wash your hands.

20 Check the resident and the restraint at least every 15 minutes.

21 Do the following at least every 2 hours:
- Remove the restraint.
- Reposition the resident.
- Meet the resident's needs for food, fluids, and elimination.
- Give skin care.
- Perform range-of-motion exercises, or ambulate the resident. Follow the care plan.
- Reapply the restraint.

22 Report your observations to the nurse. Include the care given when the restraint was removed.

Belt restraints. The belt restraint (Fig. 8-27) is used for the same reasons as the vest restraint. The belt is applied around the waist and secured to the bed or chair. It is applied over clothes, a gown, or pajamas. The resident can release the quick-release type. It is less restrictive than those that are released only by a staff member.

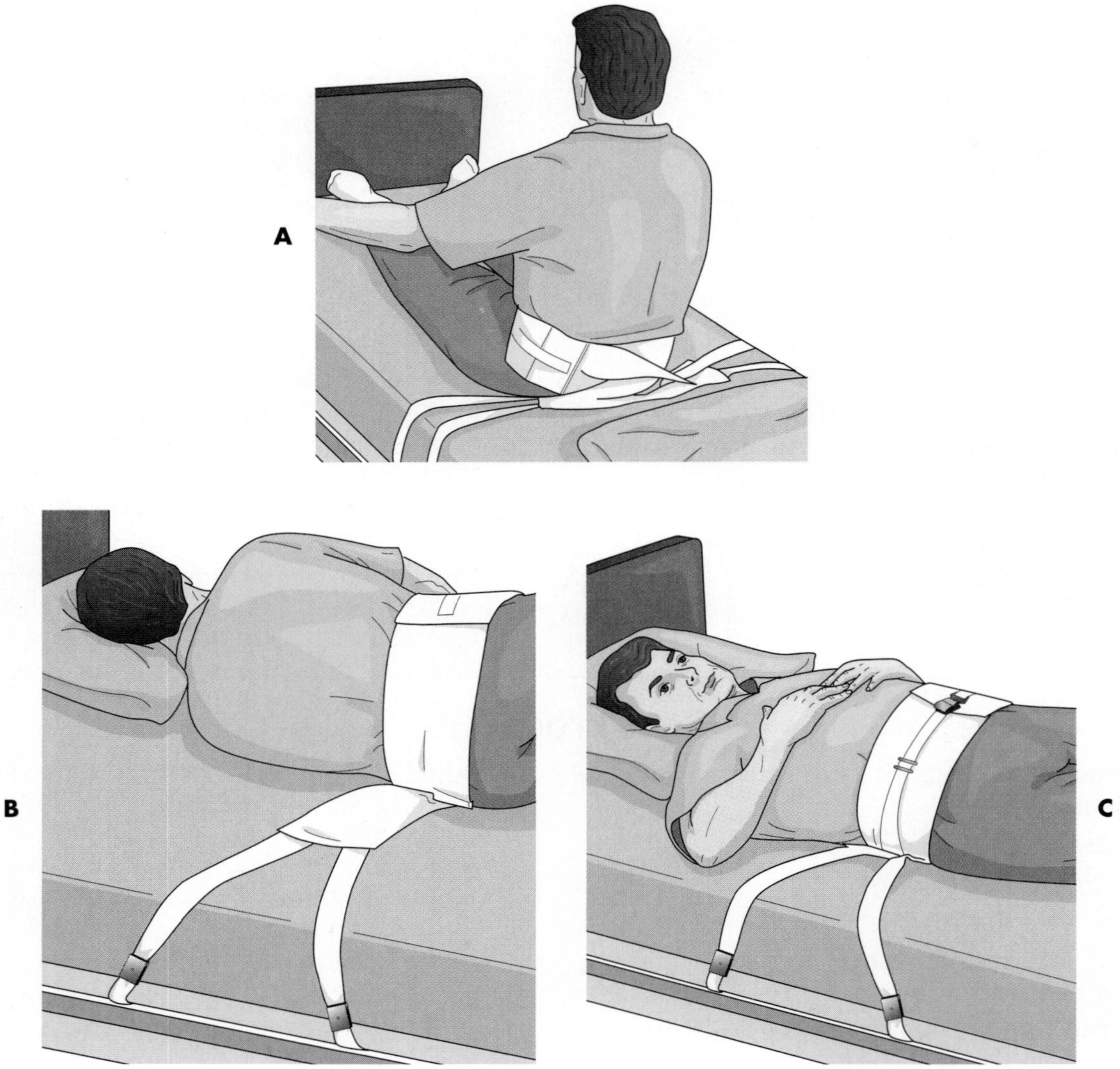

Fig. 8-27 Roll belt.

Applying a Belt Restraint

Quality of Life

Remember to:
- *Knock before entering the resident's room*
- *Address the resident by name*
- *Introduce yourself by name and title*

Pre-Procedure

1 Obtain a belt restraint. The nurse tells you the size.
2 Get help if needed.
3 Wash your hands.
4 Identify the resident. Check the ID bracelet against the assignment sheet.
5 Explain the procedure to the resident.
6 Provide for privacy.

Procedure

7 Assist the resident to a sitting position.
8 Apply the restraint with your free hand. Follow the manufacturer's instructions.
9 Remove wrinkles or creases from the front and back of the restraint.
10 Bring the ties through the slots in the belt.
11 Help the resident lie down if he or she is in bed.
12 Make sure the resident is comfortable and in good body alignment (see Chapter 10).
13 Secure the straps to the movable part of the bed frame, the bed springs, or to the chair or wheelchair. Use a center-approved knot.

Post-Procedure

14 Place the signal light within the resident's reach.
15 Unscreen the resident.
16 Wash your hands.
17 Check the resident and the restraint at least every 15 minutes
18 Do the following at least every 2 hours:
- Remove the restraint.
- Reposition the resident.
- Meet the resident's needs for food, fluids, and elimination.
- Give skin care.
- Perform range-of-motion exercises, or ambulate the resident. Follow the care plan.
- Reapply the restraint.

19 Report and record your observations and the care given.

HANDLING HAZARDOUS SUBSTANCES

The Occupational Safety and Health Administration (OSHA) requires that health care employees understand the risk of hazardous substances and how to handle them safely. A **hazardous substance** is any chemical that presents a physical hazard or a health hazard in the workplace.

Physical hazards can cause fires or explosions. Health hazards are chemicals that can cause acute or chronic health problems. Acute problems occur rapidly and last a short time. They usually occur from a short-term exposure. Chronic problems usually result from long-term exposure and occur over a long period. Health hazards can cause cancer and affect the formation and function of blood cells. They also can damage the kidneys, nervous system, lungs, skin, eyes, or mucous membranes. Birth defects, miscarriages, and fertility problems result from damage to the reproductive system.

Exposure to hazardous substances can occur under normal working conditions or during emergencies. Such emergencies include equipment failures, container ruptures, or the uncontrolled release of a hazard into the workplace. Hazardous substances include:

- Drugs used in cancer therapy (chemotherapy, anticancer drugs)
- Gases used to give anesthesia
- Gases used to sterilize equipment
- Oxygen
- Disinfectants and cleaning solutions
- Radiation used for x-rays and cancer treatments
- Mercury (found in thermometers and sphygmomanometers [see Chapter 21])

To protect employees, OSHA requires a hazard communication program. The program includes container labeling, material safety data sheets, and employee training about hazards and protective measures.

Labeling

Hazardous substance containers include bags, barrels, bottles, boxes, cans, cylinders, drums, and storage tanks. All hazardous substance containers need warning labels (Fig. 8-28). The manufacturer applies the labels. Warning labels always identify physical hazards and health hazards. Health hazards include the organs affected and potential health problems. Warning labels may include:

- Precaution measures (e.g., "do not use near open flame" or "avoid skin contact")
- What personal protective equipment to wear (Chapter 9)
- Directions about using the substance safely
- Storage and disposal information

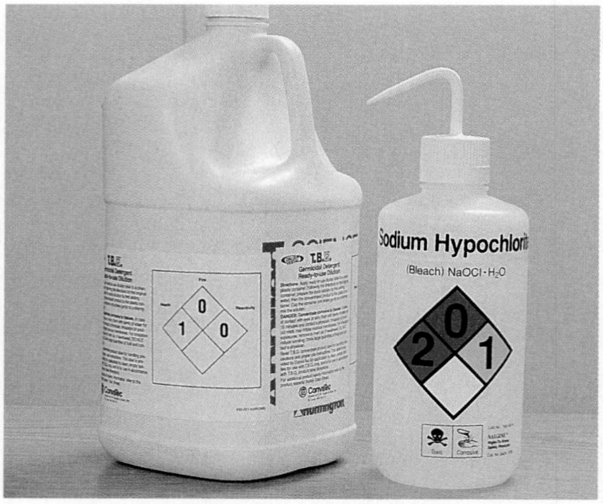

Fig. 8-28 Warning label on a hazardous substance.

Words, pictures, and symbols communicate the warnings. A container must have a label. Warning labels must not be removed or damaged in any way. If a warning label is removed or damaged, do not use the chemical. Take the container to the nurse, and explain the problem. Do not leave the container unattended.

Material Safety Data Sheets

Every hazardous substance has a material safety data sheet (MSDS). An MSDS provides detailed information about each hazardous chemical:

- The chemical name and any common names
- The ingredients contained in the substance
- Physical and chemical characteristics (appearance, color, odor, boiling point, and others)
- Potential physical effects (fire, explosion)
- Conditions that could cause a chemical reaction
- How the chemical enters the human body (inhalation, ingestion, skin contact, or absorption)
- Health hazards, including signs and symptoms
- Protective measures (how to use, handle, and store the substance)
- Emergency and first aid procedures
- Explosion information and firefighting measures (including what type of fire extinguisher to use—see p. 154)
- How to clean up a spill or leak
- Personal protective equipment needed during clean up
- How to dispose of the hazardous material
- Manufacturer information (name, address, and a telephone number for information)

Employees must have ready access to the MSDSs. They are in a binder at the specified location on each unit (Fig. 8-29). Check MSDSs before using a hazardous substance, cleaning up a leak or spill, or disposing of the substance. Also, immediately notify the nurse of a spill or leak. Do not leave a spill or leak unattended.

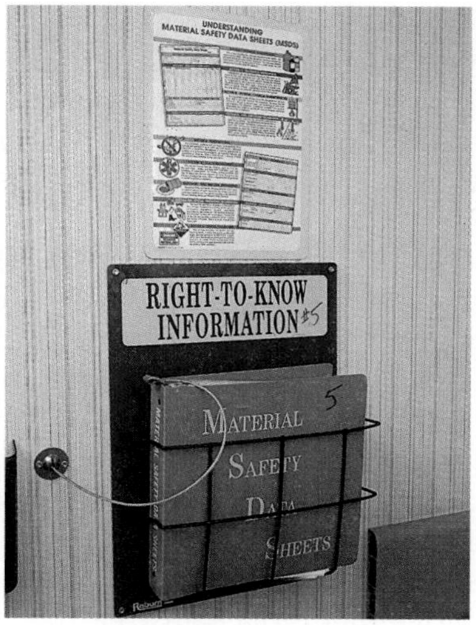

Fig. 8-29 Material safety data sheets are in a binder. The binder is available for staff use.

Employee Training

Your employer provides hazardous substance training. Information is given about the hazards, exposure risks, and protection measures. You also learn to read and use warning labels and the MSDSs.

Each hazardous substance requires specific protection measures. Box 8-6 lists general guidelines for the safe handling of hazardous substances.

Box 8-6 Safety Measures for Handling Hazardous Substances

- Read all warning labels.
- Follow the safety precautions on the warning label and MSDS.
- Make sure each container has a warning label that is not damaged.
- Use a leak-proof container to carry or transport a hazardous substance.
- Wear personal protective equipment to clean spills and leaks. The warning label or MSDS tells you what to wear (mask, gown, gloves, eye protection, safety boots).
- Clean up spills immediately. Work from clean to dirty using circular motions.
- Dispose of hazardous waste in sealed bags or containers.
- Stand behind a lead shield during x-ray or radiation therapy procedures.
- Do not enter a room while a resident is having x-rays or radiation therapy.
- Wash your hands after handling hazardous substances.
- Work in well-ventilated areas to avoid inhaling gases.
- Store hazardous substances according to the MSDS.

FIRE SAFETY

Faulty electrical equipment and wiring, overloaded electrical circuits, and smoking are major causes of fire. Fire is a constant danger. The entire health care team must prevent fires. They must act quickly and responsibly if a fire occurs.

Fire and the Use of Oxygen

Three things are needed for a fire:

- A spark or flame
- A material that will burn
- Oxygen

Air has some oxygen. However, some residents need extra oxygen. Doctors order supplemental oxygen for these residents. Supplemental oxygen is supplied in oxygen tanks or through wall outlets (see Chapter 25). Oxygen is needed for fires. Therefore special safety precautions are practiced where oxygen is used and stored:

- "No Smoking" signs are placed on the resident's door and near the bed.
- Residents and visitors are politely reminded not to smoke in the resident's room.
- Smoking materials (cigarettes, cigars, and pipes), matches, and lighters are removed from the room.
- Electrical equipment is turned off *before* being unplugged. Sparks occur when electrical appliances are unplugged while turned on.
- Wool blankets and synthetic fabrics that cause static electricity are removed from the resident's room. The resident wears a cotton gown or pajamas. Staff wear cotton uniforms.
- Electrical equipment is removed from the resident's room. This includes electric razors, heating pads, and radios.
- Materials that ignite easily are removed from the resident's room. These include oil, grease, alcohol, nail polish remover, and other hazardous substances that ignite easily.

Many centers have no-smoking policies and are smoke-free environments. No smoking is allowed inside the buildings. Signs are posted on all entry doors. However, some people ignore such policies. If a resident is receiving supplemental oxygen, remind the resident, family, and any visitors about the need for no smoking.

Box 8-7 Fire Prevention Measures

- Follow the fire safety precautions involved in the use of oxygen (see p. 153).
- Smoke only in areas where smoking is allowed. Do not smoke in resident rooms.
- Be sure all ashes, cigars, and cigarettes are extinguished before emptying ashtrays.
- Provide ashtrays to residents who are allowed to smoke.
- Empty ashtrays into a metal container partially filled with sand or water. Do not empty ashtrays into plastic containers or wastebaskets lined with paper or plastic bags.
- Supervise the smoking of residents who cannot protect themselves. This includes residents who are confused, disoriented, or sedated.
- Follow safety practices when using electrical equipment.
- Keep matches and lighters out of reach of confused and disoriented residents.
- Do not leave cooking unattended on stoves, in ovens, or in microwave ovens.
- Store flammable liquids in their original containers. Keep the containers out of residents' reach.
- Do not light matches or lighters or smoke around flammable liquids or materials.

Preventing Fires

Fire prevention measures were described in relation to burns, equipment-related accidents, and the use of oxygen. These and other fire safety measures are summarized in Box 8-7.

What To Do if a Fire Occurs

Every center has policies and procedures for fire emergencies. You must know your center's policies and procedures. Also know the location of fire alarms, fire extinguishers, and emergency exits. Centers conduct fire drills to practice emergency fire procedures.

Remember the word *RACE* when a fire occurs. That will help you remember what to do first:

- ***R*** stands for *rescue.* Rescue persons in immediate danger. Move them to a safe area.
- ***A*** stands for *alarm.* Sound the nearest fire alarm, and notify the switchboard operator.
- ***C*** stands for *confine.* Confine the fire by closing doors and windows. Turn off oxygen or electrical equipment being used in the general area of the fire.
- ***E*** stands for *extinguish.* Use a fire extinguisher on a small fire that has not spread to a larger area.

Also clear equipment from all regular and emergency exits. Remember, do not use elevators if there is a fire.

◈ **Using a fire extinguisher.** Centers require that all employees demonstrate use of a fire extinguisher. Fire departments give fire extinguishers demonstrations once or twice a year.

Different extinguishers are used for different kinds of fires: oil and grease fires; electrical fires; and paper and wood fires. A general procedure for using a fire extinguisher follows.

Using a Fire Extinguisher

Procedure

1. Pull the fire alarm.
2. Get the nearest fire extinguisher.
3. Carry the extinguisher upright.
4. Take the extinguisher to the fire.
5. Remove the safety pin (Fig. 8-30, *A*).
6. Push the top handle down (Fig. 8-30, *B*).
7. Direct the hose at the base of the fire (Fig. 8-30, *C*).

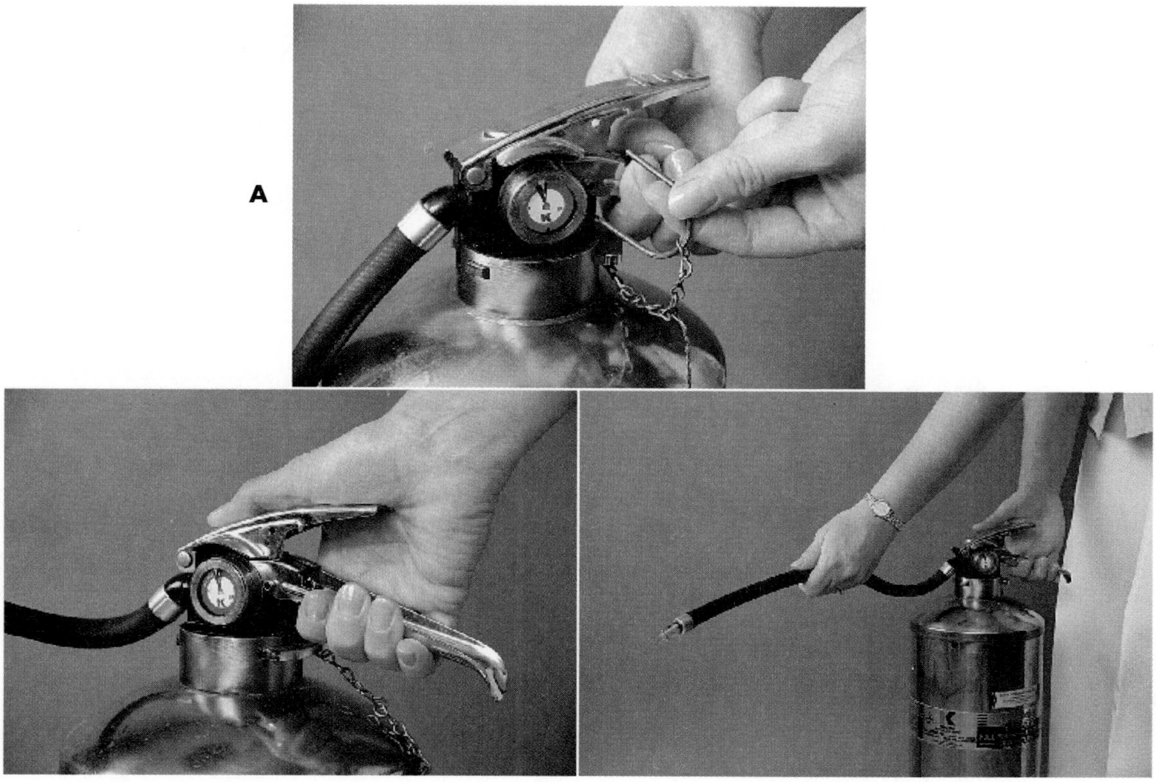

A B C

Fig. 8-30 **A,** The safety pin of the fire extinguisher is removed. **B,** The top handle is pushed down. **C,** The hose is directed at the base of the fire.

Evacuating residents. Center policies and procedures specify evacuation procedures. If evacuation is necessary, residents closest to the danger are evacuated first. Ambulatory residents are given blankets to wrap around themselves. They are escorted to a safe place by a staff member. Figures 8-31 and 8-32 show how to rescue nonambulatory residents. Once firefighters arrive, they direct rescue efforts.

A

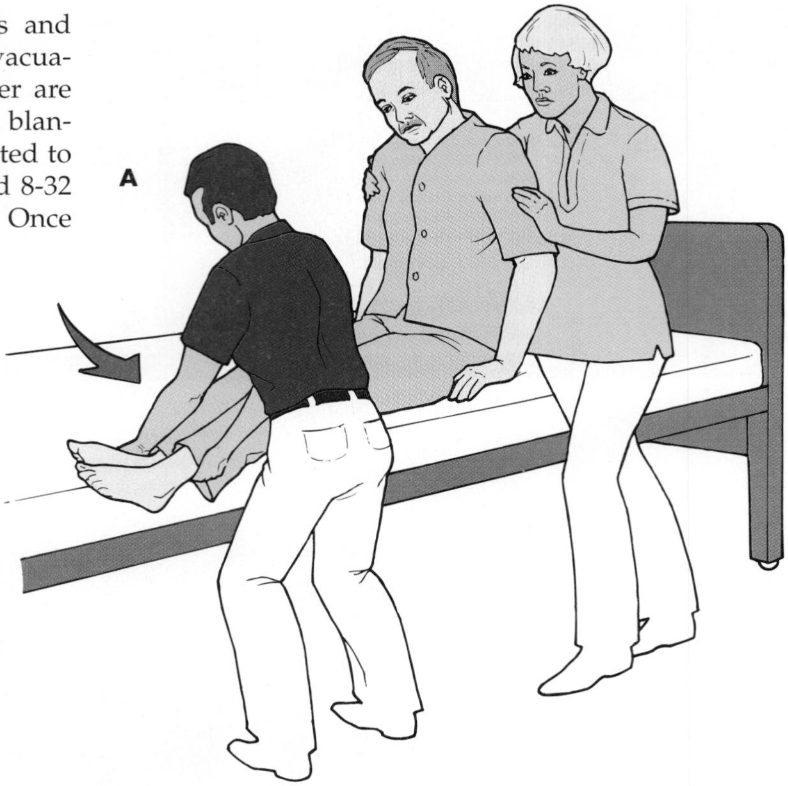

B

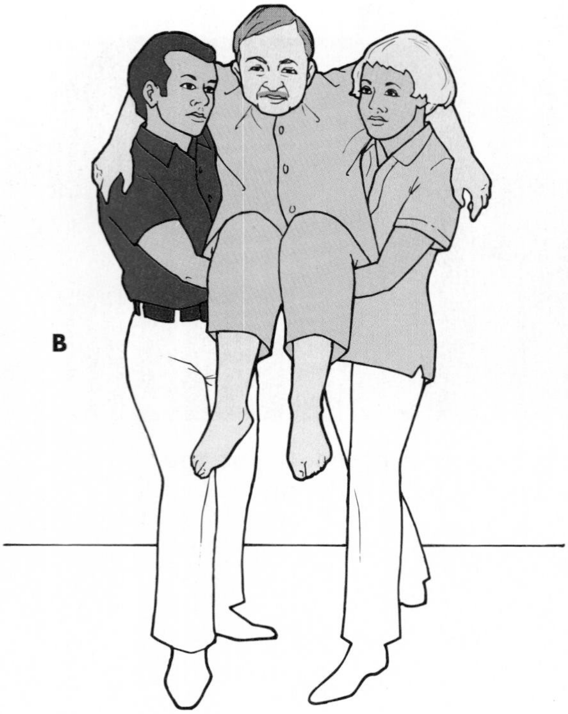

Fig. 8-31 Swing-carry technique. **A,** Assist the person to a sitting position. A co-worker grasps the person's ankles as you both turn the resident so that he sits on the side of the bed. **B,** Pull the person's arm over your shoulder. With one arm, reach across the person's back to your co-worker's shoulder. Reach under the person's knees, and grasp your co-worker's arm. Your co-worker does the same.

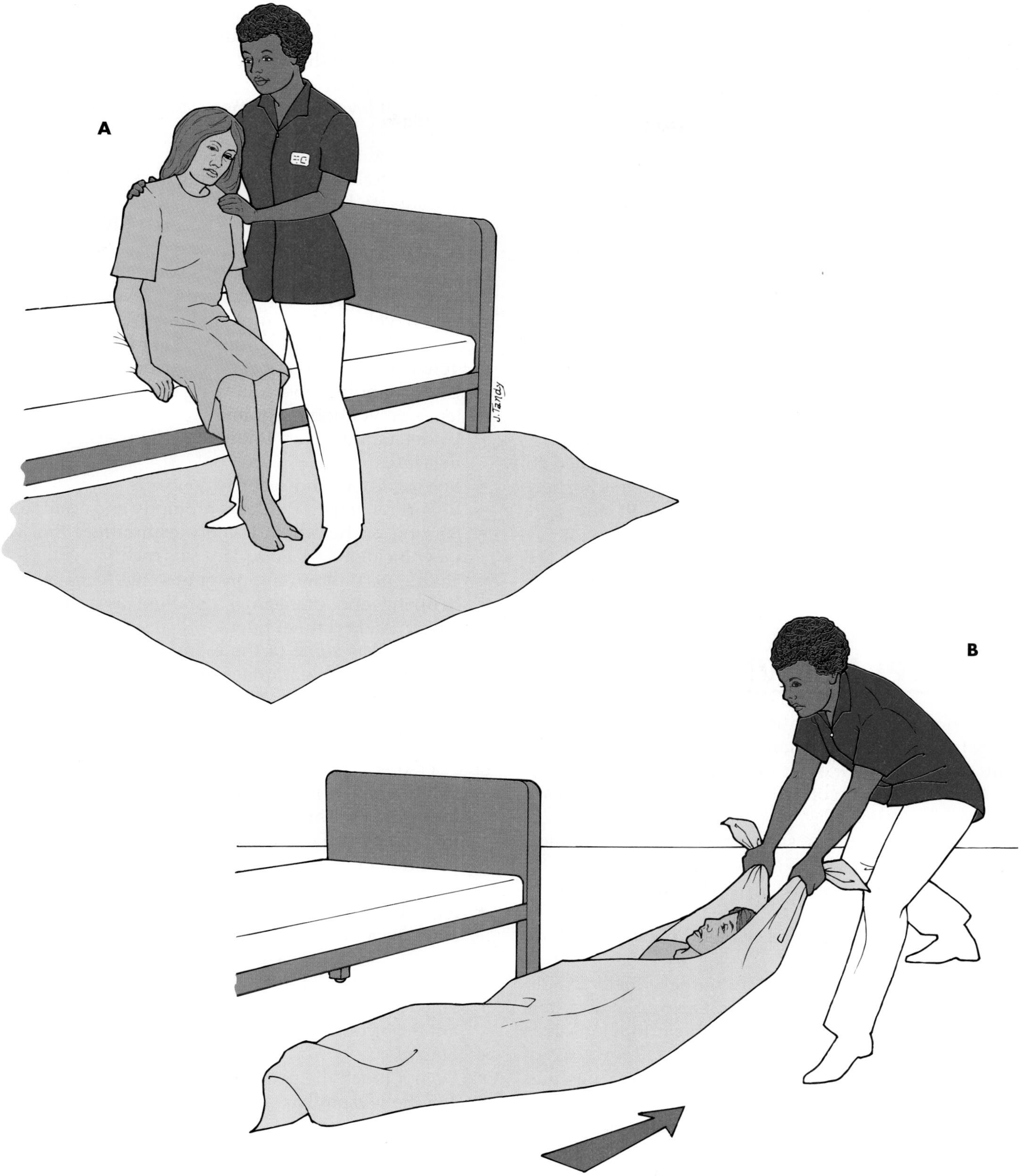

Fig. 8-32 One-rescuer carry. **A,** Spread the blanket on the floor. Make sure the blanket will extend beyond the person's head. Assist the person to sit on the side of the bed. Grasp the person under the arms, and cross your hands over her chest. Lower the person to the floor by sliding her down one of your legs. **B,** Wrap the blanket around the person. Grasp the blanket over the head area, and pull the person to a safe area.

DISASTERS

A **disaster** is a sudden catastrophic event. Many people are injured and killed, and property is destroyed. Natural disasters include tornadoes, hurricanes, blizzards, earthquakes, volcanic eruptions, floods, and some fires. Human-made disasters include auto, bus, train, and airplane accidents. They also include fires, nuclear power plant accidents, riots, explosions, and wars.

Local communities, fire and police departments, and health care facilities have disaster plans. You should know the disaster plan where you work. Also know the disaster plan of the community where you live and work.

Disaster plans include policies and procedures to deal with great numbers of people needing treatment. The plan generally provides for the discharge of residents who can go home. Certain personnel are assigned to an emergency area. Others are assigned to take equipment to the emergency area and to transport residents from the initial treatment area. Off-duty personnel may be called in to work.

A disaster may damage the center. Therefore the disaster plan includes policies and procedures for evacuating the center.

WORKPLACE VIOLENCE

According to the Occupational Safety and Health Administration (OSHA), more assaults occur in health care settings than in other industries.

Risk factors for work-related assaults in health care agencies include:

- Handguns in the possession of patients, families, and friends
- Patients as police holds (persons arrested or convicted of crimes)
- Acutely disturbed and violent persons seeking health care
- Mentally ill patients who do not take medicine, do not receive follow-up care, and are not in hospitals unless they are an immediate threat to themselves or others
- Agency pharmacies being a source of drugs and therefore a target for robberies
- Gang members and substance abusers having access to agencies as patients or visitors
- Upset, agitated, and disturbed family members and visitors
- Long emergency room waits that increase a person's agitation and frustration
- Being alone with patients during care or transport to other agency areas
- Low staff levels during meals and emergencies and at night
- Poorly lighted parking areas
- Lack of training in recognizing and managing potentially violent situations

OSHA has guidelines for violence prevention programs. The goal is to eliminate or reduce employee exposure to situations that can cause death or injury. The work site is analyzed for hazards. Prevention strategies are developed and implemented. Also, employees receive safety and health training. Your responsibilities in violence prevention programs include:

- Understanding and following the workplace violence prevention program
- Understanding and following safety and security measures
- Voicing safety and security concerns
- Reporting violent incidents promptly and accurately
- Serving on health and safety committees that review incidents of workplace violence
- Taking part in training programs that focus on recognizing and managing agitation, assaultive behavior, and criminal intent

Box 8-8 lists some of the many measures that can prevent or control workplace violence. Box 8-9, p. 160 lists personal safety practices to follow in everyday activities. In addition, you can practice the following safety measures when dealing with agitated or aggressive persons:

- Stand away from the person. Judge the length of the person's arms and legs. Stand far enough away that the person cannot hit or kick you.
- Position yourself close to the door. Do not become trapped in the room.
- Note the location of panic buttons, signal lights, alarms, closed-circuit monitors, and other security devices (see Fig. 8-33).
- Keep your hands free.
- Stay calm. Talk to the person in a calm manner. Do not raise your voice or argue, scold, or interrupt the person.
- Do not touch the person.
- Tell the person that you will get a nurse to speak to the person.
- Leave the room as soon as you can. Make sure the person is safe.
- Notify the nurse or security officer of the situation.
- Complete an incident report according to agency policy.

Box 8-8 Measures to Prevent or Control Workplace Violence

- Alarm systems, closed-circuit video monitoring (Fig. 8-33), panic buttons, hand-held alarms, cellular phones, two-way radios, and telephone systems that have a direct line to police are installed.
- Metal detectors are at entrances to identify guns, knives, or other weapons.
- Curved mirrors are at hallway intersections and hard-to-see areas.
- Bullet-resistant, shatterproof glass is at the nurses' stations, reception areas, and admitting areas.
- Waiting rooms are comfortable and reduce stress.
- Family and visitors receive information in a timely manner.
- Furniture is arranged to prevent entrapment.
- Pictures, vases, and other items that can serve as weapons are few in number.
- Staff restrooms lock and prevent access to visitors.
- Unused doors are locked, in keeping with local fire codes.
- Bright lights are inside and outside buildings.
- Burned out lights are replaced or repaired.
- Broken lights, windows, and door locks are replaced or repaired.
- Security escort services are used for walking to cars, bus stops, or train stations.
- Vehicles are locked and in good repair.
- Security officers deal with agitated, aggressive, or disruptive residents and visitors.
- Residents and visitors are restrained if they are a threat to themselves or others.
- Visiting hours and policies are enforced.
- A list of "restricted visitors" is made for residents with a history of violence or who are victims of violence. This is likely to happen only on a subacute unit.
- Access to the pharmacy and drug storage areas is controlled.
- A nurse assesses the behavioral history of new and transferred residents.
- Aggressive and agitated residents are treated in open areas. Privacy and confidentiality are maintained.
- Staff is not alone when caring for residents with agitated or aggressive behaviors.
- Jewelry that can serve as weapons is not worn (grabbing earrings and bracelets, strangulating with necklaces).
- Long hair is worn up and off the collar (see Chapter 2.) A resident can pull long hair and cause head injuries.
- Keys, scissors, pens, or other items that can serve as weapons are not visible.
- Tools or items left by maintenance personnel or visitors are removed if they can serve as weapons.
- Staff wear ID badges (without last names) that verify employment.
- A "buddy system" is used when using elevators, restrooms, and low-traffic areas.
- Uniforms fit well. Tight uniforms limit your ability to run. An attacker can grab loose uniforms.
- Shoes have good soles. Shoes that cause slipping limit your ability to run.

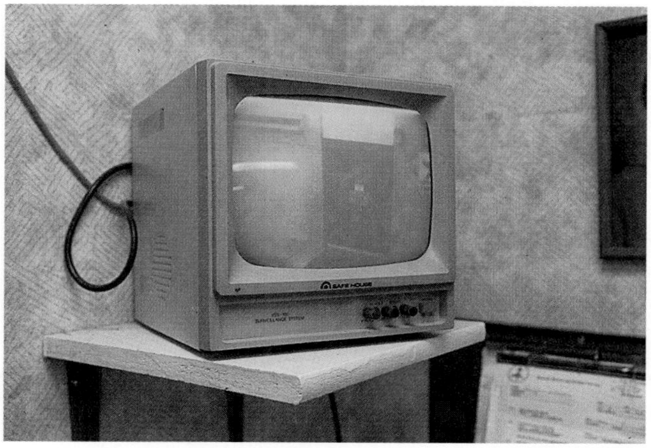

Fig. 8-33 The closed-circuit TV allows staff to monitor persons entering and leaving the center.

Box 8-9 Personal Safety Practices

- Know the area you will visit. Ask questions about the area.
- Make a "dry run" of the area. Know the route in advance. The shortest route is not always the safest.
- Have plenty of gas in your car.
- Keep your car in good working order.
- Keep a flashlight with working batteries, flares, a fire extinguisher, and a first aid kit in your car.
- Raise the hood and use the flares if the car breaks down. Stay in the car and call the police if you have a cellular phone. If someone stops by to help, ask that person to call the police.
- Check for places to park. Choose a well-lit area. If using a parking garage, park near entrances, exits, and on the lower level. Try to get close to the attendant if possible. Remember that the closest space to your destination is not always the safest for parking.
- Park your car so that you can leave quickly and easily. Park at street corners so no one can park in front of you. In parking lots, back in. You can see more from your front windshield than from the back window.
- Lock your car. However, there are times you may want to leave your car unlocked. If you need to get in the car fast, you do not want to fumble with keys. Use your judgment. Do not leave anything in the car if you leave it unlocked.
- Have your car key ready so you can get into the car quickly. Do not fumble for keys on the way to or at the car.
- Check the back seat before getting into the car. Make sure no one is in the car. Leave immediately if someone is in the car.
- Check under the car. A person hiding under the car can grab your ankle or leg. Leave immediately if someone is under the car.
- Lock car doors when you get in the car, and keep windows rolled up.
- Keep purses and other valuables under the seat or near your side. Do not leave them on the seat. They are an easy target for smash-and-grab robberies.
- Use well-lit and busy streets if you have to walk. Avoid vacant lots, alleys, wooded areas, and construction sites. Again, the shortest way is not always the safest.
- Note the location of phone booths, or carry a cellular phone. Know your location, and keep phone calls simple.
- Go to a police or fire station or a store if you think someone is following you.
- Carry money for phone calls and for bus, train, or taxi fares. Have money in your pocket to avoid fumbling with a purse or wallet.
- Stand with others and near the ticket booth if using public transportation. Sit near the driver or conductor.
- Do not hitchhike or pick up hitchhikers.
- Let someone know where you are at all times. Let someone know when you leave and when you arrive at your destination. If you do not call in when expected, the person knows something is wrong.
- Make it known that you do not carry drugs, needles, or syringes.
- Do not carry valuables with you. Leave them at home or in the car trunk. If someone wants what you have, give it. The only thing of value is *you.*
- Carry wallets and purses safely. A wallet should be in an inside coat or pants pocket. Never carry a wallet in the rear pocket. Keep a firm grip on a purse, and keep it close to your body.
- Do not wear headphones when walking. They keep you from hearing cars, trains, buses, and people around you.
- Carry a whistle or shriek alarm.
- Scream as loud and as long as you can. Keep screaming. Both men and women should scream.
- Use your car keys as a weapon. Carry them in your strong hand and have one key extended (Fig. 8-34). Hold the key firmly. If you are attacked, go for the person's face. Use the key to slash the person's face. Do not use poking motions. Also, do not try for a specific target because you might miss. Do not be shy—your attacker will not be.
- Remember that you have two arms, two hands, two feet, and two knees. This means that you can attack from four directions at once. Do not be shy—your attacker will not be. Push, pull, yank, and so on. You can attack the genital area of either a man or woman.
- Use your thumbs as weapons. Go for the eyes, and push hard.
- Carry a travel size can of aerosol hair spray. Go for the face.

Modified from McLean County Sheriff's Department, Bloomington, Ill, and the Illinois Criminal Justice Information Authority, Chicago, Ill.

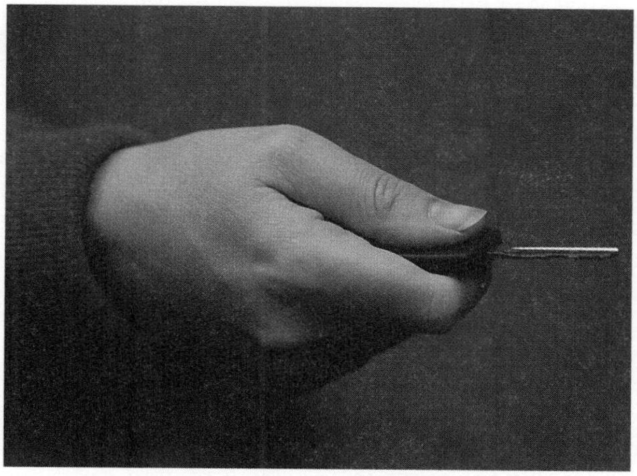

Fig. 8-34 Car keys are held to use a car key as a weapon.

RISK MANAGEMENT

Risk management involves identifying and controlling risk and safety hazards affecting the center. The intent is to protect everyone in the center (residents, visitors, and staff) and all center property from harm or danger. The person's valuables also are protected. Safety, accident and fire prevention, negligence and malpractice, and federal and state requirements are among the many issues within the scope of risk management.

Risk managers work with all departments to prevent accidents and injuries. They study incident reports, resident and staff complaints, and accident and injury investigations for patterns and trends. Risk managers also look for and correct unsafe situations. They also make policy and procedure changes and training recommendations as needed.

Clothing and Valuables

The resident's valuables must be kept safe. Often they are sent home with the family. A clothing list is completed. Each item is identified and described. The staff member and resident sign the completed list.

A valuables envelope is used for jewelry and large amounts of money. Each jewelry item is listed and described on the envelope. Describe what you see. For example, describe a ring as having a white stone with six prongs in a yellow setting. Do not assume the stone is a diamond in a gold setting. Place each jewelry item in the envelope with the resident watching. Count money with the resident. Then put it in the envelope. The envelope is sealed and signed like the clothing checklist. Give the envelope to the nurse. The nurse takes it to the safe or sends it home with the family.

Dentures, eyeglasses, contact lenses, watches, and radios are kept at the bedside. Valuables kept at the bedside are listed in the resident's record. Some residents keep money for newspapers and other personal items. The amount of money kept is noted in the resident's record. Clothing and shoes are labeled with the resident's name. Radios, blankets, and other items brought from home also are labeled.

Reporting Accidents and Errors

Immediately report accidents and errors to your supervisor. This includes accidents involving residents, visitors, or staff. You must report errors in care. Such errors include giving a resident a wrong treatment, giving a treatment to the wrong resident, or forgetting to give a treatment. Broken items owned by the resident, such as dentures or eyeglasses, are reported. Lost money or clothing is also reported. So are hazardous substance accidents and workplace violence incidents.

An *incident report* is completed. The report is completed as soon as possible after the incident. The following information is required:

- Names of those involved
- Date and time of the accident or error
- Location of the accident or error
- A complete description of what happened
- Names of witnesses
- Any other requested information

Incident reports are reviewed by the director of nursing, the administrator, and the safety or risk management committee. They look for patterns and trends of accidents or errors. For example, are falls occurring on the same shift and on the same unit? Are residents reporting lost or missing items on the same shift or same unit? The committee may recommend new policies or procedures to prevent future incidents.

Quality of Life

Most accidents can be prevented. Knowing the common safety hazards and causes of accidents, knowing who needs protection, and using common sense are all necessary to promote safety. Remember that older and disabled persons are more likely to have accidents than are healthy young adults.

Chronic illness, advanced age, physical and mental disability, medications, unfamiliar surroundings, and special equipment increase the risk of accidental injury to residents. You need to practice safety precautions and use safety devices as appropriate. Encourage residents to use handrails and special equipment, such as walkers and canes, to assist them with walking. You must always follow the resident's care plan to ensure safe care.

Identifying residents before giving care is very important. The resident's life and health can be seriously threatened if the wrong care is given or if care is omitted. Use the ID bracelet to accurately identify the resident. Having two residents on the same nursing unit with the same last name is not uncommon. Some residents may even have the same first and last names.

If restraints are ordered, they must be used for a specific medical symptom. The resident must be checked often to make sure that breathing and circulation are normal. Remember that the restrained resident depends on others for basic needs. Be sure to offer water or other fluids often. Remember that you can be charged with false imprisonment if the resident is restrained unnecessarily.

Fire is a safety hazard. Exercising safety precautions for smoking and electrical equipment helps prevent fires. Extra precautions are needed when oxygen is used. The resident who smokes presents additional fire safety concerns. Check with the nurse to find out which residents may have smoking materials at the bedside. Be sure you know where fire alarms, fire extinguishers, and emergency exits are located and what to do if there is a fire.

You must know and follow procedures for handling hazardous substances in the workplace. Physical hazards can cause fires and explosions. Exposure to some chemicals can cause acute or chronic health problems.

Workplace violence is a real danger in health care settings. You should know and practice measures to prevent and control workplace violence. Keeping the center safe for residents, visitors, and staff is everyone's job.

Circle T if the statement is true and F if the statement is false.

1 (T) F In a safe environment, a person has a very low risk of illness or injury.

2 (T) F Cleaning chemicals are kept in locked storage areas that are out of the reach of residents.

3 (T) F Aging causes body changes that place an elderly person at risk for accidents.

4 (T) F Medications are a cause of some accidents.

5 (T) F Adequate lighting helps prevent falls.

6 T (F) Bedroom slippers prevent skidding and slipping on floors.

7 T (F) The spread of infection is not a health hazard in health facilities.

8 (T) F Bed rails are kept up when the bed is in the highest horizontal position.

9 (T) F Bed rails are considered restraints by OBRA.

10 (T) F Handrails provide support for residents when walking.

11 (T) F Calling residents by name is the best way to identify them.

12 (T) F Restraints are used only for specific medical symptoms.

13 (T) F Unnecessary restraint is false imprisonment.

14 (T) F A resident (or the resident's guardian) must consent to the use of restraints.

15 T (F) You can apply restraints any time you think they are needed.

16 T (F) Geriatric chairs are restraints.

17 T (F) You can use a vest restraint to position a resident on the toilet.

18 (T) F You should be able to feel a pulse in the wrist if the arm and hand are restrained.

19 (T) F Restraints are removed every 2 hours to reposition the resident and give skin care.

20 T (F) Restrained residents are checked every 15 to 30 minutes for safety and comfort.

21 T (F) Restraints are tied to bed rails.

22 (T) F Some drugs are chemical restraints.

23 (T) F A vest restraint crosses in front.

24 T (F) Bed rails are not padded when vest restraints are used.

25 T (F) Accidents or errors in giving care are reported to the nurse at the end of the shift.

26 T (F) Smoking is allowed where oxygen is used.

Circle the BEST answer.

27 Which is *not* a risk for accidents?
A The need for eyeglasses
B Hearing impairment
C Memory problems
(D) Oriented to person, time, and place

28 A paraplegic is paralyzed
(A) From the waist down
B From the neck down
C On the right side of the body
D On the left side of the body

Continued

29 Safety measures are needed so Mrs. Hall does not fall. Which is unsafe?
A Nonglare, waxed floors
B One-color floor coverings
C Safety rails and grab bars in the bathroom
D Nonskid shoes

30 Burns are caused by the following *except*
A Smoking in bed
B Space heaters
C Bath water that is too hot
D Oxygen

31 Mrs. Hall often tries to get up without help. You should do the following *except*
A Remind her to use her signal light when she needs help.
B Check on her often.
C Help her to the bathroom at regular intervals.
D Place her chair by a wall.

32 The following can occur because of restraints. Which is the *most* serious?
A Fractures
B Strangulation
C Pressure ulcers
D Urinary tract infection

33 A belt restraint is applied to a person in bed. Where should you tie the straps?
A To the bed rails
B To the head board
C To the movable part of the bed frame
D To the foot board

34 Mrs. Hall has a restraint. You should check her and the position of the restraint
A Every 15 minutes
B Every 30 minutes
C Every hour
D Every 2 hours

35 To prevent equipment accidents, you should
A Fix broken equipment
B Use two-pronged plugs to ground electrical equipment
C Check glass and plastic items for damage
D Complete an incident report

36 You gave Mrs. Hall the wrong treatment. Which is *true?*
A You report the error to the nurse at the end of the shift.
B Action is taken only if Mrs. Hall was injured.
C You are guilty of negligence.
D You must complete an incident report.

37 All the following are needed to start a fire *except*
A A spark or flame
B A material that will burn
C Oxygen
D Carbon monoxide

38 You spilled a hazardous substance. You should do the following *except*
A Read the material safety data sheet
B Cover the spill, and go tell the RN
C Wear any needed personal protective equipment to clean up the spill
D Complete an incident report

39 The fire alarm sounds. The following are done *except*
A Turning off oxygen
B Using elevators
C Closing doors and windows
D Moving residents to a safe place

40 A resident is agitated and aggressive. You should do the following *except*
A Stand away from the resident
B Stand close to the door
C Use touch to show you care
D Talk to the resident without raising your voice

Answers to these questions are on pp. 696-697.

9 Infection Control

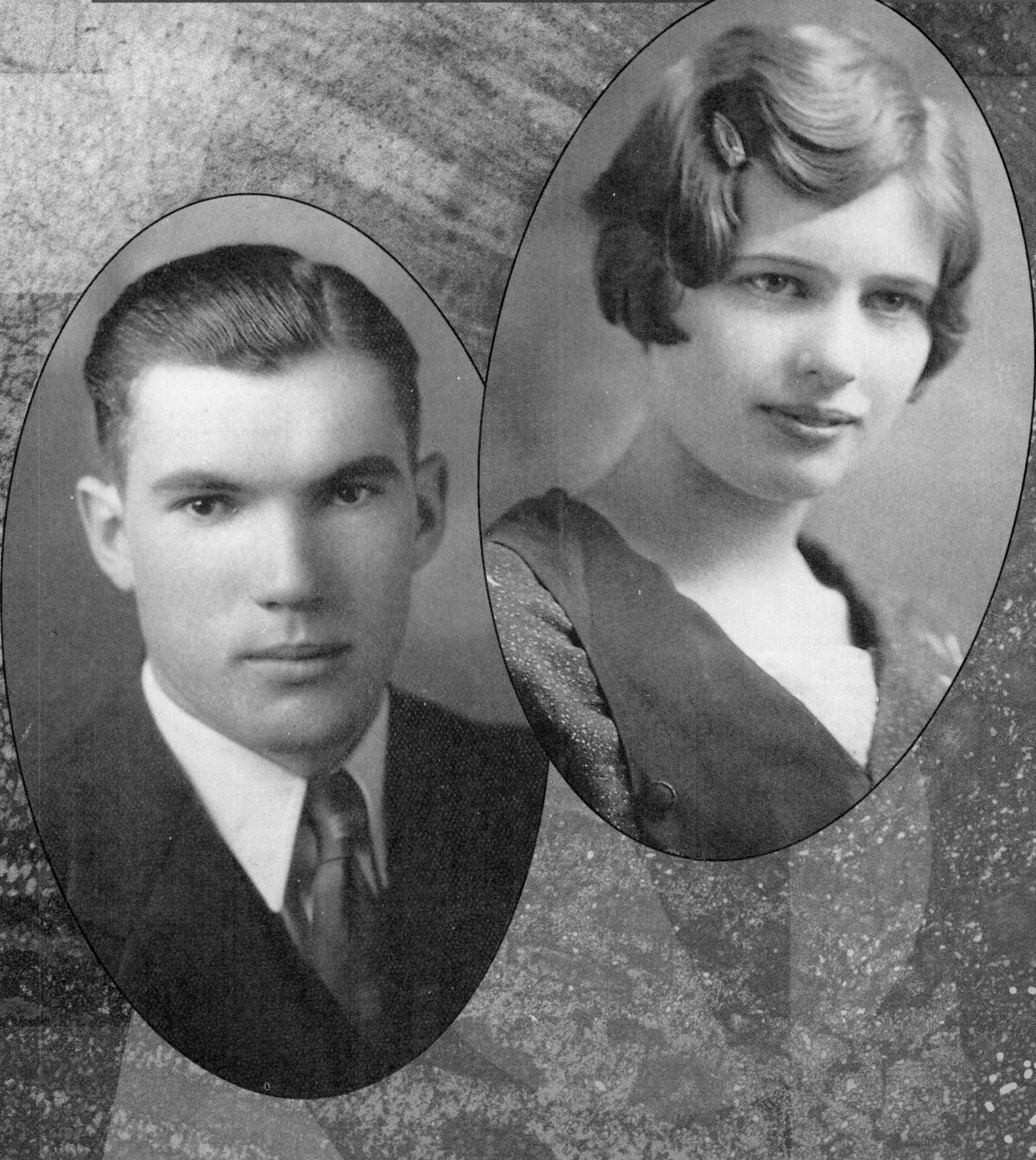

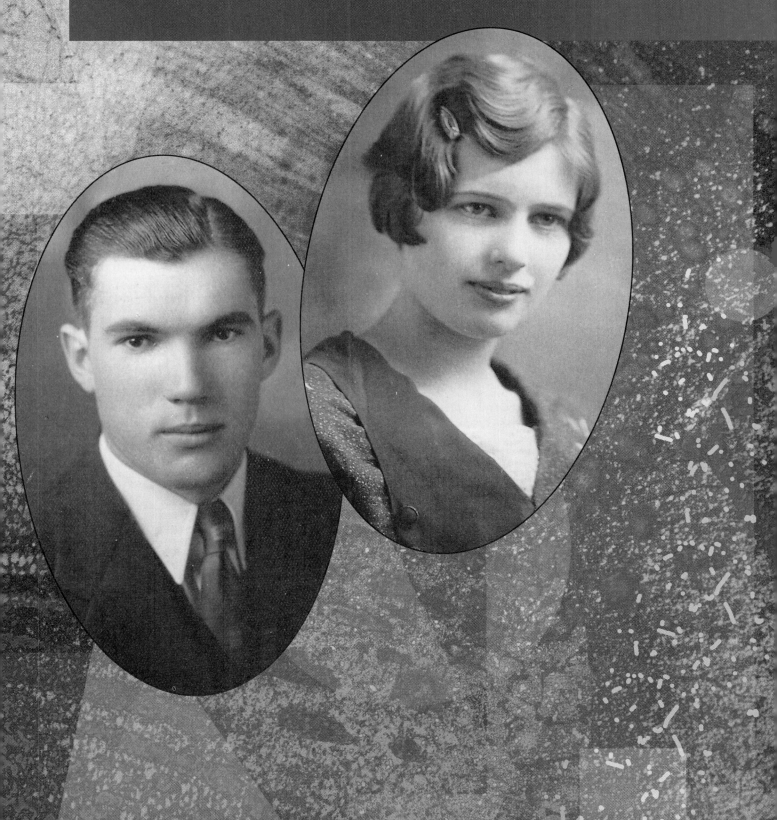

What You Will Learn

- The definition of the key terms listed in this chapter
- The difference between nonpathogens and pathogens
- What microbes need to live and grow
- The signs and symptoms of infection
- The chain of infection
- The causes of nosocomial infections and the persons at risk
- The common practices of medical asepsis
- The differences between medical asepsis, disinfection, and sterilization
- Common disinfection and sterilization methods
- How to care for equipment and supplies
- The purposes of Standard and Transmission-Based Precautions
- The Bloodborne Pathogen Standard
- The principles and practices of surgical asepsis
- The procedures described in this chapter

Key Terms

asepsis Being free of disease-producing microbes

autoclave A pressure steam sterilizer

biohazardous waste Items contaminated with blood, body fluids, secretions, or excretions and that may be harmful to others; *bio* means life, and *hazardous* means dangerous or harmful

bloodborne pathogens Pathogenic microorganisms present in human blood that can cause disease in humans

carrier A human or animal that is a reservoir for pathogens but does not have signs and symptoms of infection

clean technique Medical asepsis

communicable disease A disease caused by pathogens that spread easily; a contagious disease

contagious disease Communicable disease

contamination The process of becoming unclean

disinfection The process of destroying pathogens

germicide A disinfectant applied to skin, tissues, or nonliving objects

immunity Protection against a certain disease

infection A disease state resulting from the invasion and growth of microorganisms in the body

medical asepsis The practices used to remove or destroy pathogens and to prevent their spread from one person or place to another person or place; clean technique

microbe A microorganism

microorganism A small *(micro)* living plant or animal *(organism)* seen only with a microscope; a microbe

nonpathogen A microbe that usually does not cause an infection

normal flora Microbes that usually live and grow in a certain location

nosocomial infection An infection acquired during a stay at a health care agency

pathogen A microbe that is harmful and can cause an infection

personal protective equipment Specialized clothing or equipment (e.g. gloves, goggles, gowns) worn for protection against a hazard

reservoir The environment in which microbes live and grow; host

spore A bacterium protected by a hard shell that forms around the microbe

sterile The absence of *all* microbes

KEY TERMS—cont'd

sterile field A work area free of all pathogens and nonpathogens (including spores)

sterile technique Surgical asepsis

sterilization The process of destroying *all* microbes

surgical asepsis The practices that keep equipment and supplies free of all microbes; sterile technique

vaccine A preparation containing microbes

▲ Infection is a major safety and health hazard. Some infections are minor and cause a short illness. Others are serious and can cause death, especially in older and disabled persons. Health care workers must protect residents and themselves from infection. Do this by preventing the spread of the cause of the infection.

MICROORGANISMS

A **microorganism (microbe)** is a small *(micro)* living plant or animal *(organism)* that is seen only with a microscope. Microbes are everywhere. They are in the air, food, mouth, nose, respiratory tract, stomach, and intestines and on the skin. They are in the soil and water and on animals, clothing, and furniture. Some microbes cause infections and are harmful. They are called **pathogens.** Microbes that usually do not cause infection are **nonpathogens.**

Types of Microbes

There are five general types of microbes:
- *Bacteria* are microscopic plant life that multiply rapidly. They consist of one cell and often are called *germs.*
- *Fungi* are plants that live on other plants or animals. Mushrooms, yeasts, and molds are common fungi.
- *Protozoa* are microscopic one-celled animals.
- *Rickettsiae* are microscopic forms of life found in the tissues of fleas, lice, ticks, and other insects. They are transmitted to humans by insect bites.
- *Viruses* are extremely small microscopic organisms that grow in living cells.

Requirements of Microbes

Microbes require a **reservoir** to live and grow. The reservoir (*host*) is the environment in which the microbe lives and grows. Reservoirs are humans, plants, animals, the soil, food, water, or other material. The microbe must receive *water* and *nourishment* from the reservoir. Most microbes need *oxygen* to live. Others cannot live where there is oxygen. A *warm* and *dark* environment is needed. Most microbes grow best at body temperature and are destroyed by heat and light.

Normal Flora

Normal flora are microbes that usually live and grow in a certain area. Certain microbes are found in the respiratory tract, in the intestines, and on the skin. They are nonpathogens when in or on a natural reservoir. When a nonpathogen is transmitted from its natural site to another site or host, it becomes a pathogen. *Escherichia coli* is normally found in the large intestine. If the *E. coli* enters the urinary system, it can cause an infection.

INFECTION

An **infection** is a disease state resulting from the invasion and growth of microbes in the body. A *local infection* is in a body part. A *systemic infection* involves the whole body. The person has signs and symptoms of infection. Some or all of the signs and symptoms listed in Box 9-1 on p. 168 are present. Pathogens do not always cause an infection. The development of an infection depends on many factors.

The Chain of Infection

The chain of infection (Fig. 9-1, p. 168) is a process involving a:
- Source
- Reservoir
- Portal of exit
- Method of transmission
- Portal of entry
- Susceptible host

The *source* is a pathogen. The pathogen must have a *reservoir* where it can grow and multiply. Humans and animals are common reservoirs. If they do not have signs and symptoms of infection, they are **carriers.** Carriers can pass the pathogen to others. The pathogen must leave the reservoir. That is, it needs a *portal of exit.* Exits are the respiratory, gastrointestinal, urinary, and reproductive tracts, breaks in the skin, and the blood.

When a pathogen leaves the reservoir, it must be *transmitted* to another host. Methods of transmission include direct contact, air (airborne droplets from coughing or sneezing), food, water, animals, and insects. Microbes also are transmitted by eating and

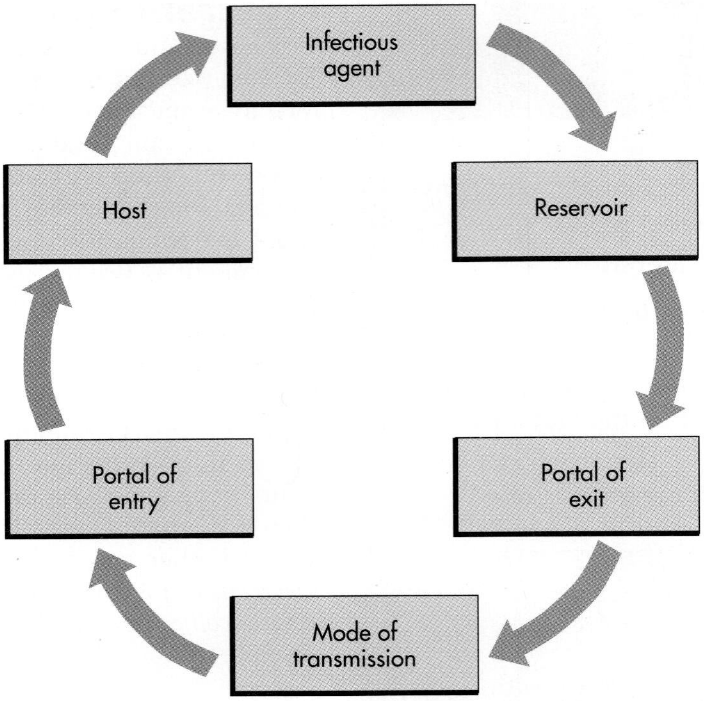

Fig. 9-1 *The chain of infection. (From Potter PA, Perry, AG:* Fundamentals of nursing: concepts, process, and practice, *ed 4, St Louis, 1997, Mosby.)*

Box 9-1 Signs and Symptoms of Infection

- Fever
- Increased pulse and respiratory rates
- Pain or tenderness
- Fatigue and loss of energy
- Loss of appetite (anorexia)
- Nausea
- Vomiting
- Diarrhea
- Rash
- Sores on mucous membranes
- Redness and swelling of a body part
- Discharge or drainage from the infected area

drinking utensils, dressings, and personal care items (Fig. 9-2). The pathogen must enter the body through a *portal of entry.* Portals of entry and exit are the same. A *susceptible host* (a person at risk for infection) is needed for the microbe to grow and multiply. The human body can protect itself from infection. A person's ability to resist infection relates to age, nutritional status, stress, fatigue, general health, medications, and the presence of disease or injury.

Nosocomial Infection

Persons can develop infections in health care settings. A **nosocomial infection** is an infection acquired during a stay at a health care agency. (*Nosocomial* comes from the Greek word for hospital.)

Nosocomial infections are caused by normal flora or by microbes transmitted to the person from another source. Remember that normal flora become pathogens when transmitted from their natural location to another site or host. For example, *E. coli* is normally in the large intestine. Feces (bowel movements) contain *E. coli.* Poor wiping after bowel movements can cause *E. coli* to enter the urinary system. The hands can also transmit *E. coli* to other body areas. If hand washing is poor, *E. coli* spreads to any body part or anything the hands touch.

Microbes can enter the body through equipment used in treatments, therapies, and diagnostic tests. Therefore equipment must be free of microbes (p. 172). Staff also can transfer microbes from one resident to another and from themselves to residents. The urinary and respiratory systems, wounds, and the bloodstream are common sites for nosocomial infections.

Older persons have difficulty fighting infections. Therefore the health care team must prevent the spread of infection. Medical and surgical asepsis, isolation precautions, and the Bloodborne Pathogen Standard all help prevent nosocomial infections.

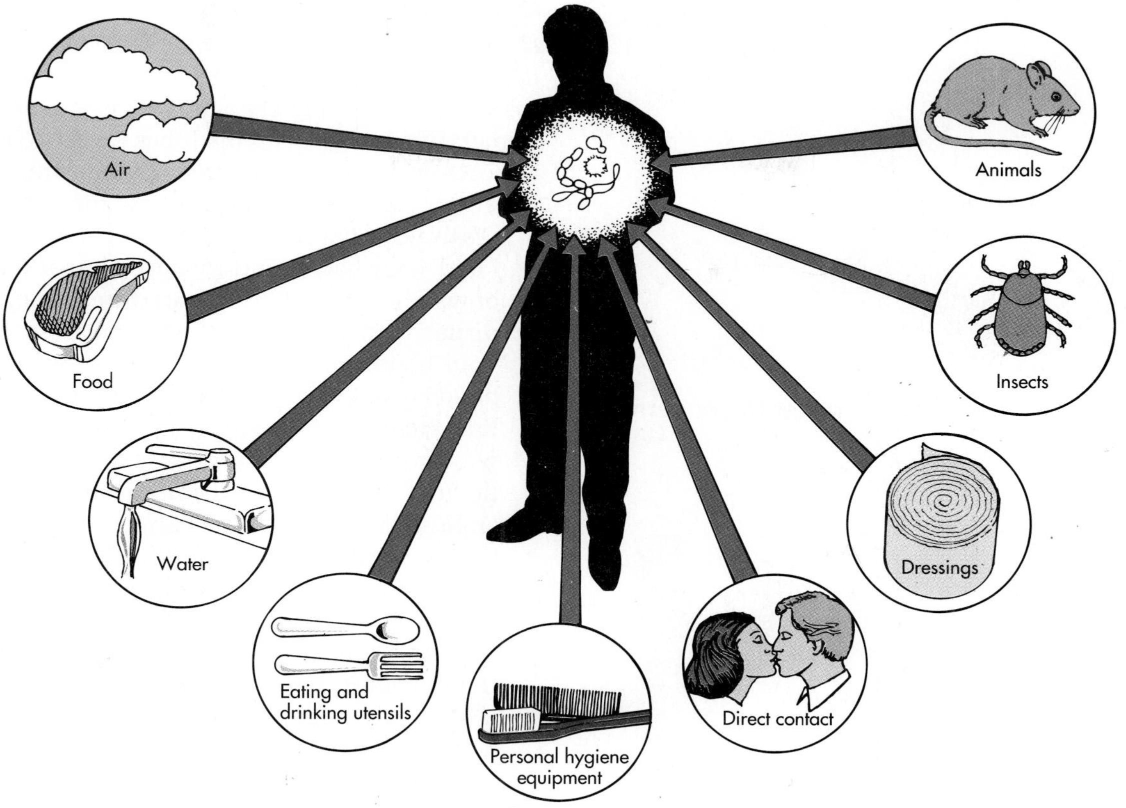

Fig. 9-2 Methods of transmitting microbes.

MEDICAL ASEPSIS

Asepsis is being free of disease-producing microbes. Microbes are everywhere. Therefore practices are needed to achieve asepsis. **Medical asepsis (clean technique)** is the practices used to remove or destroy pathogens and to prevent their spread from one person or place to another person or place. The number of pathogens is reduced.

Microbes cannot be present during surgery or when instruments are inserted into the body. Also, open wounds (cuts, burns, surgical incisions) require the absence of microbes. These provide portals of entry for microbes. **Surgical asepsis (sterile technique)** is the practices that keep equipment and supplies free of all microbes (p. 187). **Sterile** means the absence of *all* microbes—pathogens and nonpathogens. **Sterilization** is the process that destroys *all* microbes. Both pathogens and nonpathogens are destroyed.

Contamination is the process of becoming unclean. In medical asepsis, an item or area is *clean* when it is free of pathogens. The item or area is contaminated if pathogens are present. A sterile item or area is contaminated when pathogens or nonpathogens are present.

Common Aseptic Practices

Aseptic practices break the chain of infection. To prevent the spread of microbes:

- Wash your hands after urinating or having a bowel movement. Also wash your hands after changing tampons or sanitary pads.
- Wash your hands after contact with your own or another person's blood, body fluids, secretions, or excretions. This includes saliva, vomitus, urine, feces, vaginal discharge, mucus, semen, wound drainage, pus, and respiratory secretions.
- Provide all persons with their own toothbrush, drinking glass, towels, washcloths, and other personal care items.
- Cover your nose and mouth when coughing, sneezing, or blowing your nose.
- Wash your hands after coughing, sneezing, or blowing your nose.
- Bathe, wash hair, and brush your teeth regularly.
- Wash your hands before and after handling, preparing, or eating food.
- Wash fruits and raw vegetables before eating or serving them.
- Wash cooking and eating utensils with soap and water after use.

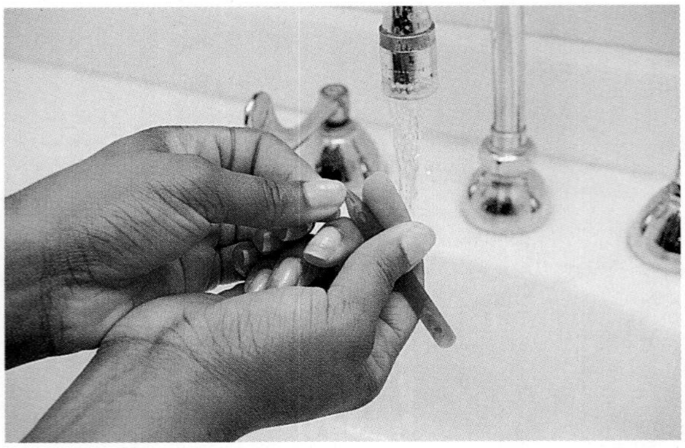

Fig. 9-3 A nail file is used to clean under the fingernails.

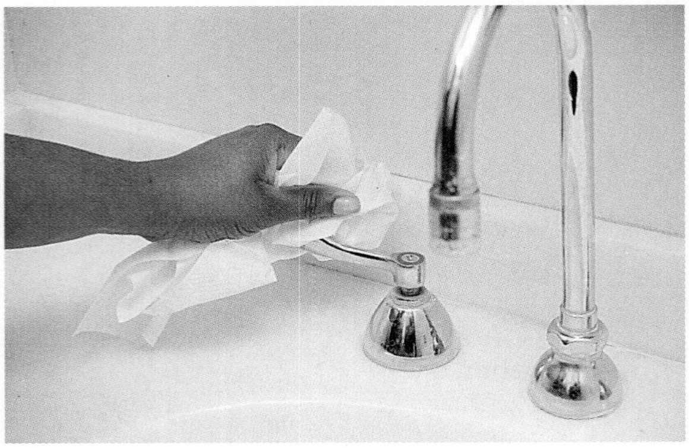

Fig. 9-4 A paper towel is used to turn off the faucet.

Handwashing

Handwashing with soap and water is the easiest and the most important way to prevent the spread of infection. Your hands are used in almost every activity. They are easily contaminated and can spread microbes if you do not practice handwashing before and after giving care. To properly wash your hands, you must follow these rules:

- Wash your hands under warm running water.
- Hold your hands and forearms lower than your elbows throughout the procedure. Your hands are dirtier than your elbows and forearms. If you hold your hands and forearms up, dirty water runs from hands to elbows. Those areas become contaminated.
- Pay attention to areas often missed during handwashing: thumbs, knuckles, sides of the hands, little fingers, and under the nails. Use a nail file or orange stick to clean under fingernails (Fig. 9-3).
- Check center policy for how long to wash your hands. At least a 10- to 15-second handwash is required. Wash your hands longer if they are visibly soiled with blood, body fluids, secretions, or excretions. Your judgment is important.
- Use a clean paper towel for each faucet to turn water off (Fig. 9-4). Faucets are contaminated. Using paper towels prevents clean hands from becoming contaminated again.
- Use a lotion after handwashing to prevent skin chapping and drying. Skin breaks can occur in chapped and dry skin. Remember that skin breaks are portals of entry for microbes.

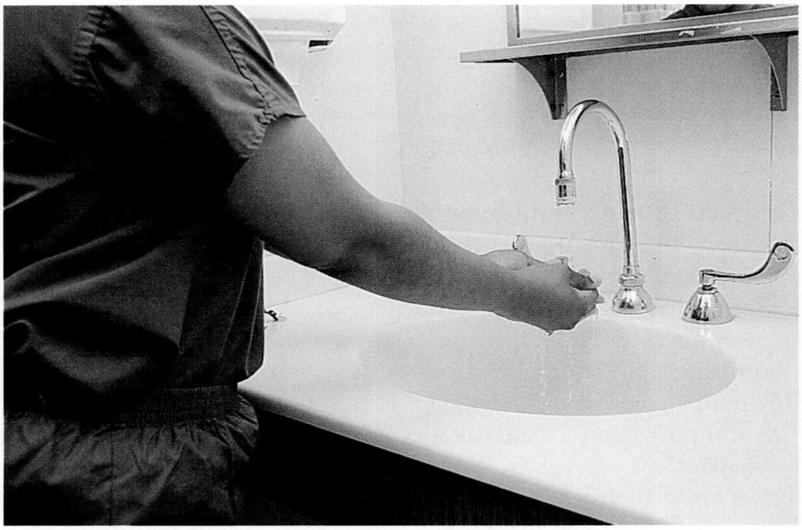

Fig. 9-5 The uniform does not touch the sink. Soap and water are within reach. Hands are lower than the elbows.

Handwashing

NNAAP™ SKILL

Procedure

1 Make sure you have soap, paper towels, orange stick or nail file, and a wastebasket. Collect missing items.

2 Push your watch up 4 to 5 inches. Also push up uniform sleeves.

3 Stand away from the sink so your clothes do not touch the sink. Stand so the soap and faucet are easy to reach (Fig. 9-5).

4 Turn on the faucet. Adjust the water until it feels warm and comfortable.

5 Wet your wrists and hands thoroughly under running water. Keep your hands lower than your elbows during the procedure (see Fig. 9-5).

6 Apply about 1 teaspoon of soap to your hands.

7 Rub your palms together, and interlace your fingers to work up a good lather (Fig. 9-6). This step should last at least 10 seconds.

8 Wash each hand and wrist thoroughly. Clean well between the fingers. Clean under the fingernails by rubbing the tips of your fingers against your palms (Fig. 9-7).

9 Use a nail file or orange stick to clean under the fingernails (see Fig. 9-3). This step is necessary for the first handwashing of the day and when your hands are highly soiled.

10 Rinse your wrists and hands well. Water should flow from the arms to the hands.

11 Repeat steps 6 through 10, if needed.

12 Dry your wrists and hands with paper towels. Pat dry.

13 Discard the paper towels.

14 Turn off faucets with clean paper towels to avoid contaminating your hands. Use a clean paper towel for each faucet.

15 Discard paper towels.

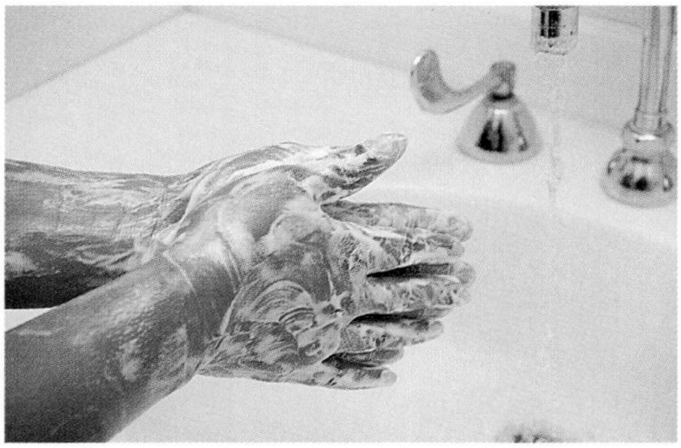

Fig. 9-6 The palms are rubbed together to work up a good lather.

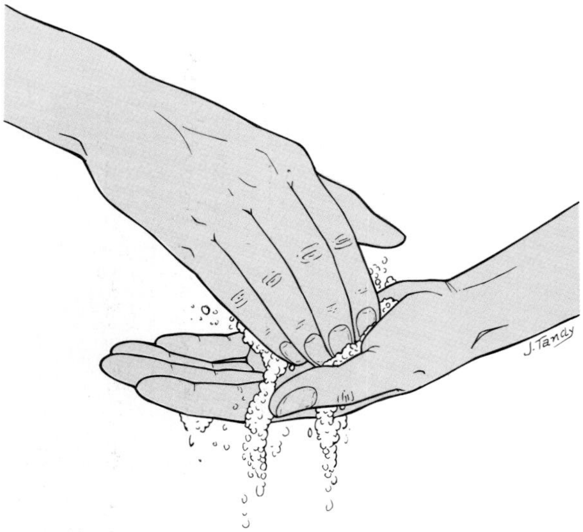

Fig. 9-7 The tips of the fingers are rubbed against the palms to clean underneath the fingernails.

Care of Supplies and Equipment

Most nursing centers have "clean" and "dirty" utility rooms. Equipment is cleaned in the "dirty" utility room before being disinfected or sterilized in the "clean" utility room. Most health care equipment is disposable (single-use). Disposable equipment is used for a resident and then discarded. However, some disposable items are used several times by a resident. Examples include disposable bedpans, urinals, wash basins, thermometers, water pitchers, and drinking cups. Items are labeled with the resident's name, room and bed number, and never "borrowed" for another resident. When used correctly, disposable items help reduce the spread of infection.

Large and costly equipment usually is not disposable. It is disinfected and sterilized before reuse. Before disinfection or sterilization, equipment is cleaned.

Cleaning. Cleaning removes debris and organic material. It also reduces the number of microbes present. Organic material includes blood, body fluids, secretions, and excretions. Follow these guidelines when cleaning equipment:

- Wear personal protective equipment (gloves, mask, gown, and protective eyewear) when cleaning items contaminated with blood, body fluids, secretions, or excretions.
- Rinse the item in cold water first. Rinsing removes organic material. Heat causes organic matter to become thick, sticky, and hard to remove.
- Wash the item with soap and hot water.
- Scrub thoroughly. Use a brush if necessary.
- Rinse the item in warm water.
- Dry the item.
- Disinfect or sterilize the item.
- Disinfect equipment and the sink used in the cleaning procedure.
- Discard personal protective equipment.

Disinfection. **Disinfection** is the process of destroying pathogens. However, spores are not destroyed. **Spores** are bacteria protected by a hard shell. Spores are killed by extremely high temperatures.

Germicides are disinfectants applied to skin, tissues, and nonliving objects. Alcohol is a common germicide.

Chemical disinfectants are used to clean nondisposable items. Such items include glass thermometers, metal bedpans, blood pressure cuffs, commodes, chairs, counter tops, tubs, wheelchairs, stretchers, and room furniture. Chemical disinfectants can burn and irritate the skin. Wear utility gloves or rubber household gloves to prevent skin irritation. These gloves are *waterproof*. Do not wear disposable gloves when using disinfectants. Some chemical disinfectants have special precautions for use or storage. Check the material safety data sheet (see Chapter 8) before handling a disinfectant.

Sterilization. Sterilizing destroys all nonpathogens and pathogens, including spores. Very high temperatures are used. Remember, microbes grow best at body temperature. They are destroyed by heat.

Boiling water, radiation, liquid or gas chemicals, dry heat, and *steam under pressure* are sterilization methods. An **autoclave** (Fig. 9-8) is a pressure steam sterilizer. Glass, surgical linens, and metal objects (such as surgical instruments and basins) are auto-

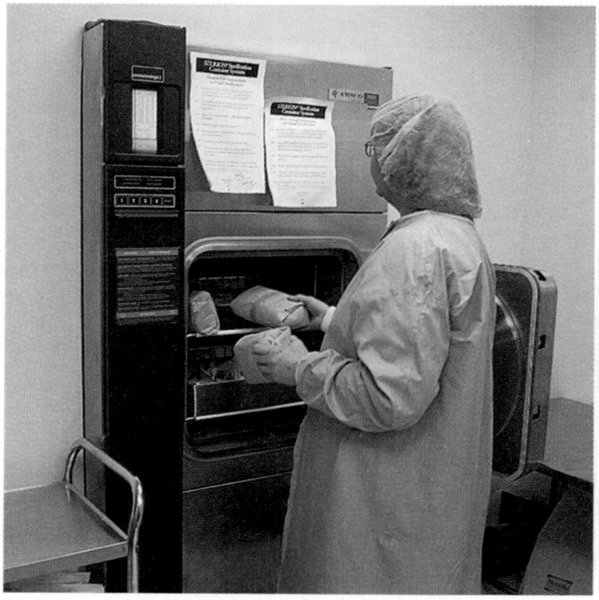

Fig. 9-8 An autoclave.

claved. High temperatures destroy plastic and rubber items. Therefore they are not autoclaved. Steam under pressure usually sterilizes objects in 30 to 45 minutes.

Other Aseptic Measures

Handwashing, cleaning, disinfection, and sterilization are important aseptic measures. However, other aseptic measures also prevent the spread of infection and microbes. These measures are listed in Box 9-2. The measures are useful in home, work, and everyday activities.

ISOLATION PRECAUTIONS

Sometimes barriers are needed to prevent the escape of pathogens. The pathogens are kept within a certain area, usually the resident's room. This requires isolation procedures.

The Centers for Disease Control and Prevention (CDC) has guidelines for isolation precautions. The guidelines recognize that all body fluids, secretions, and excretions can transmit pathogens. Two tiers of precautions are practiced—Standard Precautions and Transmission-Based Precautions.

Standard Precautions and Transmission-Based Precautions prevent the spread of a **communicable** or **contagious disease.** Communicable diseases are caused by pathogens that are spread easily.

Isolation precautions are based on *clean* and *dirty*. *Clean* areas or objects are not contaminated. Uncontaminated areas are free of pathogens. *Dirty* areas or objects are contaminated. If a *clean* area or object has contact with something *dirty*, the clean item is now dirty. *Clean* and *dirty* also depend on how the pathogen is spread.

Standard Precautions

Standard Precautions (Box 9-3, p. 174) reduce the risk of spreading pathogens and known and unknown infections. *Standard Precautions are used in the care of all residents.* They prevent the spread of infection from:

- Blood
- All body fluids, secretions, and excretions (except sweat) even if blood is not visible
- Nonintact skin (skin with open breaks)
- Mucous membranes

Transmission-Based Precautions

Some infections require precautions in addition to Standard Precautions. Transmission-Based Precautions (Table 9-1, p. 176) depend on how the pathogen is spread. You must understand how certain infections are spread (see Fig. 9-2). This helps you understand the different types of Transmission-Based Precautions.

Text continued on p. 177

BOX 9-2 ASEPTIC MEASURES

- Hold equipment and linens away from your uniform (Fig. 9-9).
- Prevent dust movement. Do not shake linens or equipment. Use a damp cloth for dusting.
- Clean from the cleanest area to the dirtiest. This prevents soiling a clean area.
- Clean away from your body. If you dust, brush, or wipe toward yourself, you transmit microbes to your skin, hair, and clothing.
- Flush urine and feces down the toilet.
- Pour contaminated liquids directly into sinks or toilets. Avoid splashing onto other areas.
- Avoid sitting on a resident's bed. You will pick up microbes and transfer them to the next surface that you sit on.
- Make sure all residents have their own personal hygiene equipment.
- Do not take equipment from one resident's room to use for another resident. Even if the item is unused, do not take it from one room to another.
- Use leakproof plastic bags for soiled tissues, linen, and other materials.
- Keep tables, counter tops, wheelchair trays, and other surfaces clean and dry.
- Label bottles with the resident's name and the date the bottle was opened.
- Keep bottles and fluid containers tightly capped or covered.
- Provide for the resident's hygiene needs (see Chapter 13). Wash contaminated areas with soap and water. Feces, urine, blood, pus, and other body fluids, secretions, or excretions may contain microbes.
- Wear personal protective equipment as needed (p. 177).

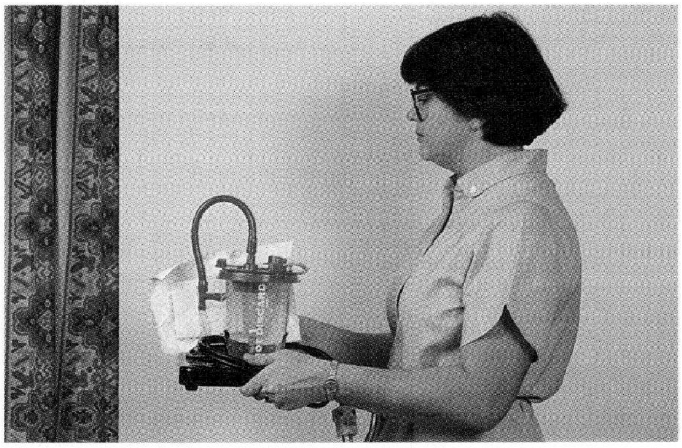

Fig. 9-9 Hold equipment away from your uniform.

Box 9-3 Standard Precautions

Handwashing

- Wash your hands after touching blood, body fluids, secretions, excretions, and contaminated items. Wash your hands even if you wore gloves.
- Wash your hands immediately after removing gloves and between resident contacts. Also wash your hands whenever needed to avoid transferring microbes to other persons or environments.
- Wash your hands between tasks and procedures on the same resident. This prevents cross-contamination of different body sites.
- Use plain soap for routine handwashing. (The nurse tells you when other agents are needed. The nurse also tells you what to use.)

Gloves

- Wear gloves when touching blood, body fluids, secretions, excretions, and contaminated items.
- Put on clean gloves just before touching mucous membranes and nonintact skin.
- Change gloves between tasks and procedures on the same resident. Also change gloves after contacting material that may be highly contaminated.
- Remove gloves promptly after use. Remove gloves before touching uncontaminated items and surfaces. Also remove gloves before going to another resident.
- Wash your hands immediately after removing gloves. This prevents the transfer of microbes to other persons or environments.

Masks, Eye Protection, and Face Shields

- Wear masks, eye protection, and face shields during procedures and tasks that are likely to cause splashes or sprays of blood, body fluids, secretions, and excretions. Masks, eye protection, and face shields protect the mucous membranes of the mouth, eyes, and nose from splashes or sprays (Fig. 9-10).

Gowns

- Wear a gown during procedures and care activities that are likely to cause splashes or sprays of blood, body fluids, secretions, or excretions. The gown protects the skin and prevents soiling of clothing.
- Remove a soiled gown as promptly as possible.
- Wash your hands after gown removal. This prevents transferring microbes to other residents or environments.

Resident-Care Equipment

- Handle used resident-care equipment carefully. Equipment may be soiled with blood, body fluids, secretions, and excretions. Prevent skin and mucous membrane exposure and clothing contamination. Also prevent the transfer of microbes to other persons and environments.
- Do not use reusable equipment for another resident. The item must be cleaned and disinfected or sterilized.
- Discard disposable (single-use) items properly.

Environmental Control

- Follow center procedures for the routine care, cleaning, and disinfecting of surfaces. This includes environmental surfaces, bed rails, bedside equipment, and other frequently touched surfaces.

Linen

- Follow center policy for used linen that is soiled with blood, body fluids, secretions, or excretions. The policy describes how to handle, transport, and process soiled linen. Prevent skin and mucous membrane exposures and clothing contamination. Also prevent the transfer of microbes to other persons and environments.

CONT'D

BOX 9-3 STANDARD PRECAUTIONS

Occupational Health and Bloodborne Pathogens

- Prevent injuries when handling needles, scalpels, and other sharp instruments or devices.
- Prevent injuries when handling sharp instruments after procedures and when cleaning used instruments.
- Prevent injuries when disposing of used needles.
- Never recap used needles. Do not manipulate them with both hands. Do not use any technique that involves directing the needle point toward any body part. Use a one-handed "scoop" technique or a mechanical device that holds the needle sheath.
- Do not remove used needles from disposable syringes by hand.
- Do not bend, break, or otherwise manipulate used needles by hand.
- Place used disposable syringes and needles, scalpel blades, and other sharp items in puncture-resistant containers.
- Place reusable syringes and needles in a puncture-resistant container for transport to the reprocessing area.
- Use resuscitation devices for mouth-to-mouth resuscitation (see Chapter 31).

Resident Placement

- A private room is used if the resident:
  - Contaminates the environment
  - Does not or cannot assist in maintaining hygiene or environmental control
- Follow the nurse's instructions if a private room is not available.

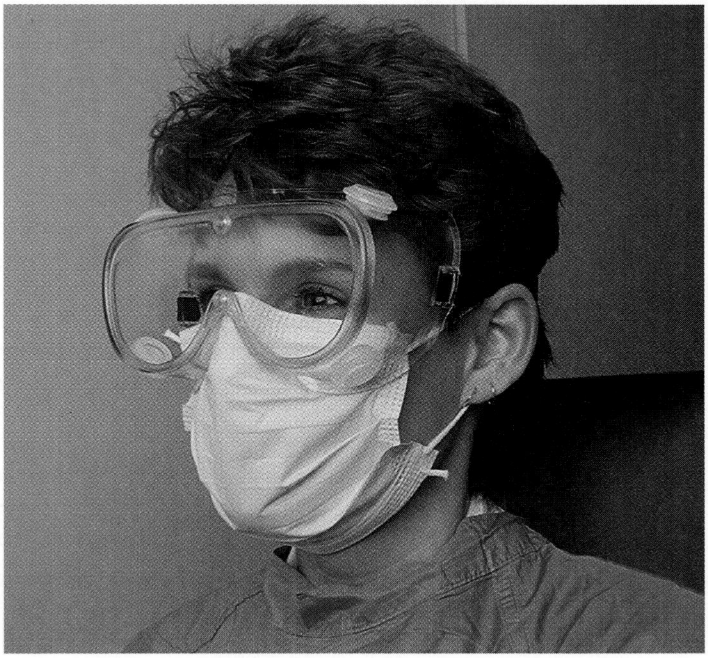

Fig. 9-10 *Goggles and a face mask protect the eyes and mucous membranes of the mouth. (From Potter PA, Perry, AG:* Fundamentals of nursing: concepts, process, and practice, *ed 4, St Louis, 1997, Mosby.)*

Table 9-1 Transmission-Based Precautions

Airborne Precautions

For known or suspected infections involving microbes transmitted by airborne droplets—measles, chickenpox, tuberculosis

Practices:
- Standard Precautions are followed.
- A private room is preferred.
- Keep the room door closed and the resident in the room.
- Wear respiratory protection (tuberculosis respirator) when entering the room of a resident with known or suspected tuberculosis.
- Do not enter the room of a resident with known or suspected measles or chickenpox if you are susceptible to these diseases.
- Wear respiratory protection (mask) if you must enter the room of a resident with known or suspected measles or chickenpox if you are susceptible to these diseases. (Respiratory protection is not needed for persons immune to measles or chickenpox.)
- Limit moving and transporting the resident from the room. The resident wears a mask if moving or transporting from the room is necessary.

Droplet Precautions

For known or suspected infections involving microbes transmitted by droplets produced by coughing, sneezing, talking, or procedures—meningitis, pneumonia, epiglottitis, diphtheria, pertussis (whooping cough), influenza, mumps, rubella, streptococcal pharyngitis, or scarlet fever

Practices:
- Standard Precautions are followed.
- A private room is preferred.
- Wear a mask when working within 3 feet of the resident. (Wear a mask on entering the room if required by center policy.)
- Limit moving and transporting the resident from the room. The resident wears a mask if moving or transporting from the room is necessary.

Contact Precautions

For known or suspected infections involving microbes transmitted by:
- *Direct contact with the resident (hand or skin-to-skin contact that occurs during care activities)*
- *Indirect contact (touching surfaces or care items in the resident's room)—gastrointestinal, respiratory, skin, or wound infections*

Practices:
- Standard Precautions are followed.
- A private room is preferred.
- Wear gloves when entering the room.
- Change gloves after having contact with infective material that may contain high concentrations of microbes.
- Remove gloves before leaving the resident's room.
- Wash your hands immediately with an agent specified by the nurse.
- Make sure your hands do not touch potentially contaminated surfaces or items after removing gloves and handwashing.
- Wear a gown on entering the room if you will have substantial contact with the resident, environmental surfaces, or items in the room.
- Wear a gown on entering the room if the resident is incontinent or has diarrhea, an ileostomy, a colostomy, or wound drainage not contained by a dressing.
- Remove the gown before leaving the resident's room. Make sure your clothing does not contact potentially contaminated surfaces in the resident's room.
- Limit moving or transferring the resident from the room. Maintain precautions if the resident is moved or transferred from the room.

Box 9-4 Rules for Isolation Precautions

- Collect all needed equipment before entering the room.
- Prevent contamination of equipment and supplies. Floors are contaminated. So is any object on the floor or that falls to the floor.
- Use mops wetted with a disinfectant solution to clean floors. Floor dust is contaminated.
- Prevent drafts. Pathogens are carried in the air by drafts.
- Use paper towels to handle contaminated items.
- Remove items from the room in sturdy, leakproof plastic bags.
- Double bag items if the outer part of the bag is or can be contaminated (p. 182).
- Follow center policy for removing and transporting disposable and reusable items.
- Return reusable dishes, eating utensils, and trays to the food service department. Discard disposable dishes, eating utensils, and trays in the waste container in the resident's room.
- Do not touch your hair, nose, mouth, eyes, or other body parts when caring for a resident in isolation.
- Do not touch any clean area or object if your hands are contaminated.
- Wash your hands if they become contaminated.
- Place clean items or objects on paper towels.
- Do not shake linen.
- Use paper towels to turn faucets on and off.
- Tell the nurse if you have any cuts, open skin areas, a sore throat, vomiting, or diarrhea.

Protective Measures

Center policies may differ from those in this text. The rules in Box 9-4 are a guide for giving safe care when isolation precautions are used.

Isolation precautions involve wearing gloves, a gown, a mask, or protective eyewear. Removing linens, trash, and equipment from the room may require double bagging. Special measures are needed to collect specimens and to transport residents on isolation precautions.

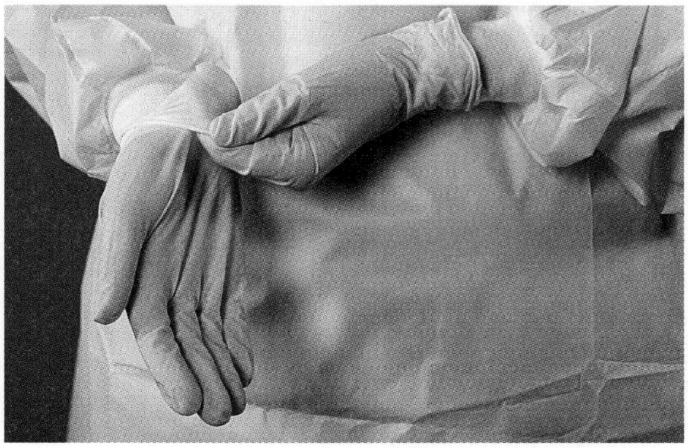

Fig. 9-11 The gloves cover the cuffs of the gown.

Wearing gloves. The skin is a natural barrier. It prevents microbes from entering the body. Small skin breaks on the hands and fingers are common. Some are very small and hard to see. Disposable gloves give added protection. They protect you from pathogens in the resident's blood, body fluids, secretions, and excretions. They also protect the resident from microbes on your hands.

Wear gloves whenever contact with blood, body fluids, secretions, excretions, mucous membranes, and nonintact skin is likely. Contact may be direct. Or contact may be with items or surfaces contaminated with blood, body fluids, secretions, or excretions.

Do not tear gloves when putting them on. Carelessness, long fingernails, and rings can tear gloves. Blood, body fluids, secretions, and excretions can enter the glove through the tear. This contaminates the hand. Remember the following about wearing gloves:

- Gloves are easier to put on when your hands are dry.
- You need a new pair for every resident.
- Remove and discard torn, cut, or punctured gloves immediately. Wash your hands and put on a new pair.
- Wear gloves only once. Discard them after use.
- Put on clean gloves just before touching mucous membranes or nonintact skin.
- Put on new gloves whenever gloves become contaminated with blood, body fluids, secretions, or excretions. You may need more than one pair of gloves for a task.
- Make sure gloves cover your wrists. If you wear a gown, gloves must cover the cuffs (Fig. 9-11).
- Remove gloves so the inside part is on the outside. The inside is considered *clean*.
- Wash your hands after removing gloves.

Removing Gloves

Procedure

1 Make sure that glove touches only glove. Do not let gloves touch skin on your wrists or arms.
2 Grasp a glove just below the cuff (Fig. 9-12, *A*).
3 Pull the glove down over your hand so it is inside out (Fig. 9-12, *B*).
4 Hold the removed glove with your other gloved hand.
5 Reach inside the other glove with the first two fingers of your ungloved hand (Fig. 9-12, *C*).
6 Pull the glove down (inside out) over your hand and the other glove (Fig. 9-12, *D*).
7 Discard the gloves. Follow center policy.
8 Wash your hands.

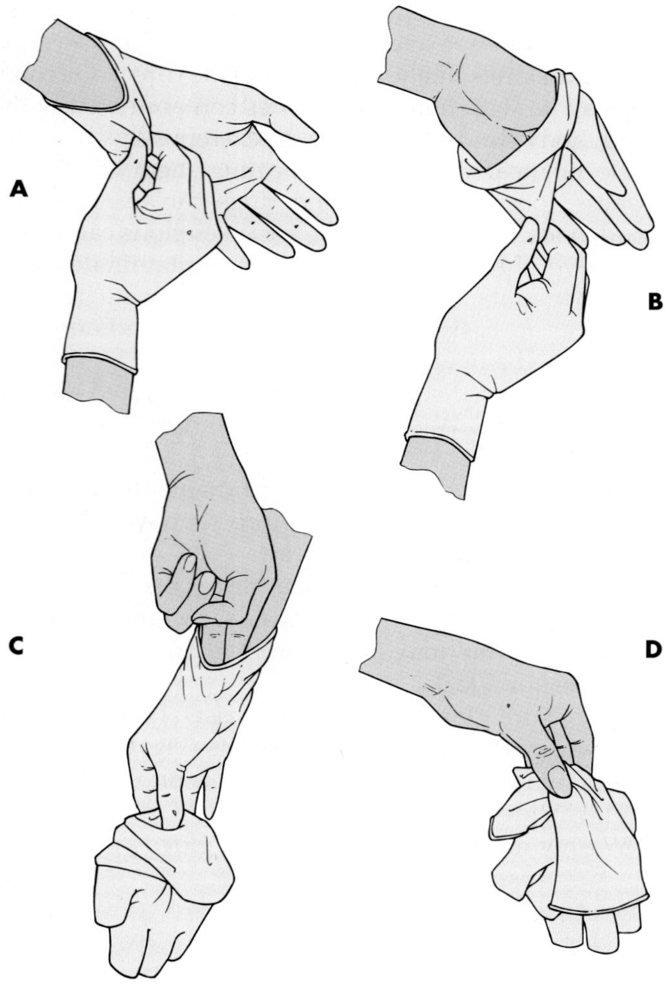

Fig. 9-12 Removing gloves. **A,** The glove is grasped below the cuff. **B,** The glove is pulled down over the hand. The glove is inside out. **C,** The fingers of the ungloved hand are inserted inside the other glove. **D,** The glove is pulled down and over the hand and glove. The glove is inside out.

Wearing protective apparel. Gowns, plastic aprons, shoe covers, boots, and leg coverings are barriers that prevent the transmission of microbes. They protect your clothes, wrists, and arms from contact with blood, body fluids, secretions, or excretions. They also protect against splashes and sprays.

Gowns must be long and large enough to completely cover clothing. The sleeves are long with tight cuffs. The gown opens at the back. It is tied at the neck and waist. The inside and neck are *clean*. The outside and waist strings are contaminated.

Gowns are used once. A wet gown is contaminated. A wet gown is removed and a dry one put on. Disposable gowns are made of paper. They are discarded after use. Reusable gowns are made of cloth. Laundering is necessary before reuse.

Donning and Removing a Gown

Procedure

1 Remove your watch and all jewelry.
2 Roll up uniform sleeves.
3 Wash your hands.
4 Put on a face mask if required.
5 Pick up a clean gown. Hold it out in front of you, and let it unfold. Do not shake the gown.
6 Put your hands and arms through the sleeves (Fig. 9-13, *A*).
7 Make sure the gown covers the front of your uniform. It should be snug at the neck.
8 Tie the strings at the back of the neck (Fig. 9-13, *B*).
9 Overlap the back of the gown. Make sure the gown covers your uniform. The gown should be snug and not hang loosely (Fig. 9-13, *C*).
10 Tie the waist strings at the back.
11 Put on the gloves.
12 Provide necessary resident care.
13 Remove and discard the gloves.
14 Remove the gown:
  a Untie the waist strings.
  b Wash your hands.
  c Untie the neck strings. Do not touch the outside of the gown.
  d Pull the gown down from the shoulder.
  e Turn the gown inside out as it is removed. Hold the gown at the inside shoulder seams and bring your hands together (Fig. 9-13, *D*).
15 Roll up the gown away from you. Keep it inside out.
16 Discard the gown. Follow center policy.
17 Wash your hands.
18 Remove the face mask. Discard it following center policy.
19 Wash your hands.
20 Open the door using a paper towel. Discard the paper towel as you leave.

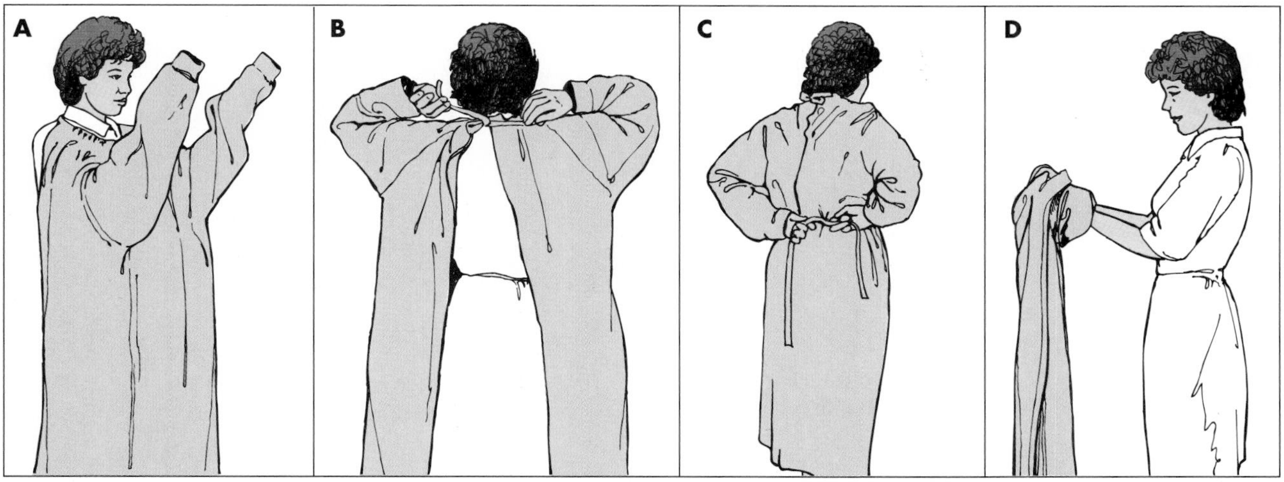

Fig. 9-13 Gowning technique. **A,** The arms and hands are put through the sleeves. **B,** The strings are tied at the back of the neck. **C,** The gown is overlapped in the back to cover the entire uniform. **D,** The gown is turned inside out as it is removed.

◈ Wearing masks and respiratory protection. Masks prevent the spread of microbes from the respiratory tract. They are used for Airborne and Droplet Precautions. Masks are worn by residents, visitors, or staff.

Disposable masks are used. A wet or moist mask is contaminated. Breathing can cause masks to become wet or moist. Apply a new mask when contamination occurs.

A mask should fit snugly over your nose and mouth. Wash your hands before putting on a mask. To remove the mask, first remove your gloves. Touch only the ties during removal. The front of the mask is contaminated.

Tuberculosis respirators (Fig. 9-14) are worn when caring for persons with tuberculosis (TB). Such protection is used for Airborne Precautions.

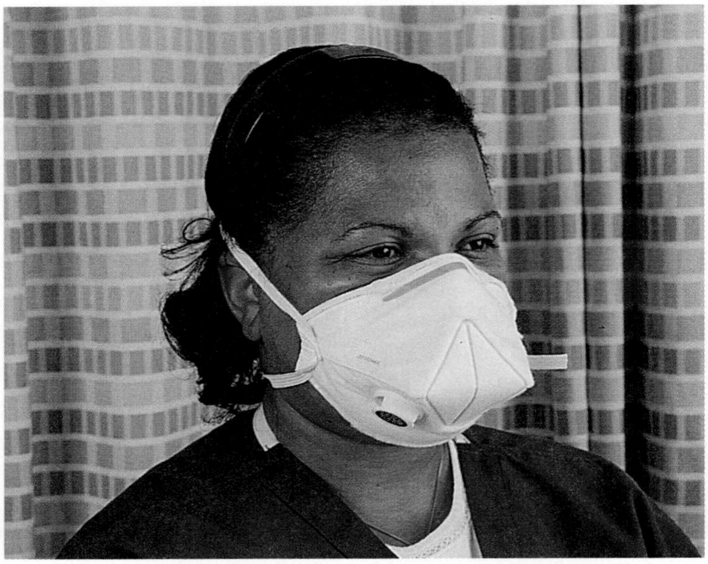

Fig. 9-14 Tuberculosis respirator.

Wearing a Mask

Procedure

1 Wash your hands.
2 Pick up the mask by its upper ties. Do not touch the part that will cover your face.
3 Place the mask over your nose and mouth.
4 Place the upper strings over your ears. Tie the strings in the back toward the top of your head (Fig. 9-15, *A*).
5 Tie the lower strings at the back of your neck (Fig. 9-15, *B*). The lower part must be under your chin.
6 Pinch the metal band around your nose if you wear glasses. The top of the mask must be snug over your nose and under the bottom edge of the glasses.
7 Wash your hands.
8 Provide necessary care. Avoid coughing, sneezing, and unnecessary talking.
9 Change the mask if it becomes moist or contaminated.
10 Remove the mask as follows:
   a Remove the gloves.
   b Untie the lower strings.
   c Untie the top strings.
   d Hold the top strings, and remove the mask.
   e Bring the strings together. The inside of the mask folds together. Do not touch the inside of the mask.
11 Discard the mask. Follow center policy.
12 Wash your hands.

A 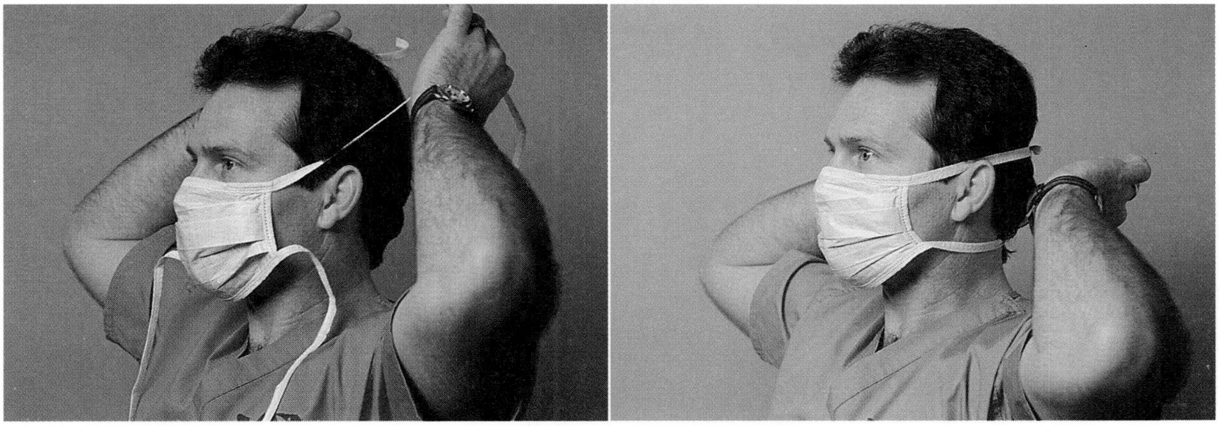 B

Fig. 9-15 *Wearing a mask.* **A,** *The upper strings are tied on the back of the head.* **B,** *The lower strings are tied at the neck. (From Potter PA, Perry, AG:* Fundamentals of nursing: concepts, process, and practice, *ed 4, St Louis, 1997, Mosby.)*

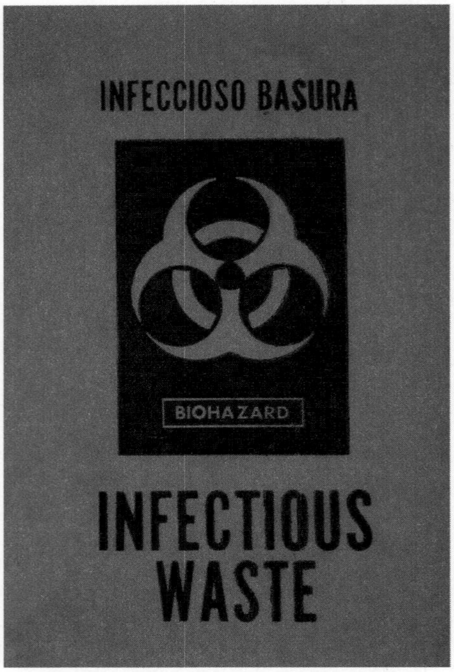

Fig. 9-16 *BIOHAZARD* symbol.

Wearing eye protection and face shields. Goggles and face shields protect the mucous membranes of your eyes, mouth, and nose from the person's pathogens. You wear goggles or face shields with face masks (see Fig. 9-10). Together they protect your eyes, nose, and mouth from splashing or spraying of blood, body fluids, secretions, or excretions. You may need such protection when giving care, cleaning instruments, or disposing of contaminated fluids.

Discard disposable eyewear after use. Reusable eyewear is cleaned before reuse. After washing reusable eyewear with soap and water, a disinfectant is used.

Bagging items. Contaminated items are bagged to remove them from the resident's room. Leak-proof plastic bags are used.

Trash is placed in a container labeled with the *BIOHAZARD* symbol (Fig. 9-16). **Biohazardous waste** is items contaminated with the resident's blood, body fluids, secretions, or excretions. (*Bio* means life, and *hazardous* means dangerous or harmful.) Linen is bagged and transported following center policy. Also follow center policy for bagging and transporting equipment and supplies.

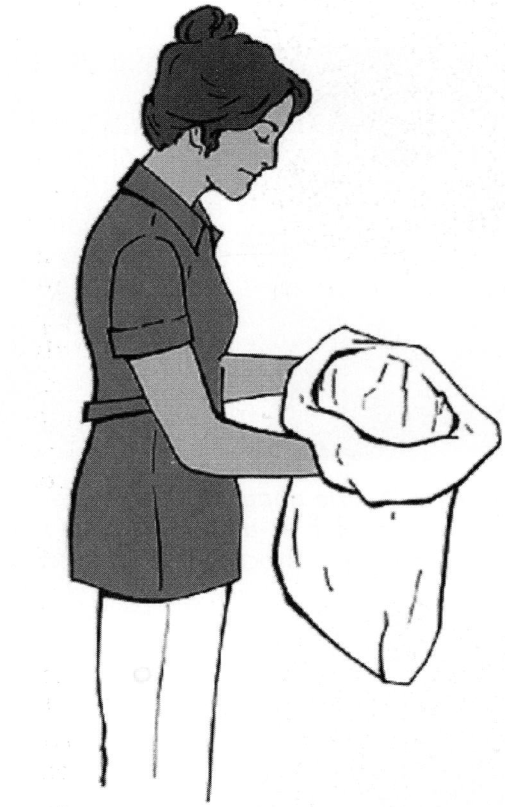

Fig. 9-17 A cuff is made on a clean bag.

One bag is usually adequate. Double bagging involves two bags. The CDC does not recommend double bagging unless the outside of the bag is soiled. Two staff members are needed for double bagging. One is inside the room. The other is at the doorway outside the room. The person in the room places contaminated items into a bag. Then the bag is sealed securely. The person outside the room holds open another bag. This bag is clean. A wide cuff is made on the clean bag to protect the hands from contamination (Fig. 9-17). The contaminated bag is placed in the clean bag at the doorway.

Collecting specimens. Specimen containers are labeled following center policy. Then the container and lid are placed on a paper towel in the resident's bathroom. Gloves are worn. Do not contaminate the outside of the container when collecting the specimen. Also avoid contamination when transferring the specimen from the collecting vessel to the container. Put the lid on securely. Some centers bag specimens for transport to the laboratory. Check center policy about applying warning labels.

Transporting residents. Residents on isolation precautions usually do not leave their rooms. However, special treatments or tests may require transporting the resident to another area. Transporting procedures vary among centers. Some require transport by bed. This prevents contaminating wheelchairs and stretchers. Other centers use wheelchairs and stretchers.

A safe transport means that other residents, staff, and visitors are protected from the infection. Follow these guidelines for safely transporting residents on isolation precautions:

- The resident wears a clean gown or pajamas and an isolation gown.
- The resident wears a mask if on Airborne or Droplet Precautions.
- Cover any draining wounds.
- Give the resident tissues and a leakproof bag. Used tissues are placed in the bag.
- Wear a gown, mask, and gloves as required by the isolation precaution.
- Place an extra layer of sheets and absorbent pads on the stretcher or wheelchair. This protects against draining body fluids.
- Do not let anyone else on the elevator. This reduces exposure to the infection.
- Alert staff in the receiving area about the isolation precautions. They wear a gown, a mask, protective eyewear, and gloves as needed.
- Disinfect the stretcher or wheelchair after use.

Psychological Impact of Isolation Precautions

The resident has love, belonging, and self-esteem needs. Too often these needs are unmet when isolation precautions are used. Visitors and staff often avoid the resident. They may need to wear a gown, a mask, protective eyewear, and gloves. This takes extra effort before entering the room. Some are unsure about what to touch. Fears about getting the disease are common. Loneliness, feeling unloved and unwanted, and rejection can occur.

Self-esteem easily suffers. The resident knows the disease can be spread to others. The resident may feel dirty and undesirable. Sometimes visitors and staff unknowingly make the resident feel ashamed and guilty about having a contagious disease.

The nurse helps the resident, visitors, and staff understand the need for isolation precautions and how they affect the resident. You can help meet the resident's need for love, belonging, and self-esteem. The following actions are helpful. Remember to disinfect or discard objects that become contaminated with infected material:

- Remember that the pathogen is undesirable—not the resident.
- Treat the resident with respect, kindness, and dignity.
- Provide newspapers, magazines, and other reading matter.
- Provide hobby materials if possible.
- Place a clock in the room.
- Encourage the resident to telephone family and friends.
- Provide a current television schedule.
- Organize your work so you can stay to visit with the resident.
- Say hello from the doorway often.

Older persons also need to see your face. This helps persons with poor vision know who you are. Personal protective equipment may increase confusion in persons who are disoriented or have dementia. Always let the resident see your face before you put on personal protective equipment. Also tell the resident who you are and what you are going to do. Report signs and symptoms of confusion to the nurse.

BLOODBORNE PATHOGEN STANDARD

The AIDS (human immunodeficiency virus [HIV]) and hepatitis B virus (HBV) are major health concerns (see Chapter 26). Health care workers care for people infected with these viruses. Therefore health care workers are at risk for exposure. The Bloodborne Pathogen Standard is intended to protect workers

Box 9-5 Bloodborne Pathogen Standard Definitions

Blood	Human blood, human blood components, and products made from human blood
Bloodborne pathogens	Pathogenic microorganisms that are present in human blood and that can cause disease in humans; these pathogens include, but are not limited to, hepatitis B virus (HBV) and human immunodeficiency virus (HIV)
Contaminated	The presence or the reasonably anticipated presence of blood or other potentially infectious materials on an item or surface
Contaminated laundry	Laundry that is soiled with blood or other potentially infectious materials or that may contain sharps
Contaminated sharps	Any contaminated object that can penetrate the skin, including, but not limited to, needles, scalpels, broken glass, broken capillary tubes, and exposed ends of dental wires
Decontamination	The use of physical or chemical means to remove, inactivate, or destroy bloodborne pathogens on a surface or item to the point where it can no longer transmit infectious particles and the surface or item is safe for handling, use, or disposal
Engineering controls	Controls that isolate or remove the bloodborne pathogen hazard from the workplace (sharps disposal containers, self-sheathing needles)
Exposure incident	A specific eye, mouth, other mucous membrane, nonintact skin, or parenteral contact with blood or other potentially infectious materials that results from the performance of an employee's duties
Handwashing facility	A facility providing an adequate supply of running water, soap, single-use towels, or hot-air drying machines
HBV	Hepatitis B virus
HIV	Human immunodeficiency virus
Occupational exposure	Reasonably anticipated skin, eye, mucous membrane, or parenteral contact with blood or other potentially infectious materials that may result from the performance of an employee's duties
Other potentially infectious materials	1. The following human body fluids: semen, vaginal secretions, cerebrospinal fluid, synovial fluid, pleural fluid, pericardial fluid, peritoneal fluid, amniotic fluid, saliva in dental procedures, any body fluid that is visibly contaminated with blood, and all body fluids in situations where it is difficult or impossible to differentiate between body fluids 2. Any unfixed tissue or organ (other than intact skin) from a human (living or dead) 3. HIV-containing cell or tissue cultures, organ cultures, and HIV- or HBV-containing culture medium or other solutions; blood, organs, or other tissues from experimental animals infected with HIV or HBV
Parenteral	Piercing mucous membranes or the skin barrier through such events as needlesticks, human bites, cuts, and abrasions
Personal protective equipment	Specialized clothing or equipment worn by an employee for protection against a hazard
Regulated waste	1. Liquid or semiliquid blood or other potentially infectious materials 2. Contaminated items that would release blood or other potentially infectious materials in a liquid or semiliquid state if compressed

CONT'D Box 9-5 Bloodborne Pathogen Standard Definitions

Regulated waste—cont'd	**3.** Items that are caked with dried blood or other potentially infectious materials that are capable of releasing these materials during handling **4.** Contaminated sharps; pathological and microbiological wastes containing blood or other potentially infectious materials
Source individual	Any individual (living or dead) whose blood or other potentially infectious materials may be a source of occupational exposure to employees; examples include, but are not limited to, the following: **1.** Hospital and clinic patients **2.** Clients in institutions for the developmentally disabled **3.** Trauma victims **4.** Clients of drug and alcohol treatment facilities **5.** Residents of hospices and nursing homes **6.** Human remains **7.** Persons who donate or sell blood or blood components
Sterilize	The use of a physical or chemical procedure to destroy all microbial life, including highly resistant bacterial endospores
Work practice controls	Controls that reduce the likelihood of exposure by altering the way the task is performed

from exposure. The standard is a regulation of the Occupational Safety and Health Administration (OSHA). OSHA is part of the U.S. Department of Labor. Box 9-5 contains the definitions used in OSHA's Bloodborne Pathogen Standard.

The AIDS and hepatitis B viruses are found in the blood. They are disease-producing pathogens. Therefore they are **bloodborne pathogens.** The viruses exit the body through blood and are transmitted to others by blood. Other potentially infectious materials (see Box 9-5) also transmit the virus. Such materials are contaminated with blood or with a body fluid that may contain blood. Potentially infectious materials may also include needles, suction equipment, soiled linens, dressings, and other equipment and items used in the resident's care.

Exposure Control Plan

Employers must have a written exposure control plan. The plan identifies those workers who have a risk of occupational exposure. That is, they may be exposed to blood or to other potentially infectious materials. In nursing centers, workers at risk usually include nurses, nursing assistants, laundry staff, housekeepers, and physical therapists. The plan also includes the actions to take when there is an exposure incident.

Staff at risk for exposure must receive free information and training. Training must occur upon employment. Retraining is done every year. Training is also required for new or changed procedures and tasks that involve exposure to bloodborne pathogens. OSHA requires that training include:

- An explanation of the Bloodborne Pathogen Standard and where to get a copy
- The causes, signs, and symptoms of bloodborne diseases
- How bloodborne pathogens are transmitted
- An explanation of the center's exposure control plan and where to get a copy
- How to know which tasks might cause occupational exposure
- The use and limitations of safe work practices, engineering controls, and personal protective equipment
- Information on the hepatitis B vaccination
- Who to contact and what to do in an emergency
- Information on reporting an exposure incident, postexposure evaluation, and follow-up
- Information on warning labels and color coding

Preventive Measures

Preventive measures help reduce the risk of occupational exposure. Such measures include hepatitis B vaccination, Standard Precautions, engineering and work practice controls, personal protective equipment, and housekeeping measures.

Hepatitis B vaccination. Hepatitis B is an inflammatory disease of the liver. It is caused by the hepatitis B virus (HBV). HBV is usually transmitted by blood and sexual contact. The hepatitis B vaccine is given to produce immunity against hepatitis B. Having **immunity** means that a person has protection against a specific disease and will not get or be affected by the disease. A vaccination involves giving a vaccine to produce immunity. A **vaccine** is a preparation containing microbes. There are vaccines for many diseases, including measles, mumps, polio, and smallpox. The microbes in the vaccine depend on the disease. The polio vaccine contains microbes that cause polio. The hepatitis B vaccine contains the virus causing hepatitis B. It provides immunity against hepatitis B.

The hepatitis B vaccination involves three injections (shots). The second injection is given 1 month after the first one. The third injection is given 6 months after the second one. The vaccination can be given before or after exposure to HBV.

Employers must make the hepatitis B vaccination available to employees within 10 working days of being hired. The employee must also receive training about the vaccination. The vaccination is free to the employee. The employer pays the cost.

An employee can refuse the vaccination. If so, the employee must sign a statement refusing the vaccine. An employee who refuses the vaccine may request and obtain the vaccination at a later date.

Methods of Control

OSHA requires engineering and work practice controls and personal protective equipment. Guidelines also are given for handling equipment and laundry.

Engineering and work practice controls

Engineering controls reduce employee exposure in the workplace. Special containers for contaminated sharps (needles, broken glass) and specimens remove and isolate the hazard from staff. Containers are puncture resistant, leakproof, and color coded in red. Or they are labeled with the *BIOHAZARD* symbol (see Fig. 9-16).

Work practice controls also reduce exposure risks. All tasks involving blood or other potentially infectious materials are done in ways that limit splattering, splashing, and spraying. Producing droplets also is avoided. OSHA requires these work practice controls:

- Do not eat, drink, smoke, apply cosmetics or lip balm, or handle contact lenses in areas of occupational exposure.
- Do not store food or drinks in refrigerators or other areas where blood or potentially infectious materials are kept.
- Wash hands after removing gloves. Wash hands as soon as possible after skin contact with blood or other potentially infectious materials.
- Never recap, bend, or remove needles by hand. When a medical procedure requires recapping, bending, or removing contaminated needles, use mechanical means (forceps) or a one-handed method.
- Never shear or break contaminated needles.
- Discard contaminated needles and sharp instruments in containers that are closable, puncture resistant, and leakproof. Containers are color coded red or have the *BIOHAZARD* symbol. Containers must be upright and not overfilled.

Personal protective equipment. Gloves, goggles, face shields, masks, laboratory coats, gowns, shoe covers, and surgical caps are examples of **personal protective equipment**. Blood or other potentially infectious material must not pass through the equipment. The equipment protects clothes, undergarments, skin, eyes, and mouth.

Personal protective equipment is free to employees. Correct sizes are available. The employer makes sure that equipment is properly cleaned, laundered, repaired, replaced, or discarded. OSHA requires these measures for safely handling and using personal protective equipment:

- Remove protective equipment before leaving the work area and when a garment becomes contaminated.
- Place used protective equipment in marked areas or containers when being stored, washed, decontaminated, or discarded.
- Wear gloves when you expect contact with blood or other potentially infectious materials. Also wear gloves when handling or touching contaminated items or surfaces. Replace worn, punctured, or contaminated gloves.
- Never wash or decontaminate disposable gloves for reuse.
- Discard utility gloves that show signs of cracking, peeling, tearing, or puncturing. Utility gloves are decontaminated for reuse if the process will not ruin them.

Equipment. Contaminated equipment is cleaned and decontaminated. Decontaminate work surfaces with an appropriate disinfectant:

- Upon completing tasks
- Immediately when there is obvious contamination
- After any spill of blood or other potentially infectious material
- At the end of the work shift when surfaces became contaminated since the last cleaning

Use a brush and dustpan or tongs to clean up broken glass. Never pick up broken glass with your hands, not even if wearing gloves. Discard broken glass into a puncture-resistant container.

Waste. Federal, state, and local laws regulate the removal of waste from the center. The Bloodborne Pathogen Standard requires special measures when discarding contaminated sharps and other regulated waste. Regulated waste includes:

- Liquid or semiliquid blood or other potentially infectious materials
- Items contaminated with blood or other potentially infectious materials
- Items caked with blood or other potentially infectious materials
- Contaminated sharps

Closable, puncture-resistant, and leakproof containers are required for regulated waste. Containers must be color coded in red or labeled with the *BIOHAZARD* symbol.

Housekeeping. The Bloodborne Pathogen Standard requires that the center be kept clean and sanitary. The employer must have a cleaning schedule. The schedule must include the methods of decontamination to be used and the tasks and procedures to be done.

Laundry. OSHA requires these precautions for contaminated laundry:

- Handle contaminated laundry as little as possible.
- Wear gloves and other needed personal protective equipment when handling contaminated laundry.
- Bag contaminated laundry where it was used.
- Mark laundry bags or containers with the *BIOHAZARD* symbol for laundry sent offsite.
- Place wet contaminated laundry in leakproof containers before transporting. The containers are color coded in red or labeled with the *BIOHAZARD* symbol.

Exposure Incidents

The exposure control plan must include the procedure for evaluating exposure incidents. An *exposure incident* is any eye, mouth, other mucous membrane, nonintact skin, or parenteral contact with blood or other potentially infectious materials. *Parenteral* means piercing the mucous membranes or the skin barrier. Piercing occurs through needlesticks, human bites, cuts, and abrasions.

Report exposure incidents at once. Medical evaluation and follow-up are free. This includes required laboratory tests. The employee's blood is tested for HBV and HIV. If the employee refuses testing, the blood sample is kept for at least 90 days. Testing is done later if the employee changes his or her mind.

Confidentiality is important. The employee is told of evaluation results. The employee is also told of any medical conditions that may need further treatment. The employee receives a written opinion of the medical evaluation within 15 days after its completion.

The source individual's blood is tested for HIV and HBV. The *source individual* is the person whose blood or body fluids are the source of an exposure incident. State laws vary about releasing the results. The employer informs the employee about any laws affecting the source's identity and test results.

SURGICAL ASEPSIS

Surgical asepsis (sterile technique) is the practices that keep equipment and supplies free of all microbes. **Sterile** means the absence of *all* microbes, including spores. Surgical asepsis is required any time the skin or sterile tissues are penetrated.

Some procedures performed by doctors and nurses require surgical asepsis. Examples include urinary catheterizations, starting IVs, suctioning, sterile dressing changes, and collecting blood specimens. Nursing assistants often assist with these procedures. Therefore you must understand the principles of surgical asepsis.

Box 9-6 Principles and Practices for Surgical Asepsis

- A sterile item can touch only another sterile item.
  - If a sterile item touches a clean item, the sterile item is contaminated.
  - If a clean item touches a sterile item, the sterile item is contaminated.
  - A sterile package that is open, torn, punctured, wet, or moist is contaminated.
  - A sterile package is contaminated after the expiration date on the package.
  - Place only sterile items on a sterile field.
  - Use sterile gloves or sterile forceps to handle other sterile items (Fig. 9-18).
  - Consider any item as contaminated if you are unsure of its sterility.
  - Do not use contaminated items. They are discarded or resterilized.
- Sterile items or a sterile field are always kept within your vision and above your waist.
  - If you cannot see an item, the item is contaminated.
  - If the item is below your waist, the item is contaminated.
  - Keep sterile gloved hands above your waist and within your sight.
  - Do not leave a sterile field unattended.
  - Do not turn your back on a sterile field.
- Airborne microbes can contaminate sterile items or a sterile field.
  - Prevent drafts by closing the door and avoiding extra movements. Ask other staff in the room to avoid extra moving.
  - Avoid coughing, sneezing, talking, or laughing over a sterile field. Turn your head away from the sterile field if you must talk.
  - Wear a mask if you need to talk during the procedure.
  - Do not assist with sterile procedures if you have a respiratory infection.
  - Do not reach over a sterile field.
- Fluid flows downward, in the direction of gravity.
  - Hold wet items down (see Fig. 9-18). If wet items are held up, fluid flows down into a contaminated area. The contaminated fluid flows back into the sterile field when the item is held up.
- The sterile field is kept dry, unless the area below it is sterile.
  - The sterile field is contaminated if it gets wet and the area below it is not sterile.
  - Avoid spilling and splashing when pouring sterile fluids into sterile containers.
- The edges of a sterile field are contaminated.
  - A 1-inch (2.5 cm) margin around the sterile field is contaminated (Fig. 9-19).
  - Place all sterile items inside the 1-inch (2.5 cm) margin of the sterile field.
  - Items outside the 1-inch (2.5 cm) margin are contaminated.
- Honesty is essential to sterile technique.
  - You know when you contaminate an item or sterile field. Be honest with yourself even if other staff members are not present.
  - Remove the contaminated item and correct the situation. If necessary, start over with sterile supplies.
  - Report the contamination to the nurse.

Principles of Surgical Asepsis

For sterile nursing procedures, regular handwashing and sterile gloves are needed. You also wear personal protective equipment as needed to prevent contact with blood, body fluids, secretions, and excretions.

For a sterile procedure, all items in contact with the person are kept sterile. If any item is contaminated, the person is at risk for infection. Therefore you must maintain a sterile field. A **sterile field** is a work area free of all pathogens and nonpathogens (including spores). Box 9-6 lists the principles and practices of surgical asepsis. Follow them to maintain a sterile field and when assisting with a sterile procedure.

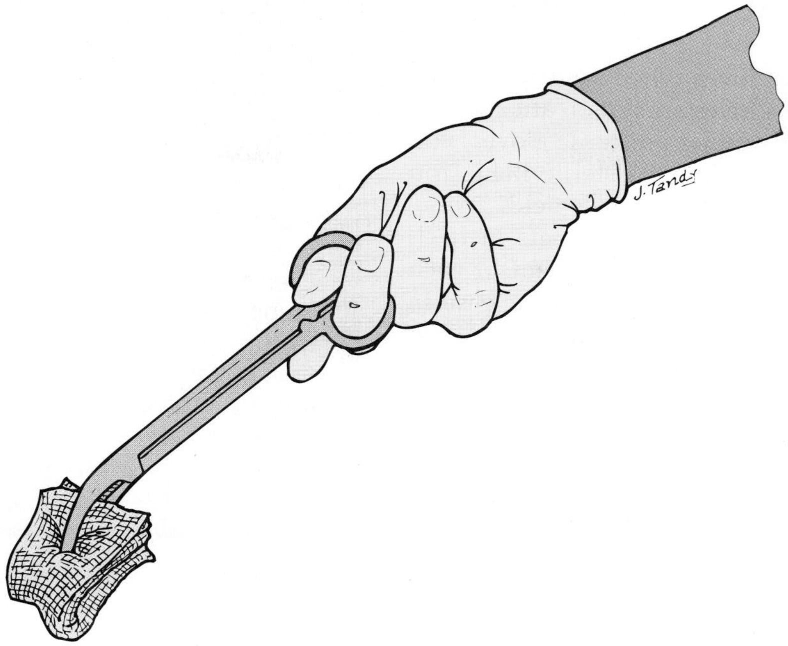

Fig. 9-18 Sterile forceps are used to handle sterile items.

Fig. 9-19 A 1-inch (2.5 cm) margin around the sterile field is considered contaminated.

Donning and Removing Sterile Gloves

You must put on sterile gloves when assisting with a sterile procedure. Sterile gloves are put on after setting up the sterile field. After putting on sterile gloves, you can handle sterile items within the sterile field. You cannot touch anything outside the sterile field.

Sterile gloves are disposable. They come in peel-back packaging. A variety of sizes lets them fit each person snugly. The insides are powdered for ease in donning the gloves. Also, the right glove and left gloves are marked on the package.

Always keep sterile gloved hands above your waist and within your vision. You can touch only items within the sterile field. If your gloves become contaminated, you must remove the gloves and put on a new pair. Also replace gloves that are torn, cut, or punctured.

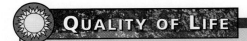

QUALITY OF LIFE

Preventing the spread of infection is the responsibility of every health care worker. You must be conscientious about your work. Your employer and your residents assume that you will practice Standard and Transmission-Based Precautions to prevent the spread of microbes and infection. Even one act of carelessness can spread microbes and endanger resident safety. The reverse is also true. You can develop the same infection that the resident has if you do not practice Standard and Transmission-Based Precautions. The simple procedure of handwashing before and after contact with a resident significantly reduces the spread of microbes.

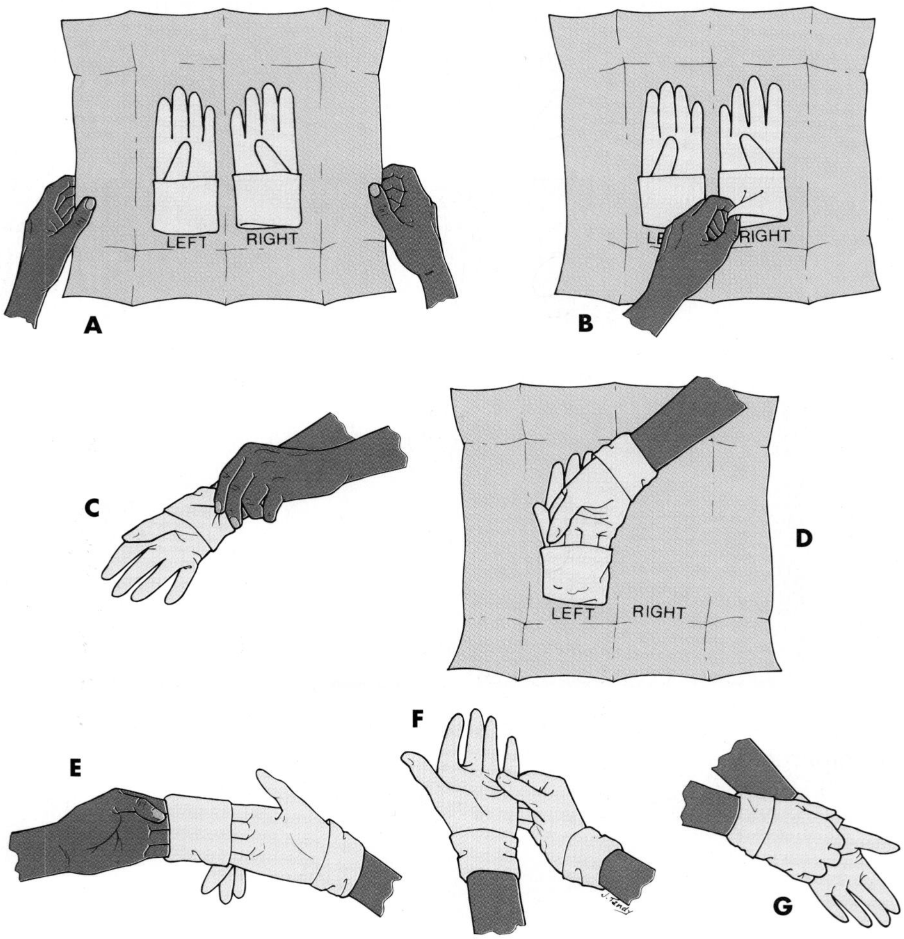

Fig. 9-20 Donning sterile gloves. **A,** Open the inner wrapper to expose the gloves. **B,** Pick up the glove at the cuff with your thumb and index finger. **C,** Slide your fingers and hand into the glove. **D,** Reach under the cuff of the other glove with your fingers. **E,** Pull on the glove. **F,** Adjust each glove for comfort. **G,** Slide your fingers under the cuffs to pull them up.

Donning and Removing Sterile Gloves

Procedure

1. Inspect the package for sterility:
   a. Check the expiration date.
   b. See if the package is dry.
   c. Check for tears, holes, punctures, and watermarks.
2. Arrange a work surface:
   a. Make sure you have enough room.
   b. Arrange the work surface at waist level and within your vision.
   c. Clean and dry the work surface.
   d. Do not reach over or turn your back on the work surface.
3. Open the package. Grasp the flaps, and gently peel the flaps back.
4. Remove the inner package. Place it on a clean work surface. Have your work surface at waist height.
5. Read any manufacturer's instructions or information on the inner packaging. The packaging may be labeled with left, right, up, and down.
6. Arrange the inner package for left, right, up, and down. Have the left glove on your left and the right glove on your right. Have the cuffs near you with the fingers pointing away.
7. Use the thumb and index finger of each hand to grasp the folded edges of the inner packaging.
8. Fold back the inner packaging to expose the gloves (Fig. 9-20, *A*). Do not touch or otherwise contaminate the inside of the package or the gloves. The inside of the inner package is a sterile field.
9. Note that each glove has a cuff about 2 to 3 inches wide. The cuffs and insides of the gloves are not sterile.
10. Put on the right glove if you are right-handed. Put on the left glove if you are left-handed:
    a. Pick up the glove with your other hand. Use your thumb and index and middle fingers (Fig. 9-20, *B*).
    b. Touch only the cuff and the inside of the glove.
    c. Turn the hand to be gloved palm side up.
    d. Lift the cuff up. Slide your fingers and hand into the glove (Fig. 9-20, *C*).
    e. Pull the glove up over your hand. If some fingers get stuck, leave them that way until the other glove is on. *Do not use your ungloved hand to straighten the glove. Do not let the outside of the glove touch any nonsterile surface.*
    f. Leave the cuff turned down.
11. Put on the other glove with your gloved hand:
    a. Reach under the cuff of the second glove with the four fingers of your gloved hand (Fig. 9-20, *D*). Keep your gloved thumb close to your gloved palm.
    b. Pull on the second glove (Fig. 9-20, *E*). Your gloved hand cannot touch the cuff or any other surface. Hold the thumb of your first gloved hand away from your gloved palm.
12. Adjust each glove with the other hand. The gloves should be smooth and comfortable (Fig. 9-20, *F*).
13. Slide your fingers under the cuffs to pull them up (Fig. 9-20, *G*).
14. Touch only sterile items.
15. Remove the gloves as in Fig. 9-12.

REVIEW QUESTIONS

Circle T if the statement is true and F if the statement is false.

1 T F Microbes are pathogens in their natural environments.

2 T F A pathogen is a microbe capable of causing an infection.

3 T F An infection results from the invasion and growth of microbes in the body.

4 T F An item is sterile if nonpathogens are present.

5 T F You hold your hands and forearms up during the handwashing procedure.

6 T F You should clean under your fingernails when washing your hands.

7 T F Disposable items help reduce the spread of infection.

8 T F Unused items in a resident's room are used for another resident.

9 T F A person has immunity against hepatitis B. The person will develop the disease.

10 T F The 1-inch edge around a sterile field is contaminated.

11 T F The inside and cuffs of sterile gloves are contaminated.

Circle the BEST answer.

12 Pathogens need the following to grow *except*
- A Water
- B Light
- C Oxygen
- D Nourishment

13 The person with an infection may have
- A Fever, nausea, vomiting, rash, and/or sores
- B Pain or tenderness, redness, and/or swelling
- C Fatigue, loss of appetite, and/or a discharge
- D All of the above

14 Microbes enter and leave the body through the following *except*
- A Respiratory tract
- B Gastrointestinal system and/or the blood
- C Reproductive system and/or urinary system
- D Intact skin

15 Which does *not* prevent nosocomial infections?
- A Handwashing before and after giving care
- B Sterilizing all items used for care
- C Surgical asepsis
- D Standard Precautions

16 When cleaning equipment, do the following *except*
- A Rinse the item in cold water before cleaning
- B Wash the item with soap and hot water
- C Use a brush if necessary
- D Clean from the dirtiest area to the cleanest

17 Isolation precautions
- A Prevent infection
- B Destroy pathogens
- C Keep pathogens within a certain area
- D Destroy pathogens and nonpathogens

18 Standard Precautions
- A Are used for all residents
- B Prevent the spread of pathogens through the air
- C Require gowns, masks, gloves, and protective eyewear
- D Involve medical and surgical asepsis

19 Gloves are worn when in contact with
- A Blood
- B Body fluids
- C Secretions and excretions
- D All of the above

20 A mask
- A Can be reused
- B Is clean on the inside
- C Is contaminated when moist
- D Should fit loosely for breathing

21 Proper use of personal protective equipment involves the following *except*
- A Washing disposable gloves for reuse
- B Removing protective equipment before leaving the work area
- C Discarding cracked or torn utility gloves
- D Wearing gloves when touching contaminated items or surfaces

22 When are contaminated work surfaces cleaned?
- A After completing a task
- B Immediately when there is obvious contamination
- C After blood or other potentially infectious material is spilled
- D All of the above

23 Goggles are
- A Always worn when using Standard Precautions
- B Worn when there is a risk of splashing blood or body fluids
- C Worn if you have an eye infection
- D All of the above

24 The Bloodborne Pathogen Standard involves the following *except*
- A Washing hands after gloves are removed
- B Discarding sharp objects into containers with the *BIOHAZARD* symbol
- C Storing food and blood in different places
- D Eating and drinking in areas of occupational exposure

25 You have been exposed to a bloodborne pathogen. Which is *true?*
- A You do not have to report the incident.
- B You pay for any required laboratory tests.
- C You can refuse HBV and HIV testing.
- D The source individual can refuse testing.

26 These statements are about surgical asepsis. Which is *false?*
- A A sterile item can touch only another sterile item.
- B Wet items are held up.
- C If you cannot see an item, it is contaminated.
- D Sterile items are kept above your waist.

Answers to these questions are on p. 697.

10 Body Mechanics

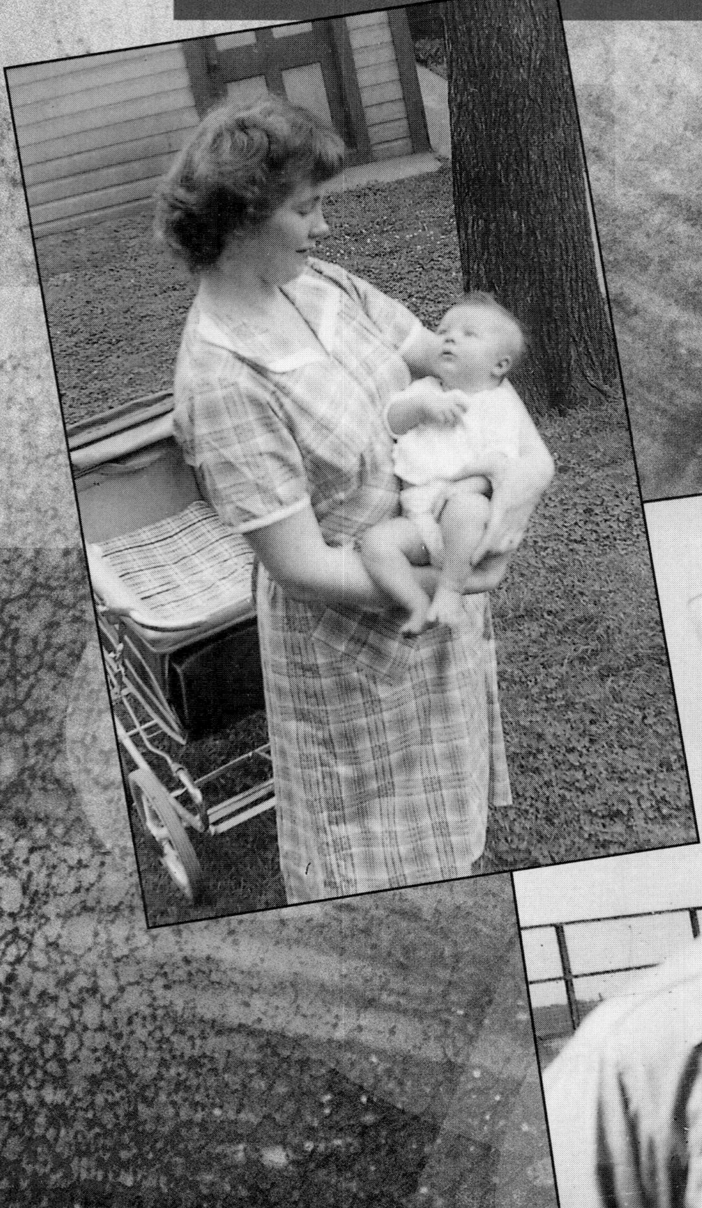

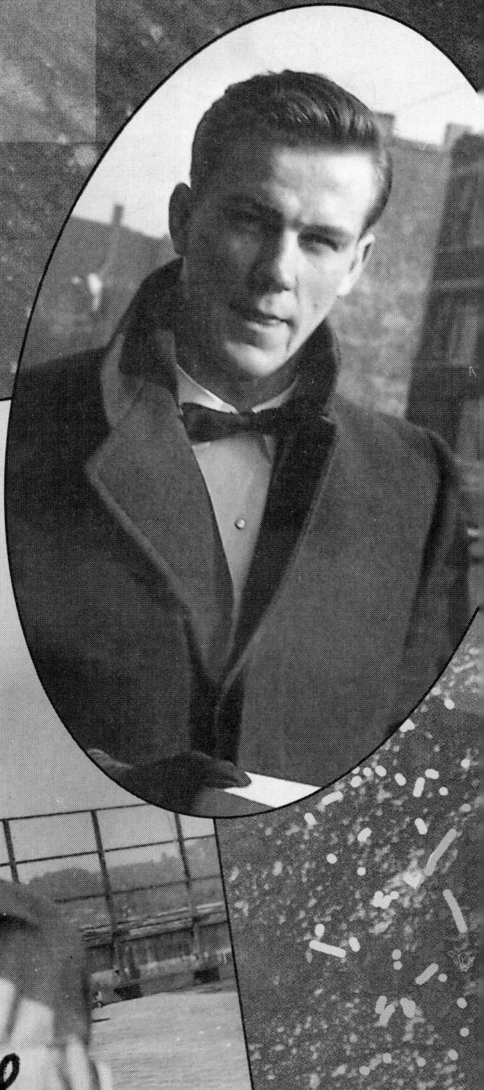

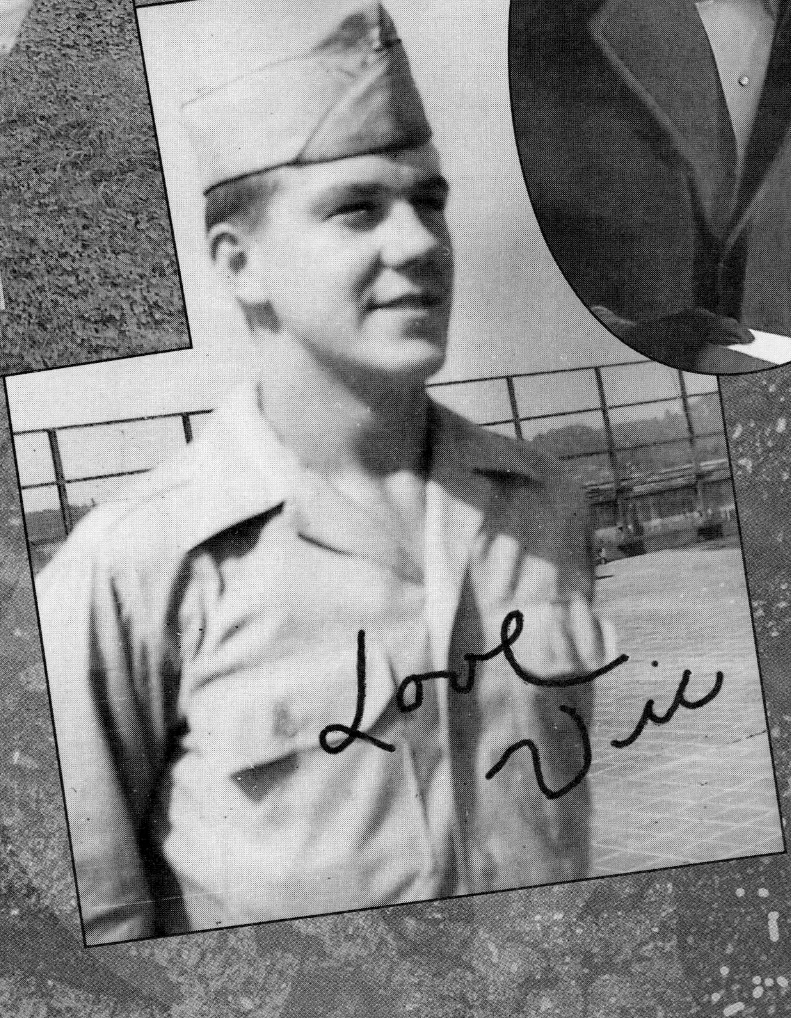

What You Will Learn

- The definition of the key terms in this chapter
- The purpose and rules of using good body mechanics
- Comfort and safety measures for lifting, turning, and moving residents in bed
- The purpose of a transfer belt (gait belt)
- How to safely transfer residents
- Why good body alignment and position changes are important for residents
- The comfort and safety measures for positioning residents in bed
- How to position residents in the basic bed positions and in a chair
- The procedures described in this chapter

Key Terms

base of support The area on which an object rests

body alignment The way in which body parts are aligned with one another; posture

body mechanics Using the body in an efficient and careful way

dorsal recumbent position The back-lying or supine position

Fowler's position A semisitting position; the head of the bed is elevated 45 to 60 degrees

friction The rubbing of one surface against another

gait belt A transfer or safety belt

lateral position The side-lying position

logrolling Turning the resident as a unit in alignment with one motion

posture The way in which body parts are aligned with one another; body alignment

prone position Lying on the abdomen with the head turned to one side

shearing When skin sticks to a surface and muscles slide in the direction the body is moving

side-lying position The lateral position

Sims' position A left side-lying position in which the upper leg is sharply flexed so that it is not on the lower leg and the lower arm is behind the person

supine position The back-lying or dorsal recumbent position

transfer belt A belt used to hold onto a resident during a transfer or when walking with the resident; a gait or safety belt

Trendelenburg's position The head of the bed is lowered, and the foot of the bed is raised

You will move and reposition residents often. Residents are moved or turned in bed or transferred from the bed to a chair, wheelchair, or stretcher. During these and other activities, you must use your body correctly. This protects you and the resident from injury.

BODY MECHANICS

Body mechanics means using the body in an efficient and careful way. It involves using good posture, balance, and the body's strongest and largest muscles to perform work. Fatigue, muscle strain, and injury can

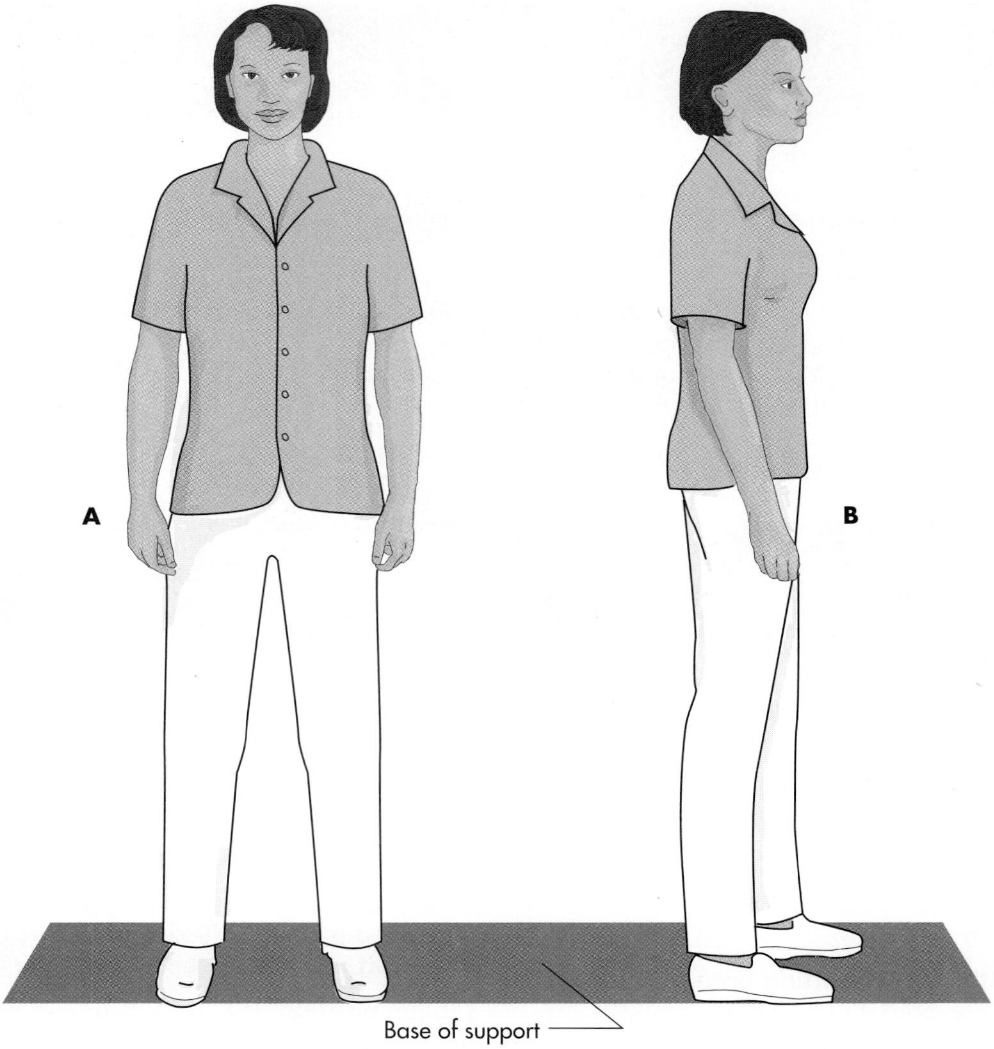

Fig. 10-1 **A,** Anterior (front) view of an adult in good body alignment with feet apart for a wide base of support. **B,** Lateral (side) view of an adult with good posture and alignment.

result from not properly using and positioning the body during activity or rest. You must be aware of your own body mechanics and those of your residents.

The body's major movable parts are the head, trunk, arms, and legs. **Posture (body alignment)** is the way the body parts are aligned with one another. Good body alignment lets the body move and function with strength and efficiency. Good alignment is necessary when standing, sitting, or lying down.

Base of support is the area on which an object rests. A good base of support is needed for balance (Fig. 10-1). When standing, your feet are your base of support. Stand with your feet apart for a wider base of support and more balance.

The strongest and largest muscles are in the shoulders, upper arms, hips, and thighs. Use these muscles to lift and move heavy objects. Otherwise, you place strain and exertion on smaller and weaker muscles. This causes fatigue and injury. *Back injuries are a major risk.* Good body mechanics involve:

- Bending your knees and squatting to lift a heavy object (Fig. 10-2). Do not bend from your waist. Bending from the waist places strain on small back muscles.
- Holding items close to your body and base of support (see Fig. 10-2). This involves upper arm and shoulder muscles. Holding objects away from your body places strain on small muscles in your lower arms.

All activities require good body mechanics. This includes cleaning, laundry, getting in and out of a car, picking up a baby, mowing, and shoveling. Follow the rules in Box 10-1 to safely and efficiently lift and move residents and heavy objects.

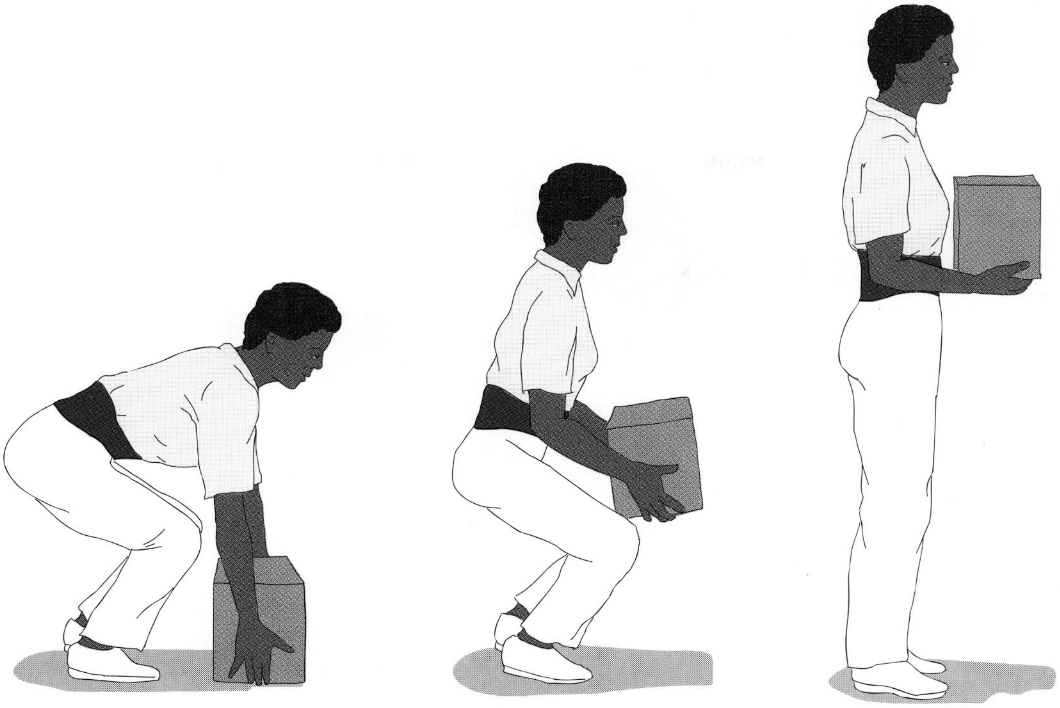

Fig. 10-2 Picking up a box using good body mechanics.

Box 10-1 Rules for Good Body Mechanics

- Keep your body in good alignment with a wide base of support.
- Use the stronger and larger muscles in your shoulders, upper arms, thighs, and hips.
- Keep objects close to your body when lifting, moving, or carrying them (see Fig. 10-2).
- Avoid unnecessary bending and reaching. Raise the bed so it is close to your waist. Adjust the overbed table so it is at your waist level.
- Face your work area. This prevents unnecessary twisting.
- Push, slide, or pull heavy objects whenever you can, rather than lifting them.
- Widen your base of support when pushing or pulling. Move your front leg forward when pushing. Move your rear leg back when pulling (Fig. 10-3, p. 198).
- Use both hands and arms to lift, move, or carry heavy objects.
- Turn your whole body when changing the direction of your movement. Move and turn your feet in the direction of the turn, instead of twisting your body.
- Work with smooth and even movements. Avoid sudden or jerky motions.
- Get help from a co-worker if the resident cannot assist with turning or moving.
- Get help from a co-worker to move heavy objects or persons. Avoid lifting or moving residents by yourself.
- Bend your hips and knees to lift heavy objects from the floor (see Fig. 10-2). Straighten your back as the object reaches thigh level. Your leg and thigh muscles work to raise the item off the floor and to waist level.
- Do not lift objects higher than chest level. Do not lift above your shoulders. Use a step stool to reach an object higher than chest level.
- Wear a body support (Fig. 10-4, p. 198) to help you use good body mechanics.

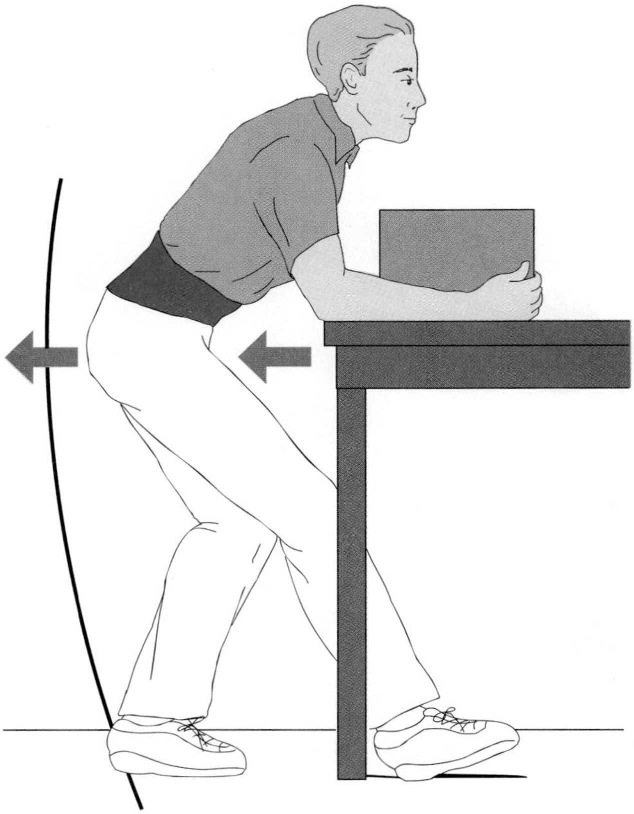

Fig. 10-3 Move your rear leg back when pulling an item.

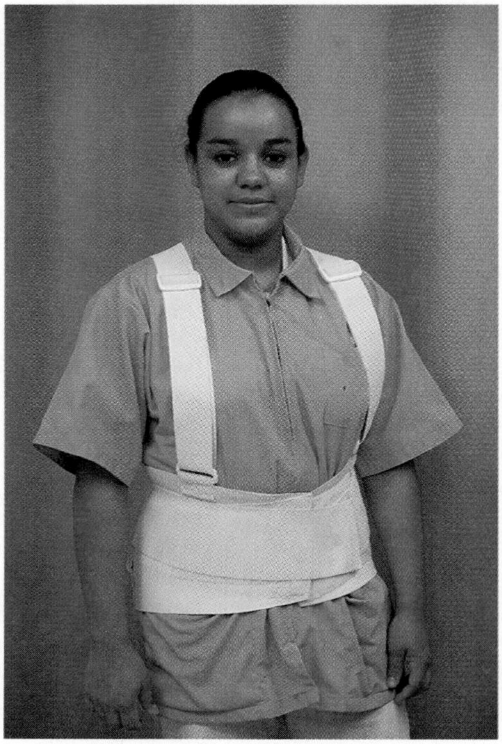

Fig. 10-4 A body support helps in using good body mechanics.

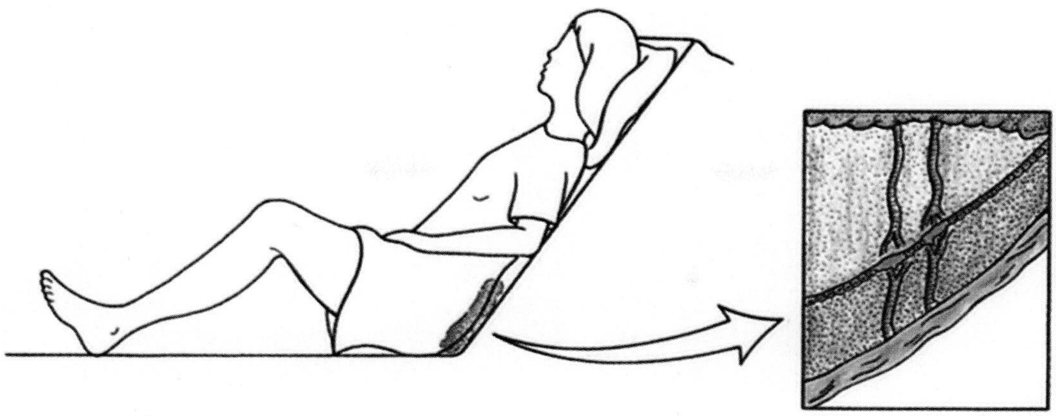

Fig. 10-5 When the head of the bed is raised to a sitting position, skin on the buttocks stays in place. However, internal structures move forward as the person slides down in bed. Skin is pinched between the mattress and hip bones.

LIFTING AND MOVING RESIDENTS IN BED

Some residents can move and turn in bed. Others need help from at least one person for position changes. Residents who are unconscious, paralyzed, on complete bedrest, in casts, or weak from illness or surgery need assistance. Sometimes more than one person or a mechanical lift is needed.

Beds are raised horizontally to give care. This reduces bending and reaching. The lowest horizontal position lets residents get out of bed with ease. You must use the bed correctly, follow the rules of body mechanics, and keep the resident in good body alignment. Also position the resident in good body alignment after moving or turning (p. 227).

Older persons are at great risk for shearing. Their skin is fragile and easily torn. You must protect the resident's skin during lifting and moving. Friction and shearing injure the skin. Both cause infection and pressure ulcers (see Chapter 14).

Friction is the rubbing of one surface against another. When moved in bed, the resident's skin rubs against the sheet. **Shearing** is when the skin sticks to a surface and muscles slide in the direction the body is moving (Fig. 10-5). Shearing occurs when the resident slides down in bed or is moved in bed. For example, when the head of the bed is raised to a sitting position, skin on the buttocks stays in place. However, the hip bones move forward as the resident slides down in bed. The skin is pinched between the mattress and the hip bones (see Fig. 10-5).

Reduce friction and shearing by rolling or lifting the resident. A cotton drawsheet (see Chapter 12) serves as a *lift sheet (turning or pull sheet)* to move the resident in bed and reduce friction. Some centers use turning pads for this purpose (p. 206).

Other comfort and safety measures are considered before moving residents in bed:

- Check with the nurse for any limits in positioning or moving the resident. These may be doctor's orders or part of the resident's care plan.
- Decide how to move the resident and how many helpers you need.
- Get enough co-workers to help you before beginning the procedure.
- Keep the resident covered and screened. This protects the right to privacy.
- Protect any tubes or drainage containers connected to the resident.
- Use caution when moving residents with severe arthritis or osteoporosis (see Chapter 26). Always ask for help when moving them to avoid causing pain or injury.

◈ Raising the Resident's Head and Shoulders

You may have to raise a resident's head and shoulders to tie the back of a gown, to turn or remove a pillow, or to give care. You can raise the resident's shoulders easily and safely by locking arms with the resident. It is best to have help with older residents to prevent pain or injury to fragile joints and bones. You also need help if the resident is heavy or hard to move.

Text continued on p. 202

Raising the Resident's Head and Shoulders by Locking Arms With the Resident

Quality of Life

Remember to:
- *Knock before entering the resident's room*
- *Address the resident by name*
- *Introduce yourself by name and title*

Pre-Procedure

1 Ask a co-worker to help if assistance is needed.
2 Wash your hands.
3 Identify the resident. Check the ID bracelet, and call the resident by name.
4 Explain what you are going to do.
5 Provide for privacy.
6 Lock the bed wheels.
7 Raise the bed to the best level for good body mechanics. Make sure the bed rails are up.

Procedure

8 Ask your helper to stand on the other side of the bed. Lower the bed rails.
9 Ask the resident to put the near arm under your near arm and behind your shoulder. His or her hand rests on top of your shoulder. If you are standing on the right side, the resident's right hand rests on your right shoulder (Fig. 10-6, *A*). If you have help, the resident does the same with your co-worker. The resident's left hand rests on your co-worker's left shoulder (Fig. 10-7, *A*).
10 Put your arm nearest to the resident under his or her arm. Your hand is on the resident's shoulder. Have your helper do the same.
11 Put your free arm under the resident's neck and shoulders (Fig. 10-6, *B*). If you have help, ask your co-worker to do the same (Fig. 10-7, *B*).
12 Help the resident pull up to a sitting or semisitting position on the count of "3" (Figs. 10-6, *C,* and 10-7, *C*).
13 Use the arm and hand that supported the resident's neck and shoulders to straighten or remove the pillow, tie the gown, etc. (Fig10-6, *D*). If you have help, your co-worker supports the resident (Fig. 10-7 *D*).
14 Help the resident lie down. Provide support with your locked arms. Support his or her neck and shoulders with your other arms.

Post-Procedure

15 Provide for comfort. Position the resident in good body alignment (p. 227).
16 Place the signal light within reach.
17 Raise or lower bed rails. Follow the care plan.
18 Lower the bed to its lowest position.
19 Unscreen the resident.
20 Wash your hands.

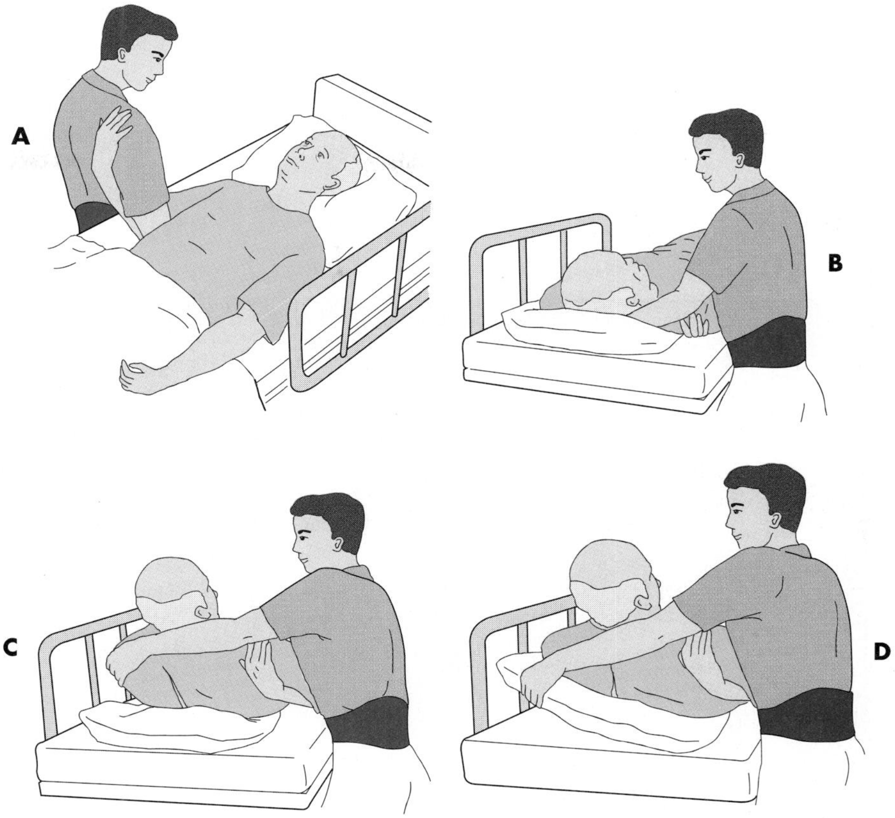

Fig. 10-6 Raise the resident's head and shoulders by locking arms with the resident. **A,** The resident's near arm is under the nursing assistant's near arm and behind the shoulder. **B,** The nursing assistant's far arm is under the resident's neck and shoulders, with the near arm under the resident's nearest arm. **C,** The resident is raised to a semisitting position by locking arms. **D,** The nursing assistant lifts the pillow while the resident is raised in a semisitting position.

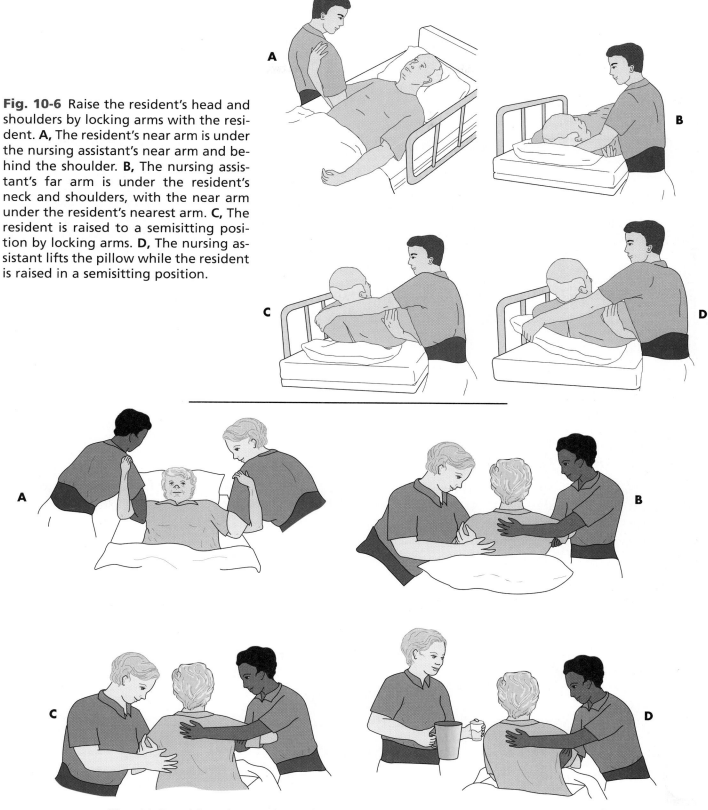

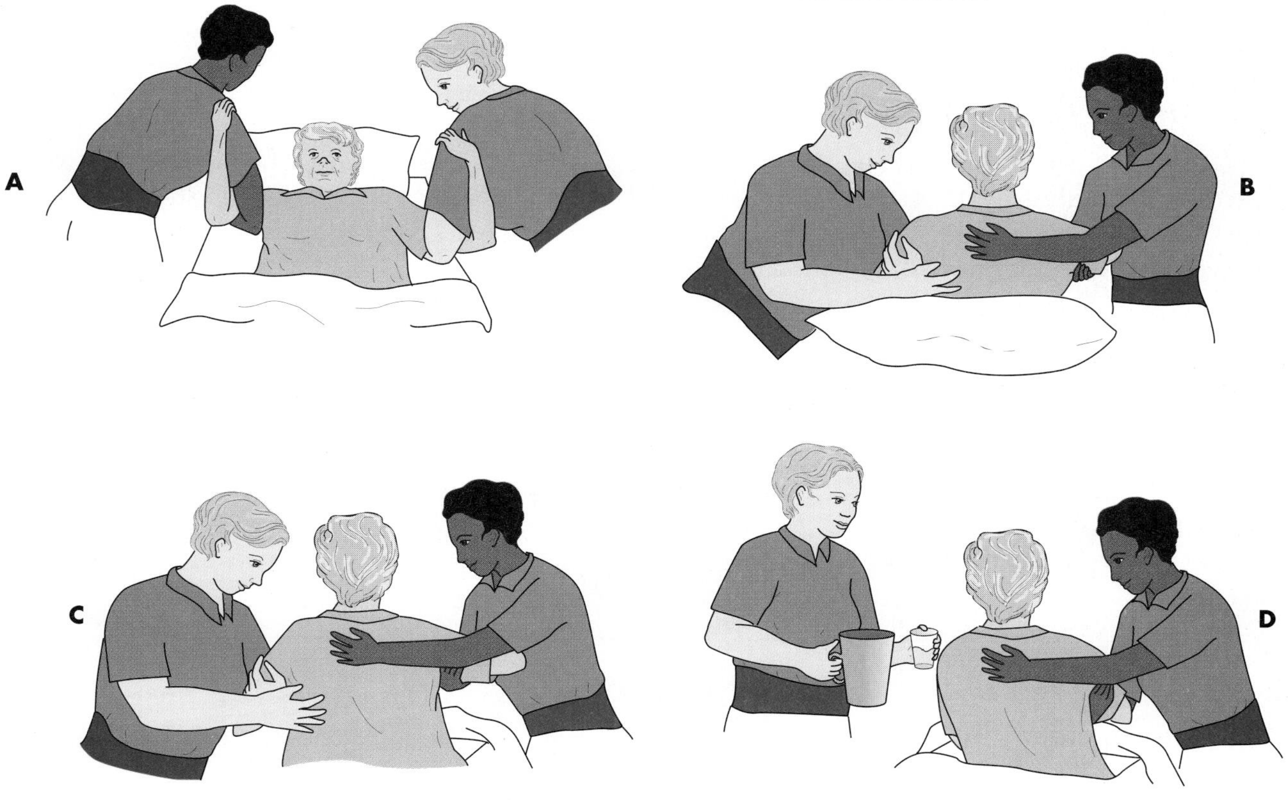

Fig. 10-7 Raising the resident's head and shoulders with assistance. **A,** Two nursing assistants lock arms with the resident. **B,** The nursing assistants have their arms under the resident's head and neck. **C,** The nursing assistants raise the resident to a semisitting position. **D,** One nursing assistant supports the resident in the semisitting position while the other gives care.

Assisting the Resident to Move Up in Bed

When the head of the bed is raised, residents often slide down toward the middle and foot of the bed (Fig. 10-8). They are moved up in bed to maintain good body alignment and comfort. Some residents can move themselves up in bed alone or with assistance. This helps their sense of independence.

You can sometimes move lightweight adults up in bed alone if they use a trapeze. However, it is best to have help to protect you and the resident from pain and injury.

Assisting the Resident to Move Up in Bed

Quality of Life

Remember to:
- *Knock before entering the resident's room*
- *Address the resident by name*
- *Introduce yourself by name and title*

Pre-Procedure

1 Wash your hands.
2 Identify the resident. Check the ID bracelet, and call the resident by name.
3 Explain what you are going to do.
4 Provide for privacy.
5 Lock the bed wheels.
6 Raise the bed to the best level for good body mechanics. Make sure the bed rails are up.

Procedure

7 Lower the head of the bed to a level appropriate for the resident. It is as flat as possible.
8 Lower the bed rail near you.
9 Place the pillow against the headboard if the resident can be without it. This prevents his or her head from hitting the headboard when moving up.
10 Stand with your feet about 12 inches apart. Point the foot nearest the head of the bed toward the head of the bed. Face the head of the bed.
11 Bend your hips and knees. Keep your back straight.
12 Place one arm under the resident's shoulders and the other under his or her thighs.
13 Ask the resident to grasp the trapeze bar and to flex both knees as in Figure 10-9.
14 Explain that you will both move on the count of "3." Ask the resident to pull up with the hands and push against the bed with the feet. Explain what you will do.
15 Move the resident to the head of the bed on the count of "3." Shift your weight from your rear leg to your front leg (Fig. 10-10).
16 Put the pillow under the resident's head and shoulders. Lock arms with him or her to complete this step.

Post-Procedure

17 Straighten linens.
18 Provide for comfort. Position the resident in good alignment (p. 227).
19 Place the signal light within reach.
20 Raise or lower bed rails. Follow the care plan.
21 Raise the head of the bed to a level appropriate for the resident.
22 Lower the bed to its lowest position.
23 Unscreen the resident.
24 Wash your hands.

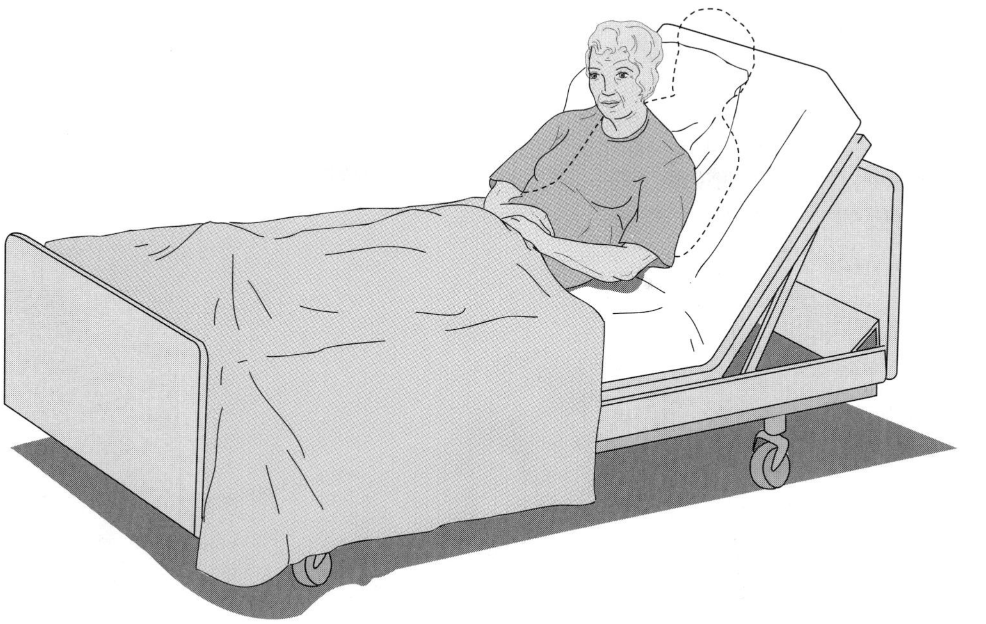

Fig. 10-8 A resident is in poor alignment after sliding down in bed.

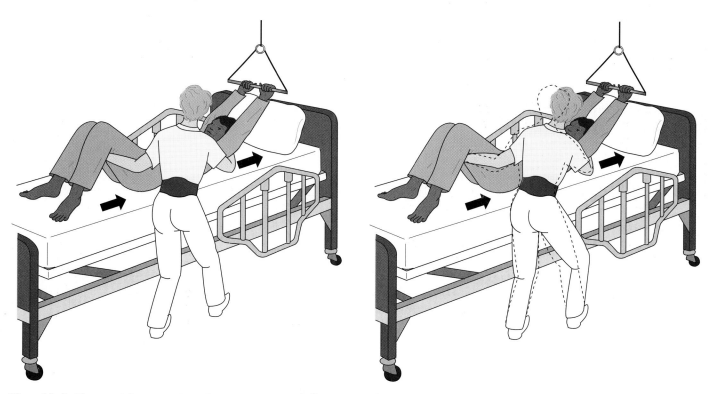

Fig. 10-9 The resident grasps the trapeze and flexes the knees. The nursing assistant has one arm under the resident's shoulder and the other under the resident's thighs.

Fig. 10-10 The nursing assistant's body weight shifts from the rear leg to the front leg.

◈ Moving the Resident Up in Bed with Assistance

You will need assistance when a resident cannot help in being moved up in bed. At least two people are needed to move heavy, weak, or very old residents. Always ask for help before starting the procedure. Also remember to help if a co-worker needs you.

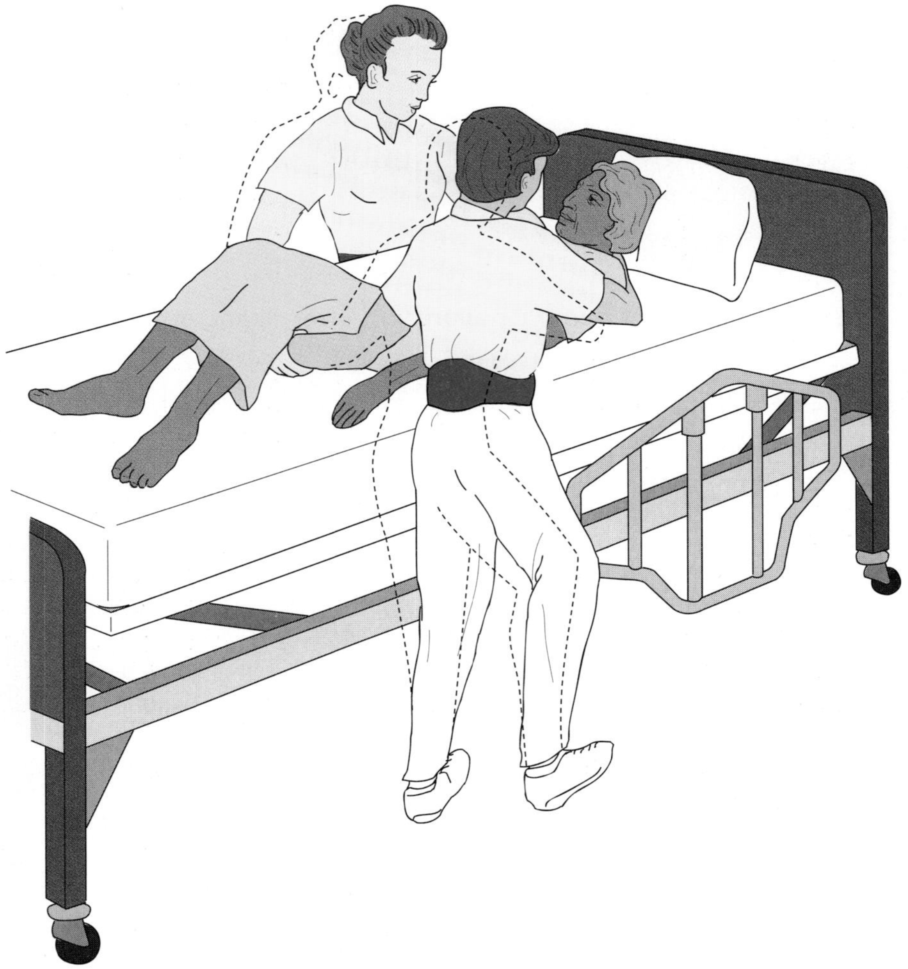

Fig. 10-11 A resident is moved up in bed by two nursing assistants. Each has one arm under the person's shoulders and the other under the buttocks. They have locked arms under the person. The person is moved up in bed as the nursing assistants shift their weight from the rear leg to the front leg.

Moving the Resident Up in Bed With Assistance

Quality of Life

Remember to:
- *Knock before entering the resident's room*
- *Address the resident by name*
- *Introduce yourself by name and title*

Pre-Procedure

1 Ask a co-worker to help you.
2 Wash your hands.
3 Identify the resident. Check the ID bracelet, and call the resident by name.
4 Explain the procedure to the resident.
5 Provide for privacy.
6 Lock the bed wheels.
7 Raise the bed to the best level for good body mechanics. Make sure the bed rails are up.

Procedure

8 Lower the head of the bed to a level appropriate for the resident. It is as flat as possible.
9 Stand on one side of the bed. Your co-worker stands on the other side.
10 Lower the bed rails.
11 Place the pillow against the headboard if the resident can be without it. This prevents his or her head from hitting the headboard when moving up.
12 Stand with a wide base of support. Point the foot near the head of the bed toward the head of the bed. Face that direction.
13 Bend your hips and knees.
14 Place one arm under the resident's shoulder and one arm under the buttocks. Your co-worker does the same. Grasp each other's forearms.
15 Have the resident flex both knees.
16 Explain that you will move on the count of "3." The resident should push against the bed with the feet if able.
17 Move the resident to the head of the bed on the count of "3." Shift your weight from your rear leg to your front leg (Fig. 10-11).
18 Repeat steps 12 through 17 if necessary.

Post-Procedure

19 Put the pillow under the resident's head and shoulders. Straighten linens.
20 Provide for comfort. Position the resident in good body alignment (p. 227).
21 Place the signal light within reach.
22 Raise or lower bed rails. Follow the care plan.
23 Raise the head of the bed to a level appropriate for the resident.
24 Lower the bed to its lowest position.
25 Unscreen the resident.
26 Wash your hands.

Moving the Resident Up in Bed With a Lift Sheet

With the help of a co-worker, you can easily and safely move a resident up in bed using a *lift sheet.* Friction and shearing are reduced, and the resident is lifted more evenly. You can use a flat sheet folded in half or a drawsheet for the lift sheet (called a *turning sheet* when used to turn a person). Some centers use *turning pads* designed for this purpose (Fig. 10-12). The lift sheet (or turning pad) is placed under the resident. It extends from the head to above the knees. Most residents should be moved up in bed with a lift sheet, particularly those who cannot move themselves.

Moving the Resident Up in Bed With a Lift Sheet

Quality of Life

Remember to:

- ***Knock before entering the resident's room***
- ***Address the resident by name***
- ***Introduce yourself by name and title***

Pre-Procedure

1 Ask a co-worker to help you.
2 Wash your hands.
3 Identify the resident. Check the ID bracelet, and call the resident by name.
4 Explain the procedure to the resident.
5 Provide for privacy.
6 Lock the bed wheels.
7 Raise the bed to the best level for good body mechanics. Make sure the bed rails are up.

Procedure

8 Lower the head of the bed to a level appropriate for the resident. It is as flat as possible.
9 Stand on one side of the bed. Your helper stands on the other side.
10 Lower the bed rails.
11 Place the pillow against the headboard if the resident can be without it.
12 Stand with a broad base of support. Point the foot near the head of the bed toward the head of the bed. Face that direction.
13 Roll the sides of the lift sheet up close to the resident.
14 Grasp the rolled-up lift sheet firmly near the resident's shoulders and buttocks (Fig. 10-13). Make sure you support the head.
15 Bend your hips and knees.
16 Slide the resident up in bed on the count of "3." Shift your weight from your rear leg to your front leg.
17 Unroll the lift sheet.

Post-Procedure

18 Put the pillow under the resident's head and shoulders. Straighten linens.
19 Provide for comfort. Position the resident in good body alignment (p. 227).
20 Place the signal light within reach.
21 Raise or lower bed rails. Follow the care plan.
22 Raise the head of the bed to a level appropriate for the resident.
23 Lower the bed to its lowest position.
24 Unscreen the resident.
25 Wash your hands.

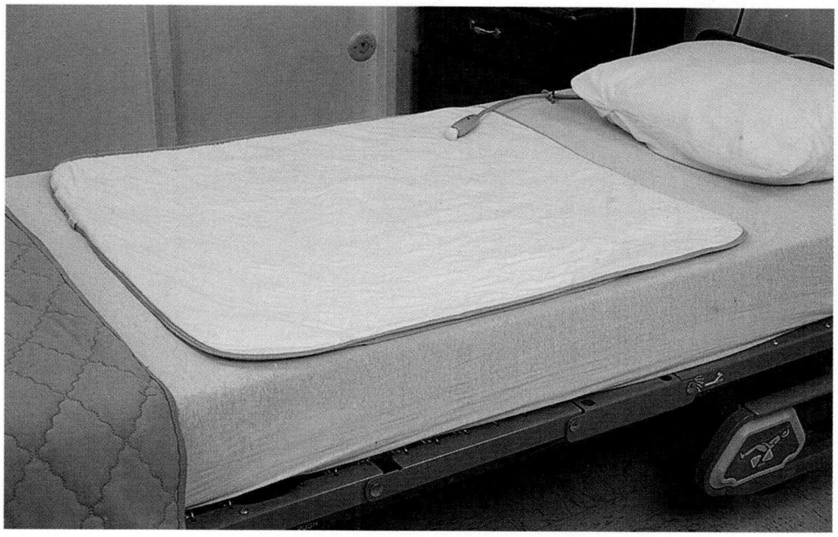

Fig. 10-12 Turning pad.

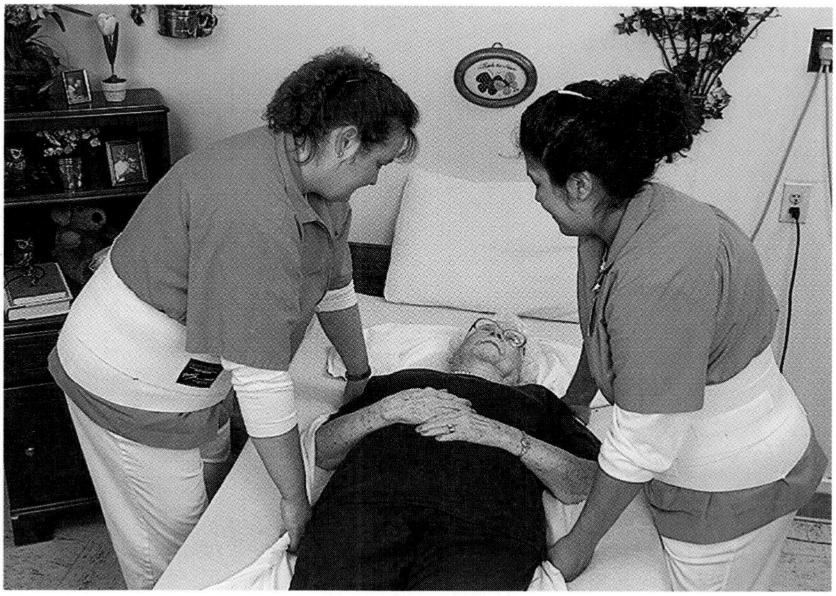

Fig. 10-13 A lift sheet is used to move the person up in bed. The lift sheet extends from the person's head to above the knees. The lift sheet is rolled close to the person and held near the shoulders and buttocks.

◈ Moving the Resident to the Side of the Bed

Residents are moved to the side of the bed for repositioning and for certain procedures such as a bed bath. A resident in the middle of the bed is moved to the side of the bed before turning. Otherwise, after turning, the resident will lay on the side of the bed rather than in the middle. Lying in the middle of the bed is necessary for good body alignment.

Sometimes you have to reach over the resident. You have to reach less if the resident is close to you.

The resident is in the back-lying position when being moved to the side of the bed. One procedure involves moving the resident in segments. One person can sometimes do this. Do not use this procedure for very old residents, those with arthritis, and those with spinal cord injuries or recovering from spinal surgery. For such cases, get help and use a lift sheet. This helps prevent pain and possible skin damage. It also prevents bone, joint, and spinal cord injury.

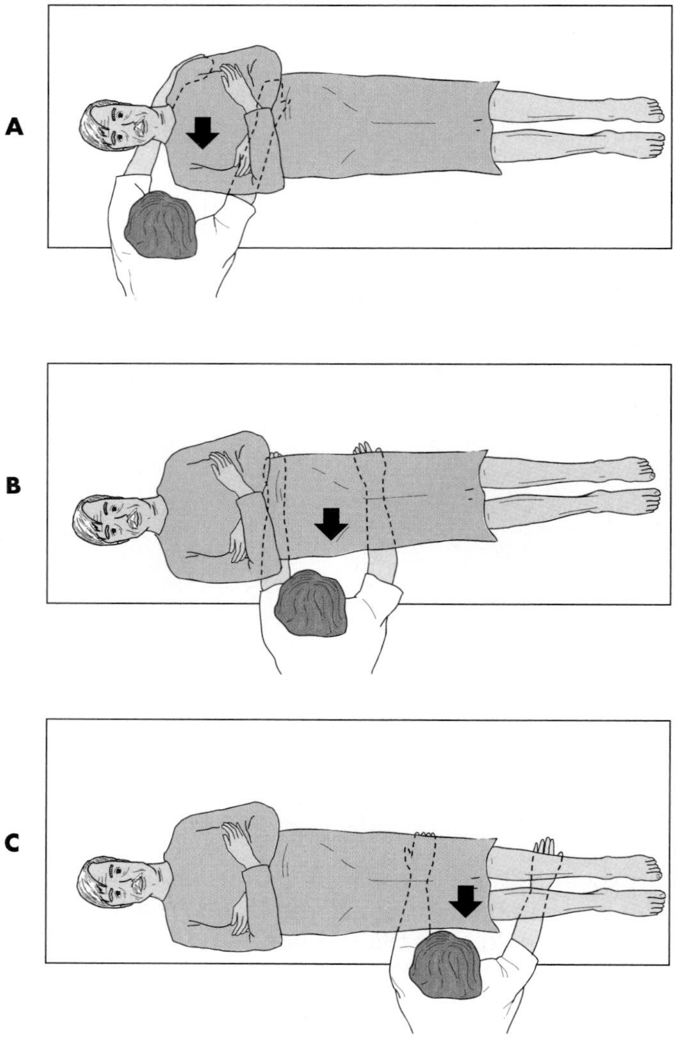

Fig. 10-14 The person is moved to the side of the bed in segments.

Moving the Resident to the Side of the Bed

Quality of Life

Remember to:
- *Knock before entering the resident's room*
- *Address the resident by name*
- *Introduce yourself by name and title*

Pre-Procedure

1 Ask a co-worker to help if you will use a lift sheet.
2 Wash your hands.
3 Identify the resident. Check the ID bracelet, and call the resident by name.
4 Explain the procedure to the resident.
5 Provide for privacy.
6 Lock the bed wheels.
7 Raise the bed to the best level for good body mechanics. Make sure bed rails are up.

Procedure

8 Lower the head of the bed to a level appropriate for the resident. It is as flat as possible.
9 Stand on the side of the bed to which you will move the resident.
10 Lower the bed rail near you. (Both bed rails are lowered for step 14).
11 Stand with your feet about 12 inches apart and with one foot in front of the other. Flex your knees.
12 Cross the resident's arms over the resident's chest.
13 *Method 1:* Moving the resident in segments:
 a Place your arm under the resident's neck and shoulders. Grasp the far shoulder.
 b Place your other arm under the midback.
 c Move the upper part of the resident's body toward you. Rock backward, and shift your weight to your rear leg (Fig. 10-14, *A*).
 d Place one arm under the resident's waist and one under the thighs.
 e Rock backward to move the lower part of the resident toward you (Fig. 10-14, *B*).
 f Repeat the procedure for the legs and feet (Fig. 10-14, *C*). Your arms are under the resident's thighs and calves.
14 *Method 2:* Moving the resident with a lift sheet:
 a Roll up the lift sheet close to the resident (see Fig. 10-13).
 b Grasp the rolled-up lift sheet near the resident's shoulders and buttocks. Make sure you support the head.
 c Rock backward on the count of "3," moving the resident toward you. Your co-worker rocks backward slightly and then forward toward you while keeping the arms straight.
 d Unroll the lift sheet.

Post-Procedure

15 Provide for comfort.
16 Position the resident in good body alignment. Follow the nurse's directions and the care plan. Reposition the pillow under the resident's head and shoulders.
17 Place the signal light within the resident's reach.
18 Raise or lower bed rails. Follow the care plan.
19 Lower the bed to its lowest position.
20 Unscreen the resident.
21 Wash your hands.

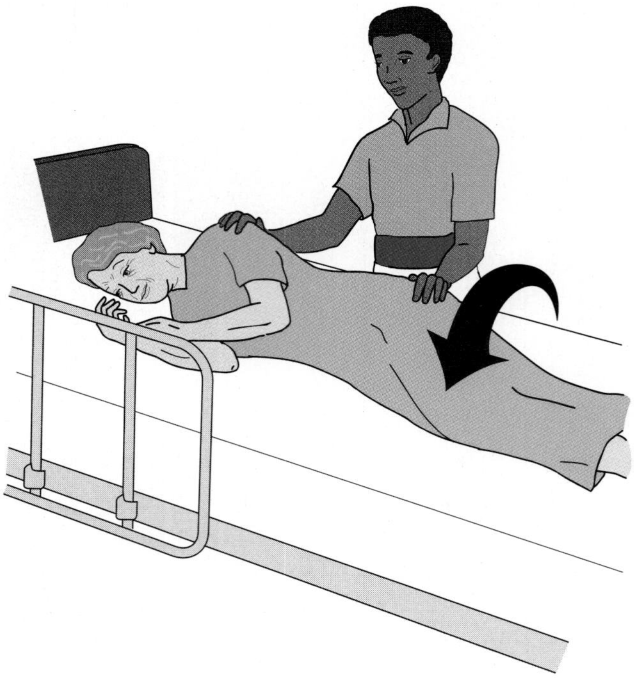

Fig. 10-15 Turning the person away from you.

Turning the Resident

Residents are turned onto their sides to prevent complications from bedrest and to receive care. Certain medical and nursing procedures require the side-lying position. Residents are turned toward or away from you. The direction depends on the resident's condition and the situation. Methods for turning residents toward or away from you are described here. However, logrolling with a lift sheet should be used for turning most residents in long-term care. It helps prevent pain in persons with arthritic spines and hips.

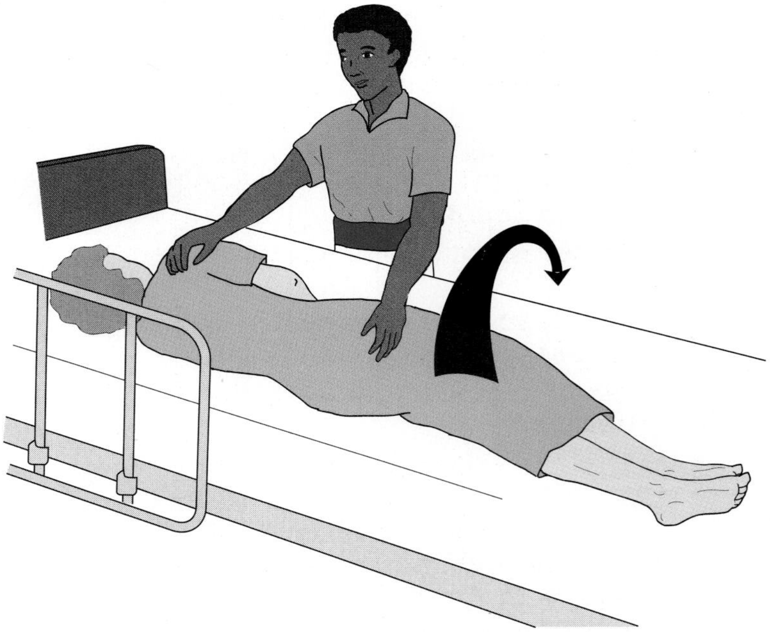

Fig. 10-16 Turning the person toward you.

Turning and Positioning the Resident

NNAAP™ SKILL

Quality of Life

Remember to:

- *Knock before entering the resident's room*
- *Address the resident by name*
- *Introduce yourself by name and title*

Pre-Procedure

1 Wash your hands.

2 Identify the resident. Check the ID bracelet, and call the resident by name.

3 Explain the procedure to the resident.

4 Provide for privacy.

5 Lock the bed wheels.

6 Raise the bed to the best level for good body mechanics. Make sure the bed rails are up.

Procedure

7 Lower the head of the bed to a level appropriate for the resident. The bed should be as flat as possible.

8 Stand on the side of the bed opposite to where you will turn the resident. The far bed rail is up.

9 Lower the bed rail near you.

10 Move the resident to the side near you. (See *Moving the Resident to the Side of the Bed,* p. 209).

11 Cross the resident's arms over his or her chest. Cross the leg near you over the far leg.

12 *Method 1:* Moving the resident away from you:

- a Stand with a wide base of support. Flex your knees.
- b Place one hand on the resident's shoulder and the other on the buttock near you.
- c Push the resident gently toward the other side of the bed (Fig. 10-15). Shift your weight from your rear leg to your front leg.

13 *Method 2:* Moving the resident toward you:

- a Raise the bed rail.
- b Go to the other side. Lower the bed rail.
- c Stand with a wide base of support. Flex your knees.
- d Place one hand on the resident's far shoulder and the other on the far hip.
- e Roll the resident toward you gently (Fig. 10-16).

Post-Procedure

14 Provide for comfort. Position the resident in good body alignment (p. 227).

15 Place the signal light within reach.

16 Raise or lower bed rails. Follow the care plan.

17 Lower the bed to its lowest position.

18 Unscreen the resident.

19 Wash your hands.

Logrolling

Logrolling is turning the resident as a unit in alignment with one motion. The back is kept in straight alignment when the resident is turned. The procedure is used to turn:

- Older persons with arthritic spines
- Persons recovering from hip fractures
- Persons with spinal cord injuries (the spine is kept straight at all times after spinal cord injury)
- Persons recovering from spinal surgery (the spine is kept straight at all times after spinal surgery)

Two workers are needed to logroll a resident. Three are needed if a resident is tall or heavy.

A

B

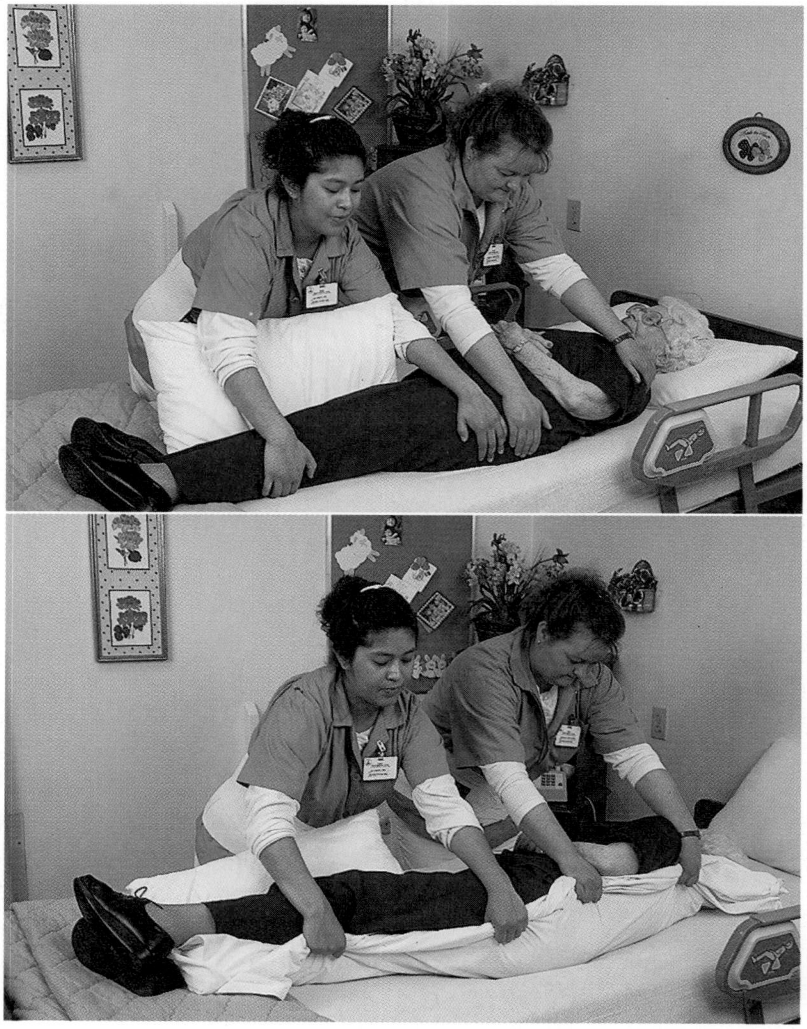

Fig. 10-17 Logrolling. **A,** A pillow is between the person's legs, and the arms are crossed on the chest. The person is on the far side of the bed. **B,** A turning sheet is used to logroll a person.

Logrolling the Resident

Quality of Life

Remember to:
- *Knock before entering the resident's room*
- *Address the resident by name*
- *Introduce yourself by name and title*

Pre-Procedure

1 Ask a co-worker to help you.
2 Wash your hands.
3 Identify the resident. Check the ID bracelet, and call the resident by name.
4 Explain the procedure to the resident.
5 Provide for privacy.
6 Lock the bed wheels.
7 Raise the bed to the best level for good body mechanics. Make sure the bed rails are up.

Procedure

8 Make sure the bed is flat.
9 Stand on the side opposite to which the resident will be turned.
10 Lower the bed rail.
11 Move the resident as a unit to the side of the bed near you. Use the lift sheet.
12 Place the resident's arms across the chest. Place a pillow between the knees.
13 Raise the bed rail. Go to the other side and lower the bed rail.
14 Position yourself near the shoulders and chest. Your co-worker stands near the buttocks and thighs.
15 Stand with a broad base of support. One foot is in front of the other.
16 Ask the resident to hold his or her body rigid.
17 Roll the resident toward you as in Fig. 10-17, *A*. Or use a turn sheet as in Fig. 10-17, *B*. Turn the resident as a unit.

Post-Procedure

18 Provide for comfort. Position the resident in good alignment. Use pillows as directed by the nurse and the care plan. The following is common:
   a One pillow against the back for support.
   b One pillow under the head and neck if allowed.
   c One pillow or folded bath blanket between the legs.
   d A small pillow under the arm and hand.
19 Place the signal light within reach.
20 Raise or lower bed rails. Follow the care plan.
21 Lower the bed to its lowest position.
22 Unscreen the resident.
23 Wash your hands.

◈ SITTING ON THE SIDE OF THE BED (DANGLING)

Residents sit on the side of the bed *(dangle)* for many reasons. Many older persons become dizzy or faint if they get out of bed too fast. They may need to sit on the side of the bed for 1 to 5 minutes before walking or transferring. Some residents increase activity in stages. They progress from bedrest, to sitting on the side of the bed, and then to sitting in a chair. Walking about in the room and then walking in the hallway are the next steps. While dangling, they cough, deep breathe, and move their legs back and forth and in circles to stimulate circulation.

Two workers may be needed to help a resident dangle. If there is a problem with balance or coordination, the resident needs support. This is especially true if the person had a stroke (see Chapter 26). Problems with sitting balance often occur after a stroke. If fainting occurs, the resident is laid down.

You must make certain observations while the resident is dangling. Take the resident's pulse and respirations. Observe for difficulty in breathing, pale skin, or cyanosis (bluish coloring to the skin). Also note complaints of dizziness or lightheadedness.

A

B

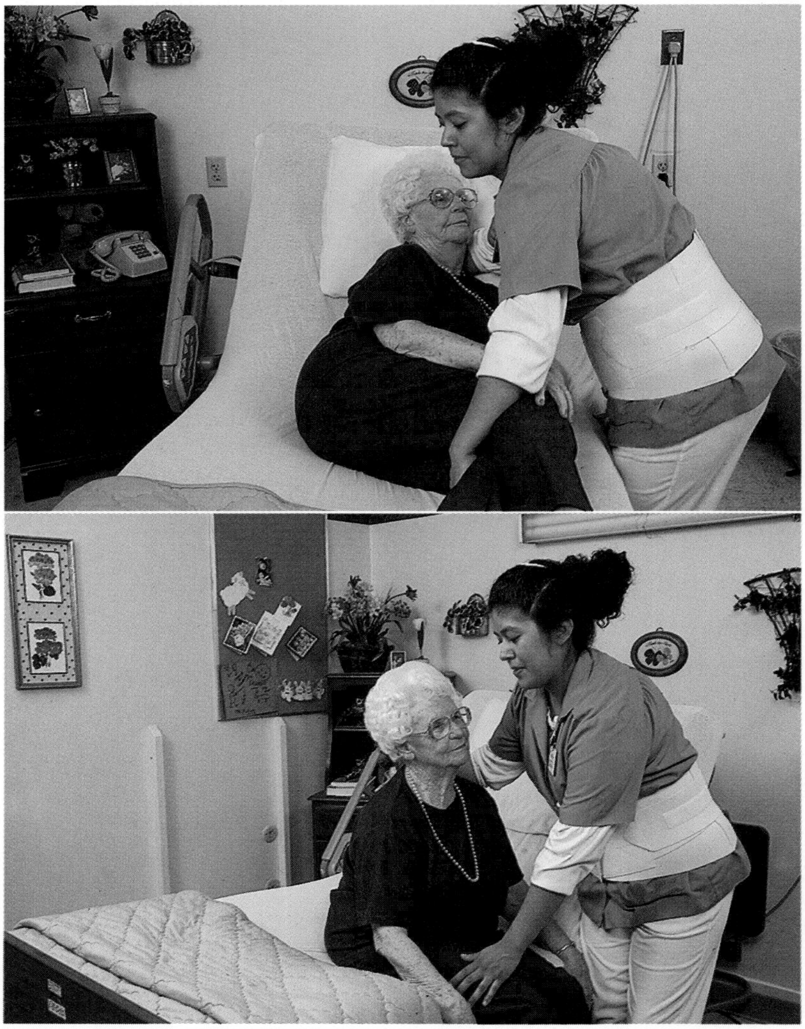

Fig. 10-18 Helping the person sit on the side of the bed. **A,** The person is supported under the shoulders and under the thighs. **B,** The person sits upright as the legs and feet are pulled over the edge of the bed.

Helping the Resident Sit on the Side of the Bed (Dangle)

Quality of Life

Remember to:
- *Knock before entering the resident's room*
- *Address the resident by name*
- *Introduce yourself by name and title*

Pre-Procedure

1. Explain the procedure to the resident.
2. Wash your hands.
3. Identify the resident. Check the ID bracelet, and call the resident by name.
4. Decide what side of the bed to use.
5. Move furniture to provide moving space.
6. Provide for privacy.
7. Position the resident in a side-lying position facing you.
8. Lock the bed wheels.
9. Raise the bed to the best level for body mechanics. Make sure the bed rails are up.

Procedure

10. Raise the head of the bed so the resident is in a sitting position.
11. Stand near the resident's waist.
12. Lower the bed rail.
13. Stand by the resident's hips. Turn so you face the far corner of the foot of the bed.
14. Stand with your feet apart. The foot closest to head of bed is in front of other foot.
15. Place one arm under the resident's shoulders to support the head and neck. Place the other arm over the resident's thighs (Fig. 10-18, *A*).
16. Pivot toward the foot of the bed while moving the resident's lower legs and feet over the side of the bed. Let the resident's upper legs swing downward. As the legs go over the edge of the mattress, the trunk is upright (Fig. 10-18, *B*).
17. Ask the resident to hold onto the edge of the mattress. This supports the resident in the sitting position.
18. Do not leave the resident alone. Provide support if necessary.
19. Ask how the resident feels. Check pulse and respirations. Help the resident lie down if necessary.
20. Reverse the procedure to return the resident to bed.
21. Lower the head of the bed after the resident returns to bed. Help him or her move to the center of the bed.

Post-Procedure

22. Provide for comfort. Position the resident in good body alignment (see p. 227).
23. Place the signal light within reach.
24. Lower the bed to its lowest position.
25. Raise or lower bed rails. Follow the care plan.
26. Return furniture to its proper places.
27. Unscreen the resident.
28. Wash your hands.
29. Report the following to the nurse:
    - How well the activity was tolerated
    - The length of time the resident dangled
    - Pulse and respiratory rates
    - The amount of assistance needed
    - Other observations or resident complaints

TRANSFERRING RESIDENTS

Residents are often moved from their bed to a chair, wheelchair, or stretcher. Some need only a little assistance. Others need help from at least one person. Some residents are transferred by at least 2 or 3 people. Ask the nurse how much assistance a resident needs. Always check the care plan. The rules of body mechanics and the safety and comfort considerations described for lifting and moving residents apply when transferring. Also, arrange the room so there is enough space for a safe transfer. Correct chair, wheelchair, or stretcher placement is necessary for a safe and efficient transfer.

Transfer Belt

A **transfer belt** is used for transferring most residents in nursing centers. The belt is used to hold onto the resident during the transfer. Remember, *if the resident needs assistance to transfer, a transfer belt is required.* The belt is applied around the resident's waist. The belt also is called a **gait belt** and is used when walking with a resident. Transfer (gait) belts help prevent falls and other injuries.

Applying a Transfer Belt

Quality of Life

Remember to:

- *Knock before entering the resident's room*
- *Address the resident by name*
- *Introduce yourself by name and title*

Procedure

1. Wash your hands.
2. Identify the resident. Check the ID bracelet, and call the resident by name.
3. Explain the procedure to the resident.
4. Provide for privacy.
5. Assist the resident to a sitting position.
6. Apply the belt around the resident's waist over clothing. Do not apply it over bare skin.
7. Tighten the belt so it is snug. It should not cause discomfort or impair breathing.
8. Make sure that a woman's breasts are not caught under the belt.
9. Place the buckle off center in the front or in the back for the resident's comfort (Fig. 10-19).

A

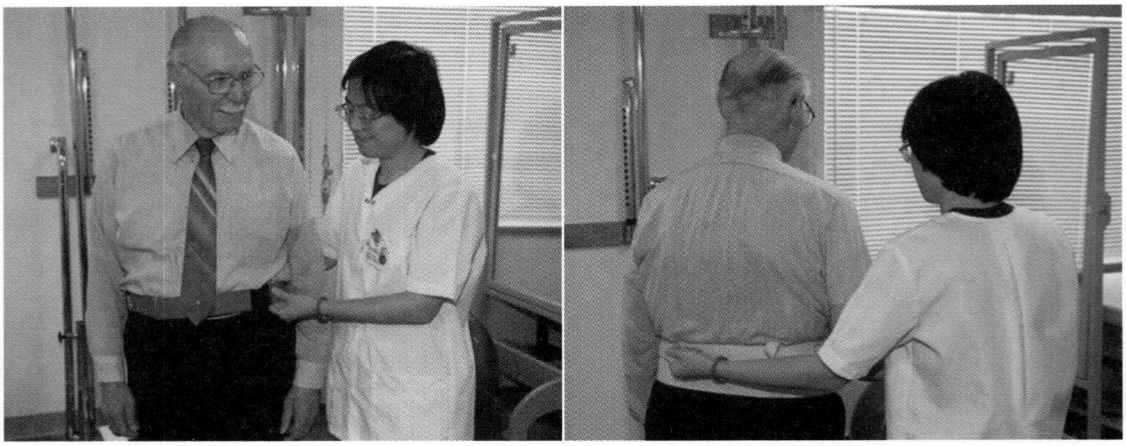

B

Fig. 10-19 Transfer belt (gait or safety belt). **A,** The belt is positioned off center in the front. **B,** The belt buckle is positioned at the back. Note the different types of transfer belts.

Transferring the Resident to a Chair Or Wheelchair

Safety is important for chair and wheelchair transfers. You must prevent falls. The resident wears shoes with nonskid soles to prevent sliding or slipping on the floor. The chair or wheelchair must support the resident's weight. The number of workers needed for a transfer depends on the resident's physical capabilities, condition, and size. This procedure is used only if the person can assist in the transfer. If the person cannot assist, a mechanical lift is used (p. 223).

Most wheelchairs or bedside chairs have vinyl seats and backs. Vinyl holds body heat. This causes the resident to become warm and to perspire more. You can cover the back and seat with a folded bath blanket. This increases the resident's comfort in the chair. Residents who use wheelchairs often have special cushions. Check with the nurse about the proper use and placement of these cushions.

Help the resident out of bed on his or her strong side. If the left side is weak and the right side strong, get the resident out of bed on the right side. In transferring, the strong side moves first and pulls the weaker side along. Transferring from the weak side is awkward and unsafe.

The nurse may want the resident's pulse taken before and after the transfer. The resident may have a severe illness and may tire with even a little exertion. The pulse rate gives some information about how the activity was tolerated. Also observe and report if the resident tires easily, complains of weakness or lightheadedness, has pain or discomfort, or has difficulty breathing (dyspnea). Report the amount of help needed and how the resident helped in the transfer.

Text continued on p. 223

Transferring the Resident to a Chair or Wheelchair

NNAAP™ SKILL

Quality of Life

Remember to:
- ***Knock before entering the resident's room***
- ***Address the resident by name***
- ***Introduce yourself by name and title***

Pre-Procedure

1. Explain the procedure to the resident.
2. Collect:
   - Wheelchair or arm chair
   - One or two bath blankets
   - Robe and nonskid shoes
   - Paper or sheet
   - Transfer belt if needed
3. Wash your hands.
4. Identify the resident. Check the ID bracelet, and call the resident by name.
5. Provide for privacy.
6. Decide which side of the bed to use. Move furniture to provide moving space.

Procedure

7. Place the chair at the head of the bed. The chair back is even with the headboard (Fig. 10-20, p. 219).
8. Place a cushion on the seat. Lock wheelchair wheels, and raise the footrests.
9. Lower the bed to its lowest position. Lock the bed wheels.
10. Fanfold top linens to the foot of the bed.
11. Place the paper or sheet under the resident's feet. Put shoes on the resident.
12. Help the resident dangle. Make sure his or her feet touch the floor.
13. Help the resident put on a robe.
14. Apply the transfer belt if it will be used.

Continued

Transferring the Resident to a Chair or Wheelchair—cont'd

NNAAP™ SKILL

Procedure—cont'd

15 Help the resident stand. Use this method if using a transfer belt. (NOTE: Most centers require the use of transfer belts when assisting residents to transfer.)
- a Stand in front of the resident.
- b Have the resident hold onto the mattress. Or ask the resident to place his or her hands on the bed by the thighs.
- c Make sure the resident's feet are flat on the floor.
- d Have the resident lean forward.
- e Grasp the transfer belt at each side.
- f Brace one knee against the resident's knee. Block his or her foot with your foot. Place your other foot slightly behind you for balance (Fig. 10-21).
- g Ask the resident to push down on the mattress and to stand on the count of "3." Pull the resident into a standing position as you straighten your knees (Fig. 10-22).

16 Use this method if a transfer belt is not used. (NOTE: Most centers require the use of transfer belts when assisting residents to transfer.)
- a Follow Step 15 a–c.
- b Place your hands under the resident's arms. Your hands are around the resident's shoulder blades (Fig. 10-23, p. 220).
- c Have the resident lean forward.
- d Brace one knee against the resident's knee. Block his or her foot with your foot. Place your other foot slightly behind you for balance.
- e Ask the resident to push down on the mattress and to stand on the count of "3." Pull the resident up into a standing position as you straighten your knees.

17 Support the resident in the standing position. Hold the transfer belt, or keep your hands around the resident's shoulder blades. Continue to block the resident's feet and knees with your feet and knees. This helps prevent falling.

18 Turn the resident so he or she can grasp the far arm of the chair. The legs will touch the edge of the chair as in Figure 10-24 on p. 220.

19 Continue to turn the resident until the other armrest is grasped.

20 Lower him or her into the chair as you bend your hips and knees (Fig. 10-25, p. 220). The resident assists by leaning forward and bending the elbows and knees.

21 Make sure the buttocks are to the back of the seat. Position the resident in good alignment.

22 Position the resident's feet on the wheelchair footrests.

23 Cover the resident's lap and legs with a bath blanket. Keep the blanket off the floor and the wheels.

24 Remove the transfer belt if used.

25 Position the chair as the resident prefers.

Post-Procedure

26 Make sure the signal light and other necessary items are within reach.

27 Unscreen the resident.

28 Wash your hands.

29 Report the following to the nurse:
- The pulse rate, if taken
- How well the activity was tolerated
- Complaints of lightheadedness, pain, discomfort, difficulty breathing, weakness, or fatigue
- The amount of help needed to transfer the resident

30 Reverse the procedure to return the resident to bed.

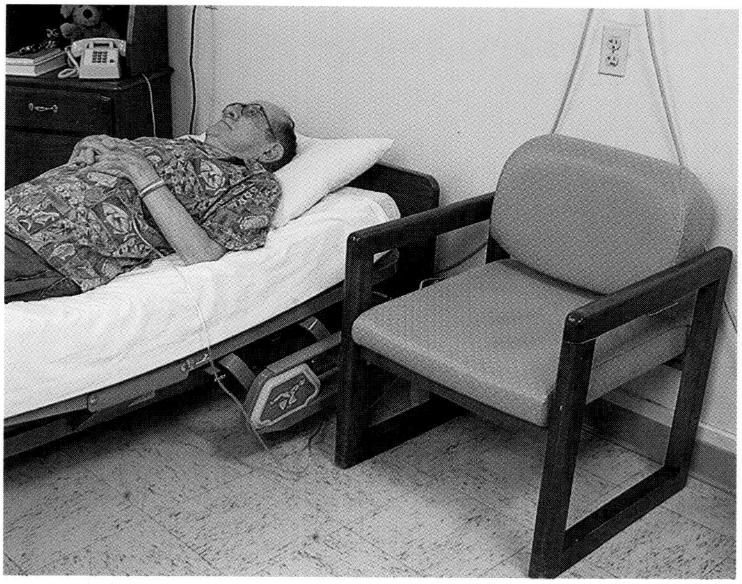

Fig. 10-20 The chair is positioned next to and even with the headboard.

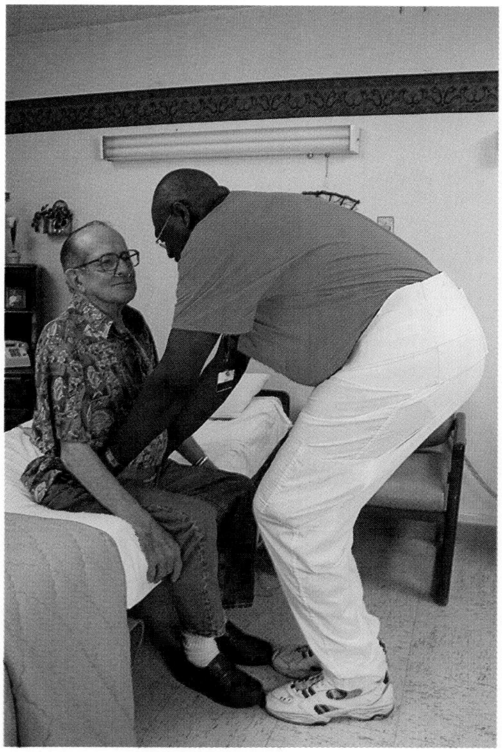

Fig. 10-21 Prevent the person from sliding or falling by blocking the person's knees and feet with your own knees and feet.

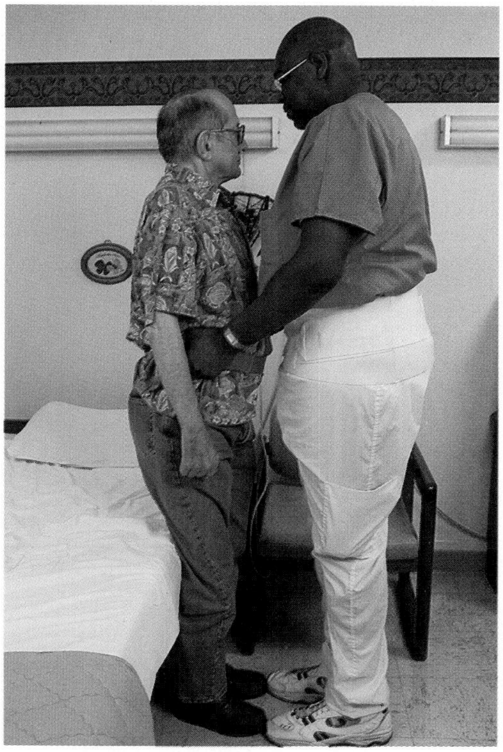

Fig. 10-22 The person is pulled up to a standing position and supported by holding the transfer belt and blocking the person's knees and feet.

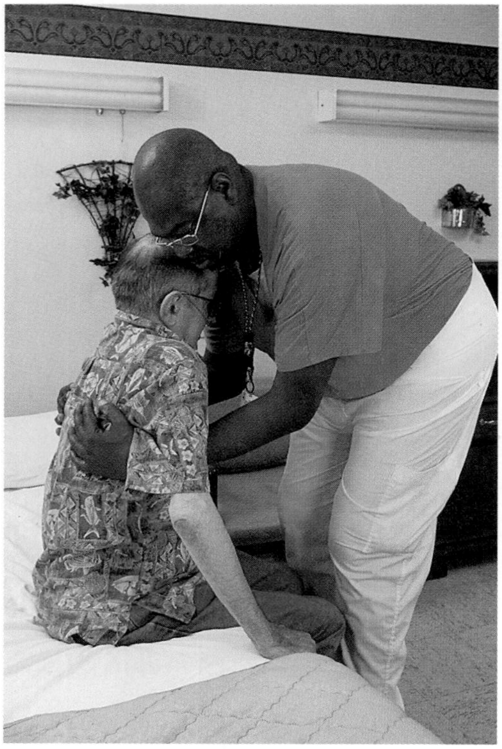

Fig. 10-23 A person being prepared to stand. The hands are placed under the person's arms and around the shoulder blades.

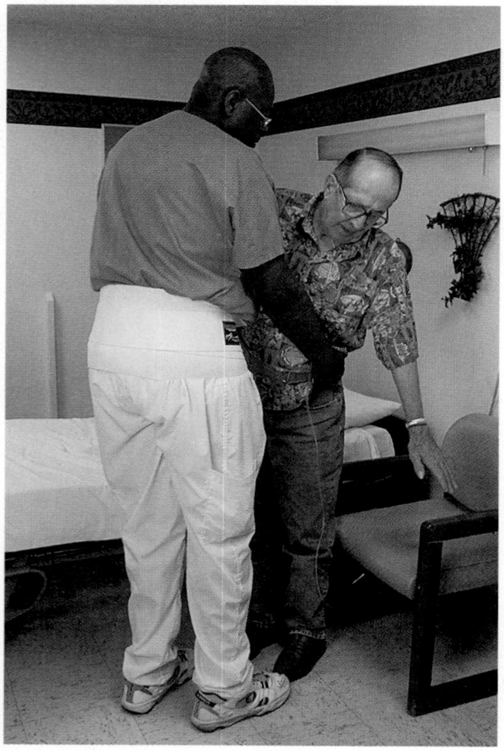

Fig. 10-24 The person is supported as he grasps the far arm of the chair. The legs are against the chair.

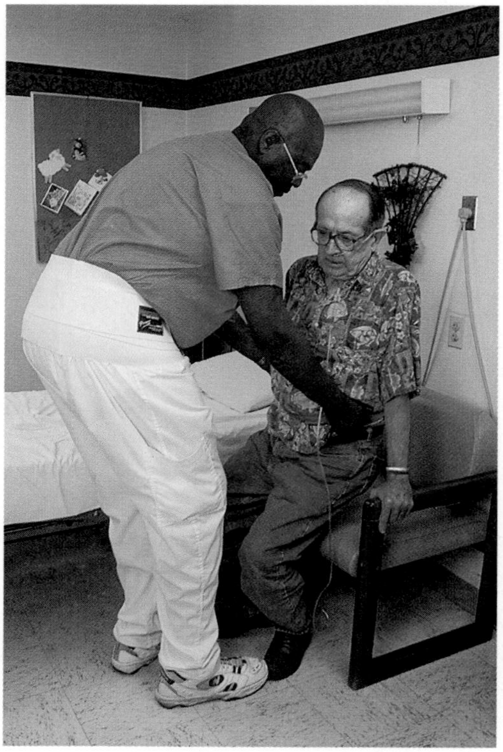

Fig. 10-25 The person holds the armrests, leans forward, and bends the elbows and knees while being lowered into the chair.

Transferring the Resident to a Wheelchair With Assistance

Quality of Life

Remember to:
- ◆ *Knock before entering the resident's room*
- ◆ *Address the resident by name*
- ◆ *Introduce yourself by name and title*

Pre-Procedure

1 Ask a co-worker to help you.
2 Explain the procedure to the person.
3 Collect:
- Wheelchair with removable armrests
- Bath blankets
- Shoes
- Cushion if used

4 Wash your hands.
5 Identify the person. Check the ID bracelet, and call the person by name.
6 Provide for privacy.
7 Decide which side of the bed to use. Move furniture to provide moving space.

Procedure

8 Fanfold top linens to the foot of the bed.
9 Assist the person to the side of the bed near you. Help him or her to a sitting position by raising the head of the bed.
10 Place the wheelchair at the side of the bed, even with the person's hips.
11 Remove the armrest near the bed. Put the cushion or a folded bath blanket on the seat.
12 Lock wheelchair and bed wheels.
13 Stand behind the wheelchair. Put your arms under the person's arms and grasp the person's forearms (Fig. 10-26, *A,* p. 222).
14 Have your co-worker grasp the person's thighs and calves (Fig. 10-26, *B,* p. 222).
15 Bring the person toward the chair on the count of "3." Lower him or her into the chair as in Figure 10-26, *C,* p. 222.
16 Make sure the person's buttocks are to the back of the seat. Position the person in good alignment.
17 Put the armrest back on the wheelchair.
18 Put the shoes on the person. Position the person's feet on the footrests.
19 Cover the person's lap and legs with a blanket. Keep the blanket off the floor and wheels.
20 Position the chair as the person prefers.

Post-Procedure

21 Make sure the signal light and other necessary items are within reach.
22 Unscreen the person.
23 Wash your hands.
24 Report the following to the nurse:
- The pulse rate, if taken
- Complaints of lightheadedness, pain, discomfort, difficulty breathing, weakness, or fatigue
- How well the activity was tolerated

25 Reverse the procedure to return the person to bed.

A

B

C

Fig. 10-26 Transferring the person to a wheelchair with two assistants. **A,** Grasp the person's forearms by putting your arms under the person's arms. **B,** Hold the thighs and calves to support the lower extremities during a transfer. **C,** Lower the person into the chair.

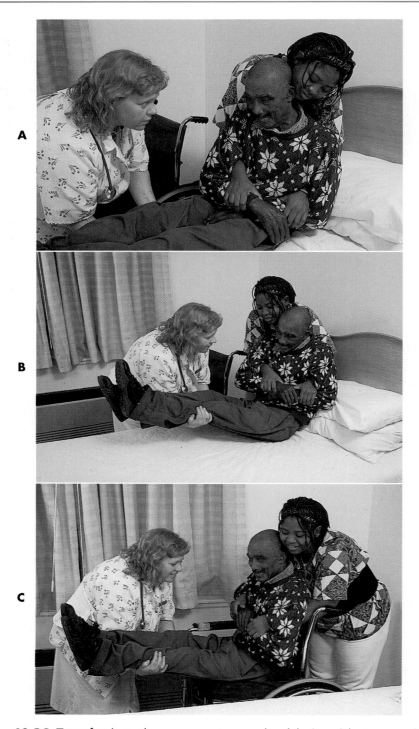

Using Mechanical Lifts

Residents who cannot help themselves are transferred with a mechanical lift. Mechanical lifts come in manual and electric types. Lifts are used for transfers to chairs, stretchers, tubs, shower chairs, toilets, whirlpools, and cars.

Lift types vary from center to center. Some centers use more than one type of lift. You have training on the proper use of each type of lift used at your center.

Before using a lift, make sure it works. Also, compare the resident's weight and the lift's weight limit. Do not use the lift if a resident's weight exceeds the lift's capacity.

At least two staff members are needed. The manufacturer's instructions are followed for a safe transfer. The following procedure is used as a guide.

Transferring the Resident Using a Mechanical Lift

Quality of Life

Remember to:
- *Knock before entering the resident's room*
- *Address the resident by name*
- *Introduce yourself by name and title*

Pre-Procedure

1. Ask a co-worker to help you.
2. Explain the procedure to the resident.
3. Collect:
   - Mechanical lift
   - Arm chair or wheelchair
   - Slippers
   - Bath blanket or cushion
4. Wash your hands.
5. Identify the resident. Check the ID bracelet, and call the resident by name.
6. Provide for privacy.

Procedure

7. Center the sling under the resident (Fig. 10-27, *A*, p. 225). Turn the resident from side to side as if making an occupied bed to position the sling (see Chapter 12). Position the sling according to the manufacturer's instructions.
8. Place the chair at the head of the bed. It should be even with the headboard and about 1 foot away from the bed. Place a folded bath blanket or cushion in the chair.
9. Lock the bed wheels, and lower the bed to its lowest position.
10. Raise the lift so it can be positioned over the resident.
11. Position the lift over the resident (Fig. 10-27, *B*, p. 225).
12. Lock the lift wheels in position.
13. Attach the sling to the swivel bar (Fig. 10-27, *C*, p. 225).
14. Raise the head of the bed to a sitting position.
15. Cross the resident's arms over the chest. Let him or her hold onto the straps or chains but not the swivel bar.
16. Pump the lift high enough until the resident and sling are free of the bed (Fig. 10-27, *D*, p. 225).
17. Ask your co-worker to support the resident's legs as you move the lift and resident away from the bed (Fig. 10-27, *E*, p. 225).

Continued

Transferring the Resident Using a Mechanical Lift—cont'd

Procedure—cont'd

18 Position the lift so that the resident's back is toward the chair.

19 Lower the resident into the chair. (Follow the manufacturer's instructions for lowering the lift.) Guide the resident into the chair as in Figure 10-27, *F.*

20 Lower the swivel bar to unhook the sling. Leave the sling under the resident unless otherwise indicated.

21 Put the slippers on the resident. Position the resident's feet on wheelchair footrests.

22 Cover the resident's lap and legs with a blanket. Keep the blanket off the floor and wheels.

23 Position the chair as the resident prefers.

Post-Procedure

24 Place the signal light and other necessary items within reach.

25 Wash your hands.

26 Report the following to the nurse:
- The pulse rate, if taken
- Complaints of lightheadedness, pain, discomfort, difficulty breathing, weakness, or fatigue
- How well the activity was tolerated

27 Reverse the procedure to return the resident to bed.

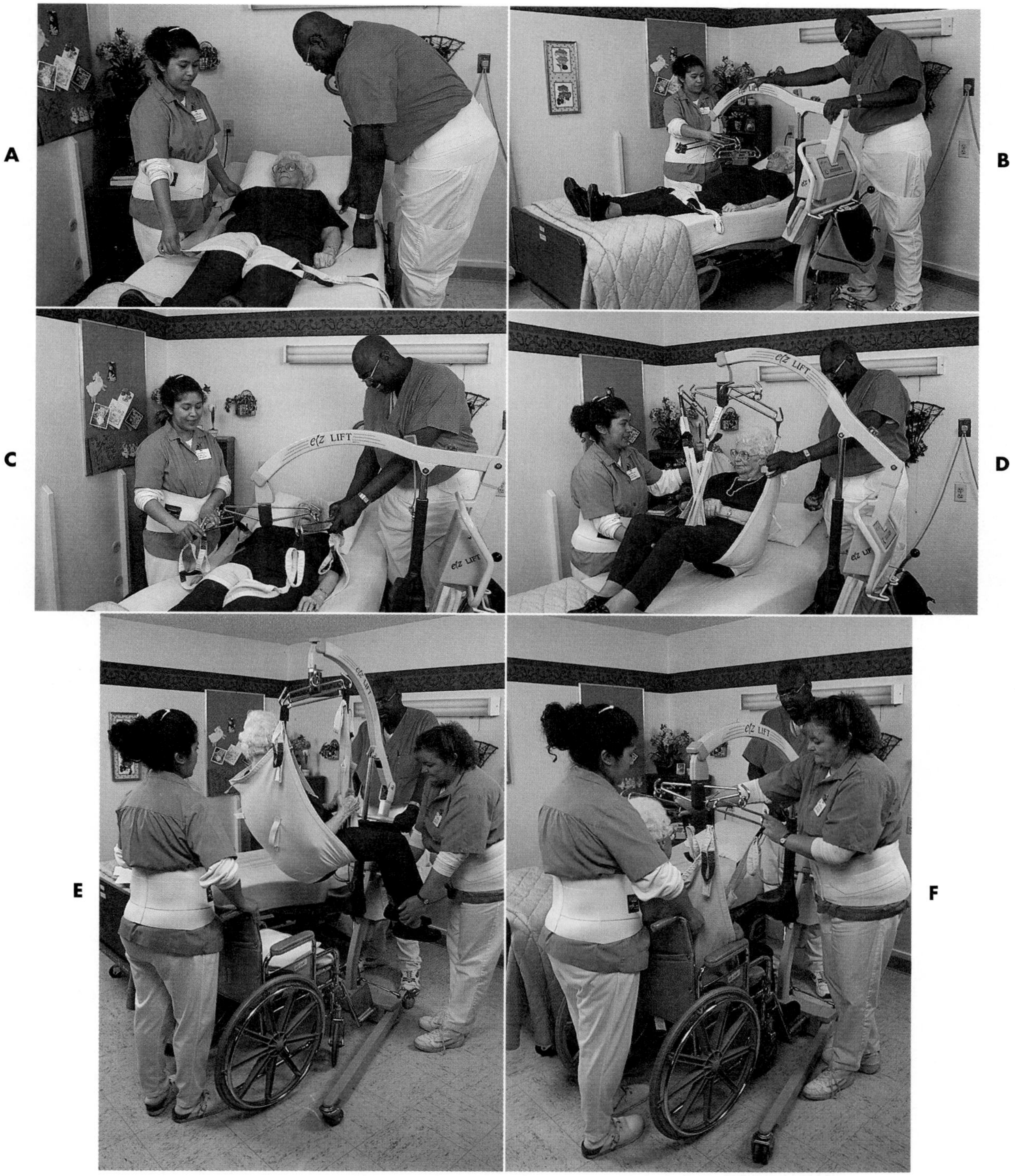

Fig. 10-27 Using a mechanical lift. **A,** The sling of the mechanical lift is positioned under the person. The lower edge of the sling is behind the person's knees. **B,** The lift is over the person. The lift's legs are spread to widen the base of support. **C,** The sling is attached to a swivel bar. **D,** The lift is raised until the sling and person are off of the bed. **E,** The person's legs are supported as the person and lift are moved away from the bed. **F,** The person is guided into a chair.

Moving the Resident to a Stretcher

Stretchers are used to transport residents within the center or to another center. They are used for residents who:

- Cannot sit up
- Must remain in a lying position
- Are seriously ill

The stretcher is covered with a folded flat sheet or bath blanket. A pillow and an extra blanket are available. The head of the stretcher is raised to a sitting or semisitting position with the nurse's permission.

Safety straps are applied once the resident is on the stretcher. The stretcher's side rails are kept up during transport. The resident is moved feet first so the co-worker at the head of the stretcher can watch the resident's breathing and color during the transport. A resident on a stretcher is never left unattended.

A drawsheet or lift sheet is used to transfer a resident from the bed to a stretcher. At least 3 workers are needed for a safe transfer. Remember to keep the resident in good body alignment and to use good body mechanics.

Transferring the Resident to a Stretcher

Quality of Life

Remember to:

- ***Knock before entering the resident's room***
- ***Address the resident by name***
- ***Introduce yourself by name and title***

Pre-Procedure

1 Ask two co-workers to help you.
2 Explain the procedure to the resident.
3 Collect:
- Stretcher covered with a sheet or bath blanket
- Bath blanket
- Pillow(s) if needed

4 Wash your hands.
5 Identify the resident. Check the ID bracelet, and call the resident by name.
6 Provide for privacy.
7 Raise the bed to its highest level.

Procedure

8 Cover the resident with a bath blanket. Fanfold top linens to the foot of the bed.
9 Loosen the cotton drawsheet on each side.
10 Lower the head of the bed so it is as flat as possible.
11 Lower the bed rail on the side to which you will move the resident.
12 Ask your co-workers to help move the resident to the side of the bed. Use the drawsheet.
13 Go to the other side of the bed. Lower the bed rail. Protect the resident from falling by holding the far arm and leg.
14 Have your co-workers position the stretcher next to the bed and stand behind the stretcher (Fig. 10-28).
15 Lock bed and stretcher wheels.
16 Roll up and grasp the drawsheet at the hip and midchest levels.
17 Ask your helpers to roll up and grasp the drawsheet. This supports the entire length of the resident's body.
18 Transfer the resident to the stretcher on the count of "3" by lifting and pulling him or her (Fig. 10-29). Make sure the resident is centered on the stretcher.
19 Place a pillow or pillows under the resident's head and shoulders, if allowed.
20 Cover the resident. Provide for comfort.
21 Fasten safety straps. Raise the rails.
22 Unlock the stretcher's wheels. Transport the resident.

Transferring the Resident to a Stretcher

Post-Procedure

23 Wash your hands.
24 Report the following to the nurse:
- The time of the transport
- Where the resident was transported
- Who went with him or her
- How the transfer was tolerated

25 Reverse the procedure to return the resident to bed.

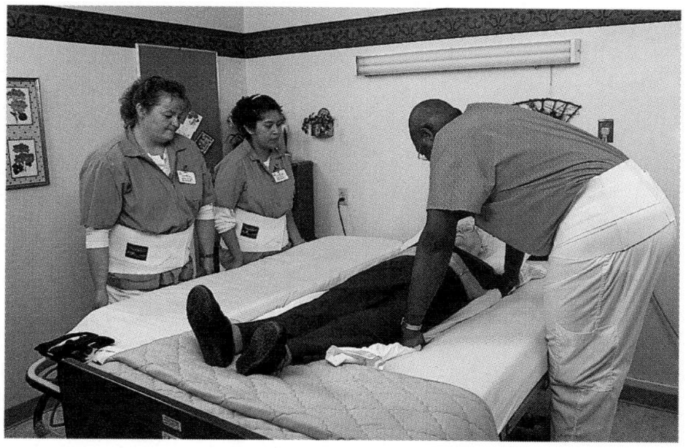

Fig. 10-28 The stretcher is against the bed and is held in place.

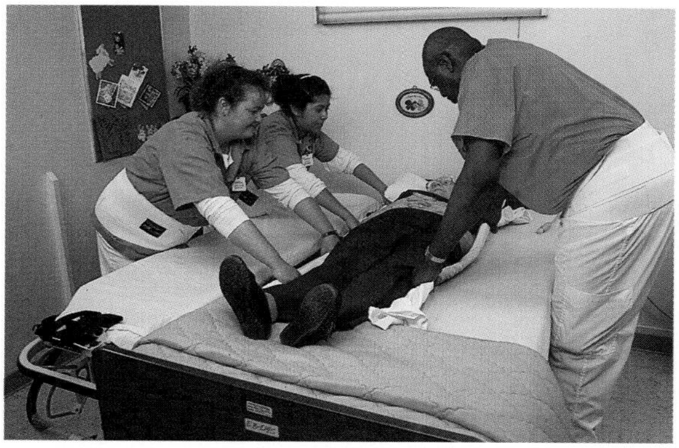

Fig. 10-29 A drawsheet is used to transfer the person from the bed to a stretcher.

POSITIONING

The resident must be properly positioned at all times. Regular position changes and good body alignment promote comfort and well-being. Breathing is easier, and circulation is promoted. Proper positioning also helps prevent many complications. These include pressure ulcers (see Chapter 14) and contractures (see Chapter 19). Residents in bed or wheelchairs are repositioned at least every 2 hours. Some residents are repositioned more often. The care plan tells you how often a resident is repositioned.

The doctor may order certain positions or position restrictions. Follow these guidelines to safely position residents:
- Ask the nurse about position changes for a resident.
- Know how often to turn a resident and to what positions.
- Use good body mechanics.
- Ask a co-worker to help you if indicated.
- Explain the procedure to the resident.
- Be gentle when moving the resident.
- Provide for privacy.
- Place the signal light within the resident's reach after positioning.
- Use pillows as directed for support and alignment.

Basic Bed Positions

Good body alignment and position changes are essential for the resident confined to bed. Some residents can change positions without help. Others need some assistance. Some depend entirely on the nursing staff for position changes.

Fowler's position. **Fowler's position** involves raising the head of the bed to a semisitting position. The head of the bed is raised between 45 and 60 degrees. Good body alignment for the Fowler's position involves keeping the spine straight, supporting the head with a small pillow, and supporting the arms with pillows (Fig. 10-30). Residents with heart and respiratory disorders usually can breathe more easily in the Fowler's position.

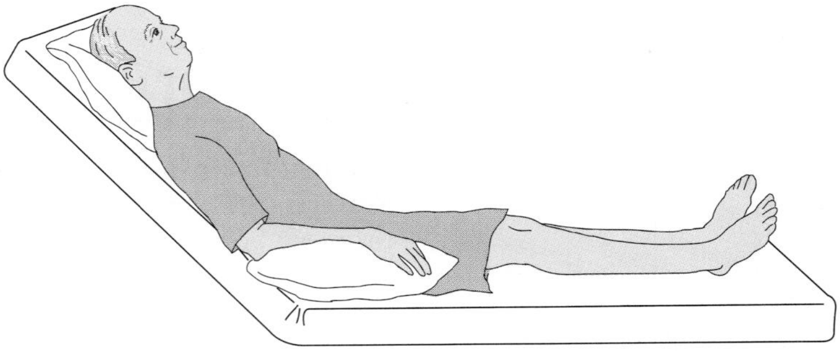

Fig. 10-30 Fowler's position. Pillows are used to maintain alignment.

Supine position. The **supine** (**dorsal recumbent**) **position** is the back-lying position. The bed is flat, the head and shoulders are supported on a pillow, and the arms and hands are placed at the side. You can support the arms with regular-size pillows. Or you can support the hands on small pillows with the palms down (Fig. 10-31).

The nurse may ask you to place a folded or rolled towel under the small of the resident's back. A small pillow is placed under the resident's thighs if requested by the nurse.

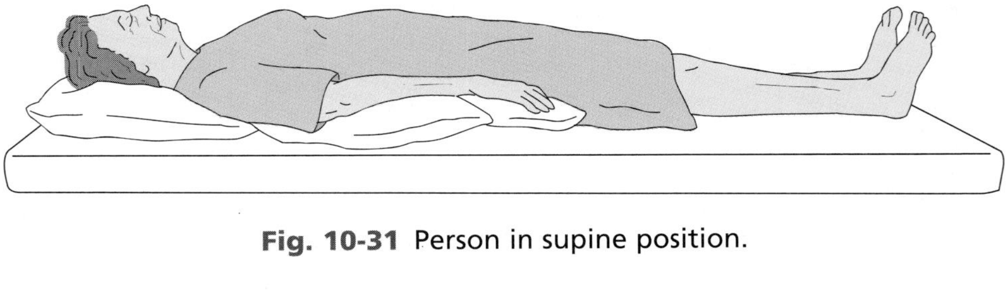

Fig. 10-31 Person in supine position.

Prone position. Residents in the **prone position** lie on their abdomen with their head turned to one side. A small pillow is placed under the resident's head, one is under the abdomen, and one is under the lower legs (Fig. 10-32). The arms are flexed at the elbows with the hands near the head.

You also can position residents with their feet hanging over the end of the mattress (Fig. 10-33). If that is done, a pillow is not needed under the lower legs.

Most older residents do not tolerate the prone position well because of limited range of motion in their necks. Check with the nurse before placing any resident in the prone position.

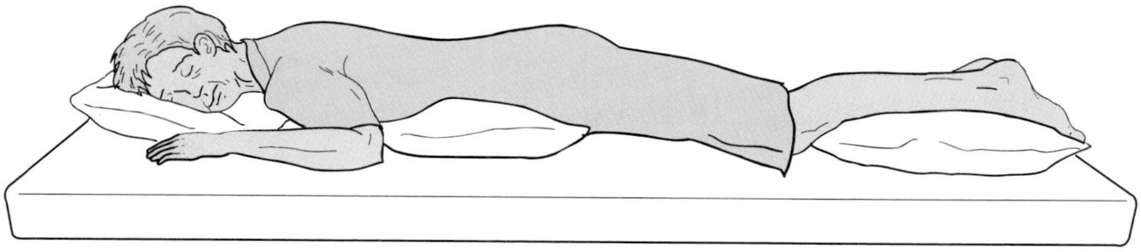

Fig. 10-32 Person in prone position.

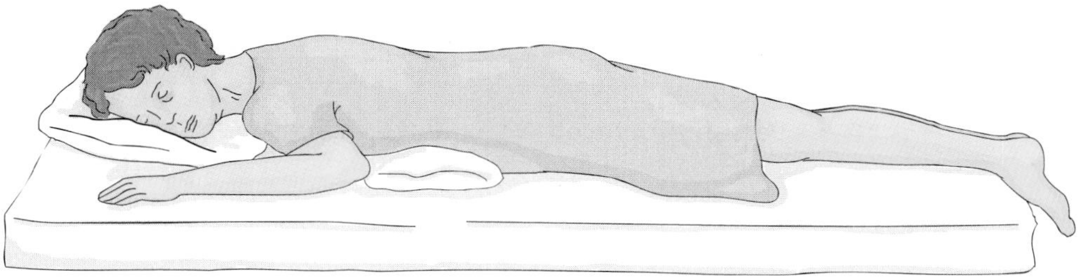

Fig. 10-33 Person in the prone position with the feet hanging over the edge of the mattress.

Lateral position. A resident in the **lateral (side-lying) position** lies on one side (Fig. 10-34). Pillows are used to maintain good alignment. Place a pillow under the resident's head and shoulders. Place the upper leg in front of the lower leg. (The nurse may ask you to position the resident so the upper leg is behind the lower leg, not on top of it.) Support the upper leg and thigh with pillows. Place a pillow against the resident's back. Help the resident to roll back against the pillow so that his or her back is at a 45-degree angle with the mattress. Place a small pillow under the upper hand and arm.

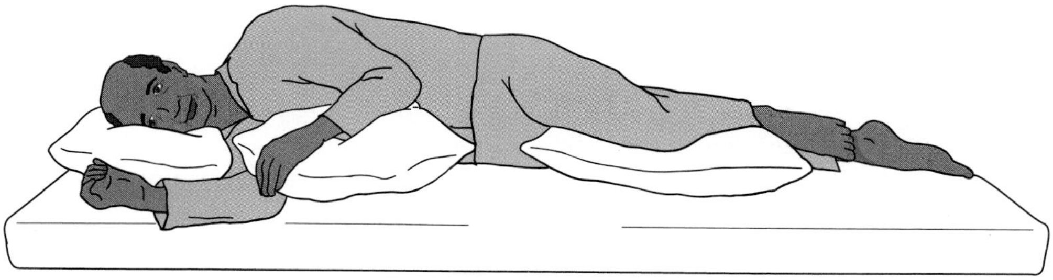

Fig. 10-34 Person in lateral position with pillows used for support.

Sims' position. The **Sims' position** is a left side-lying position. The upper leg is sharply flexed so that it is not on the lower leg. The lower arm is behind the resident (Fig. 10-35). For good body alignment, place a pillow under the resident's head and shoulder, support the upper leg with a pillow, and place a pillow under the upper arm and hand. This position usually is not comfortable for older residents. Check with the nurse before placing a resident in this position.

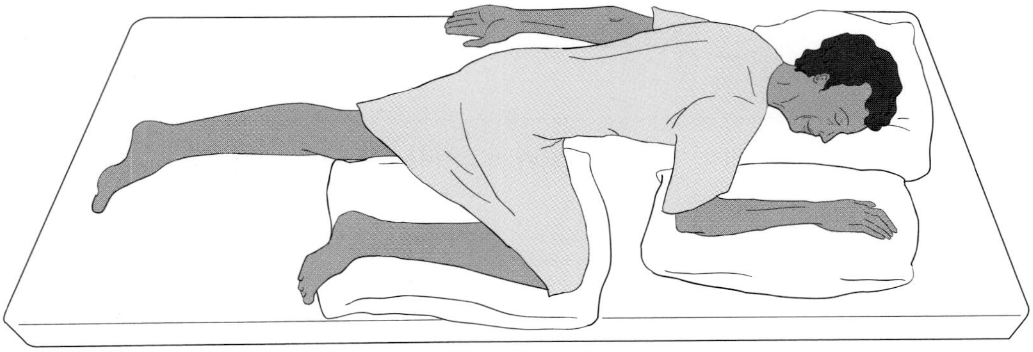

Fig. 10-35 Person supported with pillows in Sims' position.

Positioning in a Chair

Residents who sit in a chair must be able to hold their head and upper body erect. Poor alignment results if the resident cannot stay in an erect position. For good alignment, the resident's back and buttocks are against the back of the chair. Feet are flat on the floor or wheelchair footrests. Never leave the feet unsupported. Backs of knees and calves are slightly away from the edge of the seat (Fig. 10-36). With the nurse's permission, you can put a small pillow between the lower part of the resident's back and the chair. This supports the lower back. Paralyzed arms are positioned on pillows. Some residents have special foam positioners (Fig. 10-37). Ask the nurse about their proper use. Wrists are positioned at a slight upward angle.

Some residents require postural supports if they cannot keep their upper body erect (Fig. 10-38). Postural supports help keep them in good body alignment. The physical therapist, occupational therapist, and rehabilitative nurse assess the needs of residents who require postural support. They select the best product for the resident's needs. Resident safety, dignity, and function are considered.

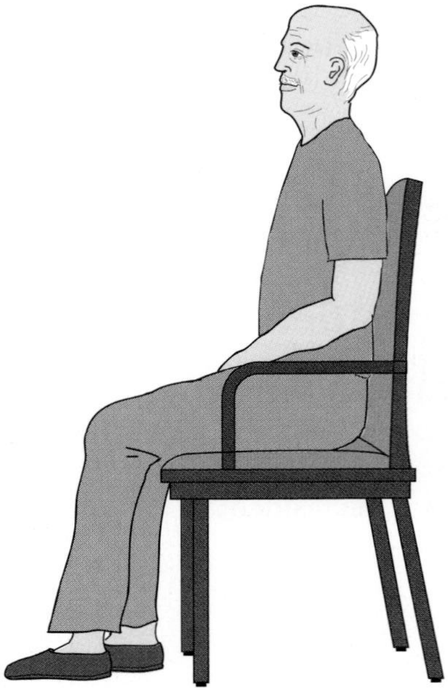

Fig. 10-36 Person positioned in a chair. The person's feet are flat on the floor, the calves do not touch the chair, and the back is straight and against the back of the chair.

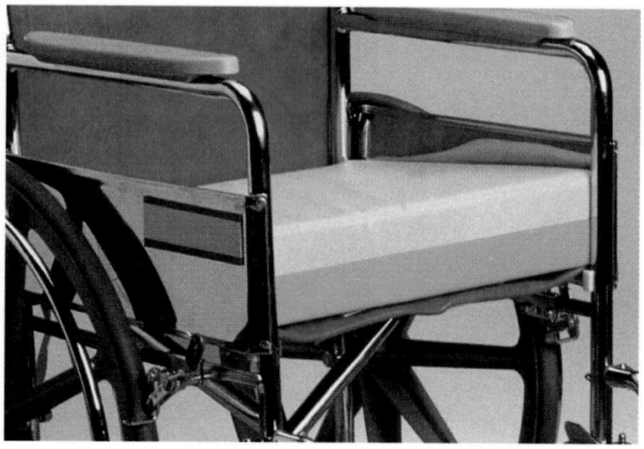

Fig. 10-37 *Foam positioner. (Courtesy J.T. Posey Co., Arcadia, Calif.)*

A

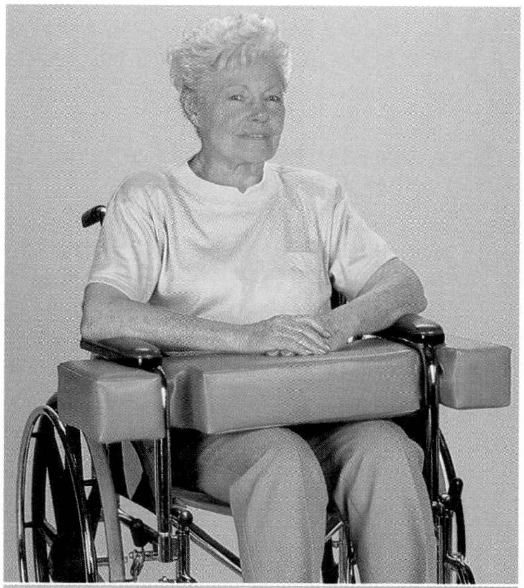

B

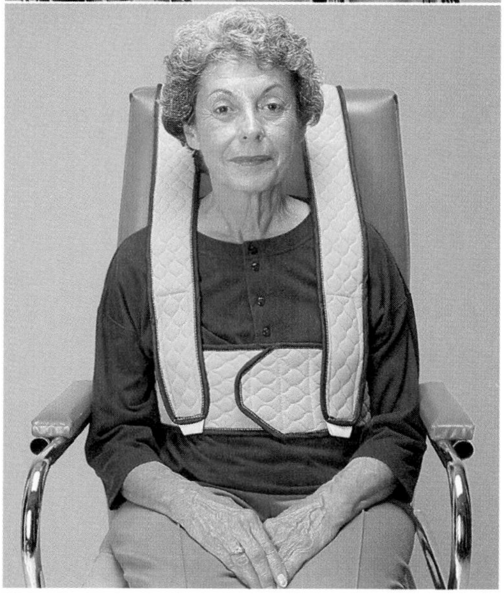

Fig. 10-38 *Postural supports.* **A,** *Pelvic holder.* **B,** *Torso support. (Courtesy J.T. Posey Co., Arcadia, Calif.)*

QUALITY OF LIFE

OBRA requires nursing centers to provide care in a manner that maintains and improves the quality of life, health, and safety of each resident. Proper body mechanics protects residents from injuries that could affect their health and ability to function.

Remember to protect residents' rights when you lift, move, transfer, and position residents. You must protect the resident's privacy at all times. Screen the resident properly, and expose only the body part involved in the procedure. Close doors, curtains, and drapes and pull window shades as needed to protect the right to privacy.

The resident's rights also are protected by allowing personal choice whenever possible. As long as the resident's safety is not affected, let the resident choose such things as bed positions, where the chair or wheelchair is positioned after transfers, and when to get up or go back to bed. Always check with the nurse and the resident's care plan to make sure the resident's choices are safe. Also let the resident help in lifting, moving, and transferring procedures to the extent possible.

The resident also has the right to be free from restraint. Bed rails are considered restraints under OBRA and are used only with the resident's consent. Many procedures in this chapter involve raising the bed for good body mechanics. Therefore the procedures in this chapter include the use of bed rails. Always check with the nurse and the resident's care plan about using bed rails. When you use bed rails, always explain to the resident why you are using them.

REVIEW QUESTIONS

Circle T if the statement is true and F if the statement is false.

1 T F Body mechanics means the way body segments are aligned with one another.

2 T F Good body mechanics help protect you and your residents from injury.

3 T F Base of support is the area on which an object rests.

4 T F Objects are held away from the body when lifting, moving, or carrying them.

5 T F Sliding the resident reduces friction and shearing.

6 T F Body mechanics involves using the small muscles of the body.

7 T F The small muscles of the body are in the back and shoulders.

8 T F Lifting the resident reduces friction.

9 T F Face the direction you are working to prevent unnecessary twisting.

10 T F When help is needed, ask a co-worker to help before starting the procedure.

11 T F Push, slide, or pull heavy objects rather than lift them.

12 T F Ask the nurse about limits in positioning or moving a resident.

13 T F The right to privacy is protected when moving, lifting, or transferring residents.

14 T F A lift sheet extends from the head to above the knees.

15 T F A resident is moved to the side of the bed before turning to the lateral position.

16 T F Logrolling is rolling the resident in segments.

17 T F A mechanical lift is used for residents with spinal cord injuries.

18 T F A transfer belt is part of a mechanical lift.

19 T F You are going to transfer Mrs. Porter from the bed to a chair. Move her from the direction of the weak side of her body.

20 T F Repositioning prevents deformities and pressure on body parts.

21 T F The head of the bed is elevated 45 to 60 degrees for the supine position.

22 T F The Sims' position is a side-lying position.

Answers to these questions are on p. 697.

11 The Resident's Unit

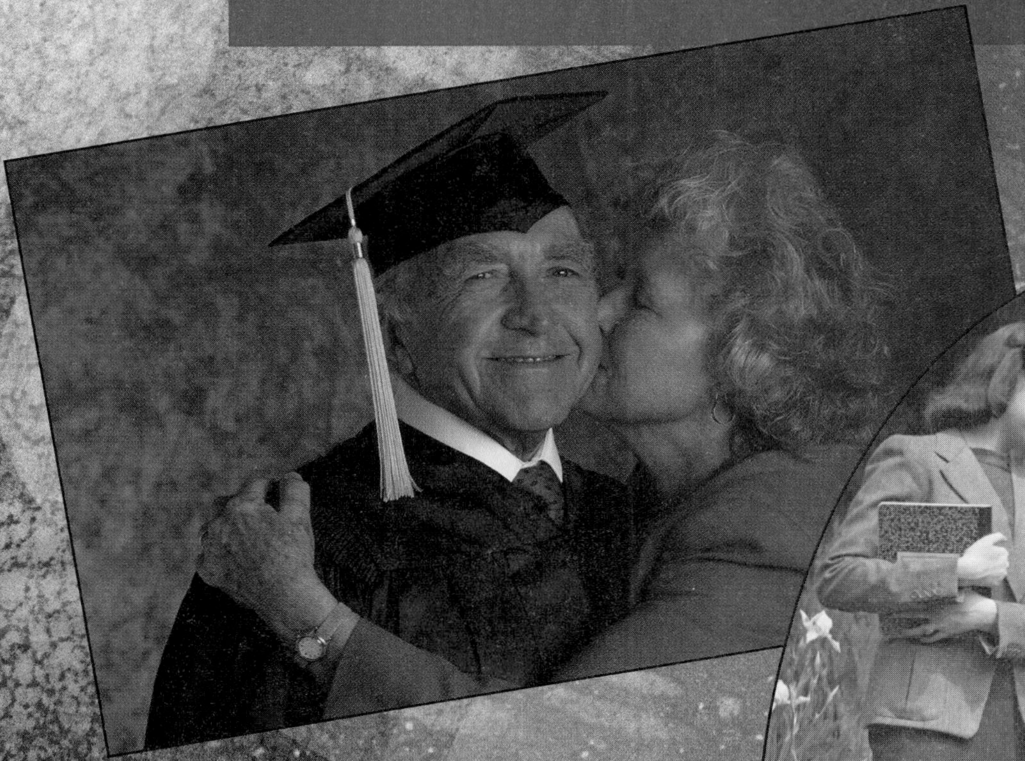

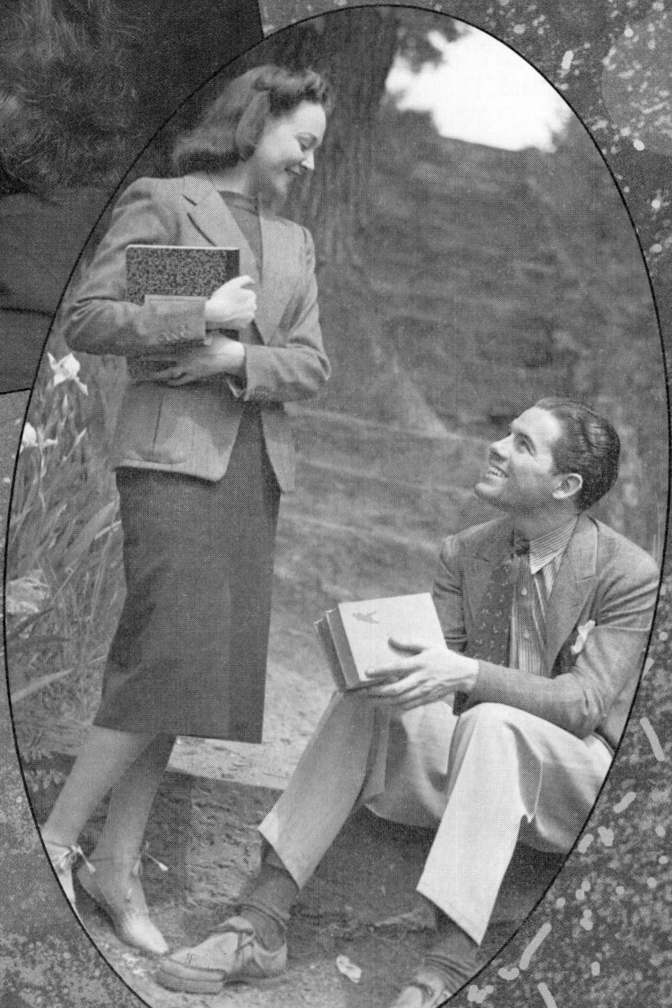

What You Will Learn

- The definition of the key terms listed in this chapter
- The temperature ranges comfortable for most people
- How to protect residents from drafts
- Measures to prevent or reduce odors in resident rooms
- How to control the common causes of noise in nursing centers
- How lighting affects the resident's comfort
- Basic bed positions
- How to use equipment in the resident's unit
- How a bathroom is equipped for the resident's use
- How to provide safety, privacy, and comfort in resident units
- Measures to help maintain the resident's unit

Key Terms

caster A small wheel made of rubber or plastic

full visual privacy The resident has the means to be completely free from public view while occupying a bed

resident unit The personal space, furniture, and equipment provided for the individual by the nursing center

reverse Trendelenburg's position The head of the bed is raised, and the foot of the bed is lowered

semi-Fowler's position The head of the bed is raised 45 degrees, and the knee portion is raised 15 degrees; or the head of the bed is raised 30 degrees, and the knee portion is not raised

Trendelenburg's position The head of the bed is lowered, and the foot of the bed is raised

Nursing center residents have very little personal or private space. Few residents have private rooms. Most must share a room with another person. Each resident has an assigned area of the room. This area is considered private. It is treated like the person's home. Residents are encouraged to keep some personal items and to arrange them as they choose. This is a challenge when space is limited. For example, a resident cannot violate the rights of other residents by taking someone else's space.

The center must also follow health and safety standards. Therefore rooms are designed to provide comfort, safety, and privacy for all residents. The intent is to have resident rooms as personal and homelike as possible.

This chapter describes the conditions that influence a person's comfort and the furnishings in a resident unit. A **resident unit** is the personal space, furniture, and equipment provided for the individual by the nursing center (Fig. 11-1). *(See Subacute Care, p. 235.)*

COMFORT

Age, illness, and activity affect a resident's comfort. So do temperature, ventilation, odors, noise, and lighting. These conditions usually are controlled to meet a person's needs.

Temperature and Ventilation

Nursing centers have heating, air conditioning, and ventilation systems. These systems maintain a comfortable temperature and provide fresh air in the rooms. A temperature range of 68° to 74° F usually is comfortable for most healthy people. What is comfortable for one person may be too hot or too cold for another. Older and chronically ill persons may need higher room temperatures. Therefore higher temperatures usually are needed in nursing centers. OBRA requires that nursing centers maintain a temperature range of 71° to 81° F. OBRA

Residents who are less active and those who cannot move about without help are usually uncomfortable

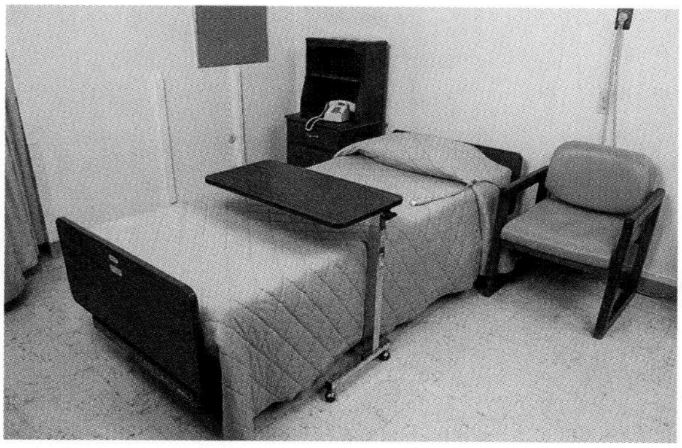

Fig. 11-1 Furniture and equipment in a typical resident unit.

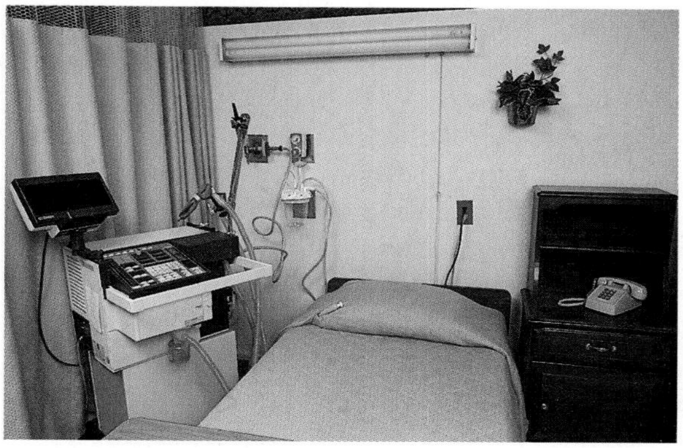

Fig. 11-2 A room in a subacute care unit.

in cool areas. Make sure that these residents are dressed warmly and that room temperatures are kept warm. Temperatures in any room used by residents must be comfortable for the residents. Remember, you are younger, more active, and healthier than the residents are.

Stale room air and lingering odors can affect comfort and rest. A good ventilation system provides fresh air and moves air in the room. Drafts are created as the air moves. Older and chronically ill persons are sensitive to drafts. You can help to protect them from drafts by:

- Making sure they have on enough clothing. Many older persons choose to wear sweaters during warm weather.
- Offering lap robes to residents in chairs and wheelchairs. Lap robes cover their legs.
- Making sure that residents in bed are covered with enough blankets.
- Moving residents from drafty areas whenever possible.

Odors

Many smells occur in nursing centers. Some are pleasant, such as the aroma of food and the scent of fresh flowers. Others are unpleasant. Draining wounds, vomitus, bowel movements, and urine cause unpleasant odors that embarrass residents. Body, breath, and smoking odors may be offensive to residents, visitors, and staff members. Some visitors and residents are quite sensitive to odors. They may become nauseated. Good nursing care and good ventilation help eliminate odors. To control odors and provide good nursing care you should:

- Check incontinent residents often (see Chapters 16 and 17).
- Change and promptly wash residents who are wet or soiled.
- Dispose of incontinence products promptly.
- Dispose of soiled linen or clothing as soon as you have finished the change.

Subacute Care

In nursing centers with subacute units, the rooms look more like hospital rooms. A person's length of stay on a subacute unit is short. The care is medically complex and focused on rehabilitation. Rooms may have piped-in wall oxygen and suction (Fig. 11-2). There are usually more medical equipment and supplies in subacute rooms. This is necessary to manage the person's complex health care needs. Remember that these persons have the same rights to privacy as other persons of the center.

- Keep soiled-linen containers closed.
- Empty and wash bedpans, bedside commodes, and emesis basins promptly.
- Empty urinals promptly.
- Use a room deodorizer when necessary (sometimes odors remain after clearing the cause of the odor). Do not use spray deodorizers around residents with breathing problems. Ask the nurse if you are unsure.
- Provide good personal hygiene for your residents to help prevent body and breath odors.

Smoking presents special problems. Make sure residents smoke only in the areas allowed. If you smoke, you must observe your center's smoking policy. Wash your hands after handling smoking materials and before giving resident care. Give careful attention to your uniforms, hair, and breath because of clinging smoke odors.

Remember that the center is the residents' home. Keep it as free of unpleasant odors as possible.

Noise

Many older and chronically ill people are sensitive to the noises and sounds around them. Common health care sounds may easily disturb residents. The clanging of metal equipment (bedpans, urinals, and wash basins) and the clatter of dishes and meal trays can be annoying. Residents may hear loud talking and laughter in hallways and at the nurses' station. They may think that staff members are talking and laughing about them. Televisions, radios, ringing telephones, buzzing signal lights, and intercoms can be irritating. So is noise from equipment that needs repair or oil. Wheels on stretchers, wheelchairs, utility carts, and other similar equipment must be oiled properly.

When in a strange environment—such as a nursing center—people try to figure out the cause and meaning of new sounds. This relates to the basic need to feel safe and secure. Residents, especially if confused, may find sounds dangerous, frightening, or irritating. As a result, they may become upset, anxious, and uncomfortable. Remember that what is noise to one person may not be noise to another. For example, a teenager's loud stereo music may be quite irritating to parents.

Nursing centers are designed to reduce noise. Drapes, carpeting, and acoustical tiles all help absorb noise. Plastic equipment has replaced some metal equipment (bedpans, urinals, and wash basins). Health care workers can reduce noise and increase resident comfort by controlling the loudness of their voices and by handling equipment carefully. Keeping equipment in good working order and promptly answering telephones, signal lights, and intercoms also decrease noise.

Lighting

Good lighting is needed for the safety and comfort of residents and health care workers. Glares, shadows, and dull lighting can cause falls, headaches, and eyestrain. People usually relax and rest better in dim light. A bright room is more cheerful and stimulating. *(See Residents With Dementia.)*

Lighting in most rooms can be adjusted to meet the changing needs of the resident. Shades are pulled or drapes drawn to control natural light. The light above the bed is adjusted to provide soft, medium, and bright lighting. Some centers also have ceiling lights over the beds. These provide very soft and low to extremely bright lighting. Residents with poor vision need very bright light to see. This is especially important at mealtime and when they are moving about the center. Bright lighting also helps when health care workers perform procedures. Always keep light controls within the resident's reach to allow for the right of personal choice.

RESIDENTS WITH DEMENTIA

In dementia care units, lighting is often adjusted to help control agitation and aggressive behavior. Soft, nonglare lights can decrease agitation and help residents to relax. Brighter lighting may improve orientation because residents can see their surroundings more clearly.

ROOM FURNITURE AND EQUIPMENT

Rooms are furnished and equipped for the resident's basic needs. The right to privacy is considered when the room is equipped. There is furniture and equipment for:

- Comfort
- Sleep
- Elimination
- Nutrition
- Personal hygiene
- Activity
- Communicating with the health care team, relatives, and friends

The Bed

Hospital beds are adjusted electrically or manually. They can be raised horizontally to give care. This reduces bending or reaching. The lowest horizontal position allows the resident to get out of bed with ease (Fig. 11-3). The head of the bed is kept flat or raised in varying degrees.

Many nursing centers have electric beds. Others use manually operated beds. Electric beds have hand controls. Staff members and residents can easily change the bed's position with the hand controls. The controls are on a side panel, attached to the bed by a cable, or on a panel at the foot of the bed (Fig. 11-4).

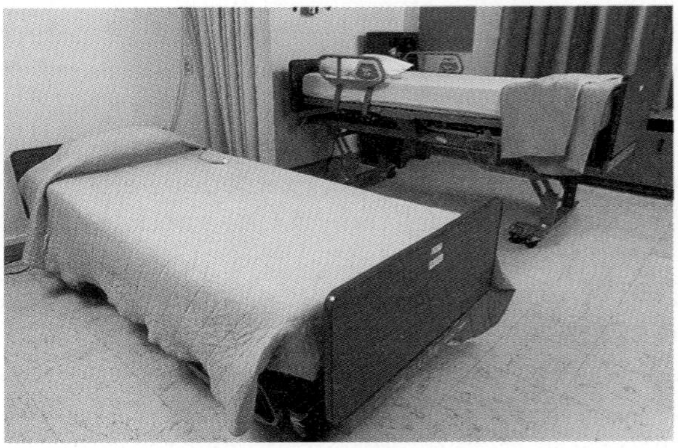

Fig. 11-3 One bed in the highest horizontal position and the other bed in the lowest horizontal position.

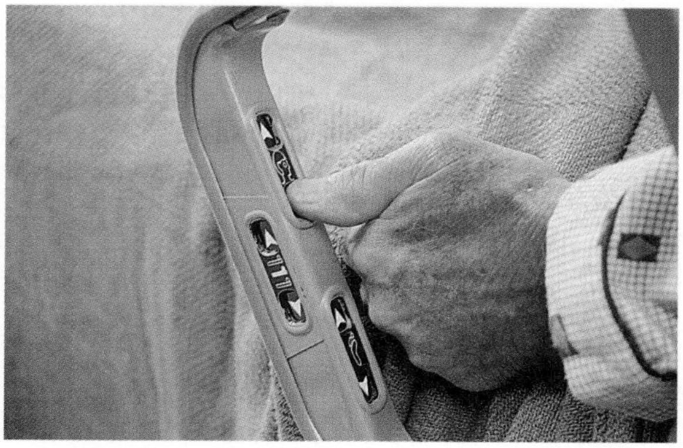

Fig. 11-4 Controls for an electric bed.

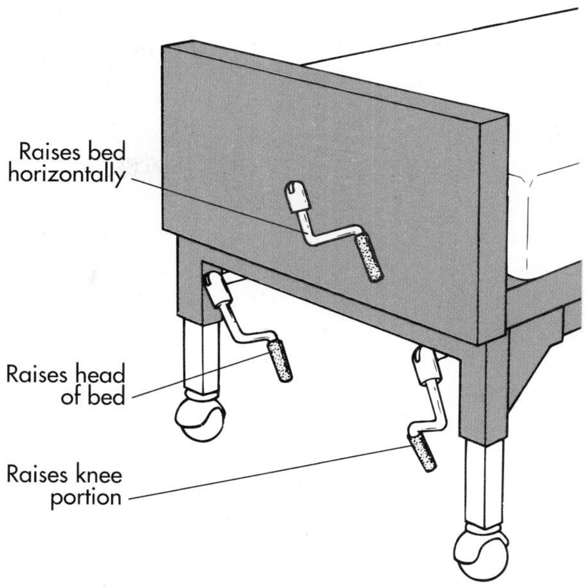

Fig. 11-5 Manually operated hospital bed.

Alert and oriented residents are taught how to use the controls. They are warned not to raise the bed to the high position and not to adjust the bed to harmful positions. They are told about any position limits or restrictions.

Most electric beds can be "locked" into any position by the staff. Often, confused residents need to have their beds locked. This prevents them from adjusting their beds to unsafe positions.

Manually operated beds have hand cranks at the foot of the bed (Fig. 11-5). The left crank raises or lowers the head of the bed. The right crank adjusts the knee portion. The center crank raises or lowers the entire bed horizontally. The cranks are pulled up during use and kept down at all other times. Cranks left in the up position are a safety hazard. Anyone walking past the cranks can bump into them.

Bed positions. There are five basic bed positions—flat, Fowler's, semi-Fowler's, Trendelenburg's, and reverse Trendelenburg's:

- **Flat**—the usual sleeping position. The position is also used after spinal cord surgery or injury and for cervical traction.
- **Fowler's position**—a semi-sitting position. The head of the bed is raised 45 to 60 degrees (Fig. 11-6). Reasons for positioning a resident in Fowler's position were described in Chapter 10.
- **Semi-Fowler's position**—the head of the bed is raised 45 degrees, and the knee portion is raised 15 degrees (Fig. 11-7). This position is comfortable and prevents residents from sliding down in bed. However, raising the knee portion can interfere with circulation in the legs. Check with the nurse before positioning a resident in the semi-Fowler's position. Some centers define semi-Fowler's position as the position in which the head of the bed is raised 30 degrees and the knee portion is *not* raised. You must know the definition used by your center so you can give safe care.

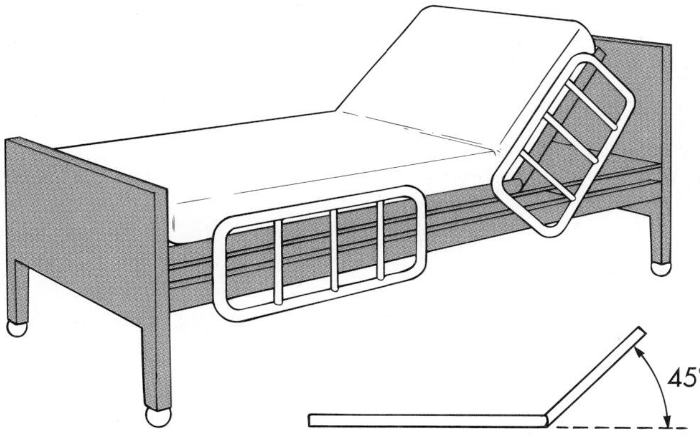

Fig. 11-6 Fowler's position.

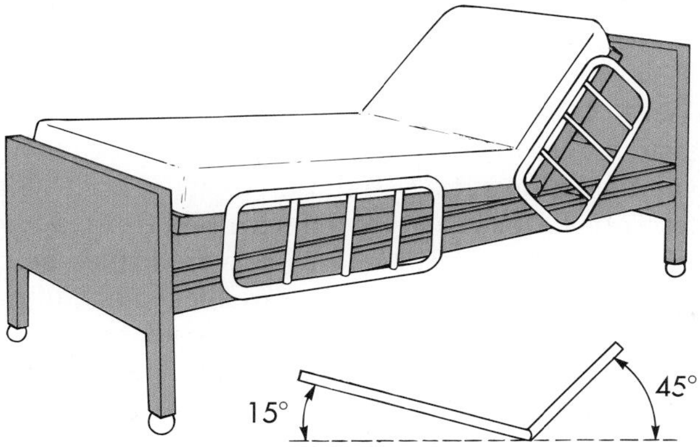

Fig. 11-7 Semi-Fowler's position.

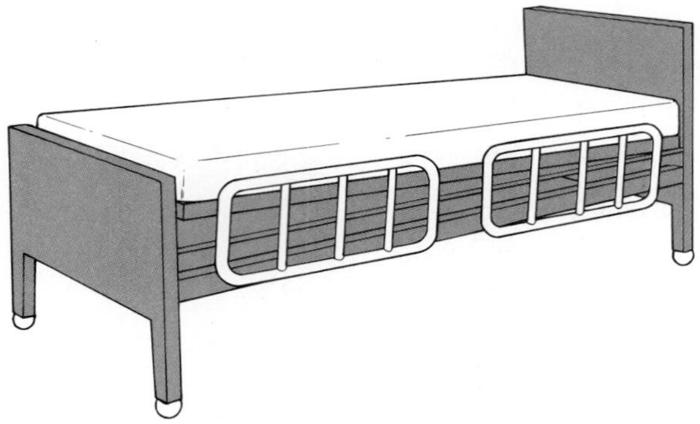

Fig. 11-8 Trendelenburg's position.

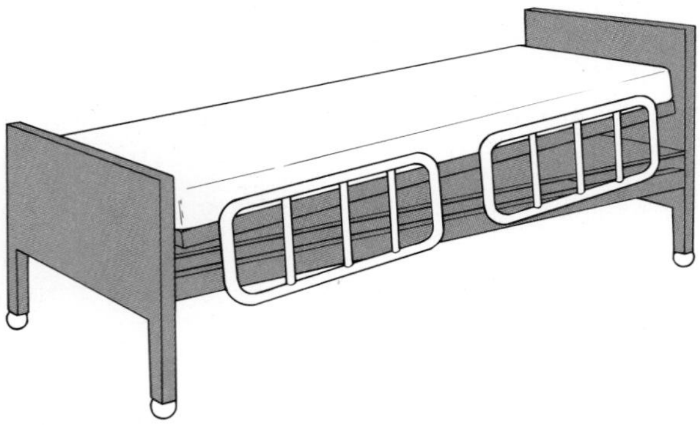

Fig. 11-9 Reverse Trendelenburg's position.

- **Trendelenburg's position**—lowering the head of the bed and raising the foot of the bed (Fig. 11-8). A doctor or nurse orders the position. Blocks are placed under the bed's lower legs, or the bed frame is tilted into Trendelenburg's position.
- **Reverse Trendelenburg's position**—the opposite of Trendelenburg's position. The head of the bed is raised, and the foot of the bed is lowered (Fig. 11-9). Blocks are put under the legs at the head of the bed, or the bed frame is tilted. This position requires a doctor's order.

Safety considerations. Bed legs have wheels or casters. A **caster** is a small wheel made of rubber or plastic that allows the bed to move easily. Each wheel or caster has a lock that prevents the bed from moving (see Fig. 8-9, p. 136). The bed wheels are locked before giving bedside care. The wheels are locked at all times except when moving the bed. Many residents get into and out of bed without help. They can be hurt if the bed moves.

The proper use of bed rails on hospital beds was discussed in Chapter 8.

The Overbed Table

The overbed table (see Fig. 11-1) is positioned over the bed by sliding the base under the bed. It is raised or lowered to a comfortable height for the resident in bed or in a chair. The overbed table is used for meals, writing, reading, and other activities.

Some overbed tables have movable tops with a storage area underneath. The storage area often is used for beauty, hair care, shaving, or other personal items. Many also have a flip-up mirror useful for personal grooming.

The nursing team uses the overbed table as a work area. Only clean and sterile items are placed on the table. Never place bedpans, urinals, or soiled linen on the overbed table. The table is cleaned after serving as a working surface.

The Bedside Stand

The bedside stand is next to the resident's bed. The stand is a storage area for the resident's personal belongings and personal care equipment. It has a top drawer and a lower cabinet with a shelf (Fig. 11-10). The drawer is used for money, eyeglasses, books, and other personal items. The top shelf is used for the wash basin, which can hold personal care items. These include soap and soap dish, powder, lotion, deodorant, towels, washcloth, bath blanket, and a clean gown or pajamas. An emesis or kidney basin (shaped like a kidney) is used to hold oral hygiene equipment. The kidney basin is stored on the top shelf or in the drawer. The bedpan and its cover, the urinal, and toilet paper are on the lower shelf.

The top of the stand often is used for tissues and other personal items. The resident may put a radio, clock, pictures, telephone, and other important items there. Some stands have a side or back rod for towels and washcloths.

Chairs

OBRA

The resident unit always has at least one chair for personal and visitor use. This is an OBRA requirement. The chair usually is an upholstered chair with armrests (Fig. 11-11). It must be comfortable for the resident. The chair also must be sturdy so it does not move easily or tip over during transfers. The resident should be able to get in and out of the chair easily. Therefore it should not be too low or too soft.

Privacy Curtains

OBRA

According to OBRA, each resident has the right to full visual privacy. **Full visual privacy** means that a resident has a means to be completely free from public view while occupying his or her bed. Rooms with more than one bed have a curtain between the resident units. The curtain is pulled around either bed to provide privacy (see Fig. 2-2, p. 28). It is *always* pulled

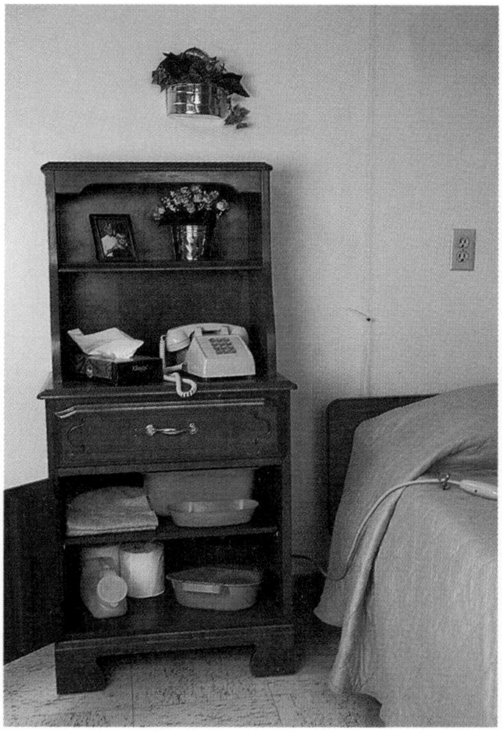

Fig. 11-10 The bedside stand is used to store personal care equipment.

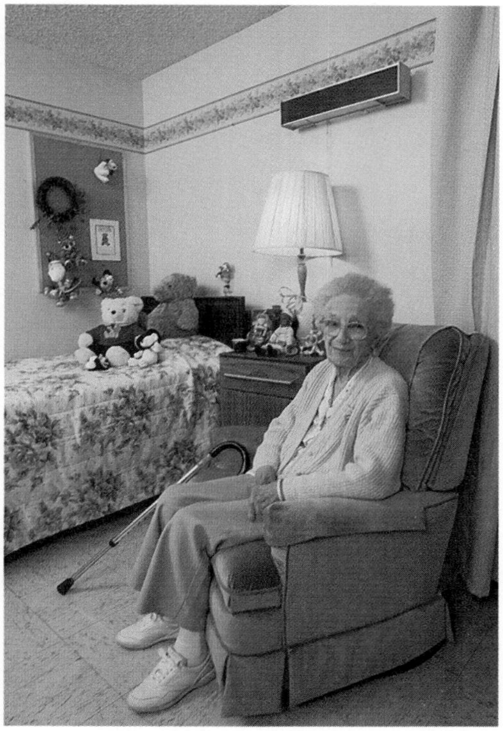

Fig. 11-11 The resident's chair provides comfort and support.

completely around the bed when care is given. Privacy curtains prevent others from seeing the resident. However, they do not block sound. Conversations can be heard.

Personal Care Equipment

Personal care equipment refers to items needed for hygiene and elimination. Most centers provide a wash basin, emesis or kidney basin, bedpan, urinal, water pitcher and glass, and soap and soap dish. Some provide powder, lotion, toothbrush, toothpaste, mouthwash, tissues, a comb, and deodorant. Usually residents bring their own oral hygiene equipment, hair care supplies, and deodorant. Some also prefer their own soap, lotion, and powder. Remember to respect the resident's personal choice in personal care products.

Call System

OBRA

The call system lets the resident signal for help. The signal light (call bell) is at the end of a long cord that is attached to the bed or chair (Fig. 11-12). It must always be within the resident's reach in his or her room, bathrooms, and shower or tub rooms. This is an OBRA requirement. The resident presses a button at the end of the signal light to get assistance. The signal light at the bedside is connected to a light above the room door (Fig. 11-13, *A*, p. 240) and to a light panel or intercom system at the nurses' station (Fig. 11-13, *B*). These tell the nursing staff that the resident needs help. The nurse or nursing assistant shuts off the light at the bedside when the help is given.

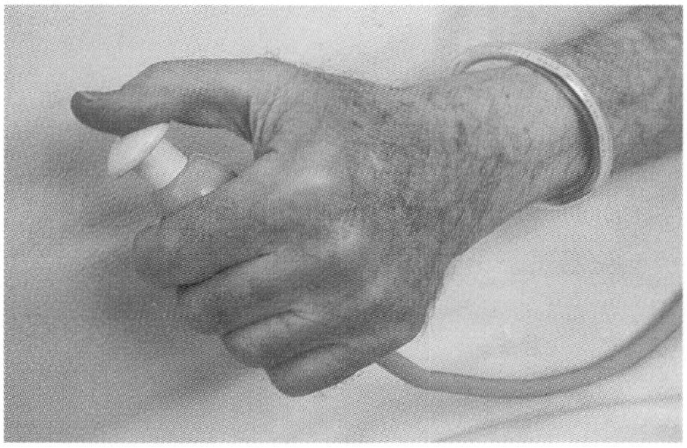

Fig. 11-12 The person presses the button of the signal light when assistance is needed.

An intercom system lets the resident and nursing staff member talk from the room to the nurses' station. The resident can tell the staff member what is needed. Hearing-impaired residents may have difficulty using an intercom.

Some residents have limited mobility in their hands. They may require a special signal light that is turned on by tapping it with a hand or fist (Fig. 11-14, p. 240). The signal light should always be on the resident's strong side. Residents are shown how to use the call system when they are admitted. Always remind residents to signal when help is needed.

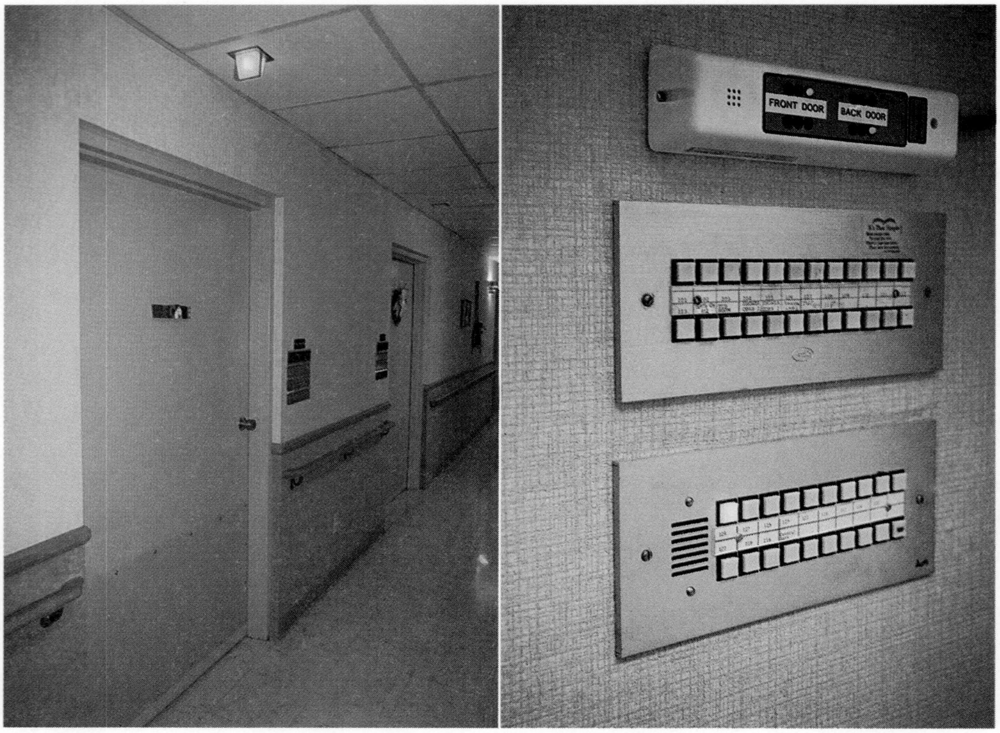

Fig. 11-13 **A,** The light above the door of the person's room. **B,** Light panel or intercom system at the nurses' station.

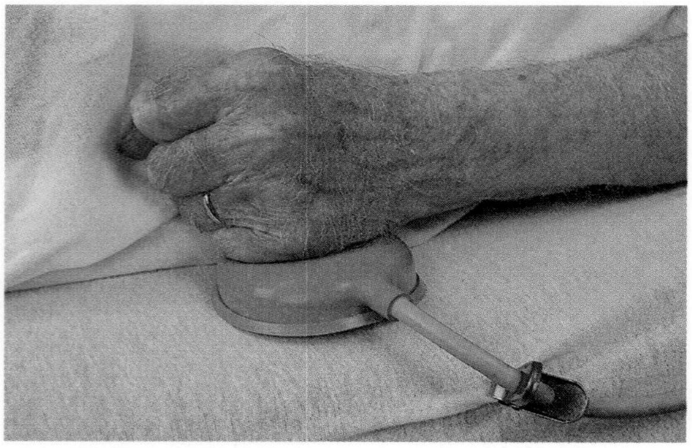

Fig. 11-14 Signal light for residents with limited hand mobility.

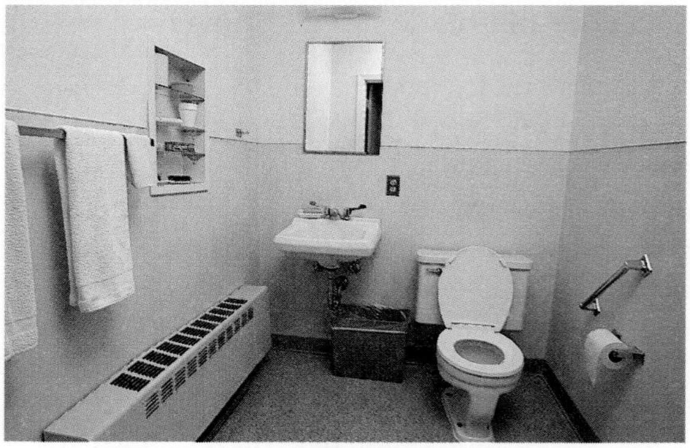

Fig. 11-15 Resident's bathroom.

Some residents cannot use the signal light. Examples include residents in a coma or very confused residents. Check the resident's care plan for any special communication measures. You must check these residents often to make sure their needs are met.

The Bathroom

Many centers have a bathroom in each room. Some have a bathroom that adjoins two resident rooms. A toilet, sink, call system, and mirror are standard equipment (Fig. 11-15). Some bathrooms have showers. For the resident's safety, grab bars are by the toilet. The resident uses them for support when sitting or getting up from the toilet. In some centers the toilet seats are higher than the standard height. The higher toilets make transfers from wheelchairs easier. They also are helpful for residents with restricted joint movement. Removable, raised toilet seats also are available.

Towel racks, toilet paper, soap, paper towel dispenser, and wastebasket also are in the bathroom. They are placed within easy reach of the resident.

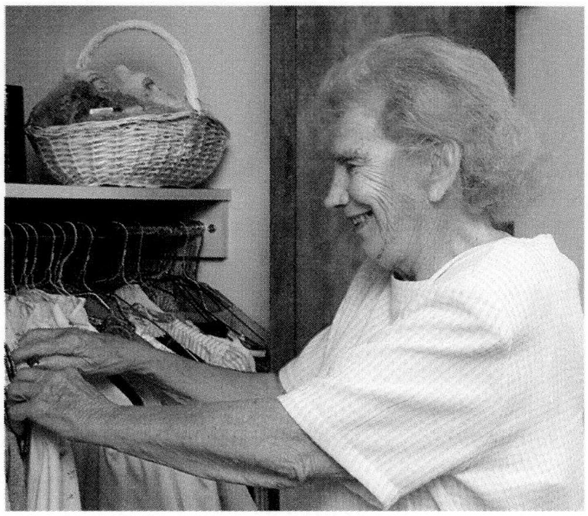

Fig. 11-16 The resident can access items in her closet.

Closet and Drawer Space

Closet and drawer space are provided for the resident's clothing. Some residents bring in another small chest of drawers for personal belongings. OBRA requires that nursing centers provide each resident with closet space. The closet space must have shelves and a clothes rack (Fig. 11-16). The resident must have free access to the closet and its contents. OBRA

Items in the closet or drawers are the resident's private property. You must not search the closet or drawers without the resident's permission.

Sometimes people hoard items. Some residents save such things as napkins, straws, food, and packets of sugar, salt, and pepper. Such hoarding can cause safety or health risks. Center representatives can inspect a person's closet or drawers if hoarding is suspected. The resident is informed of the inspection and is present when it takes place.

SUBACUTE CARE

Some rooms have equipment mounted on the wall for measuring blood pressure. Some beds are equipped with IV poles. The poles are used to hang intravenous (IV) infusion bottles or bags (see Chapter 18). The poles are stored in a special part of the bed frame. If the IV pole is not part of the bed, one is brought to the bedside when needed. Subacute care rooms also may have wall outlets for oxygen and suction (see Fig. 11-2).

Other Equipment

Nursing centers may allow residents to bring furniture or other items from home. *(See Subacute Care.)* Some residents like to bring favorite chairs and footstools. Televisions, radios, clocks, pictures, and other small items are brought from home to help the residents feel "at home" in their own units. Telephones are available in some centers.

General Rules

All health care personnel are responsible for keeping the resident unit clean, neat, safe, and comfortable. The rules in Box 11-1 will help guide you in maintaining resident units.

Box 11-1 RULES FOR MAINTAINING THE RESIDENT'S UNIT

- Make sure the resident can reach the overbed table and the bedside stand.
- Arrange personal items as the resident prefers. Make sure the resident can easily reach them.
- Keep the signal light within the resident's reach at all times.
- Meet the needs of residents who cannot use the call system.
- Provide the resident with enough tissues and toilet paper.
- Adjust lighting, temperature, and ventilation for the resident's comfort.
- Handle equipment carefully to prevent unnecessary noise.
- Reassure the resident by explaining the causes of strange noises.
- Use room deodorizers if necessary.
- Empty the resident's wastebasket as often as needed or at least once a day.
- Always treat a resident's personal items with respect.

Quality of Life

Remember that the resident once had a home or apartment with furniture, appliances, a private bathroom, and many personal belongings and treasures. Now the person lives in a strange place and probably shares a room with another person. Leaving one's home is a difficult part of growing old with poor health. Therefore it is important to make the resident's unit as homelike as possible.

The resident is allowed to bring some furniture and personal items. A chair, footstool, lamp, and small table are among the items that may be allowed. Residents always can bring such things as family photos, religious items, and books. Some may have plants to care for. The resident is allowed personal choice in arranging personal possessions. You can help the resident in choosing the best place for personal items. The health care team must make sure that residents' choices are:

- Safe
- Will not cause falls or other accidents
- Do not interfere with the rights of others

Remember that the center is now the resident's home. You and other members of the health care team must help the resident feel safe, secure, and comfortable. A homelike setting will help the resident's quality of life. OBRA serves to promote quality of life. Box 11-2 lists OBRA's requirements for resident rooms.

OBRA

Box 11-2 OBRA Requirements for Resident Rooms

- Designed for 1 to 4 residents
- Direct access to exit corridor
- Full visual privacy (privacy curtain that extends around the bed, movable screens, doors)
- At least one window to the outside
- Individual closet space with racks and shelves
- Toilet facilities in the room or nearby (includes bathing facilities)
- Call system in the room and in toilet/bathing facilities
- Bed of proper height and size
- Clean, comfortable mattress with bedding appropriate to the weather and climate
- Furniture to accommodate clothing, personal items, and a chair for visitors
- Clean and orderly room
- Odor-free room
- Room temperature between 71° and 81° F
- Acceptable noise level
- Adequate ventilation and room humidity
- Appropriate lighting
- No glares from floors, windows, and lighting
- Clean and orderly drawers, shelves, and personal items
- Pest-free room
- Hand rails in needed areas
- Bed rails only if needed
- Clean, dry floor; pathways free of clutter and furniture
- Bed in low position and locked
- Personal supplies and items labeled and stored appropriately
- Drawers free of unwrapped food
- Items within reach for use in bed or bathroom
- Space for wheelchair or walker use
- Raised toilet seat
- Stool and skidproof tub or shower

Review Questions

Circle the BEST answer.

1 Which is a comfortable temperature range for most people?
A 60° to 66° F
B 68° to 74° F
C 74° to 80° F
D 80° to 86° F

2 You can protect residents from drafts by doing the following *except*
A Making sure they wear enough clothing
B Covering them with adequate blankets
C Moving them out of drafty areas
D Having them sit by the air conditioner

3 Which does *not* prevent or reduce odors in the resident's room?
A Placing fresh flowers in the room
B Emptying bedpans promptly
C Using room deodorizers
D Practicing good personal hygiene

4 Which will *not* control noise?
A Using equipment made of plastic
B Handling dishes and metal items with care
C Speaking softly
D Talking with others in the hallway

5 The overbed table is *not* used
A For eating
B As a working surface
C To store the urinal
D To store shaving items

Circle T if the statement is true and F if the statement is false.

6 T F In Fowler's position, the head of the bed is raised 45 to 60 degrees.

7 T F The curtain is pulled around the resident's bed to provide privacy when talking.

8 T F Soft and dim lighting usually is more relaxing and comfortable.

9 T F The signal light always must be within the resident's reach except when he or she is in the bathroom.

10 T F The resident must be able to reach items in the closet.

11 T F The temperature in resident areas is adjusted so you feel comfortable.

Answers to these questions are on p. 697.

12 Bedmaking

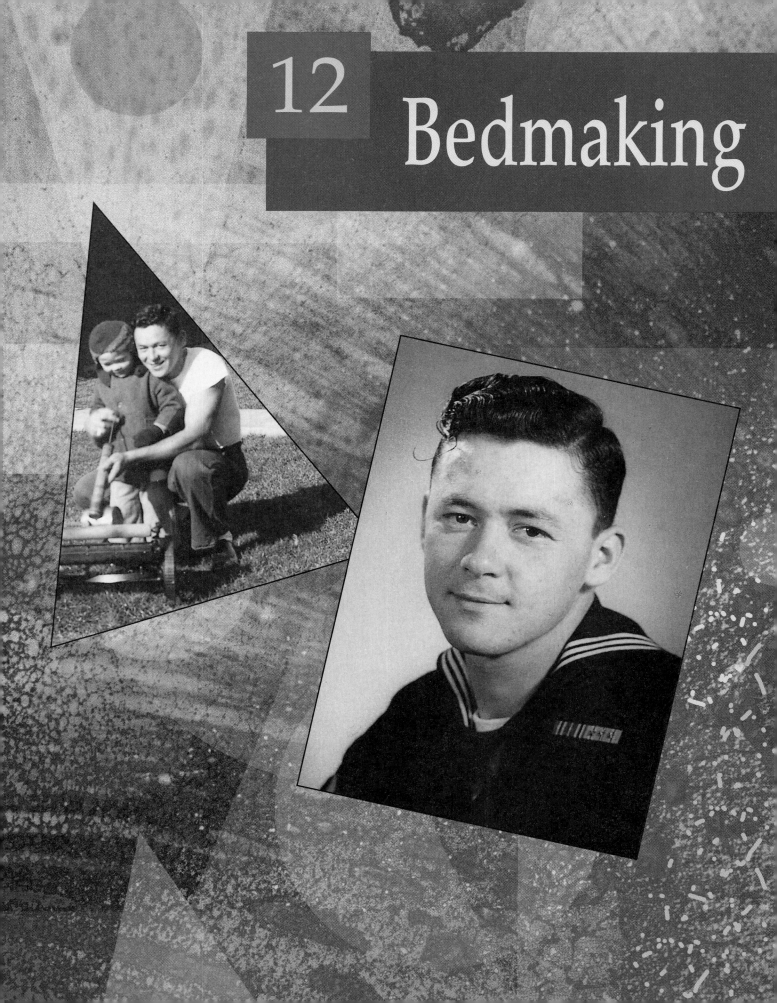

What You Will Learn

- The definition of the key terms listed in this chapter
- The differences among open, closed, occupied, and surgical beds
- When to change bed linens
- The purposes of plastic drawsheets and cotton drawsheets
- How to handle linens following the rules of medical asepsis
- The procedures described in this chapter

Key Terms

drawsheet A small sheet placed over the middle of the bottom sheet; it helps keep the mattress and bottom linens clean and dry; can be used to turn and move the person in bed; the cotton drawsheet

plastic drawsheet A drawsheet placed between the bottom sheet and the cotton drawsheet to keep the mattress and bottom linens clean and dry

▲ Most residents are out of bed most of the day. Some are in bed all the time. They are fed and bathed in bed. Some residents cannot get up to use the bathroom, and many are incontinent. Incontinent residents cannot control the passage of urine from their bladder or control bowel movements. They must have their bed linens changed often. Many treatments are done in bed.

Bedmaking is a very important part of your job. Clean, neat beds increase the resident's comfort. Residents depend on you for their comfort and well-being. By keeping beds clean, dry, and wrinkle free, you help prevent skin breakdown and pressure ulcers (see Chapter 14). These can cause residents severe pain and disability. In rare cases, death occurs.

Bed linens usually are changed every day in hospitals. In nursing centers a complete linen change is done on the resident's bath day. Older persons are less active than younger people and have drier skin. Therefore they do not need a full bath every day. The resident is scheduled for a bath or shower on certain days. The complete linen change is done after the bath or shower when the resident is up for the day. Residents like to have their bed made and room cleaned before visitors arrive.

Linens are straightened whenever they are loose or wrinkled. Check linens for crumbs after meals, and properly remove them. Also straighten linens at bedtime. Linens are changed whenever they become wet, soiled, or damp. Follow Standard Precautions and the Bloodborne Pathogen Standard for contact with the resident's blood, body fluids, secretions, or excretions.

Beds are made in the following ways:

- A *closed bed* is not being used by the resident until bedtime. A closed bed also is one that is ready for a new resident. The top linens are not folded back (Fig. 12-1, p. 246).
- An *open bed* is being used by a resident. Top linens are folded back so that the resident can get into bed. A closed bed becomes an open bed by folding back the top linens (Fig. 12-2, p. 246).
- An *occupied bed* is made with the resident in it (Fig. 12-3, p. 246).
- A *surgical bed* is made so that a resident can be moved from a stretcher to the bed. This bed is made for residents who are admitted by ambulance (Fig. 12-4, p. 246).

LINENS

Special attention is given to the care and use of linens. When handling linens and making beds, follow the rules of medical asepsis. Your uniform is considered dirty. Therefore always hold linens away from your body and uniform (Fig. 12-5, p. 246). Never shake linens in the air. Shaking them spreads microbes. Clean linens are placed on a clean surface. Never put clean or dirty linens on the floor.

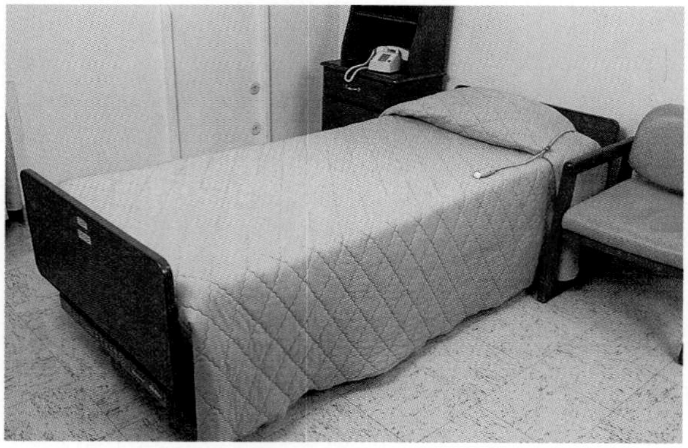

Fig. 12-1 Closed bed.

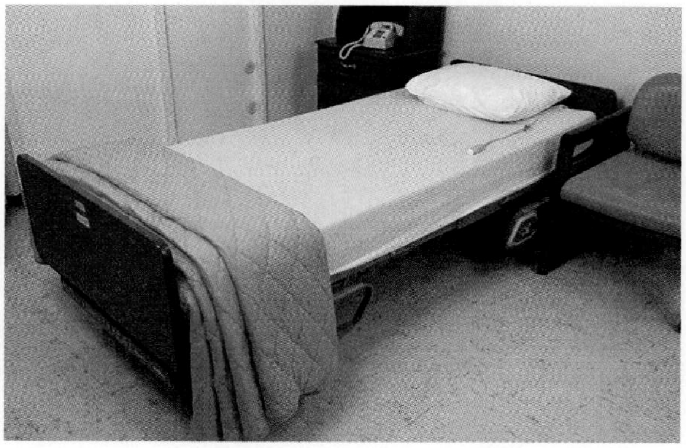

Fig. 12-2 Open bed. Top linens are folded to the foot of the bed.

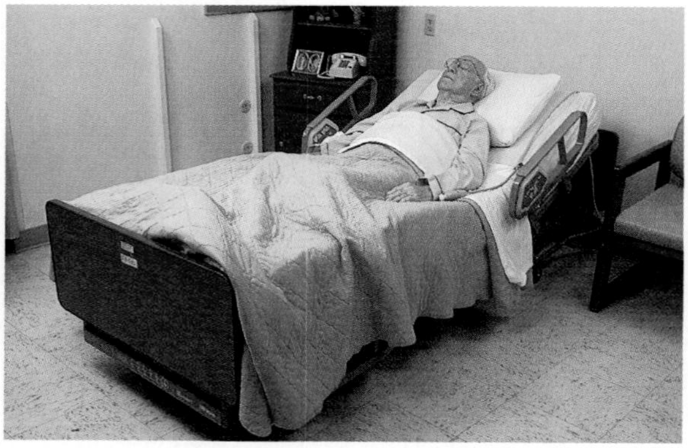

Fig. 12-3 Occupied bed.

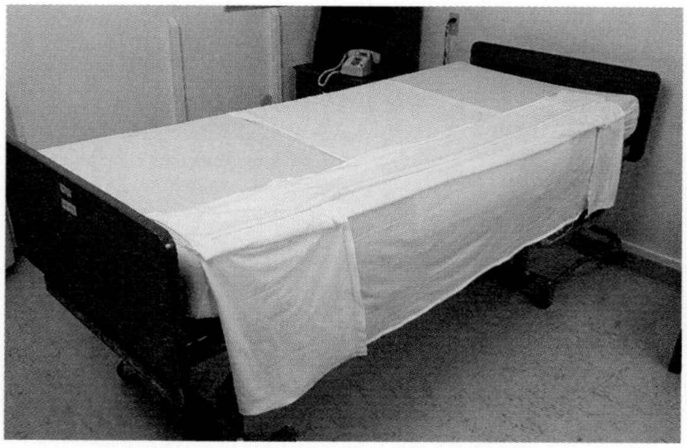

Fig. 12-4 Surgical bed.

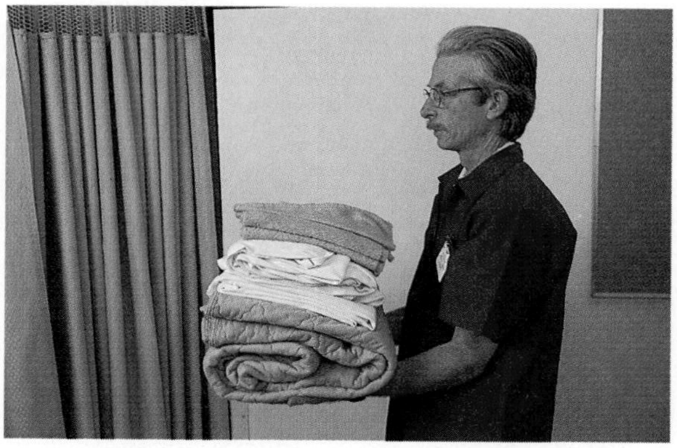

Fig. 12-5 Hold linens away from your body and uniform.

A

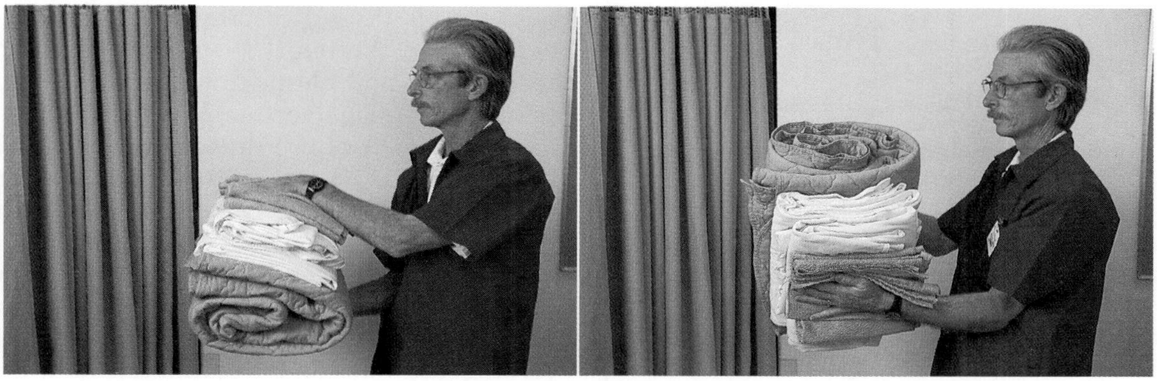

B

Fig. 12-6 A, The arm is placed over the top of the stack of linens. B, The stack of linens is turned over onto the arm. Note that linens are held away from the body.

Collect clean linens in the order of use. Be sure to collect enough linens. If the resident has 2 pillows, get 2 pillowcases. The resident may need extra blankets for warmth. Do not bring unneeded linens to a resident's room. Extra linen is considered contaminated and is not used for another resident.

You should collect linens in the order you will use them:

- Mattress pad
- Bottom sheet (flat sheet or contour sheet)
- Plastic drawsheet or disposable bed protectors
- Cotton drawsheet
- Top sheet (flat sheet)
- Blanket
- Bedspread
- Pillowcase(s)
- Bath towel(s)
- Hand towel
- Washcloth
- Hospital gown if the resident uses one
- Bath blanket

Use one arm to hold the linens and the other hand to pick them up. The item you will use first is at the bottom of your stack. (You picked up the mattress pad first; therefore it is at the bottom. The bath blanket is on top.) You need the mattress pad first. To get it on top, simply place your arm over the bath blanket. Then turn the stack over onto the arm on the bath blanket (Fig. 12-6). The arm that held the linens is now free. Place the clean linens on a clean surface.

Linens are pressed and folded to prevent the spread of microbes and to make bedmaking easy. They are pressed with a center crease. It is placed in the center of the bed from the head to the foot. The linens unfold easily.

When removing dirty linens from the bed, roll them away from you. The side of the linen that touched the resident is inside the roll. The side that has not touched the resident is on the outside (Fig. 12-7).

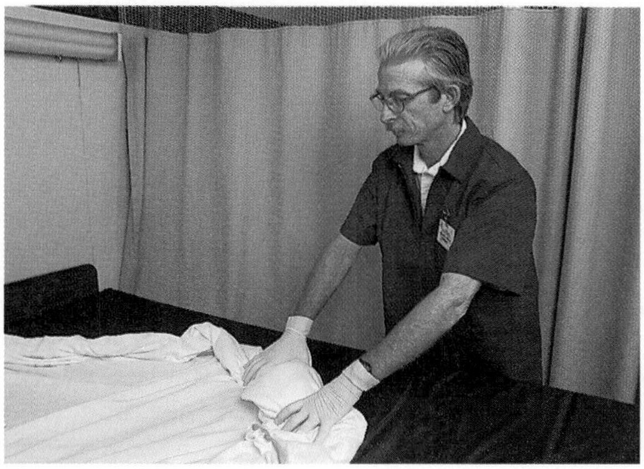

Fig. 12-7 Roll linens away from you when removing them from the bed.

Not all linens are changed every time the bed is made. The mattress pad, plastic drawsheet, blanket, and bedspread are reused for the same resident. They are reused if not soiled, wet, damp, or excessively wrinkled. Some centers use only flat sheets. The flat top sheet is reused as the bottom sheet. If a resident is discharged, all linens are removed and a closed bed is made. Make sure the bed has been washed before making it. Check your center's policy about linen changes. *Remember that wet, damp, or soiled linens are changed right away. You must wear gloves and use Standard Precautions and follow the Bloodborne Pathogen Standard.*

A bed may have a plastic drawsheet and a cotton drawsheet. A **drawsheet** is a small sheet placed over the middle of the bottom sheet. It helps keep the mattress and bottom linens clean and dry. A **plastic drawsheet** is waterproof. It protects the mattress and bottom linens from dampness and soiling. It is placed between the bottom sheet and cotton drawsheet. The cotton drawsheet protects the person from contact

Box 12-1 Rules for Bedmaking

- Use good body mechanics at all times.
- Follow the rules of medical asepsis.
- Practice Standard Precautions.
- Follow the Bloodborne Pathogen Standard.
- Wash your hands before handling clean linen and after handling dirty linen.
- Bring enough linen to the resident's room.
- Never shake linens. Shaking linens spreads microbes.
- Extra linen in a resident's room is considered contaminated. Do not use it for other residents. Put it with the dirty laundry.
- Hold linens away from your uniform. Dirty and clean linen must not touch your uniform.
- Never put dirty linens on the floor or on clean linens. Follow center policy about dirty linen.
- Keep bottom linens tucked in and wrinkle free.
- Completely cover a plastic drawsheet with a cotton drawsheet. A plastic drawsheet must not touch the resident's body.
- Straighten and tighten loose sheets, blankets, and bedspreads whenever necessary.
- Make as much of one side of the bed as possible before going to the other side. This saves time and energy.
- Change wet, damp, and soiled linens right away.

with the plastic and absorbs moisture. However, discomfort and skin breakdown may occur. The plastic retains heat, and plastic drawsheets are hard to keep tight and wrinkle free. Centers using disposable briefs (diapers) may not use drawsheets. Disposable briefs are designed to keep residents and bed linens dry. Other centers use waterproof pads instead of plastic drawsheets.

Cotton drawsheets are often used without plastic drawsheets. Plastic-covered mattresses cause some persons to perspire heavily. This increases discomfort. A cotton drawsheet reduces heat retention and absorbs moisture. Cotton drawsheets are often used as lift or turning sheets (see Chapter 10). When used for this purpose, they are not tucked in at the sides.

The bedmaking procedures that follow include plastic and cotton drawsheets so that you learn how to use them. Ask the nurse about their use.

GENERAL RULES

Your job description includes making beds. No matter what type of bed you make, safety and medical asepsis are important. Box 12-1 lists the rules for bedmaking.

◈ THE CLOSED BED

A closed bed is made if the resident will be out of bed for most of the day or after a resident is discharged. After a resident is discharged, the bed frame and mattress are cleaned before you make the bed. They are cleaned according to center policy.

Text continued on p. 254

Making a Closed Bed

Quality of Life

Remember to:
- ◆ *Knock before entering the resident's room*
- ◆ *Address the resident by name*
- ◆ *Introduce yourself by name and title*

Pre-Procedure

1 Wash your hands.

2 Collect clean linen:
- Mattress pad
- Bottom sheet
- Plastic drawsheet (optional)
- Cotton drawsheet
- Top sheet
- Blanket
- Bedspread
- Pillowcase(s)
- Bath towel(s)
- Hand towel
- Washcloth
- Hospital gown
- Bath blanket

3 Place linen on a clean surface.

4 Raise the bed for good body mechanics.

5 Make sure the bed and bed frame were cleaned if the resident was discharged. Roll linen away from you so that the surface that touched the resident is inside the roll. Wear gloves if linens are soiled. Remove and discard the gloves after removing soiled linen. Wash your hands.

Procedure

6 Move the mattress to the head of the bed.

7 Put the mattress pad on the mattress. It is even with the top of the mattress.

8 Place the bottom sheet on the mattress pad (Fig. 12-8, p. 251):
- a Unfold it lengthwise.
- b Place the center crease in the middle of the bed.
- c Position the lower edge even with the bottom of the mattress.
- d Place the large hem at the top and the small hem at the bottom.
- e Face hem stitching downward.

9 Pick the sheet up from the side to open it. Fanfold it toward the other side of the bed (Fig. 12-9, p. 251).

10 Go to the head of the bed. Tuck the top of the sheet under the mattress. Make sure the sheet is tight and smooth.

11 Make a mitered corner (Fig. 12-10, p. 251).

12 Place the plastic drawsheet on the bed about 14 inches from the top of the mattress.

13 Open the plastic drawsheet, and fanfold it toward the other side of the bed.

14 Place a cotton drawsheet over the plastic drawsheet. It must cover the entire plastic drawsheet (Fig. 12-11, p. 252).

15 Open the cotton drawsheet, and fanfold it toward the other side of the bed.

16 Tuck both drawsheets under the mattress, or tuck each in separately.

17 Go to the other side of the bed.

18 Miter the top corner of the bottom sheet.

19 Pull the bottom sheet tight so there are no wrinkles. Tuck in the sheet.

20 Pull the drawsheets tight so there are no wrinkles. Tuck both in together, or pull each tight and tuck them in separately (Fig. 12-12, p. 252).

21 Go to the other side of the bed.

22 Put the top sheet on the bed:
- a Unfold it lengthwise.
- b Place the center crease in the middle.
- c Place the large hem at the top, even with the top of the mattress.

Continued

Making a Closed Bed—cont'd

Procedure—cont'd

- d Open the sheet and fanfold the extra part toward the other side.
- e Face hem stitching outward.
- f Do not tuck the bottom in yet.
- g Never tuck top linens in on the sides.

23 Place the blanket on the bed:
- a Unfold it so the center crease is in the middle.
- b Put the upper hem about 6 to 8 inches from the top of the mattress.
- c Open the blanket, and fanfold the extra part toward the other side.
- d If steps 28 and 29 are not done, turn the top sheet down over the blanket. Hem stitching is down.

24 Place the bedspread on the bed:
- a Unfold it so the center crease is in the middle.
- b Place the upper hem even with the top of the mattress.
- c Open the bedspread, and fanfold the extra part toward the other side.
- d Make sure the bedspread facing the door is even and covers all the top linens.

25 Tuck in top linens together at the foot of the bed. They should be smooth and tight. Make a mitered corner.

26 Go to the other side.

27 Straighten all top linen, working from the head of the bed to the foot.

28 Tuck in the top linens together. Make a mitered corner.

29 Turn the top hem of the bedspread under the blanket to make a cuff (Fig. 12-13, p. 253).

30 Turn the top sheet down over the spread. Hem stitching is down. *(Steps 29 and 30 are not done in some centers. The bedspread covers the pillow. Be sure to tuck the spread under the pillow.)*

31 Place the pillow on the bed.

32 Open the pillowcase so it is flat on the bed.

33 Put the pillowcase on the pillow as in Figure 12-14 on p. 253. Fold extra pillowcase material under the pillow at the seam end of the pillowcase.

34 Place the pillow on the bed so the open end is away from the door. The seam of the pillowcase is toward the head of the bed.

Post-Procedure

35 Attach the signal light to the bed.

36 Lower the bed to its lowest position.

37 Put towels, washcloth, gown, and bath blanket in the bedside stand.

38 Wash your hands.

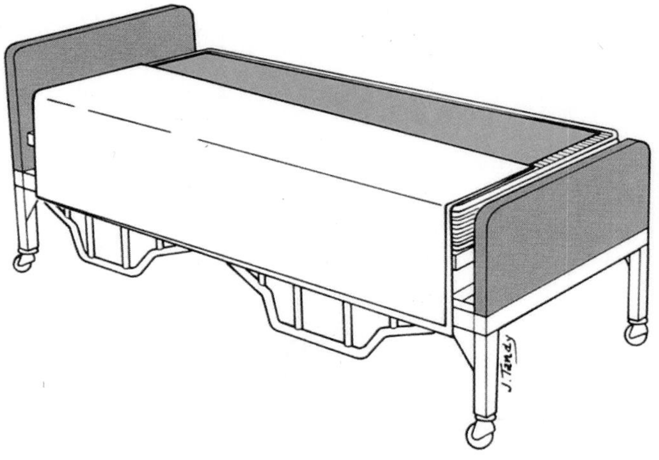

Fig. 12-8 The bottom sheet is on the bed with the center crease in the middle. The lower edge of the sheet is even with the bottom of the mattress.

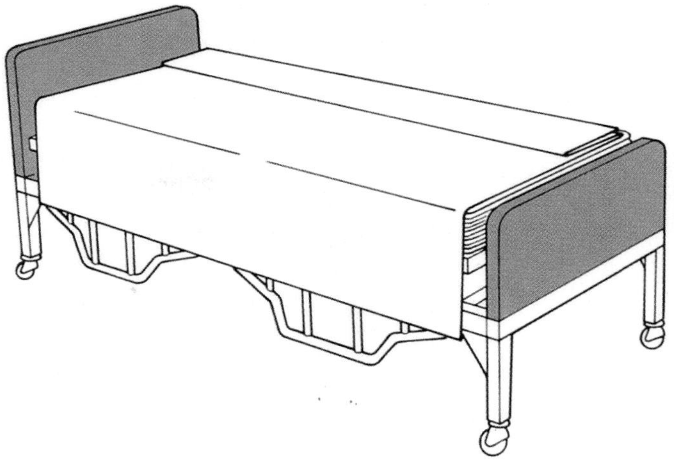

Fig. 12-9 The bottom sheet is fanfolded to the other side of the bed.

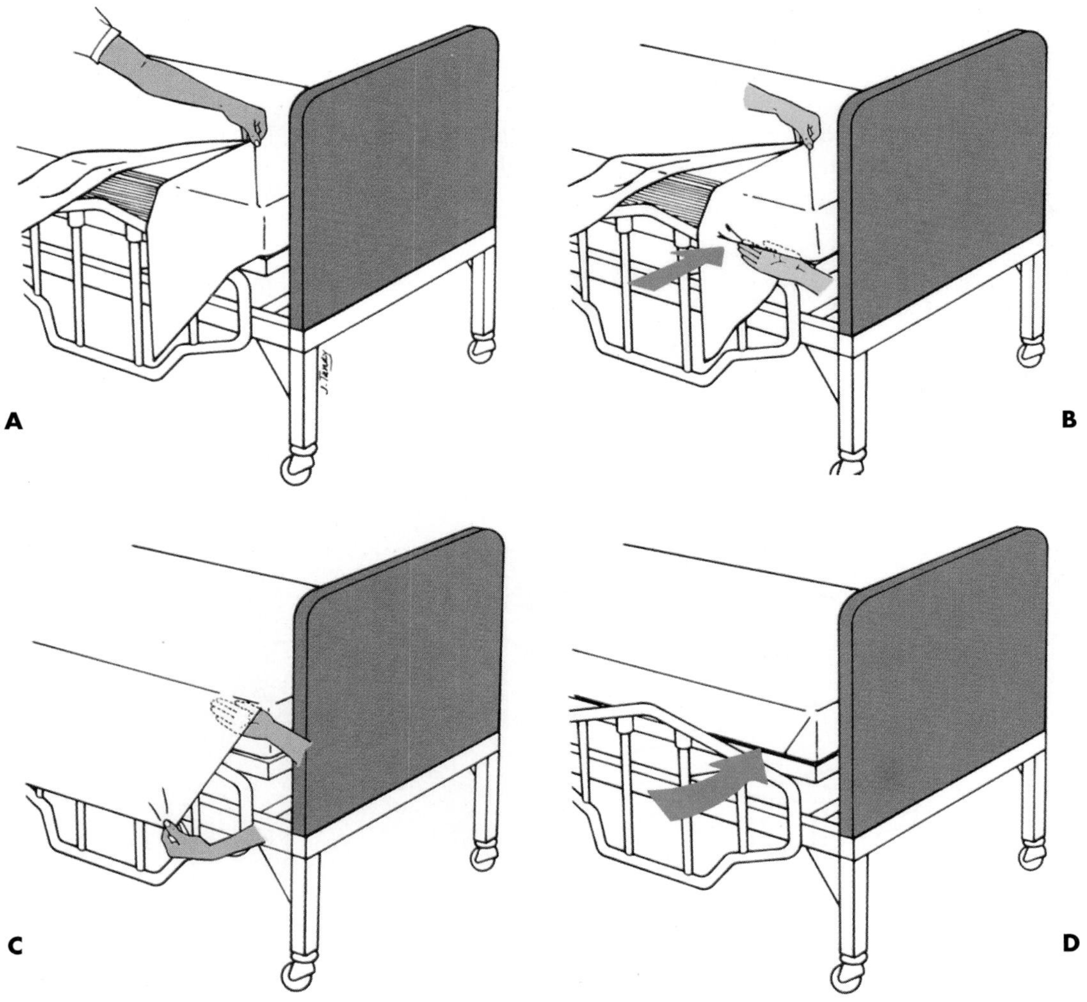

Fig. 12-10 Making a mitered corner. **A,** The bottom sheet is tucked under the mattress, and the side of the sheet is raised onto the mattress. **B,** The remaining portion of the sheet is tucked under the mattress. **C,** The raised portion of the sheet is brought off the mattress. **D,** The entire side of the sheet is tucked under the mattress.

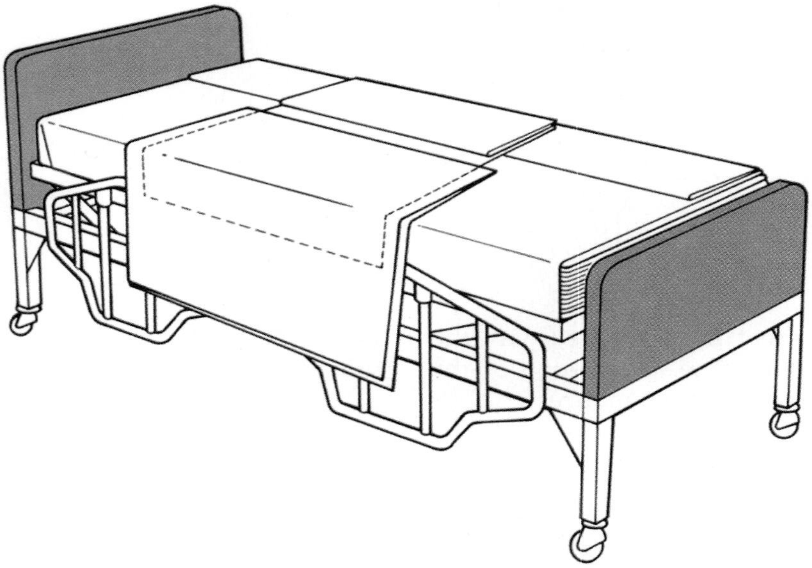

Fig. 12-11 A cotton drawsheet over the plastic drawsheet. The cotton drawsheet completely covers the plastic drawsheet.

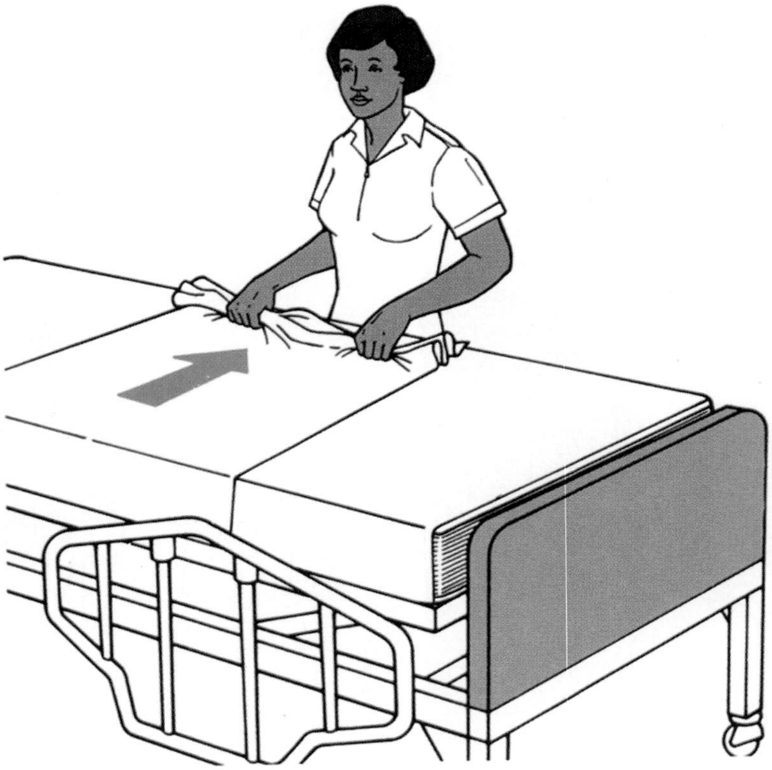

Fig. 12-12 The drawsheet is pulled tight to remove wrinkles.

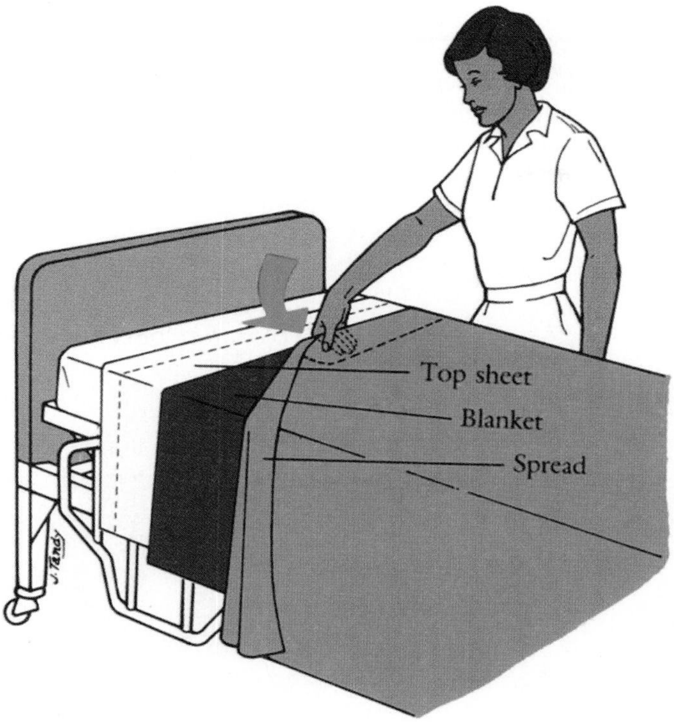

Fig. 12-13 The top hem of the bedspread is turned under the top hem of the blanket to make a cuff.

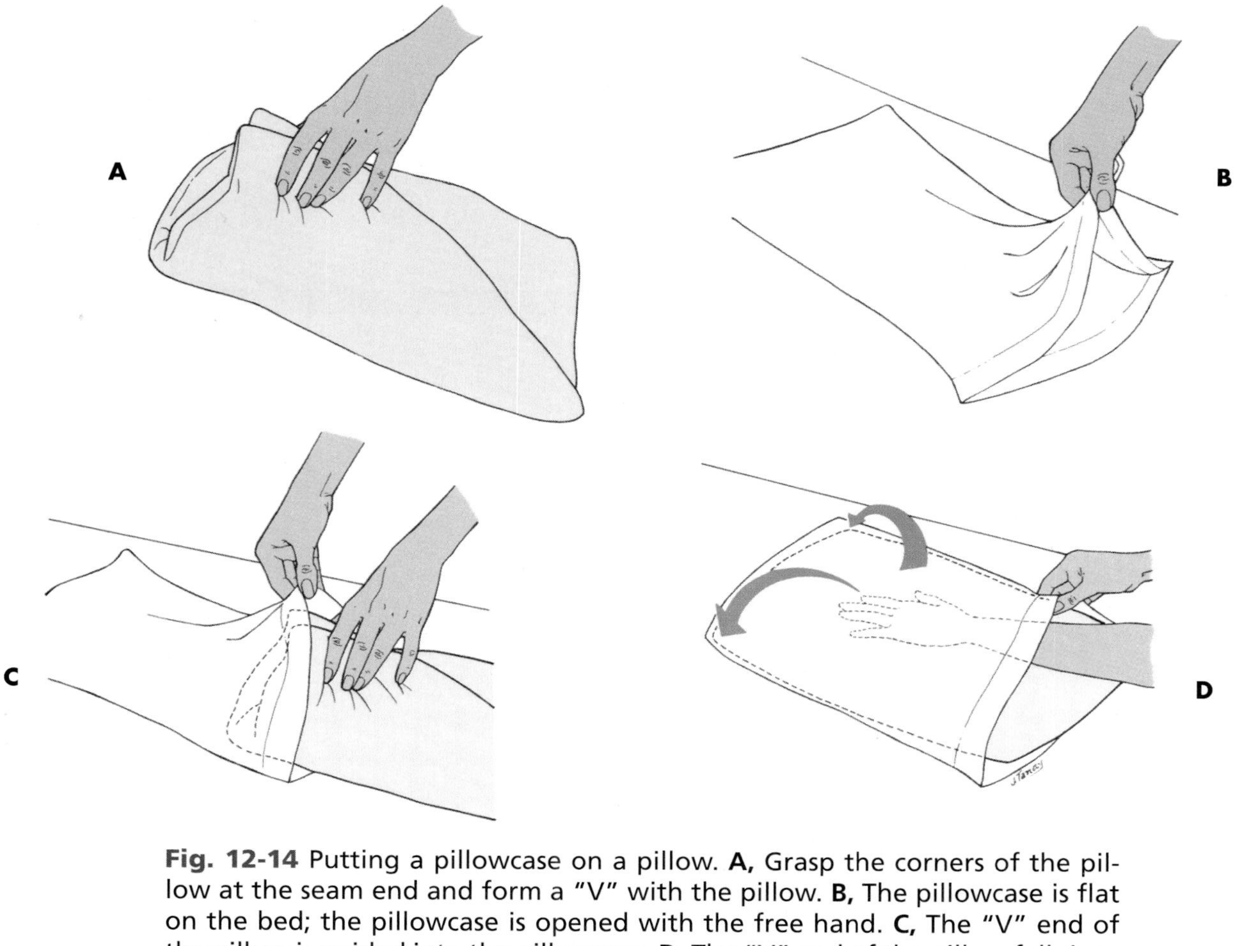

Fig. 12-14 Putting a pillowcase on a pillow. **A,** Grasp the corners of the pillow at the seam end and form a "V" with the pillow. **B,** The pillowcase is flat on the bed; the pillowcase is opened with the free hand. **C,** The "V" end of the pillow is guided into the pillowcase. **D,** The "V" end of the pillow falls into the corners of the pillowcase.

THE OPEN BED

The open bed is an unoccupied bed. The linens are folded back so the resident can get into bed with ease. An open bed is made when the resident is out of bed for a short time only. A closed bed easily becomes an open bed by folding back the top linens.

THE OCCUPIED BED

An occupied bed is made when a resident cannot be out of bed because of illness or injury. When making an occupied bed, you must keep the resident in good body alignment. You also must know of restrictions or limits in the resident's movement or positioning. Check with the nurse before you make the bed. Be sure to explain each step of the procedure to the resident before it is done. This is important even if the resident is comatose or cannot respond to you.

Text continued on p. 259

Making an Open Bed

Quality of Life

Remember to:

- ***Knock before entering the resident's room***
- ***Address the resident by name***
- ***Introduce yourself by name and title***

Procedure

1. Wash your hands.
2. Collect linen for a closed bed.
3. Make a closed bed.
4. Fanfold top linens to the foot of the bed (see Fig. 12-2).
5. Attach the signal light to the bed.
6. Lower the bed to its lowest position.
7. Put towels, washcloth, gown, and bath blanket in the bedside stand.
8. Follow center policy for dirty linen.
9. Wash your hands.

Making an Occupied Bed

NNAAP™ SKILL

Quality of Life

Remember to:

- ◆ *Knock before entering the resident's room*
- ◆ *Address the resident by name*
- ◆ *Introduce yourself by name and title*

Pre-Procedure

1 Explain the procedure to the resident.

2 Wash your hands.

3 Collect the following:
- Gloves
- Linen bag
- Clean linen (see *Making a Closed Bed*, p. 249).

4 Place linen on a clean surface.

5 Provide for privacy.

6 Remove the signal light.

7 Raise the bed for good body mechanics. Make sure the bed rails are up.

8 Lower the head of the bed to a level appropriate for the person. It should be as flat as possible.

9 Lower the bed rail near you.

10 Put on gloves. Follow Standard Precautions and the Bloodborne Pathogen Standard.

11 Loosen top linens at the foot of the bed.

12 Remove the bedspread and blanket separately. Fold them as in Figure 12-15 on p. 257 if you will reuse them.

13 Cover the resident with a bath blanket for warmth and privacy:

a Unfold a bath blanket over the top sheet.

b Ask the resident to hold onto the bath blanket. If he or she cannot, tuck the top part under the resident's shoulders.

c Grasp the top sheet under the bath blanket at the shoulders. Bring the sheet down to the foot of the bed. Remove the sheet from under the blanket (Fig. 12-16, p. 257).

Procedure

14 Move the mattress to the head of the bed.

15 Position the resident on the side of the bed away from you. Move the pillow to the far side of the bed. Adjust the pillow for the resident's comfort.

16 Loosen bottom linens from the head to the foot of the bed.

17 Fanfold bottom linens one at a time toward the resident: cotton drawsheet, plastic drawsheet, bottom sheet, and mattress pad (Fig. 12-17, p. 258). Do not fanfold the mattress pad if it will be reused.

18 Place a clean mattress pad on the bed. Unfold it lengthwise so the center crease is in the middle. Fanfold the top part toward the resident. If reusing the mattress pad, straighten and smooth any wrinkles.

19 Place the bottom sheet on the mattress pad so hem stitching is away from the resident. Unfold the sheet so the crease is in the middle. The small hem is even with the bottom of the mattress. Fanfold the top part toward the resident.

20 Make a mitered corner at the head of the bed. Tuck the sheet under the mattress from the head to the foot.

21 Pull the fanfolded plastic drawsheet toward you over the bottom sheet. Tuck excess material under the mattress. Do the following if you are using a clean plastic drawsheet (Fig. 12-18, p. 258):

a Place the plastic drawsheet on the bed about 14 inches from the mattress top.

b Fanfold the top part toward the resident.

c Tuck in the excess material.

22 Place the cotton drawsheet over the plastic drawsheet. It must cover the entire plastic drawsheet. Fanfold the top part toward the resident. Tuck in excess material.

Continued

Making an Occupied Bed—cont'd

NNAAP™ SKILL

Procedure—cont'd

23 Raise the bed rail. Go to the other side, and lower the bed rail.

24 Position the resident on the side of the bed away from you. Explain to the resident that he or she will roll over a bump. As you roll the resident, assure the resident that he or she will not fall. Adjust the pillow for the resident's comfort.

25 Loosen bottom linens. Remove soiled linen one piece at a time. Remove and discard the gloves.

26 Straighten and smooth the mattress pad.

27 Pull the clean bottom sheet toward you. Make a mitered corner at the top. Tuck the sheet under the mattress from the head to the foot of the bed.

28 Pull the drawsheets tightly toward you. Tuck both under together or tuck each in separately.

29 Position the resident supine in the center of the bed. Adjust the pillow for comfort.

30 Put the top sheet on the bed. Unfold it lengthwise. Make sure the crease is in the middle, the large hem is even with the top of the mattress, and hem stitching is on the outside.

31 Ask the resident to hold onto the top sheet so you can remove the bath blanket. You may have to tuck the top sheet under the resident's shoulders. Remove the bath blanket.

32 Place the blanket on the bed. Unfold it so the crease is in the middle. Unfold the blanket so it covers the resident. The upper hem should be 6 to 8 inches from the top of the mattress.

33 Place the bedspread on the bed. Unfold it so the center crease is in the middle and it covers the resident. The top hem is even with the mattress top.

34 Turn the top hem of the bedspread under the blanket to make a cuff.

35 Bring the top sheet down over the bedspread to form a cuff.

36 Go to the foot of the bed.

37 Lift the mattress corner with one arm. Tuck all top linens under the mattress together. Be sure the linens are loose enough to allow movement of the resident's feet. Make a mitered corner.

38 Raise the bed rail. Go to the other side and lower the bed rail.

39 Straighten and smooth top linens.

40 Tuck the top linens under the mattress as in step 37. Make a mitered corner.

41 Change the pillowcase(s).

42 Place the signal light within reach.

43 Raise or lower bed rails. Follow the care plan.

Post-Procedure

44 Raise the head of the bed to a level appropriate for the resident. Make sure the resident is comfortable.

45 Lower the bed to its lowest position.

46 Put towels, washcloth, gown, and bath blanket in the bedside stand.

47 Unscreen the resident. Thank him or her for cooperating.

48 Follow center policy for dirty linen.

49 Wash your hands.

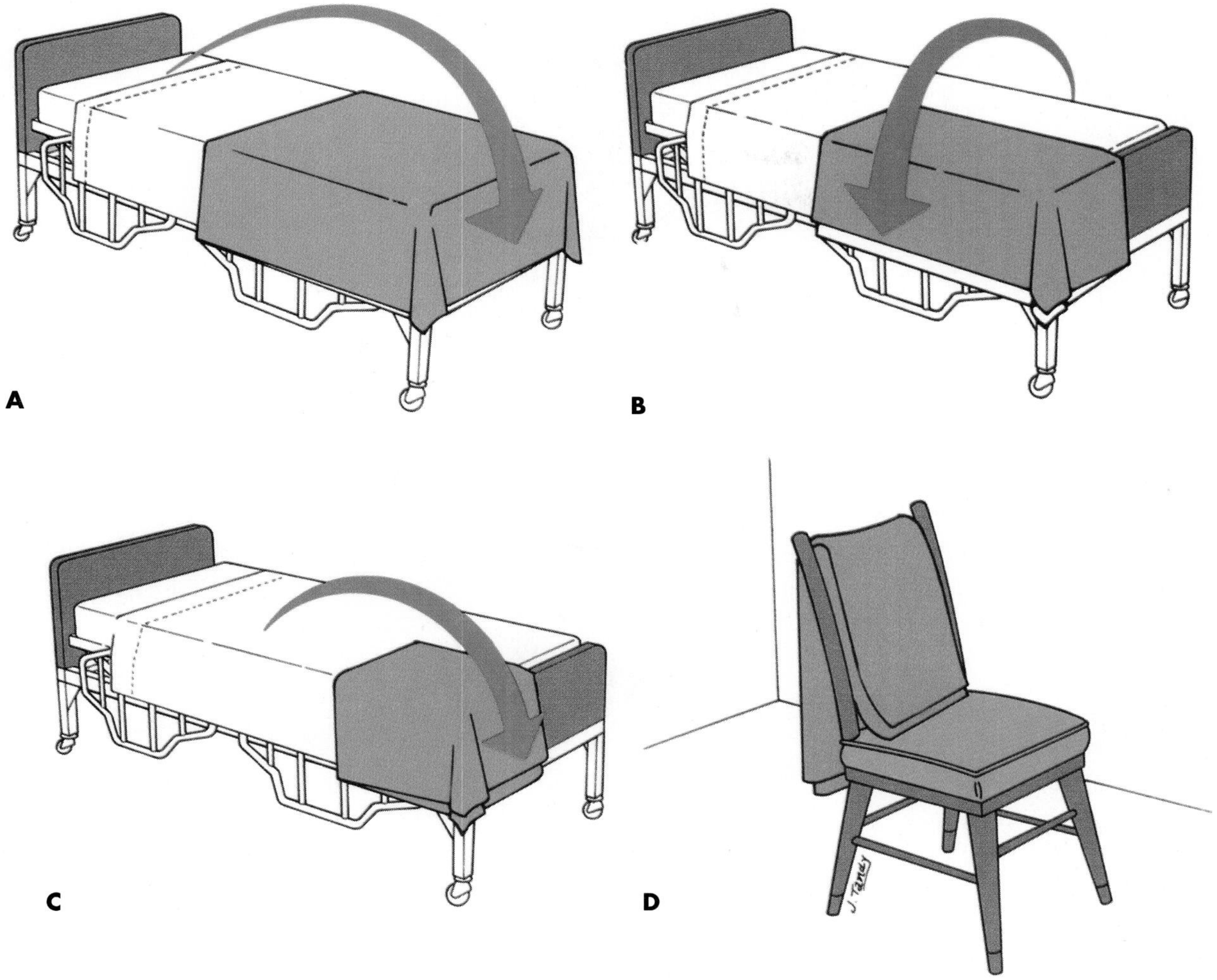

Fig. 12-15 Folding linen for reuse. **A,** The top edge of the blanket is folded down to the bottom edge. **B,** The blanket is folded from the far side of the bed to the near side. **C,** The top edge of the blanket is folded down to the bottom edge again. **D,** The folded blanket is placed over the back of a straight chair.

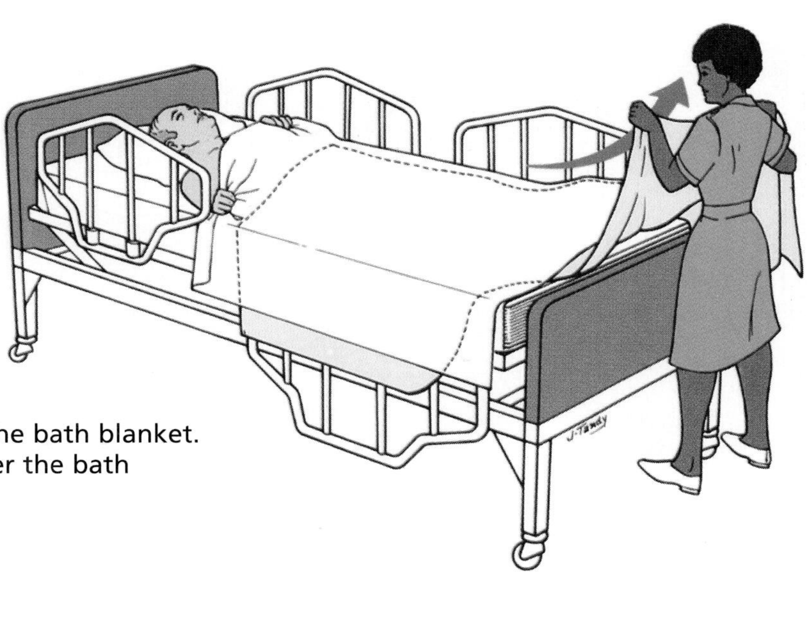

Fig. 12-16 The person holds onto the bath blanket. The top sheet is removed from under the bath blanket.

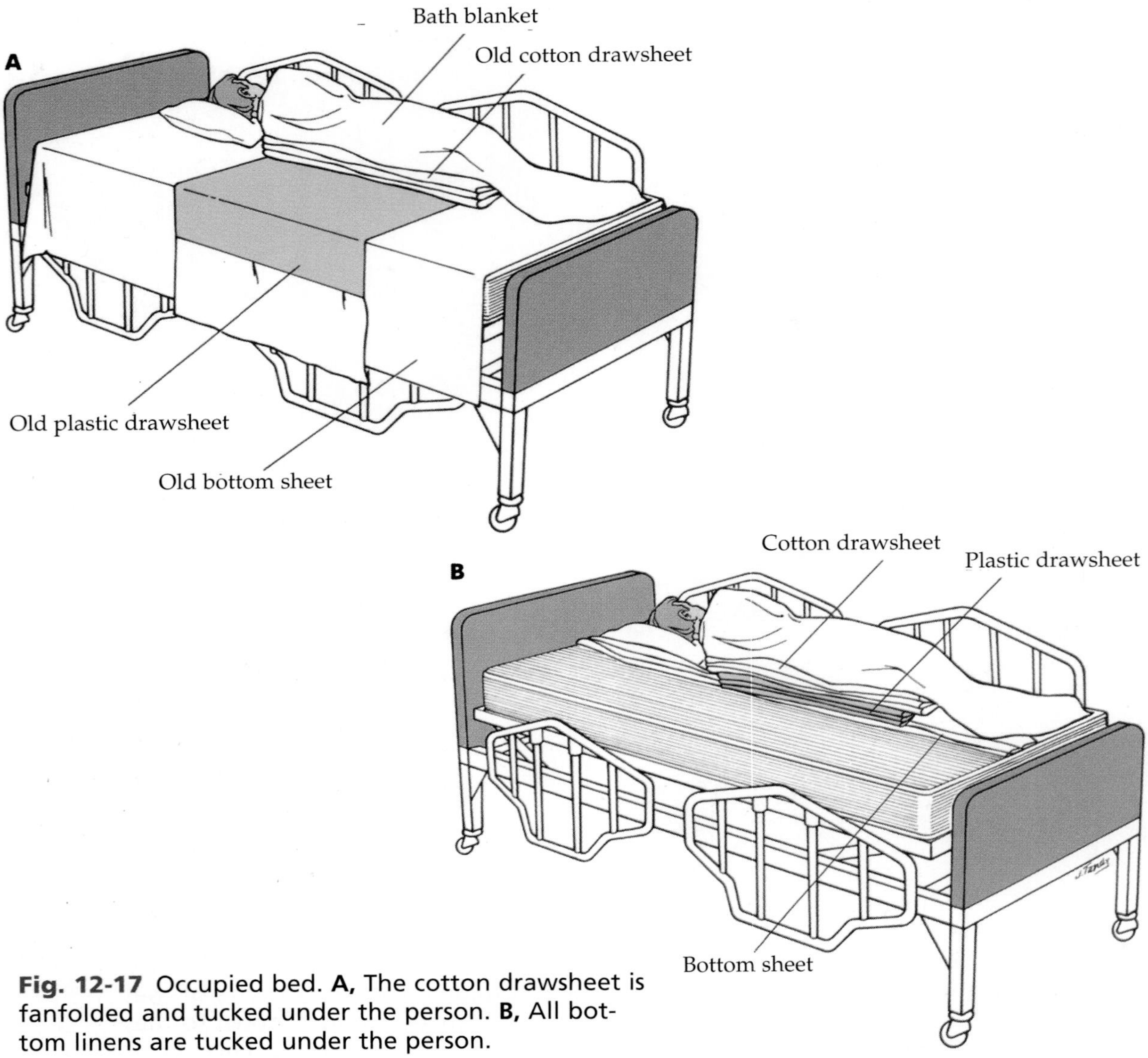

Fig. 12-17 Occupied bed. **A,** The cotton drawsheet is fanfolded and tucked under the person. **B,** All bottom linens are tucked under the person.

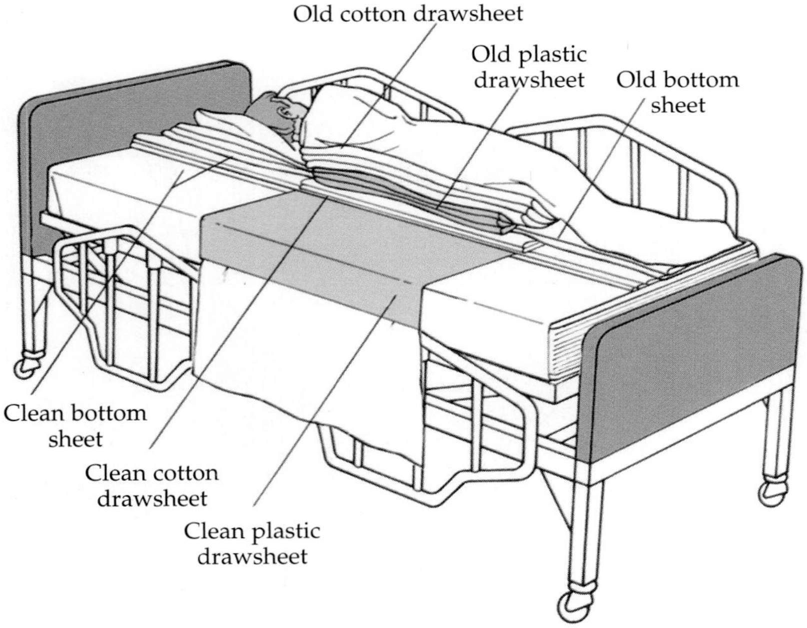

Fig. 12-18 A clean bottom sheet and plastic drawsheet are on the bed with both fanfolded and tucked under the person. The clean cotton drawsheet is put in place in step 22.

◈ THE SURGICAL BED

The surgical bed (recovery bed, postoperative bed, or anesthetic bed) is a form of the open bed. Top linens are folded so that the resident can be transferred from a stretcher to the bed. The surgical bed and its other names imply that the resident had surgery. Surgery is not performed in nursing centers. In nursing centers, surgical beds are used for residents who are arriving at the center by ambulance. They are used also when the resident is taken to a treatment room or physical therapy by stretcher or when a portable tub is used.

Making a Surgical Bed

Quality of Life

Remember to:

- ◆ ***Knock before entering the resident's room***
- ◆ ***Address the resident by name***
- ◆ ***Introduce yourself by name and title***

Pre-Procedure

1 Wash your hands.

2 Collect the following:
- Clean linen (see *Making a Closed Bed*, pp. 249-250)
- IV pole
- Tissues
- Kidney basin
- Gloves
- Laundry bag
- Other equipment as requested by the nurse

3 Place linen on a clean surface.

4 Remove the signal light.

5 Raise the bed for good body mechanics.

Procedure

6 Remove all linen from the bed. Wear gloves for contact with the resident's blood, body fluids, secretions, or excretions.

7 Make a closed bed (see *Making a Closed Bed*, p. 249). Do not tuck the top linens under the mattress.

8 Fold all top linens at the foot of the bed back onto the bed. The fold is even with the edge of the mattress (Fig. 12-19, p. 260).

9 Fanfold linen lengthwise to the side of the bed farthest from the door (Fig. 12-20, p. 260).

10 Put the pillowcase(s) on the pillow(s).

11 Place the pillow(s) on a clean surface.

12 Leave the bed in its highest position.

13 Make sure both bed rails are down.

Post-Procedure

14 Put the towels, washcloth, gown, and bath blanket in the bedside stand.

15 Place the tissues and kidney basin on the bedside stand. Place the IV pole near the head of the bed.

16 Move all furniture away from the bed. Allow enough room for the stretcher and for the staff to move about.

17 Do not attach the signal light to the bed.

18 Follow center policy for soiled linen.

19 Wash your hands.

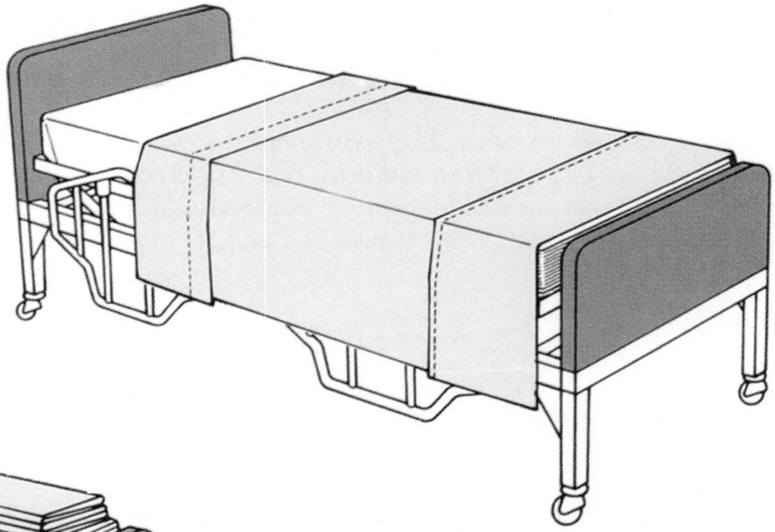

Fig. 12-19 Surgical bed. The bottom of the top linens is folded back onto the bed. The fold is even with the edge of the mattress.

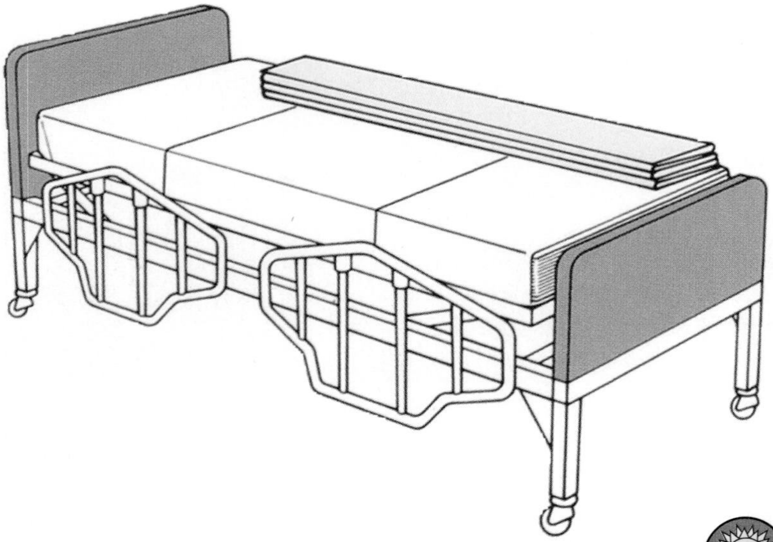

Fig. 12-20 A surgical bed with the top linens fan-folded lengthwise to the opposite side of the bed.

Quality of Life

The bed is the largest piece of equipment in the resident's unit. It is the focus of the resident's unit. The resident, family, and visitors will question the quality of care, and thus the resident's quality of life, if the bed is unmade, messy, or dirty. The bed must be neat and well made so the resident's environment is orderly and pleasant. If the resident stays in bed, you need to straighten and tighten loose sheets and other linen whenever necessary.

Some residents bring their own bedspreads, pillows, blankets, or afghans from home. Remember to use these when making the bed. Because such items are the resident's property, always handle them with care and respect. Make sure the items are properly marked with the resident's name to prevent them from becoming lost or confused with the property of other residents.

Allow the resident personal choice whenever possible. The center may use white, blue, yellow, pink, or other colored or printed linens. If so, let the resident choose which linen to use. Also, let the resident decide how many pillows or blankets to use. If possible, the resident chooses when the bed is made. The more choices you allow the resident, the greater the person's sense of usefulness and quality of life.

REVIEW QUESTIONS

Circle T if the statement is true and F if the statement is false.

1 T F Linens are changed whenever soiled, wet, or damp.

2 T F Linens are held away from your body and uniform.

3 T F Dirty linens are put on the floor.

4 T F Extra linen in a resident's room is used for another resident.

5 T F In long-term care, complete linen changes always are required for closed beds and surgical beds.

6 T F A cotton drawsheet is always used when a plastic drawsheet is used.

7 T F The hem stitching of the bottom sheet is placed downward away from the resident.

8 T F Shake linens in the air to remove crumbs from the bed.

9 T F A cotton drawsheet must completely cover the plastic drawsheet.

10 T F The upper hem of the bedspread is even with the top of the mattress.

11 T F Top linens are fanfolded to the foot of the bed for an open bed.

12 T F A resident is screened when an occupied bed is made.

13 T F When making an occupied bed, the far bed rail is up at all times.

14 T F After a surgical bed is made, it is left in its lowest position.

15 T F A cotton drawsheet is used only with a plastic drawsheet.

16 T F Nursing centers usually allow residents to bring comforters and afghans from home.

Answers to these questions are on p. 697.

13 Hygiene

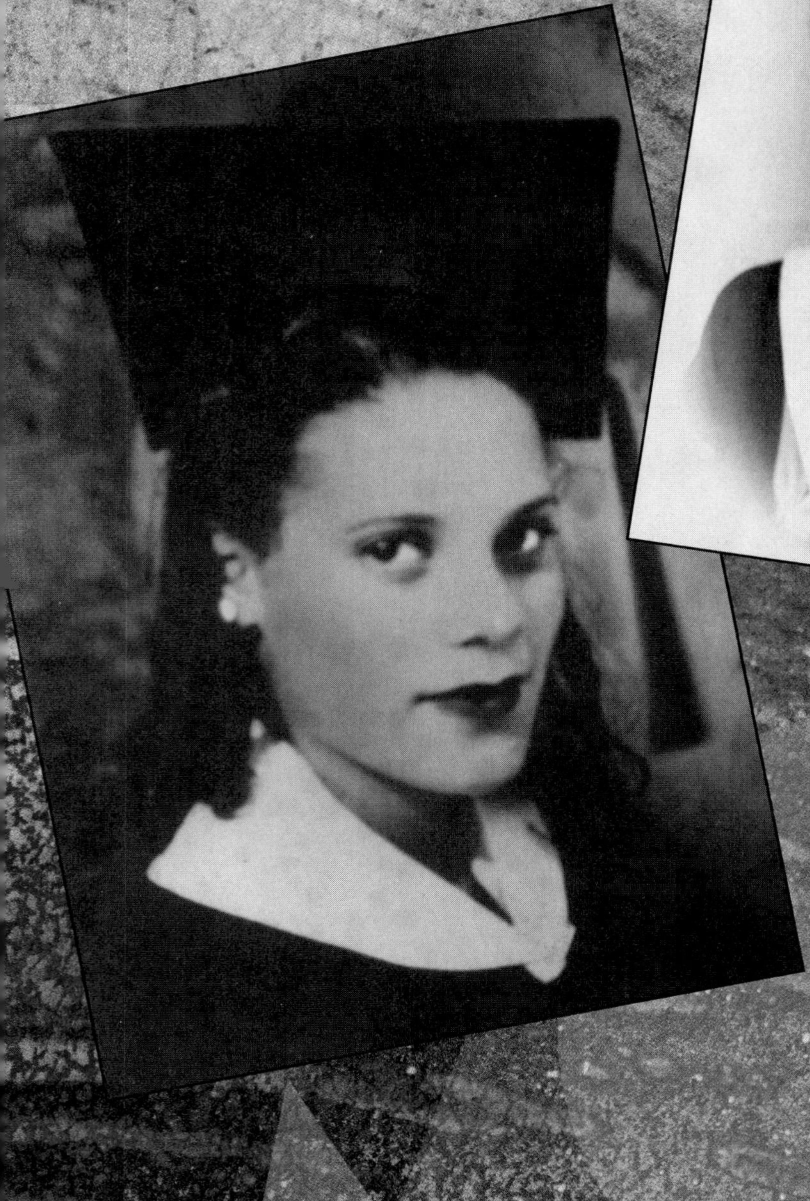

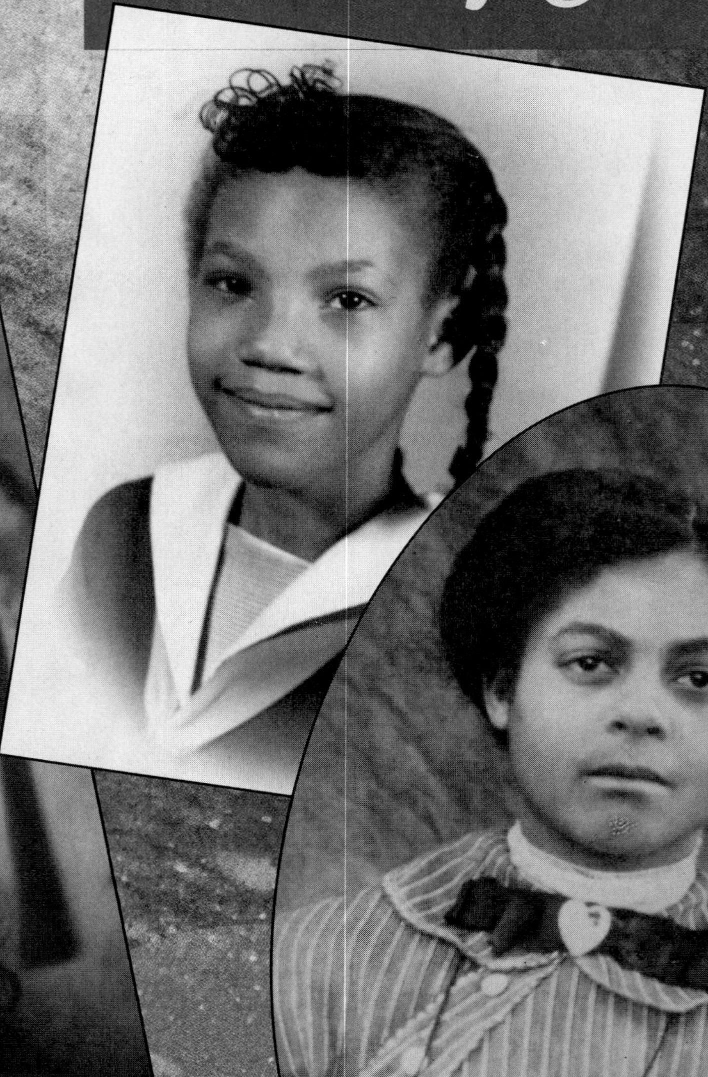

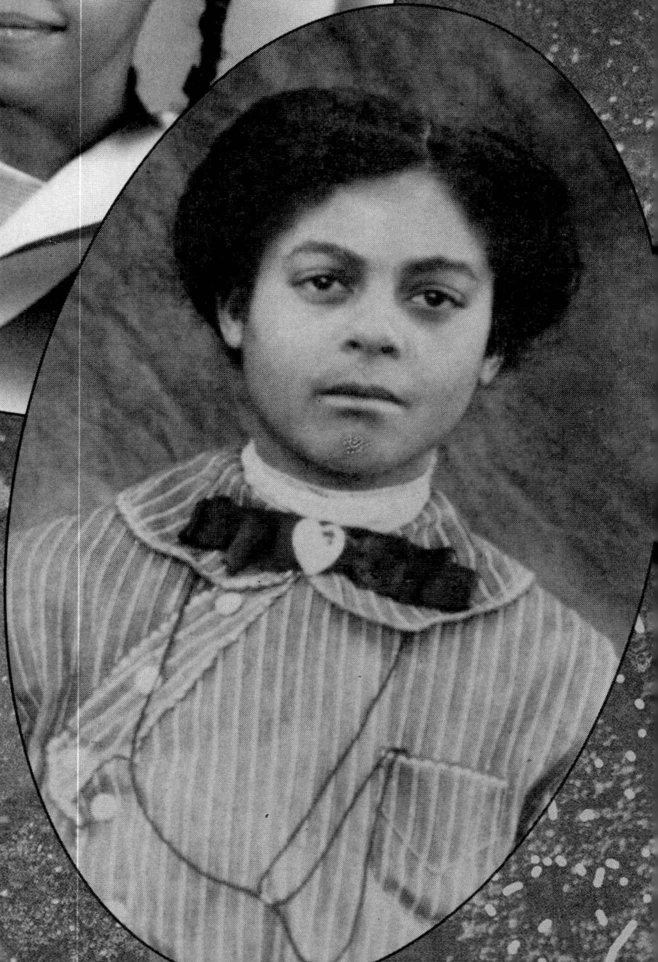

What You Will Learn

- The definition of the key terms listed in this chapter
- The importance of cleanliness and skin care
- The routine care given before and after breakfast, after lunch, and in the evening
- The importance of oral hygiene and the observations to report
- The rules for bathing and the observations to make
- The safety precautions for residents taking tub baths or showers
- The importance of hair care and shaving
- The factors that affect hair care
- Ways to shampoo a resident's hair
- The measures that are practiced when shaving a resident
- The purposes of a back massage
- The purposes of perineal care
- The procedures described in this chapter

Key Terms

AM care Routine care performed before breakfast; early morning care

aspiration Breathing fluid or an object into the lungs

early morning care AM care

HS care Care given in the evening at bedtime; evening care or PM care

morning care Care given after breakfast; cleanliness and skin care measures are more thorough at this time

oral hygiene Measures performed to keep the mouth and teeth clean; mouth care

pericare Perineal care

perineal care Cleansing the genital and anal areas; pericare

plaque A thin film that sticks to the teeth; it contains saliva, microorganisms, and other substances

PM care HS care or evening care

tartar Hardened plaque on teeth

Cleanliness and skin care promote comfort, safety, and health. The skin is the body's first line of defense against disease. Intact skin prevents microbes from entering the body and causing an infection. Likewise, mucous membranes of the mouth, genital area, and anus must be clean and intact. Besides cleansing, good hygiene prevents body and breath odors. It also promotes relaxation and increases circulation.

Culture and personal choice affect hygiene practices. *(See Caring About Culture, p. 264.)* Some people take showers. Others take tub baths. Some bathe at bedtime. Others bathe in the morning. Bathing frequency also varies. Some bathe daily or twice a day—such as before work and after work or exercise. Some people do not have water for bathing. Others cannot afford soap, deodorant, shampoo, toothpaste, or other hygiene products.

Residents often need some help with personal hygiene. Weakness from illness and the changes from aging affect the ability to practice hygiene. Many factors affect hygiene and skin care needs. They include perspiration, urinary and bowel elimination, vomiting, drainage from wounds or body openings, bedrest, and activity. The nurse uses the nursing process to help the health care team decide how to meet the resident's hygiene needs.

CARING ABOUT CULTURE

Personal Hygiene

Personal hygiene is very important to East Indian Hindus. Their religion requires at least one bath a day. Some Hindus believe that bathing after a meal causes injury. It is also believed that eye injuries can occur from a bath that is too hot. When preparing a bath, hot water can be added to cold water. However, cold water is not added to hot water. After bathing, the body is carefully rubbed dry with a towel.

Modified from Giger JN, Davidhizar RE: *Transcultural nursing: assessment and intervention,* St Louis, ed 2, 1995, Mosby.

Some residents resist your efforts to assist with hygiene. Common reasons include illness, disability, dementia, and personal choice. The health care team assesses each resident's individual needs. You must know how to approach each resident. The care plan explains the best way to work with each resident. Residents on dementia care units may require special approaches because of resistive behaviors (see Chapter 27). Always check the care plan and ask the nurse if you have questions.

DAILY CARE OF THE RESIDENT

Personal hygiene is performed as often as necessary to stay clean and comfortable. People who can care for themselves practice hygiene routinely and out of habit. For example, the teeth are brushed and face and hands washed on awakening. These and other hygiene measures are often done routinely before and after meals and at bedtime. Weak and disabled residents need help with hygiene. Routine care is given throughout the day. Remember to assist a resident with personal hygiene whenever necessary. Also remember to protect the resident's right to privacy and personal choice.

Before Breakfast

Routine care performed before breakfast is called **early morning care** or **AM care**. Night shift or day shift staff members give AM care. They get residents ready for breakfast or for special tests scheduled for early in the day. Personal hygiene measures performed at this time include:

- Assisting residents to the bathroom or offering the bedpan or urinal
- Cleaning incontinent residents and changing any soiled linen
- Helping residents wash their face and hands
- Assisting residents with oral hygiene
- Helping in brushing and combing hair
- Assisting residents to dress for breakfast in the dining room. Some are assisted into Fowler's position or to a bedside chair for breakfast.
- Assisting residents to the dining room for breakfast
- Straightening linens or making beds
- Straightening resident units

After Breakfast

Morning care is given after breakfast. Cleanliness and skin care measures are more thorough at this time. Routine morning care usually involves:

- Assisting residents to the bathroom or offering the commode, bedpan, or urinal
- Cleaning incontinent residents and changing any soiled linen
- Helping residents wash their face and hands
- Assisting with oral hygiene
- Shaving residents
- Providing showers, tub baths, or complete or partial bed baths
- Giving perineal care
- Performing range-of-motion exercises (see Chapter 19)
- Assisting residents to dress in street clothes or to change into a clean gown or pajamas
- Brushing and combing hair
- Assisting with ambulation
- Changing bed linens or making beds
- Straightening resident units

Afternoon Care

Routine personal hygiene measures are performed after lunch and the evening meal. Many residents like to have afternoon care completed before having visitors or attending activity programs. Afternoon care involves:

- Assisting residents to the bathroom or offering the commode, bedpan, or urinal before and after naps
- Cleaning incontinent residents and changing any soiled linen before and after naps
- Helping residents wash their face and hands
- Assisting residents to lie down for a nap
- Assisting residents up after the nap
- Brushing or combing hair, if necessary
- Assisting with ambulation
- Providing range-of-motion exercises
- Straightening resident units

Evening Care

Care given to residents in the evening at bedtime is called **HS care** (HS means hour of sleep) or **PM care**. Hygiene measures are performed just before the resident is ready for sleep. HS care increases comfort and the ability to relax. HS care involves:

- Assisting residents to the bathroom or offering the commode, bedpan, or urinal
- Cleaning incontinent residents and changing any dirty linen
- Helping residents wash their face and hands
- Assisting with oral hygiene
- Helping residents in street clothes to undress and put on a gown or pajamas
- Giving back massages
- Straightening resident units

ORAL HYGIENE

Oral hygiene (mouth care) keeps the mouth and teeth clean. This prevents mouth odors and infections. It also increases comfort and makes food taste better. Oral hygiene also reduces the risk for *cavities (dental caries)* and *periodontal disease (gum disease, pyorrhea).* Poor oral hygiene allows the buildup of plaque and tartar. **Plaque** is a thin film that sticks to teeth. It contains saliva, bacteria, and other substances. Plaque leads to tooth decay, or cavities. When plaque hardens it is called **tartar.** Tartar builds up at the gum line near the neck of the tooth. Tartar buildup leads to periodontal disease. The gums are red, swollen, and bleed easily. As the disease progresses, bone is destroyed and teeth loosen. Tooth loss is common.

Illness and disease often cause a bad taste in the mouth. Some drugs and diseases cause a whitish coating on the mouth and tongue. Others cause redness and swelling of the mouth and tongue. Dry mouth is common from oxygen, smoking, decreased fluid intake, and anxiety. Some drugs cause dry mouth.

The nurse assesses the resident's need for mouth care. The speech/language pathologist and the dietician may also assess the resident's need for mouth care. Oral hygiene is given on awakening, after each meal, and at bedtime. Many people also practice oral hygiene before meals.

Equipment

A toothbrush, toothpaste, dental floss, and mouthwash are needed. The toothbrush should have soft bristles. Residents with dentures need a denture cleaner, denture cup, and denture brush or regular toothbrush. Sponge swabs are used for residents with sore, tender mouths and for unconscious residents. Be careful when using sponge swabs. Check the foam pad to make sure it is tight on the stick. The resident could choke on the foam pad if it comes off the stick. Other needed items include a kidney basin, water glass, straw, tissues, towels, and gloves. Nursing unit supply rooms usually have such items. Many residents choose to bring their own oral hygiene equipment from home.

Follow Standard Precautions and the Bloodborne Pathogen Standard when giving oral hygiene. You have contact with the resident's mucous membranes. Gums may bleed during oral care. Also, the mouth contains many microbes. Pathogens spread through sexual contact may be in the mouths of some residents.

Observations

The following are reported to the nurse if observed during oral hygiene:

- Dry, cracked, swollen, or blistered lips
- Redness, swelling, irritation, sores, or white patches in the mouth or on the tongue
- Bleeding, swelling, or excessive redness of the gums
- Any loose teeth

◈ Brushing Teeth

Many residents perform oral hygiene themselves. Others need help in gathering and setting up equipment. You may have to brush the teeth of residents who are very weak or cannot use or move their arms. Some residents are too confused to brush their own teeth. You need to provide oral hygiene for them.

Assisting the Resident to Brush the Teeth

Quality of Life

Remember to:
- ◆ *Knock before entering the resident's room*
- ◆ *Address the resident by name*
- ◆ *Introduce yourself by name and title*

Pre-Procedure

1 Explain the procedure to the resident.
2 Wash your hands.
3 Collect the following:
- Toothbrush
- Toothpaste or dentifrice
- Mouthwash (or solution specified on the care plan)
- Dental floss
- Water glass with cool water
- Straw
- Kidney basin
- Face towel
- Paper towels

4 Place the paper towels on the overbed table. Arrange items on top of them.
5 Identify the resident. Check the ID bracelet, and call the resident by name.
6 Provide for privacy.
7 Raise the head so the resident can brush with ease.

Procedure

8 Lower the bed rail (if used).
9 Place the towel over the resident's chest. This protects the gown and linens from spills.
10 Place the overbed table in front of the resident. Adjust table height for the resident.
11 Allow the resident to perform oral hygiene. This includes brushing the teeth, rinsing the mouth, and using mouthwash or other specified solution.
12 Remove the towel when the resident is done.
13 Move the overbed table next to the bed. Lower it to a level appropriate for the resident.

Post-Procedure

14 Provide for comfort.
15 Place the signal light within reach.
16 Raise or lower bed rails. Follow the care plan.
17 Clean and return items to their proper place.
18 Wipe off the overbed table with the paper towels and discard them.
19 Unscreen the resident.
20 Follow center policy for dirty linen.
21 Wash your hands.
22 Report your observations to the nurse.

Brushing the Resident's Teeth

Quality of Life

Remember to:
- ◆ *Knock before entering the resident's room*
- ◆ *Address the resident by name*
- ◆ *Introduce yourself by name and title*

Pre-Procedure

1 Explain the procedure to the resident.
2 Wash your hands.
3 Collect gloves and items listed in *Assisting the Resident to Brush the Teeth* (p. 266).
4 Place the paper towels on the overbed table. Arrange items on top of them.
5 Identify the resident. Check the ID bracelet, and call the resident by name.
6 Provide for privacy.
7 Raise the bed to the best level for good body mechanics. Make sure bed rails are up.

Procedure

8 Lower the bed rail near you.
9 Raise the head of the bed so the resident can sit comfortably. If the person cannot sit up, position him or her in a side-lying position on the side near you.
10 Place the towel over the resident's chest. This protects the gown and linens from spills.
11 Position the overbed table so you can reach it with ease. Adjust the height as needed.
12 Put on the gloves.
13 Apply toothpaste to the toothbrush.
14 Hold the toothbrush over the kidney basin. Pour some water over the brush.
15 Brush the resident's teeth gently as shown in Figure 13-1 on p. 268.
16 Brush the resident's tongue gently, if needed.
17 Let the resident rinse the mouth with water. Hold the kidney basin under the resident's chin (Fig. 13-2, p. 268). Repeat this step as necessary.
18 Floss the resident's teeth (see *Flossing the Resident's Teeth*, p. 269).
19 Let the resident use mouthwash or other specified solution. Hold the kidney basin under the chin.
20 Remove the towel when done.
21 Remove and discard the gloves.

Post-Procedure

22 Provide for comfort.
23 Place the signal light within reach.
24 Lower the bed to its lowest position.
25 Raise or lower bed rails. Follow the care plan.
26 Clean and return equipment to its proper place.
27 Wipe off the overbed table with the paper towels and discard them.
28 Lower the overbed table to a level appropriate for the resident.
29 Unscreen the resident.
30 Follow center policy for dirty linen.
31 Wash your hands.
32 Report your observations to the nurse.

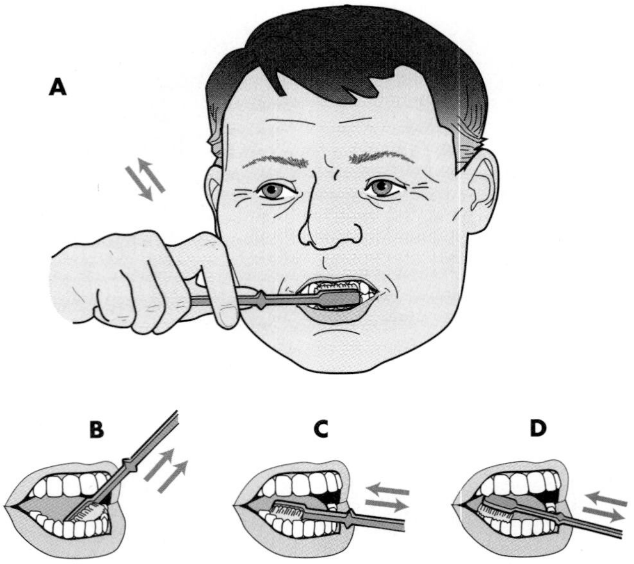

Fig. 13-1 Brushing teeth. **A,** Position the brush at a 45-degree angle to the gums. Brush with short strokes. **B,** Position the brush at a 45-degree angle against the inside of the front teeth. Brush from the gum to the crown of the tooth with short strokes. **C,** Hold the brush horizontally against the inner surfaces of the teeth. Brush back and forth. **D,** Position the brush on the biting surfaces of the teeth. Brush back and forth.

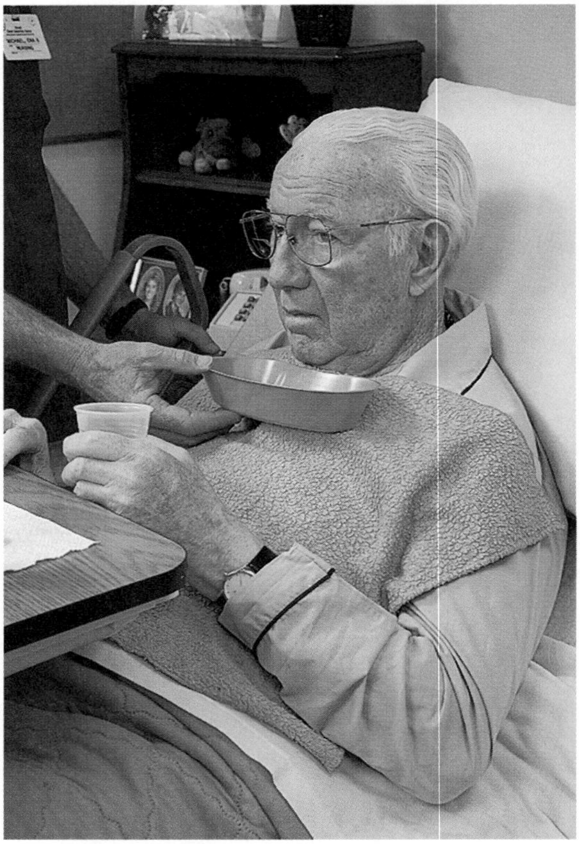

Fig. 13-2 The kidney basin is held under the person's chin.

Flossing

Flossing is a preventive measure. It removes plaque and tartar from the teeth. These substances cause serious gum disease that leads to loosening and loss of teeth. Flossing also removes food from between the teeth. It is usually done after brushing but can be done at other times. Some people floss after meals. If flossing is done only once a day, bedtime is the best time to floss.

You will need to floss for any resident who cannot tend to oral hygiene. Some older persons have never flossed their teeth. Respect their wishes if they refuse to have it done. Report the refusal to the nurse so the information is noted on the resident's care plan.

Flossing the Resident's Teeth

Quality of Life

Remember to:
- ◆ ***Knock before entering the resident's room***
- ◆ ***Address the resident by name***
- ◆ ***Introduce yourself by name and title***

Pre-Procedure

1 Explain to the resident what you are going to do.

2 Wash your hands.

3 Collect the following:
- Kidney basin
- Water glass with cool water
- Dental floss
- Face towel
- Paper towels
- Gloves

4 Place the paper towels on the overbed table. Arrange items on top of them.

5 Identify the resident. Check the ID bracelet, and call the resident by name.

6 Provide for privacy.

7 Raise the bed to the best level for good body mechanics. Make sure bed rails are up.

Procedure

8 Lower the bed rail near you.

9 Raise the head of the bed so the resident can sit comfortably. If the resident cannot sit up, position him or her in a side-lying position near you.

10 Place the towel over the resident's chest.

11 Position the overbed table so you can reach it with ease. Adjust the height as needed.

12 Put on the gloves.

13 Break off an 18-inch piece of floss from the dispenser.

14 Hold the floss between the middle fingers of each hand (Fig. 13-3, *A,* p. 270).

15 Stretch the floss with your thumbs.

16 Start at the upper back tooth on the right side, and work around to the left side.

17 Move the floss gently up and down between the teeth (Fig. 13-3, *B,* p. 270). Move floss up and down from the top of the crown to the gum line.

18 Move to a new section of floss after every second tooth.

Continued

Flossing the Resident's Teeth—cont'd

Procedure—cont'd

19 Floss the lower teeth. Hold the floss with your index fingers (Fig. 13-3, *C*, p. 270). Use up and down motions, and go under the gums as for the upper teeth. Start on the right side, and work around to the left side.

20 Let the resident rinse his or her mouth. Hold the kidney basin under the chin. Repeat rinsing as necessary.

21 Remove the towel when done.

22 Remove and discard the gloves.

Post-Procedure

23 Follow steps 22 through 32 for *Brushing the Resident's Teeth*, p. 267.

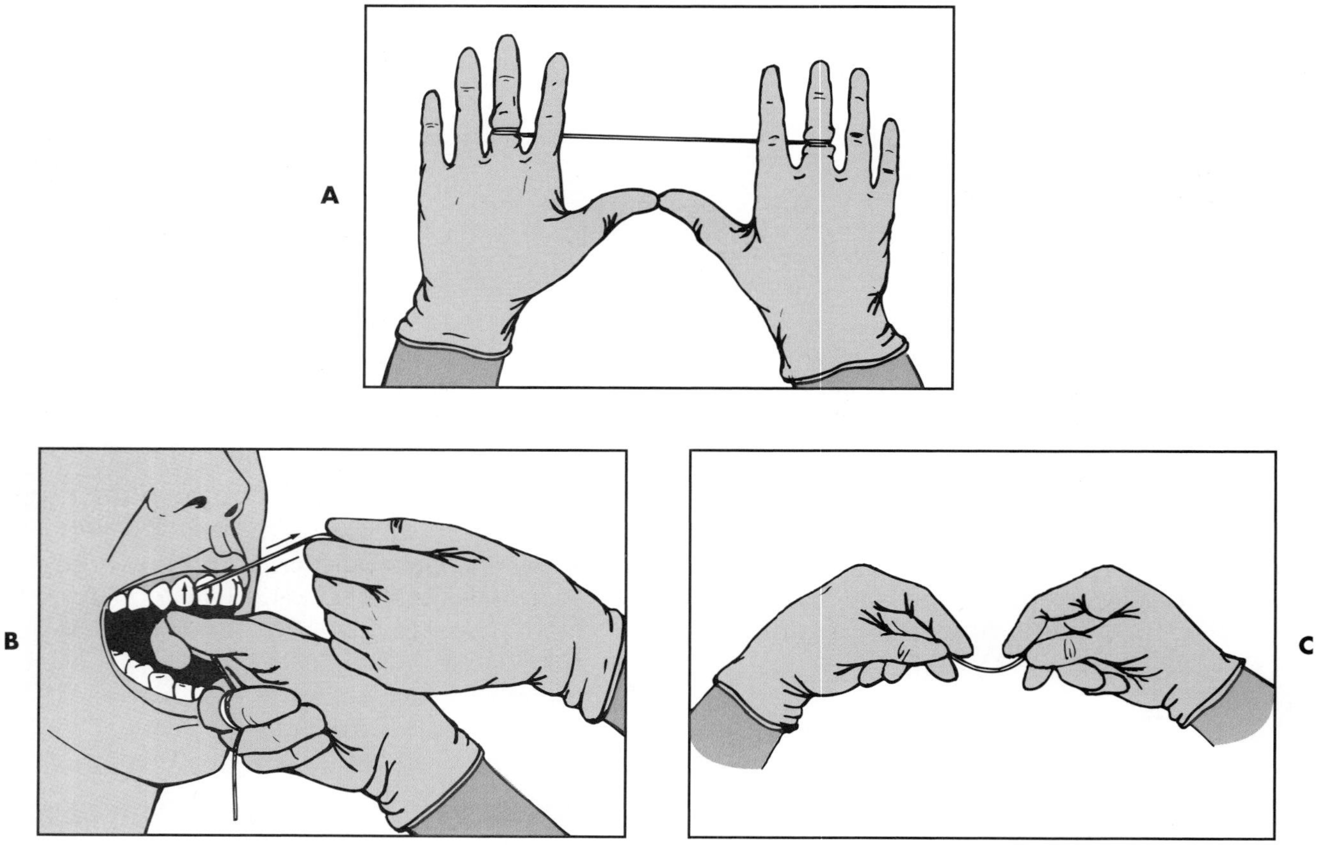

Fig. 13-3 Flossing teeth. **A,** Dental floss is held between the middle fingers to floss the upper teeth. **B,** Floss is moved in up-and-down motions between the teeth. Floss is moved up and down from the crown to the gum line. **C,** Floss is held with the index fingers to floss the lower teeth.

◈ Mouth Care for the Unconscious Resident

Unconscious residents need special mouth care. They cannot eat and drink, and they breathe with their mouths open. Many receive supplemental oxygen. These factors cause the mouth to dry and crusts to form on the tongue and mucous membranes. Good mouth care helps keep the mouth clean and moist. It also helps prevent infection.

The care plan tells you what cleaning agent to use. If you have questions, ask the nurse. Use sponge swabs to apply the cleaning agent. Apply a lubricant (check the care plan) to the lips after cleaning to prevent cracking.

Unconscious persons usually cannot swallow. Protect them from choking and aspiration. **Aspiration** is the breathing of fluid or an object into the lungs. It can cause pneumonia and death. To prevent aspiration, position the resident on one side with the head turned well to the side (Fig. 13-4). In this position, excess fluid runs out of the mouth. This reduces the risk of aspiration. Using only a small amount of fluid also reduces the risk of aspiration. Sometimes oral suctioning (see Chapter 25) is part of the procedure.

The resident's mouth is kept open with a padded tongue blade. (If there are none in the supply area, make a padded tongue blade as in Figure 13-5.) Do not use your fingers to hold the mouth open. The resident can bite down on them. The bite breaks the skin and creates a portal of entry for microbes. An infection could develop.

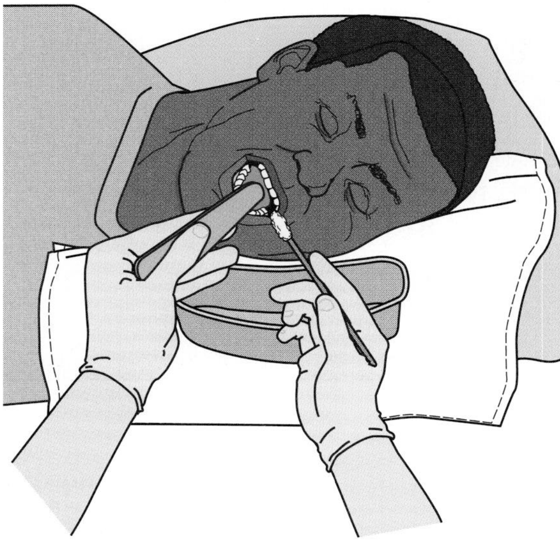

Fig. 13-4 The head of the unconscious person is turned well to the side to prevent aspiration. A padded tongue blade is used to keep the mouth open while cleaning the mouth with swabs.

Unconscious persons cannot speak or respond to what is happening. However, they may be able to hear. Always assume that unconscious persons can hear. Explain what you are doing step by step. Also tell the resident when you are done and when you are leaving the room.

Mouth care is given at least every 2 hours. The health care team assesses the resident's needs and then writes a care plan. Check with the nurse and the resident's care plan. They tell you how often to do oral hygiene and what to use. Unconscious residents are also repositioned at least every 2 hours. Combining mouth care, skin care, and other comfort measures increases their comfort and safety. You may need help from a coworker when caring for an unconscious resident.

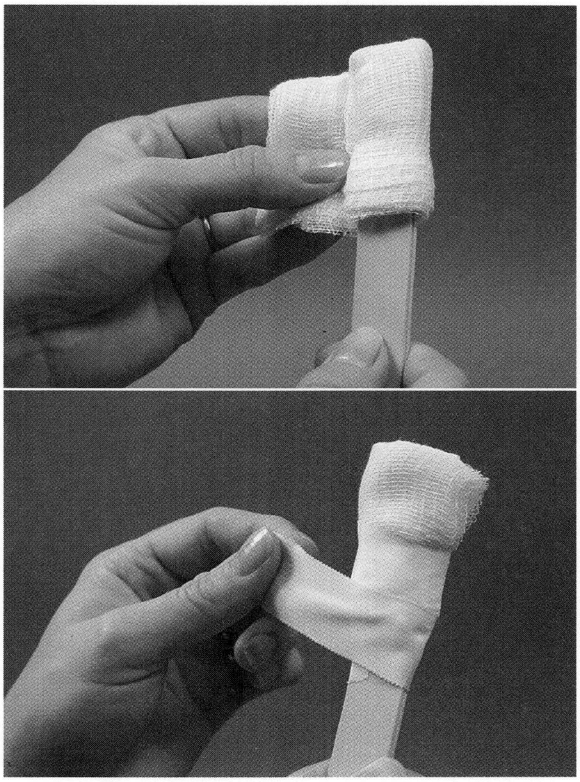

A

B

Fig. 13-5 Padded tongue blade. **A,** Place two wooden tongue blades together, and wrap gauze around the top half. **B,** Tape the gauze in place.

Providing Mouth Care for the Unconscious Resident

NNAAP™ SKILL

Quality of Life

Remember to:
- ◆ *Knock before entering the resident's room*
- ◆ *Address the resident by name*
- ◆ *Introduce yourself by name and title*

Pre-Procedure

1 Wash your hands.

2 Collect the following:
- Cleaning agent (check the care plan)
- Sponge swabs
- Padded tongue blade
- Water glass with cool water
- Face towel
- Kidney basin
- Lubricant for lips
- Paper towels
- Gloves

3 Place the paper towels on the overbed table. Arrange items on top of them.

4 Identify the resident. Check the ID bracelet, and call the resident by name.

5 Explain the procedure to the resident.

6 Provide for privacy.

7 Raise the bed to the best level for good body mechanics. Make sure bed rails are up.

Procedure

8 Lower the bed rail near you.

9 Put on the gloves.

10 Position the resident in a side-lying position on the side toward you. Turn his or her head well to the side.

11 Place the towel under the resident's face.

12 Place the kidney basin under the chin.

13 Position the overbed table so you can reach it. Adjust the height as needed.

14 Separate the upper and lower teeth with the padded tongue blade. Be gentle. Never use force. If you have problems, ask the nurse to assist you.

15 Clean the mouth. Use the sponge swabs moistened with the cleaning agent (see Fig. 13-4).

a Clean the chewing and inner surfaces of the teeth.

b Clean the outer surfaces of the teeth.

c Swab the roof of the mouth, the inside of the cheeks, and the lips.

d Swab the tongue.

e Moisten a clean swab with water, and swab the mouth to rinse.

f Place used swabs in the kidney basin.

16 Apply lubricant to the lips.

17 Remove the towel.

18 Remove and discard the gloves.

19 Explain that the procedure is done and that you will reposition him or her.

20 Reposition the resident.

21 Raise the bed rail. Make sure both bed rails are up.

Post-Procedure

22 Place the signal light within reach.

23 Lower the bed to its lowest position.

24 Clean and return equipment to its proper place. Discard disposable items.

25 Unscreen the resident.

26 Tell the resident that you are leaving the room.

27 Follow center policy for dirty linen.

28 Wash your hands.

29 Report your observations to the nurse.

Denture Care

Dentures are cleaned for residents who cannot do so themselves. Mouth care is given and dentures are cleaned as often as natural teeth. Remember that dentures are the resident's property. They are costly. You must handle them very carefully. Lost or damaged dentures are reported to the nurse immediately.

Dentures are slippery when wet. They easily break or chip if dropped onto a hard surface such as floors or sinks. You must hold them firmly. During cleaning, firmly hold them over a basin of water lined with a towel. Hot water causes them to warp. Do not use hot water to clean or store dentures. If dentures are not worn, store them in a container of cool water. Otherwise, dentures can dry out and warp.

Dentures are generally removed at bedtime. Some people choose not to wear their dentures. Others wear dentures for eating and remove them after meals. Remind residents not to wrap dentures in tissues or napkins. Otherwise they are easily discarded.

Many residents clean their own dentures. However, some need help collecting and cleaning items. They also may need help getting to the bathroom.

Providing Denture Care

NNAAP™ SKILL

Quality of Life

Remember to:
- ***Knock before entering the resident's room***
- ***Address the resident by name***
- ***Introduce yourself by name and title***

Pre-Procedure

1 Explain the procedure to the resident.
2 Wash your hands.
3 Collect the following:
- Denture brush or toothbrush
- Denture cup labeled with the resident's name and room number
- Denture cleaner or toothpaste
- Water glass with cool water
- Straw
- Mouthwash (or other specified solution)
- Kidney basin
- Two face towels
- Gauze squares
- Gloves

4 Identify the resident. Check the ID bracelet, and call the resident by name.
5 Provide for privacy.

Procedure

6 Lower the bed rail (if used).
7 Place a towel over the resident's chest.
8 Put on the gloves.
9 Ask the resident to remove the dentures. Carefully place them in the kidney basin.
10 Remove the dentures using gauze if the resident cannot do so. (The gauze lets you get a good grip on the slippery dentures.)
   a Grasp the upper denture with your thumb and index finger (Fig. 13-6, p. 274). Move the denture up and down slightly to break the seal. Gently remove the denture once the seal is broken. Place it in the kidney basin.
   b Remove the lower denture by grasping it with your thumb and index finger. Turn it slightly, and lift it out of the resident's mouth. Place it in the kidney basin.
11 Follow the care plan for raising bed rails.
12 Take the kidney basin, denture cup, brush, and denture cleaner or toothpaste to the sink.
13 Line the sink with a towel, and fill the sink with water.
14 Rinse each denture under warm running water. Return them to the denture cup.

Continued

Providing Denture Care—cont'd

NNAAP™ SKILL

Procedure—cont'd

15 Apply denture cleaner or toothpaste to the brush.

16 Brush the dentures as in Figure 13-7.

17 Rinse dentures under cool running water. Handle them carefully; do not drop them.

18 Place them in the denture cup. Fill it with cool water until the dentures are covered.

19 Clean the kidney basin.

20 Bring the denture cup and kidney basin to the bedside table.

21 Lower the bed rail if up.

22 Position the resident for oral hygiene.

23 Assist the resident to rinse his or her mouth with mouthwash (or specified solution). Hold the kidney basin under the chin.

24 Ask the resident to insert the dentures. Insert them if the resident cannot:

- a Grasp the upper denture firmly with your thumb and index finger. Raise the upper lip with the other hand, and insert the denture. Use your index fingers to gently press on the denture to make sure it is securely in place.
- b Grasp the lower denture securely with your thumb and index finger. Pull down slightly on the lower lip, and insert the denture. Gently press down on it to make sure it is in place.

25 Put the denture cup in the top drawer of the bedside stand if the dentures are not reinserted.

26 Remove the towel.

27 Remove the gloves.

Post-Procedure

28 Provide for comfort.

29 Place the signal light within reach.

30 Raise or lower bed rails. Follow the care plan.

31 Unscreen the resident.

32 Clean and return equipment to its proper place. Discard disposable items.

33 Follow center policy for dirty linen.

34 Wash your hands.

35 Report your observations to the nurse.

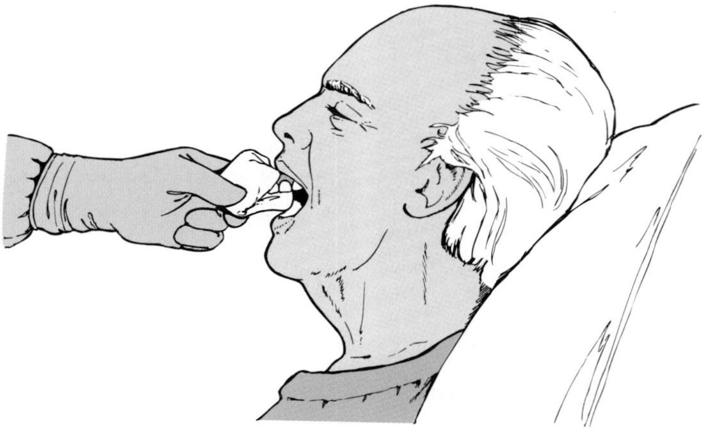

Fig. 13-6 Remove the upper denture by grasping it with the thumb and index finger of one hand. Use a piece of gauze to grasp the slippery denture.

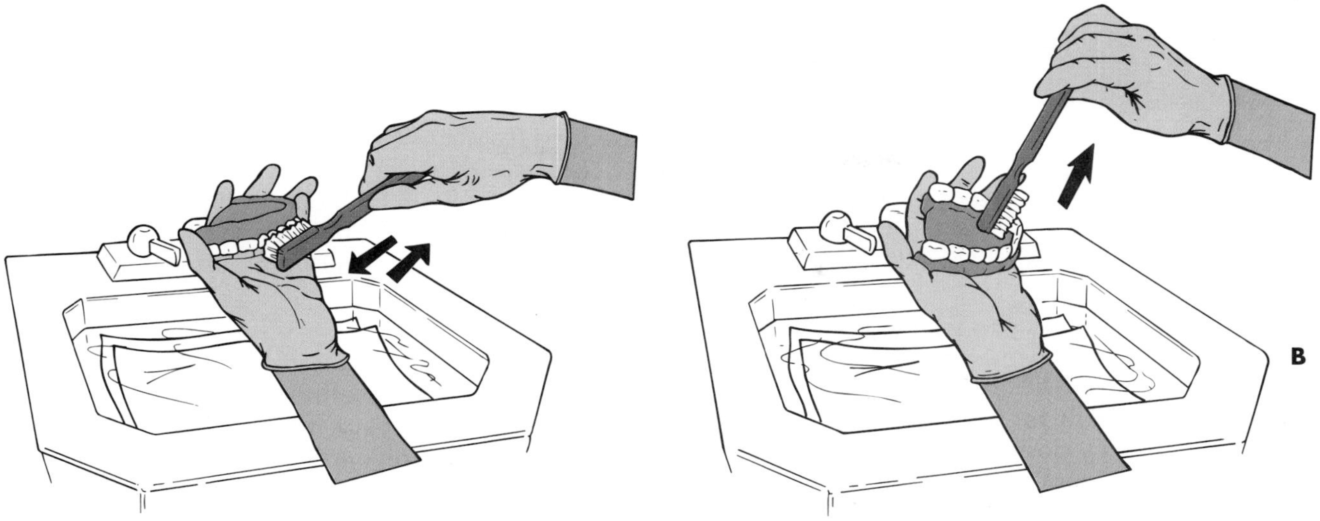

Fig. 13-7 Cleaning dentures. **A,** Brush the outer surfaces of the upper denture with back-and-forth motions. Note that the denture is held over the sink, which is filled halfway with water and lined with a towel. **B,** Position the brush vertically to clean the inner surfaces of the denture. Use upward strokes.

BATHING

Bathing cleans the skin. It also cleans the mucous membranes of the genital and anal areas. Microbes, dead skin, perspiration, and excess oils are removed. A bath is refreshing and relaxing. Circulation is stimulated and body parts exercised. You make important observations during the bath. The bath also gives you time to get to know the resident.

A resident may get a complete or partial bed bath, a tub bath, or a shower. The method depends on the resident's condition, self-care abilities, and personal choice. *(See Residents With Dementia.)* In nursing centers, bathing usually occurs after breakfast or the evening meal. You should respect the resident's choice of bath time whenever possible.

Bathing frequency is a personal matter. Some people bathe daily. Others take a complete bath only once or twice a week. Personal choice, weather, physical activity, and illness affect how often a person bathes. Illness usually increases the need for bathing because of fever and increased perspiration. Other illnesses and dry skin may require bathing every 2 or 3 days.

Age affects bathing frequency. Dry skin occurs with aging. Soap also dries the skin. Dry skin is easily damaged. Therefore older persons usually need a complete bath once a week. Partial baths are taken the other days. Some bathe daily but do not always use soap. Thorough rinsing is essential when using soap. Lotions and oils help keep the skin soft.

The rules for bed baths, showers, and tub baths are listed in Box 13-1 on p. 276.

RESIDENTS WITH DEMENTIA

Residents with dementia are often threatened by bathing procedures. They do not understand what is happening or why and may fear harm or danger. Therefore they may resist care and become agitated and combative. They may shout at the caregiver and cry out for help.

The rules in Box 13-1 on p. 276 apply when bathing residents with dementia. The resident's care plan will also include measures to help the resident through the bathing procedure. Such measures may include:

- Not rushing the person
- Using a calm, pleasant voice
- Diverting the person's attention (see Chapter 27)
- Calming the person and trying the bath later

BOX 13-1 RULES FOR BATHING

- The care plan tells you what type of bath a resident is to have. Find out which skin care products to use. Allow personal choice whenever possible.
- Collect necessary items before starting the procedure.
- Protect the resident's privacy. Properly screen the resident, and close doors, shades, or drapes.
- Cover the resident for warmth and privacy.
- Reduce drafts by closing doors and windows.
- Protect the resident from falling.
- Use good body mechanics at all times.
- Make sure water temperature is not too hot, particularly for older persons.
- Keep soap in the soap dish between latherings. This prevents the water from becoming too soapy. If a tub bath is taken, it reduces the chance of slipping and falls.
- Wash from the cleanest to the dirtiest areas.
- Encourage the resident to help as much as is safely possible.
- Rinse the skin thoroughly to remove the soap.
- Pat the skin dry to avoid irritating or breaking the skin.
- Bathe the skin whenever fecal material or urine is on the skin. Follow Standard Precautions and the Bloodborne Pathogen Standard.

Skin Care Products

There are many kinds of skin care products. Some clean the skin. Others protect the skin from drying or friction. The products used depend on personal choice and cost.

Soaps cleanse the skin. They remove dirt, dead skin, skin oil, some microbes, and perspiration. However, they tend to dry and irritate skin. Dry skin is itchy, uncomfortable, and easily injured. Skin must be rinsed well to remove all soap.

Soap is not needed for every bath. Plain water can clean the skin. Plain water often is used for older persons because of their dry skin. Those with dry skin may prefer soaps that contain bath oils. Soaps are not used if a resident has very dry skin.

Bath oils keep the skin soft and prevent drying. Some soaps contain bath oils, or liquid bath oil can be added to bath water. Showers and tubs become slippery from bath oils. Safety precautions are needed to prevent falls.

Creams and lotions protect the skin from the drying effect of air and evaporation. They do not feel greasy but leave an oily film on the skin. Most are scented. Lotion is used for the back massage. Applying lotion to bony parts helps prevent skin breakdown. You can apply lotion to the elbows, knees, and heels after the bath or shower.

Powders absorb moisture and prevent friction when two skin surfaces rub together. They usually are applied under the breasts, under the arms, and in the groin area. Sometimes powders are applied between the toes. Powder is applied to dry skin in a thin, even layer. Excessive powder causes caking and crusts that can irritate the skin. Powders are not used near persons with respiratory diseases. Inhaling the powder can further irritate the airway and lungs.

Deodorants and antiperspirants are applied to the axillae (underarms) after bathing. *Deodorants* mask and control body odors. *Antiperspirants* reduce perspiration. Deodorants and antiperspirants are not applied to irritated skin. They do not take the place of bathing.

Observations

Observe the skin during bathing procedures. Report the following observations to the nurse:

- The color of the skin, lips, nail beds, and sclera (whites of the eyes)
- The location and description of rashes
- Dry skin
- Bruises or open skin areas
- Pale or reddened areas, particularly over bony parts
- Drainage or bleeding from wounds or body openings
- Swelling of the feet and legs
- Corns or calluses on the feet
- Skin temperature
- Complaints of pain or discomfort

The Complete Bed Bath

The *complete bed bath* involves washing the resident's entire body in bed. Residents who are unconscious, paralyzed, in casts or traction, or weak from illness or surgery usually need bed baths. You give complete bed baths to residents who cannot bathe themselves.

Ask the nurse about a resident's ability to assist in the bath. Also ask about any limits in activity or position. You also should check the resident's care plan and ask the resident for any personal choices about bathing. Remember to follow Standard Precautions and the Bloodborne Pathogen Standard.

Many residents have never had a bed bath. They may be embarrassed to have another person see their bodies. Some residents may fear being exposed. Each resident must get an explanation about how a bed bath is given and how the body is covered to protect privacy.

Text continued on p. 283

Giving a Complete Bed Bath

NNAAP™ SKILL

Quality of Life

Remember to:
- ◆ *Knock before entering the resident's room*
- ◆ *Address the resident by name*
- ◆ *Introduce yourself by name and title*

Pre-Procedure

1 Identify the resident. Check the ID bracelet, and call the resident by name.
2 Explain the procedure to the resident.
3 Offer the bedpan or urinal (see Chapter 16). Provide for privacy.
4 Wash your hands.
5 Collect clean linen for a closed bed. Place linen on a clean surface.
6 Collect the following:
- Wash basin
- Soap dish with bar or liquid soap
- Bath thermometer
- Orange stick or nail file
- Washcloth
- Two bath towels and two face towels
- Bath blanket
- Gown or pajamas
- Items for oral hygiene
- Body lotion
- Talcum powder
- Deodorant or antiperspirant
- Brush and comb
- Other toilet articles if requested
- Paper towels
- Gloves

Procedure

7 Arrange items on the overbed table. Adjust the height as needed. Use the bedside stand if necessary.
8 Close doors and windows to prevent drafts.
9 Provide for privacy.
10 Raise the bed to the best level for good body mechanics. Make sure bed rails are up.
11 Remove the signal light, and lower the bed rail near you.
12 Provide oral hygiene.
13 Remove top linens, and cover the resident with a bath blanket (see *Making an Occupied Bed,* p. 255).
14 Lower the head of the bed to a level appropriate for the resident. Keep it as flat as possible. Let the resident have at least one pillow.
15 Place paper towels on the overbed table.
16 Raise the bed rail near you. Fill the wash basin.

Continued

Giving a Complete Bed Bath—cont'd

NNAAP™ SKILL

Procedure—cont'd

17 Fill the wash basin 2/3 (two-thirds) full with water. Water temperature should be 110° F to 115° F (43° C to 46° C) for adults. These higher water temperatures are needed because the water cools rapidly. (Measure the water temperature with the bath thermometer. Some states require testing bath water by dipping your elbow into the basin.)

18 Place the basin on the overbed table on top of the paper towels.

19 Lower the bed rail.

20 Place a face towel over the resident's chest.

21 Make a mitt with the washcloth (Fig. 13-8, p. 280). Use a mitt throughout the procedure.

22 Wash around the resident's eyes with water. Do not use soap. Gently wipe from the inner aspect with a corner of the mitt (Fig. 13-9, p. 280). Clean around the far eye first. Repeat this step for around the near eye.

23 Ask the resident if you should use soap to wash the face.

24 Wash the face, ears, and neck. Rinse and dry the skin well using the towel on the chest.

25 Help the resident move to the side of the bed nearest you.

26 Remove the gown. Do not expose the resident.

27 Place a bath towel lengthwise under the far arm.

28 Support the arm with your palm under the resident's elbow. His or her forearm rests on your forearm.

29 Wash the arm, shoulder, and underarm (axilla) with long, firm strokes (Fig. 13-10, p. 281). Rinse and pat dry.

30 Place the basin on the towel. Put the resident's hand into the water (Fig. 13-11, p. 281). Wash it well. Clean under fingernails with an orange stick or nail file.

31 Encourage the resident to exercise the hand and fingers.

32 Remove the basin, and dry the hand well. Cover the arm with the bath blanket.

33 Repeat steps 27 to 32 for the near arm.

34 Place a bath towel over the chest crosswise. Hold the towel in place, and pull the bath blanket from under the towel to the waist.

35 Lift the towel slightly, and wash the chest (Fig. 13-12, p. 281). Do not expose the resident. Rinse and pat dry, especially under breasts.

36 Move the towel lengthwise over the chest and abdomen. Do not expose the resident. Pull the bath blanket down to the pubic area.

37 Lift the towel slightly, and wash the abdomen (Fig. 13-13, p. 281). Rinse and pat dry.

38 Pull the bath blanket up to the shoulders, covering both arms. Remove the towel.

39 Change the water if it is soapy or cool. (Measure bath water temperature as in step 17.) Raise the bed rail before you leave the bedside. Lower it when you return.

40 Uncover the far leg. Do not expose the genital area. Place a towel lengthwise under the foot and leg.

41 Bend the knee and support the leg with your arm. Wash it with long, firm strokes. Rinse and pat dry.

42 Place the basin on the towel near the foot.

43 Lift the leg slightly. Slide the basin under the foot.

Giving a Complete Bed Bath—cont'd

NNAAP™ SKILL

Procedure—cont'd

44 Place the foot in the basin (Fig. 13-14, p. 282). Use an orange stick or nail file to clean under toenails if necessary. Do the following if the resident cannot bend the knees:
- Place a bath towel under the leg and foot.
- Wash the leg with long, firm strokes. Rinse and pat dry.
- Wash the foot. Carefully separate the toes. Rinse and pat dry.
- Clean under toenails with an orange stick or nail file if necessary.

45 Remove the basin, and dry the leg. Cover the foot with the bath blanket. Remove the towel.

46 Repeat steps 40 to 45 for the near leg.

47 Change the water. (Measure bath water temperature as in step 17.) Raise the bed rail before leaving the bedside. Lower it when you return.

48 Turn the resident onto the side away from you. Keep him or her covered with the bath blanket.

49 Uncover the back and buttocks. Do not expose the resident. Place a towel lengthwise on the bed along the back.

50 Wash the back, working from the back of the neck to the lower end of the buttocks. Use long, firm, continuous strokes (Fig. 13-15, p. 282). Rinse and dry well.

51 Give a back massage (see p. 290). (The resident may prefer to have the back massage after the bath.)

52 Turn the resident onto his or her back.

53 Change the water for perineal care. (Measure bath water temperature as in step 17. Also, some states require changing gloves and handwashing at this time.) Raise the bed rail before you leave the bedside. Lower it when you return.

54 Let the resident wash the genital area. Adjust the overbed table so he or she can reach the wash basin, soap, and towels with ease. Place the signal light within reach. Ask the resident to signal when finished. Make sure the resident understands what to do. Answer the signal light promptly. Provide perineal care if the resident cannot do so (see *Perineal Care*, pp. 292-295).

55 Give a back massage if you have not already done so.

56 Apply deodorant or antiperspirant.

57 Put a clean gown or pajamas on the resident.

58 Comb and brush the hair.

59 Make the bed. Attach the signal light.

Post-Procedure

60 Provide for comfort.

61 Lower the bed to its lowest position.

62 Raise or lower bed rails. Follow the care plan.

63 Empty and clean the wash basin. Return it and other supplies to their proper place.

64 Wipe off the overbed table with the paper towels and discard them.

65 Unscreen the resident.

66 Follow center policy for dirty linen.

67 Wash your hands.

68 Report your observations to the nurse (p. 276).

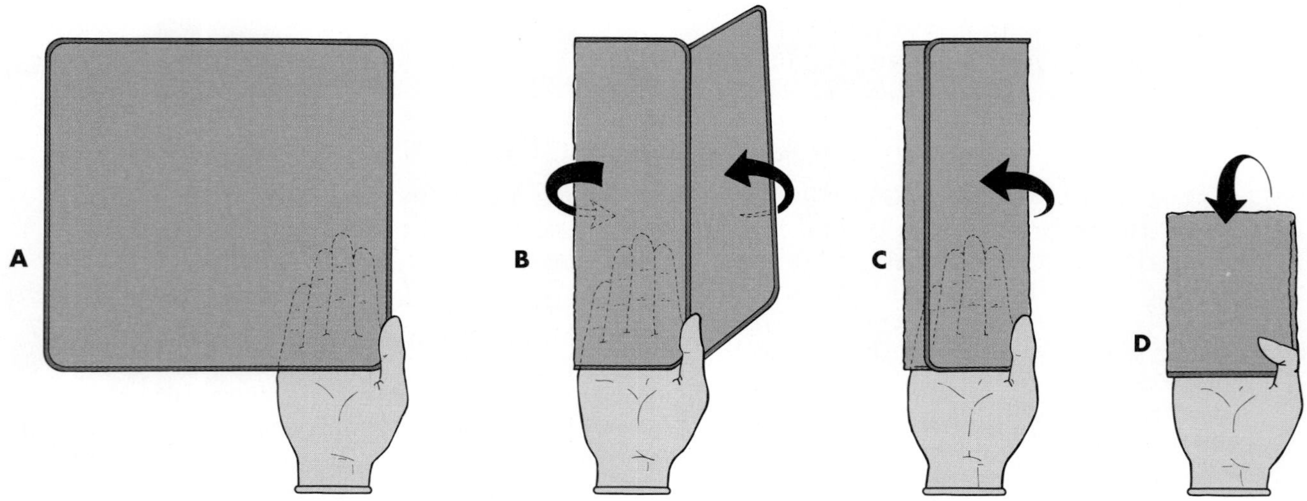

Fig. 13-8 Making a mitted washcloth. **A,** Make a mitt with a washcloth by grasping the near side of the washcloth with your thumb. **B,** Bring the washcloth around and behind your hand. **C,** Fold the side of the washcloth over your palm as you grasp it with your thumb. **D,** Fold the top of the washcloth down and tuck it under next to your palm.

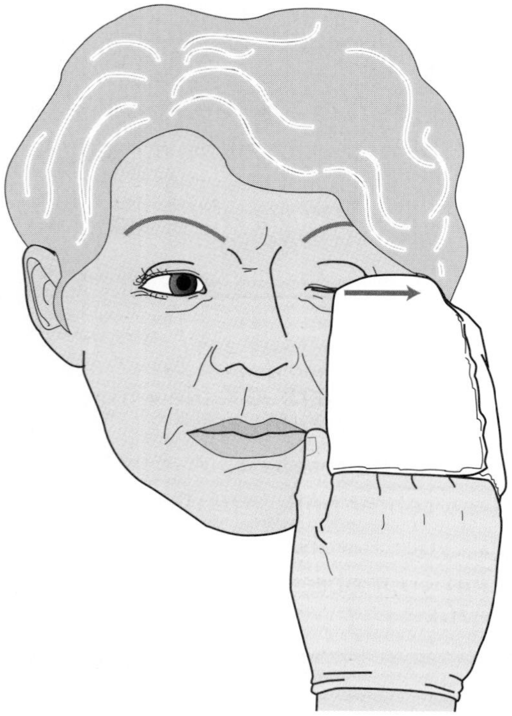

Fig. 13-9 Wash around the person's eyes with a mitted washcloth. Wipe from the inner to the outer aspect of the eye.

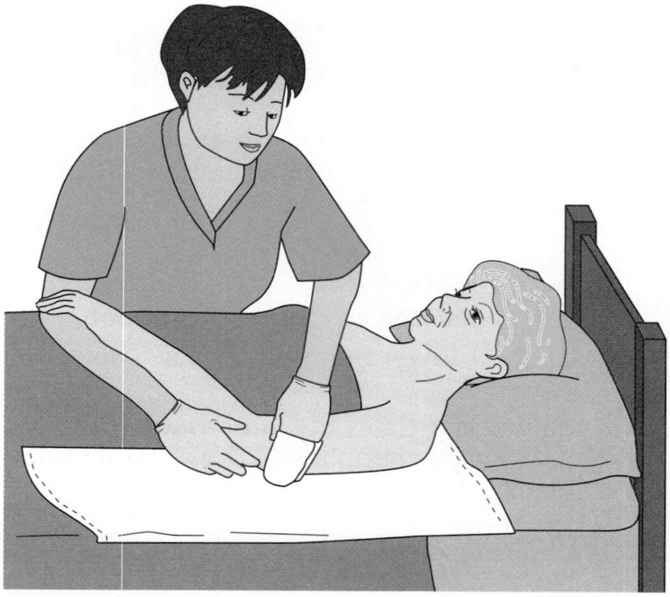

Fig. 13-10 Wash the person's arm with firm, long strokes using a mitted washcloth.

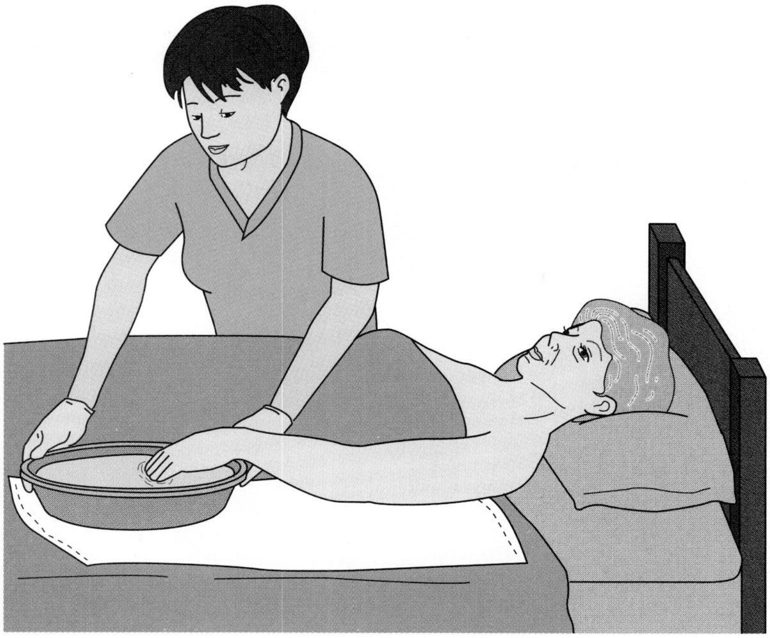

Fig. 13-11 The person's hands are washed by placing the wash basin on the bed.

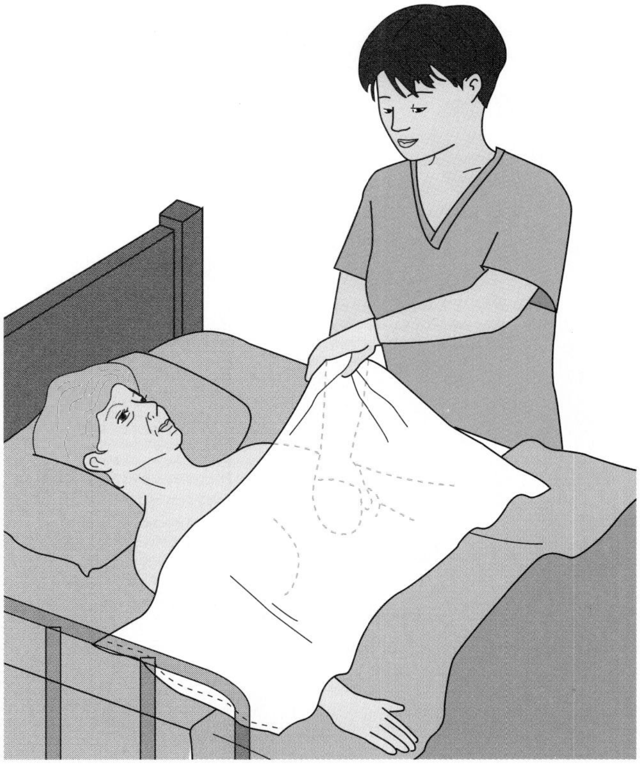

Fig. 13-12 The person's breasts are not exposed during the bath. A bath towel is placed horizontally over the chest area. The towel is lifted slightly to reach under to wash the breasts and chest.

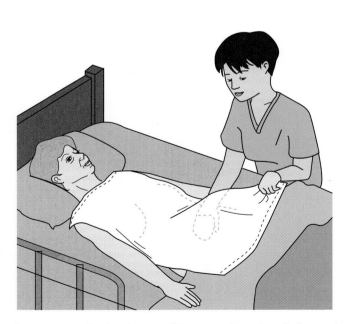

Fig. 13-13 The bath towel is turned so that it is vertical to cover the breasts and abdomen. The towel is lifted slightly to bathe the abdomen. The bath blanket covers the pubic area.

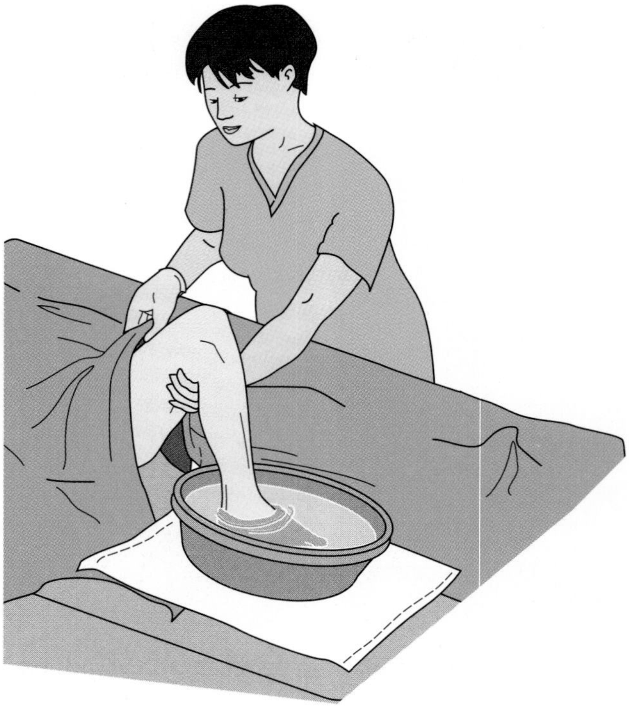

Fig. 13-14 The foot is washed by placing it in the wash basin on the bed.

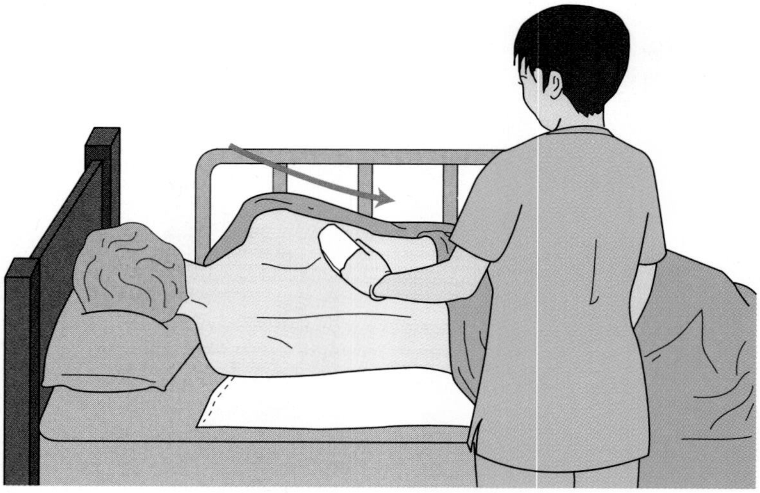

Fig. 13-15 The back is washed with long, firm, continuous strokes. Note that the person is in a side-lying position. A towel is placed lengthwise on the bed to protect the linens from water.

The Partial Bath

The *partial bath* involves bathing the resident's face, hands, axillae (underarms), back, buttocks, and perineal area. These areas develop odors or cause discomfort if not clean. Some residents can bathe themselves in bed or at the sink. You assist as needed, particularly in washing the back. You give partial bed baths to residents unable to bathe themselves.

The rules for bathing (see Box 13-1) apply when giving a partial bed bath. The considerations involved in giving a complete bed bath also apply.

Giving a Partial Bath

Quality of Life

Remember to:
- *Knock before entering the resident's room*
- *Address the resident by name*
- *Introduce yourself by name and title*

Pre-Procedure

1 Follow steps 1 through 9 in *Giving a Complete Bed Bath*, p. 277.

Procedure

2 Make sure the bed is in the lowest position.
3 Assist with oral hygiene. Adjust the height of the overbed table to an appropriate level.
4 Remove top linen. Cover the resident with a bath blanket.
5 Place the paper towels on the overbed table.
6 Fill the wash basin with water. Water temperature should be 110° F to 115° F (43° C to 46° C). (Measure the water temperature with the bath thermometer. Some states require testing bath water by dipping your elbow into the basin.)
7 Place the basin on the overbed table on top of the paper towels.
8 Raise the head of the bed so the resident can bathe comfortably. Assist him or her to sit at the bedside if allowed this position.
9 Position the overbed table so the resident can easily reach the basin and supplies.
10 Help the resident remove the gown or pajamas.
11 Ask the resident to wash easy-to-reach body parts (Fig. 13-16, p. 284). Explain that you will wash the back and those areas that cannot be reached.
12 Place the signal light within reach. Ask the resident to signal if help is needed or when bathing is complete.
13 Leave the room after washing your hands.
14 Return when the signal light is on. Knock before entering.
15 Change the bath water. (Measure bath water temperature as in step 6.)
16 Ask what was washed. Wash areas the resident could not reach. The face, hands, axillae, back, buttocks, and genital and rectal areas (perineal area) are washed for the partial bath.
17 Give a back massage.
18 Apply deodorant or antiperspirant.
19 Help the resident put on clean clothes, a gown, or pajamas.
20 Assist with hair care.
21 Assist him or her to a chair. Otherwise, turn the resident onto the side away from you.
22 Make the bed.
23 Lower the bed to its lowest position.
24 Assist the resident to return to bed.

Continued

Giving a Partial Bath—cont'd

Post-Procedure

25 Provide for comfort.
26 Place the signal light within reach.
27 Raise or lower bed rails. Follow the care plan.
28 Empty and clean the basin. Return the basin and supplies to their proper place.
29 Wipe off the overbed table with the paper towels and discard them.
30 Unscreen the resident.
31 Follow center policy for dirty linen.
32 Wash your hands.
33 Report your observations to the nurse (p. 276).

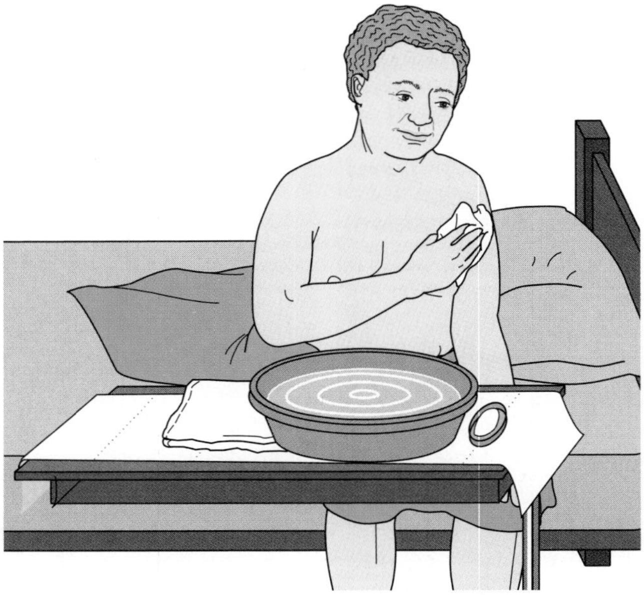

Fig. 13-16 The person is bathing himself in bed. Necessary equipment is within his reach.

◈ The Tub Bath

Many people prefer tub baths to showers. Most residents find them relaxing. However, safety is important. Falls are risks when getting in and out of the tub. Burns caused by hot water also are risks. A tub bath can cause a resident to feel faint, weak, or tired. These are greater risks for residents who were on bedrest. A bath should last no longer than 20 minutes. Do not let a resident take a tub bath without the nurse's approval.

You need to reserve the tub room. The tub must be cleaned before it is used. This prevents the spread of microbes and infection. The resident's safety is important. You must prevent slipping, falls, and chills (Box 13-2).

Changes in this procedure may be necessary for some residents. If the resident is very weak or large, two staff members are needed to safely perform the procedure. Check the care plan and with the nurse for any special instructions before assisting a resident with a tub bath or shower.

Some centers have portable tubs. The sides are lowered to transfer the resident from the bed to the tub (Fig. 13-17). After the transfer, the sides are raised into position. The resident is then transported to the tub room. The tub is filled and the resident bathed in the usual manner.

Box 13-2 Safety Rules for Tub Baths and Showers

- Place a bath mat in the tub or on the shower floor unless there are nonskid strips or a nonskid surface.
- Place needed items within the resident's reach. This includes the signal light.
- Drain the tub before the resident gets out of the tub. Keep the resident covered to protect from exposure and chilling.
- Have the resident use safety bars when getting in and out of the tub.
- Avoid using bath oils. They make tub and shower surfaces slippery.
- Do not leave the resident unattended in the tub or shower.
- Have the resident use safety bars for support when getting in or out of the tub or shower.

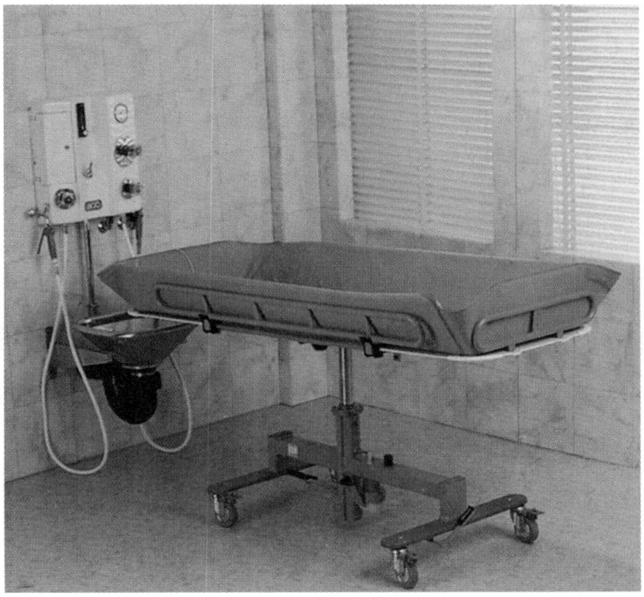

Fig. 13-17 Portable tub.The sides can be lowered to transfer the resident from the bed to the tub. *(Courtesy Arjo, Inc, Morton Grove, Illinois.)*

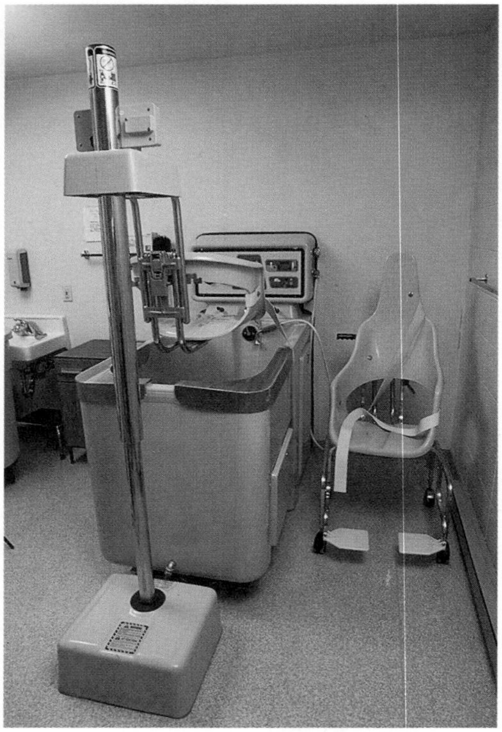

Fig. 13-18 The whirlpool tub has a hydraulic lift.

Whirlpool tubs have a special hydraulic lift (Fig. 13-18). A resident is placed in a special wheeled chair at the bedside and taken to the tub room. The chair is attached to the lift and unlocked from the wheeled base. The chair and resident are lifted into the tub. The tub has a whirlpool action that cleans the resident. The nursing assistant washes the upper portion of the resident's body. Make sure to carefully wash under breasts, between skin folds, and in the perineal area. Carefully dry these areas after the bath.

Some tubs have special gurneys (stretchers) for residents who cannot sit up. The resident is transferred from the bed to the gurney and wheeled into the tub room. The resident is lowered into a tub on the gurney (Fig. 13-19).

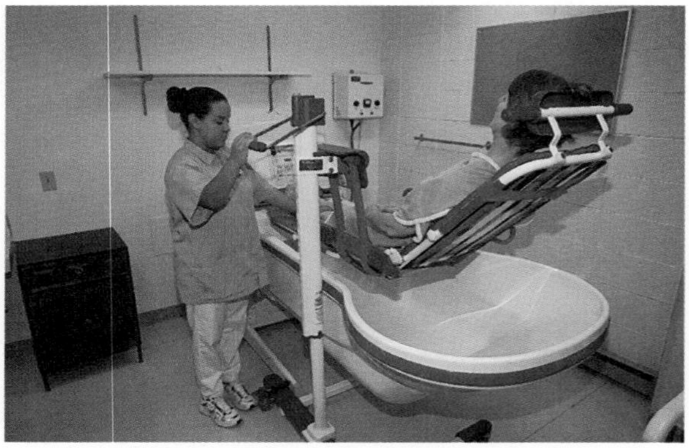

Fig. 13-19 A resident can be placed on a special gurney that is lowered into the tub. The tub has whirlpool action.

◈ The Shower

Most nursing centers have shower rooms with shower stalls or shower cabinets (Fig. 13-20). These have advantages over bathtub-shower units. The resident does not have to step into the tub. The resident walks into the shower cabinet. With a shower stall, the resident simply walks into the stall or is wheeled in on a shower chair. Shower chairs have wheels on the legs. A round open area on the plastic seat lets water drain off the chair (see Fig. 13-20). The chair can be used to transport the resident to and from the shower room. The wheels are locked during the shower to prevent the chair from moving.

The shower room may have more than one stall or cabinet. You must protect the resident's right to privacy. Remember that the resident has the right not to have his or her body seen by others. Make sure you properly screen and cover the resident.

You need to protect residents from falls and chills during showers (see Box 13-2). Encourage the use of handrails for support while the resident is showering. Like tubs, shower stalls and cabinets have nonskid surfaces. If not, a bathmat is used. Never let weak or unsteady residents stand in the shower. They need to use a shower chair. Privacy also is protected. Remember to close doors and the shower curtain. Never leave a resident alone in the shower room. Stay in the shower room in case the resident needs help or becomes weak or faint. Residents are not allowed to shower unless the nurse gives approval.

Text continued on p. 290

A 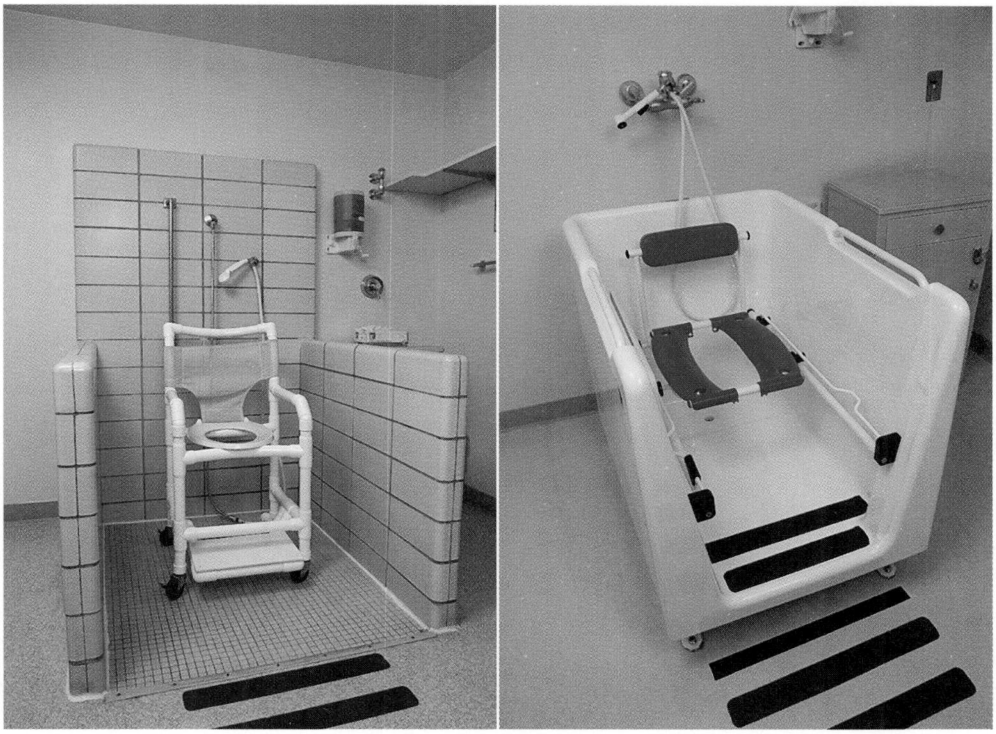 B

Fig. 13-20 A, Shower stall. Note the shower chair. **B,** Shower cabinet.

Assisting With a Tub Bath or Shower

Quality of Life

Remember to:
- *Knock before entering the resident's room*
- *Address the resident by name*
- *Introduce yourself by name and title*

Pre-Procedure

1 Reserve the bathtub or shower if necessary.
2 Identify the resident. Check the ID bracelet, and call the resident by name.
3 Explain the procedure to the resident.
4 Wash your hands.
5 Collect the following:
- Washcloth and two bath towels
- Bar or liquid soap
- Bath thermometer (for a tub bath)
- Clean gown or pajamas
- Deodorant and other toilet articles as requested
- Robe and nonskid slippers or shoes
- Rubber bath mat if needed
- Disposable bath mat

Procedure

6 Place items in the bathroom or shower room in the space provided or on a chair.
7 Clean the tub or shower if needed.
8 Place a rubber bath mat in the tub or on the shower floor. Do not block the drain.
9 Place a disposable bath mat on the floor in front of the tub or shower.
10 Put the *occupied* sign on the door.
11 Return to the resident's room. Provide for privacy.
12 Help the resident sit on the side of the bed.
13 Help the resident put on a robe and slippers.
14 Assist the resident to the bathroom or shower room. Use a wheelchair if necessary.
15 *For a tub bath:*
  a Have the resident sit on the chair by the tub.
  b Fill the tub halfway with warm water (105° F; 41° C.) (Fig. 13-21). Measure water temperature with the bath thermometer, or check the digital display (see Fig. 8-3, p. 132).

For a shower:
  a Turn on the shower.
  b Adjust water temperature and pressure.

16 Help the resident remove slippers, robe, and gown.
17 Assist the resident into the tub or shower. If using a shower chair, place it in position and lock the wheels.
18 Assist with washing if necessary. Remember that the bath should not last longer than 20 minutes.
19 Do not leave the resident unattended in the tub or shower room.
20 Place a towel across the chair.
21 Turn off the shower.
22 Help the resident out of the tub or shower and onto the chair.
23 Help the resident dry off. Pat gently. Remember to dry under breasts, between skin folds, in the perineal area, and between toes.

Assisting With a Tub Bath or Shower—cont'd

Procedure—cont'd

24 Assist with lotion, deodorant, or antiperspirant as needed.

25 Help the resident to dress, or put on a clean gown or pajamas, a bathrobe, and slippers or shoes.

26 Help the resident return to the room. Assist the person into bed if indicated.

27 Provide a back massage if the resident returns to bed.

28 Assist with hair care and other grooming needs as requested by the resident.

Post-Procedure

29 Provide for comfort.

30 Raise or lower bed rails. Follow the care plan.

31 Place the signal light within reach.

32 Clean the tub or shower. Remove soiled linen, and discard disposable items. Put the *unoccupied* sign on the door. Return supplies to their proper place.

33 Follow center policy for dirty linen.

34 Wash your hands.

35 Report your observations to the nurse (p. 276).

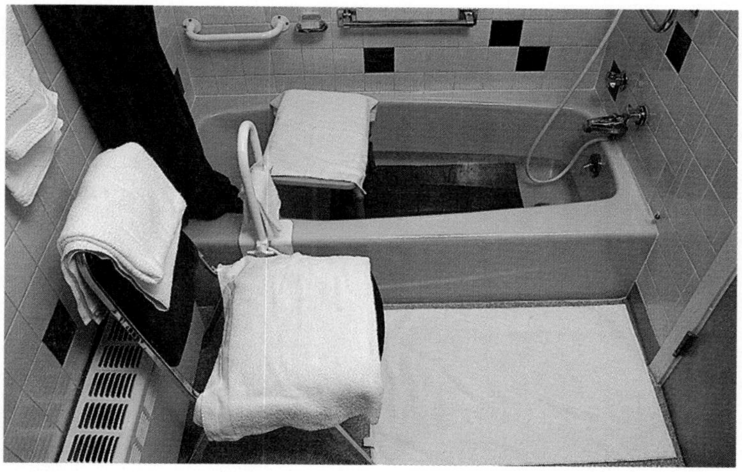

Fig. 13-21 A bath mat is in the tub, the tub is filled halfway with water, and a floor mat is in front of the tub.

◈ THE BACK MASSAGE

The back massage (back rub) relaxes muscles and stimulates circulation. Massages are normally given after the bath and with HS care. It should last 3 to 5 minutes. Observe the skin before starting the procedure. Look for breaks in the skin, bruises, reddened areas, and other signs of skin breakdown.

Lotion reduces friction when giving the massage. It is warmed before being applied. Warm lotion by placing the bottle in the bath water or holding it under warm water. You can warm lotion also by rubbing some between your hands.

The prone position is best for a massage. However, the side-lying position is often more comfortable for older or disabled persons. Use firm strokes, and always keep your hands in contact with the resident's skin. After the massage, apply some lotion to the elbows, knees, and heels to keep the skin soft. These bony areas are at risk for skin breakdown.

Some residents should not have back massages as described in this procedure. They are dangerous for those with certain heart diseases, back injuries, back surgeries, skin diseases, and some lung disorders. Check with the nurse before giving a back massage to residents with these conditions.

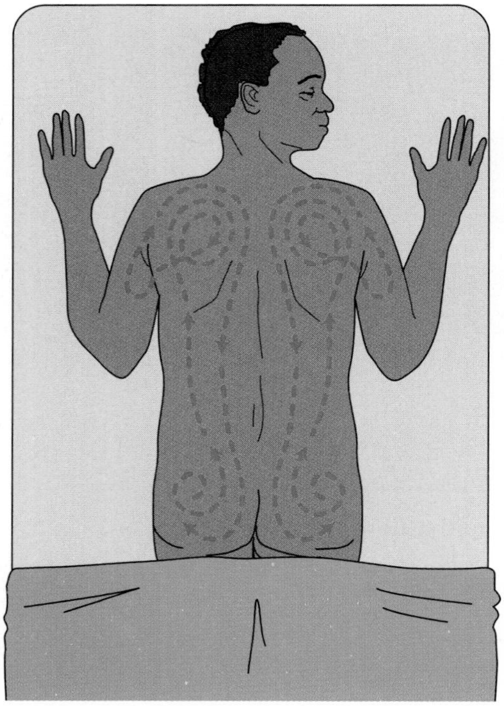

Fig. 13-22 The person lies in the prone position for a back massage. Stroke upward from the buttocks to the shoulders, down over the upper arms, back up the upper arms, across the shoulders, and down the back to the buttocks.

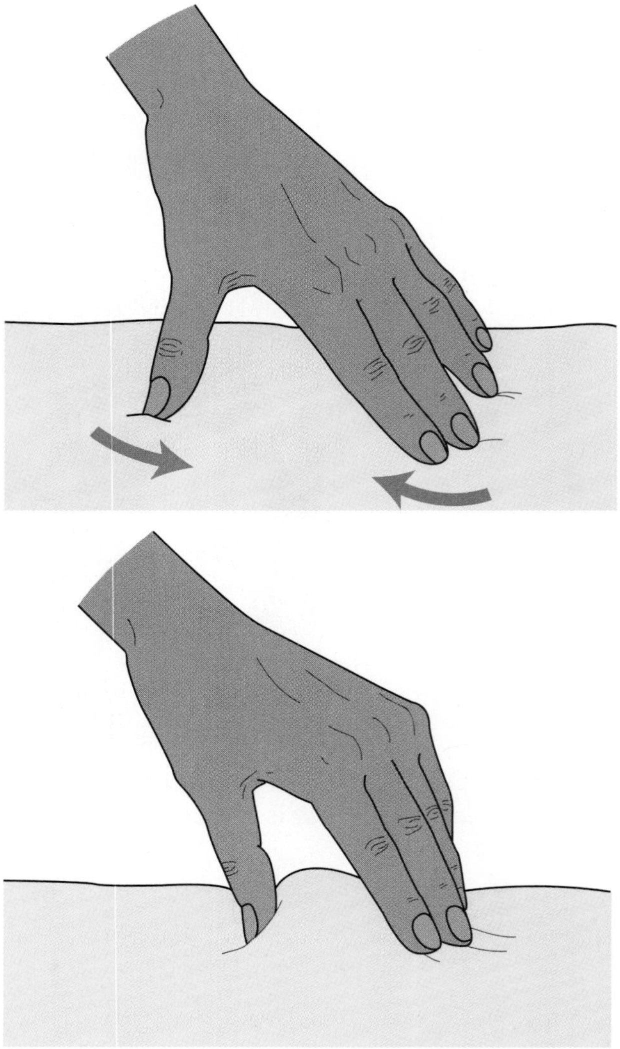

Fig. 13-23 Kneading is done by picking up tissue between the thumb and fingers.

Giving a Back Massage

Quality of Life

Remember to:
- ◆ *Knock before entering the resident's room*
- ◆ *Address the resident by name*
- ◆ *Introduce yourself by name and title*

Pre-Procedure

1 Identify the resident. Check the ID bracelet, and call the resident by name.
2 Explain the procedure to the resident.
3 Wash your hands.
4 Collect the following:
- Bath blanket
- Bath towel
- Lotion

5 Provide for privacy.
6 Raise the bed to the best level for good body mechanics. Make sure bed rails are up.

Procedure

7 Lower the bed rail near you.
8 Position the resident in the prone or side-lying position with the back toward you.
9 Expose the back, shoulders, upper arms, and buttocks. Cover the rest of the body with the bath blanket.
10 Lay the towel on the bed along the back.
11 Warm some lotion between your hands.
12 Explain that the lotion may feel cool and wet.
13 Apply lotion to the lower back area.
14 Stroke up from the buttocks to the shoulders. Then stroke down over the upper arms. Stroke up the upper arms, across the shoulders, and down the back to the buttocks (Fig. 13-22). Use firm strokes. Keep your hands in contact with the resident's skin.
15 Repeat step 14 for at least 3 minutes.
16 Knead by grasping skin between your thumb and fingers (Fig. 13-23). Knead half of the back starting at the buttocks and moving up to the shoulder. Then knead down from the shoulder to the buttocks. Repeat on the other half of the back.
17 Apply lotion to bony areas. Use circular motions with the tips of your index and middle fingers. (Do not massage bony areas that are reddened. See Chapter 14.)
18 Use fast movements to stimulate and slow movements to relax the resident.
19 Stroke with long, firm movements to end the massage. Tell the resident you are finishing.
20 Cover the resident. Remove the towel and bath blanket.

Post-Procedure

21 Provide for comfort.
22 Lower the bed to its lowest position.
23 Raise or lower bed rails. Follow the care plan.
24 Place the signal light within reach.
25 Return lotion to its proper place.
26 Unscreen the resident.
27 Follow center policy for dirty linen.
28 Wash your hands.
29 Report your observations to the nurse.

◈ PERINEAL CARE

Perineal care (pericare) involves cleaning the genital and anal areas. These areas are warm, moist, and dark. They provide a place for microbes to grow. The genital and anal areas are cleaned to prevent infection and odors and to promote comfort.

Perineal care is done at least daily during the bath. The procedure is done also whenever the area is soiled with urine or feces. Residents with certain disorders need perineal care more often. This is indicated on the care plan. Ask the nurse if you have questions.

Residents do their own perineal care if able. Otherwise, it is given by nursing staff. Many people and nursing staff find the procedure embarrassing, especially when given to the other sex. People may not know the terms *perineum* and *perineal.* Most understand *privates, private parts, crotch, genitals,* or the *area between your legs.* Use terms the resident understands. The term also must be in good taste professionally.

Standard Precautions, medical asepsis, and the Bloodborne Pathogen Standard are followed. Work from the cleanest area to the dirtiest. The urethral area is the cleanest, the anal area the dirtiest. Therefore clean from the urethra to the anal area. The perineal area is very delicate and easily injured. Use warm water, not hot. Washcloths are used if pericare is part of the bath. The nurse may ask you to use disposable towelettes, cotton balls, or swabs at other times. The area is rinsed thoroughly. Pat dry after rinsing to reduce moisture and promote comfort.

Giving Female Perineal Care

NNAAP™ SKILL

Quality of Life

Remember to:
- ◆ ***Knock before entering the resident's room***
- ◆ ***Address the resident by name***
- ◆ ***Introduce yourself by name and title***

Pre-Procedure

1 Explain the procedure to the resident.

2 Wash your hands.

3 Collect the following:
- Soap dish with bar or liquid soap
- At least four washcloths
- Bath towel
- Bath blanket
- Bath thermometer
- Waterproof pad
- Gloves
- Paper towels

4 Arrange items on the overbed table.

5 Identify the resident. Check the ID bracelet, and call her by name.

6 Provide for privacy.

7 Raise the bed to the best level for good body mechanics. Make sure bed rails are up.

Procedure

8 Lower the bed rail near you.

9 Cover the resident with a bath blanket. Move top linens to the foot of the bed.

10 Position the resident on her back.

11 Position the waterproof pad under her buttocks.

12 Drape the resident as in Figure 13-24 on p. 294.

13 Raise the bed rail.

14 Fill the wash basin. Water temperature is about 105° F to 109° F (41° C to 43° C).

15 Place the basin on the overbed table on top of the paper towels.

Giving Female Perineal Care—cont'd

NNAAP™ SKILL

Procedure—cont'd

16 Lower the bed rail.

17 Help the resident flex her knees and spread her legs. If the resident cannot flex her knees, help her spread her legs as much as possible with her knees straight.

18 Put on the gloves.

19 Fold the corner of the bath blanket between the resident's legs onto her abdomen.

20 Wet the washcloths. Squeeze out excess water from washcloths before using them.

21 Apply soap to a washcloth.

22 Separate the labia. Clean downward from front to back with one stroke (Fig. 13-25, p. 294).

23 Repeat steps 21 and 22 until the area is clean. Use a different part of the washcloth for each stroke. Use more than one washcloth if needed.

24 Rinse the perineum with a clean washcloth. Separate the labia. Stroke downward from front to back. Repeat the step as necessary. Use a different part of the washcloth for each stroke. Use more than one washcloth if needed.

25 Pat the area dry with the towel.

26 Fold the blanket back between her legs.

27 Help the resident lower her legs and turn onto her side away from you.

28 Apply soap to a washcloth.

29 Clean the rectal area. Clean from the vagina to the anus with one stroke (Fig. 13-26, p. 294).

30 Repeat steps 28 and 29 until the area is clean. Use a different part of the washcloth for each stroke. Use more than one washcloth if needed.

31 Rinse the rectal area with a washcloth. Stroke from the vagina to the anus. Repeat the step as necessary using a different part of the washcloth for each stroke. Use more than one washcloth if needed.

32 Pat the area dry with the towel.

33 Remove and discard the gloves.

Post-Procedure

34 Position the resident so she is comfortable.

35 Return linens to their proper position, and remove the bath blanket.

36 Lower the bed to its lowest position.

37 Raise or lower bed rails. Follow the care plan.

38 Place the signal light within reach.

39 Empty and clean the wash basin.

40 Return the basin and supplies to their proper place.

41 Wipe off the overbed table with the paper towels and discard them.

42 Unscreen the resident.

43 Follow center policy for dirty linen.

44 Wash your hands.

45 Report your observations to the nurse:
- Any odors
- Redness, swelling, discharge, or irritation
- Complaints of pain, burning, or other discomfort

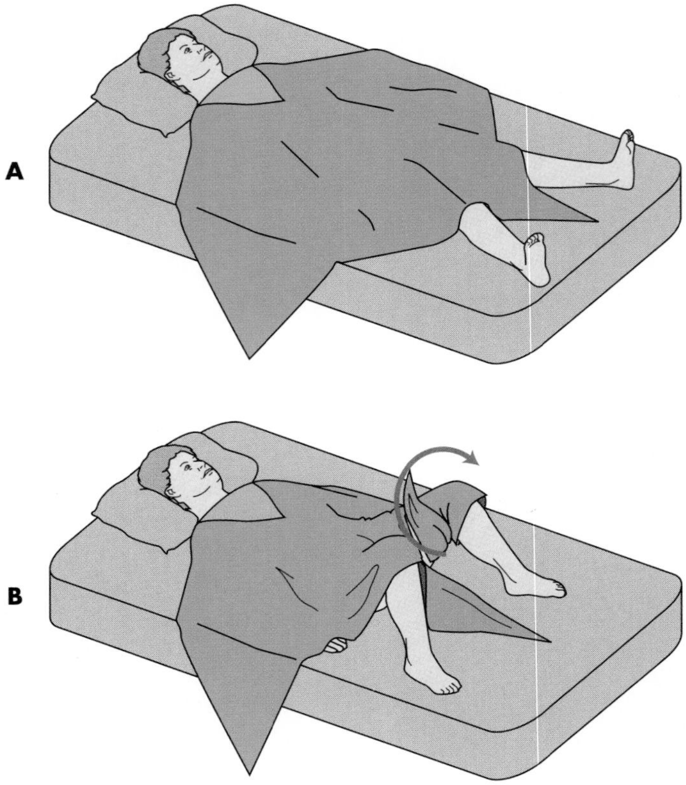

Fig. 13-24 Draping for perineal care. **A,** Drape the person for perineal care by positioning the bath blanket like a diamond: one corner is at the neck, there is a corner at each side, and one corner is between the person's legs. **B,** Wrap the blanket around the leg by bringing the corner around under the leg and over the top. Tuck the corner under the hip.

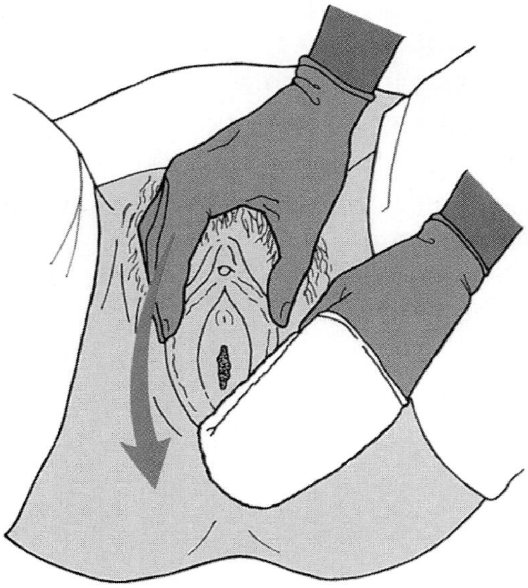

Fig. 13-25 Separate the labia with one hand to give female perineal care. Use a mitted washcloth to cleanse between the labia with downward strokes.

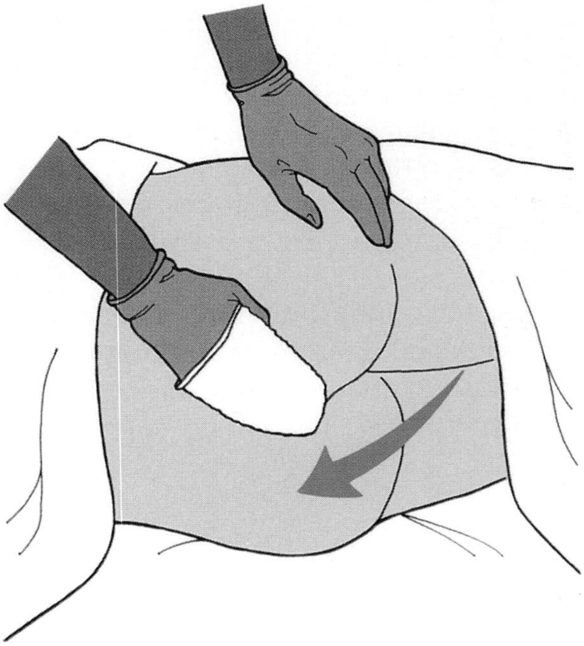

Fig. 13-26 The rectal area is cleaned by wiping from the vagina to the anus. The side-lying position allows the anal area to be cleaned more thoroughly.

Giving Male Perineal Care

NNAAP™ SKILL

Quality of Life

Remember to:
- *Knock before entering the resident's room*
- *Address the resident by name*
- *Introduce yourself by name and title*

Procedure

1 Follow steps 1 through 21 in *Giving Female Perineal Care*, pp. 292-293.

2 Retract the foreskin if the resident is uncircumcised (Fig. 13-27).

3 Grasp the penis.

4 Clean the tip using a circular motion. Start at the urethral opening and work outward (Fig. 13-28). Repeat this step as necessary. Use a different part of the washcloth each time.

5 Rinse the area with another washcloth.

6 Return the foreskin to its natural position.

7 Clean the shaft of the penis with firm downward strokes. Rinse the area.

8 Help the resident flex his knees and spread his legs. If the resident cannot flex his knees, help him spread his legs as much as possible with knees straight.

9 Clean the scrotum, and rinse well. Observe for redness and irritation in the skin folds.

10 Pat dry the penis and scrotum.

11 Fold the bath blanket back between his legs.

12 Help him lower his legs and turn onto his side away from you.

13 Clean the rectal area (see *Giving Female Perineal Care*). Rinse and dry well.

14 Remove and discard the gloves.

Post-Procedure

15 Follow steps 34 through 45 in *Giving Female Perineal Care*.

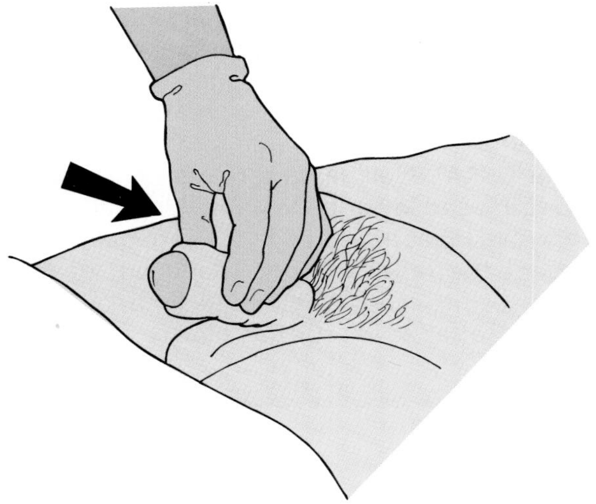

Fig. 13-27 The foreskin of the uncircumcised male is pulled back for perineal care. It is returned to the normal position immediately after cleaning.

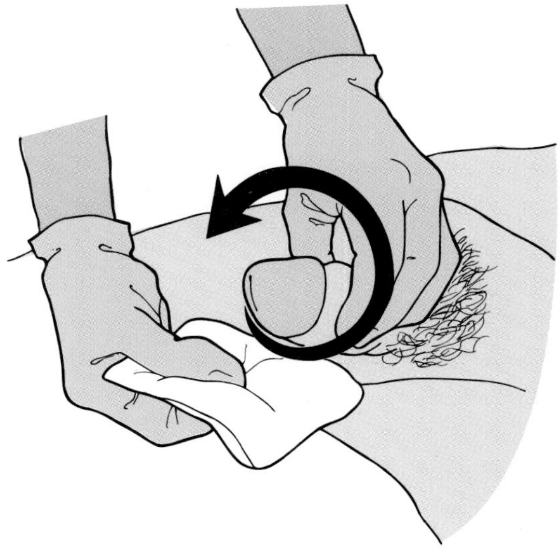

Fig. 13-28 The penis is cleaned with circular motions starting at the urethra.

QUALITY OF LIFE

Remember that resident rights are protected by OBRA. Such rights are intended to improve the resident's quality of life, health, and safety. You must provide personal hygiene in a manner that maintains or improves the resident's quality of life, health, and safety. You must protect the resident's rights when performing personal hygiene activities.

The right to privacy and confidentiality is very important. The resident is not exposed during personal hygiene. Ask visitors to leave the room when care is to be given. A family member or friend may want to help give care. The resident must give permission for this. Remember to close doors, privacy curtains, shades, and drapes before starting procedures. Only the body part involved in the procedure is exposed. Remember to properly cover residents who are taken to and from tub or shower rooms. If the shower room has more than one shower stall, you must protect the resident from being exposed to others who are present.

Residents also have the right to personal choice. This means that they have the right to be involved in planning their care and treatment. Hygiene is a very personal matter. Whenever possible, the resident is allowed to make choices. Residents are involved in deciding when and how personal hygiene is done. The resident is allowed personal choice in such matters as bath time, the products to use, what to wear, and hair styling.

Residents have the right to keep and use personal possessions. You will handle the resident's property in personal hygiene procedures. Dentures and eyeglasses are protected from loss or breakage. If jewelry or religious medals are removed for care, make sure you protect them from loss, damage, or theft.

Freedom from restraint is another resident right. Bed rails are considered physical restraints under OBRA. Hygiene procedures include steps on raising and lowering bed rails. Bed rails must always be up as indicated in the care plan. They prevent the resident from falling out of bed when giving care. When used, bed rails are lowered after lowering the bed to its lowest position.

REVIEW QUESTIONS

Circle T if the statement is true and F if the statement is false.

1 T F Cleanliness and skin care are needed for comfort, safety, and health.

2 T F Mrs. Hart asks for a back massage as part of HS care. You can tell her that back massages are given during morning care.

3 T F Mrs. Hart's toothbrush has hard bristles. They are good for oral hygiene.

4 T F Unconscious residents are supine for mouth care.

5 T F You use your fingers to keep an unconscious person's mouth open for oral hygiene.

6 T F Mrs. Hart has a lower denture. It is washed in warm water over a hard surface.

7 T F Bath oils cleanse and soften the skin.

8 T F Powders absorb moisture and prevent friction.

9 T F Deodorants reduce the amount of perspiration.

10 T F You can give permission for showers but not for tub baths.

11 T F Weak residents can be left alone in the shower if they are sitting.

12 T F A back massage relaxes muscles and stimulates circulation.

13 T F Perineal care helps prevent infection.

14 T F Foreskin is returned to its normal position after giving male perineal care.

15 T F Bed rails are raised to prevent the resident from falling out of bed when giving care.

Circle the BEST answer.

16 Oral hygiene is part of
- A AM care and HS care
- B Morning care
- C Care given after lunch
- D All of the above

17 You brush Mrs. Hart's teeth and note the following. Which do you report to the nurse?
- A Bleeding, swelling, or redness of the gums
- B Irritations, sores, or white patches in the mouth or on the tongue
- C Lips that are dry, cracked, swollen, or blistered
- D All of the above

18 Which is *not* a purpose of bathing?
- A Increasing circulation
- B Promoting drying of the skin
- C Exercising body parts
- D Refreshing and relaxing the resident

19 Soaps do the following *except*
- A Remove dirt and dead skin
- B Remove pigment
- C Remove skin oil and perspiration
- D Dry the skin

20 Which action is *wrong* when bathing Mrs. Hart?
- A Cover her for warmth and privacy.
- B Rinse her skin thoroughly to remove all soaps.
- C Wash from the dirtiest to cleanest area.
- D Pat her skin dry.

21 Water for Mrs. Hart's complete bed bath is at least
- A 100° F
- B 105° F
- C 110° F
- D 120° F

22 You are going to give Mrs. Hart a back massage. Which is *false?*
- A The massage should last about 5 minutes.
- B Lotion is warmed before being applied.
- C Your hands are always in contact with the skin.
- D The side-lying position is best.

Answers to these questions are on p. 697.

14

Skin and Nail Care

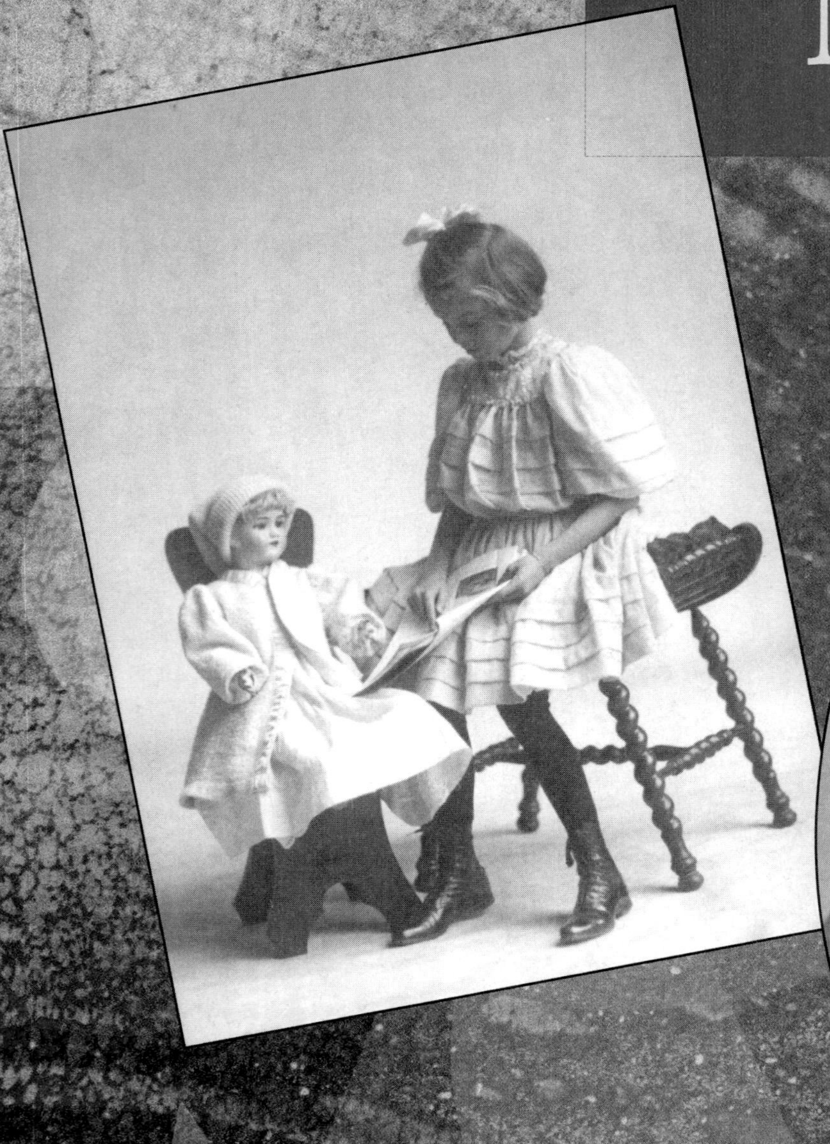

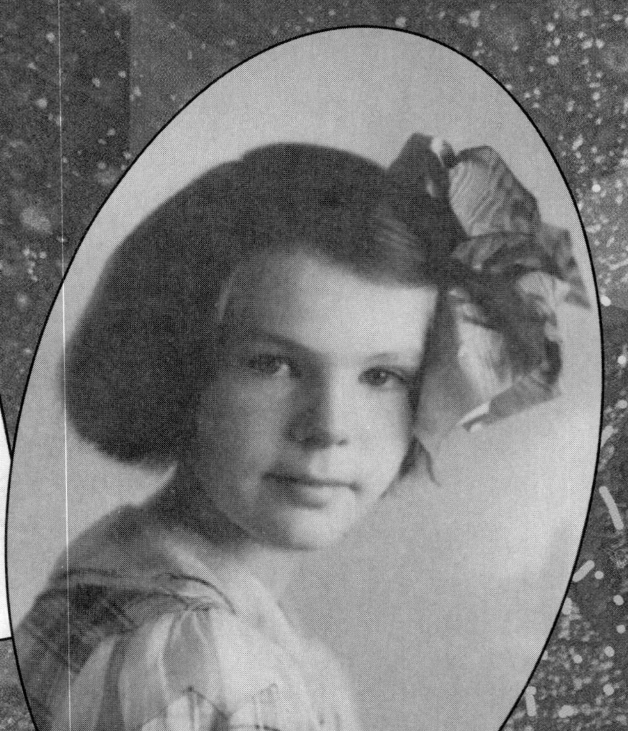

What You Will Learn

- The definition of the key terms listed in this chapter
- The importance of providing good skin care for all residents
- The residents at risk for common skin problems
- The causes of skin tears and how to prevent them
- The signs, symptoms, and causes of pressure ulcers
- The pressure points of the body in the prone, supine, lateral, Fowler's, and sitting positions
- How to prevent pressure ulcers
- The causes of circulatory ulcers and how to prevent them
- How to care for residents with common types of skin breakdown
- How to give foot and nail care
- The different types of wounds
- The process, types, and complications of wound healing
- The observations to make about a wound
- The different types of wound drainage
- How to meet the basic needs of persons with wounds
- The procedures described in this chapter

Key Terms

abrasion A partial-thickness wound caused by the scraping away or rubbing of the skin

arterial ulcer An open wound on the lower legs and feet caused by decreased blood flow through the arteries

bed sore A pressure ulcer, decubitus ulcer, or pressure sore

chronic wound A wound that does not heal easily

circulatory ulcer An open wound on the lower legs and feet caused by a decrease in blood flow through arteries and veins; vascular wound

clean-contaminated wound A wound occurring from the surgical entry of the urinary, reproductive, respiratory, or gastrointestinal system

clean wound A wound that is not infected; microbes have not entered the wound

closed wound A wound in which tissues are injured but the skin is not broken

contaminated wound A wound with a high risk of infection

contusion A closed wound caused by a blow to the body

decubitus ulcer A pressure ulcer, pressure sore, or bed sore

dehiscence The separation of wound layers

dirty wound An infected wound

edema Swelling caused by fluid collecting in tissues

embolus A blood clot that travels through the vascular system until it lodges in a distant vessel

evisceration The separation of the wound along with the protrusion of abdominal organs

full-thickness wound The dermis, epidermis, and subcutaneous tissue are penetrated; muscle and bone may be involved

gangrene A condition in which there is death of tissue

incision An open wound with clean, straight edges; usually intentionally produced with a sharp instrument

infected wound A wound that contains large amounts of bacteria and that shows signs of infection; a dirty wound

intentional wound A wound created for therapy

laceration An open wound with torn tissues and jagged edges

open wound The skin or mucous membrane is broken

Continued

KEY TERMS—cont'd

partial-thickness wound A wound in which the dermis and epidermis of the skin are broken

penetrating wound An open wound in which the skin and underlying tissues are pierced

phlebitis Inflammation *(itis)* of a vein *(phleb)*

podiatrist A foot *(pod)* doctor

pressure sore A bed sore, decubitus ulcer, or pressure ulcer

pressure ulcer Any injury caused by unrelieved pressure; a decubitus ulcer, bedsore, or pressure sore

puncture wound An open wound made by a sharp object; entry of the skin and underlying tissues; may be intentional or unintentional

purulent drainage Thick green, yellow, or brown drainage

sanguineous drainage Bloody drainage *(sanguis)*

serosanguineous drainage Thin, watery drainage *(sero)* that is blood-tinged *(sanguineous)*

serous drainage Clear, watery fluid (serum)

skin tear A break or rip in the skin that separates the epidermis from underlying tissue

stasis ulcer An open wound on the lower legs and feet caused by poor blood return through the veins; venous ulcer

thrombus A blood clot

trauma An accident or violent act that injures the skin, mucous membranes, bones, and internal organs

unintentional wound A wound resulting from trauma

vascular wound A circulatory ulcer

venous ulcer A stasis ulcer

wound A break in the skin or mucous membrane

Skin and nail care are very important to a resident's overall health and quality of life. The skin is the body's first line of defense against changes in the environment. It protects the body from microbes, which cause infection. It also helps regulate the body's temperature. Providing good skin and nail care to residents every day is one of your most important jobs.

Older and disabled persons are at great risk for skin breakdown and nail problems. Their skin is easily injured. Causes include age-related changes in the skin, chronic disease, and general debility. The health care team carefully assesses the resident's potential for skin breakdown. (See Box 14-1 for common causes of skin breakdown.)The nurse uses the nursing process to help the health care team keep the resident's skin and nails healthy. Some centers have a skin care team to manage all skin problems. Team members usually include an RN, a physical therapist, and a dietician. The care plan gives specific skin care instructions for the individual resident. You must use great care when moving, bathing, dressing, and undressing residents to prevent injury to the skin. Always follow the care plan.

SKIN TEARS

A **skin tear** is a break or rip in the skin that separates the epidermis (top layer of skin) from the underlying tissue (see Figure 6-4, p. 96). The hands, arms, and

Box 14-1 Common Causes of Skin Breakdown

- Age-related changes in the skin
- Dryness
- Fragile and weak capillaries
- General thinning of the skin
- Loss of fatty layer under the skin
- Decreased sensation to touch, heat, and cold
- Decreased mobility
- Sitting in a chair or lying in bed most or all of the day
- Chronic diseases (diabetes, high blood pressure)
- Diseases that decrease circulation
- Poor nutrition and poor hydration
- Incontinence
- Moisture in dark areas of the body (skin folds, under breasts, and perineal areas)
- Pressure on bony parts (Fig. 14-1)
- Poor care of fingernails or toenails
- Friction and shearing

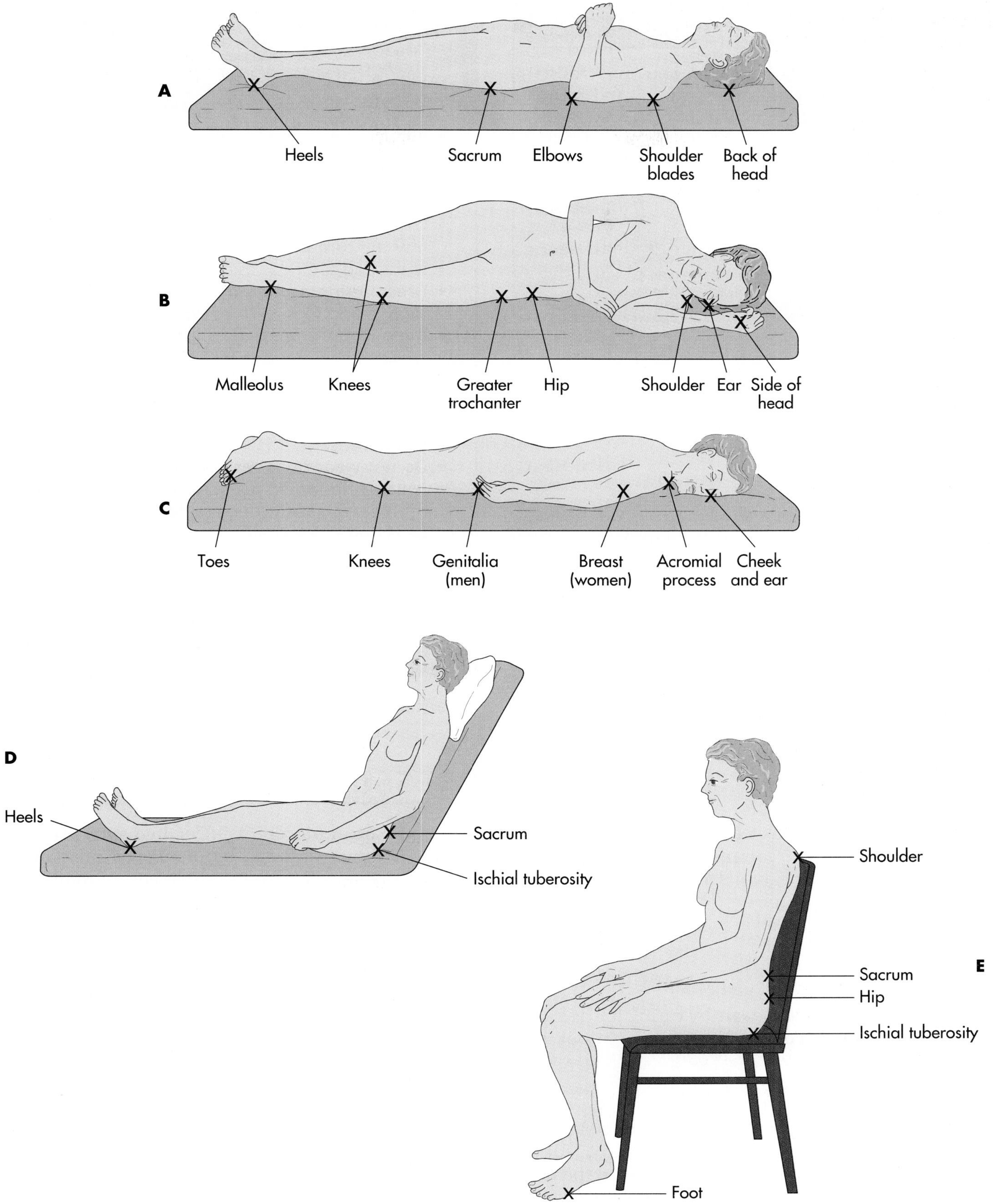

Fig. 14-1 Pressure points. **A,** The supine position. **B,** The lateral position. **C,** The prone position. **D,** Fowler's position. **E,** The sitting position.

RESIDENTS WITH DEMENTIA

Some residents are confused and may resist care at times. They may move quickly and without warning. Or they may pull away from you during care. Some residents try to hit or kick caregivers. These unexpected movements can cause skin tears. When giving care to a resident who resists care, ask the nurse for help. Never force care on a resident. See Chapter 27 for approaches to use when caring for residents who are confused and resist care. Always follow the care plan.

lower legs are common sites for skin tears. Many residents have very thin and fragile skin. Even a small amount of pressure can cause a skin tear.

Causes

Skin tears are caused by shearing (see Chapter 10), pulling, or direct pressure on the skin. For example, a skin tear can occur by bumping a hand, arm, or leg on a bed rail, wheelchair foot pedal, or other hard surface. A caregiver can cause a skin tear by holding on to a resident's arm or leg too tightly when moving the person. Buttons or zippers pulled across fragile skin can also cause a skin tear. Skin tears are painful. They provide a portal of entry for microbes. You must notify the nurse immediately if you cause or find a skin tear on a resident. (*See Residents With Dementia.*)

Residents at Risk

Residents at risk for skins tears are those who:

- Require moderate to complete help in moving
- Have poor nutrition
- Have poor hydration
- Have altered mental awareness
- Are very thin

Prevention

You can help prevent skin tears by caring for residents carefully and safely. Follow the measures in Box 14-2 to prevent skin tears.

Treatment

The doctor and the skin care team direct skin tear treatment. Special dressings may be ordered. Elastic wraps protect the skin from injury and help the healing process (p. 318). You must be very careful when providing care to decrease the risk of further injury. Check the care plan and ask the nurse for specific instructions.

BOX 14-2 MEASURES TO PREVENT SKIN TEARS

- Follow the care plan for moving, dressing, and bathing residents.
- Keep residents' skin well lubricated. Follow the care plan.
- Offer fluids to keep residents hydrated. Follow the care plan.
- Dress and undress residents carefully.
- Dress residents in soft clothing with long sleeves and legs, such as sweat suits.
- Keep your fingernails short and smoothly filed.
- Keep residents' fingernails and toenails short and smoothly filed. If you are not allowed to trim toenails, report long and rough toenails to the nurse.
- Do not wear rings with large stones.
- Follow the safety rules in Chapter 10 when lifting and transferring residents to and from beds and wheelchairs.
- Be patient and stay calm when caring for confused or agitated residents or those who resist care.
- Pad bed rails and wheelchair arms and foot pedals. Follow the care plan.

PRESSURE ULCERS

A **pressure ulcer (decubitus ulcer, bed sore, pressure sore)** is any injury caused by unrelieved pressure. It usually occurs over a bony prominence. Prominence means to stick out. Therefore a bony prominence is an area where the bone sticks out or projects out from the flat surface of the body. The shoulder blades, elbows, hip bones, sacrum, knees, ankle bones, heels, and toes are bony prominences (see Figure 14-1).

Causes

Pressure, friction, and shearing are common causes of skin breakdown and pressure ulcers. Other factors include breaks in the skin, poor circulation to an area, moisture, dry skin, and irritation by urine and feces.

Pressure occurs when the skin over a bony prominence is squeezed between hard surfaces. The bone itself is one hard surface. The other is usually the mattress or chair seat. The squeezing or pressure prevents blood flow to the skin and underlying tissues. Lack of

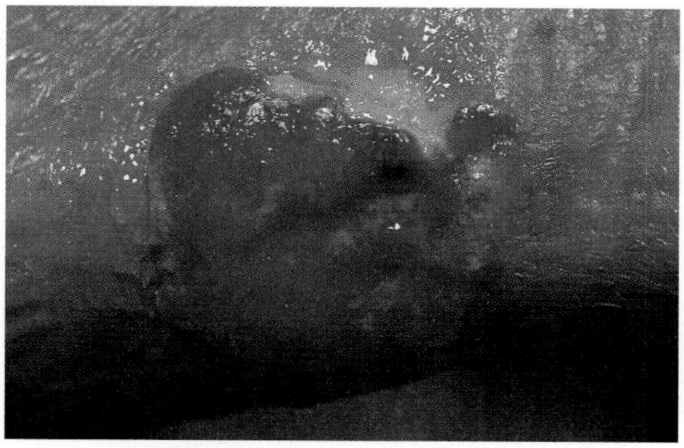

Fig. 14-2 A pressure ulcer.

blood flow means oxygen and nutrients cannot get to the cells. Therefore the involved skin and tissues die (Fig. 14-2).

Friction scrapes the skin. An open area, the scrape is a portal of entry for microbes. The open area needs to heal. A good blood supply to the area is necessary. Infection is prevented so healing occurs. A poor blood supply or an infection can lead to a pressure ulcer.

Shearing is when the skin sticks to a surface (usually the bed or chair) and deeper tissues move downward (see Fig. 10-5, p. 199). This occurs when a resident is sitting in a chair or in Fowler's position. Shearing occurs when the resident slides down in the bed or chair. Blood vessels and tissues are damaged. Therefore blood flow to the area is reduced.

Residents at Risk

The nurse uses the nursing process to identify residents at risk for pressure ulcers. Residents at risk for pressure ulcers are those who:

- Are confined to bed or chair
- Require moderate to complete help in moving
- Have loss of bowel or bladder control
- Have poor nutrition
- Have poor hydration
- Have altered mental awareness
- Have problems sensing pain or pressure
- Have circulatory problems
- Are older, obese, or very thin

Signs of Pressure Ulcers

The first sign of a pressure ulcer is pale skin or a reddened area. Color changes may be difficult to notice in residents with dark skin. The resident may complain of pain, burning, or tingling in the area. Some do not feel anything unusual. Box 14-3 describes the four stages of pressure ulcer development.

Box 14-3 Stages of Pressure Ulcers

Stage 1	The skin is red. The color does not return to normal when the skin is relieved of pressure (Fig. 14-3, *A*, p. 304).
Stage 2	The skin cracks, blisters, or peels (Fig. 14-3, *B*, p. 304). There may be a shallow crater.
Stage 3	The skin is gone, and the underlying tissues are exposed (Fig. 14-3, *C*, p. 304). The exposed tissue is damaged. There may be drainage from the area.
Stage 4	Muscle and bone are exposed and damaged (Fig. 14-3, *D*, p. 304). Drainage is likely.

Sites

Pressure ulcers usually occur over bony areas. The bony areas are called *pressure points* because they bear the weight of the body in a certain position. Pressure from body weight can reduce the blood supply to the area. Figure 14-1 shows the pressure points for the bed positions and the sitting position. In obese people, pressure ulcers can develop in areas where skin is in contact with skin. Friction results when this occurs. Pressure ulcers can develop between abdominal folds, the legs, and the buttocks and under the breasts.

Prevention

Preventing pressure ulcers is much easier than trying to heal them. Good nursing care, cleanliness, and skin care are essential. Any resident at risk for developing a pressure ulcer should be placed on a pressure-reducing surface. Such surfaces include foam, air, alternating air, gel, or water mattresses. The health care team decides which surface is best for each resident. The measures listed in Box 14-4 on p. 305 help prevent skin breakdown and pressure ulcers.

OBRA and JCAHO require that the health care team develop an individualized plan of care to prevent pressure ulcers in residents at risk. You must know and follow the care plan. OBRA

Treatment

The doctor directs pressure ulcer treatment. Wound care products, drugs, treatments, and special equipment are ordered to promote healing. The nurse and the care plan tell you about a resident's treatment. (*See Subacute Care, p. 306.*) The following protective devices are often ordered to prevent and treat pressure ulcers and other types of skin breakdown.

Text continued on p. 306

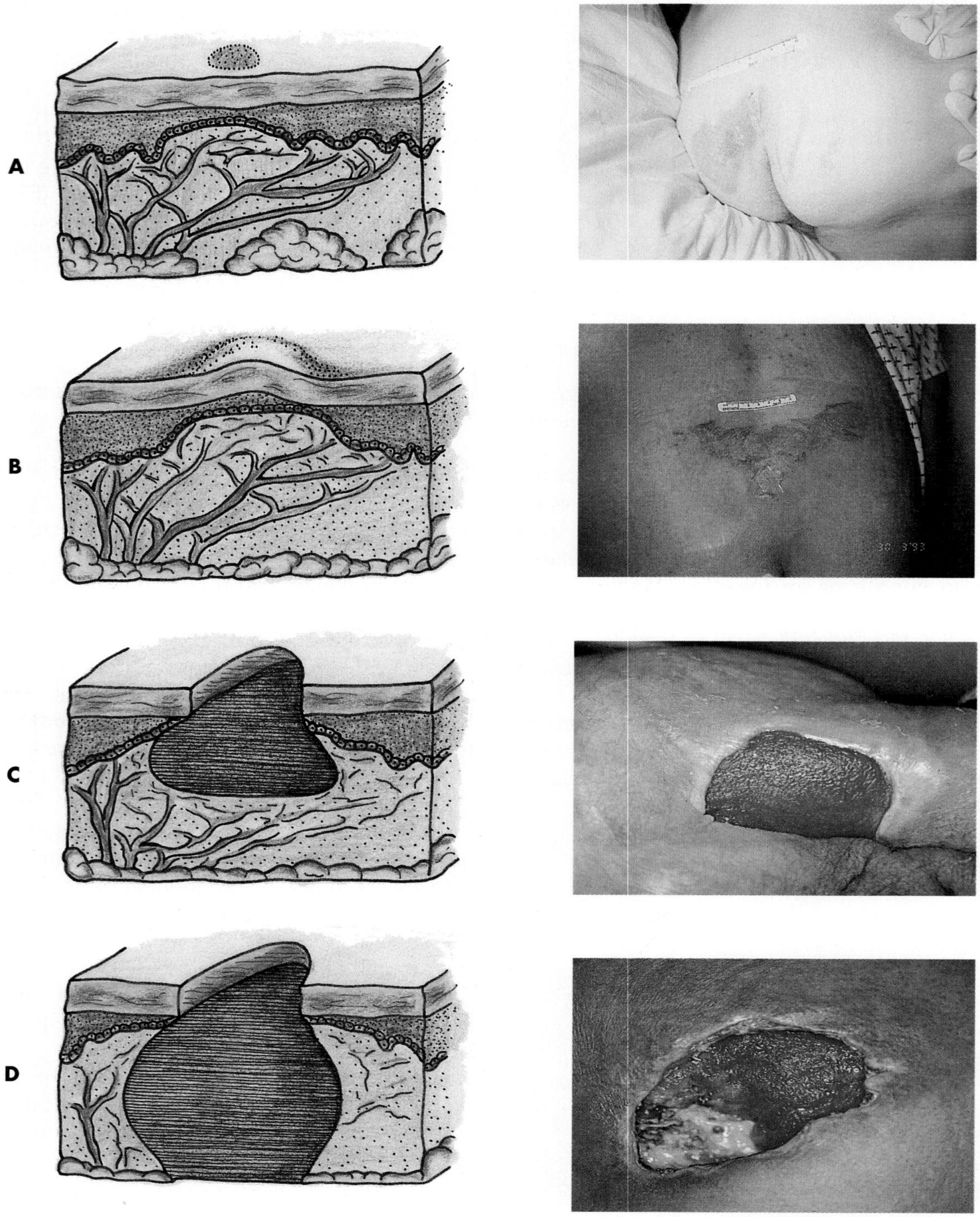

Fig. 14-3 Stages of a pressure ulcer. **A,** Stage 1. **B,** Stage 2. **C,** Stage 3. **D,** Stage 4. *(Courtesy Laurel Wiersma-Bryant, RN, MSN, Clinical Nurse Specialist, Barnes-Jewish Hospital, St Louis, Mo.)*

Box 14-4 Measures to Prevent Pressure Ulcers

- Reposition the resident at least every 2 hours or as scheduled in the resident's care plan. Some residents are repositioned every 15 minutes. Use pillows for support as instructed by the nurse. The 30-degree lateral position is recommended (Fig. 14-4).
- Prevent shearing and friction during lifting and moving procedures.
- Prevent shearing by not raising the head of the bed more than 30 degrees. Follow the care plan.
- Prevent friction by applying a thin layer of cornstarch to the bottom sheets.
- Provide good skin care. Make sure skin is clean and dry after bathing. The skin is free of moisture from urine, feces, perspiration, and wound drainage.
- Minimize skin exposure to moisture. Check incontinent residents (those without bowel or bladder control) often. Also check residents who perspire heavily and those with wound drainage. Change linens and clothing as needed, and provide good skin care.
- Check with the nurse before using soap. Remember that soap can dry and irritate the skin.
- Apply a moisturizer to dry areas such as the hands, elbows, legs, ankles, and heels. The nurse tells you what to use and the areas that need attention.
- Give a back massage when repositioning the resident. Do not massage bony areas.
- Keep linens clean, dry, and free of wrinkles.
- Apply powder where skin touches skin.
- Do not irritate the skin. Avoid scrubbing or vigorous rubbing when bathing or drying the resident.
- Avoid massaging over pressure points. *Never rub or massage reddened areas.*
- Use pillows and blankets to prevent skin from being in contact with skin and to reduce moisture and friction.
- Keep the heels off the bed. Use pillows or other devices as instructed by the nurse. Place the pillows or devices under the lower legs from midcalf to the ankles.
- Use protective devices as instructed by the nurse and the care plan (pp. 306-307).
- Remind residents sitting in a chair to shift their position every 15 minutes. This decreases pressure on bony points.
- Report any signs of skin breakdown or pressure ulcers immediately to the nurse.

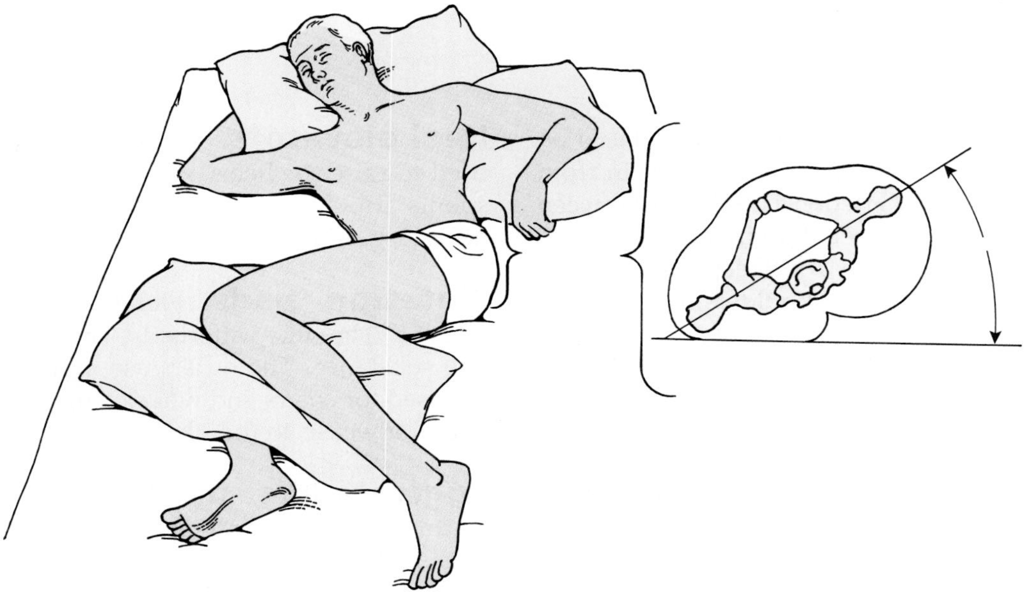

Fig. 14-4 The 30-degree lateral position. Pillows are placed under the head, shoulder, and leg. This position inclines (lifts up) the hip to avoid pressure on the hip. The person does not lie on the hip as in the side-lying position. *(From Potter PA, Perry, AG:* Fundamentals of nursing: concepts, process, and practice, *ed 4, St Louis, 1997, Mosby.)*

SUBACUTE CARE

You may see other beds on subacute and rehabilitation units. One type allows repositioning without moving the patient. Depending on the bed, the patient is turned to the prone or supine position or tilted various degrees. Body alignment does not change. Pressure points change as the position changes. There is little friction.

Some beds constantly rotate from side to side. These beds are useful for patients with spinal cord injuries. They are also used for patients receiving respiratory rehabilitation.

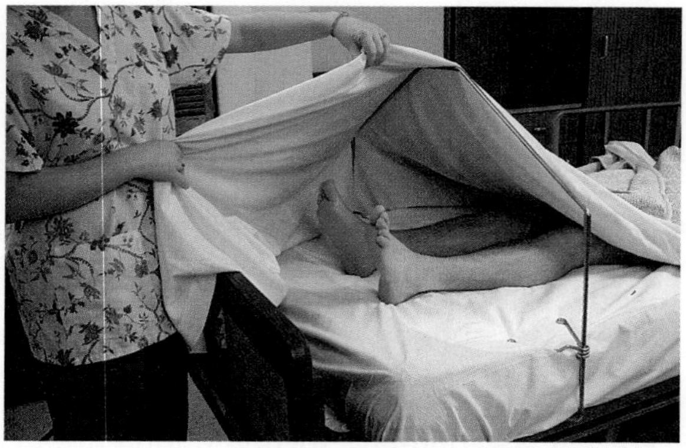

Fig. 14-6 A bed cradle is placed on top of the bed. Linens are brought over the top of the cradle to keep them off the feet.

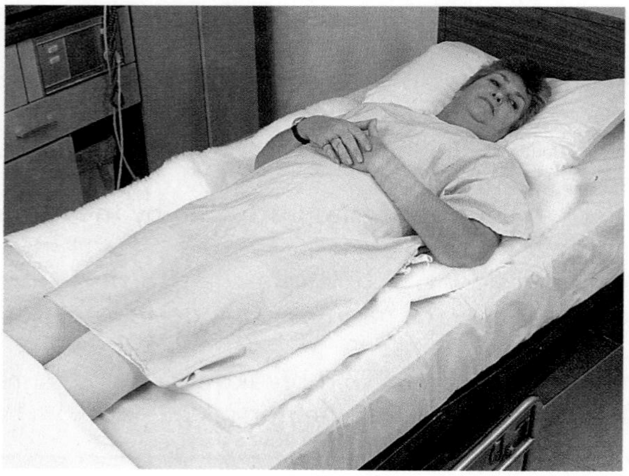

Fig. 14-5 Sheepskin.

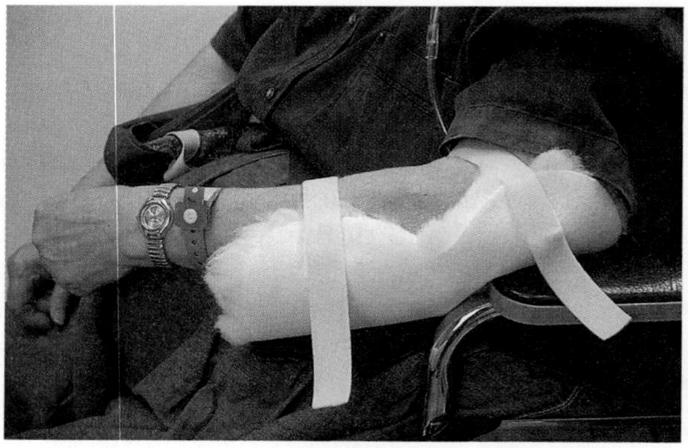

Fig. 14-7 Elbow protector.

Sheepskin. Sheepskin (lamb's wool) is placed on the bottom sheet (Fig. 14-5). It protects the skin from the irritating bed linens. Friction is reduced between the skin and the bottom sheet. Air circulates between the tufts to help keep the skin dry. Sheepskin comes in many sizes for use under the shoulders, buttocks, or heels. It can also be placed in chair seats.

Bed cradle. A bed cradle (Anderson frame) is a metal frame placed on the bed and over the resident. Top linens are brought over the cradle to prevent pressure on the legs and feet (Fig. 14-6). Top linens are tucked in at the bottom of the mattress and mitered. They are also tucked under both sides of the mattress to protect the resident from air drafts and chilling.

Elbow protectors. Elbow protectors are made of foam rubber or sheepskin. They fit the shape of the elbow (Fig. 14-7) and are secured in place with straps. Friction is prevented between the bed and the elbow.

Heel elevators. Pillows or special cushions are used to raise the heels off the bed. Special braces and splints also are used to keep pressure away from the heels (Fig. 14-8).

Flotation pads. Flotation pads or cushions (Fig. 14-9) are like waterbeds. They are made of a gel-like substance. The outer case is heavy plastic. They are used for chairs and wheelchairs. The pad is placed in a pillowcase so the plastic does not touch the skin.

Eggcrate-like mattress. The eggcrate-like mattress is a foam pad that looks like an egg carton (Fig. 14-10). Peaks in the mattress distribute the resident's weight more evenly. The eggcrate-like mattress is placed on top of the regular mattress. Only a bottom sheet covers the eggcrate-like mattress. Before the bottom sheet is put on, the eggcrate-like mattress is put in a special cover. The cover protects against moisture and soiling.

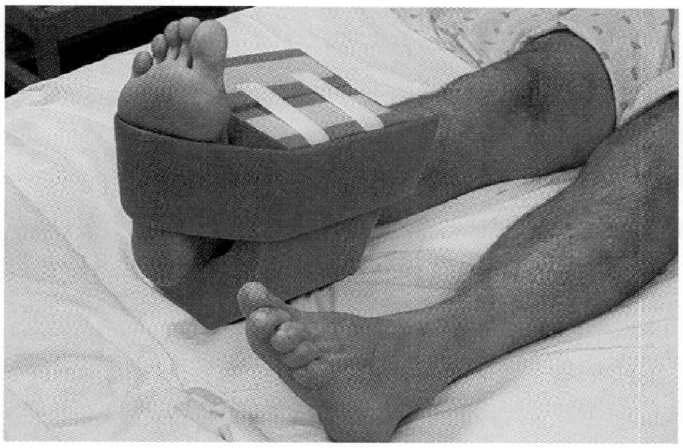

Fig. 14-8 Heel elevator.

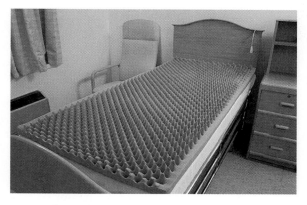

Fig. 14-10 Eggcrate-like mattress.

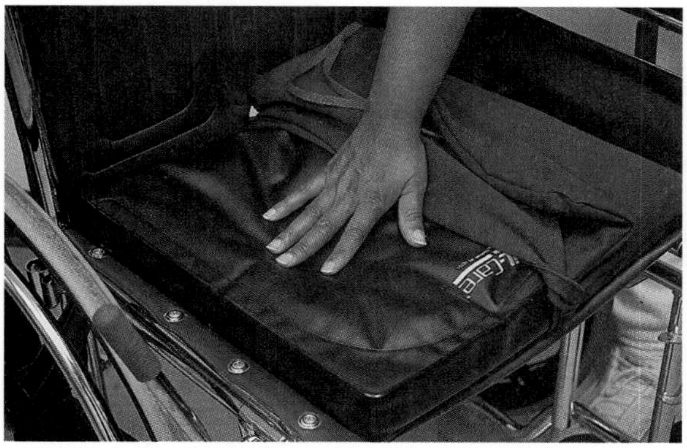

Fig. 14-9 Flotation pad.

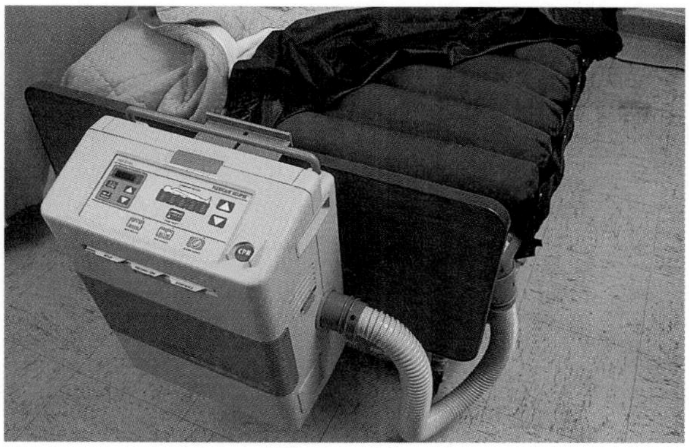

Fig. 14-11 Air flotation bed.

Special beds. Some beds have air flowing through the mattress (Fig. 14-11). The *person floats* on the mattress. Body weight is distributed evenly. There is little pressure on bony parts.

Other equipment. Trochanter rolls and footboards are also used to prevent and treat pressure ulcers. These are described in Chapter 19.

LEG AND FOOT ULCERS

Some residents have diseases that affect the blood flow to and from the legs and feet. They require special skin care. Poor circulation to and from the legs and feet can lead to pain, open wounds, and edema. **Edema** is swelling caused by fluid collecting in tissues. Infection and gangrene can result from the open wound and poor circulation. **Gangrene** is a condition in which there is death of tissue (see Chapter 26.)

The doctor directs the resident's care. The nurse uses the nursing process to help the health care team develop and carry out the right plan of care. Preventing skin breakdown on the legs and feet is very important.

Circulatory Ulcers

Circulatory ulcers (vascular wounds) are wounds caused by a decrease in blood flow through arteries or veins. Older residents with certain diseases affecting the blood vessels are at risk for these ulcers on the legs and feet. These wounds are often painful. They are difficult to heal and require special care by the entire health care team.

Stasis Ulcers

Stasis ulcers (venous ulcers) are wounds on the legs and feet caused by poor blood return to the heart from the legs and feet (Fig. 14-12, p. 308). The valves in the veins do not close efficiently. Therefore the veins do not pump blood back to the heart normally. This

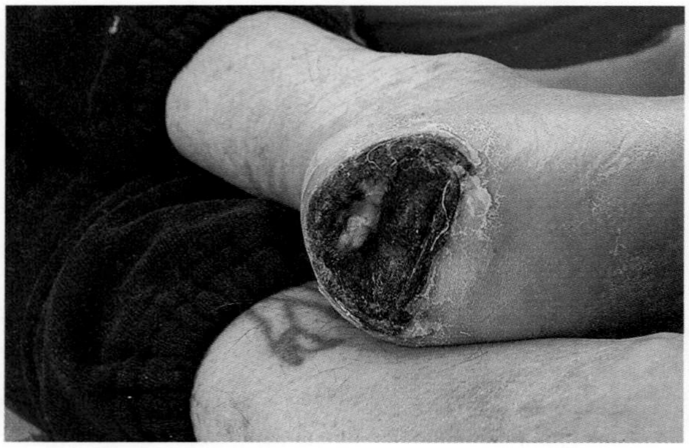

Fig. 14-12 Stasis ulcer.

Box 14-5 Measures for Preventing Stasis Ulcers

- Apply elastic stockings or elastic wraps according to the care plan.
- Remind residents not to sit with legs crossed.
- Do not use elastic, rubberband-type garters to hold the resident's socks or hose in place.
- Do not dress residents in tight clothing.
- Provide good skin care daily. Make sure areas between the toes are clean and dry.
- Avoid injury to legs and feet when providing resident care.
- Keep linens clean, dry, and free of wrinkles.
- Walk residents and exercise residents' legs to increase venous blood flow. Follow the resident's care plan.
- Reposition the resident at least every 2 hours. Follow the resident's care plan.
- Encourage residents to elevate the legs. Follow the resident's care plan.
- Make sure the resident wears comfortable socks and shoes.
- Do not irritate the skin. Avoid scrubbing or vigorous rubbing when bathing or drying the resident.
- Avoid massaging over pressure points. *Never rub or massage reddened areas.*
- Keep the heels off the bed. Use pillows or other devices as instructed by the nurse. Place the pillows or devices under the lower legs from midcalf to the ankles.
- Use protective devices as instructed by the nurse (p. 306). Follow the care plan.
- Report any signs of skin breakdown or pressure ulcers immediately to the nurse.

causes blood and fluid to collect in the legs and feet. Edema occurs in the legs and feet. Small veins in the skin can rupture. Remember, hemoglobin gives blood its red color. When the veins rupture, hemoglobin is released into the tissues. This causes the skin to turn brown. The skin also is dry, leathery, and hard. Residents often complain of itching.

Ulcers occur from skin injury. Scratching itching skin is a common cause of injury. Or the ulcers occur spontaneously. Stasis ulcers are painful and make walking difficult. Stasis ulcers weep fluid. The ulcer is an open wound. Infection is a great risk.

Causes. Some chronic diseases cause blood and fluid to collect in the legs and feet. The skin is more prone to injury and slow to heal. Even a small injury may lead to an ulcer. The problem is made worse by smoking, obesity, inactivity, and long periods with the legs down. Pressure under the knees also makes the problem worse.

Residents at risk. Risk factors for the development of stasis ulcers include:

- History of blood clots or varicose veins
- Decreased mobility
- Obesity
- Injury to the legs or feet
- Advanced age
- Surgery on bones and joints of the legs
- **Phlebitis** (inflammation *[itis]* of a vein *[phleb]*)

Sites. Stasis ulcers are found on the lower legs and feet. The heels and inner aspect of the ankles are common sites for stasis ulcers. These sites are observed carefully.

Prevention. Preventing skin breakdown caused by poor venous circulation is very important. Stasis ulcers are hard to heal once they develop. The nurse uses the nursing process to help the care team develop a plan to prevent skin breakdown. Box 14-5 lists the measures for preventing stasis ulcers.

Residents at risk have routine professional foot care (p. 314). Toenails, corns, and calluses are treated. (Nursing assistants do not cut toenails for residents with diseases that affect venous circulation.)

The doctor may order elastic support stockings or special elastic wraps. They promote comfort and circulation by providing support and pressure to the veins. They also promote healing and prevent injury. They must be applied properly. Otherwise severe discomfort, skin irritation, and circulatory complications occur.

◈ **Elastic stockings.** Elastic stockings often are ordered for residents with circulatory disorders and heart disease. They also are indicated for residents on bedrest. These residents are at risk for developing blood clots (thrombi). A blood clot is called a **thrombus.**

Blood clots can form if blood flow is sluggish. They are more likely to form in deep leg veins (Fig. 14-13, *A,* p. 310). A thrombus can break loose and travel through the bloodstream. It then becomes an embolus. An **embolus** is a blood clot that travels through the vascular system until it lodges in a distant vessel (Fig. 14-13, *B*). An embolus from a vein can eventually lodge in the lung *(pulmonary embolus).* A pulmonary embolus can cause severe respiratory problems and death.

Elastic stockings are also known as *antiembolism stockings* or *antiembolic* (*AE*) stockings. They help prevent the development of thrombi. The elastic exerts pressure on the veins, promoting venous blood flow to the heart.

Stockings come in many sizes. Thigh-high and knee-high lengths are available. The nurse measures the resident to determine the proper size. The stockings are removed at least twice a day. They are applied before the resident gets out of bed.

Applying Elastic Stockings

NNAAP™ SKILL

Quality of Life

Remember to:

- *Knock before entering the resident's room*
- *Address the resident by name*
- *Introduce yourself by name and title*

Pre-Procedure

1 Explain the procedure to the resident.
2 Wash your hands.
3 Obtain elastic stockings in the correct size.
4 Identify the resident. Check the ID bracelet against the assignment sheet.
5 Provide for privacy.
6 Raise the bed to the best position for good body mechanics. Make sure bed rails are up.
7 Lower the bed rail near you.

Procedure

8 Position the resident supine.
9 Expose the legs. Fanfold top linens toward the resident.
10 Turn the stocking inside out down to the heel (Fig. 14-14, *A,* p. 310).
11 Slip the foot of the stocking over the toes, foot, and heel (Fig. 14-14, *B,* p. 310).
12 Grasp the stocking top. Slip it over the foot and heel, and pull it up the leg. It turns right side out as it is pulled up. The stocking should be even and snug (Fig. 14-14, *C,* p. 310).
13 Make sure the stocking is not twisted and has no creases or wrinkles.
14 Repeat steps 10 through 13 for the other leg.

Post-Procedure

15 Return top linens to their proper position.
16 Provide for comfort.
17 Lower the bed to its lowest position.
18 Raise or lower bed rails. Follow the care plan.
19 Place the signal light within reach.
20 Unscreen the resident.
21 Wash your hands.
22 Tell the nurse that the stockings were applied.

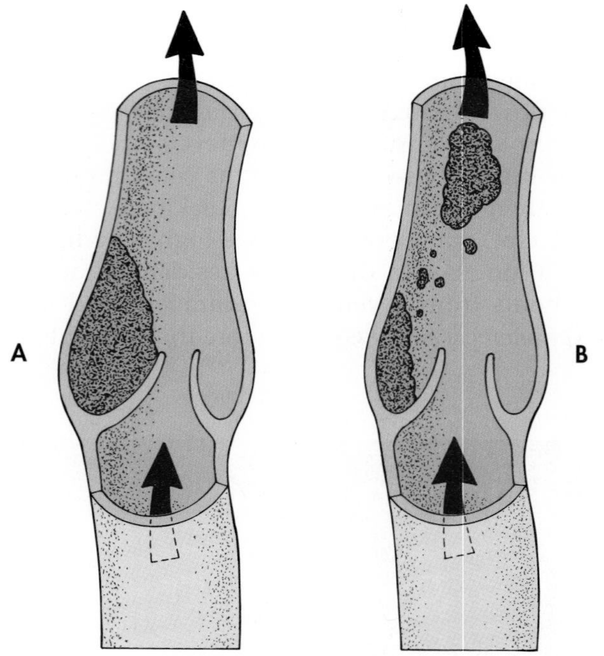

Fig. 14-13 A, A blood clot is attached to the wall of a vein. The arrows show the direction of blood flow. **B,** Part of the thrombus has broken off and is an embolus. The embolus will travel in the bloodstream until it lodges in a distant vessel.

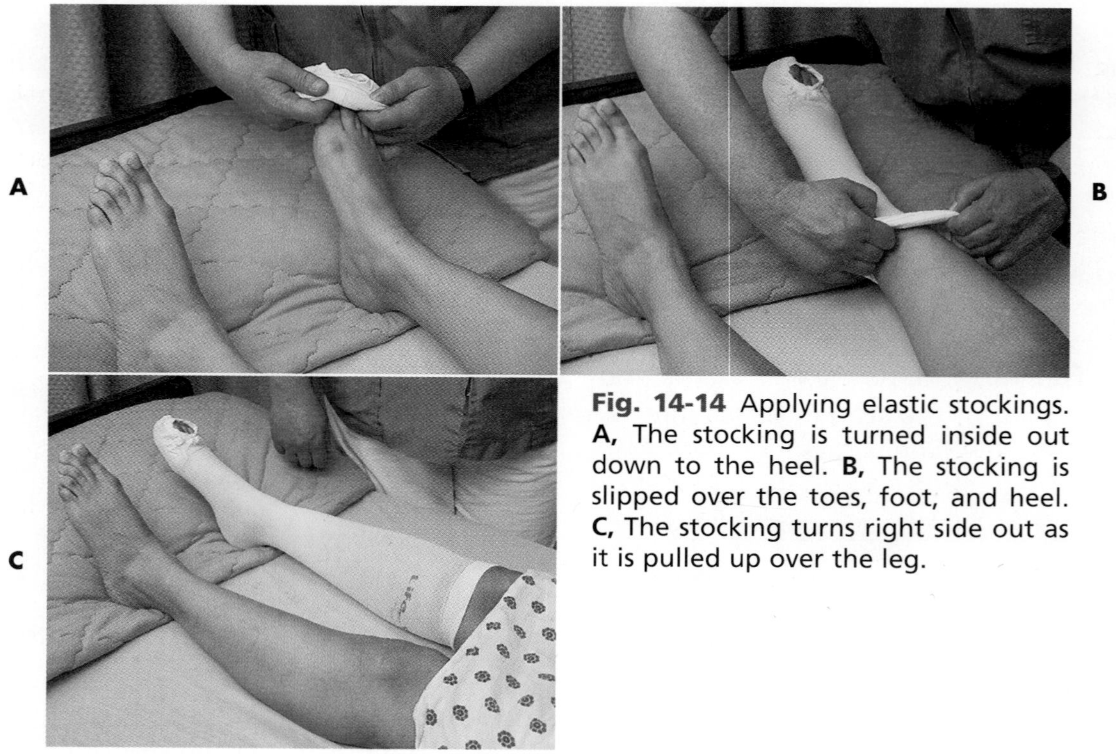

Fig. 14-14 Applying elastic stockings. **A,** The stocking is turned inside out down to the heel. **B,** The stocking is slipped over the toes, foot, and heel. **C,** The stocking turns right side out as it is pulled up over the leg.

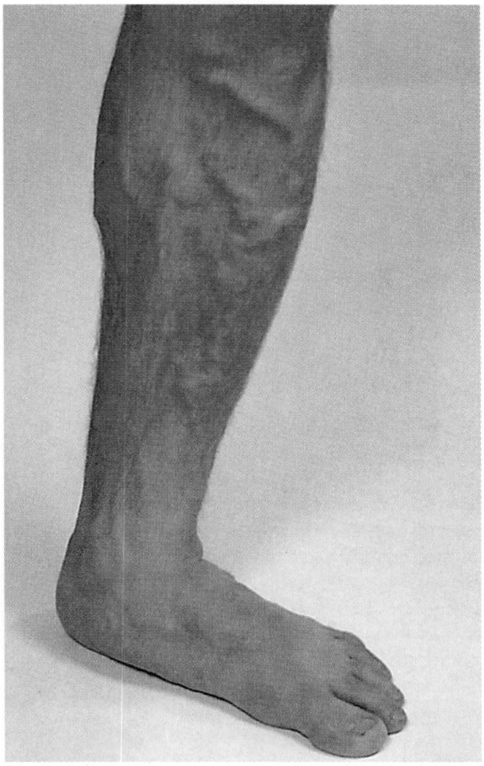

Fig. 14-15 Varicose veins. *(From Belch J, et al:* Color atlas of peripheral vascular diseases, *ed 2, London, 1996, Wolfe Medical Publishers.)*

Elastic bandages. Elastic bandages have the same purposes as elastic stockings. They also provide support and reduce swelling from injuries. In addition, they can hold dressings in place. They are applied to the upper or lower extremities.

Elastic bandages may be ordered for residents with varicose veins. Varicose veins are veins under the skin that have become dilated (wide) and bulging (Fig. 14-15).

The bandage is applied from the lower (distal) part of the extremity to the top (proximal) part. The nurse tells you what area to bandage. Some centers do not let nursing assistants apply elastic bandages. Make sure that you know the center's policy.

You need to follow these rules when applying elastic bandages:

- Obtain the elastic bandage in the proper length and width.
- Make sure the extremity is in good alignment.
- Face the resident during the procedure.
- Leave fingers or toes exposed if possible. This allows for circulation checks.
- Apply the bandage with firm, even pressure.
- Check the color and temperature of the extremity every hour.
- Reapply a loose, wrinkled, moist, or soiled bandage.

Treatment. The doctor directs stasis ulcer treatment. Some centers also have skin teams to manage the care of stasis ulcers. The doctor may order drugs to decrease swelling and to treat or prevent infection. Medicated leg wrappings and other wound care products are often part of the treatment plan. The equipment used to treat pressure ulcers also is used to treat stasis ulcers. Preventing further injury is important. Move and transfer residents carefully to avoid bumping the legs and feet.

Applying Elastic Bandages

Quality of Life

Remember to:
- ◆ *Knock before entering the resident's room*
- ◆ *Address the resident by name*
- ◆ *Introduce yourself by name and title*

Pre-Procedure

1 Explain the procedure to the resident.
2 Wash your hands.
3 Collect the following:
   - Elastic bandage as directed by the nurse
   - Tape, metal clips, or safety pins (follow center policy)
4 Identify the resident. Check the ID bracelet against the assignment sheet.
5 Provide for privacy.
6 Raise the bed to the best level for good body mechanics. Make sure bed rails are up.

Procedure

7 Lower the bed rail near you.
8 Help the resident to a comfortable position. Expose the part you will bandage.
9 Make sure the area is clean and dry.
10 Hold the bandage so that the roll is up and the loose end is on the bottom (Fig. 14-16, *A,* p. 311).
11 Apply the bandage to the smallest part of the wrist, foot, ankle, or knee.
12 Make two circular turns around the part (Fig. 14-16, *B,* p. 311).
13 Make overlapping spiral turns in an upward direction. Each turn overlaps about 2/3 (two thirds) of the previous turn (Fig. 14-16, *C,* p. 311).
14 Apply the bandage smoothly with firm, even pressure. The bandage should not be tight.
15 Pin, tape, or clip the end of the bandage to hold it in place. (Do not put tape around entire part.) Make sure the pin or clip is not under the part.
16 Check the fingers or toes for coldness or cyanosis. Also check for complaints of pain, numbness, or tingling. Remove the bandage if any are noted. Report your observations to the nurse.

Post-Procedure

17 Provide for comfort.
18 Place the signal light within reach.
19 Lower the bed.
20 Raise or lower bed rails. Follow the care plan.
21 Unscreen the resident.
22 Wash your hands.
23 Report the following to the nurse:
   - The time the bandage was applied
   - The site of the application
   - Any other observations

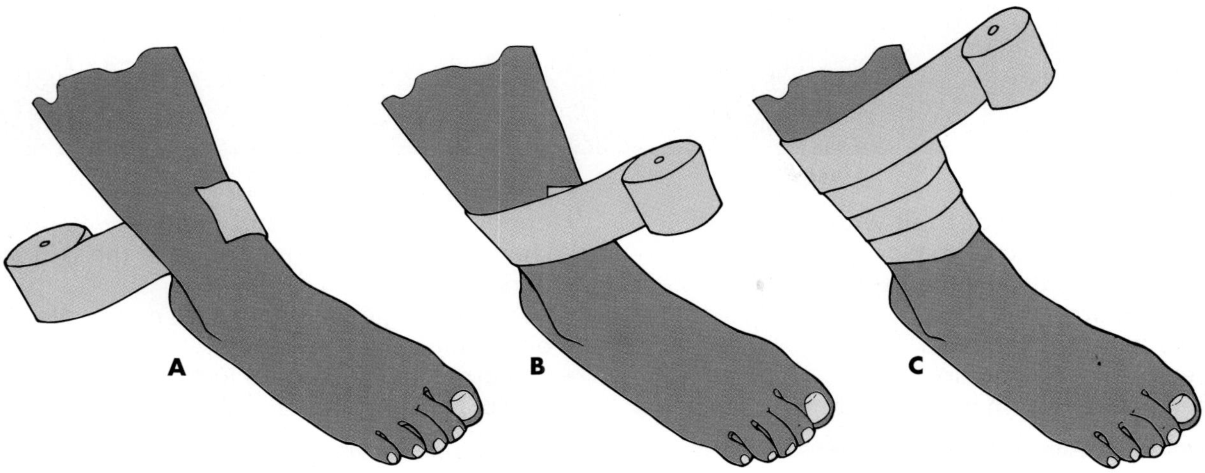

Fig. 14-16 **A,** The roll of the elastic bandage is up, and the loose end is on the bottom. **B,** The bandage is applied to the smallest part with two circular turns. **C,** The bandage is applied with spiral turns in an upward direction.

Arterial Ulcers

Arterial ulcers are open wounds on the lower legs and feet caused by poor blood flow through the arteries. The leg and foot may feel cold and look blue and shiny. The ulcer is often painful when the resident is resting. The pain is usually worse at night.

Causes. Arterial ulcers are caused by diseases or injuries that decrease arterial blood flow to the legs and feet. High blood pressure and diabetes are common causes. Some narrowing of the arteries also occurs as people age (see Chapter 7).

Residents at risk. Risk factors for the development of arterial ulcers include:

- History of diabetes
- History of high blood pressure
- Smoking
- Advanced age

Sites. Arterial ulcers are found between the toes or on the tops of the toes. They are also found on the outer side of the ankle. Areas of the feet exposed to pressure from poorly fitting shoes are common sites. The heels are common sites on residents who are on bedrest.

Prevention. The nurse uses the nursing process to prevent arterial ulcers. Box 14-6 on p. 314 lists preventive measures. The resident's care plan lists specific instructions for foot care.

Residents at risk for arterial ulcers also have routine professional foot care (p. 314). Toenails, corns, and calluses are treated. (Nursing assistants do not cut toenails for residents with diseases that affect arterial circulation.)

Treatment. The doctor directs arterial ulcer treatment. It involves treating the disease process that causes the problem. Drugs to control edema and pain are ordered. Drugs to clean and dress wounds are part of the treatment plan. Exercise and walking schedules are ordered. Always check the care plan with the nurse before giving care to residents with leg and foot wounds. Be very careful not to cause further injury.

Box 14-6 Measures for Preventing Arterial Ulcers

- No smoking.
- Remind residents not to sit with legs crossed.
- Avoid exposure to cold.
- Do not use elastic band garters to hold socks and hose in place.
- Make sure shoes fit well.
- Keep feet clean and dry.
- Keep pressure from heels and other bony points.
- Keep pressure from under the knees.
- Check residents' legs and feet daily. Report any changes in skin color or breaks in the skin to the nurse.
- Avoid massaging over pressure points. *Never rub or massage reddened areas.*
- Use protective devices as instructed by the nurse (p. 306). Follow the care plan.

CARE OF NAILS AND FEET

Nails and feet need special attention to prevent infection, injury, and odors. Hangnails, ingrown nails (nails that grow in at the side), and nails torn away from the skin cause breaks in the skin. These breaks let microbes enter the body. Long or broken nails can scratch the skin or snag clothing. Dirty feet, socks, or stockings can harbor microbes and cause foot odors.

Nails are easier to trim and clean right after they are soaked. After a tub bath or shower is also a good time because the nails already are soft. Nail clippers are used to cut nails. Do not use scissors. Extreme caution is taken to prevent damage to surrounding tissue when nails are clipped and trimmed. Nursing assistants do not cut or trim nails if a resident:

- Has diabetes
- Has a disease that decreases circulation to the legs and feet
- Takes drugs that affect how the blood clots
- Has very thick nails
- Has ingrown toenails

The RN or a **podiatrist** (foot *[pod]* doctor) must cut toenails and provide foot care for these residents. Always check the care plan before trimming a resident's nails. Some centers do not allow nursing assistants to cut or trim toenails. You must follow center policy.

Fig. 14-17 Nail and foot care. The feet soak in a foot basin. The fingers soak in a kidney basin.

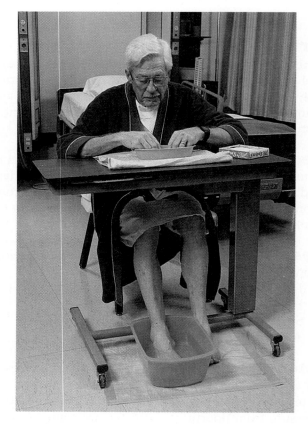

Giving Nail and Foot Care

NNAAP™ SKILL

Quality of Life

Remember to:
- ◆ *Knock before entering the resident's room*
- ◆ *Address the resident by name*
- ◆ *Introduce yourself by name and title*

Pre-Procedure

1 Explain the procedure to the resident.
2 Wash your hands.
3 Collect the following:
- Wash basin
- Bath thermometer
- Bath towel
- Face towel
- Washcloth
- Kidney basin
- Nail clippers
- Orange stick
- Emery board or nail file
- Lotion or petroleum jelly
- Paper towels
- Disposable bath mat

4 Arrange the equipment on the overbed table.
5 Identify the resident. Check the ID bracelet against the assignment sheet.
6 Provide for privacy.
7 Assist the resident to the bedside chair. Place the signal light within reach.

Procedure

8 Place the bath mat under the resident's feet.
9 Fill the basin. Water temperature should be 109° F (42° C) or as directed by the nurse.
10 Place the wash basin on the floor on the towel. Help the resident put the feet into the basin.
11 Position the overbed table in front of the resident. It should be low and close to the resident.
12 Fill the kidney basin. See step 9 for water temperature.
13 Place the kidney basin on the overbed table on top of the paper towels.
14 Put the resident's fingers into the basin. Position the arms so that he or she is comfortable (Fig. 14-17).
15 Let the feet and fingernails soak for 15 to 20 minutes. Rewarm the water in 10 to 15 minutes.
16 Clean under fingernails with the orange stick.
17 Remove the kidney basin. Dry fingers thoroughly.
18 Clip fingernails straight across with nail clippers (Fig. 14-18, p. 316).
19 Shape nails with an emery board or nail file.
20 Push cuticles back with a washcloth or orange stick (Fig. 14-19, p. 316).
21 Move the overbed table from in front of the resident.
22 Scrub calloused areas of the feet with the washcloth.
23 Remove the feet from the basin. Dry thoroughly, especially between the toes.
24 Check between toes for cracks and sores.
25 Apply lotion or petroleum jelly to the tops and soles of the feet. Do not apply between the toes. (If allowed to clip toenails, follow the same procedure as for clipping fingernails.)

Continued

Giving Nail and Foot Care—cont'd

NNAAP™ SKILL

Post-Procedure

26 Help the resident back to bed (if indicated). Provide for comfort.
27 Place the signal light within reach.
28 Raise or lower bed rails. Follow the care plan.
29 Put socks and shoes or slippers on residents who will stay up.
30 Clean and return equipment and supplies to their proper places. Discard disposable supplies.
31 Unscreen the resident.
32 Follow center policy for soiled linen.
33 Wash your hands.
34 Report your observations to the nurse:
- Reddened, irritated, or calloused areas
- Breaks in the skin
- Corns on top of and between toes
- Very thick nails
- Loose nails

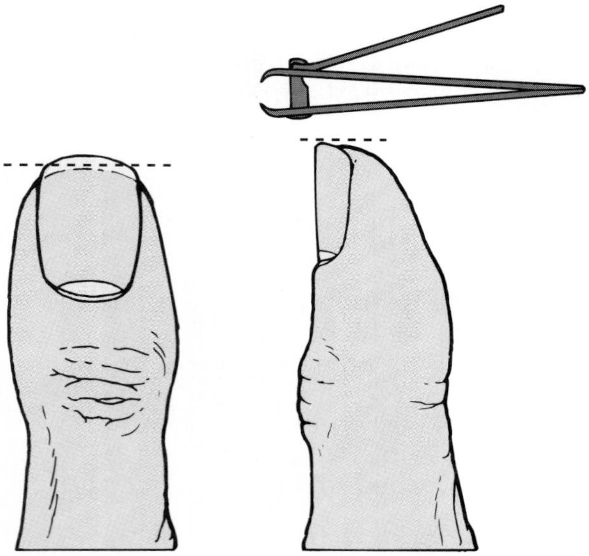

Fig. 14-18 Fingernails are clipped straight across. A nail clipper is used.

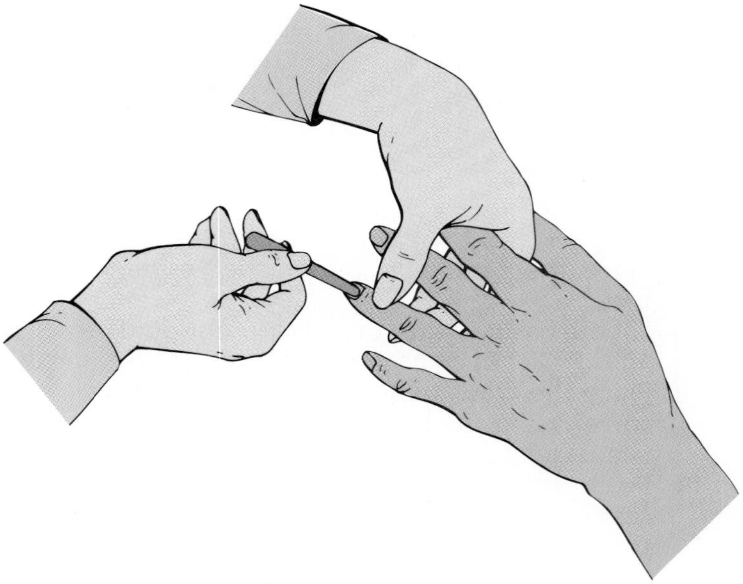

Fig. 14-19 The cuticle is pushed back with an orange stick.

WOUND CARE

A **wound** is a break in the skin or mucous membrane. Wounds result from many causes. A surgical incision leaves a wound. Often wounds result from **trauma**—an accident or violent act that injures the skin, mucous membranes, bones, and internal organs. Falls, vehicle accidents, gun shots, stabbings, and other violent acts are sources of trauma. Human and animal bites, burns, and frostbite are other types of trauma. Pressure ulcers are wounds that occur from poor skin care and immobility. Circulatory ulcers occur from decreased blood flow through the arteries or veins.

The wound is a portal of entry for microorganisms. Thus infection is a major threat. Wound care involves preventing infection and preventing further injury to the wound and surrounding tissues. Preventing blood loss and pain also are important. (*See Subacute Care, p. 317.*)

Box 14-7 Types of Wounds

Intentional and Unintentional Wounds

- **Intentional wounds**—are created for therapy. Surgical incisions and venipunctures for starting intravenous (IV) therapy or for collecting blood specimens are examples.
- **Unintentional wounds**—result from trauma (falls, vehicle accidents, gun shots, stabbings, and other violent acts).

Open and Closed Wounds

- **Open wound**—when the skin or mucous membrane is broken. Intentional and most unintentional wounds are open.
- **Closed wound**—tissues are injured but the skin is not broken (bruises, twists, and sprains).

Clean and Dirty Wounds

- **Clean wound**—is not infected and microbes have not entered the wound. Closed wounds are usually clean. So are intentional wounds created under surgically aseptic conditions. In addition, the urinary, respiratory, and gastrointestinal systems are not entered.
- **Clean-contaminated wound**—occurs from the surgical entry of the urinary, reproductive, respiratory, or gastrointestinal system. These systems are not sterile and contain normal flora.
- **Contaminated wound**—has a high risk of infection. Unintentional wounds are generally contaminated. Wound contamination also occurs from breaks in surgical asepsis and spillage of intestinal contents. Tissues may show signs of inflammation.
- **Infected wound (dirty wound)**—contains large amounts of bacteria and shows signs of infection. Examples include old wounds, surgical incisions into infected areas, and traumatic injuries that rupture the bowel.
- **Chronic wound**—one that does not heal easily. Pressure ulcers and circulatory ulcers are examples.

Partial- and Full-Thickness Wounds *(describe wound depth)*

- **Partial-thickness wound**—the dermis and epidermis of the skin are broken.
- **Full-thickness wound**—the dermis, epidermis, and subcutaneous tissue are penetrated. Muscle and bone may be involved.

Cause

- **Abrasion**—a partial-thickness wound caused by the scraping away or rubbing of the skin.
- **Contusion**—a closed wound caused by a blow to the body.
- **Incision**—an open wound with clean, straight edges; usually intentionally produced with a sharp instrument.
- **Laceration**—an open wound with torn tissues and jagged edges.
- **Penetrating wound**—an open wound in which the skin and underlying tissues are pierced.
- **Puncture wound**—an open wound made by a sharp object; entry of the skin and underlying tissues may be intentional or unintentional.

Subacute Care

Centers with subacute care units often provide specialized wound care. Residents may need subacute care because of poor or delayed wound healing. Others have complications from wound healing. You will provide care for these residents. You may be asked to assist the nurse with wound care. A basic knowledge of wounds and how they heal will help you provide quality care.

Types of Wounds

Wounds are described in many ways. They are intentional or unintentional, open or closed, clean or dirty, and partial-thickness or full-thickness (Box 14-7).

Wound Healing

The healing process has three phases:

- *Inflammatory phase* (3 days). Bleeding stops, and a scab forms over the wound. The scab prevents microbes from entering the wound. Blood supply to the wound increases. The blood brings nutrients and healing substances. Because of the increased blood supply, signs and symptoms of inflammation appear: redness, swelling, heat or warmth, and pain. Loss of function may occur.
- *Proliferative phase* (day 3 to day 21). Proliferate means to multiply rapidly. During this phase, tissue cells multiply to repair the wound.

Continued

SUBACUTE CARE—CONT'D

- *Maturation phase* (day 21 to 1 or 2 years). The scar gains strength. The red, raised scar eventually becomes thin and pale.

Types of wound healing. The healing process occurs through primary intention, secondary intention, or tertiary intention. With *primary intention (first intention, primary closure),* the wound edges are brought together. This closes the wound. Sutures (stitches), staples, clips, or adhesive strips hold the wound edges together. Special glues are now available to doctors for wound closings.

Secondary intention (second intention) is used for contaminated and infected wounds. Wounds are cleaned and dead tissue removed. Wound edges are not brought together, and the wound gaps. Healing occurs naturally. However, healing takes longer and leaves a larger scar. The threat of infection is great.

Tertiary intention (third intention, delayed intention) involves leaving a wound open and then closing it later. Thus tertiary intention combines secondary and primary intention. Infection and poor circulation are common reasons for tertiary intention.

Complications of wound healing. Many factors affect the healing process and increase the risk of complications. The type of wound is one factor. Other factors include the person's age, general health, nutrition, and life-style. Good circulation is important. Age, smoking, circulatory disease, and diabetes all affect circulation. Certain medications (Coumadin and heparin) can prolong bleeding. Tissue growth and repair require adequate protein in the diet. Infection is a risk for persons with immune system changes and for those taking antibiotics.

Persons may need subacute care because of:

- *Infection*—Wound contamination can occur during or after the injury. Trauma is a common source of contaminated wounds. Surgical wounds can be contaminated during or after surgery. An infected wound appears inflamed (reddened) and has drainage. The wound is painful and tender. The person has a fever.
- *Dehiscence*—**Dehiscence** is the separation of the wound layers (Fig. 14-20, p. 321). Separation may involve the skin layer or underlying tissues. Abdominal wounds are most commonly affected. Coughing, vomiting, and abdominal distention place stress on the wound. The person often describes the sensation of the wound popping open.
- *Evisceration*—**Evisceration** is the separation of the wound along with the protrusion of abdominal organs (Fig. 14-21, p. 321). Causes are the same as for dehiscence.

Dehiscence and evisceration are surgical emergencies. The wound is covered with large sterile dressings saturated with sterile saline. You must notify the nurse immediately and assist in preparing the resident for emergency transport to the hospital.

Wound appearance. During the healing process, doctors and nurses routinely observe the wound and its drainage. They observe for healing and complications. Certain observations are made when giving wound care. Box 14-8 on p. 321 lists the wound observations that the nurse makes. You will also make these observations when assisting the nurse with wound care.

Wound drainage. During injury and the inflammatory phase of wound healing, fluid and cells escape from the tissues. The amount of drainage may be small or large, depending on wound size and location. Bleeding and infection also affect the amount and kind of drainage. Wound drainage is observed and measured. Major types of wound drainage are as follows:

- **Serous drainage**—clear, watery fluid (Fig. 14-22, *A,* p. 321). The fluid in a blister is serous. *Serous* comes from the word *serum,* which is the clear, thin, fluid portion of the blood. Serum does not contain blood cells or platelets.
- **Sanguineous drainage**—bloody drainage (Fig. 14-22, *B,* p. 321). Sanguineous comes from the Latin word *sanguis,* which means blood. The amount and color of sanguineous drainage is important. Hemorrhage is suspected when a large amount is present. Bright drainage indicates fresh bleeding. Older bleeding is darker.
- **Serosanguineous drainage**—thin, watery drainage *(sero)* that is blood-tinged *(sanguineous)* (Fig. 14-22, *C,* p. 321).
- **Purulent drainage**—thick drainage that is green, yellow, or brown (Fig. 14-22, *D,* p. 321)

Drainage must leave the wound for healing to occur. If drainage is trapped inside the wound, underlying tissues swell. The wound may heal at the skin level, but underlying tissues do not close. This can lead to infection and other complications.

When a large amount of drainage is expected, the doctor inserts a drain. A *penrose drain* is a rubber tube that drains onto a dressing (Fig. 14-23,

Subacute Care—cont'd

p. 322). Because the penrose drain opens onto the dressing, it is an open drain and a portal of entry for microbes.

Closed drainage systems prevent microbes from entering the wound. A drainage tube is placed in the wound and attached to suction. The Hemovac (Fig. 14-24, p. 322) and Jackson-Pratt (Fig. 14-25, p. 322) systems are examples. Other systems are used depending on the type of wound, its size, and its location.

Drainage is measured by the nurse in three ways:

- Noting the number and size of dressings with drainage. The amount and kind of drainage is described. Are dressings saturated? Is drainage on just part of the dressing? If so, which part? Is drainage through some or all layers of the dressing?
- Weighing dressings before applying them to the wound. The weight of each dressing is noted. Dressings are weighed after removal. The weight of the dry dressing is subtracted from the weight of the wet dressing (wet dressings weigh more).
- Measuring the amount of drainage in the collecting receptacle if closed drainage is used.

Dressings

Wound dressings have many functions. They protect wounds from injury and microbes. Drainage is absorbed and removed along with dead tissue. Dressings can promote comfort and cover unsightly wounds. They also provide a moist environment for wound healing. When bleeding is a problem, pressure dressings help control bleeding.

The type and size of dressing used depends on many factors. These include the type of wound, its size, and location; amount of drainage; and the presence or absence of infection. The dressing's function and the frequency of dressing changes are other factors. The doctor and RN choose the best type of dressing for each wound.

Types of dressings. Dressings are described by the material used and application method. Many products are available for dressing wounds. The following are common types of wound dressings:

- Gauze—comes in squares, rectangles, pads, and rolls (Fig. 14-26, p. 322). Gauze dressings absorb moisture.
- Nonadherent gauze—is a gauze dressing with a nonstick surface. The dressing does not stick to the wound and removes easily without injuring tissue.
- Transparent adhesive film—prevents fluids and bacteria from reaching the wound but air can. The wound is kept moist. Drainage is not absorbed. The transparent film allows wound observation.

Some dressings contain special agents to promote wound healing. If you assist with the dressing change, the RN explains its use to you.

Dressing application methods involve dry and wet dressings:

- *Dry-to-dry dressing*—usually called a *dry dressing.* A dry gauze dressing is placed over the wound. Additional dressings are placed on top of the first dressing as needed. Drainage is absorbed by the dressing and is removed with the dressing. A dry dressing can stick to the wound. The dressing is removed carefully to prevent tissue injury and discomfort.
- *Wet-to-dry dressing*—a gauze dressing saturated with a solution is applied over the wound. Additional dressings are applied as needed. These dressings are also moistened with solution. The solution softens dead tissue in the wound. The dead tissue is absorbed by the dressing and is removed with the dressing. The dressings are removed when dry.
- *Wet-to-wet dressing*—a gauze dressing saturated with solution is placed in the wound. The dressing is kept moist.

Securing dressings. Dressings must be secure over wounds. Bacteria can enter the wound and drain-age can escape if the dressing is dislodged. Tape and Montgomery ties are commonly used to secure dressings. Binders also hold dressings in place (p. 320).

- ***Tape*** Adhesive, paper, plastic, and elastic tapes are available. Adhesive tape sticks well to the skin. However, the adhesive part can remain on the skin and is hard to remove. The adhesive can irritate the skin. Sometimes skin is removed with the tape, causing an abrasion. Many people are allergic to adhesive tape. Paper and plastic tapes are nonallergenic. This means that they do not cause allergic reactions. Elastic tape allows movement of the body part. The RN and the doctor choose the type of tape used.
- ***Montgomery ties*** Montgomery ties (Fig. 14-27, p. 322) are used for large dressings and when frequent dressing changes are needed. A Montgomery tie consists of an adhesive strip and a cloth tie. When the dressing is in place, the adhesive strips are placed on both sides of the

Continued

SUBACUTE CARE—CONT'D

dressing. Then the cloth ties are secured over the dressing. Two or three Montgomery ties are needed on each side. The cloth ties are undone for the dressing change. The adhesive strips are not removed unless soiled.

Applying dressings. The nurse is responsible for applying dressings. You may be asked to assist. Always follow Standard Precautions and the Bloodborne Pathogen Standard.

Binders

Binders are applied to the abdomen, chest, or perineal areas. Binders promote healing because they:

- Support wounds and hold dressings in place
- Reduce or prevent swelling by promoting circulation
- Promote comfort
- Prevent injury

You may care for residents with the following types of binders:

- *Straight abdominal binders*—provide abdominal support and hold dressings in place (Fig. 14-28, p. 323).
- *Breast binders*—support the breasts after breast surgery (Fig. 14-29, p. 323).
- *T binders*—are used to secure dressings in place after rectal and perineal surgeries. The single T binder is used for women (Fig. 14-30, *A*, p. 323). The double T binder is used for men (Fig. 14-30, *B*, p. 323). If perineal dressings are large, women may need double T binders.

Wound Care and the Person's Basic Needs

The wound, which can affect the person's basic needs, is only one aspect of the person's care. You must remember that it is the *person* who has the wound.

The person is recovering from surgery or trauma. The wound is a source of pain and discomfort. The wound and the pain may interfere with breathing and moving. Turning, repositioning, and ambulating may be painful. You must handle the person gently and allow pain medications to take effect before giving care.

Good nutrition is needed for healing. However, pain and discomfort can affect the person's appetite. So can odors from wound drainage. Remove soiled dressings promptly from the room, use room deodorizers, and keep drainage containers out of the person's sight. If the person has a taste for certain foods or beverages, report this information to the nurse.

Infection is always a threat. You must practice Standard Precautions and follow the Bloodborne Pathogen Standard. The wound and the person are observed carefully for signs and symptoms of infection.

Delayed healing is a risk for persons who are elderly or obese or who have poor nutrition. Poor circulation and diabetes also affect healing. These conditions are risk factors for infection.

Many fears affect the person's sense of safety and security. The person fears scarring, disfigurement, delayed healing, and infection. Fears about the wound "popping" open are common. Costly medical bills are other concerns. Continued subacute care, home care, or long-term care may be needed.

Victims of violence have many other concerns. Future attacks, finding and convicting the attacker, and fear for family members are common concerns. Victims of domestic violence, child abuse, and elderly abuse often hide the true source of their injuries.

The person's wound may be large or small. It may be visible to others—on the face, arms, or legs—or hidden by clothing. Wound drainage may have unpleasant odors. The wound may be extensive and disfiguring. It may affect the person's ability to perform sexually or the person's sense of being sexually attractive. The amputation of a finger, hand, arm, toe, foot, or leg can affect the person's function, everyday activities, and job. Eye injuries can affect vision. Abdominal trauma and surgery can affect eating and elimination.

Whatever the location or size of the wound, physical function and body image are affected. The person's sense of love and belonging and self-esteem are affected. You must be sensitive to the person's feelings. The person may be sad and tearful or angry and hostile. Adjustment may be difficult and rehabilitation necessary. You must be gentle and kind, give thoughtful care, and practice good communication techniques. Other health team members—therapists, social workers, psychiatrists, and the clergy—may be involved in the person's care.

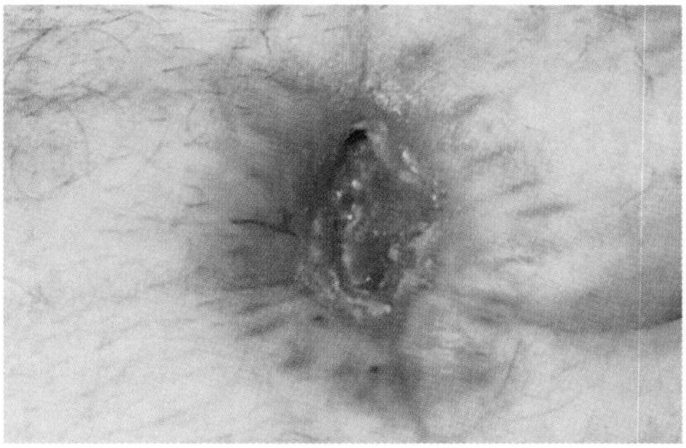

Fig. 14-20 Wound dehiscence. *(Courtesy Morison M:* A colour guide to the nursing management of wounds, *London, 1992, Wolfe Medical Publishers.)*

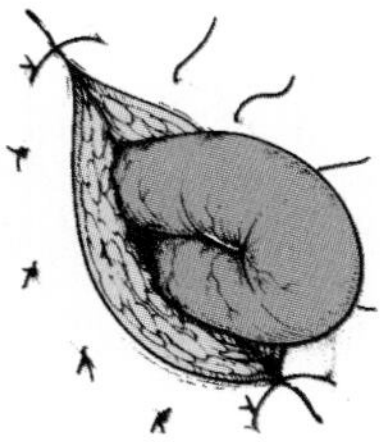

Fig. 14-21 Wound evisceration. *(From* Mosby's medical, nursing, & allied health dictionary, *ed 4, St Louis, 1994, Mosby.)*

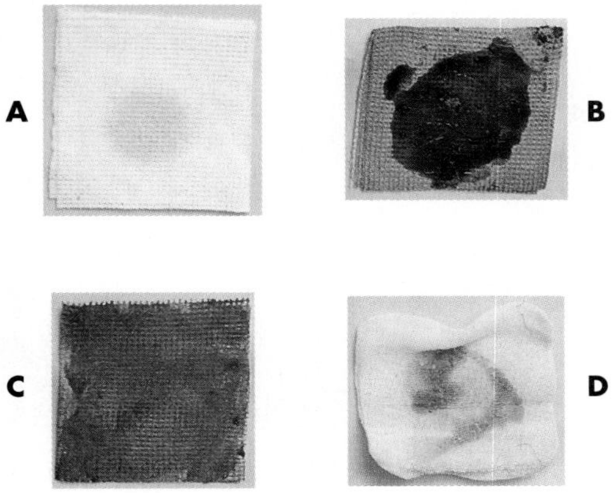

Fig. 14-22 Wound drainage. **A,** Serous drainage. **B,** Sanguineous drainage. **C,** Serosanguineous drainage. **D,** Purulent drainage. *(From Potter PA, Perry AG:* Fundamentals of nursing: concepts, process, and practice, *ed 4, St Louis, 1997, Mosby.)*

Box 14-8 Wound Observations

- **Wound location**
  - Multiple wounds may exist from surgery or trauma.
- **Wound size and depth (measure in centimeters)**
  - Size: measured from top to bottom and side to side.
  - Depth: (1) measured by very carefully inserting a gloved finger or a sterile swab inside the deepest part of the wound; (2) the gloved finger or swab is removed. Measure the distance on the gloved finger or swab. *Only the RN measures wound depth.*
  - The same ruler is used when measuring the wound.
- **Wound appearance**
  - Is the wound red and swollen?
  - Is the area around the wound warm to touch?
  - Are sutures, staples, or clips intact or broken?
  - Are wound edges closed or separated? Did the wound break open?
- **Drainage**
  - Is the drainage serous, sanguineous, serosanguineous, or purulent?
  - What is the amount of drainage?
- **Odor**
  - Does the wound or drainage have an odor?
- **Surrounding skin**
  - Is surrounding skin intact?
  - What is the color of surrounding skin?
  - Are surrounding tissues swollen?

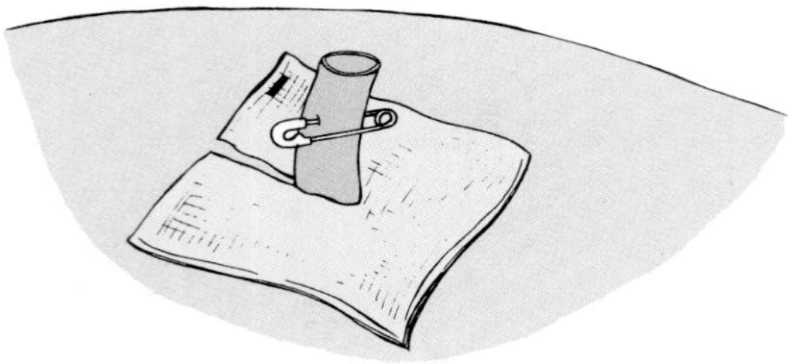

Fig. 14-23 A penrose drain. The safety pin prevents the drain from slipping into the wound. *(From Potter PA, Perry, AG:* Fundamentals of nursing: concepts, process, and practice, *ed 4, St Louis, 1997, Mosby.)*

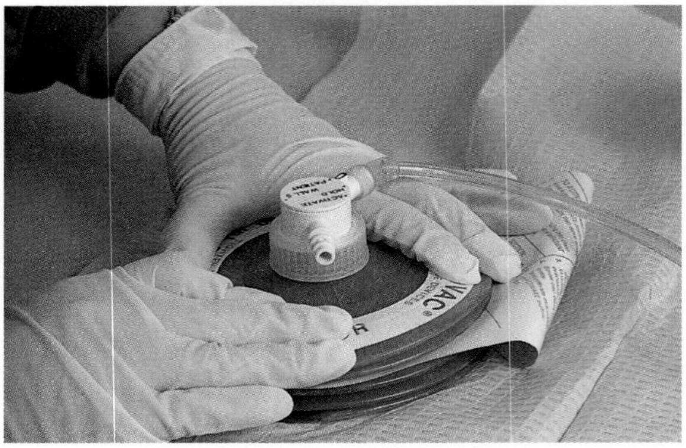

Fig. 14-24 A Hemovac. Drains are sutured to the wound and connected to the reservoir. *(From Elkin MK, Perry AG, Potter PA:* Nursing interventions and clinical skills, *1996, Mosby.)*

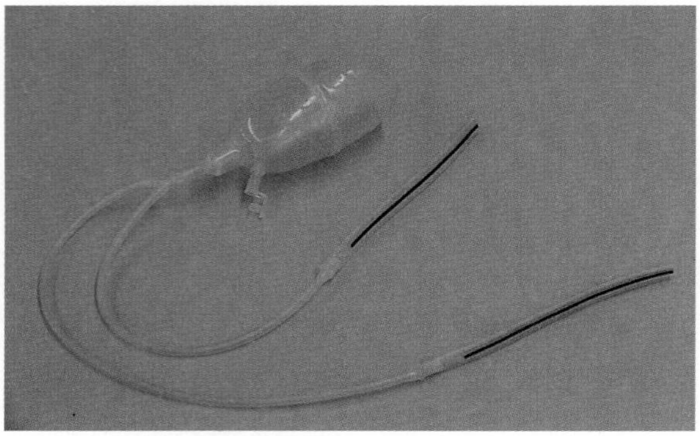

Fig. 14-25 The Jackson-Pratt drainage system. *(From Elkin MK, Perry AG, Potter PA:* Nursing interventions and clinical skills, *1996, Mosby.)*

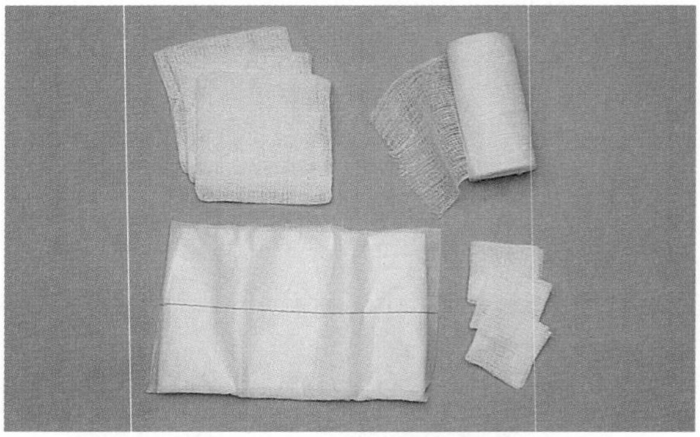

Fig. 14-26 Gauze dressings. **A,** 4 × 4. **B,** Gauze roll. **C,** Abdominal pad (ABD). **D,** 2 × 2.

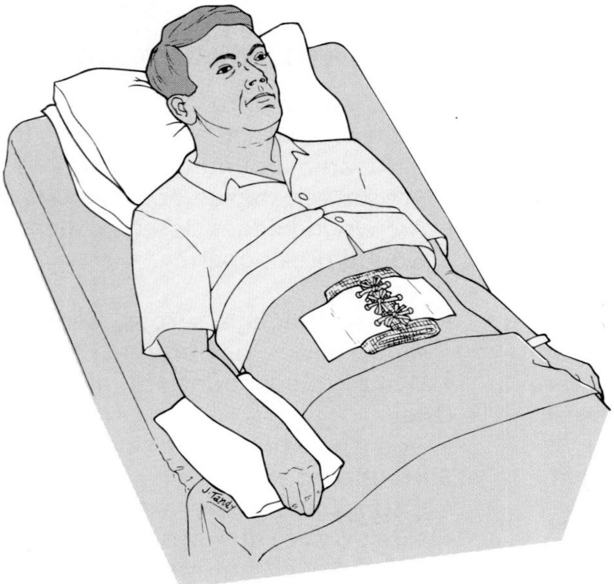

Fig. 14-27 Montgomery ties.

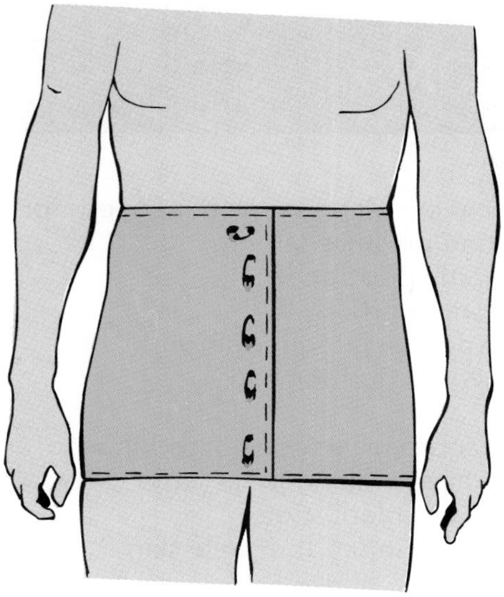

Fig. 14-28 Straight abdominal binder.

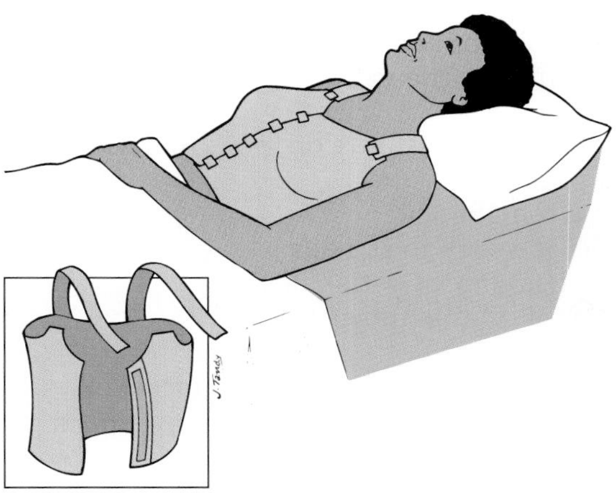

Fig. 14-29 Breast binder.

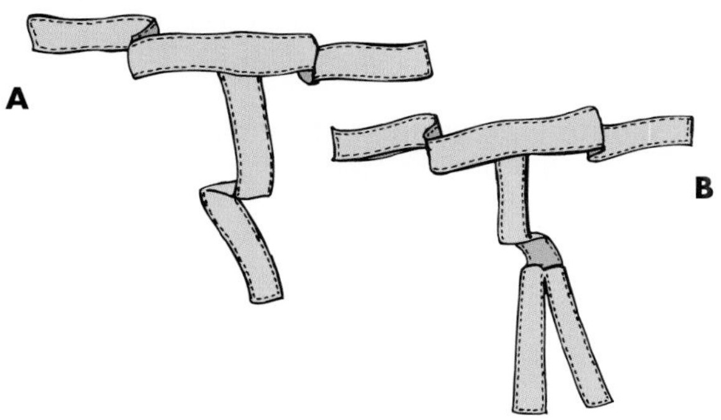

Fig. 14-30 **A,** Single T binder. **B,** Double T binder.

Quality of Life

Remember that providing good skin and nail care is important for a resident's overall comfort and quality of life. Residents have the right to have care provided in a way that promotes healthy skin and prevents skin breakdown. OBRA and JCAHO require the health care team to develop an individualized plan of care for each resident. It must ensure that the resident receives the right skin care. Sometimes special skin care products, protective devices, and special stockings or bandages are necessary. It is everyone's job to keep the resident's skin healthy.

The skin is the body's first line of defense against changes in the environment. The skin is kept clean and intact. This promotes comfort and prevents infection. Providing good skin and nail care to residents is one of your most important jobs. Older persons require special skin care because their skin is thin and frail. Good nail and foot care is an important part of skin care. You must follow center policy and the resident's care plan when providing nail and foot care. Report reddened areas, breaks in the skin, corns, very thick nails, and loose nails to the nurse.

Residents who spend long periods in bed are at risk for pressure ulcers, skin breakdown, and thrombi (blood clots). Many residents have diseases that cause poor arterial or venous circulation. This increases their risk for developing open wounds on the lower legs and feet. Care of the legs and feet for residents with circulatory problems is directed by the doctor. You must be very careful not to injure the resident's skin during care.

Circle T if the statement is true and F if the statement is false.

1 (T) F Good nutrition and hydration can help prevent skin breakdown.

2 (T) F White or reddened skin is the first sign of a pressure ulcer.

3 (T) F Pressure ulcers usually occur over bony areas.

4 (T) F Poor nursing care can lead to the development of pressure ulcers.

5 (T) F Shearing and friction can cause pressure ulcers.

6 T (F) You should hold agitated residents tightly by the arms to help them dress and undress.

Circle the BEST answer.

7 Which will *not* prevent skin tears?
A Keeping your nails trimmed and smoothly filed
B Dressing residents in soft clothing with long legs and sleeves
(C) Hurrying when lifting and transferring residents
D Padding wheelchair foot pedals

8 Which does *not* prevent pressure ulcers?
A Repositioning the resident every 2 hours
B Applying lotion to dry areas
(C) Scrubbing and rubbing the skin
D Keeping bed linens clean, dry, and free of wrinkles

9 Which are *not* used to treat pressure ulcers?
A Special beds
B Waterbeds and flotation pads
(C) Plastic drawsheets and waterproof pads
D Heel elevators and elbow protectors

10 Which position is recommended for preventing pressure ulcers?
A Supine position
B Prone position
(C) 30-degree lateral position
D Fowler's position

11 Mr. Moore wears elastic stockings to
A Reduce swelling in his legs
(B) Prevent blood clots
C Prevent injury to fragile skin
D All of the above

12 When applying an elastic bandage
(A) The extremity needs to be in good body alignment
B The fingers or toes are covered if possible
C It is applied from the largest to the smallest part of the extremity
D It is applied from the upper to the lower part of the extremity

13 Nursing assistants do not cut toenails if a resident
A Is diabetic
B Has very thick nails
C Has ingrown toenails
(D) All of the above

14 You can help prevent stasis ulcers by
A Using elastic, rubberband-type garters to hold socks in place
B Keeping residents in bed as much as possible
C Encouraging residents to sit with legs down
(D) Avoiding injury to residents' legs and feet when providing care

15 Which decreases a resident's risk for arterial ulcers?
A Smoking
(B) Routine professional foot care
C A history of diabetes
D Advanced age

16 The skin and underlying tissues are pierced. This is
A A penetrating wound
B An incision
C A contusion
D An abrasion

17 A wound appears red and swollen. The area around the wound is warm to touch. These signs are characteristics of
A The inflammatory phase of wound healing
B The proliferative phase of wound healing
C Healing by primary intention
D Healing by secondary intention

18 A wound is healing by primary intention. While assisting with a dressing change you note that the wound is separating. This is called
A Dehiscence
B Tertiary intention
C Evisceration
D Proliferation

19 You note a clear, watery drainage from a wound. This drainage is called
A Purulent drainage
B Serous drainage
C Seropurulent drainage
D Serosanguineous drainage

20 A dressing does the following *except*
A Protect the wound from injury
B Absorb drainage
C Provide a moist environment for wound healing
D Support the wound and reduce swelling

Answers to these questions are on p. 698.

15 Grooming

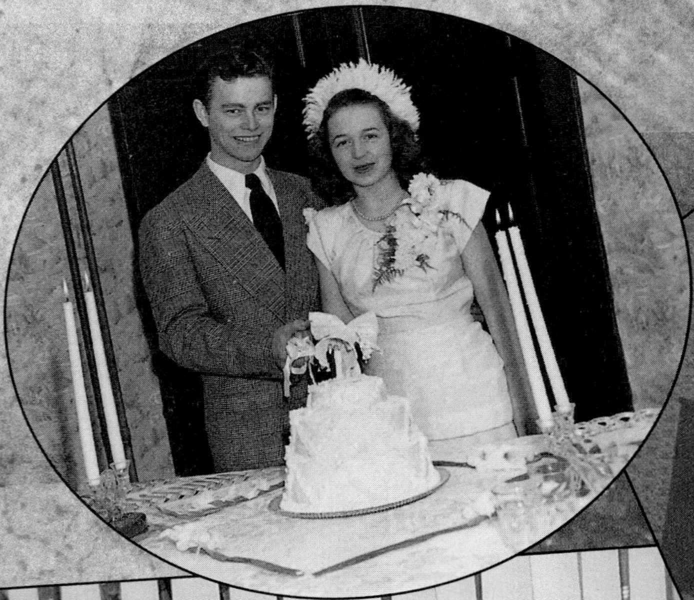

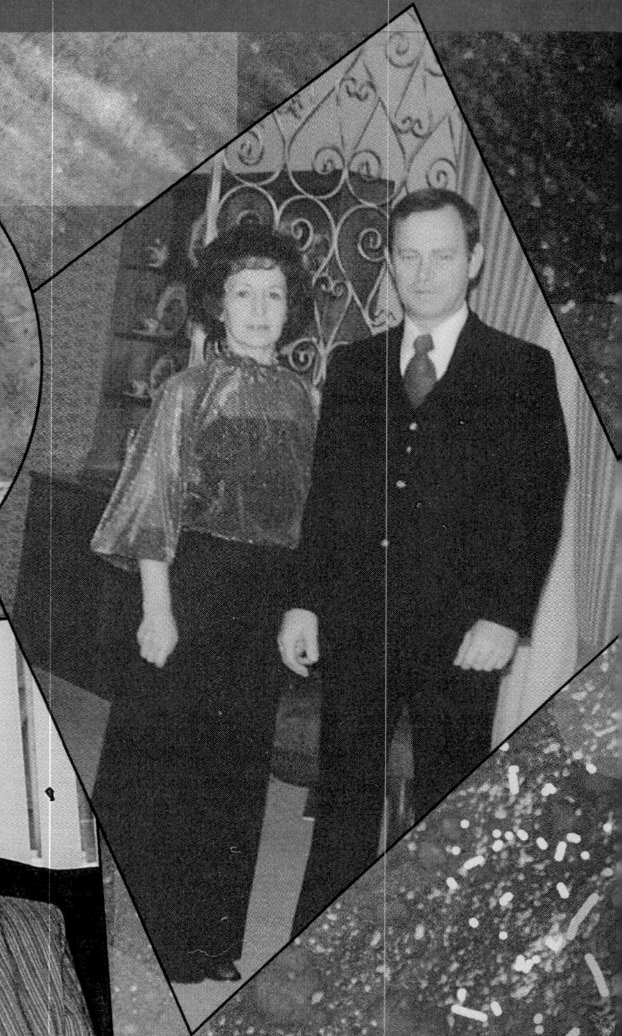

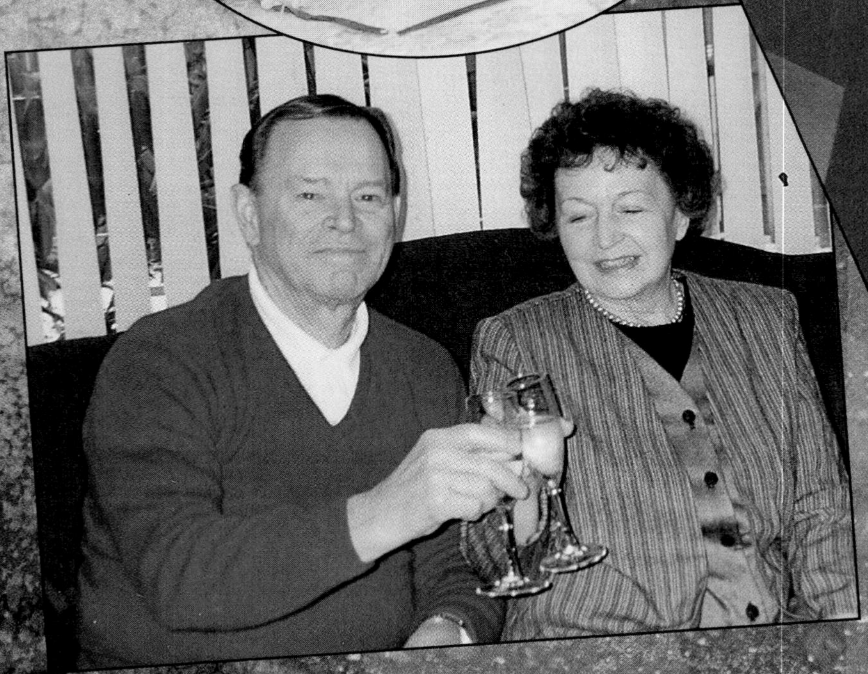

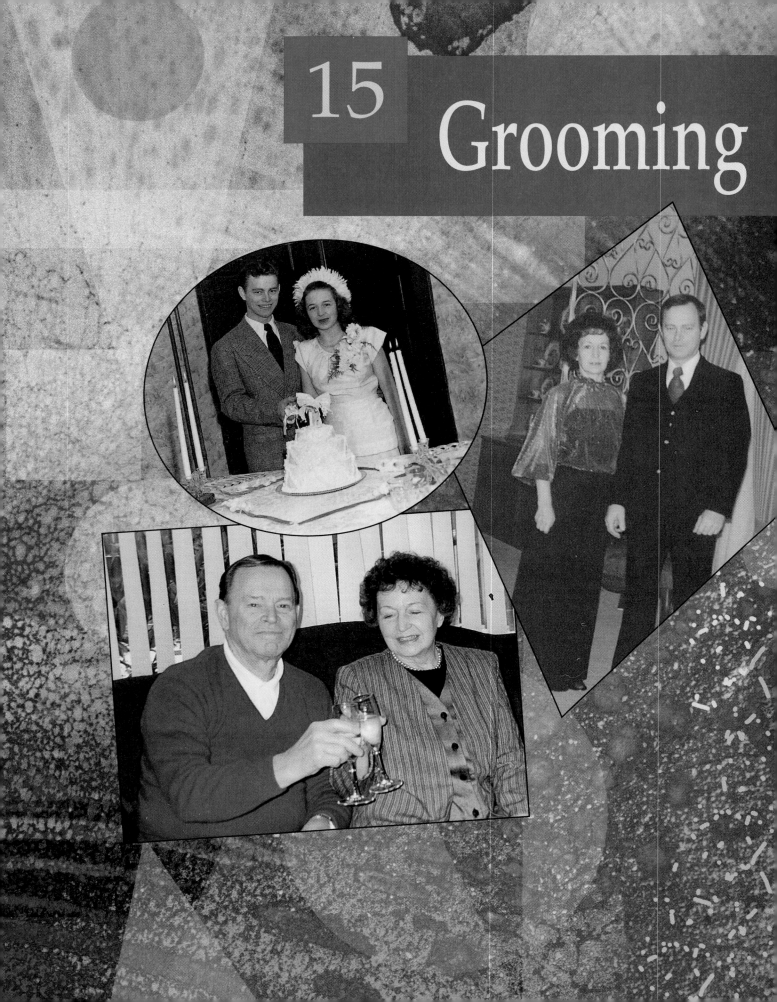

What You Will Learn

- The definition of the key terms listed in this chapter
- The importance of hair care and shaving
- The factors that affect hair care
- Ways to shampoo a resident's hair
- The measures practiced when shaving a resident
- How to dress and undress residents
- The procedures described in this chapter

Key Terms

alopecia Hair loss

anticoagulant A drug that thins the blood and slows down clotting time; it is given to prevent blood clotting

dandruff The excessive amount of dry, white flakes from the scalp

hirsutism Excessive body hair in women and children

pediculosis (lice) The infestation with lice

pediculosis capitis The infestation of the scalp (*capitis*) with lice

pediculosis corporis The infestation of the body (*corporis*) with lice

pediculosis pubis The infestation of the pubic (*pubis*) hair with lice

Cleanliness and skin care meet basic physical, safety, and security needs. Clean and intact skin protects against infection. Bathing and back massage promote circulation, exercise, comfort, and relaxation. For many people, being clean is necessary for love and belonging and self-esteem needs.

Hair care, shaving, and nail care also are important to many residents. They vary in how much attention they give to such matters. Some want only clean hair. Others want hair styled in a certain way. Clean hands are enough for some people. Others want nails clean, manicured, and polished. Shaving and beard grooming are important to many men. Likewise, many women shave their legs and underarms.

HAIR CARE

Appearance and mental well-being are affected by how the hair looks and feels. Some residents are unable to care for their own hair. You need to assist them with hair care whenever necessary. Some centers have a barber and a beautician to cut and shampoo hair. However, you assist with daily hair care.

The nurse uses the nursing process to help the health care team meet the resident's hair care needs. They consider the resident's culture, personal choice, skin and scalp condition, health history, and self-care ability. These terms are common in care plans:

- **Alopecia** means hair loss. Hair loss may be complete or partial. Male pattern baldness occurs with aging and is the result of heredity. Hair also thins in some women with aging. Cancer treatments (radiation therapy to the head and chemotherapy) often cause alopecia in both men and women. Skin disease is another cause. Other causes include stress, poor nutrition, pregnancy, some drugs, and hormone changes. Except for hair loss from aging, the hair grows back in many cases.
- **Hirsutism** is excessive body hair in women and children. It is the result of heredity and an abnormal amount of male hormones.

- **Dandruff** is the excessive amount of dry, white flakes from the scalp. Itching often occurs. Sometimes the eyebrows and ear canals are involved. Medicated shampoos correct the problem.
- **Pediculosis (lice)** is the infestation with lice. Lice are parasites. Lice bites cause severe itching in the affected body area. **Pediculosis capitis** is the infestation of the scalp *(capitis)* with lice. **Pediculosis pubis** is the infestation of the pubic *(pubis)* hair with lice. Both head and pubic lice attach their eggs to hair shafts. **Pediculosis corporis** is the infestation of the body *(corporis)* with lice. Lice eggs attach to clothing and furniture. Lice easily spread to other persons through clothing, furniture, bed linen, and sexual contact. Medicated shampoos, lotions, and creams are used to treat lice. Thorough bathing is necessary. So is washing clothing and linen in hot water. Report any signs of lice to the nurse immediately.

Brushing and Combing Hair

Brushing and combing hair are part of early morning, morning, and afternoon care. They are also done whenever needed. Encourage residents to do their own hair care. However, provide assistance as necessary. You must provide hair care for residents who cannot do it themselves. Let the resident choose how hair is brushed, combed, and styled.

Long hair easily mats and tangles during bedrest. Daily brushing and combing helps prevent this problem. Braiding does too. Do not braid hair without the resident's permission. Never cut hair to remove mats or tangles.

Brushing brings scalp oils along the hair shaft. Scalp oils help keep hair soft and shiny. Brushing and combing keep hair from tangling and matting. When brushing and combing hair, start at the scalp. Then brush or comb to the hair ends.

Talk to the nurse if the resident has matted or tangled hair. The nurse may have you comb or brush through the matting and tangling. To do this, take a small section of hair near the ends. Then comb or brush through to the hair ends. Working up to the scalp, add small sections of hair. Comb or brush through each longer section to the hair ends. Finally, brush or comb from the scalp to the hair ends. *Never cut matted or tangled hair.*

Special measures are needed for curly, coarse, and dry hair. Use a wide-tooth comb for curly hair. Start at the neckline. Work upward, lifting and fluffing hair outward. Continue until you reach the forehead. Wetting the hair or applying a conditioner or petroleum jelly makes combing easier. The resident may have certain practices or use special hair care products. The nurse asks the resident about personal preferences and routine hair care measures. These become part of the resident's care plan. The resident can guide you when giving hair care.

When giving hair care, protect the resident's gown or clothing by placing a towel across the shoulders. If giving hair care when the resident is in bed, do so before changing the pillowcase. If done after a linen change, place a towel across the pillow for falling hair.

Brushing and Combing the Resident's Hair

Quality of Life

Remember to:
- *Knock before entering the resident's room*
- *Address the resident by name*
- *Introduce yourself by name and title*

Pre-Procedure

1 Identify the resident. Check the ID bracelet, and call the resident by name.
2 Explain the procedure to the resident. Ask the resident how to style his or her hair.
3 Collect the following:
- Comb and brush
- Bath towel
- Other toilet items as requested

4 Arrange items on the bedside stand.
5 Wash your hands.
6 Provide for privacy.

Procedure

7 Lower the bed rail (if used).
8 Help the resident to the chair. (If a resident is in bed, raise the bed to the best position for good body mechanics. Make sure side rails are up. Lower the bed rail near you, and position the resident in semi-Fowler's position if allowed.)
9 Place the towel across the resident's shoulders. Place the towel across the pillow if the resident is in bed.
10 Ask the resident to remove eyeglasses. Put them in the glass case. Put the glass case in the bedside stand.
11 Part the hair into 2 main sections (Fig. 15-1, *A,* p. 330). Then divide one side into 2 sections (Fig. 15-1, *B,* p. 330).
12 Brush the hair. Start at the scalp, and brush toward the hair ends (Fig. 15-2, p. 330).
13 Style the hair as the resident prefers.
14 Remove the towel.
15 Let the resident put eyeglasses on again.

Post-Procedure

16 Provide for comfort.
17 Raise or lower bed rails. Follow the care plan.
18 Place the signal light within reach.
19 Unscreen the resident.
20 Clean and return equipment to its proper place.
21 Follow center policy for dirty linen.
22 Wash your hands.

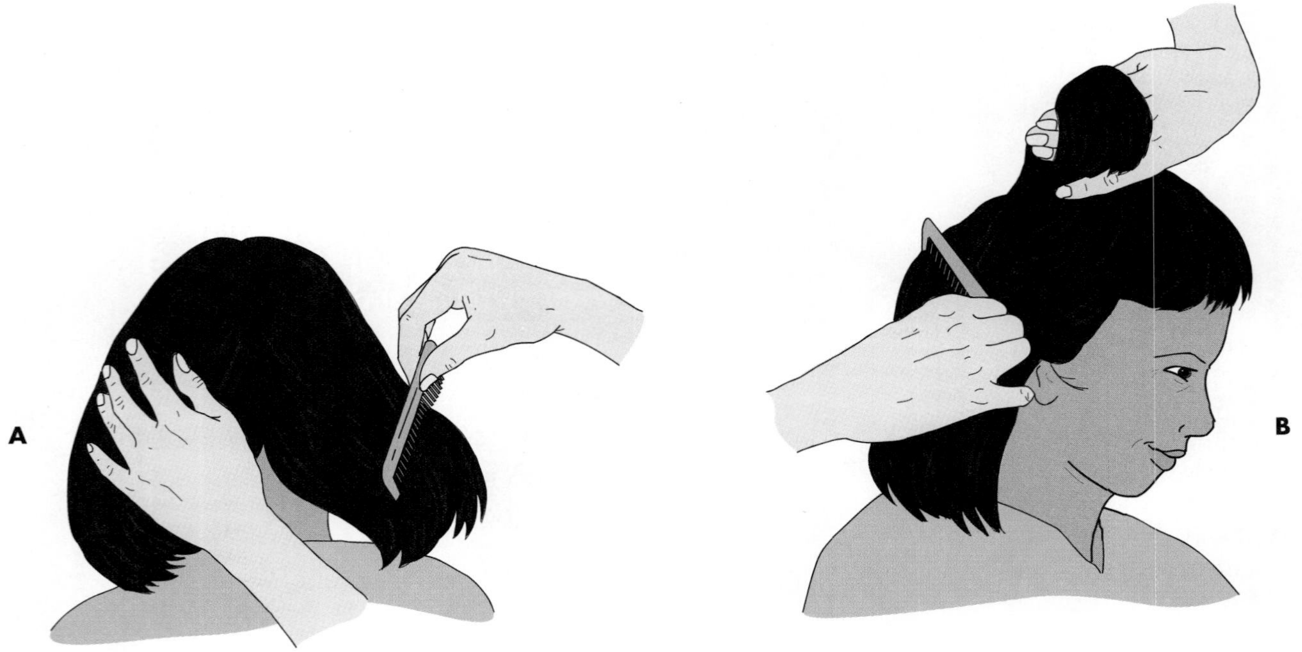

Fig. 15-1 Parting the hair. **A,** Part hair down the middle, and divide it into two main sections. **B,** Then part the main section into two smaller sections.

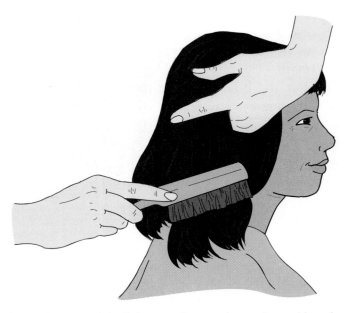

Fig. 15-2 Brush hair by starting at the scalp and brushing down to the hair ends.

Shampooing

Residents usually need help shampooing. Shampooing usually is done weekly on the resident's bath or shower day. Some residents use special shampoos or conditioners. Others may have a doctor's order for a medicated shampoo. Ask the nurse about the type of shampoo or conditioner to use. If a woman has her hair done by the beautician, do not shampoo her hair. Protect her hair with a shower cap during the tub bath or shower. Check the care plan for specific information.

There are several shampooing methods. The method used depends on the resident's condition, safety factors, and personal choice. The health care team decides which method to use. Hair is dried and styled as quickly as possible after shampooing. Women may want hair curled or rolled up before drying. Check with the nurse before curling or rolling up a resident's hair.

Shampooing during the shower or tub bath. The resident's hair usually is shampooed during the shower or tub bath. A hand-held shower nozzle is used. The resident tips his or her head back to keep shampoo and water out of the eyes. This is especially important if a medicated shampoo is used. Support the back of the resident's head with one hand as you shampoo with the other. Some residents cannot tip their head back. Have them lean forward and hold a folded washcloth over the eyes. Support the resident's forehead with one hand as you shampoo with the other. Be sure that the resident can breathe easily. If a medicated shampoo or conditioner is used, return it to the nurse. Never leave it at the bedside unless instructed to do so.

Shampooing at the sink. Some people want to sit in front of a sink for a shampoo. This is done at the resident's request and with the nurse's permission. Many older or disabled residents have limited range-of-motion in their neck and upper back. They do not tolerate this procedure.

The resident sits in a chair or wheelchair facing away from the sink. A folded towel placed over the edge of the sink protects the resident's neck. The resident's head is tilted back over the edge of the sink. A water pitcher or hand-held nozzle is used to wet and rinse the hair.

Shampooing a resident on a stretcher
Hair is washed with the resident on a stretcher (Fig. 15-3). The stretcher is positioned in front of the sink. A pillow is placed under the resident's head and neck. The head is tilted over the edge of the sink. The water pitcher or hand-held nozzle is used to wet and rinse the hair. Remember to lock the stretcher wheels and use the safety straps. Make sure the far side rail is up. Do not use this method for residents with limited range-of-motion in the neck or upper back. Check with the nurse before using this method.

Shampooing a resident in bed. This method is used for residents who cannot sit in a chair or be shampooed on a stretcher. The resident's head and shoulders are moved to the edge of the bed if this position is allowed. A rubber or plastic trough is placed under the resident's head to protect the linens and mattress from water. The trough also drains water into a basin placed on a chair next to the bed (Fig. 15-4). Use a water pitcher to wet and rinse the hair.

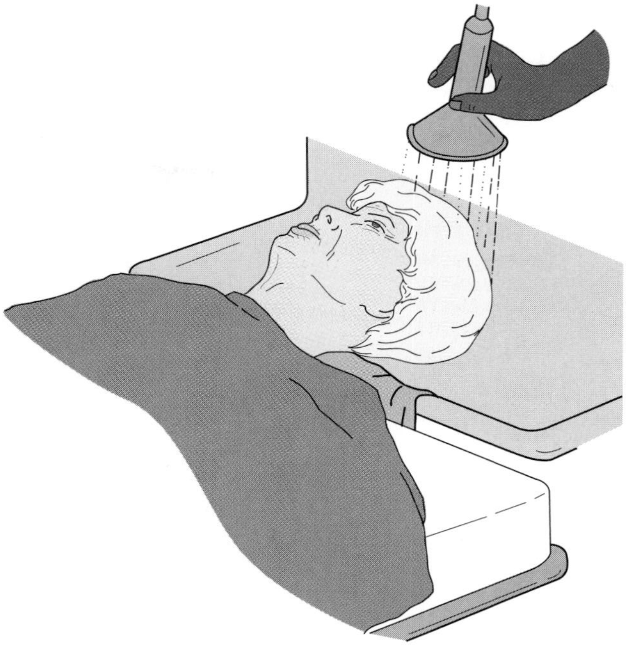

Fig. 15-3 Shampooing while the person is on a stretcher. The stretcher is in front of the sink.

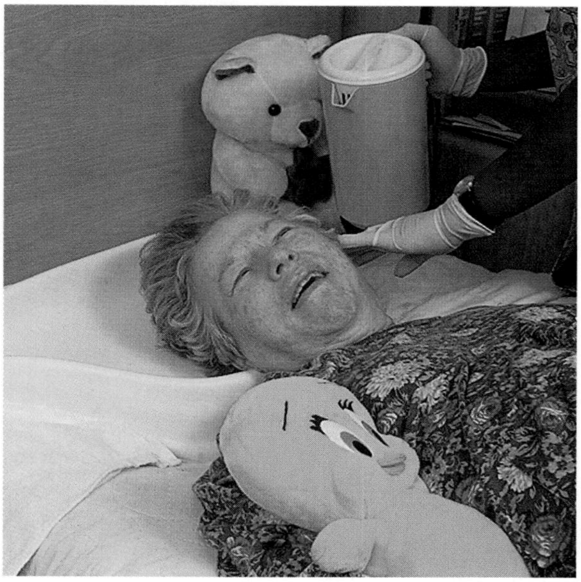

Fig. 15-4 A trough is used when shampooing a person in bed. The trough is directed to the side of the bed so water drains into a collecting basin.

Shampooing the Resident's Hair

NNAAP™ SKILL

Quality of Life

Remember to:
- ◆ *Knock before entering the resident's room*
- ◆ *Address the resident by name*
- ◆ *Introduce yourself by name and title*

Pre-Procedure

1 Explain the procedure to the resident.
2 Wash your hands.
3 Collect the following:
- Two bath towels
- Face towel or washcloth folded lengthwise
- Shampoo
- Hair conditioner if requested
- Bath thermometer
- Pitcher or hand-held nozzle
- Equipment for the shampoo in bed (if needed)
  - Trough
  - Basin or pail
  - Waterproof bed protector
- Comb and brush
- Hair dryer

4 Arrange equipment where you can reach it with ease.
5 Identify the resident. Check the ID bracelet against the assignment sheet.
6 Provide for privacy.

Procedure

7 Position the resident for the method you are going to use.
8 Place a bath towel across the shoulders or across the pillow under the resident's head.
9 Brush and comb hair thoroughly to remove snarls and tangles.
10 Raise side rails on the bed or stretcher if you need to leave to get water.
11 Obtain water. Measure water temperature with the bath thermometer. Water temperature should be about 110° F (43° C to 44° C) or as directed by the nurse.
12 Lower the bed rail.
13 Ask the resident to hold the face towel or washcloth over the eyes. Make sure it does not slip down over the nose or mouth.
14 Use the pitcher or nozzle to wet the hair completely.
15 Use a small amount of shampoo.
16 Work up a lather with both hands. Start at the hairline, and work toward the back of the head.
17 Massage the scalp with your fingertips. Do not scratch the scalp with your fingernails.
18 Rinse the hair.
19 Repeat steps 15 through 18.
20 Rinse the hair thoroughly.
21 Apply conditioner and rinse as directed on the container.
22 Wrap the resident's head with a bath towel.
23 Dry his or her face with the towel or washcloth used to protect the eyes.
24 Help the resident raise his or her head if appropriate.
25 Rub the hair and scalp with the towel. Use the second towel if the first becomes too wet.
26 Comb hair to remove snarls and tangles. A woman may want her hair curled or rolled up.
27 Dry the hair as quickly as possible.

Shampooing the Resident's Hair—cont'd

NNAAP™ SKILL

Post-Procedure

28 Provide for comfort.
29 Raise or lower bed rails. Follow the care plan.
30 Place the signal light within reach.
31 Clean and return equipment to its proper place. Discard disposable items.
32 Follow center policy for dirty linen.
33 Wash your hands.

SHAVING

Many men want a clean-shaven face for comfort and mental well-being. Coarse facial hair is common in many older women. They may want such hair shaved off. Younger women usually shave their legs and underarms.

Some residents use an electric shaver. They usually are required to have their own electric shaver. If the center's shaver is used for residents, the shaver is cleaned between each use. Follow center policy for cleaning electric shavers. Also practice the safety precautions for using electrical equipment.

Some residents like a blade shaver (razor blade). *(See Residents With Dementia.)* Razor blades can cause nicks or cuts. Always wear gloves and practice Standard Precautions to prevent contact with the resident's blood. Residents should have their own blade shaver. If not, a disposable shaver is used. Remember that razor blades are extremely sharp. You must protect the resident and yourself from nicks or cuts. Follow the Bloodborne Pathogen Standard. Dispose of used razor blades and disposable shavers in a sharps container. Follow center policy for disposal of sharps.

An **anticoagulant** is a drug that thins the blood and slows down clotting time. It is given to prevent blood clotting. Therefore nicks or cuts can cause serious bleeding problems. Residents can bleed easily from even a small nick or cut. Avoid using a razor blade to shave these residents. An electric shaver is safer for them. Check the resident's care plan, and ask the nurse what type of shaver to use.

RESIDENTS WITH DEMENTIA

Avoid using a razor blade when shaving residents with dementia. These residents may not understand what you are doing. They may resist care and move suddenly. This increases the risk for serious nicks and cuts. Electric razors are safer for these residents.

The beard and skin are softened before shaving with a blade. Soften the beard by applying a warm washcloth or face towel to the face for a few minutes. Then lather the face with soap and water or shaving cream. Take care not to cut or irritate the skin while shaving. Women's legs and underarms are shaved after the bath when the skin is soft. Soap and water, shaving cream, or lotion also can provide lather for shaving legs and underarms.

Box 15-1 on p. 334 lists the rules that are followed when shaving the face or legs and underarms.

Box 15-1 Rules for Shaving

- Never use blade razors to shave residents receiving anticoagulant drugs.
- Follow Standard Precautions and the Bloodborne Pathogen Standard.
- Protect the bed linens. Place a towel under the part being shaved.
- Soften the skin before shaving.
- Encourage the resident to do as much for himself or herself as safely possible.
- Hold the skin taut as necessary.
- Shave in the direction of hair growth when shaving the face and underarms.
- Shave upward, starting at the ankle, when shaving legs.
- Rinse the body part thoroughly.
- Apply direct pressure to any nicks or cuts.
- Report nicks and cuts to the nurse immediately.

Caring for Mustaches and Beards

Beards and mustaches need daily care. Food can collect in hair; so can mouth and nose drainage. Daily washing and combing usually are enough. Ask the resident how to groom his beard or mustache. *Never trim or shave a beard or mustache without the person's consent.*

Shaving Female Legs and Underarms

Many women shave their legs and underarms. This practice varies among cultures. Some women shave only the lower legs. Others shave to midthigh, and others shave the entire leg.

Legs and underarms are shaved after bathing when the skin is soft. Soap and water or a shaving cream provides lather. Needed shaving items are collected with the bath items. Use the kidney basin to rinse the razor rather than using the bath water.

Shaving underarms and legs is similar to shaving the face. See Box 15-1.

Shaving the Resident With a Blade Shaver

Quality of Life

Remember to:
- ◆ ***Knock before entering the resident's room***
- ◆ ***Address the resident by name***
- ◆ ***Introduce yourself by name and title***

Pre-Procedure

1 Explain the procedure to the resident.
2 Wash your hands.
3 Collect the following:
- Wash basin
- Bath towel
- Face towel
- Washcloth
- Bath thermometer
- Disposable razor
- Mirror
- Shaving cream, soap, or lotion
- Shaving brush
- After-shave lotion (male residents only)
- Tissues
- Paper towels
- Gloves

4 Arrange the equipment on the overbed table.
5 Identify the resident. Check the ID bracelet against the assignment sheet.
6 Provide for privacy.
7 Raise the bed to the best level for good body mechanics. Make sure the bed rails are up.
8 Fill the basin with water. Measure water temperature with the bath thermometer. Water temperature should be about 115° F (46°C).
9 Place the basin on the overbed table on top of the paper towels.
10 Lower the bed rail near you.

Shaving the Resident With a Blade Shaver—cont'd

Procedure

11 Position the resident in a semi-Fowler's position if allowed. Or position the person on his or her back.

12 Adjust lighting to clearly see the resident's face.

13 Place the bath towel over the chest.

14 Position the overbed table within easy reach and at a comfortable working height.

15 Tighten the razor blade to the razor.

16 Wash the resident's face. Do not dry.

17 Place a washcloth or face towel in the basin and wet thoroughly. Wring it out.

18 Apply the washcloth or towel to the resident's face for a few minutes.

19 Put on the gloves.

20 Apply shaving cream with your hands. Or use a shaving brush to apply lather.

21 Hold the skin taut with one hand.

22 Shave in the direction of hair growth. Use shorter strokes around the chin and lips (Fig. 15-5).

23 Rinse the razor often, and wipe with tissues.

24 Apply direct pressure to any bleeding area.

25 Wash off any remaining shaving cream or soap. Dry with a towel.

26 Apply after-shave lotion if requested.

Post-Procedure

27 Move the overbed table to the side of the bed.

28 Provide for comfort.

29 Place the signal light within reach.

30 Lower the bed to its lowest position.

31 Raise or lower bed rails. Follow the care plan.

32 Clean and return equipment and supplies to their proper place.

33 Discard disposable items. Remove and discard the gloves.

34 Wipe off the overbed table with the paper towels. Position the table for the resident's ease. Discard paper towels.

35 Unscreen the resident.

36 Follow center policy for dirty linen.

37 Wash your hands.

38 Report any nicks or bleeding to the nurse.

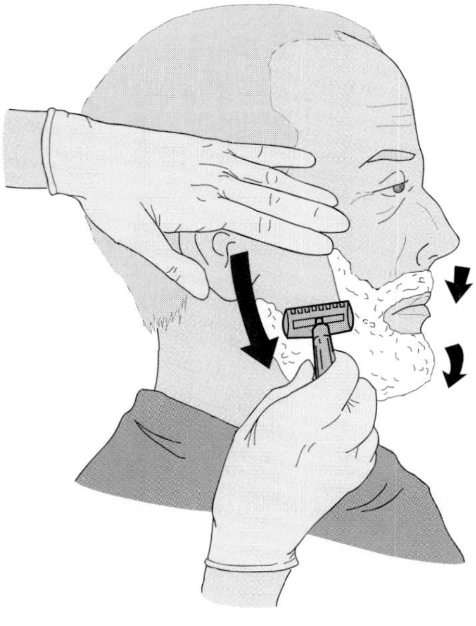

Fig. 15-5 Shave in the direction of hair growth. Use longer strokes on the larger areas of the face. Use short strokes around the chin and lips.

SUBACUTE CARE

Some patients wear a hospital gown. Gowns usually are worn for IV therapy. This is more common on subacute units. Hospital gowns are put on and removed in a certain way (p. 342).

CHANGING CLOTHING AND HOSPITAL GOWNS

Dressing and undressing occur at least daily. Residents change from gowns or pajamas into clothing after morning care. *(See subacute Care.)* They undress and put on a gown or pajamas at bedtime. Incontinent residents may have more frequent clothing changes. Some residents cannot dress and undress themselves. Others need some help. Changing is easier for residents who can move their arms and legs. Arm or leg injuries or paralysis also requires special measures.

Certain rules are followed when changing hospital gowns or clothing:

- Provide for privacy. Do not expose the resident.
- Encourage the resident to do as much as possible.
- Allow the resident personal choice in selecting clothes. Make sure the resident chooses the proper undergarments.
- Remove clothing from the strong or "good" side first.
- Put clothing on the weak side first.
- Support the arm or leg when removing or putting on a garment.

Undressing the Resident

QUALITY OF LIFE

Remember to:

- ◆ *Knock before entering the resident's room*
- ◆ *Address the resident by name*
- ◆ *Introduce yourself by name and title*

Pre-Procedure

1 Explain the procedure to the resident.
2 Wash your hands.
3 Get a bath blanket.
4 Identify the resident. Check the ID bracelet, and call the resident by name.
5 Provide for privacy.
6 Raise the bed to a level for good body mechanics. Make sure bed rails are up.
7 Lower the bed rail on the resident's weak side.
8 Position the resident supine.
9 Cover the resident with the bath blanket. Fanfold linens to the foot of the bed. Do not expose the resident.

Procedure

10 Remove garments that open in the back:
  a Raise the head and shoulders (see *Raising the Resident's Head and Shoulders by Locking Arms With the Resident,* p. 200). Or turn him or her onto the side away from you.
  b Undo buttons, zippers, ties, or snaps.
  c Bring the sides of the garment to the resident's sides (Fig. 15-6, p. 338). Do the following if he or she is in a side-lying position. Tuck the far side under the resident. Fold the near side onto the chest (Fig. 15-7, p. 338).
  d Position the resident supine.

Undressing the Resident—cont'd

Procedure—cont'd

- e Slide the garment off the shoulder on the strong side. Remove the garment from the arm (Fig. 15-8, p. 338).
- f Repeat step 10e for the weak side.

11 Remove garments that open in the front:
- a Undo buttons, zippers, snaps, or ties.
- b Slide the garment off the shoulder and arm on the strong side.
- c Raise the resident's head and shoulders. Bring the garment over to the weak side (Fig. 15-9, p. 338). Lower the resident's head and shoulders.
- d Remove the garment from the weak side.
- e Do the following if you cannot raise the resident's head and shoulders:
  - 1 Turn the resident toward you. Tuck the removed part of the garment under the resident.
  - 2 Turn him or her onto the side away from you.
  - 3 Pull the side of the garment out from under the person. Make sure he or she will not lie on it when supine.
  - 4 Return the resident to the supine position.
  - 5 Remove the garment from the weak side.

12 Remove pullover garments:
- a Undo any buttons, zippers, ties, or snaps.
- b Remove the garment from the strong side.
- c Raise the resident's head and shoulders. Or turn him or her onto the side away from you. Bring the garment up the resident's neck (Fig. 15-10, p. 338).
- d Remove the garment from the weak side.
- e Bring the garment over the resident's head.
- f Position the resident in the supine position.

13 Remove pants or slacks:
- a Remove shoes or slippers.
- b Position the resident supine.
- c Undo buttons, zippers, ties, snaps, or buckles.
- d Remove the belt if one is worn.
- e Ask the resident to lift the buttocks off the bed. Slide the pants down over the hips and buttocks (Fig. 15-11, p. 339). Have the resident lower the hips and buttocks.
- f Do the following if the resident cannot raise the hips off the bed:
  - 1 Turn the resident toward you.
  - 2 Slide the pants off the hip and buttock on the strong side (Fig. 15-12, p. 339).
  - 3 Turn the resident away from you.
  - 4 Slide the pants off the hip and buttock on the weak side (Fig. 15-13, p. 339).
  - 5 Slide the pants down the legs and over the feet.

Post-Procedure

14 Dress the resident *(see Dressing the Resident, p. 340).*

15 Help the resident get out of bed if he or she is to be up.

16 Do the following for the resident who will stay in bed:
- a Cover the resident, and remove the bath blanket.
- b Provide for comfort.
- c Lower the bed to its lowest position.
- d Raise or lower the bed rails. Follow the care plan.
- e Place the signal light within reach.

17 Unscreen the resident.

18 Follow center policy for dirty linen.

19 Report your observations to the nurse.

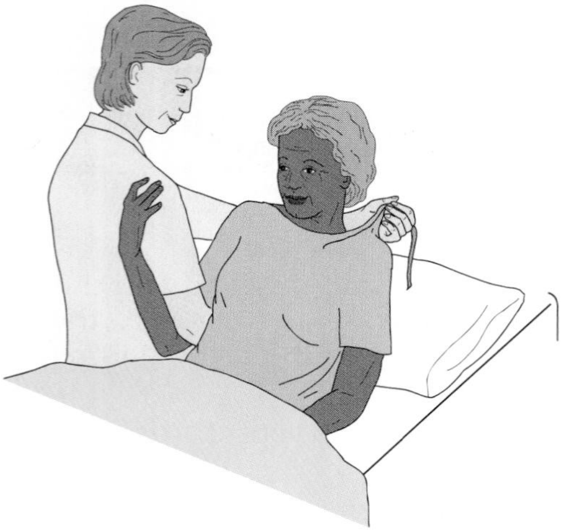

Fig. 15-6 The sides of the garment are brought from the back to the sides of the person.

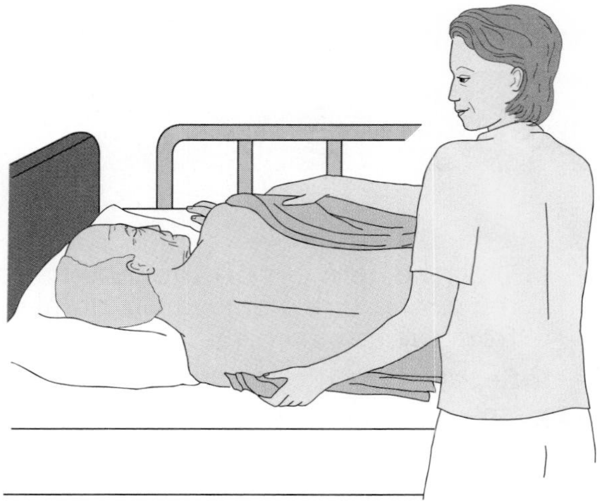

Fig. 15-7 A garment that opens in back is removed from the person in the side-lying position. The far side of the garment is tucked under the person. The near side is folded onto the person's chest.

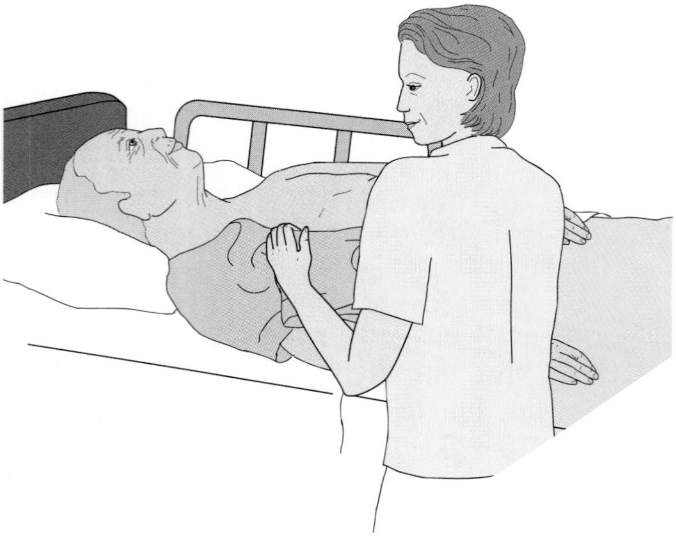

Fig. 15-8 The garment is removed from the strong side first.

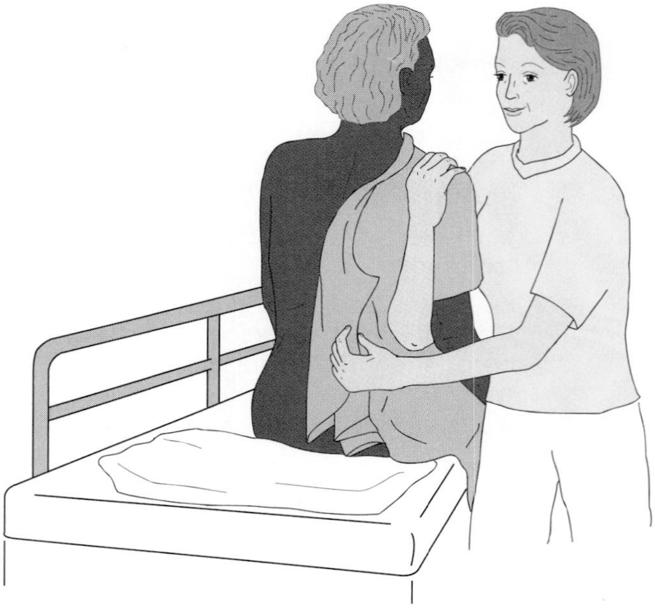

Fig. 15-9 A front-opening garment is removed with the person's head and shoulders raised. The garment is removed from the strong side first. Then it is brought around the back to the weak side.

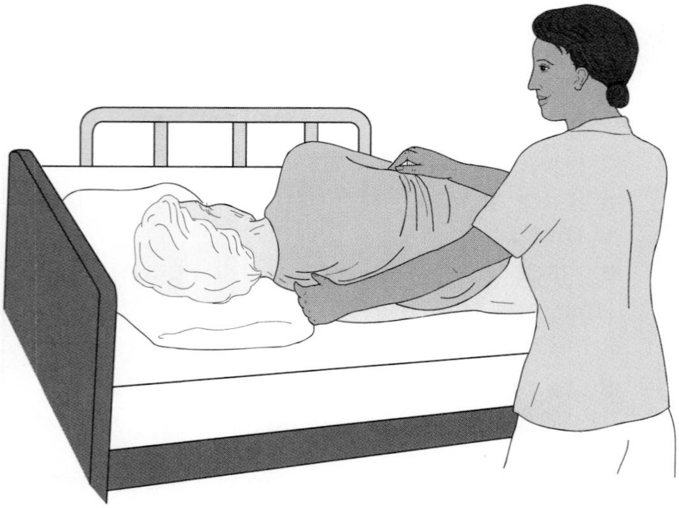

Fig. 15-10 A pullover garment is removed from the strong side first. Then the garment is brought up to the person's neck so that it can be removed from the weak side.

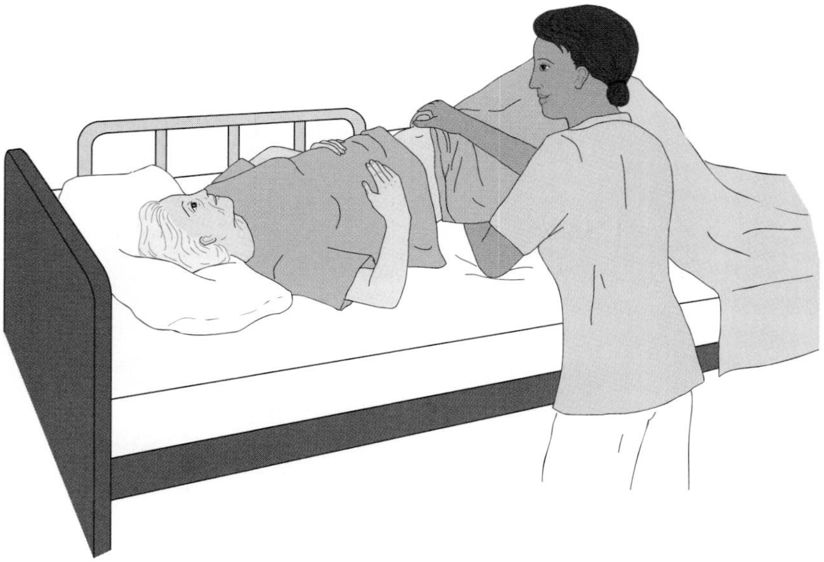

Fig. 15-11 The person lifts the hips and buttocks for removing the pants. The pants are slid down over the hips and buttocks.

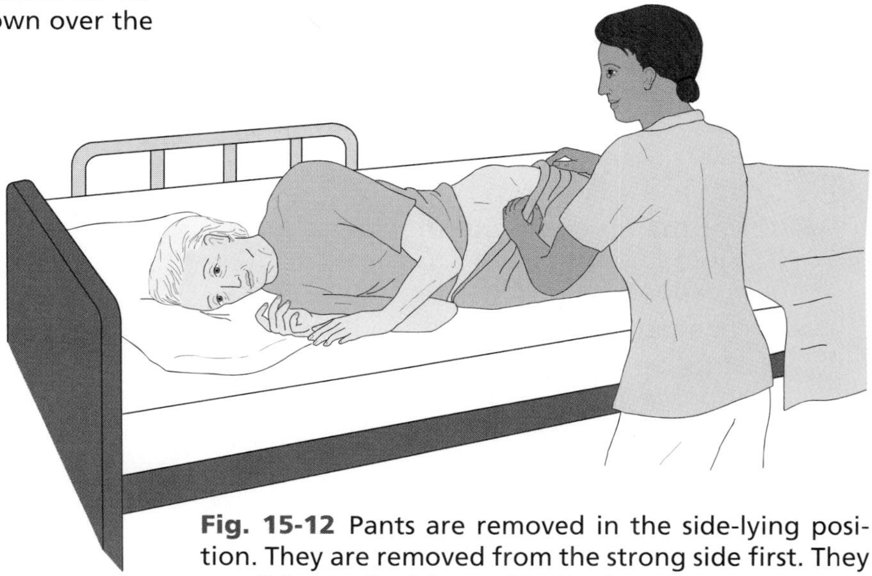

Fig. 15-12 Pants are removed in the side-lying position. They are removed from the strong side first. They are slid over the hips and buttocks.

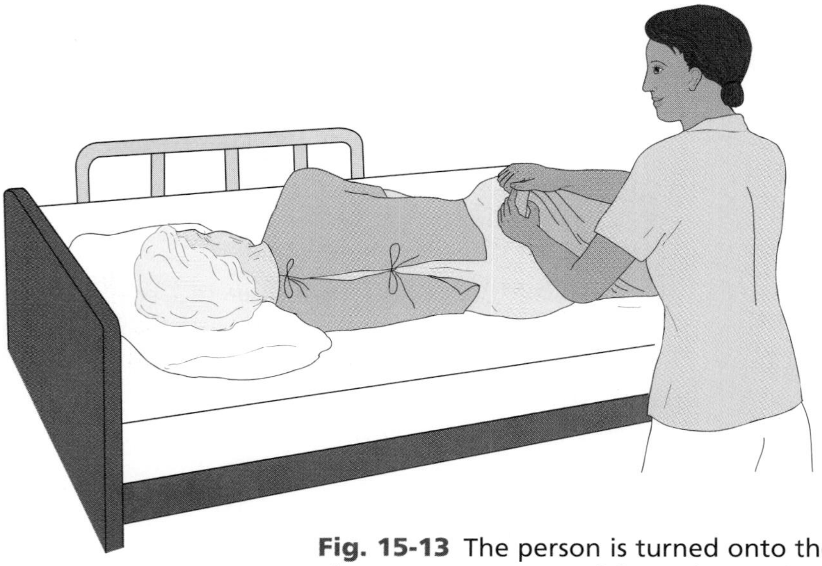

Fig. 15-13 The person is turned onto the other side. The pants are removed from the weak side.

Dressing the Resident

NNAAP™ SKILL

Quality of Life

Remember to:
- ◆ ***Knock before entering the resident's room***
- ◆ ***Address the resident by name***
- ◆ ***Introduce yourself by name and title***

Pre-Procedure

1 Explain the procedure to the resident.
2 Wash your hands.
3 Get a bath blanket and necessary clothing.
4 Identify the resident. Check the ID bracelet, and call the resident by name.
5 Provide for privacy.
6 Raise the bed to the best level for good body mechanics. Make sure the bed rails are up.
7 Undress the resident (see *Undressing the Resident,* pp. 336-337).
8 Lower the bed rail on the resident's strong side.
9 Position the resident supine.

Procedure

10 Cover the resident with the bath blanket. Fanfold linens to the foot of the bed. Do not expose the resident.
11 Put on garments that open in the back:
  a Slide the garment onto the arm and shoulder of the weak side.
  b Slide the garment onto the arm and shoulder of the strong side.
  c Raise the resident's head and shoulders.
  d Bring the sides of the garment to the back.
  e Do the following if the resident is in a side-lying position:
    1 Turn the resident toward you.
    2 Bring the side of the garment to the resident's back (Fig. 15-14, *A*).
    3 Turn the resident away from you.
    4 Bring the other side of the garment to the resident's back (Fig. 15-14, *B*).
  f Fasten buttons, snaps, ties, or zippers.
  g Position the resident supine.
12 Put on garments that open in the front:
  a Slide the garment onto the arm and shoulder on the weak side.
  b Raise the head and shoulders by locking arms with the resident. Bring the side of the garment around to the back. Lower the resident to the supine position. Slide the garment onto the arm and shoulder of the strong arm.
  c Do the following if the resident cannot raise the head and shoulders:
    1 Turn the resident toward you.
    2 Tuck the garment under him or her.
    3 Turn the resident away from you.
    4 Pull the garment out from under the resident.
    5 Turn the resident back to the supine position.
    6 Slide the garment over the arm and shoulder of the strong arm.
  d Fasten buttons, snaps, ties, or zippers.
13 Put on pullover garments:
  a Position the resident supine.
  b Bring the neck of the garment over the head.
  c Slide the arm and shoulder of the garment onto the weak side.
  d Raise the resident's head and shoulders.
  e Bring the garment down.
  f Slide the arm and shoulder of the garment onto the strong side.
  g Do the following if the resident cannot assume a semisitting position:
    1 Turn the resident toward you.
    2 Tuck the garment under the resident.

Dressing the Resident—cont'd

NNAAP™ SKILL

Procedure—cont'd

3 Turn the resident away from you.
4 Pull the garment out from under him or her.
5 Return the resident to the supine position.
6 Slide the arm and shoulder of the garment onto the strong side.

h Fasten buttons, snaps, ties, or zippers.

14 Put on pants or slacks:

a Slide the pants over the feet and up the legs.
b Ask the resident to raise the hips and buttocks off the bed.
c Bring the pants up over the buttocks and hips.
d Ask the resident to lower the hips and buttocks.
e Do the following if the resident cannot raise the hips and buttocks:

1 Turn the resident onto the strong side.
2 Pull the pants over the buttock and hip on the weak side.
3 Turn the resident onto the weak side.
4 Pull the pants over the buttock and hip on the strong side.
5 Position the resident supine.

f Fasten buttons, ties, snaps, the zipper, and belt buckle.

15 Put socks and shoes or slippers on the resident.

Post-Procedure

16 Help the resident get out of bed if he or she is to be up.

17 Do the following for the resident who will stay in bed:

a Cover the resident, and remove the bath blanket.
b Provide for comfort.
c Lower the bed to its lowest position.
d Raise or lower the bed rails. Follow the care plan.
e Place the signal light within reach.

18 Unscreen the resident.

19 Follow center policy for dirty linen.

20 Report your observations to the nurse.

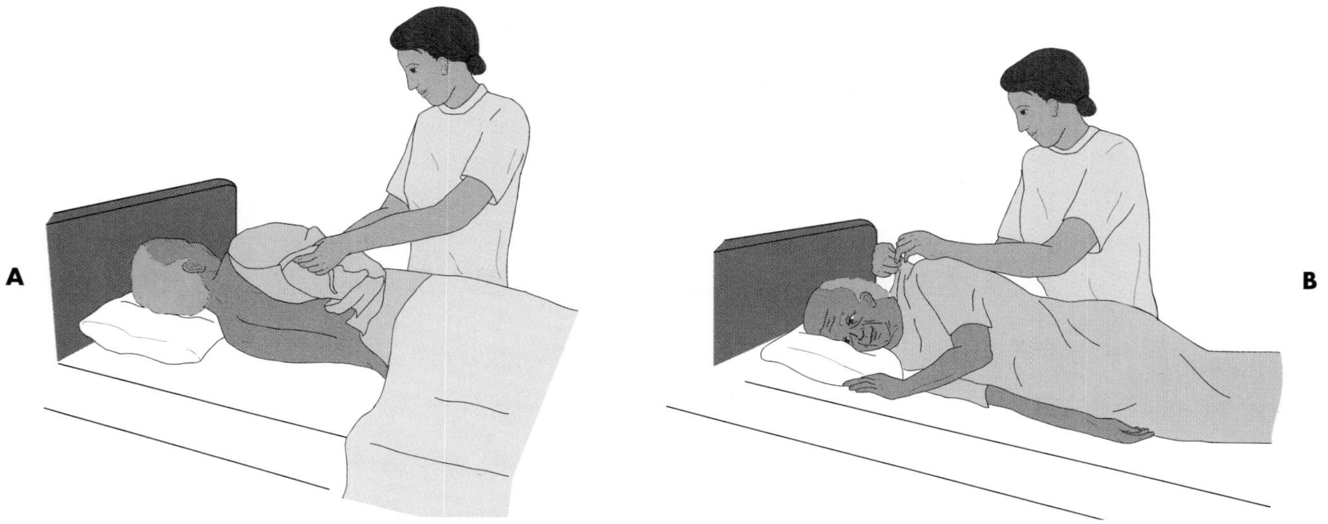

Fig. 15-14 Putting on garments that open in the back. **A,** The side-lying position can be used to put on garments that open in the back. Turn the person toward you after the garment is put on the arms. The side of the garment is brought to the person's back. **B,** Then turn the person away from you. The other side of the garment is brought to the back and fastened.

Changing the Gown of a Resident With an IV

Quality of Life

Remember to:
- *Knock before entering the resident's room*
- *Address the resident by name*
- *Introduce yourself by name and title*

Pre-Procedure

1 Explain the procedure to the resident.
2 Wash your hands.
3 Get a clean gown.
4 Identify the resident. Check the ID bracelet, and call the resident by name.
5 Provide for privacy.
6 Raise the bed to the best level for good body mechanics. Make sure bed rails are up.
7 Lower the bed rail near you.

Procedure

8 Untie the back of the gown. Free parts that the resident is lying on.
9 Remove the gown from the arm with no IV.
10 Gather up the sleeve of the arm with the IV. Slide it over the IV site and tubing. Remove the arm and hand from the sleeve (Fig. 15-15, *A*).
11 Keep the sleeve gathered. Slide your arm along the tubing to the bag (Fig. 15-15, *B*).
12 Remove the IV bag from the pole. Slide the bag and tubing through the sleeve (Fig. 15-15, *C*). Do not pull on the tubing.
13 Hang the IV bag on the pole.
14 Gather the sleeve of the clean gown that will go on the arm with the IV infusion.
15 Remove the bag from the pole. Quickly slip the gathered sleeve over the bag at the shoulder part of the gown (Fig. 15-15, *D*). Hang the bag on the pole.
16 Slide the gathered sleeve over the tubing, hand, arm, and IV site. Then slide the sleeve onto the resident's shoulder.
17 Put the other side of the gown on, and fasten the back.

Post-Procedure

18 Provide for comfort.
19 Place the signal light within reach.
20 Lower the bed to its lowest position.
21 Raise or lower bed rails. Follow the care plan.
22 Unscreen the resident.
23 Follow center policy for dirty linen.
24 Wash your hands.
25 Ask the nurse to check the IV flow rate.

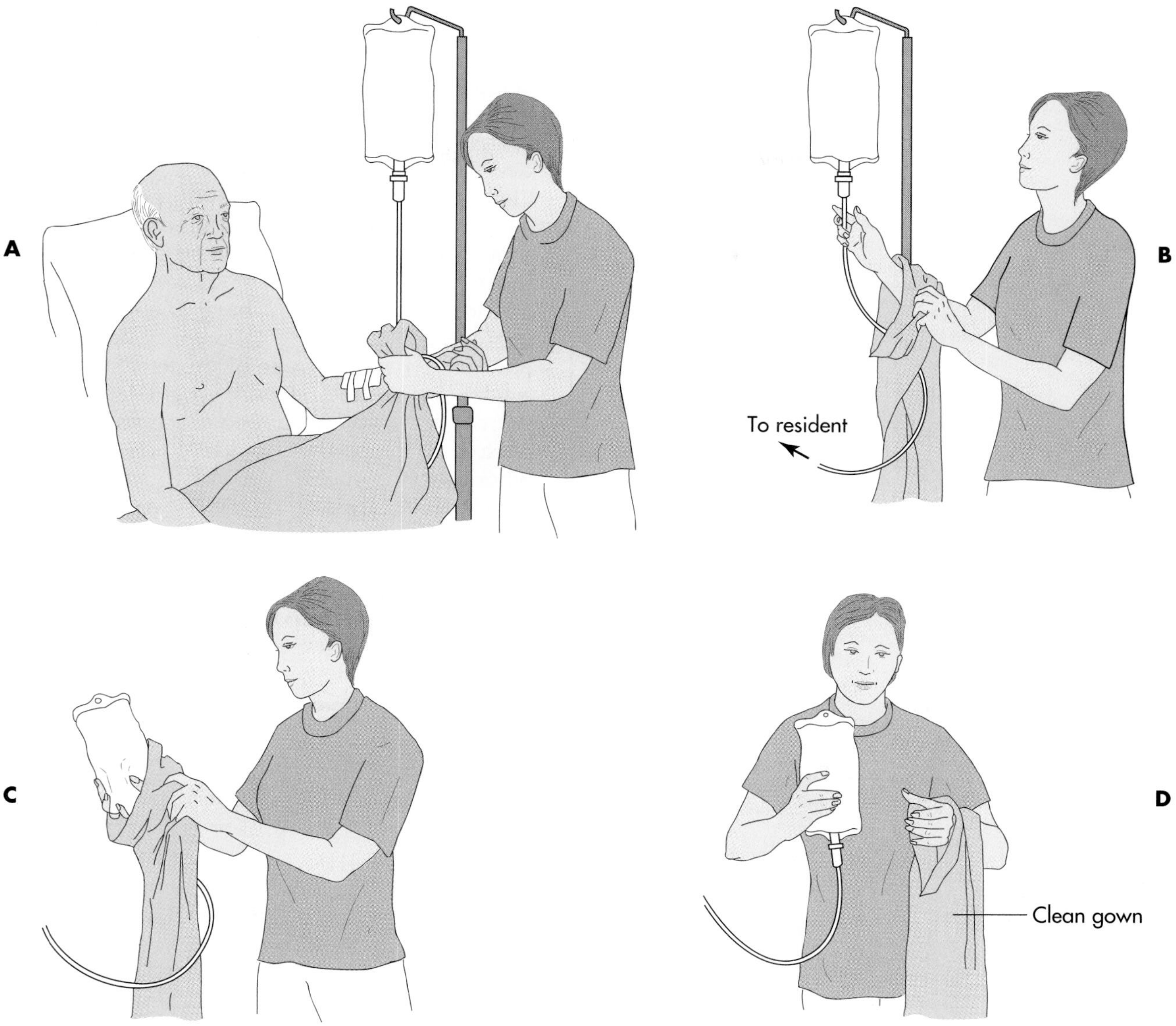

Fig. 15-15 Changing a hospital gown. **A,** The gown is removed from the good arm. The sleeve on the arm with the IV is gathered up, slipped over the IV site and tubing, and removed from the arm and hand. **B,** The gathered sleeve is slipped along the IV tubing to the bag. **C,** The IV bag is removed from the pole and passed through the sleeve. **D,** The gathered sleeve of the clean gown is slipped over the IV bag at the shoulder part of the gown.

QUALITY OF LIFE

Personal care and grooming measures are important for physical comfort. They also help the person's body image and self-esteem needs. Good grooming is important to many people. Clean hair and nails and wearing clean clothes all help a person feel good mentally. A clean-shaven face or a well-groomed beard or mustache affects a man's sense of well-being.

The resident may not have energy for some procedures. The nurse tells you what care to give and when it is to be given. Personal choice is encouraged and allowed whenever possible. Personal care and grooming practices vary from person to person. Always provide assistance whenever it is necessary.

You must carefully handle the resident's personal hygiene products, shaver, hair dryer, brush and comb, perfumes, and other personal care items. The resident's clothing also needs your attention. Do not break zippers, tear clothing, or lose buttons. Remember to treat all of the resident's property with care and respect.

REVIEW QUESTIONS

Circle the BEST answer.

1 You read the word *alopecia* in Mr. Polk's medical record. The term means
- A Excessive body hair
- B Dry, white flakes from the scalp
- C An infestation of lice
- D Hair loss

2 Which prevents hair from matting and tangling?
- A Bedrest
- B Daily brushing and combing
- C Daily shampooing
- D Cutting long hair

3 You are going to brush a woman's hair. The hair is not matted or tangled. When brushing the hair, start at
- A The forehead and brush backward
- B The hair ends
- C The scalp
- D The back of the neck and brush forward

4 Brushing is important to keep the hair
- A Soft and shiny
- B Clean
- C Free from pediculosis
- D All of the above

5 Mr. Polk wants his hair washed. You should
- A Wash his hair during his shower
- B Wash his hair at the sink
- C Shampoo him in bed
- D Follow the nurse's instructions

6 When shaving Mr. Polk, you need to do the following *except*
- A Practice Standard Precautions
- B Follow the Bloodborne Pathogen Standard
- C Shave in the opposite direction of hair growth
- D Make sure the skin is soft before shaving

7 Mr. Polk is nicked during shaving. Your first action is to
- A Wash your hands
- B Apply direct pressure
- C Tell the nurse
- D Apply a bandage

8 Mr. Polk has a mustache and beard. You think he would be more comfortable without the facial hair. You can shave his beard and mustache.
- A True
- B False

9 Clothing is removed from the strong side first.
- A True
- B False

10 The person is allowed to choose what to wear.
- A True
- B False

Answers to these questions are on p. 698.

16 Urinary Elimination

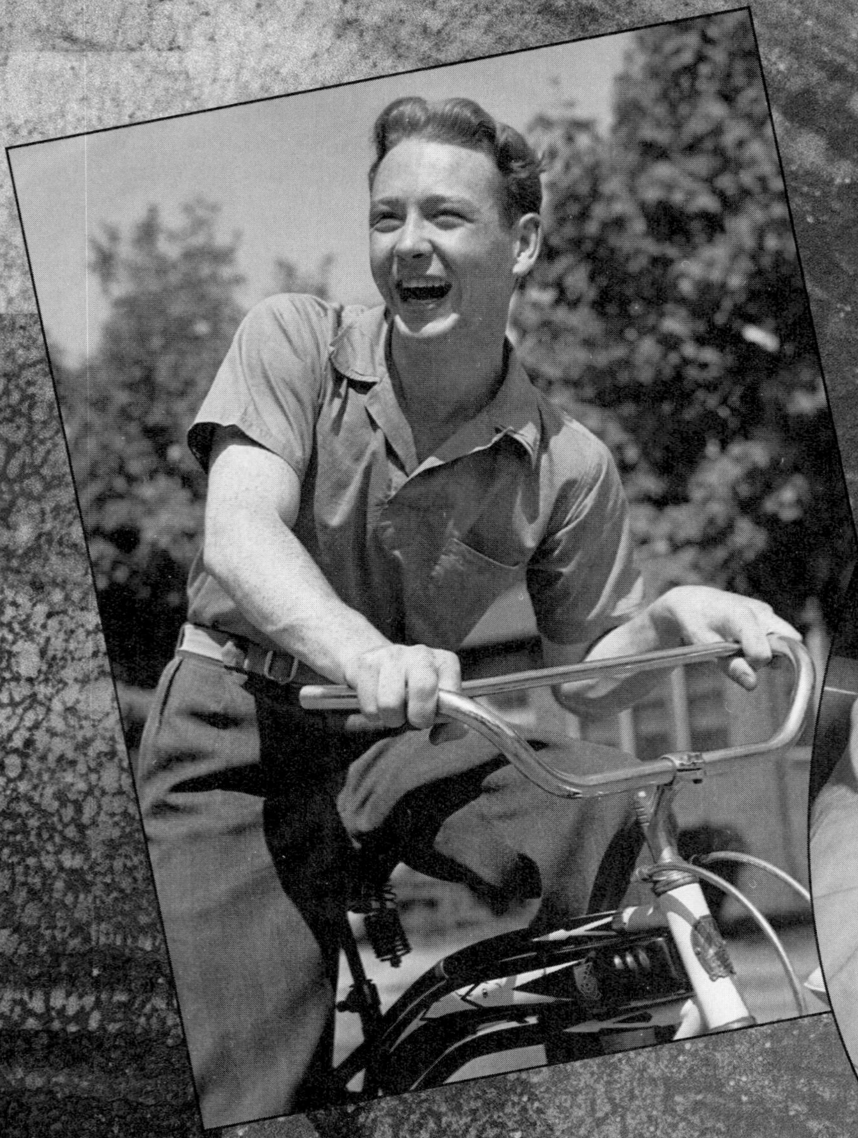

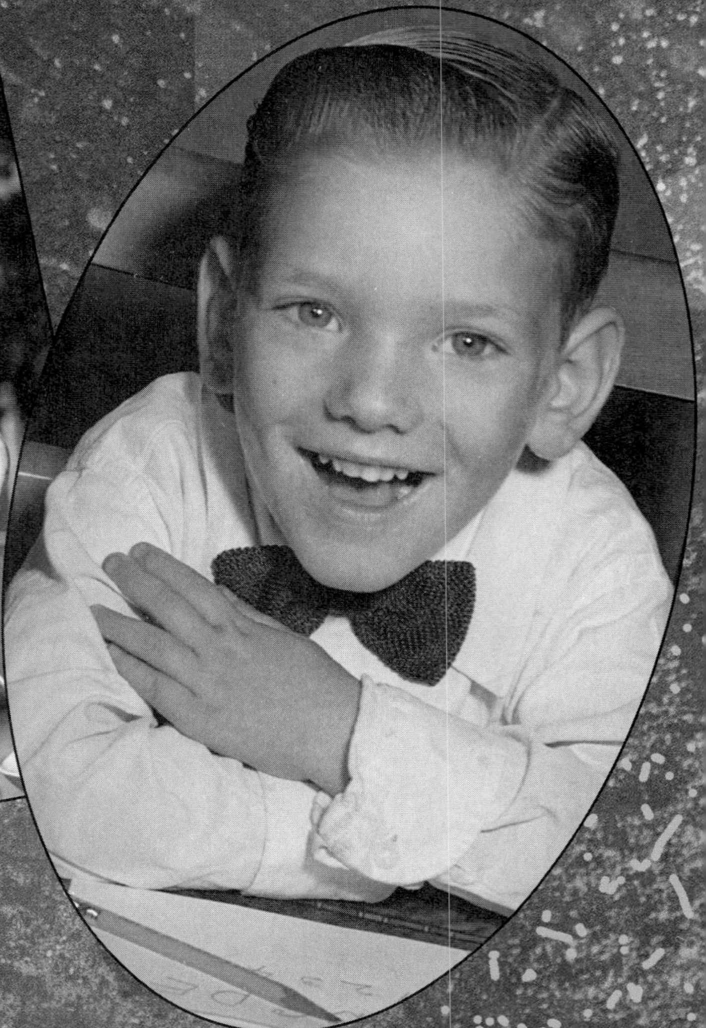

WHAT YOU WILL LEARN

- The definition of the key terms listed in this chapter
- The characteristics of normal urine
- The rules for maintaining normal urinary elimination
- The observations to make about urine
- The care required for urinary incontinence
- Why catheters are used
- The rules for caring for residents with catheters
- The differences between straight, indwelling, and condom catheters
- Two methods of bladder training
- The rules for collecting and testing urine specimens
- How to care for the resident with a ureterostomy
- The purpose of dialysis
- The procedures described in this chapter

KEY TERMS

acetone Ketone bodies that appear in the urine because of the rapid breakdown of fat for energy

catheter A tube used to drain or inject fluid through a body opening

catheterization The process of inserting a catheter

dialysis An artificial way to remove waste and excess fluid from the blood

dysuria Painful or difficult *(dys)* urination *(uria)*

functional incontinence The involuntary, unpredicted loss of urine from the bladder

glucosuria Sugar *(glucose)* in the urine *(uria)*; glycosuria

glycosuria Sugar *(glycos)* in the urine *(uria)*; glucosuria

hematuria Blood *(hemat)* in the urine *(uria)*

hemodialysis Removal of waste and fluid from the body by filtering the blood (*hemo*) through an artificial kidney called a *dialyzer*

ketone body Acetone

micturition The process of emptying urine from the bladder; urination or voiding

mixed incontinence A combination of urge and stress incontinence

nocturia Frequent urination *(uria)* at night *(noct)*

oliguria Scant amount *(olig)* of urine *(uria)*; usually less than 500 ml in 24 hours

ostomy Surgical creation of an artificial opening

overflow incontinence The loss of urine when the bladder is too full

peritoneal dialysis A process that uses the lining of the abdominal cavity (the *peritoneal membrane*) to remove waste from the body

polyuria The production of abnormally large amounts *(poly)* of urine *(uria)*

reflex incontinence The loss of urine at predictable intervals; unconscious incontinence

stoma An artificial opening to the outside of the body

stress incontinence The loss of small amounts of urine with exercise and certain movements

unconscious incontinence Reflex incontinence

ureterostomy An artificial opening *(stomy)* between the ureter *(uretero)* and abdomen

urge incontinence The involuntary loss of urine after feeling a strong need to void

urinary frequency Voiding at frequent intervals

Continued

KEY TERMS—cont'd

urinary incontinence The inability to control the loss of urine from the bladder

urinary urgency The need to void immediately

urination The process of emptying urine from the bladder; micturition or voiding

voiding Urination or micturition

Eliminating waste is a physical need. The respiratory, digestive, integumentary, and urinary systems all remove body wastes. The digestive system rids the body of solid wastes. The lungs rid the body of carbon dioxide. Sweat contains water and other substances. Blood contains waste products from body cells burning food for energy. The urinary system removes waste products from the blood and maintains the body's water balance (see Chapter 6).

NORMAL URINATION

The healthy adult excretes about 1500 ml (milliliters) (3 pints) of urine a day. Many factors affect urine production. They include age, disease, the amount and kinds of fluid ingested, dietary salt, and drugs. Some substances increase urine production. Examples are coffee, tea, alcohol, and some drugs. A diet high in salt causes the body to retain water. Body temperature and perspiration also influence urine production. When water is retained, less urine is produced.

Urination, micturition, and **voiding** mean the process of emptying urine from the bladder. Urination patterns depend on many factors. The amount of fluid ingested, personal habits, and available toilet facilities affect frequency. So do activity, work, and illness. People usually urinate at bedtime, after getting up, and before meals. Some people urinate every 2 to 3 hours. The need to urinate at night disturbs sleep.

MAINTAINING NORMAL URINATION

OBRA requires centers to provide care in a way that ensures that residents maintain the highest level of independence. The care team must assess the elimination needs of residents. The team then develops a plan of care to ensure that these needs are met. Residents often need help to maintain normal elimination. Some need help getting to the bathroom. Others use a bedpan, urinal, or commode. Follow the rules in Box 16-1 to help residents maintain normal urination. OBRA

What to Report to the Nurse

Urine is normally pale yellow, straw colored, or amber. It is clear with no particles. A faint odor is normal. Observe urine for color, clarity, odor, amount, and particles. Some foods normally affect urine color. Red food dyes, beets, blackberries, and rhubarb cause red-colored urine. Carrots and sweet potatoes cause bright yellow urine. Certain drugs cause changes in urine color. Asparagus causes a urine odor.

Ask the nurse to observe any urine that looks or smells abnormal. Report complaints of urgency, burning on urination, or dysuria. **Dysuria** means painful or difficult *(dys)* urination *(uria)*. Also report any problems described in Table 16-1. The nurse uses the information for the nursing process.

◈ Bedpans

Bedpans are used when residents cannot be out of bed. Women use a bedpan for voiding and bowel movements. Men use it only for bowel movements. Bedpans are made of plastic or stainless steel. Stainless steel bedpans often are cold. They are warmed with water and dried before use.

A *fracture pan* has a thinner rim and is only about ½-inch deep at one end (Fig. 16-1, p. 350). The smaller end is placed under the buttocks (Fig. 16-2, p. 350). Fracture pans are used for residents with casts or those in traction. Residents with limited range of motion in their back may also use a fracture pan.

Follow medical asepsis, Standard Precautions, and the Bloodborne Pathogen Standard when handling bedpans and their contents.

Text continued on p. 353

Box 16-1 Rules for Maintaining Urinary Elimination

- Practice medical asepsis and Standard Precautions. Also follow the Bloodborne Pathogen Standard.
- Provide fluids as instructed by the nurse.
- Follow the resident's normal voiding routines and habits. Check with the nurse and the care plan.
- Help the resident to the bathroom when the request is made. Or provide the commode, bedpan, or urinal. The need to void may be urgent.
- Help the resident assume a normal position for voiding if possible. Women sit or squat; men stand.
- Warm the bedpan or urinal.
- Cover the resident for warmth and privacy.
- Provide for privacy. Pull the curtain around the bed, close room and bathroom doors, and pull drapes or window shades. Leave the room if the resident can be alone.
- Tell the resident that running water, flushing the toilet, or playing music can mask urination sounds. Some residents are embarrassed about voiding with others close by.
- Remain nearby if the resident is weak or unsteady.
- Place the signal light and toilet tissue within reach.
- Allow the resident enough time to void. Do not rush the resident.
- Promote relaxation. Some people like to read when eliminating.
- Run water in a nearby sink if the resident has difficulty starting the urine stream, or place the resident's fingers in some warm water.
- Provide perineal care as needed.
- Have the resident wash his or her hands after voiding. Provide a wash basin, soap, washcloth, and towel. Assist as necessary.
- Offer the bedpan or urinal at regular times. Some people are embarrassed or are too weak to ask.

Table 16-1 Common Urinary Elimination Problems

	Definition	Causes
dysuria	Painful or difficult *(dys)* urination *(uria)*	Urinary tract infection, trauma, urinary tract obstruction
hematuria	Blood *(hemat)* in the urine *(uria)*	Kidney disease, urinary tract infection, trauma
nocturia	Frequent urination *(uria)* at night *(noct)*	Excessive fluid intake, kidney disease, disease of the prostate
oliguria	Scant amount *(olig)* of urine *(uria)*, usually less than 500 ml in 24 hours	Inadequate fluid intake, shock, burns, kidney diease, heart failure
polyuria	The production of abnormally large amounts *(poly)* of urine *(uria)*	Drugs, excessive fluid intake, diabetes mellitus, hormone imbalance
urinary frequency	Voiding at frequent intervals	Excessive fluid intake, bladder infections, pressure on the bladder, drugs
urinary incontinence	Inability to control the loss of urine from the bladder	Trauma, disease, urinary tract infections, reproductive or urinary tract surgeries, aging, fecal impaction, constipation, not getting to the bathroom
urinary urgency	The need to void immediately	Urinary tract infection, fear of incontinence (p. 356), full bladder, stress

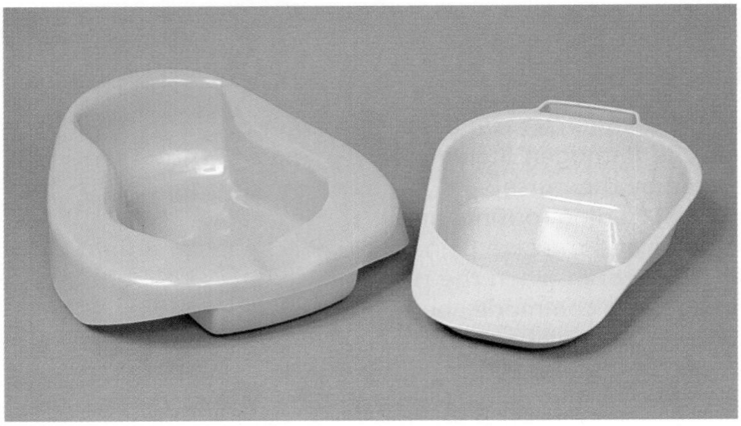

Fig. 16-1 The regular bedpan and the fracture pan.

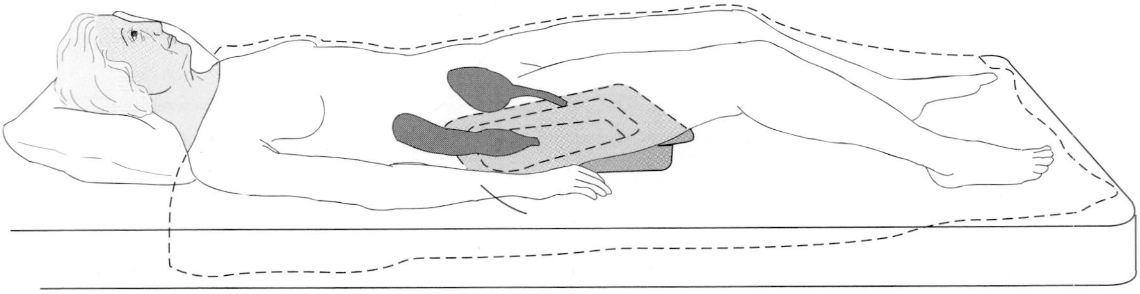

Fig. 16-2 A person positioned on a fracture pan. The smaller end is placed under the buttocks.

Giving the Bedpan

Quality of Life

Remember to:
- *Knock before entering the resident's room*
- *Address the resident by name*
- *Introduce yourself by name and title*

Pre-Procedure

1 Provide for privacy.
2 Put on gloves.
3 Collect the following:
- Bedpan
- Bedpan cover
- Toilet tissue

4 Arrange equipment on the chair or bed.
5 Explain the procedure to the resident.
6 Raise the bed to the best level for good body mechanics. Make sure bed rails are up.

Giving the Bedpan—cont'd

NNAAP™ SKILL

Procedure

7 Warm and dry the bedpan if necessary.
8 Lower the bed rail near you.
9 Position the resident supine. Raise the head of the bed slightly.
10 Fold the top linens and gown out of the way. Keep the lower body covered.
11 Ask the resident to flex the knees and raise the buttocks by pushing against the mattress with his or her feet.
12 Slide your hand under the lower back, and help him or her raise the buttocks.
13 Slide the bedpan under the resident (Fig. 16-3, p. 352).
14 Do the following if the resident cannot assist in getting on the bedpan:
   a Turn the resident onto the side away from you.
   b Place the bedpan firmly against the buttocks (Fig. 16-4, *A,* p. 352).
   c Push the bedpan down and toward the resident (Fig. 16-4, *B,* p. 352).
   d Hold the bedpan securely. Turn the resident onto the back. Make sure the bedpan is centered under the resident.
15 Return top linens to their proper position.
16 Raise the head of the bed so the resident is in a sitting position.
17 Make sure the resident is correctly positioned on the bedpan (Fig. 16-5, p. 352).
18 Raise the bed rail.
19 Place the toilet tissue and signal light within reach.
20 Ask the resident to signal when done or when help is needed.
21 Remove the gloves, and wash your hands.
22 Leave the room, and close the door.
23 Return when the resident signals. Knock before entering.
24 Lower the bed rail and the head of the bed.
25 Put on gloves.
26 Ask the resident to raise the buttocks. Remove the bedpan. Or hold the bedpan securely, and turn him or her onto the side away from you.
27 Clean the genital area if the resident cannot do so. Clean from front to back with toilet tissue. Use fresh tissue for each wipe. Provide perineal care if necessary.
28 Cover the bedpan. Take it to the bathroom or dirty utility room. Raise the bed rail before leaving the bedside.
29 Note the color, amount, and character of urine or feces.
30 Empty and rinse the bedpan. Clean it with a disinfectant.
31 Return the bedpan and clean cover to the bedside stand.
32 Remove soiled gloves. Wash your hands, and put on clean gloves.
33 Help the resident wash the hands.
34 Remove the gloves.

Post-Procedure

35 Provide for comfort.
36 Place the signal light within reach.
37 Lower the bed to its lowest position.
38 Raise or lower bed rails. Follow the care plan.
39 Unscreen the resident.
40 Follow center policy for soiled linen.
41 Wash your hands.
42 Report your observations to the nurse.

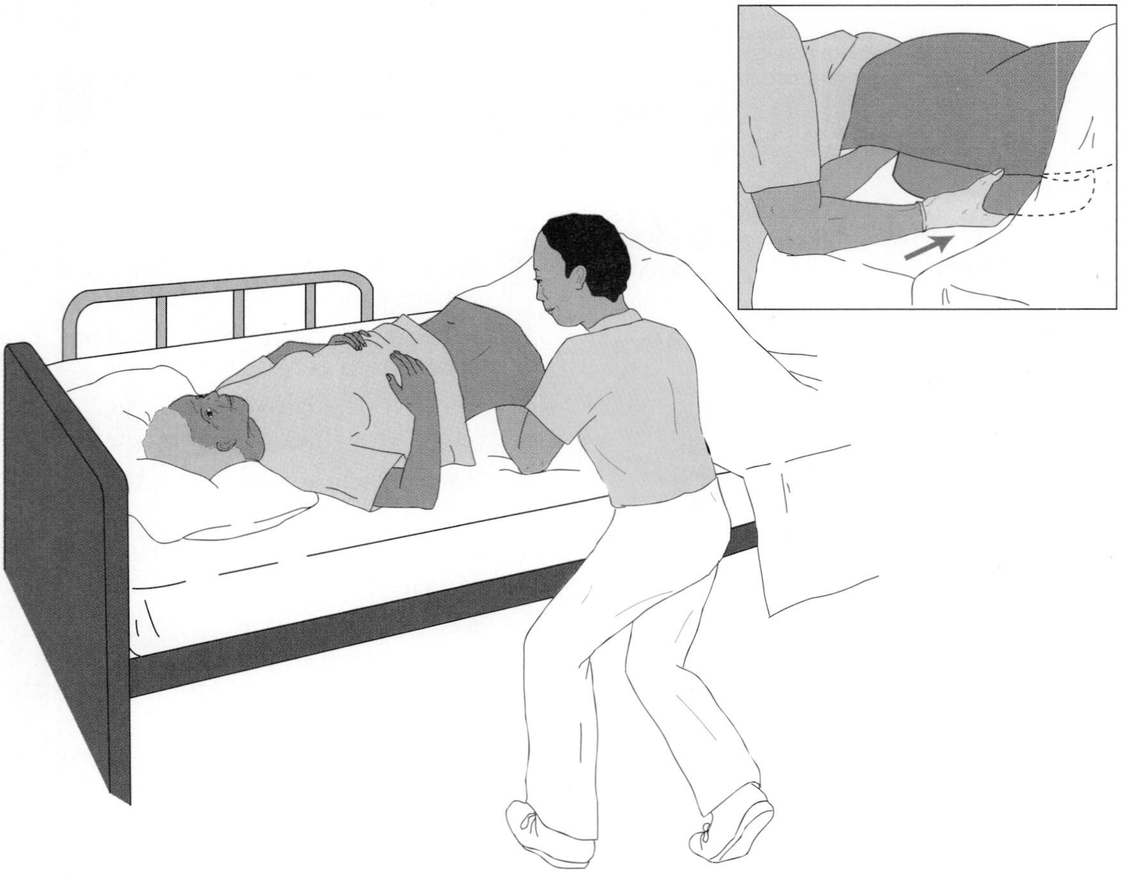

Fig. 16-3 The person raises the buttocks off the bed with help. The bedpan is slid under the person.

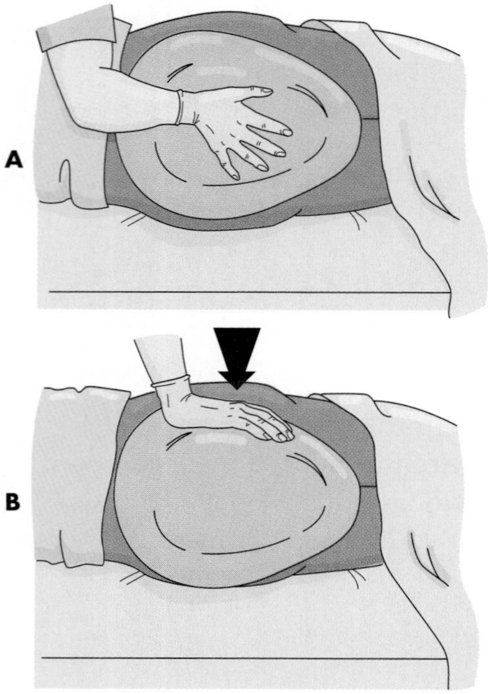

Fig. 16-4 Positioning the resident on a bedpan. **A,** Position the person on one side, and place the bedpan firmly against the buttocks. **B,** Push downward on the bedpan and toward the person.

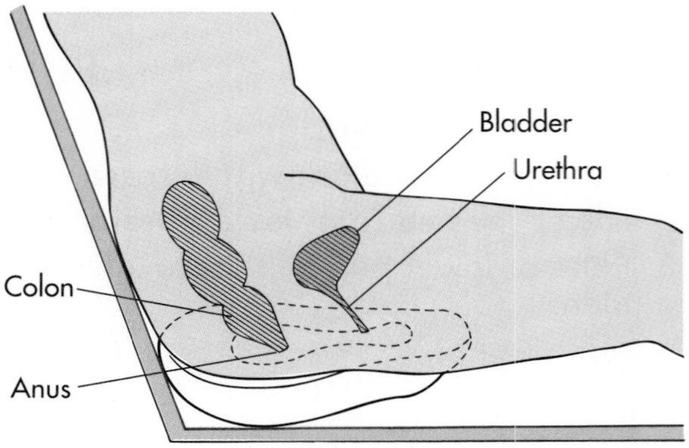

Fig. 16-5 The person is positioned on the bedpan so the urethra and anus are directly over the opening.

Urinals

Men use a urinal to void (Fig. 16-6). Urinals are made of the same materials as bedpans. Plastic urinals have a cap at the top and a hook-type handle. The urinal hooks to the bed rail within the man's reach. The man stands to use the urinal if possible. He may also use it sitting on the side of the bed or lying in bed. Some men stand with the support of 1 or 2 people. You may have to place and hold the urinal for some men.

Remind men to hang the urinal on the bed rail and to signal when the urinal needs emptying. Discourage them from placing the urinal on the overbed table and bedside stand. The overbed table is used for eating and as a work surface. Bedside stands are used for supplies. For these reasons, table surfaces must not be contaminated with urine.

Follow medical asepsis, Standard Precautions, and the Bloodborne Pathogen Standard when handling urinals and their contents. Empty urinals promptly to prevent odors and the spread of microbes. A filled urinal spills easily, causing safety hazards. Also, it is an unpleasant sight and a source of odor. Urinals are cleaned like bedpans.

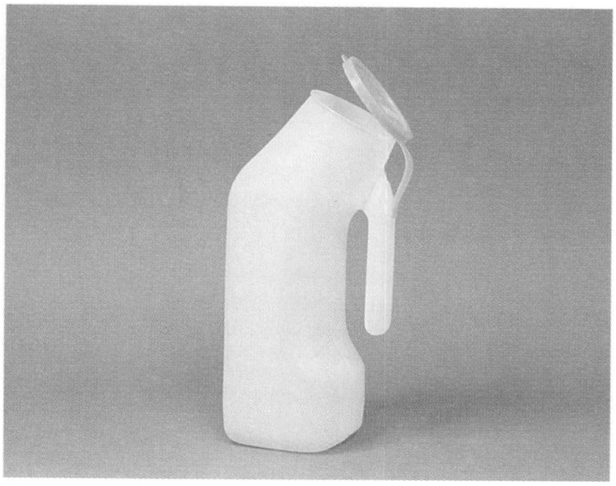

Fig. 16-6 A urinal.

Giving the Urinal

Quality of Life

Remember to:

- ***Knock before entering the resident's room***
- ***Address the resident by name***
- ***Introduce yourself by name and title***

Pre-Procedure

1 Provide for privacy.
2 Determine if the resident will stand or stay in bed.
3 Put on gloves.

Procedure

4 Give him the urinal if he is in bed. Remind him to tilt the bottom down to prevent spills.
5 Do the following if he is going to stand:
 a Help him sit on the side of the bed.
 b Put nonskid shoes or slippers on him.
 c Assist him to a standing position.
 d Provide support if he is unsteady.
 e Give him the urinal.
6 Position the urinal between his legs if necessary. Position his penis in the urinal if he cannot hold the urinal.
7 Cover him to provide for privacy.
8 Place the signal light within reach. Ask him to signal when done or when he needs help.
9 Remove the gloves, and wash your hands.
10 Leave the room, and close the door.

Continued

Giving the Urinal—cont'd

Procedure—cont'd

11 Return when he signals for you. Knock before entering.
12 Put on gloves.
13 Cover the urinal. Take it to the bathroom or dirty utility room.
14 Note the color, amount, and character of the urine.
15 Empty the urinal, and rinse it with cold water. Clean it with a disinfectant.
16 Return the urinal to the bedside stand.
17 Remove soiled gloves. Wash your hands, and put on clean gloves.
18 Help the resident wash his hands.
19 Remove the gloves.

Post-Procedure

20 Provide for comfort.
21 Place the signal light within reach.
22 Raise or lower bed rails. Follow the care plan.
23 Unscreen him.
24 Follow center policy for soiled linen.
25 Wash your hands.
26 Report your observations to the nurse.

Commodes

A bedside commode is a portable chair or wheelchair with an opening for a bedpan or container (Fig. 16-7). Residents unable to walk to the bathroom often use a commode. The commode allows a normal position for elimination. The arms and back of the commode support the resident and help prevent falls.

Some commodes are wheeled into the bathroom and placed over the toilet. This provides privacy and safety for residents who cannot walk to the bathroom or who cannot sit unsupported on the toilet. The container is removed if the commode is used with the toilet. Make sure the wheels are locked after the commode is positioned over the toilet.

It is not safe to leave some residents alone on the commode. You will find this information in the care plan and your assignment sheet. If you have questions, ask the nurse before leaving a resident alone on the commode.

The bedpan or commode container is cleaned after use like the regular bedpan.

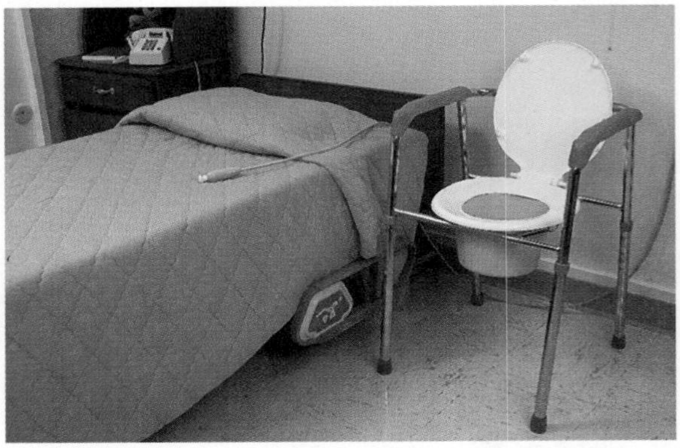

Fig. 16-7 The bedside commode has a toilet seat with a container. The container slides out from under the toilet seat for emptying.

Helping the Resident to the Commode

Quality of Life

Remember to:
- *Knock before entering the resident's room*
- *Address the resident by name*
- *Introduce yourself by name and title*

Pre-Procedure

1 Explain the procedure to the resident.
2 Provide for privacy.
3 Put on gloves.
4 Collect the following:
- Commode
- Toilet tissue
- Bath blanket

Procedure

5 Bring the commode next to the bed. Remove the chair seat and lid from the container.
6 Help the resident sit on the side of the bed.
7 Help him or her put on a robe and slippers.
8 Assist the resident to the commode.
9 Place a bath blanket over his or her lap for warmth.
10 Place the toilet tissue and signal light within reach.
11 Ask him or her to signal when done or when help is needed. (If it is not safe to leave the resident alone, you must stay with the resident. Be respectful and provide as much privacy as possible.)
12 Remove the gloves, and wash your hands.
13 Leave the room, and close the door.
14 Return when the resident signals. Knock before entering.
15 Put on the gloves.
16 Help the resident clean the genital area if indicated. Remove the gloves.
17 Help the resident back to bed. Remove the robe and slippers. Raise the bed rail according to the care plan.
18 Put on clean gloves. Cover and remove the container from the commode. Clean the commode if necessary.
19 Take the container to the bathroom or dirty utility room.
20 Check urine and feces for color, amount, and character. Measure urine if intake and output (I&O) is ordered (see Chapter 18.) Collect a specimen if one is needed (p. 366).
21 Clean and disinfect the container.
22 Return the container to the commode. Return other supplies to their proper place.
23 Return the commode to its proper place.
24 Remove soiled gloves. Wash your hands, and put on clean gloves.
25 Help the resident wash the hands.
26 Remove the gloves.

Post-Procedure

27 Provide for comfort.
28 Place the signal light within reach.
29 Raise or lower bed rails. Follow the care plan.
30 Unscreen the resident.
31 Follow center policy for soiled linen.
32 Wash your hands.
33 Report your observations to the nurse.

URINARY INCONTINENCE

Urinary incontinence is the involuntary loss of urine from the bladder. It may be temporary or permanent. There are different types of incontinence:

- **Urge incontinence** is the involuntary loss of urine after feeling a strong need to void. The resident cannot stop urinating and cannot get to the bathroom in time. Urinary frequency, urinary urgency, and nighttime voidings are common. Urinary tract infections, decreased bladder capacity, alcohol and caffeine intake, and increased fluid intake are causes.
- **Stress incontinence** is the loss of small amounts of urine with exercise and certain movements. Urine loss is usually small (less than 50 ml). Often called *dribbling*, stress incontinence occurs with laughing, sneezing, coughing, lifting, or other activities. Late pregnancy and obesity are other causes. The problem is common in women. Pelvic muscles weaken after multiple pregnancies and with aging.
- **Mixed incontinence** is a combination of urge and stress incontinence. This type is more common in older women.
- **Overflow incontinence** is the loss of urine when the bladder is too full. The resident feels like the bladder is never completely empty. Much time is spent trying to void. However, the resident only dribbles or has a weak stream of urine. Small amounts of urine are lost during the day and night. Nocturia is common. Fecal impaction, diabetes, and spinal cord injury are causes. Prostate enlargement is a common cause in men.
- **Functional incontinence** is the involuntary, unpredicted loss of urine. The resident does not have nervous system or urinary system injuries. The resident cannot use the bathroom, bedpan, urinal, or commode in time. Immobility, some drugs, restraints, unanswered signal lights, not having a signal light within reach, and not knowing where to find the bathroom also are causes. So is difficulty removing clothes. Confusion and disorientation are other causes.
- **Unconscious or reflex incontinence** is the loss of urine at predictable intervals. Urine is lost when the bladder is full. The resident does not know the bladder is full and has no urge to void. Central nervous system disorders and injuries are common causes.

Incontinence is embarrassing. Clothing gets wet, odors develop, and the resident is uncomfortable. Skin irritation, infection, and skin breakdown can occur. Falling is a risk as the resident tries to get to the bathroom quickly. Loss of independence, social isolation, decreased self-esteem, and depression also can occur as a result of incontinence.

The nurse uses the nursing process to help the health care team meet the resident's needs. Follow the nurse's instructions and the care plan. Nursing measures depend on the type of incontinence. The resident's care plan may include some of the nursing measures listed in Box 16-2. Good skin care and dry clothing and linens are always essential. Following the rules for maintaining normal urinary elimination prevents incontinence in some people. Others need bladder training programs (p. 366). Sometimes a catheter is ordered. Some residents wear garment protectors (Fig. 16-8). Incontinence drawsheets help keep the resident dry. The drawsheet has two layers and a waterproof back. Fluid passes through the first layer and is absorbed by the lower layer. A variety of incontinence products are available. The nurse selects products best suited to the resident's needs. You must follow center procedures for proper use of these products.

Incontinence is linked to abuse, mistreatment, and neglect. Caring for these residents is stressful. They need frequent care and may wet again just after you gave skin care and changed a wet gown and linens. Do not lose patience. Their needs are great, and your role is to meet their needs. If you find yourself short tempered and impatient, discuss the problem with the nurse immediately. Remember that the resident has the right to be free from abuse, mistreatment, and neglect. The incontinence is beyond the resident's control. It is not something the resident chooses to let happen. Kindness, empathy, understanding, and patience are very important. *(See Residents With Dementia.)*

RESIDENTS WITH DEMENTIA

Caring for the urinary elimination needs of residents with dementia is often very stressful. These residents may urinate in inappropriate places. Trashcans, planters, and heating vents are examples. Some residents remove incontinence products and throw them on the floor or in the toilet. Others resist your efforts to keep them clean and dry. The health care team must work together to provide safe care for these residents. Special approaches are found in the person's care plan. You may need the help of a co-worker to keep residents clean and dry. If you have questions, ask the nurse for help. Remember that all residents have the right to safe care and to be treated with respect.

Box 16-2 Nursing Measures for Residents With Urinary Incontinence

- Keep records of the resident's voidings. This includes incontinent episodes and successful use of the toilet, commode, bedpan, or urinal.
- Answer sginal lights promptly. The resident may have an urgent need to void.
- Promote normal urinary elimination (see Box 16-1).
- Promote normal bowel elimination (see Chapter 17).
- Encourage urination at scheduled intervals.
- Follow the resident's bladder training program (p. 366).
- Encourage the resident to wear clothing that is easy to remove. Incontinence can occur as the resident is trying to deal with buttons, zippers, and undergarments.
- Encourage the resident to do pelvic muscle exercises as instructed by the nurse.
- Help prevent urinary tract infections by:
  - Encouraging adequate fluid intake as directed by the nurse.
  - Encouraging the resident to wear cotton underpants.
  - Keeping perineal areas clean.
- Decrease fluid intake before bedtime.
- Provide good skin care.
- Provide dry gowns and linens.
- Observe the skin for signs of breakdown (see Chapters 13 and 14).
- Use incontinence products as directed by the nurse.

A

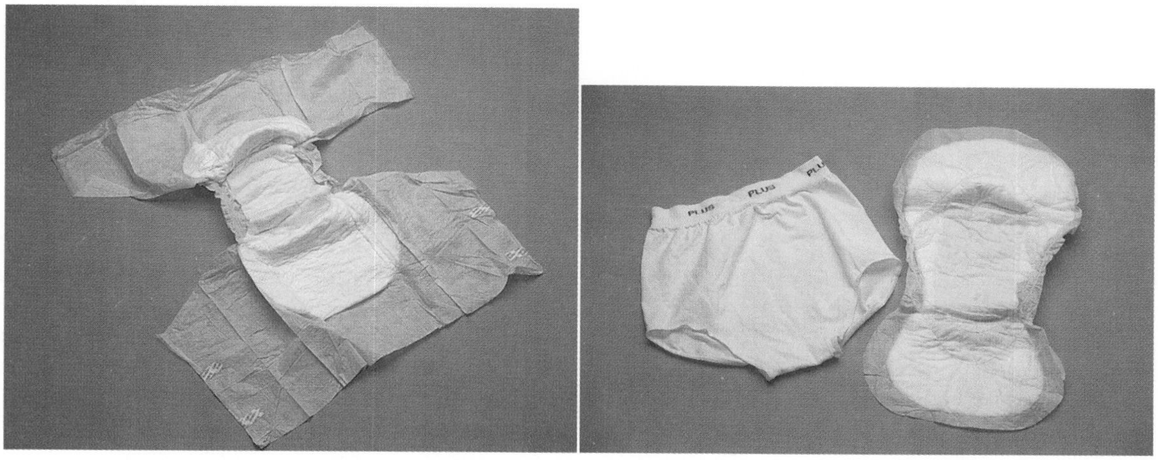

B

Fig. 16-8 Disposable garment protectors. **A,** Complete incontinence brief. **B,** Pant liner and undergarment.

◈ CATHETERS

A **catheter** is a rubber or plastic tube used to drain or inject fluid through a body opening. Inserted through the urethra into the bladder, a urinary catheter drains urine. A *straight catheter* drains the bladder and is removed. An *indwelling catheter* (*retention* or *Foley catheter*) is left in the bladder so urine drains constantly into a drainage bag. A balloon near the tip of the catheter is inflated after the catheter is inserted. The balloon prevents the catheter from slipping out of the bladder (Fig. 16-9). Tubing connects the catheter to the collection bag. Catheter insertion **(catheterization)** is done by a nurse or doctor.

Catheters often are used before, during, and after surgery to keep the bladder empty. This reduces the risk of accidental bladder injury during surgery. After surgery, a full bladder causes pressure on nearby organs.

Catheters also allow hourly urinary output measurements. They are a last resort for incontinence. Catheters do not treat the cause of incontinence. And the risk of infection is high. However, some residents have wounds and pressure ulcers that need protection from urine. Catheters can protect the wounds and pressure ulcers from contamination with urine.

Some residents are too weak or disabled to use the bedpan, commode, or toilet. Dying residents are an example. For these residents, catheters can promote comfort. Also, the resident is protected from incontinence.

Catheters are inserted for diagnostic purposes. They are used to collect sterile urine specimens. Another test involves inserting a catheter to see how much urine is left in the bladder *(residual urine)*. The catheter is inserted after the resident voids.

You will care for residents with indwelling catheters. The rules listed in Box 16-3 promote their comfort and safety.

Text continued on p. 364

Box 16-3 Caring for Residents With Indwelling Catheters

- Follow the rules of medical asepsis, Standard Precautions, and the Bloodborne Pathogen Standard.
- Make sure urine flows freely through the catheter or tubing. Tubing should not have kinks. The resident should not lie on the tubing.
- Keep the drainage bag below the bladder. This prevents urine from flowing backward into the bladder. Attach the drainage bag to the bed frame. *Never attach the drainage bag to the bed rail.* Otherwise the drainage bag is higher than the bladder when the bed rail is raised.
- Coil the drainage tubing on the bed, and pin or tape it to the bottom linen (Fig. 16-10).
- Secure the catheter to the inner thigh as in Figure 16-10. Or secure it to the man's abdomen. This prevents excessive movement of the catheter and reduces friction at the insertion site. Secure the catheter with tape or other devices as ordered by the nurse.
- Check for leaks. Check the site where the catheter connects to the drainage bag. Report any leaks to the nurse immediately.
- Provide catheter care if ordered. Catheter care is done daily or twice a day (see *GIving Catheter Care*, p. 360). Some centers consider perineal care to be sufficient. Catheter care is sometimes needed after bowel movements and when vaginal drainage is present.
- Provide perineal care daily and after bowel movements.
- Empty the drainage bag at the end of the shift or at time intervals as directed by the nurse. Measure and record the amount of urine (see *Emptying a Urinary Drainage Bag*, p. 362). Report increases or decreases in the amount of urine.
- Use a separate measuring container for each resident. This prevents the spread of microbes from one resident to another.
- Do not the let the drain on the drainage bag touch any surface.
- Report complaints to the nurse immediately. These include complaints of pain, burning, the need to urinate, or irritation. Also report the color, clarity, and odor of urine and the presence of particles.
- Encourage fluid intake as instructed by the nurse.

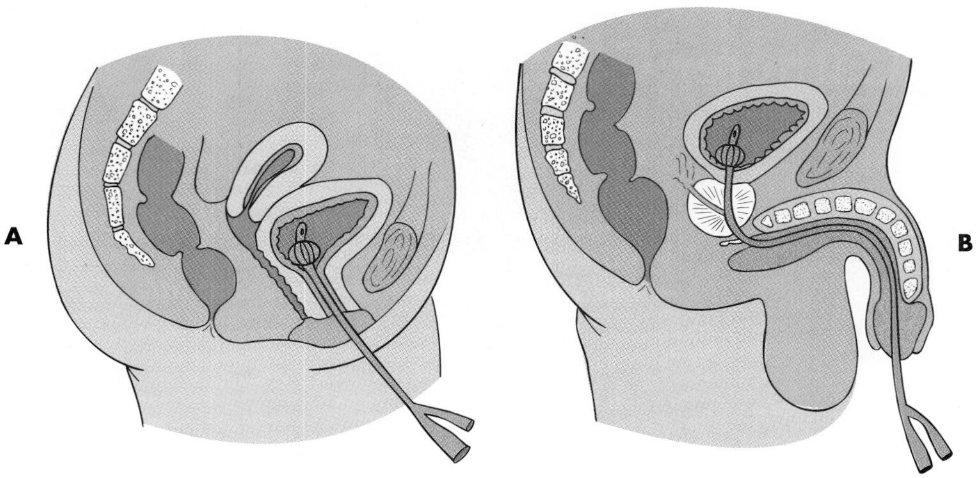

Fig. 16-9 Indwelling catheter. **A,** Indwelling catheter in the female bladder. The inflated balloon at the top prevents the catheter from slipping out through the urethra. **B,** Indwelling catheter with the balloon inflated in the male bladder.

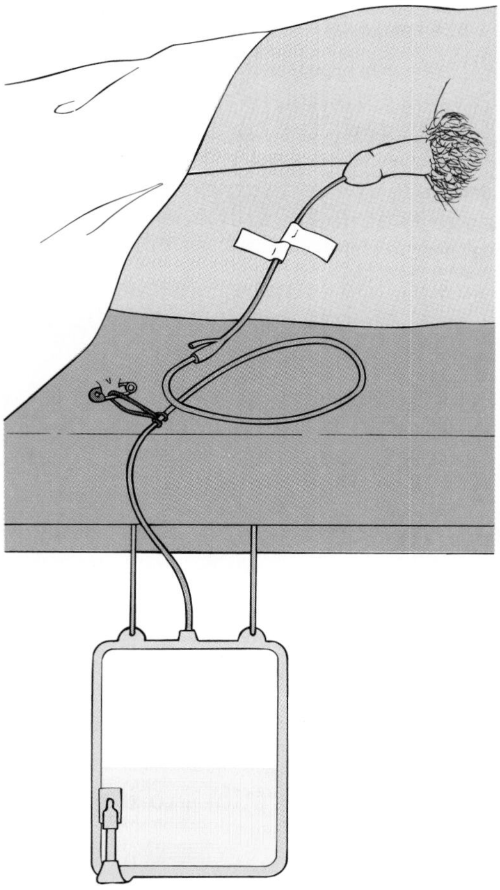

Fig. 16-10 The drainage tubing is coiled on the bed and pinned to the bottom linens so urine flows freely. A rubber band is placed around the tubing with a clove hitch. The safety pin is passed through the loops and pinned to the linens. The catheter is taped to the inner thigh. Enough slack is left on the catheter to prevent friction at the urethra.

Giving Catheter Care

NNAAP™ SKILL

Quality of Life

Remember to:
- ◆ *Knock before entering the resident's room*
- ◆ *Address the resident by name*
- ◆ *Introduce yourself by name and title*

Pre-Procedure

1 Explain the procedure to the resident.

2 Wash your hands.

3 Collect the following:
- Equipment for perineal care (p. 292)
- Gloves
- Bed protector
- Bath blanket

4 Identify the resident. Check the ID bracelet against the assignment sheet.

5 Provide for privacy.

6 Raise the bed to the best level for good body mechanics. Make sure bed rails are up.

Procedure

7 Lower the bed rail near you.

8 Put on the gloves.

9 Cover the resident with a bath blanket. Fanfold top linens to the foot of the bed.

10 Drape the resident for perineal care (see Fig. 13-24, p. 294).

11 Fold back the bath blanket between the legs to expose the genital area.

12 Place the bed protector under the buttocks. Ask the resident to flex the knees and raise the buttocks off the bed by pushing against the mattress with the feet.

13 Perform perineal care (see *Female Perineal Care* or *Male Perineal Care,* pp. 292-295).

14 Separate the labia (female) or retract the foreskin (uncircumcised male) as in Figure 16-11. Check for crusts, abnormal drainage, or secretions.

15 Clean the catheter from the meatus down the catheter about 4 inches (Fig. 16-12). Use soap and water and a clean washcloth. Avoid tugging or pulling on the catheter. Repeat, if necessary, with a clean washcloth.

16 Make sure the catheter is secured properly. Coil and secure tubing (see Fig. 16-10).

17 Remove the bed protector.

18 Cover the resident, and remove the bath blanket.

19 Remove the gloves.

Post-Procedure

20 Provide for comfort.

21 Place the signal light within reach.

22 Raise or lower bed rails. Follow the care plan.

23 Lower the bed to its lowest position.

24 Clean and return equipment to its proper place. Discard disposable items. (Wear gloves for this step).

25 Unscreen the resident.

26 Follow center policy for soiled linen.

27 Wash your hands.

28 Report your observations to the nurse.

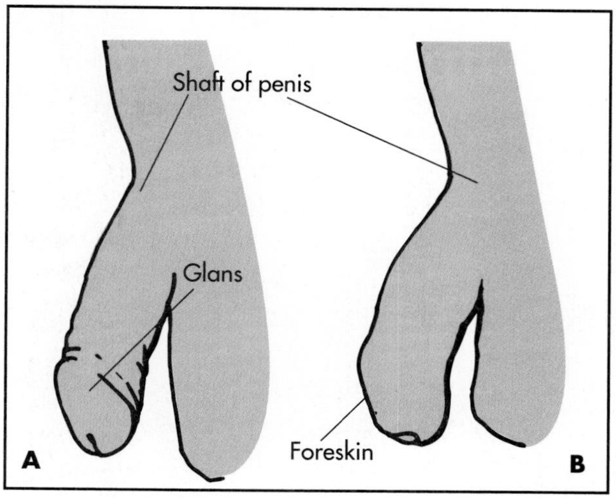

Fig. 16-11 **A,** Circumcised male. **B,** Uncircumcised male.

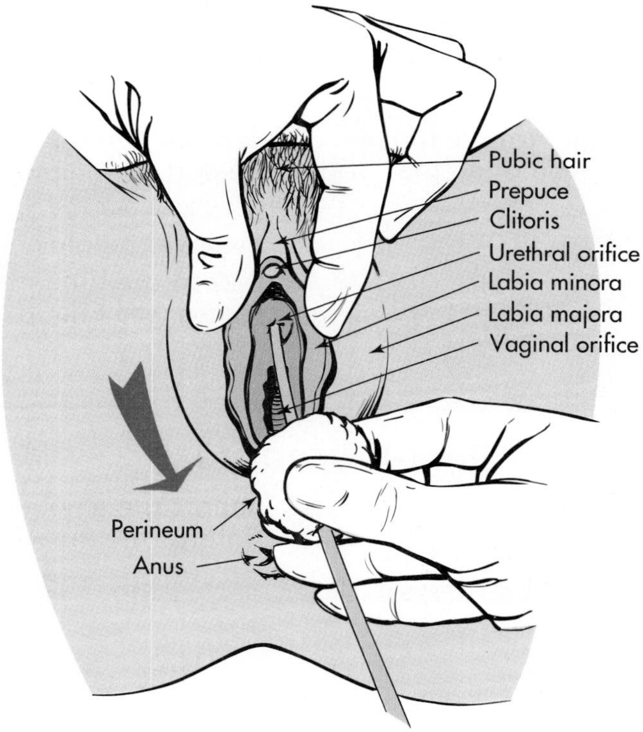

Fig. 16-12 The catheter is cleaned beginning at the meatus. About 4 inches of the catheter is cleaned.

Emptying a Urinary Drainage Bag

Quality of Life

Remember to:
- *Knock before entering the resident's room*
- *Address the resident by name*
- *Introduce yourself by name and title*

Pre-Procedure

1 Collect equipment:
- Graduate (measuring container)
- Gloves
- Paper towels

2 Wash your hands.

3 Explain the procedure to the resident.

4 Identify the resident. Check the ID bracelet against the assignment sheet.

5 Provide for privacy.

Procedure

6 Put on the gloves.

7 Place a paper towel on the floor. Place the measuring container on top of the paper towel.

8 Position measuring container (graduate) so urine is collected when you open the drain.

9 Open the clamp on the bottom of the drainage bag.

10 Let all urine drain into the graduate. Do not let the drain touch the graduate (Fig. 16-13).

11 Close the clamp. Replace the clamped drain in the holder on the bag (see Fig. 16-10).

12 Measure urine.

13 Remove and discard the paper towel.

14 Rinse the graduate, and return it to its proper place.

15 Remove the gloves, and wash your hands.

16 Record the time and amount on the I&O record (see Chapter 18).

Post-Procedure

17 Unscreen the resident.

18 Report the amount and other observations to the nurse (Fig. 16-14).

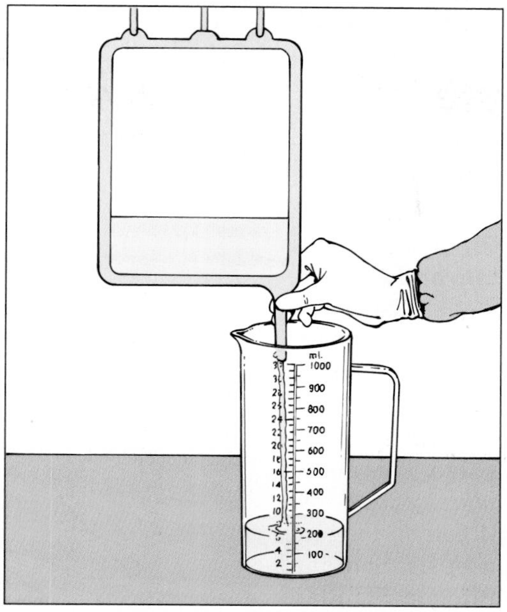

Fig. 16-13 The clamp on the drainage bag is opened, and the drain is directed into the measuring container. The drain must not touch the inside of the container.

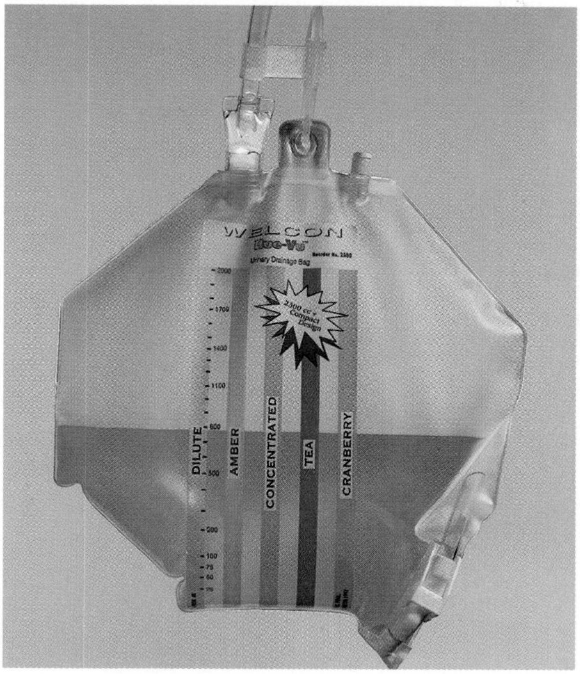

Fig. 16-14 This urinary drainage bag has a comparison chart for the color of urine. *(Courtesy Welcon, Inc., Fort Worth, Tex.).*

◈ The Condom Catheter

Condom catheters (external catheter, urinary sheath) are often used for incontinent men. A condom catheter is a soft, rubber sheath that slides over the penis. Tubing connects the condom catheter and the drainage bag. Many men prefer a leg bag (Fig. 16-15).

A new condom catheter is applied daily. The manufacturer's instructions are followed. The penis is thoroughly washed with soap and water and dried before applying a new catheter. The penis also is observed for reddened or open areas. These are reported to and observed by the nurse before a new catheter is applied.

Elastic tape secures the catheter in place. Elastic tape expands when the penis changes size. This allows blood flow to the penis. *Never used adhesive tape to secure catheters. It does not expand. Blood flow to the penis is cut off, injuring the penis.* Medical asepsis, Standard Precautions, and the Bloodborne Pathogen Standard are followed when removing or applying condom catheters.

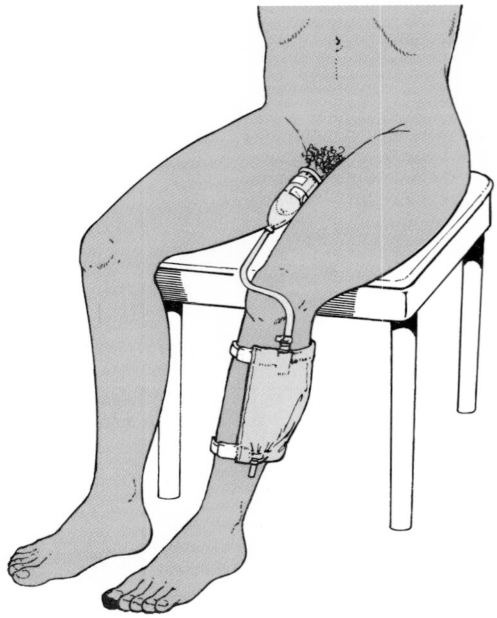

Fig. 16-15 A condom catheter attached to a leg bag.

Applying a Condom Catheter

Quality of Life

Remember to:
- ◆ ***Knock before entering the resident's room***
- ◆ ***Address the resident by name***
- ◆ ***Introduce yourself by name and title***

Pre-Procedure

1. Explain the procedure to the resident.
2. Wash your hands.
3. Collect the following:
   - Condom catheter
   - Elastic tape
   - Drainage bag or leg bag
   - Basin of warm water
   - Soap
   - Towel and washcloths
   - Bath blanket
   - Gloves
   - Bed protector
   - Paper towels
4. Arrange paper towels and equipment on the overbed table.
5. Provide for privacy.
6. Raise the bed to the best level for good body mechanics. Make sure bed rails are up.

Procedure

7. Lower the bed rail near you.
8. Cover the resident with a bath blanket. Bring top linens to the foot of the bed.
9. Ask the resident to raise his buttocks off the bed. Or turn him onto his side away from you.
10. Slide the bed protector under his buttocks.
11. Have the resident lower his buttocks, or turn him onto his back.
12. Bring top linens up to cover his knees and lower legs.

Applying a Condom Catheter—cont'd

Procedure—cont'd

13 Secure the drainage bag to the bed frame, or have a leg bag ready. Close the drain.

14 Raise the bath blanket to expose the genital area.

15 Put on the gloves.

16 Remove the condom catheter:

- a Remove the tape and roll the sheath off the penis.
- b Disconnect the drainage tubing from the condom.
- c Discard the tape and condom.

17 Provide perineal care (see *Male Perineal Care,* p. 295). Observe the penis for skin breakdown or irritation.

18 Remove the protective backing from the condom. This exposes the adhesive strip.

19 Hold the penis firmly. Roll the condom onto the penis. Leave a 1-inch space between the penis and the end of the catheter (Fig. 16-16).

20 Secure the condom with elastic tape. Apply tape in a spiral (Fig. 16-17). Do not apply tape completely around the penis.

21 Connect the condom to the drainage tubing. Coil excess tubing on the bed as shown in Figure 16-10, or attach a leg bag.

22 Remove the bed protector.

23 Remove the gloves.

24 Return top linens, and remove the bath blanket.

Post-Procedure

25 Provide for comfort.

26 Place the signal light within reach.

27 Raise or lower bed rails. Follow the care plan.

27 Lower the bed to its lowest position.

29 Wash your hands. Put on clean gloves.

30 Clean and return the wash basin and other equipment. Return items to their proper place.

31 Unscreen the resident.

32 Measure and record the amount of urine in the bag. Discard the collection bag and disposable items.

33 Remove the gloves, and wash your hands.

34 Report your observations to the nurse.

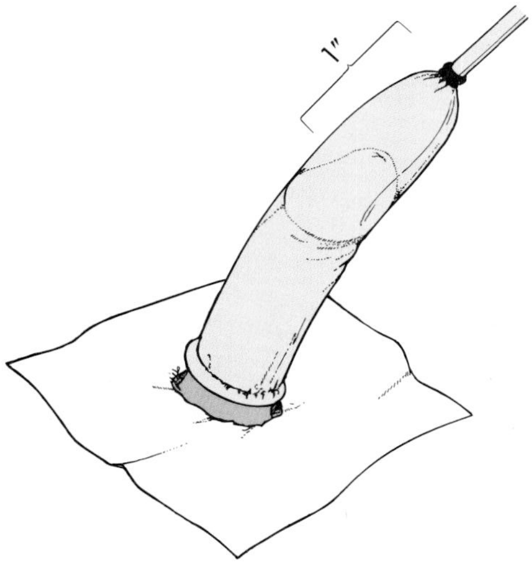

Fig. 16-16 A condom catheter applied to the penis. There is a 1-inch space between the penis and the end of the catheter.

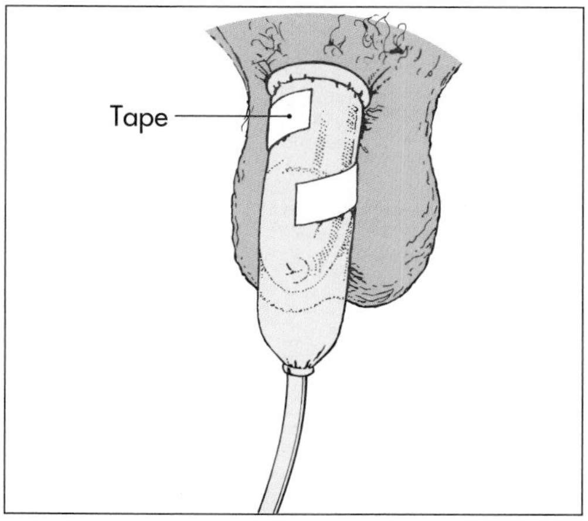

Fig. 16-17 Tape is applied in spiral fashion to secure the condom catheter to the penis.

BLADDER TRAINING

Bladder training programs are developed for some residents with urinary incontinence. Some residents need bladder training after indwelling catheter removal. The nurse uses the nursing process to help the health care team develop an individualized bladder training program when appropriate. Voluntary control of urination is the goal. Good bladder control promotes comfort and increases self-esteem. The bladder training program is part of the care plan. You assist with bladder training as directed by the nurse. Successful bladder training can help improve the resident's quality of life.

There are two basic methods for bladder training. With one, the resident uses the toilet, commode, bedpan, or urinal at scheduled times. The resident is given 15 or 20 minutes to start voiding. The rules for maintaining normal urination are followed. The normal position for urination is assumed if possible. Privacy is important. Helping the resident relax and providing positive reinforcement can help the resident succeed.

The second method is used with catheters. Clamping the catheter prevents urine from draining out of the bladder. Usually the catheter is clamped for 1 hour at first. Eventually it is clamped for 3 to 4 hours at a time. Urine drains from the bladder when the catheter is unclamped. When the catheter is removed, urination is encouraged every 3 to 4 hours.

COLLECTING URINE SPECIMENS

Urine specimens (samples) are collected for urine tests. Doctors use test results to make a diagnosis or evaluate treatment. Each specimen sent to the laboratory needs a requisition slip. The slip has the resident's identifying information and the required test. Box 16-4 lists the rules to follow when collecting specimens.

Box 16-4 Rules for Collecting Urine Specimens

- Follow the rules of medical asepsis, Standard Precautions, and the Bloodborne Pathogen Standard.
- Use a clean container for each specimen.
- Use a container appropriate for the specimen.
- Label the container accurately. Write the resident's full name, room and bed number, the date, and time the specimen was collected. Some centers have preprinted labels with this information. If preprinted labels are used, place a label on the container.
- Do not touch the inside of the container or lid.
- Collect the specimen at the time specified.
- Ask the resident not to have a bowel movement during specimen collection. The specimen must not contain feces.
- Ask the resident to put toilet tissue in the toilet or wastebasket. The specimen must not contain tissue.
- Take the specimen and requisition slip to the storage area. The specimen container should be in a plastic bag.

The Random Urine Specimen

The random urine specimen is collected for a urinalysis. No special measures are needed. It is collected at any time. Many residents can collect the specimen themselves. Weak and very ill residents need assistance.

Collecting a Random Urine Specimen

Quality of Life

Remember to:
- *Knock before entering the resident's room*
- *Address the resident by name*
- *Introduce yourself by name and title*

Pre-Procedure

1 Explain the procedure to the resident.
2 Wash your hands.
3 Collect the following:
- Bedpan and cover, urinal, or specimen pan
- Specimen container and lid
- Label
- Gloves
- Plastic bag

Procedure

4 Fill out the label. Put it on the container.
5 Put the container and lid in the bathroom.
6 Identify the resident. Check the ID bracelet against the requisition slip.
7 Provide for privacy.
8 Put on the gloves.
9 Ask the resident to urinate in the receptacle. Remind him or her to put toilet tissue into the wastebasket or toilet, not in the bedpan or specimen pan.
10 Take the receptacle to the bathroom.
11 Measure urine if I&O is ordered (see Chapter 18).
12 Pour about 120 ml (4 oz) of urine into the specimen container. Dispose of excess urine.
13 Place the lid on the specimen container. Put the container in the plastic bag.
14 Clean and return the receptacle to its proper place.
15 Help the resident wash the hands.
16 Remove the gloves.

Post-Procedure

17 Provide for comfort.
18 Place the signal light within reach.
19 Raise or lower bed rails. Follow the care plan.
20 Unscreen the resident.
21 Wash your hands.
22 Report your observations to the nurse.
23 Take the specimen and the requisition slip to the storage area.

The Midstream Specimen

The midstream specimen is also called a *clean-voided specimen* or a *clean-catch specimen.* The perineal area is cleaned before collecting the specimen. This reduces the number of microbes in the urethral area during specimen collection. The resident starts to void into the toilet, bedpan, urinal, or commode. Then the stream is stopped and a sterile specimen container positioned. The resident voids into the container until the specimen is obtained.

Stopping the stream of urine is hard for many people. You may need to position and hold the specimen container in place after the resident starts to void.

Collecting a Midstream Specimen

Quality of Life

Remember to:

- ***Knock before entering the resident's room***
- ***Address the resident by name***
- ***Introduce yourself by name and title***

Pre-Procedure

1 Explain the procedure to the resident.

2 Wash your hands.

3 Collect the following:
- Clean-voided specimen kit with sterile specimen container
- Label
- Antiseptic solution
- Disposable gloves
- Sterile gloves (if not part of the kit)
- Bedpan, urinal, or commode if the resident cannot use the bathroom
- Plastic bag
- Supplies for perineal care

4 Label the container with the requested information.

5 Identify the resident. Check the ID bracelet against the requisition slip.

6 Provide for privacy.

Procedure

7 Let the resident complete perineal care if able. Place the signal light within reach.

8 Provide perineal care if the resident cannot.

9 Open the sterile kit using sterile technique (see Chapter 9).

10 Put on the sterile gloves.

11 Pour the antiseptic solution over the cotton balls.

12 Open the sterile specimen container. Do not touch the inside of the container or lid. Set the lid down so the inside is up.

13 Clean the perineum with cotton balls if the resident cannot:

a Female:
- Spread the labia with your thumb and index finger. Use your nondominant hand. (This hand is now contaminated and must not touch anything sterile.)
- Clean down the urethral area from front to back. Use a clean cotton ball for each stroke.
- Keep the labia separated to collect the urine specimen (steps 15 and 16).

b Male:
- Hold the penis with your nondominant hand.
- Clean the penis starting at the meatus. Use a cotton ball, and clean in a circular motion.
- Keep holding the penis until the specimen is collected (steps 15 and 16).

14 Ask the resident to start urinating into the toilet, bedpan, commode, or urinal.

15 Pass the specimen container into the stream of urine. Keep the labia separated (Fig. 16-18, p. 369).

16 Collect about 30 to 60 ml of urine (1 to 2 oz).

Collecting a Midstream Specimen—cont'd

Procedure—cont'd

17 Remove the specimen container before the resident stops urinating.

18 Release the labia or penis.

19 Let the resident finish urinating into the toilet, bedpan, commode, or urinal.

20 Put the lid on the specimen container. Touch only the outside of the container or lid.

21 Wipe the outside of the container.

22 Place the container in a plastic bag.

23 Provide toilet tissue after the resident finishes urinating.

24 Remove and empty the bedpan, commode container, or urinal.

25 Clean the bedpan, urinal, or commode container and other equipment. Return equipment to its proper place.

26 Remove soiled gloves. Wash your hands, and put on clean gloves.

27 Let the resident wash his or her hands.

28 Remove the gloves.

Post-Procedure

29 Follow steps 17-23 in *Collecting a Random Urine Specimen.*

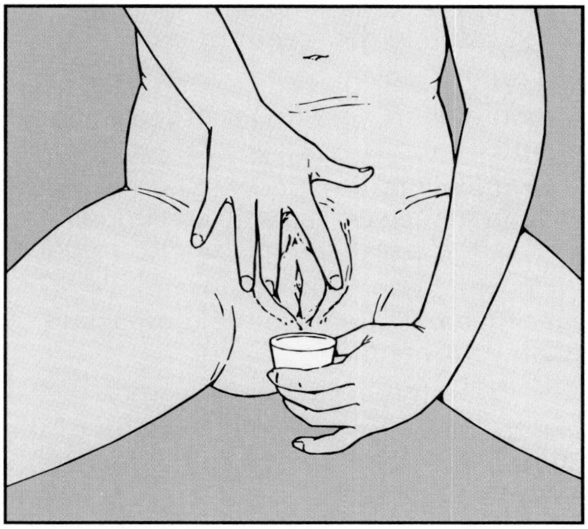

Fig. 16-18 The labia are separated to collect a midstream specimen. *(From Potter PA, Perry AG:* Fundamentals of nursing: concepts, process, and practice, *ed 4, St Louis, 1997, Mosby.)*

The 24-Hour Urine Specimen

All urine voided during a 24-hour period is collected for a 24-hour urine specimen. Urine is chilled on ice or refrigerated during the collection period. This prevents the growth of microbes. A preservative is added to the collection container for some tests.

The resident voids to begin the test; this voiding is discarded. *All* voidings during the next 24 hours are collected. The resident and nursing staff must clearly understand the procedure and test period. The rules for collecting urine specimens are followed.

Collecting a 24-Hour Urine Specimen

Quality of Life

Remember to:
- ◆ *Knock before entering the resident's room*
- ◆ *Address the resident by name*
- ◆ *Introduce yourself by name and title*

Pre-Procedure

1 Review the procedure with the nurse.
2 Explain the procedure to the resident.
3 Wash your hands.
4 Collect the following:
- Urine container for a 24-hour collection
- Preservative from the laboratory if needed
- Bucket with ice if needed
- Two 24-hour urine specimen labels
- Funnel
- Bedpan, urinal, commode, or specimen pan
- Gloves
- Measuring container

Procedure

5 Label the specimen container.
6 Identify the resident. Check the ID bracelet against the requisition slip.
7 Arrange equipment in the resident's bathroom or dirty utility room.
8 Place one 24-hour specimen label in the bathroom or dirty utility room. Place the other near the bed.
9 Put on the gloves.
10 Offer the bedpan or urinal, or assist the resident to the bathroom or bedside commode.
11 Ask the resident to void.
12 Discard the specimen, and note the time. This starts the 24-hour collection period.
13 Clean the bedpan, urinal, commode, or specimen pan.
14 Remove the gloves. Wash your hands.
15 Mark the time the test began and the time it ends on the room and bathroom labels. Also mark the specimen container.
16 Ask the resident to use the bedpan, urinal, commode, or specimen pan when voiding during the next 24 hours. Tell the resident to signal after voiding. Remind him or her not to have a bowel movement at the same time and not to put toilet tissue in the receptacle.
17 Put on the gloves.
18 Measure all urine if I&O is ordered (see Chapter 18).
19 Pour urine into the specimen container using the funnel. Do not spill any urine. Restart the test if you spill or discard urine.
20 Clean the bedpan, urinal, commode, or specimen pan. Remove the gloves, and wash your hands.
21 Add ice to the bucket as necessary.
22 Ask the resident to void at the end of the 24-hour period. Pour the urine into the specimen container.
23 Thank the resident for cooperating.

Post-Procedure

24 Provide for comfort.
25 Place the signal light within reach.
26 Raise or lower bed rails. Follow the care plan.
27 Remove the labels from the room and bathroom. Clean and return equipment to its proper place. Discard disposable items.
28 Wash your hands.
29 Report your observations to the nurse.
30 Take the specimen and requisition slip to the storage area.

◈ The Double-Voided Specimen

Fresh-fractional urine specimen is another term for a double-voided specimen. The resident voids twice. The first time the bladder is emptied of "stale" urine. "Fresh" urine collects in the bladder after the first voiding. In 30 minutes the resident voids again. The second voiding is usually a very small or "fractional" amount of urine.

Fresh-fractional specimens are used to test urine for glucose and ketones (p. 373).

Collecting a Double-Voided Specimen

Quality of Life

Remember to:

- ◆ *Knock before entering the resident's room*
- ◆ *Address the resident by name*
- ◆ *Introduce yourself by name and title*

Pre-Procedure

1. Explain the procedure to the resident.
2. Wash your hands.
3. Collect the following:
   - Bedpan, urinal, commode, or disposable specimen pan
   - Two specimen containers
   - Urine testing equipment
   - Gloves
4. Identify the resident. Check the ID bracelet against the assignment sheet.
5. Provide for privacy.

Procedure

6. Put on the gloves.
7. Offer the bedpan or urinal, or assist the resident to the bathroom or commode.
8. Ask the resident to urinate.
9. Take the receptacle to the bathroom.
10. Measure urine if I&O is ordered (see Chapter 18). Pour some urine into the specimen container.
11. Test the specimen in case you cannot obtain a second specimen (p. 373). Discard the urine.
12. Clean the receptacle. Remove the gloves.
13. Return the receptacle to its proper place.
14. Help the resident wash the hands.
15. Ask the resident to drink an 8-ounce glass of water.
16. Make sure the resident is comfortable, the bed rails are up if needed, and the signal light is within reach.
17. Unscreen the resident.
18. Wash your hands.
19. Return to the room in 20 to 30 minutes.
20. Repeat steps 5 through 18.
21. Report the results of the second test and any other observations to the nurse.

Straining Urine

Stones (calculi) can develop in the kidneys, ureters, or bladder. Stones vary in size. Some are pinhead size; others are the size of an orange. Stones causing severe pain and damage to the urinary system may require surgical removal. Some stones exit the body through urine. Therefore all of the resident's urine is strained. Passed stones are sent to the laboratory for examination.

Straining Urine

Quality of Life

Remember to:
- ***Knock before entering the resident's room***
- ***Address the resident by name***
- ***Introduce yourself by name and title***

Pre-Procedure

1 Explain the procedure to the resident. Also explain that the urinal, bedpan, commode, or specimen pan is used for voiding.
2 Wash your hands.
3 Collect the following:
- Strainer or 4 × 4 gauze
- Specimen container
- Urinal, bedpan, commode, or specimen pan
- Two labels stating that all urine is strained
- Gloves
- Plastic bag

4 Identify the resident. Check the ID bracelet against the assignment sheet.

Procedure

5 Arrange items in the resident's bathroom.
6 Place one label in the bathroom. Place the other near the bed.
7 Put on the gloves.
8 Offer the bedpan or urinal. Or assist the resident to the bedside commode or bathroom.
9 Provide for privacy, and remove the gloves.
10 Tell the resident to signal after voiding.
11 Put on gloves.
12 Place the strainer or gauze into the specimen container.
13 Pour urine into the specimen container. Urine passes through the strainer or gauze (Fig. 16-19).
14 Remove the strainer and discard the urine.
15 Place the strainer or gauze in the container if any crystals, stones, or particles appear.
16 Help the resident clean the perineal area if necessary.
17 Clean and return equipment to its proper place.
18 Removed soiled gloves. Wash your hands, and put on clean gloves.
19 Help the resident wash the hands.
20 Remove the gloves.

Straining Urine—cont'd

Post-Procedure

21 Provide for comfort.
22 Place the signal light within reach.
23 Raise or lower bed rails. Follow the care plan.
24 Unscreen the resident.
25 Label the specimen container with the requested information. Put the container in the plastic bag. (Wear gloves for this step).
26 Wash your hands.
27 Report your observations to the nurse.
28 Take the specimen and requisition slip to the storage area.

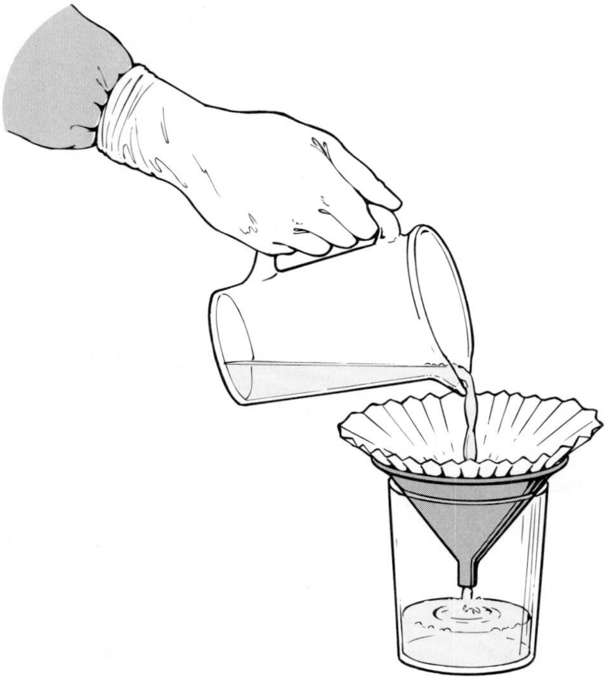

Fig. 16-19 A disposable strainer is placed in a specimen container. Urine is poured through the strainer into the specimen container.

TESTING URINE

The nurse may ask you to do simple urine tests. You can test for pH, glucose, ketones, and blood using reagent strips:

- *Testing for pH*—Urine pH measures whether urine is acidic or alkaline. Changes in normal pH (4.6 to 8.0) occur from illness, foods, and medications. A routine urine specimen is needed.
- *Testing for glucose and ketones—Diabetes mellitus* is a chronic disease in which the pancreas fails to secrete enough insulin (see Chapter 26). The body needs insulin to use sugar for energy. Sugar builds up in the blood if it cannot be used. Some sugar appears in the urine. **Glucosuria** or **glycosuria** means sugar *(glucos, glycos)* in the urine *(uria)*. The diabetic person may also have **acetone (ketones)** in the urine. These appear in urine because of the rapid breakdown of fat for energy. The body uses fat for energy if it cannot use sugar. Urine is also tested for ketones. The doctor orders the type and frequency of urine tests. They are usually done four times a day: 30 minutes before each meal (ac) and at bedtime (HS). The doctor uses the test results to regulate the person's medication and diet. Double-voided specimens are best for testing urine for sugar and ketones.
- *Testing for blood*—normal urine is free of blood. Injury and disease can cause blood *(hemat)* to appear in the urine *(uria)*. This is called **hematuria.** Sometimes blood is seen in the urine. At other times it is unseen *(occult)*. A routine urine specimen is needed.

Using Reagent Strips

Reagent strips have different sections that change color when they react with urine. To use a reagent strip, dip the strip into urine. Then compare the strip with the color chart on the bottle (Fig. 16-20). The nurse gives you specific instructions for the urine test ordered. You must read the manufacturer's instructions before you begin.

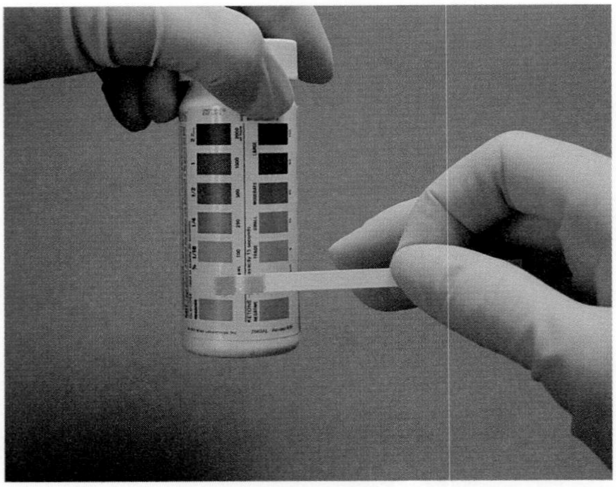

Fig. 16-20 Reagent strip for sugar and ketones.

Testing Urine With Reagent Strips

Quality of Life

Remember to:
- *Knock before entering the resident's room*
- *Address the resident by name*
- *Introduce yourself by name and title*

Pre-Procedure

1 Explain the procedure to the person.
2 Wash your hands.
3 Identify the person. Check the ID bracelet against the assignment sheet.

Procedure

4 Put on the gloves.
5 Collect the following:
- Urine specimen (routine specimen for pH and occult blood; double-voided specimen for sugar and ketones)
- Reagent strip as ordered
- Gloves

6 Remove a strip from the bottle. Put the cap on the bottle immediately. Make sure it is tight.
7 Dip the strip test areas into the specimen.
8 Remove the strip after the correct amount of time (see the manufacturer's instructions).
9 Tap the strip gently against the container to remove excess urine.
10 Wait the required amount of time (see the manufacturer's instructions).
11 Compare the strip with the color chart on the bottle. Read the results.
12 Discard disposable items and the specimen.

Post-Procedure

13 Clean and return equipment to its proper place.
14 Remove the gloves, and wash your hands.
15 Report the results and other observations to the nurse.

THE RESIDENT WITH A URETEROSTOMY

Sometimes it is necessary to surgically remove the urinary bladder. Cancer and bladder injuries are common causes. When the bladder is removed, a new pathway is necessary for urine to exit the body. The new pathway is called a *urinary diversion.* There are many types of urinary diversions. Often an ostomy is involved. An **ostomy** is the surgical creation of an artificial opening. A **ureterostomy** is the surgical creation of an artificial opening *(stomy)* between the ureter *(uretero)* and the abdomen. The opening is called a **stoma** (Fig. 16-21). The nurse provides stoma care in the early postoperative period. You may care for residents who have a long-standing ureterostomy.

The resident with a ureterostomy wears a pouch (Fig. 16-22). The pouch is a disposable plastic bag applied over the stoma. Urine drains through the stoma into the pouch. The pouch is replaced anytime it leaks. Leakage can cause skin irritation, breakdown, and infection. Follow Standard Precautions and the Bloodborne Pathogen Standard when giving stoma care. If able, the resident assists with his or her care.

Residents with a ureterostomy require good skin care. It is very important to prevent skin breakdown. You must always report any changes in the skin around the stoma to the nurse. Before changing an ostomy pouch, make sure that:

- Your state allows nursing assistants to perform the procedure.
- The procedure is in your job description.
- You have the necessary education and training.
- You have reviewed the procedure with the nurse.
- The nurse is available to answer questions and to supervise you.

A

B

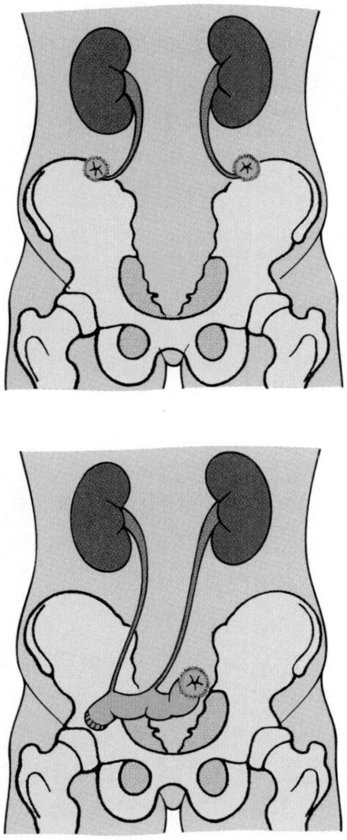

Fig. 16-21 Ureterostomies. **A,** Both ureters are brought through the skin onto the abdomen. The person has two stomas. **B,** The ileal conduit. A small section of the small intestine (ileum) is resected (removed) from the intestine. One end is sutured closed. The other end is brought through the skin onto the abdomen to form a stoma. The ureters are attached to the resected ileum. *(From Beare PA, Myers JL:* Principles and practices of adult health nursing, *ed 3, St Louis, 1998, Mosby.)*

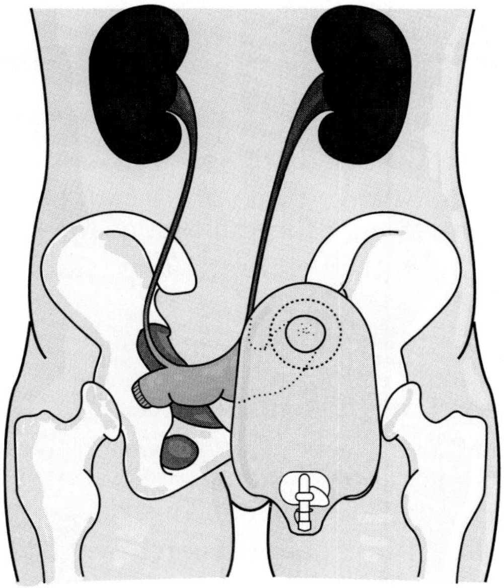

Fig. 16-22 Ureterostomy pouch.

Changing a Ureterostomy Pouch

Quality of Life

Remember to:
- ◆ ***Knock before entering the resident's room***
- ◆ ***Address the resident by name***
- ◆ ***Introduce yourself by name and title***

Pre-Procedure

1 Explain the procedure to the resident.

2 Wash your hands.

3 Collect the following:
- Clean pouch with skin barrier
- Skin barrier (if not part of the pouch)
- Pouch clamp, clip, or wire closure
- Clean ostomy belt (if used)
- Skin barrier as ordered
- 4 to 8 gauze squares
- Adhesive remover
- Cotton balls
- Bedpan with cover
- Waterproof pad
- Bath blanket
- Toilet tissue
- Wash basin
- Bath thermometer
- Prescribed soap or cleansing agent
- Pouch deodorant
- Paper towels
- Gloves
- Disposable bag

4 Arrange your work area.

5 Identify the resident. Check the ID bracelet against the assignment sheet.

6 Provide for privacy.

7 Raise the bed to the best level for good body mechanics. Make sure bed rails are up.

Procedure

8 Lower the bed rail near you.

9 Cover the resident with a bath blanket. Fanfold linens to the foot of the bed.

10 Place the waterproof pad under the buttocks.

11 Put on the gloves.

12 Disconnect the pouch from the belt if one is worn. Remove the belt.

13 Remove the pouch gently. Gently push the skin down and away from the skin barrier. Place the pouch in the bedpan.

14 Place 1 or 2 gauze squares over the stoma to absorb urine.

15 Wipe around the stoma with toilet tissue or a gauze square. Place soiled tissue or gauze in the bedpan.

16 Moisten a cotton ball with adhesive remover. Clean around the stoma to remove any remaining skin barrier. Clean from the stoma outward.

17 Cover the bedpan, and take it to the bathroom. (Raise the bed rail before you leave the bedside.)

18 Measure urine. Ask the nurse to observe abnormal urine. Then empty the pouch and bedpan into the toilet. Note the color, amount, clarity, and odor of urine. Put the pouch in the disposable bag.

19 Remove the gloves. Wash your hands, and put on clean gloves.

20 Fill the wash basin with warm water. Place the basin on the overbed table on top of the paper towels. Lower the bed rail near you.

21 Clean the skin around the stoma with water. Rinse and pat dry. Use soap or other cleansing agent as directed by the nurse.

22 Observe the stoma and skin around the stoma. Report any irritation or skin breakdown to the nurse.

23 Apply the skin barrier if is a separate device.

24 Put a clean ostomy belt on the person if a belt is worn.

Changing a Ureterostomy Pouch—cont'd

Procedure—cont'd

25 Add deodorant to the new pouch.
26 Remove the gauze square used to absorb urine from the stoma.
27 Remove adhesive backing on the pouch.
28 Center the pouch over the stoma. Make sure the drain points downward.
29 Press around the skin barrier so the pouch seals to the skin. Apply gentle pressure from the stoma outward.
30 Maintain pressure for 1 to 2 minutes.
31 Connect the belt to the pouch (if a belt is worn).
32 Remove the waterproof pad.
33 Cover the resident. Remove the bath blanket.

Post-Procedure

34 Provide for comfort.
35 Raise or lower bed rails. Follow the care plan.
36 Lower the bed to its lowest position.
37 Place the signal light within reach.
38 Unscreen the resident.
39 Clean the bedpan, wash basin, and other equipment.
40 Return equipment to its proper place.
41 Discard the disposable bag according to center policy. Follow center policy for soiled linen.
42 Remove the gloves, and wash your hands.
43 Report your observations to the nurse.

DIALYSIS

Some people may have a disease that causes the kidneys to fail (see Chapter 26). Common causes of kidney failure include diabetes, high blood pressure, and inflammation of the kidneys. When the kidneys fail, little or no urine is produced. This causes body waste and excess fluid to collect in the blood. If this waste and fluid are not removed, the person will die. **Dialysis** is a process that removes excess fluid and waste from the blood. Dialysis allows people to live, work, and enjoy life even though their kidneys do not work properly.

There are two main methods of dialysis. **Hemodialysis** removes waste and fluid by filtering the blood through an artificial kidney called a *dialyzer* (Fig. 16-23). **Peritoneal dialysis** uses the lining of the abdominal cavity (the *peritoneal membrane*) to remove waste from the blood (Fig. 16-24, p. 378). The procedure is ordered by a doctor and performed by an RN with special training.

Dialysis is usually done in the hospital or in special dialysis centers. (*See Subacute Care, p. 378.*) Residents who need dialysis are transported to a dialysis center 2 to 3 times a week. Residents who receive dialysis often require a special diet and fluid restrictions. You will get specific instructions from the nurse and the care plan.

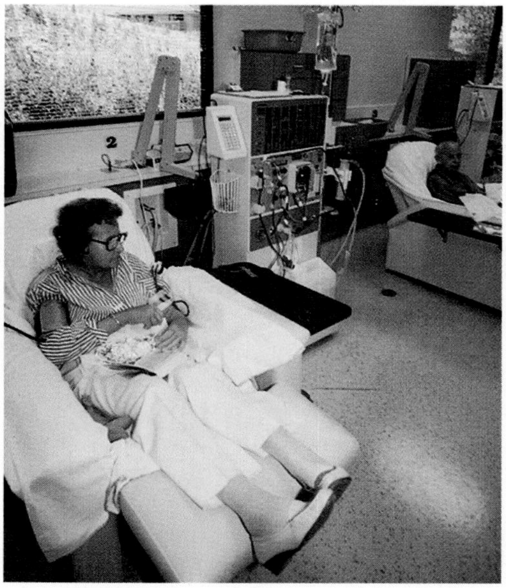

Fig. 16-23 Dialysis machine. *(Courtesy Fresinius USA, Walnut Creek, Calif.)*

SUBACUTE CARE

Dialysis is done in some subacute care units. An RN does the procedure. You may be asked to assist with positioning and the patient's comfort during the procedure. Follow Standard Precautions and the Bloodborne Pathogen Standard. Patients receiving dialysis are often very ill and need a great deal of skilled nursing care.

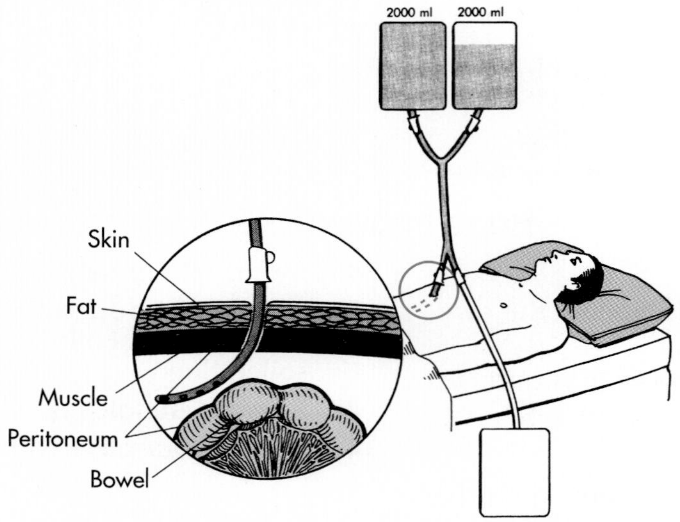

Fig. 16-24 Peritoneal dialysis system. *(From Phipps WJ, Cassmeyer VL, Sands JK, Lehman, MK:* Medical-surgical nursing: concepts and clinical practice, *ed 5, St Louis, 1995, Mosby.)*

QUALITY OF LIFE

Elimination is a very private act. People usually do not urinate in front of others. Unfortunately, illness, disease, and aging can affect this very private act. Residents often depend on the nursing staff to assist with elimination needs. Some are so weak and disabled that they cannot be left alone to use the bathroom, commode, bedpan, or urinal.

You must do all you can to protect the resident's privacy. Pull privacy curtains, and close doors, shades, and drapes. If you must stay in the room, position yourself so that the resident has as much privacy as possible. You might stand just outside the bathroom door in case the resident needs you. Perhaps it is safe to stand on the other side of the privacy curtain. The nurse helps you with ways to protect the resident's privacy.

Privacy and confidentiality are important for incontinent residents. Remember that incontinence is embarrassing and affects the resident's self-esteem. Only those involved in the resident's care need to know about the incontinence.

Incontinence has been linked to abuse, mistreatment, and neglect of residents. Caring for these residents is often very stressful. They need frequent care and may wet again just after you give incontinent care. You must not lose patience with these residents. Their needs are great, and your role is to meet their needs. If you find yourself becoming short tempered and impatient, discuss the situation with the nurse immediately. The nurse may need to reassign you to other residents for a while. Residents have the right to be free from abuse, mistreatment, or neglect. *Remember that incontinence is beyond the resident's control. It is not something he or she chooses to let happen.* Kindness, empathy, understanding, and patience are very important.

REVIEW QUESTIONS

Circle the BEST answer.

1 Which is *false?*
A Urine is normally clear and yellow or amber in color.
B Urine normally has an ammonia odor.
C Micturition usually occurs before going to bed and on rising.
D A person normally voids about 1500 ml a day.

2 Which is *not* a rule for maintaining normal elimination?
A Help the resident assume a normal position for urination.
B Provide for privacy.
C Help the resident to the bathroom or commode, or provide the bedpan or urinal as soon as requested.
D Always stay with the resident who is on a bedpan.

3 The best position for using a bedpan is
A Fowler's position
B The supine position
C The prone position
D The side-lying position

4 After a man uses the urinal, he should
A Put the urinal on the bedside stand
B Use the signal light
C Put the urinal on the overbed table
D Empty the urinal

5 Urinary incontinence
A Is always permanent
B Requires good skin care
C Is treated with an indwelling catheter
D Requires tests for sugar and ketones

6 A resident has an indwelling catheter. Which is *incorrect?*
A Keep the drainage bag above the level of the bladder.
B Make sure the drainage tubing is free of kinks.
C Coil the drainage tubing on the bed.
D Tape the catheter to the inner thigh.

7 A resident has an indwelling catheter. Which is *false?*
A Tape any leaks at the connection site.
B Follow the rules of medical asepsis and Standard Precautions.
C Empty the drainage bag at the end of each shift.
D Report complaints of pain, burning, the need to urinate, or irritation immediately.

8 Mr. Cooper has a condom catheter. You apply elastic tape
A Completely around the penis
B To the inner thigh
C To the abdomen
D In a spiral fashion

9 The goal of bladder training is to
A Remove the catheter
B Allow the resident to walk to the bathroom
C Gain voluntary control of urination
D Heal the stoma

10 You can prevent functional incontinence by doing all of the following *except*
A Answering the signal light promptly
B Keeping the signal light within the resident's reach
C Catheterizing the resident
D Following the rules for normal elimination

11 When collecting a urine specimen, you should do the following *except*
A Label the container with the requested information
B Use the correct container
C Collect the specimen at the time specified
D Use sterile supplies

12 The perineum is cleaned immediately before collecting a:
A Random specimen
B Midstream specimen
C 24-hour urine specimen
D Double-voided specimen

REVIEW QUESTIONS—cont'd

13 A 24-hour urine specimen involves
- A Collecting all urine voided by a resident during a 24-hour period
- B Collecting a random specimen every hour for 24 hours
- C A catheterization
- D Testing the urine for sugar and acetone

14 Straining urine is done to find
- A Hematuria
- B Stones
- C Nocturia
- D Urgency

15 Which specimen is best for sugar and acetone testing?
- A A random urine specimen
- B A midstream urine specimen
- C A 24-hour urine specimen
- D A double-voided specimen

16 When caring for a resident with a ureterostomy, you must do the following *except*
- A Provide good skin care
- B Change the pouch whenever it leaks
- C Report any changes in the skin around the stoma to the nurse
- D Provide incontinent briefs

17 Mr. Parker is receiving dialysis. Which is *true?*
- A He may need a special diet.
- B He needs to drink a lot of fluid.
- C His kidneys work properly.
- D He wears a pouch to collect urine.

Answers to these questions are on p. 698.

17 Bowel Elimination

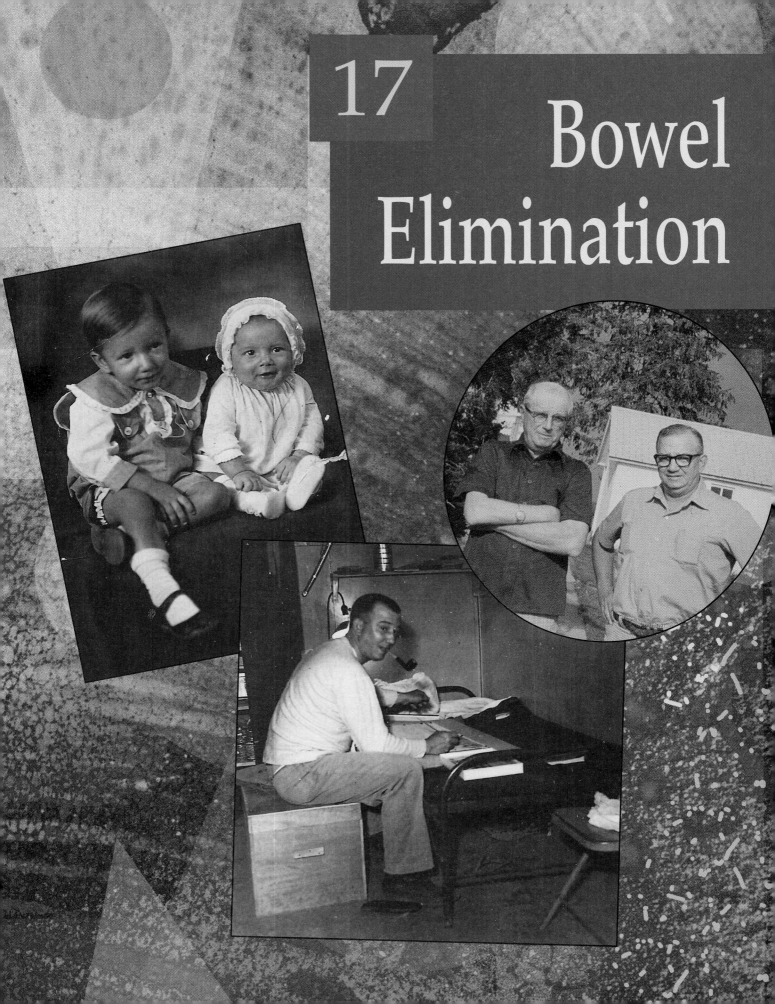

What You Will Learn

- The definition of the key terms listed in this chapter
- The normal pattern and frequency of bowel movements
- The observations about defecation to report to the nurse
- The factors that affect bowel elimination
- Common bowel elimination problems
- Measures to promote comfort and safety during defecation
- The purpose of bowel training
- Why enemas are given
- The common enema solutions
- The rules for administering enemas
- The purpose of rectal tubes
- How to care for a resident with an ostomy
- Why stool specimens are collected
- The procedures described in this chapter

Key Terms

bowel movement (BM) Defecation

chyme partially digested food and fluids

colostomy An artificial opening *(stomy)* between the colon *(colo)* and abdominal wall

constipation The passage of a hard, dry stool

defecation The process of excreting feces from the rectum through the anus; a bowel movement

dehydration The excessive loss of water from tissues

diarrhea The frequent passage of liquid stools

enema The introduction of fluid into the rectum and lower colon

fecal (anal) incontinence The inability to control the passage of feces and gas through the anus

fecal impaction The prolonged retention and accumulation of feces in the rectum

feces The semisolid mass of waste products in the colon

flatulence The excessive formation of gas or air in the stomach and intestines

flatus Gas or air in the stomach or intestines passed through the anus

ileostomy An artificial opening *(stomy)* between the ileum (small intestine; *ileo*) and the abdominal wall

melena A black, tarry stool

ostomy Surgical creation of an artificial opening

peristalsis The alternating contraction and relaxation of intestinal muscles

stoma An opening; see colostomy and ileostomy

stool Excreted feces

suppository A cone-shaped solid medication that is inserted into a body opening; it melts at body temperature

Like urinary elimination, bowel elimination is a basic physical need. Bowel elimination is the excretion of wastes from the gastrointestinal system. Many factors affect bowel elimination. They include privacy, personal habits, age, diet, exercise and activity, fluids, and drugs. Problems easily occur. Promoting normal bowel elimination is important. You will assist residents in meeting their elimination needs.

NORMAL BOWEL MOVEMENT

Foods and fluids normally are taken in through the mouth and are partially digested in the stomach. The partially digested foods and fluids are called **chyme.** Chyme passes from the stomach and into the small intestine. Further digestion and absorption of nutrients occur as chyme passes through the small bowel. The chyme eventually enters the large intestine (large bowel or colon) where fluid is absorbed. There chyme becomes less fluid and more solid in consistency. **Feces** refers to the semisolid mass of waste products in the colon.

Feces move through the intestines by **peristalsis**—the alternating contraction and relaxation of intestinal muscles. Feces move through the large intestine to the rectum. Feces are stored in the rectum until excreted from the body. **Defecation (bowel movement [BM])** is the process of excreting feces from the rectum through the anus. **Stool** is the term for excreted feces.

The frequency of bowel movements varies from person to person. Some have a bowel movement every day. Others have one every 2 to 3 days. Some people have 2 or 3 bowel movements a day. The elimination pattern also involves the time of day. Many people defecate after breakfast, others in the evening. Many older persons expect to have a bowel movement every day. The slightest irregularity concerns them. The nurse provides resident teaching about normal elimination.

Stools are normally brown in color. Bleeding in the stomach and small intestine causes black or tarry stools. Bleeding in the lower colon and rectum causes red-colored stools. So do beets. A diet high in green vegetables can cause green stools. Diseases and infection can also cause clay-colored or white, pale, orange-colored, or green-colored stools.

Stools are normally soft, formed, moist, and shaped like the rectum. They have a characteristic odor. The odor is from bacterial action in the intestines. Certain foods and drugs also cause odors.

What to Report to the Nurse

The nurse uses your observations for the nursing process. Therefore stools are carefully observed before disposal. Ask the nurse to observe abnormal stools. You need to observe stools and report the following to the nurse: color, amount, consistency, odor, shape, size, frequency of defecation, and any complaints of pain.

FACTORS AFFECTING BOWEL ELIMINATION

Normal, regular defecation is affected by many factors. The following factors affect the frequency, consistency, color, and odor of stools. The nurse considers these factors when using the nursing process to meet the resident's elimination needs. Normal, regular elimination is the goal:

- *Privacy*—Like voiding, bowel elimination is a private act. Lack of privacy prevents many people from defecating despite having the urge. Bowel movement odors and sounds are embarrassing. Imagine having to use a bedpan or commode for bowel movement in a semiprivate room. Some residents ignore the urge to defecate to avoid having a bowel movement in the presence of others.
- *Personal Habits*—Many people routinely have a bowel movement after breakfast. Some drink a hot beverage, read a book or newspaper, or take a walk. These activities relax the person. Defecation is easier when a person is relaxed rather than tense.
- *Diet*—A well-balanced diet and bulk are needed. High-fiber foods leave a residue that provides needed bulk. Fruits, vegetables, and whole grain cereals are high in fiber. Many older people do not eat enough fruits and vegetables. Some do not have teeth, or their dentures fit poorly. Therefore they cannot chew these foods. Some people think that they cannot digest fruits and vegetables and refuse to eat them. Bran often is added to cereal, prunes, or prune juice in nursing centers. These foods are a good source of fiber and help prevent constipation. Certain foods can cause constipation and diarrhea (pp. 384-385). Milk causes constipation in some people and diarrhea in others. Chocolate and other foods can cause similar reactions. Gas-forming foods stimulate peristalsis. This aids defecation. Gas-forming foods include onions, beans, cabbage, cauliflower, radishes, and cucumbers. Older persons often avoid gas-forming foods. Gas may cause "stomach aches" or "bloating."

- *Fluids*—Feces contain water. Stool consistency depends on the amount of water absorbed in the large intestine. The amount of fluid ingested, urine output, and vomiting are factors. Feces become hard and dry when large amounts of water are absorbed or when fluid intake is poor. Hard, dry feces move through the intestines at a slower rate. Constipation can occur. Drinking 6 to 8 glasses of water every day promotes normal bowel elimination. Warm fluids—coffee, tea, hot cider, and warm water—increase peristalsis.
- *Activity*—Exercise and activity maintain muscle tone and stimulate peristalsis. Irregular elimination and constipation often occur from inactivity and bedrest. Inactivity may result from disease, surgery, injury, and aging.
- *Medications*—Drugs can prevent constipation or control diarrhea. Other drugs have diarrhea or constipation as side effects. Drugs for pain relief often cause constipation. Antibiotics, used to fight or prevent infection, often cause diarrhea. Diarrhea occurs when the antibiotics kill normal flora in the large intestine. Normal flora is necessary in forming stools.
- *Aging*—Aging and illness also can slow down the passage of feces through the intestine. This results in constipation. For some people, the changes from aging and illness cause loss of bowel control (see *Fecal Incontinence*, p. 385). Older persons do not always completely empty the rectum. They often need to use the bathroom, commode, or bedpan again. This usually occurs about 30 to 45 minutes after the first bowel movement.
- *Disability*—Many paraplegic and quadriplegic residents lack voluntary control of bowel movements. Defecation occurs whenever feces enter the rectum. Bowel training programs are common for these residents (p. 386). The goal is to have a bowel movement at the same time each day. This keeps the rectum empty and prevents fecal incontinence.

COMMON PROBLEMS

Many factors affect normal bowel elimination. Common problems include constipation, fecal impaction, diarrhea, fecal incontinence, and flatulence.

Constipation

Constipation is the passage of a hard, dry stool. The person usually strains to have a bowel movement. Stools are large or marble-size. Large stools cause pain as they pass through the anus. Constipation occurs when feces move through the intestine slowly. This allows more time for water absorption. Common causes include a low-fiber diet, ignoring the urge to defecate, decreased fluid intake, inactivity, drugs, aging, and certain diseases. Dietary changes, fluids, activity, enemas, and drugs prevent or relieve constipation.

Fecal Impaction

A **fecal impaction** is the prolonged retention and accumulation of feces in the rectum. Feces become hard or puttylike in consistency. Fecal impaction results if constipation is not relieved. The person cannot defecate. More water is absorbed from the already hardened feces. Liquid seeping from the anus is a sign of fecal impaction. Liquid feces pass around the hardened fecal mass in the rectum.

The person tries several times to have a bowel movement. Abdominal discomfort, nausea, and rectal pain are common. Older persons also may have poor appetite or mental confusion. Report these signs and symptoms to the nurse.

The nurse does a digital examination to check for an impaction. (Digital refers to the finger.) This is done by inserting a gloved finger into the rectum and feeling for a hard mass (Fig. 17-1). The mass is felt in the lower rectum. Sometimes it is higher in the colon and out of reach. The digital examination often produces the urge to defecate. The doctor may order drugs and enemas to remove the impaction. Sometimes the nurse removes the fecal mass with a gloved finger. *This is called digital removal of an impaction.*

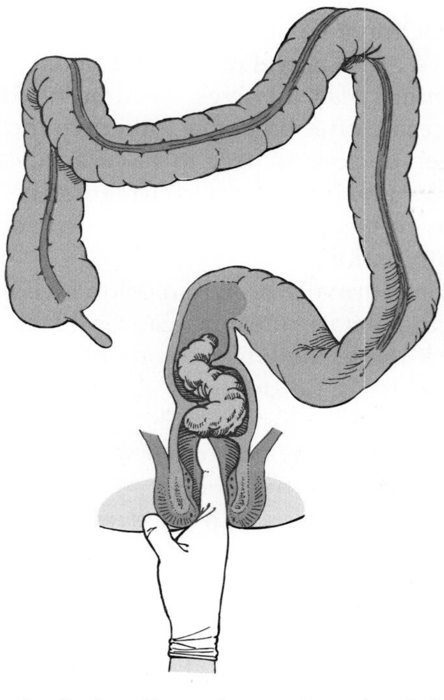

Fig. 17-1 An index finger is used to check for a fecal impaction.

Diarrhea

Diarrhea is the frequent passage of liquid stools. Feces move through the intestines rapidly. This reduces the time for fluid absorption. The need to defecate is urgent. Some people cannot get to a bathroom in time. Abdominal cramping, nausea, and vomiting also may occur.

Causes of diarrhea include infections, certain drugs, irritating foods, and microbes in food and water. Diet or drugs reduce peristalsis. Nursing measures include promptly assisting the person to the bathroom or providing the commode or bedpan. Stools require prompt disposal to reduce odors and prevent the spread of microbes. Good skin care is essential. Liquid feces are very irritating to the skin. So is the frequent wiping of the anal area with toilet tissue. Skin breakdown and pressure ulcers are risks if cleanliness and good skin care are not practiced.

Fluid lost through diarrhea is replaced. Otherwise, dehydration occurs. **Dehydration** is the excessive loss of water from tissues. Signs and symptoms include pale or flushed skin, dry skin, coated tongue, oliguria (scant amount of urine), thirst, weakness, dizziness, and confusion. Falling blood pressure and increased pulse and respirations are serious signs. The nurse uses the nursing process to meet the resident's fluid needs. The doctor orders intravenous fluids in severe cases.

Microbes often cause diarrhea. Preventing the spread of infection is important. Always practice Standard Precautions when in contact with stools.

Death is a risk from unrecognized and untreated dehydration. The amount of body water decreases with aging. Therefore diarrhea is very serious in older persons. Report any signs of diarrhea to the nurse immediately. Ask the nurse to observe the stool.

Fecal Incontinence

Fecal incontinence (anal incontinence) is the inability to control the passage of feces and gas through the anus. Causes include intestinal diseases and nervous system diseases and injuries. Fecal impaction, diarrhea, and some drugs are other causes. Persons with mental health problems or dementia (Chapters 26 and 27) may not recognize the need or act of defecating. (*See Residents With Dementia.*) Fecal incontinence also can result from unanswered signal lights when the person needs to use the bathroom, commode, or bedpan. When in a new setting, some people cannot find the bathroom in time.

Good skin care is required. A bowel training program may be developed. Assisting the person to the bathroom or providing the bedpan or commode after meals or every 2 to 3 hours may be helpful. Waterproof pads or incontinence products keep linens and clothes clean. Fecal incontinence affects the person emotionally. Frustration, embarrassment, anger, and humiliation are common emotions.

Fecal incontinence in older persons is caused by changes in the body as a result of aging or chronic illness. These residents may need bowel training programs.

Residents With Dementia

Residents with dementia may smear feces on themselves, furniture, and walls. They also may resist caregiver efforts to keep them clean. Use the same approaches for residents with dementia who are incontinent of urine (see Chapter 16). You must be patient and follow the care plan. Ask for help from co-workers. If you have questions, ask the nurse.

Flatulence

Gas and air are normally found in the stomach and intestines. They are expelled through the mouth (belching, eructating) and anus. Gas and air passed through the anus is called **flatus. Flatulence** is the excessive formation of gas or air in the stomach and intestines. Common causes are:

- Swallowing air while eating and drinking. This includes chewing gum, eating fast, drinking through a straw, and drinking carbonated beverages. Tense or anxious people may swallow large amounts of air when drinking.
- Bacterial action in the intestines
- Gas-forming foods (onions, beans, cabbage, cauliflower, radishes, and cucumbers)
- Constipation
- Bowel and abdominal surgeries
- Drugs that decrease peristalsis

If flatus is not expelled, the intestines distend. That is, they swell or enlarge from the pressure of the gases. Abdominal cramping or pain, shortness of breath, and a swollen abdomen occur. "Bloating" is a common complaint. Walking and the left side-lying position often produce flatus. Doctors may order enemas, drugs, or rectal tubes to relieve flatulence.

COMFORT AND SAFETY DURING ELIMINATION

Certain measures help promote normal bowel elimination. The nurse uses the nursing process to meet the person's elimination needs. The care plan may include measures that involve diet, fluids, and exercise. The actions listed in Box 17-1 on p. 386 are routinely practiced to promote comfort and safety during bowel elimination.

Box 17-1 Comfort and Safety During Bowel Elimination

- Assist the resident to the toilet or commode, or provide the bedpan as soon as requested. Whenever possible, wheel the resident into the bathroom on the commode. Place it over the toilet. This provides privacy for the resident who cannot walk to the bathroom or sit safely on the toilet.
- Provide for privacy. Ask visitors to leave the room. Close doors, pull curtains around the bed, and pull window curtains or shades. Remember, defecation is a private act. Leave the room if the resident can be alone.
- Make sure the bedpan is warm.
- Position the resident in a normal sitting or squatting position.
- Cover the resident for warmth and privacy.
- Allow enough time for defecation.
- Place the signal light and toilet tissue within the resident's reach.
- Stay nearby if the resident is weak or unsteady.
- Provide perineal care.
- Dispose of feces promptly. This reduces odors and prevents the spread of microbes.
- Let the resident wash the hands after defecating and wiping with toilet tissue.
- Assist the resident to the bathroom or commode or offer the bedpan after meals if the resident has the problem of incontinence.
- Practice Standard Precautions, and follow the Bloodborne Pathogen Standard.

BOWEL TRAINING

Bowel training has two goals. One is to gain control of bowel movements. The other is to develop a regular pattern of elimination. Fecal impaction, constipation, and fecal incontinence are prevented.

The urge to defecate is usually felt after a meal, particularly breakfast. The time of day that the resident usually has a bowel movement is noted on the care plan. Toilet, commode, or bedpan use is offered at this time. Other factors that promote elimination are included in the care plan and bowel training program. These include a high-fiber diet, increased fluids, warm fluids, activity, and privacy. The nurse tells you about a resident's bowel training program.

The doctor may order a suppository to stimulate defecation. A **suppository** is a cone-shaped, solid medication that is inserted into a body opening. It melts at body temperature. A nurse inserts a rectal suppository into the rectum (Fig. 17-2). A bowel movement occurs about 30 minutes later. Enemas are sometimes ordered.

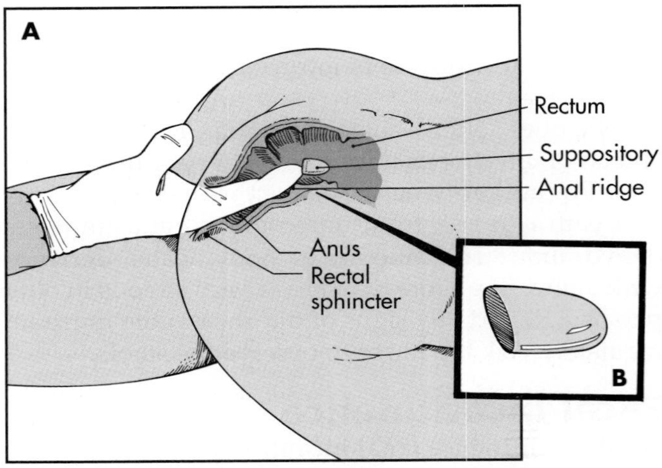

Fig. 17-2 **A,** A rectal suppository. **B,** The suppository is inserted into the rectum.

ENEMAS

An **enema** is the introduction of fluid into the rectum and lower colon. Doctors order enemas. They are given to remove feces and to relieve constipation or fecal impaction. They are also ordered to clean the bowel of feces before certain surgeries, x-ray procedures, or childbirth. Sometimes enemas are ordered to relieve flatulence and intestinal distention. Bowel training programs can involve enemas.

Enemas are usually safe procedures. Many people give themselves enemas at home. However, enemas are dangerous for older persons and those with certain heart and kidney diseases. Comfort and safety measures are practiced when giving an enema. The rules in Box 17-2 also are followed.

Some states allow nursing assistants to give enemas. Others do not. Before giving an enema, make sure that:

- Your state allows nursing assistants to perform the procedure

Box 17-2 Comfort and Safety Measures for Giving Enemas

- Solution temperature for adults is 105° F (40.5° C). Measure the temperature with a bath thermometer.
- The amount of solution given depends on the enema's purpose. Adults generally receive 500 to 1000 ml. The doctor orders the amount of solution to be given.
- The left Sims' position or the left side-lying position is preferred.
- The enema bag is raised 12 inches above the anus.
- The lubricated enema tubing is inserted only 6 inches into the rectum. Inserting the tube any deeper can injure the intestine.
- The solution is given slowly. Usually it takes 10 to 15 minutes to give 750 to 1000 ml.
- The solution should be retained in the bowel for a certain length of time. The length of time depends on the amount and type of solution. Ask the nurse how long the resident should retain the enema solution.
- The enema tube is held in place while giving the solution.
- The bathroom must be vacant when the resident has the urge to defecate. Make sure another resident will not use the bathroom.
- The nurse observes the enema results.
- Standard Precautions and the Bloodborne Pathogen Standard are followed.

- The procedure is in your job description
- You have the necessary education and training
- You review the procedure with the nurse
- A nurse is available to answer questions and to supervise you

Enema Solutions

The enema solution is ordered by the doctor. The solution ordered depends on the purpose of the enema:

- *Tap-water* enema—obtained from a faucet.
- *Soapsuds enema (SSE)*—add 5 ml of Castile soap to 1000 ml of tap water.
- *Saline enema*—a solution of salt and water. Add 2 teaspoons of table salt to 1000 ml of tap water.
- *Oil-retention enema*—mineral oil or a commercial oil-retention enema is used.
- *Commercial enema*—contains about 120 ml (4 ounces) of solution.

Other enema solutions may be ordered. Consult with the nurse and use the center's procedure manual to safely prepare and give uncommon enemas. Do not administer enemas that contain drugs. Nurses give these enemas.

◈ The Cleansing Enema

Cleansing enemas clean the bowel of feces and flatus. They are sometimes given before some surgeries and x-rays. The doctor orders a soapsuds, tap-water, or saline enema. The doctor may order *enemas until clear*. This means that enemas are given until the return solution is clear and free of feces. Ask the nurse how many enemas to give. Center policy may allow repeating enemas only 2 or 3 times.

Tap-water enemas can be dangerous. The large intestine may absorb some of the water into the bloodstream. This creates a fluid imbalance in the body. Only one tap-water enema is given. Do not repeat the enema. Repeated enemas increase the risk of excessive fluid absorption.

Soapsuds enemas are very irritating to the bowel's mucous lining. Repeated enemas can damage the bowel. Using more than 5 ml (1 teaspoon) of Castile soap or using stronger soaps can also damage the bowel.

The saline enema solution is similar to body fluid. However, some of the salt solution may be absorbed. This too can cause a fluid imbalance. When there is excess salt in the body, the body retains water.

Text continued on p. 391

Giving a Cleansing Enema

Quality of Life

Remember to:
- *Knock before entering the resident's room*
- *Address the resident by name*
- *Introduce yourself by name and title*

Pre-Procedure

1 Explain the procedure to the resident.
2 Wash your hands.
3 Collect the following:
- Bedpan or commode
- Disposable enema kit (enema bag, tube, clamp, and waterproof pad); for adults, the tube size is #22 to #30 (22 to 30 Fr)
- Bath thermometer
- Waterproof pad
- Water-soluble lubricant
- Gloves
- Material for enema solution: 5 ml (1 teaspoon) Castile soap or 2 teaspoons of salt
- Toilet tissue
- Bath blanket
- IV pole
- Robe and nonskid shoes or slippers
- Specimen container if needed
- Paper towels

4 Identify the resident. Check the ID bracelet against the assignment sheet.
5 Provide for privacy.
6 Raise the bed to the best level for good body mechanics. Make sure bed rails are up.

Procedure

7 Lower the bed rail near you.
8 Cover the resident with a bath blanket. Fanfold top linens to the foot of the bed.
9 Position the IV pole so the enema bag is 12 inches above the anus.
10 Raise the bed rail.
11 Prepare the enema:
 a Close the clamp on the tube.
 b Adjust water flow until it is lukewarm.
 c Fill the enema bag to the 1000-ml mark or as otherwise ordered.
 d Measure water temperature. For adults it should be 105° F (40.5° C).
 e Prepare the enema solution:
 - Saline enema: add 2 teaspoons of salt
 - Soapsuds enema: add 5 ml (1 teaspoon) of Castile soap
 - Tap-water enema: add nothing to the water

 f Stir the solution with the bath thermometer. Scoop off any suds (SSE).
 g Seal the top of the bag.
 h Hang the bag on the IV pole.
12 Lower the bed rail.
13 Position the resident in the left Sims' position or in a left side-lying position.
14 Place a waterproof pad under the buttocks.
15 Put on the gloves.
16 Expose the anal area.
17 Place the bedpan behind the resident.
18 Position the enema tube in the bedpan. Open the clamp. Let solution flow through the tube to remove air. Clamp the tube.
19 Lubricate the tube with the lubricant. Lubricate 6 inches from the tip.
20 Separate the buttocks to see the anus.
21 Ask the resident to take a deep breath through the mouth.

Giving a Cleansing Enema—cont'd

Procedure—cont'd

22 Insert the tube gently 6 inches into the rectum when the resident is exhaling (Fig. 17-3, p. 390). Stop if the resident complains of pain or if you feel resistance.
23 Check how much solution is in the enema bag.
24 Unclamp the tube, and administer the solution slowly (Fig. 17-4, p. 390).
25 Ask the resident to take slow, deep breaths. This helps the resident relax while the enema is given.
26 Clamp the tube if the resident needs to defecate, has abdominal cramping, or starts to expel solution. Unclamp when symptoms subside.
27 Give the amount of solution ordered. Stop if the resident cannot tolerate the procedure.
28 Clamp the tube before it is empty. This prevents air from entering the bowel.
29 Hold several thicknesses of toilet tissue around the tube and against the anus. Remove the tube.
30 Discard the soiled toilet tissue into the bedpan.
31 Wrap the tubing tip with paper towels and place it inside the enema bag.
32 Help the resident onto the bedpan. Raise the head of the bed. Or assist the resident to the bathroom or commode. The resident wears a robe and shoes or slippers when up. The bed is in the lowest position.
33 Place the signal light and toilet tissue within reach. Remind the resident not to flush the toilet.
34 Discard disposable items.
35 Remove the gloves, and wash your hands.
36 Leave the room if the resident can be left alone.
37 Return when the resident signals. Knock before entering.
38 Observe enema results for amount, color, consistency, and odor.
39 Put on the gloves.
40 Obtain a stool specimen if ordered (p.399).
41 Provide perineal care as needed.
42 Remove the bed protector.
43 Empty, clean, and disinfect the bedpan or commode. Flush the toilet after the nurse observes the results. Return items to their proper place. Remove the gloves, and wash your hands.
44 Help the resident wash the hands. Wear gloves for this step if necessary.
45 Return top linens, and remove the bath blanket.

Post-Procedure

46 Provide for comfort.
47 Place the signal light within reach.
48 Lower the bed to its lowest position.
49 Raise or lower bed rails. Follow the care plan.
50 Unscreen the resident.
51 Follow center policy for soiled linen and used supplies.
52 Wash your hands.
53 Report your observations to the nurse.

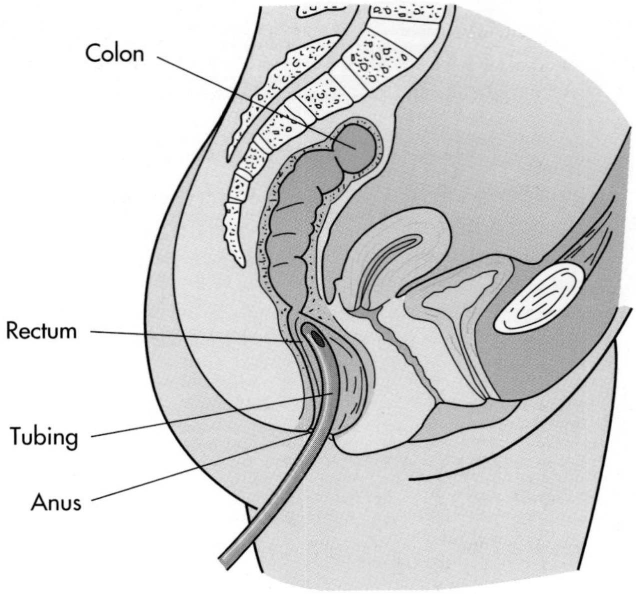

Fig. 17-3 The enema tubing is inserted 6 inches into the adult.

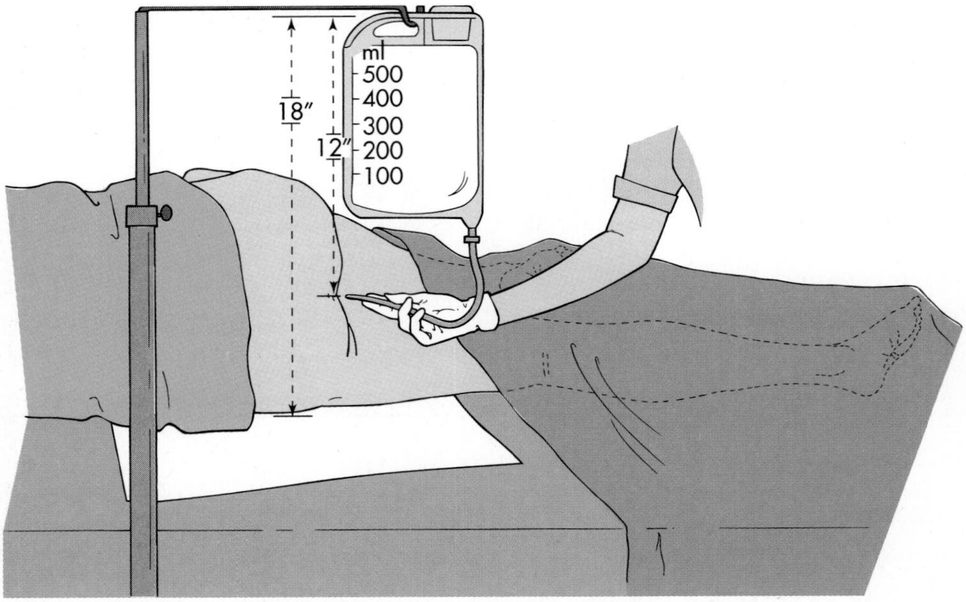

Fig. 17-4 An enema is given in the left Sims' position. The IV pole is positioned so that the enema bag is 12 inches above the anus and 18 inches above the mattress.

The Commercial Enema

Commercial enemas irritate and distend the rectum. This causes defecation. They are often ordered for constipation or when complete cleansing of the bowel is not indicated.

A manufacturer prepares and packages the commercial enema. It is ready to give. The solution is usually given at room temperature. However, the nurse may have you warm the enema in a basin of warm water.

To give the enema, squeeze and roll up the plastic bottle from the bottom. Do not release pressure on the bottle. Otherwise solution is drawn from the rectum back into the bottle. Encourage the resident to retain the solution until feeling the urge to defecate. Remaining in the left Sims' or side-lying position helps retain the enema longer.

Giving a Commercial Enema

Quality of Life

Remember to:

- *Knock before entering the resident's room*
- *Address the resident by name*
- *Introduce yourself by name and title*

Pre-Procedure

1 Explain the procedure to the resident.
2 Wash your hands.
3 Collect the following:
- Commercial enema
- Bedpan or commode
- Waterproof pad
- Toilet tissue
- Gloves
- Robe and nonskid shoes or slippers
- Bath blanket

4 Identify the resident. Check the ID bracelet against the assignment sheet.
5 Provide for privacy.
6 Raise the bed to the best level for good body mechanics. Make sure the bed rails are up.

Procedure

7 Lower the bed rail near you.
8 Cover the resident with a bath blanket. Fanfold top linens to the foot of the bed.
9 Position the resident in the left Sims' or left side-lying position.
10 Place the waterproof pad under the buttocks.
11 Put on the gloves.
12 Expose the anal area.
13 Position the bedpan near the resident.
14 Remove the cap from the enema bottle tip.
15 Separate the buttocks to see the anus.
16 Ask the resident to take a deep breath through the mouth.
17 Insert the enema tip 2 inches into the rectum when the resident is exhaling (Fig. 17-5, p. 392). Insert the tip gently.
18 Squeeze and roll the bottle gently. Release pressure on the bottle after you remove the tip from the rectum.
19 Put the bottle into the box, tip first.
20 Help the resident onto the bedpan; raise the head of the bed. Or assist the resident to the bathroom or commode. The resident wears a robe and shoes or slippers when up. The bed is in the lowest position.
21 Place the signal light and toilet tissue within reach. Remind the resident not to flush the toilet.

Continued

Giving a Commercial Enema—cont'd

Procedure—cont'd

22 Discard used disposable items. Remove the gloves, and wash your hands.
23 Leave the room if the resident can be left alone.
24 Return when the resident signals. Knock before entering.
25 Observe enema results for amount, color, consistency, and odor.
26 Put on gloves.
27 Help the resident clean the perineal area if indicated.
28 Remove the bed protector.
29 Empty, clean, and disinfect the bedpan or commode. Flush the toilet after the nurse observes the results. Return equipment to its proper place. Remove the gloves, and wash your hands.
30 Help the resident wash the hands. Wear gloves for this step if necessary.

Post-Procedure

31 Follow steps 46 through 53 in *Giving a Cleansing Enema*.

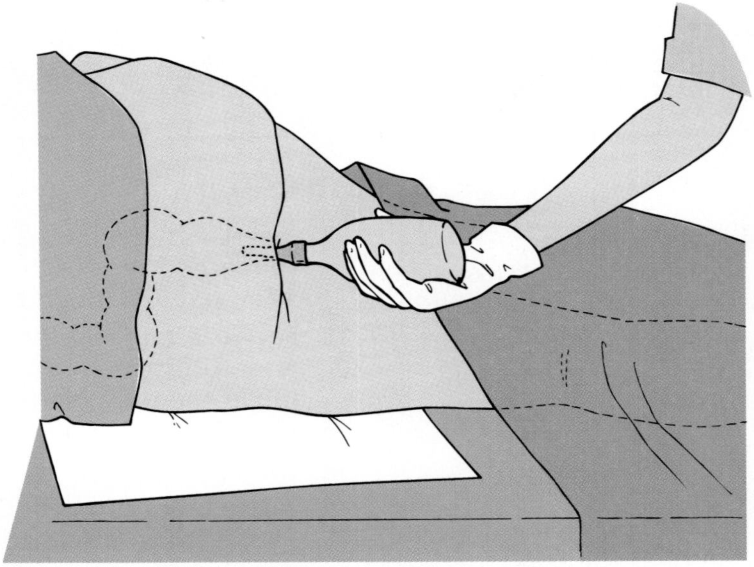

Fig. 17-5 The tip of the commercial enema is inserted 2 inches into the rectum.

The Oil-Retention Enema

Oil-retention enemas are given for constipation or fecal impactions. The oil is retained for 30 to 60 minutes to soften feces and lubricate the rectum. This allows feces to pass with ease. Most oil-retention enemas are commercially prepared.

Giving an Oil-Retention Enema

Quality of Life

Remember to:

- *Knock before entering the resident's room*
- *Address the resident by name*
- *Introduce yourself by name and title*

Pre-Procedure

1 Explain the procedure to the resident.

2 Wash your hands.

3 Collect the following:
- Commercial oil-retention enema
- Waterproof pad
- Gloves
- Bath blanket

4 Identify the resident. Check the ID bracelet against the assignment sheet.

5 Provide for privacy.

6 Raise the bed to the best level for good body mechanics. Make sure bed rails are up.

Procedure

7 Lower the bed rail near you.

8 Cover the resident with a bath blanket. Fanfold top linens to the foot of the bed.

9 Position the resident in the left Sims' or left side-lying position.

10 Place a waterproof pad under the buttocks.

11 Put on the gloves.

12 Expose the anal area.

13 Remove the cap from the enema tip.

14 Separate the buttocks to see the anus.

15 Ask the resident to take a deep breath through the mouth.

16 Insert the tip 2 inches into the rectum when the resident is exhaling. Insert the tip gently.

17 Squeeze and roll the bottle slowly and gently. Release pressure on the bottle after you remove the tip from the rectum.

18 Put the bottle in the box, tip first.

19 Cover the resident. Leave him or her in the Sims' or left side-lying position.

20 Encourage him or her to retain the enema for the time ordered.

21 Place additional waterproof pads on the bed if needed.

22 Remove the gloves.

23 Lower the bed to its lowest position.

24 Raise or lower bed rails. Follow the care plan.

25 Provide for comfort.

26 Place the signal light within reach.

27 Check the resident often.

Post-Procedure

28 Follow steps 46 through 53 in *Giving a Cleansing Enema.*

◈ RECTAL TUBES

A rectal tube is inserted into the rectum to relieve flatulence and intestinal distention. Flatus passes from the body without effort or straining. The rectal tube is inserted 6 inches into the adult rectum. It is left in place for 20 to 30 minutes. This helps prevent rectal irritation. It can be reinserted every 2 to 3 hours. The nurse tells you when to insert the tube and how long to leave it in place. *Rectal tubes are not used after rectal surgery.*

Size #22 to #30 (22 to 30 Fr) tubes are used for adults. Often the tube is connected to a flatus bag or to a container with water (Fig. 17-6). The bag inflates as gas passes into it. If connected to a container with water, the water bubbles as gas passes through the tube into the water. For this system, the rectal tube is attached to connecting tubing. The connecting tubing attaches to the water container.

Feces may be expelled along with flatus. If a flatus bag is not used, place the open end of the tube in a folded waterproof pad.

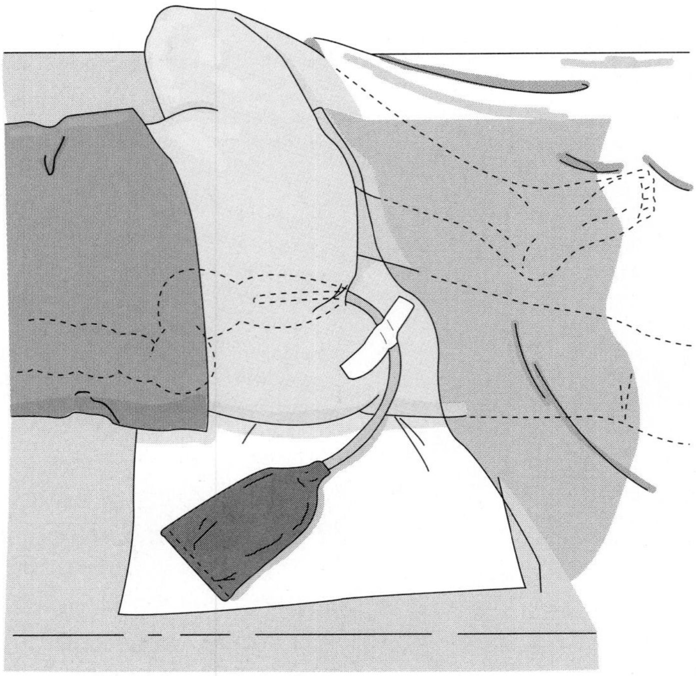

Fig. 17-6 The tube is inserted 6 inches into the adult rectum. The rectal tube is taped to the buttocks. The flatus bag rests on the bed.

Inserting a Rectal Tube

Quality of Life

Remember to:
- ◆ *Knock before entering the resident's room*
- ◆ *Address the resident by name*
- ◆ *Introduce yourself by name and title*

Pre-Procedure

1 Explain the procedure to the resident.
2 Wash your hands.
3 Collect the following:
- Disposable rectal tube with flatus bag
- Water-soluble lubricant
- Tape
- Gloves
- Waterproof pad

4 Identify the resident. Check the ID bracelet against the assignment sheet.
5 Provide for privacy.
6 Raise the bed to the best level for good body mechanics. Make sure bed rails are up.

Procedure

7 Lower the bed rail near you.
8 Position the resident in the left Sims' or left side-lying position.
9 Place the waterproof pad under the buttocks.
10 Put on the gloves.
11 Expose the anal area.
12 Lubricate the tip of the tube. Lubricate 6 inches.
13 Separate the buttocks to see the anus.
14 Ask the resident to take a deep breath through the mouth.
15 Insert the tube 6 inches into the rectum when the resident is exhaling. Stop if resident complains of pain or if you feel resistance. Insert the tube gently.
16 Tape the rectal tube to the buttocks.
17 Position the flatus bag so it rests on the bed protector (see Fig. 17-6).
18 Cover the resident.
19 Leave the tube in place no longer than 30 minutes.
20 Lower the bed to its lowest position. Place the signal light within reach. Raise or lower bed rails. Follow the care plan.
21 Remove the gloves, and wash your hands.
22 Leave the room. Check the resident often.
23 Return to the room in 30 minutes. Knock before entering the room.
24 Put on gloves, and remove the tube. Wipe the rectal area.
25 Wrap the rectal tube and flatus bag in the bed protector. Remove the bed protector.
26 Ask the resident about the amount of gas expelled.

Post-Procedure

27 Provide for comfort.
28 Place the signal light within reach.
29 Unscreen the resident.
30 Discard disposable items. Follow center policy for soiled linen.
31 Remove the gloves, and wash your hands.
32 Report your observations to the nurse.

THE RESIDENT WITH AN OSTOMY

Sometimes surgical removal of part of the intestines is necessary. Cancer, bowel diseases, and trauma (such as stab or bullet wounds) are common reasons for intestinal surgery. An ostomy is sometimes necessary. An **ostomy** is the surgical creation of an artificial opening. The opening is called a **stoma.** The resident wears a pouch over the stoma to collect feces and flatus. Stomas do not have nerve endings and are not painful. You will not hurt the resident when touching the stoma.

Some states let nursing assistants change ostomy pouches. Before changing an ostomy pouch, make sure that:

- Your state allows nursing assistants to perform the procedure
- The procedure is in your job description
- You have the necessary education and training
- You review the procedure with the nurse
- A nurse is available to answer questions and to supervise you

Colostomy

A **colostomy** is the surgical creation of an artificial opening *(stomy)* between the colon *(colo)* and abdominal wall. Part of the colon is brought out onto the abdominal wall and a stoma made. Feces and flatus pass through the stoma rather than the anus. Colostomies are permanent or temporary. If the colostomy is permanent, the diseased part of the colon is removed. A temporary colostomy gives the diseased or injured bowel time to heal. After healing, surgery is done to reconnect the bowel.

The colostomy site depends on the site of disease or injury (Fig. 17-7). Stool consistency depends on the colostomy site. Stool consistency ranges from liquid to formed. The more colon remaining to absorb water, the more solid and formed the stool. If the colostomy is near the beginning of the colon, stools are liquid. A colostomy near the end of the large intestine results in formed stools.

Feces irritate the skin. Skin care prevents skin breakdown around the stoma. The skin is washed and dried when the pouch is removed. Then a skin barrier is applied around the stoma. The skin barrier prevents feces from coming in contact with the skin. The skin barrier is part of the pouch or a separate device.

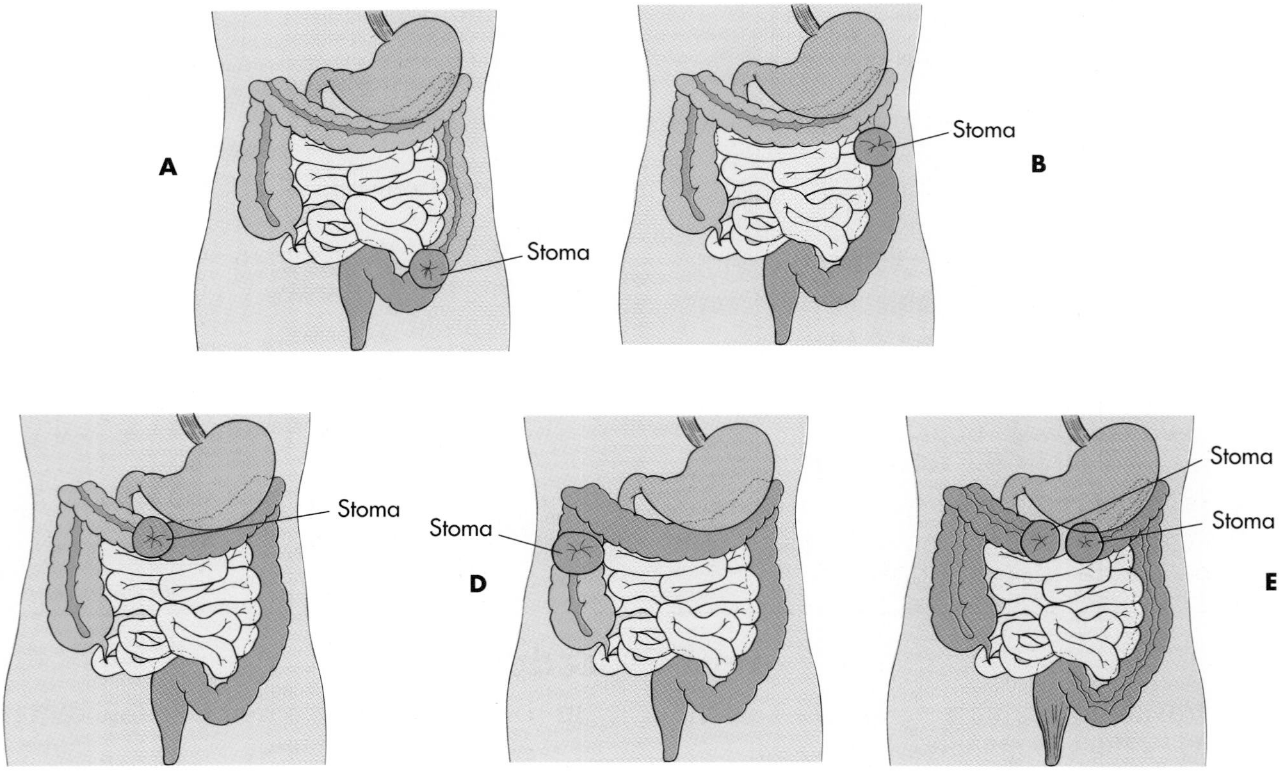

Fig. 17-7 Colostomy sites. Shading shows the part of the bowel that has been surgically removed. **A,** Sigmoid colostomy. **B,** Descending colostomy. **C,** Transverse colostomy. **D,** Ascending colostomy. **E,** Double-barrel colostomy. Two stomas are created: one allows for the excretion of fecal material; the other is for the introduction of medicine to help the bowel heal. This type of colostomy is usually temporary.

Ileostomy

An **ileostomy** is the surgical creation of an artificial opening *(stomy)* between the ileum (small intestine [*ileo*]) and the abdominal wall. Part of the ileum is brought out onto the abdominal wall and a stoma made. The entire large intestine is removed (Fig. 17-8). Liquid feces drain constantly from an ileostomy. Water is not absorbed because the colon was removed. Feces in the small intestine contain digestive juices that are very irritating to the skin. The ileostomy pouch must fit well so feces do not touch the skin. Good skin care is essential.

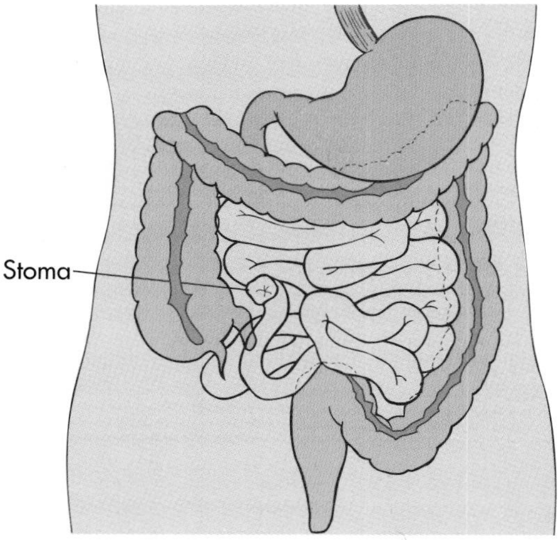

Fig. 17-8 An ileostomy. The entire large intestine is surgically removed.

◈ **Ostomy pouches.** The pouch has an adhesive backing that is applied to the skin. Sometimes pouches are secured to ostomy belts (Fig. 17-9). Many pouches have a drain at the bottom that is closed with a clip, a clamp, or a wire closure. The drain is opened to empty the pouch of feces (see Fig. 17-9). The pouch is emptied when half full. It is also opened when the bag balloons or bulges with flatus. The drain is wiped with toilet tissue before it is closed.

The pouch is changed every 3 to 7 days and any time it leaks. Some residents want the pouch changed whenever soiling occurs. Some residents manage their colostomy without help. Use Standard Precautions and the Bloodborne Pathogen Standard when assisting with ostomy care.

Odors are prevented. Good hygiene is essential. The pouch is emptied when feces are present. Avoiding gas-forming foods also controls odors. Special deodorants can be put into the pouch. The nurse tells you what to use.

The resident can wear regular clothes with an ostomy pouch. However, tight undergarments can interfere with feces being expelled into the pouch. Also, bulging from feces or flatus is often noticeable with tight clothes.

As with intact intestines, peristalsis increases after eating. Therefore stomas are usually quieter before breakfast. That is, expelling feces is less likely at this time. If the resident takes a shower or bath with the pouch off, it is best done before breakfast. Showers and baths are delayed 1 or 2 hours after applying a new pouch.

Do not flush pouches down the toilet. Follow center policy for disposing of used pouches.

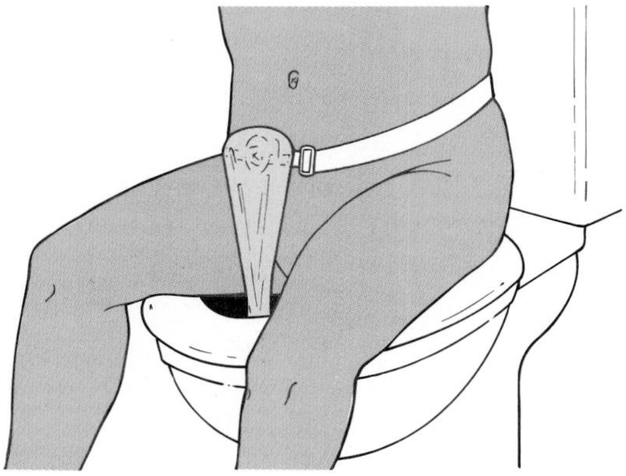

Fig. 17-9 The ostomy pouch is secured to an ostomy belt. The pouch is emptied by directing it into the toilet and unclamping the end.

Changing an Ostomy Pouch

Quality of Life

Remember to:
- ◆ *Knock before entering the resident's room*
- ◆ *Address the resident by name*
- ◆ *Introduce yourself by name and title*

Pre-Procedure

1 Explain the procedure to the resident.

2 Wash your hands.

3 Collect the following:
- Clean pouch with skin barrier
- Skin barrier (if not part of the pouch)
- Pouch clamp, clip, or wire closure
- Clean ostomy belt (if used)
- Skin barrier as ordered
- Gauze squares or washcloths
- Adhesive remover
- Cotton balls
- Bedpan with cover
- Waterproof pad
- Bath blanket
- Toilet tissue
- Wash basin
- Bath thermometer
- Prescribed soap or cleansing agent
- Pouch deodorant
- Paper towels
- Gloves
- Disposable bag

4 Arrange your work area.

5 Identify the resident. Check the ID bracelet against the assignment sheet.

6 Provide for privacy.

7 Raise the bed to the best level for good body mechanics. Make sure bed rails are up.

Procedure

8 Lower the bed rail near you.

9 Cover the resident with a bath blanket. Fanfold linens to the foot of the bed.

10 Place the waterproof pad under the buttocks.

11 Put on the gloves.

12 Disconnect the pouch from the belt if one is worn. Remove the belt.

13 Remove the pouch gently. Gently push the skin down and away from the skin barrier. Place the pouch in the bedpan.

14 Wipe around the stoma with toilet tissue or a gauze square. This removes mucus and feces. Place soiled tissue or gauze in the bedpan.

15 Moisten a cotton ball with adhesive remover. Clean around the stoma to remove any remaining skin barrier. Clean from the stoma outward.

16 Cover the bedpan, and take it to the bathroom. (Raise the bed rail before you leave the bedside.)

17 Measure feces as directed by the nurse. Ask the nurse to observe abnormal feces. Then empty the pouch and bedpan into the toilet. Note the color, amount, consistency, and odor of feces. Put the pouch in the disposable bag.

18 Remove the gloves, and wash your hands. Put on clean gloves.

19 Fill the wash basin with warm water. Place the basin on the overbed table on top of the paper towels. Lower the near bed rail.

20 Clean the skin around the stoma with water. Rinse and pat dry. Use soap or other cleansing agent as directed by the nurse.

21 Apply the skin barrier if it is a separate device.

22 Put a clean ostomy belt on the resident if a belt is worn.

23 Add deodorant to the new pouch.

24 Remove adhesive backing on the pouch.

Changing an Ostomy Pouch—cont'd

Procedure—cont'd

25 Center the pouch over the stoma. Make sure the drain points downward.
26 Press around the skin barrier so the pouch seals to the skin. Apply gentle pressure from the stoma outward.
27 Maintain pressure for 1 to 2 minutes.
28 Connect the belt to the pouch (if a belt is worn).
29 Remove the waterproof pad.
30 Remove the gloves.
31 Cover the resident. Remove the bath blanket.

Post-Procedure

32 Provide for comfort.
33 Raise or lower bed rails. Follow the care plan.
34 Lower the bed to its lowest position.
35 Place the signal light within reach.
36 Unscreen the resident.
37 Clean the bedpan, wash basin, and other equipment. Wear gloves for this step.
38 Return equipment to its proper place.
39 Discard the disposable bag according to center policy. Follow center policy for soiled linen.
40 Remove the gloves, and wash your hands.
41 Report your observations to the nurse.

STOOL SPECIMENS

When internal bleeding is suspected, feces are checked for blood. Stools are also studied for fat, microbes, worms, and other abnormal contents. The rules for collecting urine specimens (see Chapter 16) apply when collecting stool specimens. Standard Precautions and the Bloodborne Pathogen Standard are followed.

The stool specimen must not be contaminated with urine. Some tests require a warm stool. The specimen is taken to the laboratory immediately if a warm stool is needed.

Text continued on p. 402

Collecting a Stool Specimen

Quality of Life

Remember to:
- *Knock before entering the resident's room*
- *Address the resident by name*
- *Introduce yourself by name and title*

Pre-Procedure

1 Explain the procedure to the resident.
2 Wash your hands.
3 Collect the following:
- Bedpan and cover (two bedpans if the resident needs to urinate) or bedside commode
- Urinal
- Specimen pan for the toilet or commode
- Specimen container and lid
- Tongue blade
- Disposable bag
- Gloves
- Toilet tissue
- Laboratory requisition slip
- Plastic bag

Procedure

4 Label the container with the requested information.
5 Identify the resident. Check the ID bracelet with the requisition slip.
6 Provide for privacy.
7 Offer the bedpan or urinal for voiding.
8 Assist the resident onto the bedpan or to the toilet or commode. Place the specimen pan under the toilet seat (Fig. 17-10). The resident wears a robe and nonskid shoes or slippers when up.
9 Ask the resident not to put toilet tissue in the bedpan, commode, or specimen pan. Provide a disposable bag for toilet tissue.
10 Place the signal light and toilet tissue within reach. Raise or lower bed rails. Follow the care plan.
11 Wash your hands, and leave the room.
12 Return when the resident signals. Knock before entering.
13 Lower the bed rail near you if up.
14 Put on the gloves. Provide perineal care if necessary.
15 Use a tongue blade to transfer about 2 tablespoons of feces from the bedpan, commode, or specimen pan to the specimen container (Fig. 17-11).
16 Put the lid on the specimen container. Do not touch the inside of the lid or container. Place the container in the plastic bag.
17 Place the tongue blade in the disposable bag.
18 Empty, clean, and disinfect the bedpan, commode container, or specimen pan. Remove the gloves, and wash your hands.
19 Return equipment to its proper place.
20 Help the resident wash the hands. Wear gloves for this step if necessary.

Post-Procedure

21 Provide for comfort.
22 Place the signal light within reach.
23 Make sure the bed is in its lowest position. Raise or lower bed rails. Follow the care plan.
24 Unscreen the resident.
25 Take the specimen and requisition slip to the nurse.
26 Wash your hands.
27 Report your observations to the nurse.

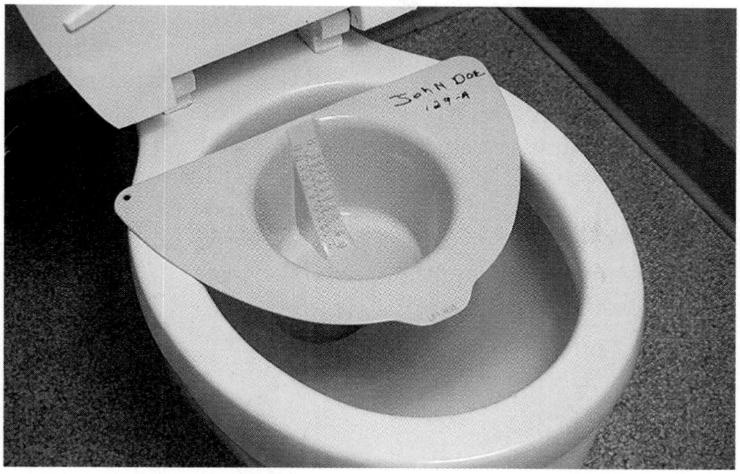

Fig. 17-10 A specimen pan is placed in the toilet for a stool specimen.

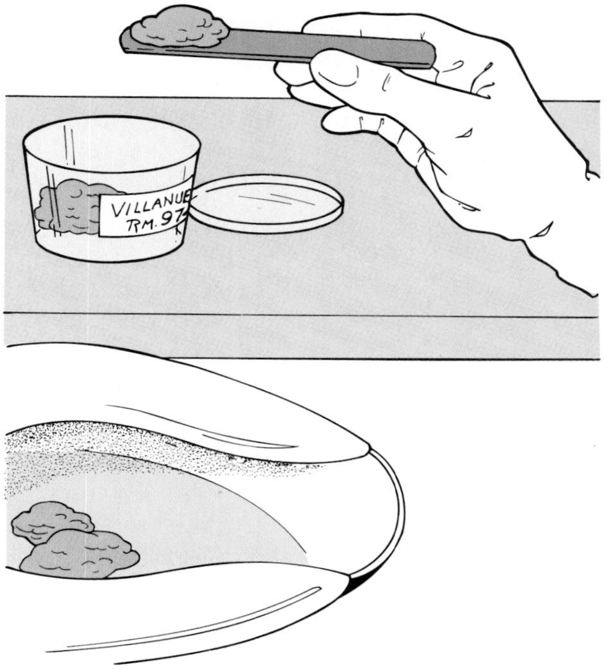

Fig. 17-11 A tongue blade is used to transfer a small amount of stool from the bedpan to the specimen container.

Testing Stools for Blood

Blood can appear in stools for many reasons. Ulcers, colon cancer, and hemorrhoids are common causes. Often blood is visible. Blood is usually seen if bleeding is low in the gastrointestinal (GI) tract. Stools are black and tarry if there is bleeding in the stomach or upper GI tract. **Melena** is a black, tarry stool.

Sometimes bleeding occurs in very small amounts. It is hard to detect such bleeding by just observing the stools. Therefore stools are often tested for the presence of *occult blood.* Occult means *hidden* or *unseen.* The test is commonly done to screen for colon cancer.

There are many types of tests. You must follow the manufacturer's instructions for the test ordered. Also follow Standard Precautions and the Bloodborne Pathogen Standard. The nurse tells you when to collect the specimen. Many factors can affect the test results. One is eating red meat. Therefore the resident cannot eat red meat for 3 days before the test. Bleeding from hemorrhoids and menstrual periods also affect the test results.

Testing a Stool Specimen for Blood

Quality of Life

Remember to:
- *Knock before entering the resident's room*
- *Address the resident by name*
- *Introduce yourself by name and title*

Pre-Procedure

1 Explain the procedure to the resident.

2 Wash your hands.

Procedure

3 Collect a stool specimen (see *Collecting a Stool Specimen*).

4 Collect the following:
- Paper towel
- Hemoccult test kit (includes developer)
- Tongue blades
- Gloves

5 Put on the gloves.

6 Open the test kit.

7 Use a tongue blade to obtain a small amount of stool.

8 Apply a thin smear of stool on box A on the test paper (Fig. 17-12, *A*).

9 Use another tongue blade to obtain some feces from another part of the specimen.

10 Apply a thin smear of stool on box B on the test paper (Fig. 17-12, *B*).

11 Close the test packet.

12 Turn the test packet to the other side. Open the flap. Apply developer to boxes A and B. Follow the manufacturer's instructions (Fig. 17-12, *C*).

13 Wait the amount of time noted in the manufacturer's instructions. Time can vary from 10 to 60 seconds.

14 Note and record the color changes (Fig. 17-12, *D*). Follow the manufacturer's instructions.

15 Dispose of the test packet.

16 Discard the tongue blade.

17 Dispose of the specimen.

Post-Procedure

18 Remove the gloves, and wash your hands.

19 Report the test results and your observations to the nurse.

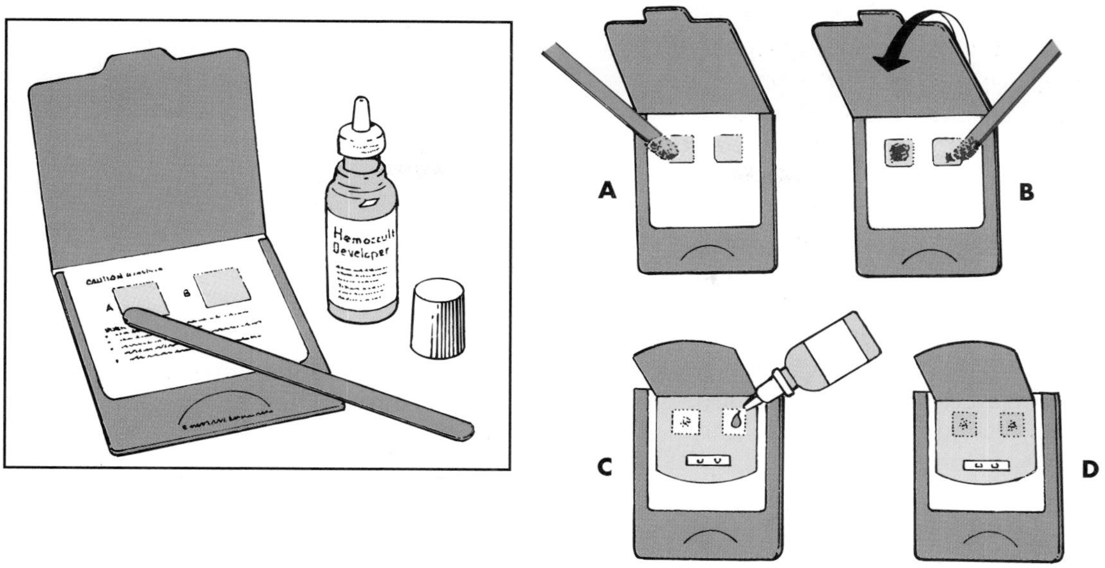

Fig. 17-12 Testing for occult blood. **A,** Stool is smeared on box A. **B,** Stool is smeared on box B. **C,** Developer is applied to boxes A and B. **D,** Color changes are noted.

QUALITY OF LIFE

Like urinary elimination, bowel elimination is a very private act. Odors occur with defecation. Therefore people are even more sensitive about their privacy. You must do all you can to protect the resident's right to privacy. Otherwise, normal bowel elimination can be affected. Constipation and fecal impaction could result.

Residents have the right to personal choice. Residents with an ostomy are allowed to manage their own care if able. Some have had their ostomy a long time. They may have special routines or care measures. Their choices in ostomy care are followed.

Quality of life considerations described for urinary elimination (see Chapter 16) apply for bowel elimination. As always, do all you can to protect the resident's rights. Your role in assisting residents with bowel elimination is like that for urinary elimination. Bowel control is important to people. So are the hygiene practices that follow bowel movements. Physical and mental well-being are closely related to maintaining normal bowel function. The personal routines related to defecation also affect well-being.

Normal bowel elimination is not always possible. Constipation, fecal impaction, diarrhea, fecal incontinence, and flatulence are common problems. The doctor may order enemas, rectal tubes, drugs, or diet changes to relieve the problem. The nurse may ask you to give an enema or insert a rectal tube. You need to completely understand the nurse's instructions and the procedure.

REVIEW QUESTIONS

Circle the BEST answer.

1 Which is *false?*
A A resident must have a bowel movement every day.
B Stools are normally brown, soft, and formed.
C Diarrhea occurs when feces move through the intestines rapidly.
D Constipation results when feces move through the large intestine slowly.

2 The prolonged retention and accumulation of feces in the rectum is called
A Constipation
B Fecal impaction
C Diarrhea
D Anal incontinence

3 Which will *not* promote comfort and safety for bowel elimination?
A Asking visitors to leave the room
B Helping the resident assume a sitting position
C Offering the bedpan after meals
D Telling the resident that you will return very soon

4 Bowel training is aimed at
A Gaining control of bowel movements and developing a regular elimination pattern
B Ostomy control
C Preventing fecal impaction, constipation, and anal incontinence
D All of the above

5 Which is *not* used for a cleansing enema?
A Soap suds
B Saline
C Oil
D Tap water

6 Which is *false?*
A Enema solutions should be 105° F (40.5° C).
B The left Sims' position is used for an enema.
C The enema bag is held 12 inches above the anus.
D The enema solution is administered rapidly.

7 In adults, the enema tube is inserted
A 2 inches
B 4 inches
C 6 inches
D 8 inches

8 The oil-retention enema is retained for
A 10 to 15 minutes
B 15 to 30 minutes
C 30 to 60 minutes
D 60 to 90 minutes

9 Rectal tubes are left in place no longer than
A 60 minutes
B 30 minutes
C 20 minutes
D 10 minutes

10 Which statement about ostomies is *false?*
A Good skin care around the stoma is essential.
B Deodorants can control odors.
C The resident wears a pouch.
D Fecal material is always liquid.

11 A resident wears an ostomy pouch. It is usually emptied
A Every 4 to 6 hours
B Every morning
C Every 3 to 7 days
D When ½ full

12 You note a black, tarry stool. This is called
A Melena
B Feces
C Hemostool
D Occult blood

Answers to these questions are on p. 698.

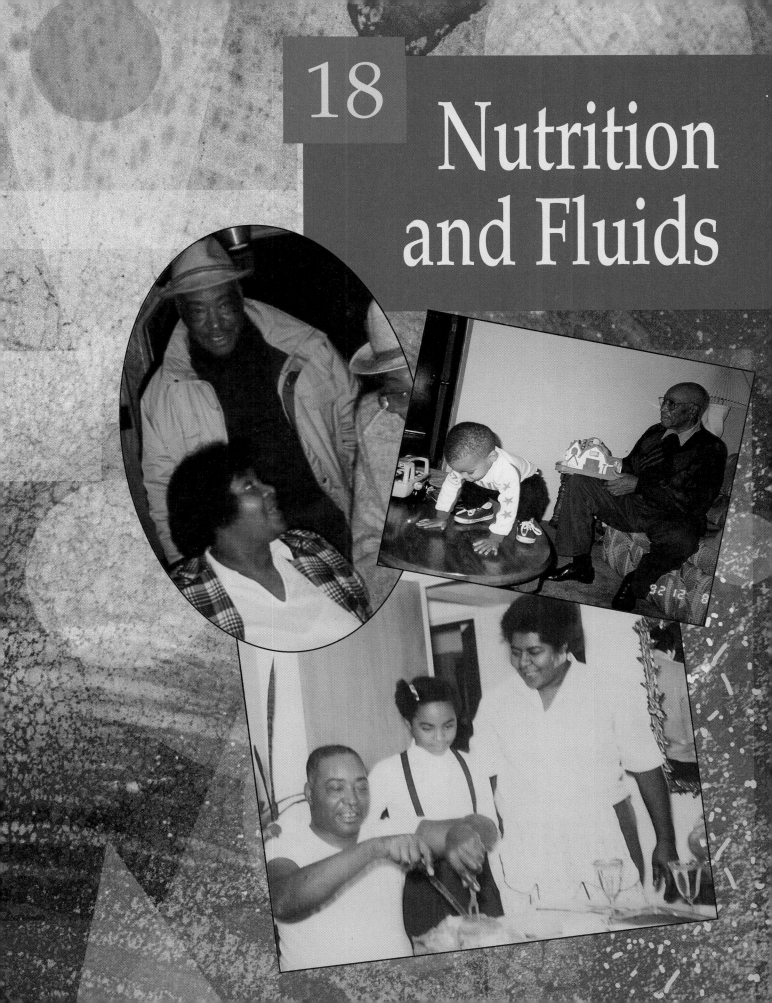

18 Nutrition and Fluids

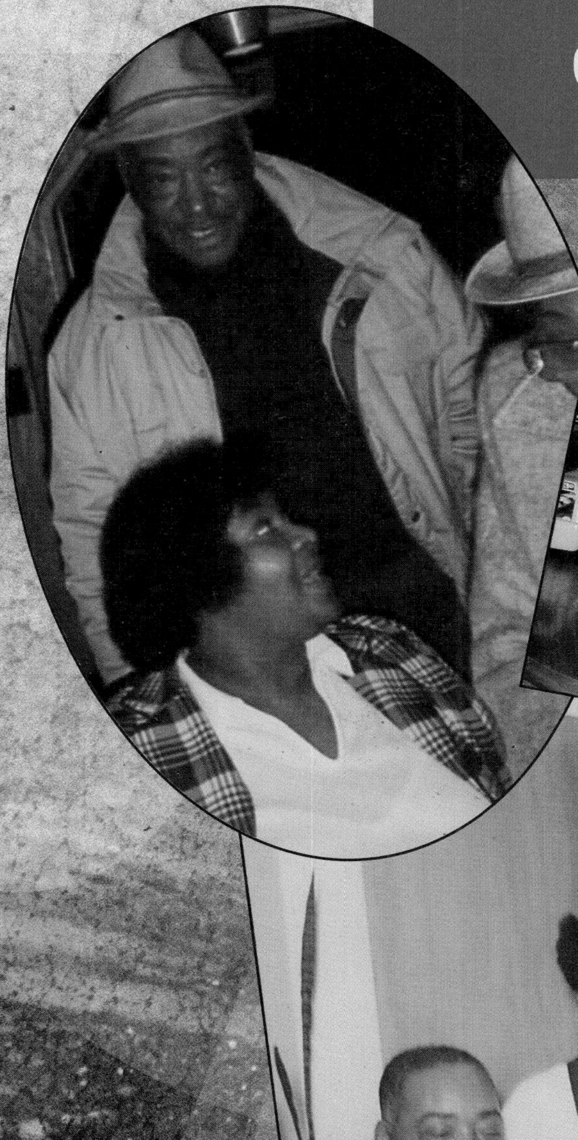

WHAT YOU WILL LEARN

- The definition of the key terms listed in this chapter
- The purpose and use of the Food Guide Pyramid
- The importance and major sources of protein, carbohydrates, and fats
- The functions and sources of vitamins and minerals
- Factors that affect eating and nutrition
- The purpose of special diets
- Normal adult fluid requirements
- Common causes of dehydration
- The purpose of between-meal nourishments
- The purpose of enteral nutrition and necessary comfort measures
- The signs and symptoms of aspiration
- How to prevent aspiration and regurgitation
- Your responsibilities when "encourage fluids," "restrict fluids," and "nothing by mouth (NPO)" are ordered
- The purpose of intake and output records
- What is counted as fluid intake
- How to promote the resident's quality of life
- The procedures described in this chapter

KEY TERMS

anorexia The loss of appetite

aspiration Breathing fluid or an object into the lungs

calorie The amount of energy produced from the burning of food by the body

Daily Reference Values (DRVs) The maximum daily intake values for total fat, saturated fat, cholesterol, sodium, carbohydrate, and dietary fiber

Daily Value (DV) How a serving fits into the daily diet; it is expressed in a percentage based on a daily diet of 2000 calories

dehydration A decrease in the amount of water in body tissues

dysphagia Difficulty or discomfort *(dys)* in swallowing *(phagia)*

edema Swelling of body tissues with water

enteral nutrition Giving nutrients through the gastrointestinal tract *(enteral)*

gastrostomy An opening *(stomy)* into the stomach *(gastro)*

gavage Tube feeding

graduate A calibrated container used to measure fluid

intravenous therapy Fluid administered through a needle inserted into a vein (IV or IV infusion)

jejunostomy An opening *(stomy)* into the middle part of the small intestine *(jejunum)*

nasogastric (NG) tube A tube inserted through the nose *(naso)* into the stomach *(gastro)*

nasointestinal tube A tube inserted through the nose into the duodenum or jejunum of the small intestine

nutrient A substance that is ingested, digested, absorbed, and used by the body

nutrition The many processes involved in the ingestion, digestion, absorption, and use of foods and fluids by the body

KEY TERMS—cont'd

percutaneous endoscopic gastrostomy (PEG) tube A tube inserted into the stomach *(gastro)* through a stab or puncture wound *(stomy)* made through *(per)* the skin *(cutaneous)*; a lighted instrument *(scope)* allows the doctor to see inside a body cavity or organ *(endo)*

regurgitation The backward flow of food from the stomach into the mouth

The need for food and water is a basic physical need. Food and water are necessary for life. The amount and quality of foods and fluids in the diet affect physical and mental well-being. Older and disabled persons may have special dietary needs. A poor diet and poor eating habits increase the risk for infection and chronic diseases. Chronic illnesses may become worse. Healing problems and changes in physical and mental function also are related to poor diet and eating habits. Poor physical and mental function increase the risk for accidents and injuries.

Eating and drinking also provide pleasure. They often are a part of social activity with family and friends. A friendly, social setting at mealtimes is important (Fig. 18-1). People may eat poorly if they eat alone or in an unpleasant setting.

Many factors affect dietary practices. They include culture, finances, and personal choice. (*See Caring About Culture.*) Dietary practices also include selecting, preparing, and serving food. The nurse considers these factors when using the nursing process to help the health care team meet the resident's nutritional needs. The dietitian has an important role in developing the nutritional care plan.

BASIC NUTRITION

Nutrition is the many processes involved in the ingestion, digestion, absorption, and use of foods and fluids by the body. Good nutrition is needed for growth, healing, and maintaining body functions. Selected foods must provide a well-balanced diet and correct calorie intake. A high-fat and high-calorie diet causes weight gain and obesity. When fewer calories than needed are consumed, weight loss occurs.

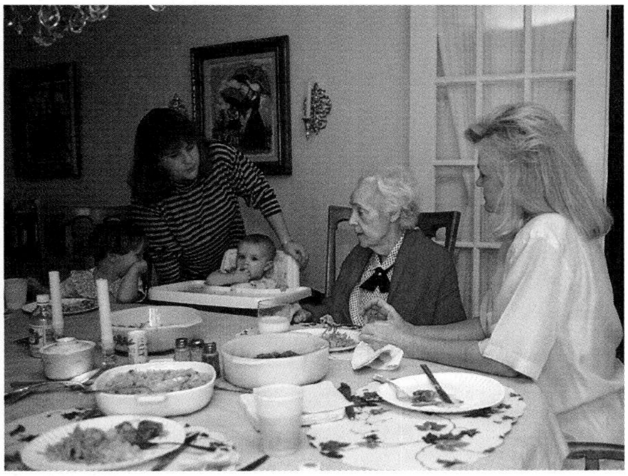

Fig. 18-1 Meals are more enjoyable when shared with family and friends.

CARING ABOUT CULTURE

Mealtime Practices

Unlike Americans, many cultural groups have their main meal at midday. For example, the Austrians have their main meal at midday and eat a light meal in the early evening and at the end of the day. Persons from Brazil also eat their main meal at noon. They have a light meal around 8 pm. A main meal at noon is common also in Finland, France, Germany, Greece, and Iran. In South Korea, breakfast is the main meal of the day.

(Modified from Geissler EM: *Pocket guide to cultural assessment,* ed 2, St Louis, 1998, Mosby.)

Foods and fluids contain nutrients. A **nutrient** is a substance that is ingested, digested, absorbed, and used by the body. Many nutrients are needed for body functions. Nutrients are grouped into fats, proteins, carbohydrates, vitamins, and minerals.

Fats, proteins, and carbohydrates give the body fuel for energy. The amount of energy provided by a nutrient is measured in calories. A **calorie** is the amount of energy produced from the burning of food by the body:

- 1 gram of fat supplies the body with 9 calories
- 1 gram of protein provides 4 calories
- 1 gram of carbohydrate supplies 4 calories

Food Guide Pyramid

In 1992 the U.S. Dept. of Agriculture (USDA) released its *Food Guide Pyramid*. The Food Guide Pyramid promotes wise food choices (Fig. 18-2, p. 408). The pyramid has 6 food groups:

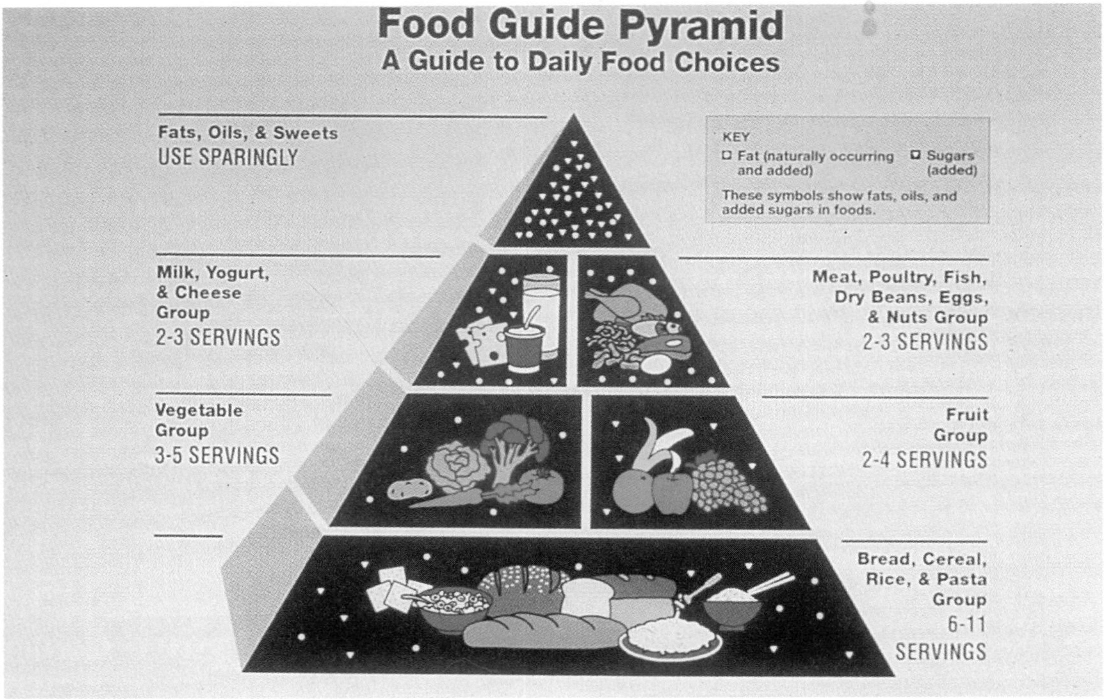

Fig. 18-2 Food Guide Pyramid. *(Courtesy U.S. Dept. of Agriculture, Washington, D.C.)*

- Bread, cereal, rice, and pasta
- Vegetables
- Fruits
- Milk, yogurt, and cheese
- Meat, poultry, fish, dry beans, eggs, and nuts
- Fats, oils, and sweets

The pyramid suggests eating more foods at the bottom level (level 1) and lesser amounts at each level moving to the top (level 4). The Food Guide Pyramid encourages a low-fat diet. More bread, cereal, rice, and pasta (level 1) and more vegetables and fruits (level 2) are eaten. Foods from the milk, yogurt, and cheese group are eaten in moderate amounts. So are foods from the meat, poultry, fish, beans, eggs, and nut group (level 3). Fats, oils, and sweets (level 4) are used sparingly.

Foods from the five food groups in levels 1, 2, and 3 are needed daily. These foods contain varying amounts of the essential nutrients. No one food or food group contains every nutrient needed by the body.

Note the small circles and triangles in the pyramid (see Fig. 18-2). The circles are for fat and the triangles for sugar. Some sugar and fat naturally occur in all foods. They appear in all levels of the pyramid. There are fewer fats and sugars at levels 1 and 2. The food groups in those levels are low in sugar and fat. More servings are allowed from these groups than the others. The result is a low-fat diet. Level 4 foods contain more fat and calories than do foods at level 1. As you move up the Food Guide Pyramid, fat and calorie amounts increase.

Box 18-1 Dietary Guidelines for Americans

- Eat a variety of foods.
- Maintain a healthy weight.
- Choose a diet low in fat, saturated fat, and cholesterol.
- Choose a diet with plenty of vegetables, fruits, and grain products.
- Use sugars only in moderation.
- Use salt and sodium only in moderation.
- If you drink alcoholic beverages, do so in moderation.

The pyramid is for everyone older than 2 years. Better health is the goal. Many diseases are related to diet and the kinds of food eaten. They include heart disease, high blood pressure, stroke, diabetes, and certain cancers. Following the Dietary Guidelines for Americans reduces the risk for such diseases. Box 18-1 lists the guidelines developed by the U.S. Dept. of Agriculture and the U.S. Dept. of Health and Human Services.

Breads, cereals, rice, and pasta group

This group forms the base of the pyramid. More servings are allowed from this group than any other group. The USDA recommends 6 to 11 servings a day

Box 18-2 Food Guide Pyramid Serving Sizes

Bread, Cereals, Rice, and Pasta Group
1 slice of bread = 1 serving
1 ounce of ready-to-eat cereal = 1 serving
½ cup of cooked cereal, rice, or pasta = 1 serving

Vegetable Group
1 cup raw leafy vegetables = 1 serving
½ cup other cooked or chopped raw vegetables = 1 serving
¾ cup vegetable juice = 1 serving

Fruit Group
1 medium apple, orange, or banana = 1 serving
½ cup chopped, cooked, or canned fruit = 1 serving
¾ cup fruit juice = 1 serving

Milk, Cheese, and Yogurt Group
1 cup of milk or yogurt = 1 serving
½ to 1 ounce cheese = 1 serving
2 ounces process cheese = 1 serving

Meat, Poultry, Fish, Dry Beans, Eggs, and Nuts Group
2 to 3 ounces cooked lean meat, poultry, or fish = 1 serving
½ cup cooked dry beans = 1 serving
1 egg = 1 serving
2 tablespoons peanut butter = 1 serving

Fats, Oils, and Sweets Group
Use sparingly

(Box 18-2). All foods in the group come from grain (e.g., wheat, oats, rice). Protein, carbohydrates, iron, thiamin, niacin, and riboflavin are the main nutrients in this group. There are small amounts of fats and sugars.

Foods such as pies, cakes, cookies, pastries, doughnuts, and muffins are made from grains. However, they are also made with fats and sugars. They are high-fat food choices, depending on the amount of fat and sugar added.

Vegetable group. The USDA recommends 3 to 5 servings a day from this group (see Box 18-2). Vegetables provide fiber, vitamins A and C, carbohydrates, and minerals. They are naturally low in fat. A variety of vegetables are eaten: dark green and yellow vegetables, tomatoes, potatoes, and vegetable juices.

Vegetables can become high in fat from food preparation. French fries are very high in fat compared with a baked or boiled potato. Butter, oil, mayonnaise, salad dressing, sour cream, and sauces are often added to vegetables. These toppings are high in fat. Low-fat toppings, used in small amounts, help keep vegetables low in fat.

Fruit group. Fruits naturally contain some sugar and are low in fat. The USDA recommends 2 to 4 servings of fruit daily (see Box 18-2). Fruits provide carbohydrates, vitamins A and C, potassium, and other minerals. This group includes all fruits and fruit juices. Fresh fruits and juices are best. Frozen or canned fruits should be unsweetened. Often they are sweetened or syrupy and therefore higher in sugar and calories.

Milk, yogurt, and cheese group. Milk and milk products are high in protein, carbohydrates, fat, calcium, and riboflavin. The USDA recommends 2 to 3 servings daily from the milk group—milk, cheese, and yogurt (see Box 18-2). Children and breast-feeding mothers need 3 servings a day.

Skim milk has less fat than whole milk. One cup of skim milk has only a trace of fat (86 calories); 1 cup of whole milk has 8 grams of fat. One cup of whole milk has about 150 calories—72 of the calories come from fat. Other low-fat foods in this group include cheeses made with skim milk, low or nonfat yogurt, and ice milk rather than ice cream.

Meat, poultry, fish, dry beans, eggs, and nuts group. This food group is higher in fat than the milk, fruit, vegetable, and bread groups. The USDA recommends 2 to 3 servings a day (see Box 18-2). Protein, fat, iron, and thiamin are the main nutrients found in this group.

Serving size is very important for a well-balanced diet. This is very important for meat, poultry, and fish because they contain many calories. Culture, appetite, personal choice, and the recipe used are some factors affecting serving size. A quarter-pound hamburger, a 12-ounce steak, a 10-ounce lobster tail, and a quarter of a chicken are servings offered by restaurants. *One serving* in this group is 2 to 3 ounces of boned meat, fish, or poultry. A 12-ounce steak is 4 to 6 servings from this group!

Remember that foods in this group are high in fat. The more fat, the more calories. Wise food choices lower fat intake from this group. Fish and shellfish are low in fat. Chicken and turkey have less fat than veal,

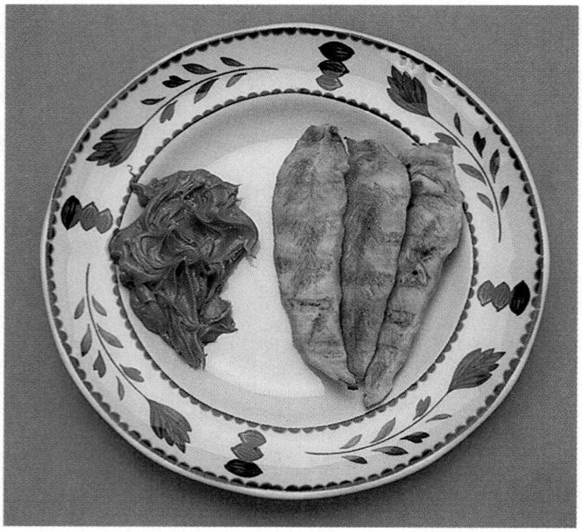

Fig. 18-3 Two tablespoons of peanut butter (1 serving) equals this 3-ounce chicken breast (1 serving).

beef, pork, and lamb. Skinless chicken and turkey are even lower in fat. Veal is lower in fat than beef. Lean cuts of beef and pork should be used. Egg yolks have more fat than egg whites. Low-fat egg substitutes can be used for cooking and baking.

Food preparation is also important. Trim fat from meat and poultry. Remove skin from poultry. Roasting, broiling, and baking are better than frying. Gravies and sauces also add fat.

Nuts and peanut butter have the most fat in this group. Use them wisely. As shown in Figure 18-3, 1 serving of peanut butter (2 tablespoons) equals 1 meat serving (2 to 3 ounces)! Peas and cooked dry beans are very low in fat. Use them often.

Fats, oils, and sweets group. This group is at the top of the pyramid. The USDA recommends that they be used sparingly and as little as possible. Fats, oils, and sweets (foods with added sugar) have little nutritional value. However, they are very high in calories. Foods in this group include cooking oils, shortening, butter, margarine, salad dressing, soft drinks, sour cream, cream cheese, and frosting. They also include all candy, many desserts (cookies, cakes, pies, ice cream), jelly and jam, syrup, and alcohol.

You can buy many low-fat or nonfat foods. Use food labels to determine fat content.

Nutrients

No one food or food group has every essential nutrient. A well-balanced diet consists of servings from the five food groups in levels 1, 2, and 3 of the Food Guide Pyramid. It ensures an adequate intake of the essential nutrients:

- **Protein**—the most important nutrient, it is needed for tissue growth and repair. Protein sources include meat, fish, poultry, eggs, milk and milk products, cereals, beans, peas, and nuts.
- **Carbohydrates**—provide energy and fiber for bowel elimination. They are found in fruits, vegetables, breads, cereals, and sugar. Carbohydrates are broken down into sugars during digestion. The sugars are then absorbed into the bloodstream. The fiber is not digested. It provides the bulky part of chyme for elimination.
- **Fats**—provide energy and add flavor to food and help the body use certain vitamins. Fat sources include the fat in meats, lard, butter, shortening, salad and vegetable oils, milk, cheese, egg yolks, and nuts. Dietary fat not needed by the body is stored as body fat (adipose tissue).
- **Vitamins**—do not provide calories but are essential nutrients. The body can store vitamins A, D, E, and K. Vitamin C and the B complex vitamins are not stored. They must be ingested daily. Each vitamin is needed for certain body functions. The lack of a specific vitamin results in signs and symptoms of an illness. Table 18-1 lists the sources and major functions of common vitamins.
- **Minerals**—are used for many body processes. They are needed for bone and tooth formation, nerve and muscle function, fluid balance, and other body processes. Table 18-2 on p. 412 lists the major functions and dietary sources of common minerals.

Food Labels

The Nutrition Labeling and Education Act of 1990 (NLEA) requires food labeling for almost all foods (Fig. 18-4, p. 412). Food labels are useful for planning a healthy diet and for following special diets ordered by the doctor (p. 417). The food label (Fig. 18-5, p. 413) has information about:

- Serving size and how the serving fits into the daily diet
- Total number of calories per serving and the number of calories from fat
- The total amount of fat and the amount of saturated fat
- Amount of cholesterol, sodium, and protein
- Total amount of carbohydrates and the amount of dietary fiber and sugars
- Amount of vitamins A and C
- Amount of calcium and iron

Table 18-1 Functions and Sources of Common Vitamins

Vitamin	Major Functions	Sources
Vitamin A	Growth; vision; healthy hair, skin, and mucous membranes; resistance to infection	Liver, spinach, green leafy and yellow vegetables, yellow fruits, fish liver oils, egg yolk, butter, cream, and whole milk
Vitamin B_1 (thiamin)	Muscle tone; nerve function; digestion; appetite; normal elimination; carbohydrate use	Pork, fish, poultry, eggs, liver, breads, pastas, cereals, oatmeal, potatoes, peas, beans, soybeans, peanuts
Vitamin B_2 (riboflavin)	Growth; healthy eyes; protein and carbohydrate metabolism; healthy skin and mucous membranes	Milk and milk products, liver, green leafy vegetables, eggs, breads, and cereals
Vitamin B_3 (niacin)	Protein, fat, and carbohydrate metabolism; nervous system function; appetite; digestive system function	Meat, pork, liver, fish, peanuts, breads and cereals, green vegetables, dairy products
Vitamin B_{12}	Formation of red blood cells; protein metabolism; nervous system functioning	Liver, meats, poultry, fish, eggs, milk, cheese
Folic acid	Formation of red blood cells; functioning of the intestines; protein metabolism	Liver, meats, fish, poultry, green leafy vegetables, whole grains
Vitamin C (ascorbic acid)	Formation of substances that hold tissues together; healthy blood vessels, skin, gums, bones, and teeth; wound healing; prevention of bleeding; resistance to infection	Citrus fruits, tomatoes, potatoes, cabbage, strawberries, green vegetables, melons
Vitamin D	Absorption and metabolism of calcium and phosphorus; healthy bones	Fish liver oils, milk, butter, liver, exposure to sunlight
Vitamin E	Normal reproduction; formation of red blood cells; muscle function	Vegetable oils, milk, eggs, meats, cereals, green leafy vegetables
Vitamin K	Blood clotting	Liver, green leafy vegetables, egg yolk, cheese

How a serving fits into the daily diet is called the **Daily Value (DV)**. The Daily Value is expressed in a percent (%). The percent is based on a daily diet of 2000 calories. Some food labels show the maximum daily intake values for total fat, saturated fat, cholesterol, sodium, carbohydrate, and dietary fiber. These are **Daily Reference Values (DRVs)**. The DV and DRVs are used as follows:

- No more than 30% of the calories in the daily diet should come from fat.
- Based on a 2000-calorie diet, the diet should have no more than 65 grams of fat.
- The food label in Figure 18-5 shows that one serving has 13 grams of fat, or 20% of the Daily Value.
- The person can have 52 more grams of fat (80%) that day.

Table 18-2 Functions and Sources of Common Minerals

Mineral	Major Functions	Sources
Calcium	Formation of teeth and bones; blood clotting; muscle contraction; heart function; nerve function	Milk and milk products, green leafy vegetables, whole grains, egg yolks, dried peas and beans, nuts
Phosphorus	Formation of bones and teeth; use of proteins, fats, and carbohydrates; nerve and muscle function	Meat, fish, poultry, milk and milk products, nuts, egg yolks, dried peas and beans
Iron	Allows red blood cells to carry oxygen	Liver, meat, eggs, green leafy vegetables, breads and cereals, dried peas and beans, nuts
Iodine	Thyroid gland function; growth; and metabolism	Iodized salt, seafood, and shellfish
Sodium	Fluid balance; nerve and muscle function	Almost all foods
Potassium	Nerve function; muscle contraction; heart function	Fruits, vegetables, cereals, meats, dried peas and beans

Fig. 18-4 Food labels are required on most foods.

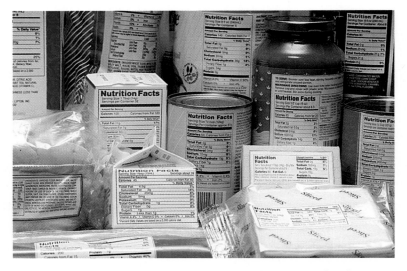

Nutrition Facts
Serving Size 1 cup (228g)
Servings Per Container 2

Amount Per Serving

Calories 260 Calories from Fat 120

	% Daily Value*
Total Fat 13g	**20%**
Saturated Fat 5g	**25%**
Cholesterol 30mg	**10%**
Sodium 660mg	**28%**
Total Carbohydrate 31g	**10%**
Dietary Fiber 0g	**0%**
Sugars 5g	
Protein 5g	

Vitamin A 4% • Vitamin C 2%
Calcium 15% • Iron 4%

* Percent Daily Values are based on a 2,000 calorie diet. Your daily values may be higher or lower depending on your calorie needs:

	Calories:	2,000	2,500
Total Fat	Less than	65g	80g
Sat Fat	Less than	20g	25g
Cholesterol	Less than	300mg	300mg
Sodium	Less than	2,400mg	2,400mg
Total Carbohydrate		300g	375g
Dietary Fiber		25g	30g

Calories per gram:
Fat 9 • Carbohydrate 4 • Protein 4

Fig. 18-5 Information contained on a food label. *(From U.S. Food and Drug Administration:* FDA consumer: an FDA consumer special report, *May 1993).*

FACTORS THAT AFFECT EATING AND NUTRITION

Meeting a resident's nutritional needs requires a team approach. The doctor, dietician, nurse, speech/language pathologist, occupational therapist, and nursing assistant develop and carry out the nutritional care plan. The resident is always part of the team. Sometimes the family is also involved. The team must know the resident's likes and dislikes and lifelong habits. What a person eats is influenced by many factors. Some begin during infancy and continue throughout life. Others develop later.

Culture

Culture influences dietary practices, food choices, and food preparation *(see Caring About Culture)*. Frying, baking, smoking, or roasting food and eating raw food are cultural practices. The use of sauces and spices also relates to culture.

CARING ABOUT CULTURE

Food Practices

Food practices vary among cultural groups. Rice and beans are protein sources in Mexico. Rice is also common in the Philippines. It is preferred with every meal. A diet high in starch and fat is common in Poland. Potatoes, rye, and wheat are common. However, a low-fat diet is common in China. Although the diet in China is low in fat, it is high in sodium. The high-sodium content is from the use of soy sauce and dried and preserved foods.

Although eating beef is common in the United States, beef is not eaten in India. Organ meats are common in England.

Modified from Geissler EM: *Pocket guide to cultural assessment,* ed 2, St Louis, 1998, Mosby.

Religion

Selecting, preparing, and eating food often involve religious practices (Box 18-3, p. 414). Members of a religious group may follow all, some, or none of the dietary practices of their faith. You must respect the resident's religious practices.

Finances

People with limited incomes often buy the cheaper carbohydrate foods. Their diets often lack protein and certain vitamins and minerals.

Appetite Appetite relates to the desire for food. When hungry, a person seeks food and eats until the appetite is satisfied. Aromas and thoughts of food can also stimulate the appetite. However, loss of appetite **(anorexia)** can occur. Illness, medications, unpleasant thoughts or sights, anxiety, pain, and depression are some causes of anorexia. Older persons may have loss of appetite from decreased senses of taste and smell.

Personal Choice

The like or dislike of certain foods is a personal matter. Food preferences begin in childhood. They are influenced by the kinds of food served in the home. As a child grows older, new foods are introduced through school and social events. Many people decide whether they like or dislike a certain food by the way it looks, how it is prepared, its smell, or recipe ingredients. Usually food preferences expand with age and social experiences.

Food choices also are influenced by body reactions. People usually avoid foods that cause allergic reactions, nausea, vomiting, diarrhea, indigestion, gas, or headaches.

Box 18-3 Religion and Dietary Practices

Adventist (Seventh Day Adventist)
- Coffee, tea, and alcohol are not allowed.
- Beverages with caffeine (colas) are not allowed.
- Some groups forbid eating meat.

Baptist
- Some groups forbid coffee, tea, and alcohol.

Christian Scientist
- Alcohol and coffee are not allowed.

Church of Jesus Christ of Latter Day Saints (Mormon)
- Alcohol and hot drinks, such as coffee and tea, are not allowed.
- Meat is not forbidden, but members are encouraged to eat meat infrequently.

Greek Orthodox Church
- Wednesdays, Fridays, and Lent are days of fasting.
- Meat and dairy products are usually avoided during days of fast.

Islam (Muslim or Moslem)
- All pork and pork products are forbidden.
- Alcohol is not allowed except for medical reasons.

Judaism (Jewish Faith)
- Foods must be kosher (prepared according to Jewish law).
- Meat of kosher animals (cows, goats, and sheep) can be eaten.
- Chickens, ducks, and geese are kosher fowls.
- Kosher fish have scales and fins, such as tuna, sardines, carp, and salmon.
- Shellfish cannot be eaten.
- Milk, milk products, and eggs from kosher animals and fowl are acceptable.
- Milk and milk products cannot be eaten with or immediately after eating meat.
- Milk and milk products can be eaten 6 hours after eating meat.
- Milk and milk products can be a part of the same meal with meat—they are served separately and before the meat.
- Kosher foods are not prepared in utensils used to prepare nonkosher foods.
- Breads, cakes, cookies, noodles, and alcoholic beverages are not consumed during Passover.

Roman Catholic
- Fasting for 1 hour before receiving Holy Communion.
- Fasting from meat on Ash Wednesday and Good Friday—some may continue to fast from meat on Fridays.

Nursing centers allow residents some choice in the foods served. Meals must be balanced. Residents are encouraged to choose food from the five food groups. They make personal choices from food menus (Fig. 18-6). Some centers involve resident groups in planning special meals. Often residents plan holiday meals—Christmas, St. Patrick's Day, Easter, Fourth of July, Labor Day, and Thanksgiving. They also plan such events as picnics, pizza parties, and ice cream socials (Fig. 18-7, p. 416). Remember that residents have the right to personal choice.

MENU—WEEK 3

Tuesday

Juice Oatmeal w/raisins Egg in a souffle cup Hash browned potatoes Toast	Roast ham w/sweet potatoes OR Meat loaf w/gravy Cabbage w/green peppers Cottage cheese salad Cornbread Frosted brownie	Chicken croquettes w/gravy OR BBQ mini franks Cook's choice soup Broccoli cuts Bread slice Cinnamon applesauce

Wednesday

Juice Malt O'Meal Waffles Ham	Baked chicken w/orange sauce Baked potato OR Beef stroganoff w/noodles Baby lima beans Cole slaw w/carrots Pumpkin cake	Ravioli w/roll OR Tuna melt Beef barley soup Italian blend vegetables Banana half

Thursday

Juice Cream of wheat Scrambled eggs Toast	Beef stew w/biscuit OR Fried chicken w/mashed potatoes & gravy Peach half w/cottage cheese Peas & carrots Poke cake	Deviled ham on pumpernickel sandwich OR Fruit plate w/cottage cheese Muffin Cream of chicken soup Salad fruits

Friday

Juice Cream of rice Egg in a souffle cup Raisin toast	Oven fried fish OR Roast Turkey w/gravy Cranberry sauce O'Brien potatoes Winter mix vegetables Red Jello w/oranges Vanilla pudding w/crushed Oreos	Hot ham & cheese on a bun OR Beef & potato casserole Chicken noddle soup Corn Apricots

Saturday

Juice Oatmeal French toast Bacon	Chicken Tetrazzini OR Pepper steak w/sauteed peppers & onions Mashed potatoes Francois blend vegetables Spinach salad Lemon surprise dessert	Chicken salad sandwich on raisin bread OR Chef salad Broccoli cheese soup Diced peaches & pears

Sunday

Juice Malt O'Meal Biscuits in gravy	Roast beef w/gravy Baked potatoes Cauliflower w/cheese sauce Tossed salad Cheesecake tart	Fish sandwich on a bun w/lettuce and tomato OR Ham & cheese omelet Beef vegetable soup Tropical fruit Ice cream

Monday

Juice Cream of wheat Egg in a souffle cup English muffin	Chicken & dumplings w/gravy OR Stuffed cabbage w/tomato sauce Mashed potatoes Scandinavian vegetable blend Butterscotch pudding	Spaghetti casserole OR Chicken Philly sandwich on a bun w/onions and peppers Cream of mushroom soup Broccoli cuts Ambrosia

SERVING TIME—TOWER DINING ROOM		**SERVING TIME—MANOR DINING ROOM**	
Breakfast	**7:30 a.m.**	**Breakfast**	**7:00 a.m.**
Dinner	**12:15 p.m.**	**Dinner**	**12:30 p.m.**

Fig. 18-6 Choosing from a menu protects the right to personal choice. *(Courtesy Bonell Good Samaritan Center, Greeley, Colo.)*

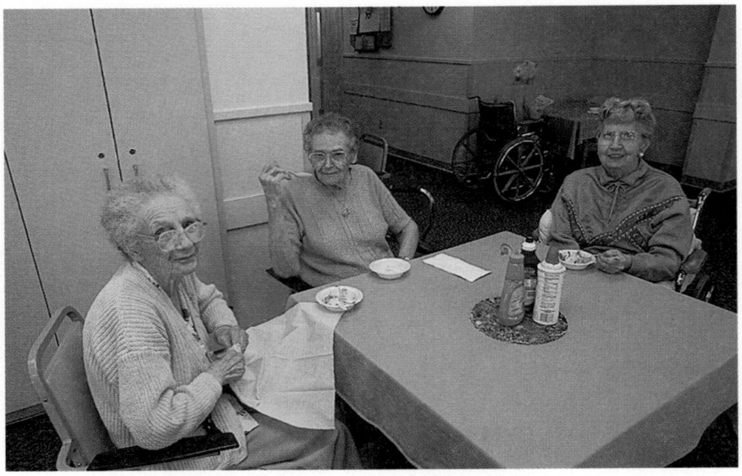

Fig. 18-7 Residents enjoying an ice cream social.

Illness

Appetite usually decreases during illness and recovery from injuries. However, nutritional needs increase at these times. The body must fight infection, heal tissue, and replace lost blood cells. Nutrients lost through vomiting and diarrhea need replacement. Some diseases and drugs cause a sore mouth, which makes eating painful. Tooth loss or poor-fitting dentures affects chewing. Protein foods (the meat group) may be hard to chew.

Age

Many changes occur in the gastrointestinal system. As people age, difficulty in swallowing often occurs. Dysphagia can result. **Dysphagia** is difficulty or discomfort *(dys)* in swallowing *(phagia)*. It can result from stroke, dementia, or other nervous system disorders. Taste and smell dull, and appetite decreases. Secretion of digestive juices decreases. As a result, fried and fatty foods are hard to digest and may cause indigestion.

Dry, fried, and fatty foods are avoided. This helps swallowing and digestion problems. Good oral hygiene and denture care improve the ability to taste. It might be necessary to avoid high-fiber foods even though they help prevent constipation. High-fiber foods are hard to chew and can irritate the intestines. High-fiber foods include apricots, celery, and fruits and vegetables with skins and seeds. Foods providing soft bulk often are ordered for persons with chewing problems or constipation. These foods include whole-grain cereals and cooked fruits and vegetables.

Older persons need fewer calories than younger people do. Energy levels and daily activity levels are lower. The diet must include foods that contain calcium to prevent musculoskeletal changes. Protein is needed for tissue growth and repair. However, the diet of some older persons may lack protein. High-protein foods often are costly.

OBRA DIETARY REQUIREMENTS

OBRA has the following requirements for food served in nursing centers: OBRA

- Each person's nutritional and special dietary needs must be met.
- Residents must receive a well-balanced diet. The diet must be nourishing and taste good. Food must be well seasoned. It must not be too salty or too sweet.
- Food must be appetizing. It must have an appealing aroma and be attractive.
- Hot food must be served hot and cold food served cold. Centers have special food servers to keep food at the correct temperature. Food is served promptly. Otherwise, hot food will cool and cold food will warm.
- Food must be prepared to meet the person's individual needs. Some persons need food cut, ground, or chopped. Others have special diets ordered by the doctor. OBRA
- Each person must receive at least 3 meals a day and be offered a bedtime snack.
- The center must provide any special eating equipment and utensils that are needed (Fig. 18-8). They allow the person to eat independently. The speech/language therapist and occupational therapist teach

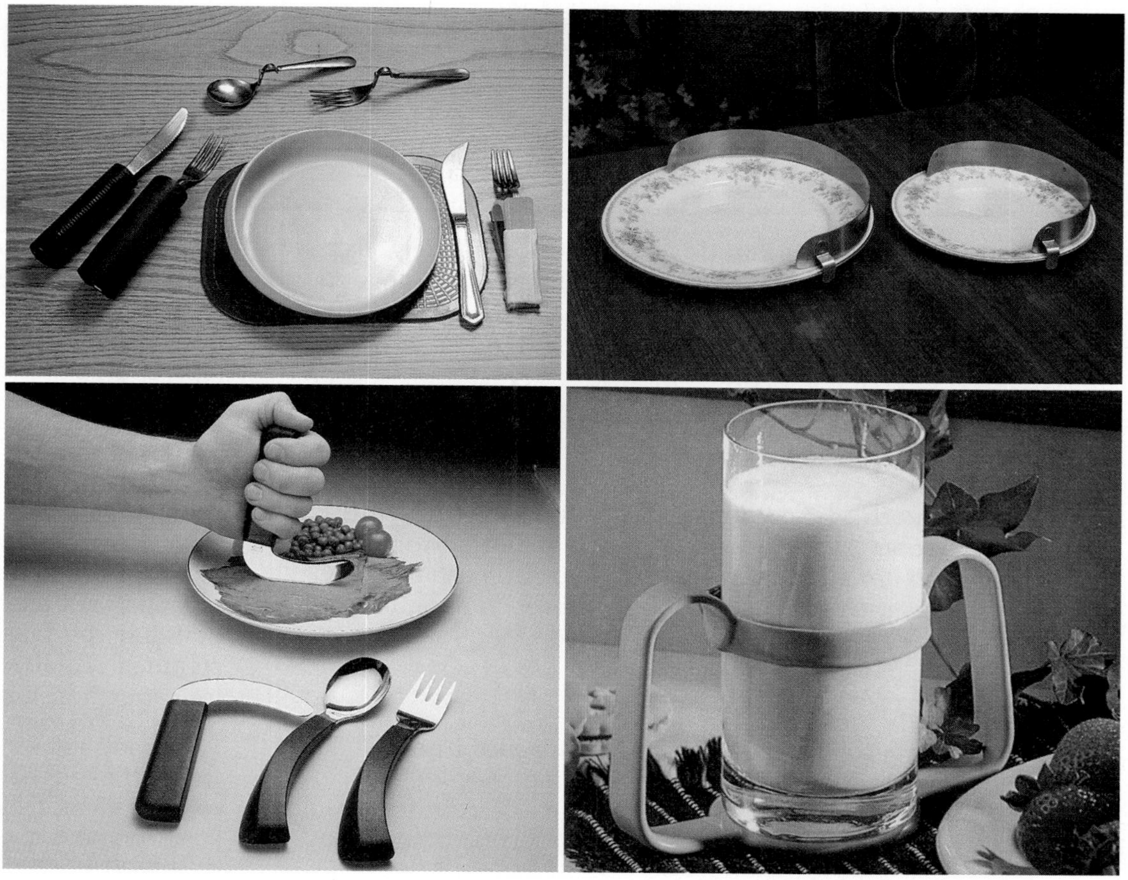

Fig. 18-8 Eating utensils for persons with special needs. **A,** The curved fork fits over the hand. The rounded plate helps keep food on the plate. Special grips and swivel handles are helpful for some persons. **B,** Plate guards help keep food on the plate. **C,** Knives with rounded blades are rocked back and forth to cut food. The person does not need a fork in one hand and a knife in the other. **D,** Glass holder. *(Courtesy Bissell Healthcare Corp.; Fred Sammons, Inc.)*

the person how to use the item. You must make sure needed equipment is available for the resident. Disease or injury can affect the hands, wrists, and arms.

SPECIAL DIETS

Doctors may order special diets. Such diets are ordered because of a nutritional deficiency or a disease. They also are ordered to eliminate or decrease certain substances in the diet or to control weight. The doctor, nurses, and dietitian work together to meet the resident's nutritional needs. They consider the need for dietary changes, personal choices, religion, culture, and eating problems. Food allergies and sensitivities also are considered.

Many residents do not need special diets. Many centers use *general diet, regular diet,* and *house diet* to mean no dietary restrictions or changes. Special or therapeutic diets are ordered for residents with diabetes or diseases of the heart, kidneys, gallbladder, liver, stomach, or intestines. Residents with pressure ulcers or other wounds will likely have high-protein diets. Added protein is needed for healing. Bran may be added to the diet of older and disabled persons. It provides fiber necessary for good bowel health.

Some residents need special textured foods in their diets. A *dysphagia diet* is ordered for residents with difficulty swallowing. In this diet, food thickness is changed to meet the resident's needs (p. 422). Others need all foods pureed.

Allergies, obesity, and other disorders also require therapeutic diets. Table 18-3 on pp. 418-420 summarizes the common therapeutic diets.

The sodium-restricted diet, diabetic diet, and dysphagia diet are commonly ordered. They are described in greater detail.

Text continued on p. 420

Table 18-3 Common Therapeutic Diets

Diet	Description	Use	Foods Allowed
Clear liquid	Clear liquids that do not leave a residue; nonirritating and non-gas-forming	Postoperatively, acute illness, infection, and nausea and vomiting	Water, tea, and coffee (without milk or cream); carbonated beverages; gelatin; clear fruit juices (apple, grape, and cranberry); fat-free clear broth; hard candy, sugar, and Popsicles
Full liquid	Foods that are liquid at room temperature or that melt at body temperature	Advance from clear liquid diet postoperatively; for stomach irritation, fever, and nausea and vomiting	All foods allowed on a clear liquid diet; custard; eggnog; strained soups; strained fruit and vegetable juices; milk; creamed cereals; plain ice cream and sherbet
Soft	Semisolid foods that are easily digested	Advance from full liquid diet; chewing difficulties, gastrointestinal disorders, and infections	All liquids; eggs (not fried); broiled, baked, or roasted meat, fish, or poultry that is chopped or shredded; mild cheeses (American, Swiss, cheddar, cream, and cottage); strained fruit juices; refined bread (no crust) and crackers; cooked cereal; cooked or pureed vegetables; cooked or canned fruit without skin or seeds; pudding; plain cakes
Low residue	Foods that leave a small amount of residue in the colon	Diseases of the colon and diarrhea	Coffee, tea, milk, carbonated beverages, strained fruit juices; refined bread and crackers; creamed and refined cereal; rice; cottage and cream cheese; eggs (not fried); plain puddings and cakes; gelatin; custard; sherbet and ice cream; strained vegetable juices; canned or cooked fruit without skin or seeds; potatoes (not fried); strained cooked vegetables; plain pasta; *no raw fruits and vegetables*

CONT'D
TABLE 18-3
COMMON THERAPEUTIC DIETS

Diet	Description	Use	Foods Allowed
High fiber	Foods that increase the amount of residue in the colon to stimulate peristalsis	Constipation and colon disorders	All fruits and vegetables; whole wheat bread; whole grain cereals; fried foods; whole grain rice; milk, cream, butter, and cheese; meats
Bland	Foods that are mechanically and chemically nonirritating and low in roughage; foods served at moderate temperatures; no strong spices or condiments	Ulcers, gallbladder disorders, and some intestinal disorders; postoperatively after abdominal surgery	Lean meats; white bread; creamed and refined cereals; cream or cottage cheese; gelatin, plain puddings, cakes, and cookies; eggs (not fried); butter and cream; canned fruits and vegetables without skin and seeds; strained fruit juices; potatoes (not fried); pastas and rice; strained or soft-cooked carrots, peas, beets, spinach, squash, and asparagus tips; creamed soups from allowed vegetables; no fried foods
High calorie	Calorie intake is increased to about 4000; includes three full meals and between-meal snacks	Weight gain and some thyroid imbalances	Dietary increases in all foods
Low calorie	Calorie intake is reduced below the minimum daily requirements	Weight reduction	Foods low in fats and carbohydrates and lean meats; avoid butter, cream, rice, gravies, salad oils, noodles, cakes, pastries, carbonated and alcoholic beverages, candy, potato chips, and similar foods
High iron	Foods that are high in iron	Anemia; following blood loss; for women during the reproductive years	Liver and other organ meats; lean meats; egg yolks; shellfish; dried fruits; dried beans; green leafy vegetables; lima beans; peanut butter; enriched breads and cereals

Continued

CONT'D TABLE 18-3 COMMON THERAPEUTIC DIETS

Diet	Description	Use	Foods Allowed
Low fat (low cholesterol)	Foods low in fat and foods prepared without adding fat	Heart disease, gallbladder disease, disorders of fat digestion, and liver disease	Skim milk or buttermilk; cottage cheese (no other cheeses allowed); gelatin; sherbet; fruit; lean meat, poultry, and fish (baked, broiled, or roasted); fat-free broth; soups made with skim milk; margarine; rice, pasta, breads and cereals; vegetables; potatoes
High protein	Aid and promote tissue healing	For burns, high fever, infection, and some liver diseases	Meat, milk, eggs, cheese, fish, poultry; breads and cereals; green leafy vegetables
Sodium restricted	A certain amount of sodium is allowed; sodium restriction ranges from mild to severe	Heart disease, fluid retention, and some kidney diseases	Fruits and vegetables and unsalted butter are allowed; adding salt at the table is not allowed; highly salted foods and foods high in sodium are not allowed; the use of salt during cooking may be restricted
Consistent-carbohydrate diabetes meal plan	The amount of carbohydrates, protein, and fat is regulated	Diabetes mellitus	Determined by nutritional and energy requirements

The Sodium-Restricted Diet

The average amount of sodium in the daily diet is 3000 to 5000 mg. The body needs only half this amount. Healthy people excrete excess sodium in the urine. However, heart and kidney diseases cause the body to retain the extra sodium. So do some drugs.

Sodium-restricted diets are ordered for residents with heart disease. They also may be ordered for those with liver or kidney disease or hypertension (high blood pressure) or for those taking certain drugs. Sodium causes the body to retain water. If there is too much sodium, the body retains more water. Body tissues swell with water, and there is excess fluid in the blood vessels. The increased fluid in the tissues and bloodstream forces the heart to work harder. In other words, the workload of the heart increases. With heart disease, the extra workload can cause serious problems or death. Restricting the amount of sodium in the diet decreases the amount of sodium in the body. The body retains less water. Less water in the tissues and blood vessels reduces the heart's workload.

Sodium-restricted diets range from mild to severe. The doctor orders the amount of restriction. Some residents on sodium-restricted diets will return home. They need to know which foods are high in sodium and which are low in sodium. They also need to know how to calculate the amount of sodium in the diet. The nurse or dietitian teaches the resident and family about the diet:

- *2000- to 3000-mg sodium diet*. This is called the *low-salt* or *no added salt diet*. Sodium restriction is "mild." All high-sodium foods are omitted (Box 18-4). A minimum amount of salt is used in cooking. Salt is not added to foods at the table.

Box 18-4 High-Sodium Foods

Bread, Cereal, Rice, and Pasta Group
- Saltine crackers
- Baking powder biscuits
- Muffins
- Bisquick
- Pretzels
- Salted crackers
- Quick breads (corn bread, nut bread)
- Pancakes
- Waffles
- Instant cooked cereal
- Processed bran cereals
- Rice
- Noodle mixes
- Corn chips and other salted snacks

Vegetable Group
- Sauerkraut
- Tomato juice
- V-8 juice
- Vegetables in creams or sauces
- Frozen vegetables processed with salt or sodium
- Bloody Mary mixes
- Potato chips
- French fries
- Instant potatoes
- Pickles
- Relishes

Fruit Group
- No restrictions

Milk, Yogurt, and Cheese Group
- Buttermilk
- Cheese
- Commercial dips made with sour cream

Meat, Poultry, Fish, Dry Beans, Eggs, and Nuts Group
- Bacon
- Ham
- Sausage
- Salt pork
- Hot dogs
- Luncheon meats
- Corned or chopped beef
- Organ meats
- Shellfish
- Sardines
- Herring
- Anchovies
- Caviar
- Kosher meats
- Canned tuna
- Canned salmon
- Mackerel
- Salted nuts or seeds
- Peanut butter

Fats, Oils, and Sweets
- Salad dressings
- Mayonnaise
- Baked desserts

Other
- Mineral water
- Club soda
- Canned soups
- Bouillon cubes
- Dried soup mixes
- Olives
- Salted popcorn
- Frozen or canned dinners
- Salt
- Baking powder
- Baking soda
- Celery, onion, garlic, and other seasoning salts
- Meat tenderizers
- Worcestershire sauce
- Soy sauce
- Mustard
- Catsup
- Horseradish
- Sauces: chili, tomato, steak, barbecue

Modified from Lewis SM, Collier IC, Heitkemper MM: *Medical-surgical nursing: assessment & management of clinical problems,* ed 4, St. Louis, 1996, Mosby.

- *1000-mg sodium diet.* Sodium restriction is "moderate." Food is cooked without salt. Foods high in sodium are omitted from the diet. Vegetables high in sodium are restricted in amount. Salt-free products, such as salt-free bread, are used. Diet planning is necessary.
- *500-mg sodium diet.* Sodium restriction is "strict." Restrictions for the less-restricted diets are followed. Only fresh vegetables are allowed. Vegetables high in sodium are omitted (see Box 18-4). Milk is limited to 2 cups per day, and only 1 egg per day is allowed. Meat is limited to 4 ounces per day. Diet planning is essential.

Medical Nutrition Therapy for Diabetes Mellitus

Medical nutrition therapy (MNT) is necessary for people with diabetes mellitus. Diabetes mellitus is a chronic disease caused by a lack of insulin (see Chapter 26). The pancreas produces and secretes insulin. Insulin allows the body to use sugar. If there is not enough insulin, sugar builds up in the bloodstream rather than being used by cells for energy. Diabetes is usually treated with insulin or drugs, diet, and exercise.

Carbohydrates are broken down into sugar during digestion. For the person with diabetes, the amount of carbohydrates is controlled. Only the amount of carbohydrates needed is ingested. The doctor determines the amount of carbohydrate a person should have. The dietician develops a *consistent-carbohydrate diabetes meal plan* for the person. The meal plan also specifies a certain amount of fat and protein to meet the person's needs. The person's age, gender, activity, and weight are considered.

The person ingests a consistent amount of carbohydrate each day. The amount is the same at each breakfast, each lunch, each dinner, and for each snack. The amount of carbohydrate at each meal is not the same, but the amount ingested each day is the same. The person must eat only what is allowed and all that is allowed. Otherwise the person gets too many or too few carbohydrates.

Meal and snack times also are consistent from day to day. You must serve the person's meals and snacks on time. The person must eat at regular times to maintain a certain blood sugar level. Always check the tray to see what the person ate. Report to the nurse what the person did and did not eat. If all food was not eaten, a between-meal nourishment is needed (p. 434). The nourishment makes up for what was not eaten at the regular meal. The amount of insulin given also depends on the resident's daily food intake. You must inform the nurse of any change in a diabetic resident's eating habits.

The Dysphagia Diet

The dysphagia diet is ordered for residents who have difficulty swallowing (Table 18-4). Food thickness is changed to meet the resident's needs. The doctor, speech/language pathologist, occupational therapist, dietician, and nurse work together to choose the right food thickness.

Some residents are aware of their swallowing problem and can describe it. A *slow swallow* means the resident has difficulty getting enough food and fluids for good nutrition and hydration. An *unsafe swallow* also is common. This means that food enters the airway (aspiration). **Aspiration** is the breathing of fluid or an object into the lungs (p. 436).

You play an important role in meeting the nutritional needs of the resident with dysphagia. Some need assistance with eating. Often you will feed residents with dysphagia. You must know the signs and symptoms of swallowing problems to ensure the resident's safety (Box 18-5). The position of the resident's head and neck while eating also is important. A swallow guide is used under the direction of a speech language/pathologist and is part of the resident's care plan (Fig. 18-9, p. 424). The swallow guide gives specific directions on how to feed the resident.

Aspiration precautions also are followed when feeding these residents (Box 18-6, p. 425). The speech/language pathologist will teach you aspiration precautions. Report to the nurse any changes in how the resident eats. You must report if the resident chokes, coughs, or has difficulty breathing during or after meals.

FLUID BALANCE

After oxygen, water is the most important physical need for survival. Death can result from inadequate water intake or from excessive fluid loss. Water enters the body through fluids and foods. Water is lost through urine and feces. It also is lost through the skin (perspiration) and through the lungs (expiration). Fluid balance is important for health. There must be a balance between the amount of fluid taken in and the amount lost.

The amount of fluid taken in and the amount lost must be equal. If fluid intake exceeds fluid output (the amount lost), body tissues swell with water. This is called **edema**. Edema is common in persons with heart and kidney diseases. **Dehydration** is a decrease in the amount of water in body tissues. It results when fluid output exceeds intake. Inadequate fluid intake, vomiting, diarrhea, bleeding, excessive sweating, and increased urine production are common causes of dehydration.

Table 18-4 Dysphagia Diet

Consistency Type	Description
Puree	No lumps; mounds when placed on a plate. May be as thick as mashed potatoes.
Thickened liquid	No lumps; puree with diluted milk, gravy, or broth to the consistency of baby food peaches. In some foods, this consistency is formed when the food is pureed and thickener is added to make the correct consistency (e.g., many fruits). Does not mound significantly when placed on a plate. May also be called *creamy* or *sauce*. May need to stir before serving if the food settles. This consistency is still spoonable (baby food consistency)—not drinkable from a glass. Served in a bowl.
Medium thick	Consistency of nectar or V-8 juice (does not hold its shape in container). Stir right before serving. (Some beverages of this thickness do not look very thick!)
Extra thick	Consistency of honey. Mounds a bit on the spoon but drinkable from a cup. May need to stir before serving.
Yogurt-like consistency (spoonable)	Consistency of yogurt; definitely holds its shape and must be spooned.

Box 18-5 Signs and Symptoms of a Swallowing Problem (Dysphagia)

- The resident avoids foods that need chewing.
- Food spills out of the resident's mouth while eating.
- Food gets "pocketed" or "squirreled" in the resident's cheeks.
- The resident eats slowly, especially solid foods.
- The resident complains that food will not go down or that food is stuck.
- The resident frequently coughs or chokes before, during, or after swallowing.
- Regurgitation of food occurs after meals (p. 438).
- The resident spits out food suddenly and almost violently.
- Food comes up through the resident's nose.
- The resident has vocal hoarseness—especially after eating.
- After swallowing, the resident sounds like he or she is gargling while talking or breathing.
- The resident excessively drools saliva.
- The resident complaints of frequent heartburn.
- The resident's appetite is decreased.
- The resident has unexplained weight loss.
- The resident has recurrent pneumonia.

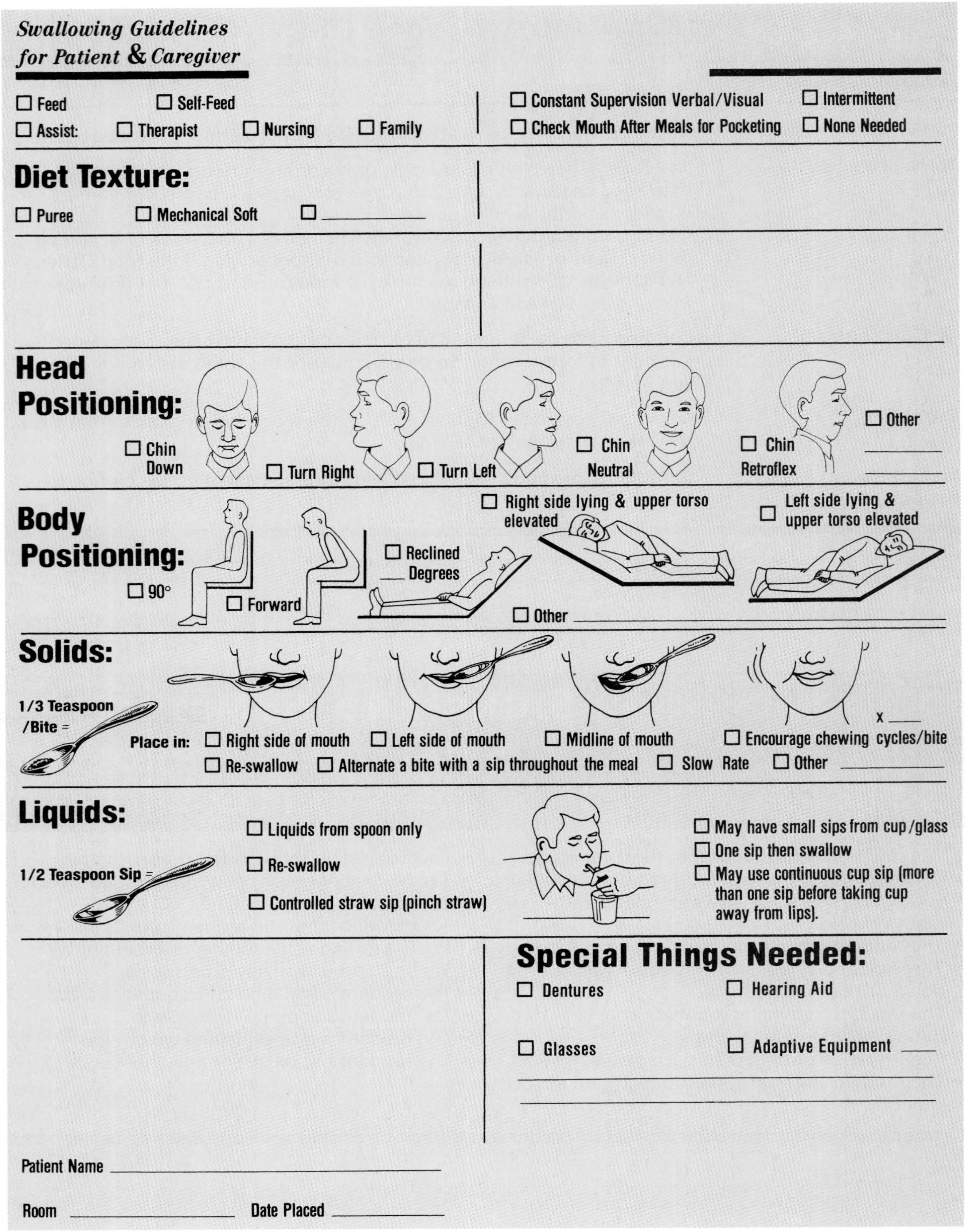

Swallowing Guidelines for Patient & Caregiver

☐ Feed ☐ Self-Feed
☐ Assist: ☐ Therapist ☐ Nursing ☐ Family

☐ Constant Supervision Verbal/Visual ☐ Intermittent
☐ Check Mouth After Meals for Pocketing ☐ None Needed

Diet Texture:

☐ Puree ☐ Mechanical Soft ☐ ________

Head Positioning:

☐ Chin Down ☐ Turn Right ☐ Turn Left ☐ Chin Neutral ☐ Chin Retroflex ☐ Other ________

Body Positioning:

☐ 90° ☐ Forward ☐ Reclined ___ Degrees ☐ Right side lying & upper torso elevated ☐ Left side lying & upper torso elevated ☐ Other ________

Solids:

1/3 Teaspoon /Bite =

Place in: ☐ Right side of mouth ☐ Left side of mouth ☐ Midline of mouth ☐ Encourage chewing cycles/bite x ____

☐ Re-swallow ☐ Alternate a bite with a sip throughout the meal ☐ Slow Rate ☐ Other ________

Liquids:

1/2 Teaspoon Sip =

☐ Liquids from spoon only
☐ Re-swallow
☐ Controlled straw sip (pinch straw)

☐ May have small sips from cup/glass
☐ One sip then swallow
☐ May use continuous cup sip (more than one sip before taking cup away from lips).

Special Things Needed:

☐ Dentures ☐ Hearing Aid
☐ Glasses ☐ Adaptive Equipment ____

Patient Name ________

Room ________ Date Placed ________

Fig. 18-9 Sections of a swallowing guidelines form. *(Excerpted from "Swallow-guide." Courtesy Interactive Therapeutics, Inc., Stow, Ohio. For more information regarding the complete form call 800-253-5111.)*

Box 18-6 Aspiration Precautions

- Check the care plan for special instructions before helping residents with meals or snacks.
- Raise the head of the bed or have the resident sit in a chair at 90 degrees when eating meals and snacks. Support the upper back, shoulders, and neck with a pillow as recommended by the speech/language pathologist or occupational therapist.
- Watch the resident closely for an active swallow or signs of aspiration during meals and snacks.
- Visually check the resident's mouth after each meal and snack for pocketing. Check for food in the cheeks, under the tongue, or on the roof of the mouth. Remove any food present. Report your observations to the nurse.
- Allow residents to remain in a seated position for at least 30 minutes after each meal and snack. For residents eating in bed, lower the head of the bed between 45 degrees and 60 degrees. The resident maintains this position for at least 30 minutes after eating.
- Provide mouth care after each meal and snack.

Normal Requirements

An adult needs 1500 ml of water daily to survive. About 2000 to 2500 ml of fluid per day is required to maintain normal fluid balance. The water requirement increases with hot weather temperatures, exercise, fever, and illness. Excessive fluid loss also increases the water requirement. Older persons may have a decreased sense of thirst. Their body needs water, but they may not feel thirsty. You need to offer water often. Some residents have special fluid orders. The nurse gives you needed information.

Special Orders

The doctor may order the amount of fluid that a resident can have during a 24-hour period. This is done to maintain fluid balance. Special orders for a resident are noted in the care plan. The information also is shared during the end-of-shift report. Common orders are:

- *Encourage fluids*—the person needs to drink an increased amount of fluid. The *encourage fluids* order includes the specific amount of fluid to be ingested. Records are kept of the amount taken in. The resident is given a variety of fluids allowed on the diet. Fluids are kept within the person's reach and served at the correct temperature. Fluids are offered regularly to residents who cannot feed themselves.
- *Restrict fluids*—fluids are restricted to a specific amount. Water is offered in small amounts and in small containers. The water pitcher is removed from the room or kept out of sight. Accurate intake records are kept. You must give the resident frequent oral hygiene to help keep mucous membranes of the mouth moist.
- *Nothing by mouth*—the resident cannot eat or drink anything. NPO is the abbreviation for the Latin term *nil per os,* which means nothing by mouth. NPO often is ordered before residents are to have some laboratory tests or x-ray procedures, as well as in the treatment of certain illnesses. Residents who are tube fed may be NPO. An NPO sign is posted above the bed. The water pitcher and glass are removed. Frequent oral hygiene is important, but the resident must not swallow any fluid. The NPO status begins at midnight before scheduled laboratory tests or x-ray examinations.

Intake and Output Records

The doctor or nurse may order fluid intake and output (I&O) measurements. This order involves keeping records. I&O records are used to evaluate fluid balance and kidney function. They help in evaluating and planning medical treatment. They also are necessary when fluid intake is encouraged or restricted.

All fluids taken by mouth are measured, and the amount is recorded. IV fluids and tube feedings also are measured. The obvious fluids are measured: water, milk, coffee, tea, juices, soups, and soft drinks. Soft and semisolid foods such as ice cream, sherbet, custard, pudding, creamed cereals, gelatin, and Popsicles also are measured. Output includes urinary output, vomitus, diarrhea, and wound drainage.

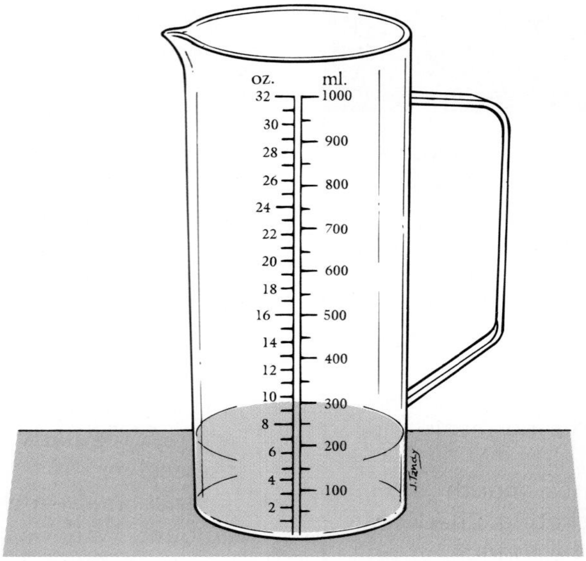

Fig. 18-10 A graduate calibrated in milliliters.

Measuring intake and output.

Intake and output are measured in milliliters (ml) or in cubic centimeters (cc). These metric system measurements are equal in amount. One ounce equals 30 ml. A pint is about 500 ml. A quart is about 1000 ml. You need to know the size of the bowls, dishes, cups, pitchers, glasses, and other containers used to serve fluids. Most I&O records have tables for use in measuring intake.

A container called a **graduate** is used to measure fluids. You will use it to measure leftover fluids, urine, vomitus, and drainage from suction (see Chapter 14). The graduate is like a measuring cup (it shows calibrations for amounts). Some graduates are marked in ounces and in milliliters or cubic centimeters (Fig. 18-10). Plastic urinals and emesis basins often are calibrated.

An I&O record is kept at the bedside. Whenever fluid is ingested or output measured, the amount is recorded in the correct column (Fig. 18-11). The amounts are totaled at the end of the shift. The nurse records the amount in the resident's record. The resident's I&O also is communicated to the oncoming shift during the end-of-shift report. The nurse is responsible for recording any intake through IV therapy or enteral feedings (p. 434).

The purpose of measuring intake and output and how to help in the process are explained to the resident. Some residents measure and record their intake. The urinal, commode, bedpan, or specimen pan is used for urination. Remind the resident not to put toilet tissue into the container. Also remind the resident not to urinate in the toilet.

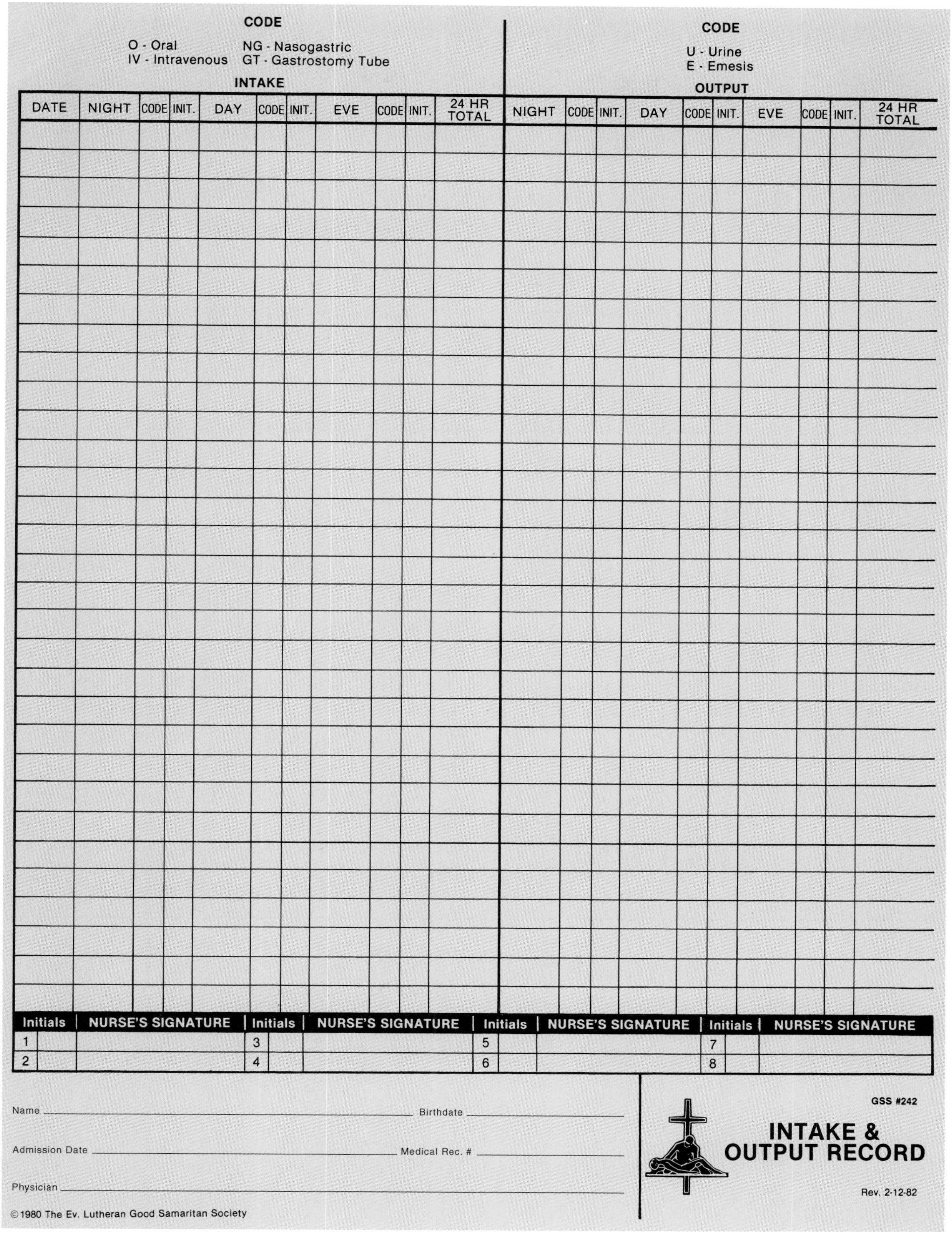

CODE

O - Oral NG - Nasogastric
IV - Intravenous GT - Gastrostomy Tube

INTAKE

CODE

U - Urine
E - Emesis

OUTPUT

DATE	NIGHT	CODE	INIT.	DAY	CODE	INIT.	EVE	CODE	INIT.	24 HR TOTAL	NIGHT	CODE	INIT.	DAY	CODE	INIT.	EVE	CODE	INIT.	24 HR TOTAL

Initials	NURSE'S SIGNATURE	Initials	NURSE'S SIGNATURE	Initials	NURSE'S SIGNATURE	Initials	NURSE'S SIGNATURE
1		3		5		7	
2		4		6		8	

Name ______ Birthdate ______

Admission Date ______ Medical Rec. # ______

Physician ______

©1980 The Ev. Lutheran Good Samaritan Society

GSS #242

INTAKE & OUTPUT RECORD

Rev. 2-12-82

Fig. 18-11 An intake and output record. *(Courtesy Evangelical Lutheran Good Samaritan Society, Sioux Falls, SD)*

Measuring Intake and Output

NNAAP™ SKILL

Quality of Life

Remember to:
- *Knock before entering the resident's room*
- *Address the resident by name*
- *Introduce yourself by name and title*

Pre-Procedure

1 Explain the procedure to the resident.
2 Wash your hands.
3 Collect the following:
   - Intake and output (I&O) record
   - Two I&O labels
   - Graduate
   - Gloves

Procedure

4 Place the I&O record at the bedside or on the room door (follow center policy).
5 Place one label in the bathroom. Place the other in the appropriate place near the bed
6 Measure intake as follows:
   a Wash your hands.
   b Put on gloves.
   c Pour liquid remaining in a container into the graduate.
   d Measure the amount at eye level.
   e Check the amount of the serving on the I&O record.
   f Subtract the remaining amount from the full serving amount. Record the amount.
   g Repeat steps 6c through 6f for each liquid. Total the amounts from each liquid. Record the total amount and time on the I&O record.
7 Measure output as follows:
   a Wash your hands.
   b Put on gloves.
   c Pour fluid into the graduate.
   d Measure the amount at eye level.
   e Record the amount on the I&O record.
   f Dispose of fluid in the toilet.
   g Rinse and return the graduate to its proper place.
   h Clean and rinse the bedpan, urinal, emesis basin, or other drainage container. Return it to its proper place.

Post-Procedure

8 Remove the gloves.
9 Wash your hands.
10 Report your observations to the nurse.

◈ ASSISTING THE RESIDENT WITH FOOD AND FLUIDS

Weakness, illness, and confusion can affect a resident's appetite and ability to eat. So can unpleasant odors, sights, and sounds. An uncomfortable position, the need for oral hygiene, or the need to use the bathroom also affects appetite. Residents vary in mental and physical abilities. Some are alert and oriented and enjoy being together for meals. Others like to eat in their room. Others are confused and noisy at mealtime. Some residents are incontinent or have other odor problems. Some are too weak or ill to be out of their rooms for meals. Because of these different situations, centers have special dining programs.

In a *social dining program*, residents eat in a dining room. There are 4 to 6 persons at a table (Fig. 18-12). Tables have a tablecloth or placemats. Food is served as in a restaurant. This program is for residents who are oriented and can feed themselves. Sometimes quietly confused residents are included if they can feed themselves and do not disrupt other residents.

Family dining is like social dining except that food is served differently. Food is placed in bowls and on platters. Residents serve themselves from these dishes as they would at home.

Assistive dining programs are common. The dining room has circular or horseshoe-shaped dining tables. Residents who need to be fed are seated around these tables. Nursing assistants sit at the center of the table and feed as many as 4 residents (Fig. 18-13). The program has two advantages. Very confused residents are with others at mealtime. Each nursing assistant can feed several residents at one time. This allows prompt feeding of residents with food at the correct temperature.

Some centers have dining areas where residents can dine with guests. The resident can have a family meal with a spouse, children, grandchildren, relatives, or friends. The dietary department provides the meal or it is brought by the guests. Holidays, birthdays, anniversaries, and other special events are celebrated.

Comfort is important during meals. The setting must be free of unpleasant sights, sounds, and odors. Some centers have *low stimulation dining programs*. These programs are designed to prevent unnecessary distractions during meals. Together the nurse, speech/language pathologist, occupational therapist, and nursing assistant decide on the best seating arrangement for each resident. Sometimes a one-to-one dining assistance program is needed.

Meals are more pleasant if residents are properly prepared. Residents should have oral care and use the bathroom before going to the dining area. Make sure incontinent residents are clean and dry. Also make sure that dentures, eyeglasses, and hearing aids are in place. To increase mealtime enjoyment and comfort, remove unpleasant equipment from the room. Helping residents assume a comfortable eating position also is important.

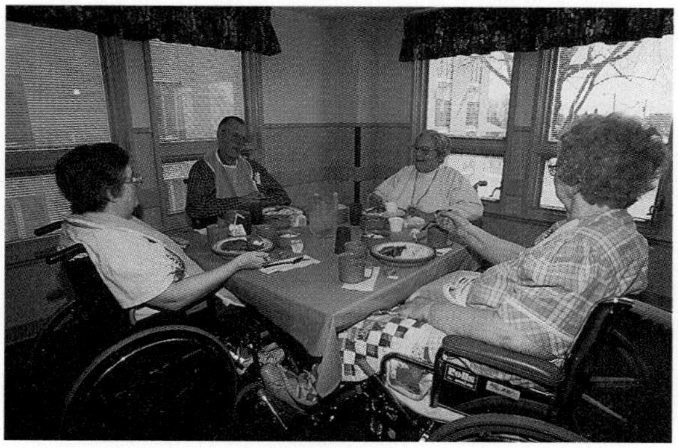

Fig. 18-12 Residents enjoy a pleasant meal in the dining room.

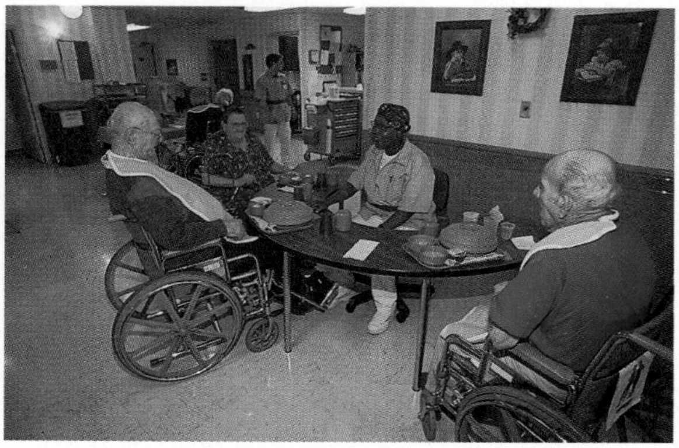

Fig. 18-13 Special dining tables are used for assistive dining programs. The nursing assistant feeds 3 residents at one time. Residents are in the company of others.

Getting the Resident Ready for Meals

Quality of Life

Remember to:
- *Knock before entering the resident's room*
- *Address the resident by name*
- *Introduce yourself by name and title*

Pre-Procedure

1 Explain to the resident that it is mealtime.
2 Wash your hands.
3 Collect the following:
   a Equipment for oral hygiene
   b Bedpan or urinal and toilet tissue
   c Wash basin
   d Soap
   e Washcloth
   f Towel
   g Gloves
4 Provide for privacy.

Procedure

5 Make sure the resident's eyeglasses and hearing aid are in place.
6 Assist with oral hygiene (follow Standard Precautions). Make sure dentures are in place.
7 Offer the bedpan or urinal, or assist the resident to the bathroom. Make sure the incontinent resident is clean and dry. Follow Standard Precautions for this step.
8 Help the resident with handwashing.
9 Do the following for residents who will eat in bed:
   a Raise the head of the bed to a comfortable sitting position.
   b Position the overbed table in front of the resident. Make sure it is clean.
   c Place the signal light within reach.
   d Unscreen the resident.
10 Do the following for residents who can sit in a chair:
   a Make sure the resident is comfortable in a chair or wheelchair.
   b Remove items from the overbed table. Make sure it is clean.
   c Position the overbed table in front of the resident. Adjust the height as needed.
   d Place the signal light within reach.
   e Unscreen the resident.
11 Assist residents in special dining programs to the correct dining area. Follow center procedure for the dining programs.

Post-Procedure

12 Return to the room.
13 Clean and return equipment to its proper place. Use Standard Precautions.
14 Straighten the room. Eliminate unpleasant noise, odors, or equipment.
15 Wash your hands.

◈ Serving Meal Trays

Meals are served in containers that keep foods hot or cold as appropriate. You serve meal trays after preparing residents for the meal and assisting them to the dining area. Trays are served promptly. OBRA requires that food be at the desired temperature when the resident receives it.

OBRA

Trays are served in the order assigned by the health care team. All residents seated at the same table are served at the same time. If a tray is not served within 15 minutes, food temperature is rechecked. If food is not at the right temperature, you must get another tray. Temperature guides and food thermometers are available in resident dining rooms. Some centers let you reheat hot foods in a microwave oven. Always check the food temperature after reheating. Food that is too hot can burn the resident.

Serving Meal Trays

Quality of Life

Remember to:

- ◆ *Knock before entering the resident's room*
- ◆ *Address the resident by name*
- ◆ *Introduce yourself by name and title*

Pre-Procedure

1 Wash your hands.

Procedure

2 Make sure the tray is complete and accurate. Check items on the tray with the dietary card.

3 Identify the resident. Check the ID bracelet against the dietary card.

4 Have the resident in a sitting position if possible.

5 Place the tray within the resident's reach. If the overbed table is used, position it and adjust the height as necessary.

6 Remove food covers. Open milk cartons and cereal boxes, cut meat, and butter bread as needed (Fig. 18-14, p. 432).

7 Place the napkin, clothes protector, and silverware within reach.

8 Measure and record intake if ordered (p. 428). Note the amount and type of foods eaten (p. 434).

9 Remove the tray.

10 Assist the resident with oral hygiene. (Wear gloves for this step.)

11 Check for and remove any food left in the mouth (pocketing).

12 Clean any spills, and change soiled linen.

13 Help the person return to bed if indicated.

Post-Procedure

14 Assist the resident with handwashing.

15 Provide for comfort.

16 Place the signal light within reach.

17 Raise or lower bed rails. Follow the care plan.

18 Follow center policy for soiled linen.

19 Wash your hands.

20 Report your observations to the nurse.

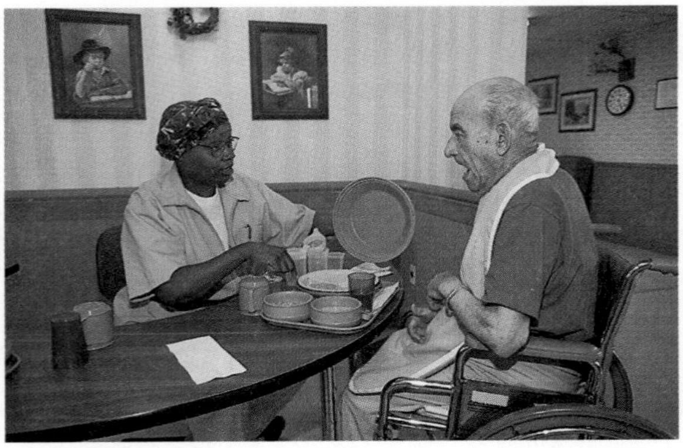

Fig. 18-14 Open cartons and other containers for the resident.

Residents With Dementia

Residents with dementia may become easily distracted during meals. It is difficult for some residents to sit long enough to finish a meal. Others forget how to use eating utensils. Some residents resist your efforts to assist them with eating. A confused resident may throw or spit food at the caregiver. You must be patient. A quiet and calm dining area often is helpful. Special schedules are helpful for some residents. They eat small amounts more often than 3 times a day. Individual approaches are found in the resident's care plan. Ask the nurse for help if you feel upset or impatient. Remember, all residents have the right to be treated with dignity and respect.

Feeding the Resident

Some residents cannot feed themselves. (*See Residents With Dementia.*) Weakness, paralysis, casts, confusion, and other limitations can make self-feeding impossible. These residents are fed. When feeding a resident, assume a comfortable position. Relax so the resident does not feel rushed. Many people pray before eating. Allow time and privacy for prayer. This shows respect and care for the resident.

Ask the resident about the order in which to offer foods and fluids. Spoons are used to feed residents. They are less likely to cause injury. The spoon should be only one-third full. The portion is chewed and swallowed easily. Some residents need even smaller portions. Special instructions are in the resident's care plan.

Also remember to offer the resident fluids during the meal. Fluids help the person chew and swallow.

Residents who cannot feed themselves often are angry, humiliated, and embarrassed at their dependence on others. Some are depressed or resentful or may refuse to eat. Let these residents feed themselves as much as possible. Give them "finger foods" (bread, cookies, crackers) if they can manage them. If they are strong enough, let them hold their milk or juice glasses (never hot drinks). Assist them to drink if necessary. Never exceed the limits ordered by the doctor. Be supportive. Encourage them to keep trying even if food is spilled.

Visually impaired persons are often keenly aware of food aromas. Often they can identify some foods served. Always tell the resident what foods and fluids are on the tray. When feeding a visually impaired person, always describe what you are offering. For residents who feed themselves, describe foods and fluids and their place on the tray. Use the numbers on a clock to identify the location of foods (Fig. 18-15).

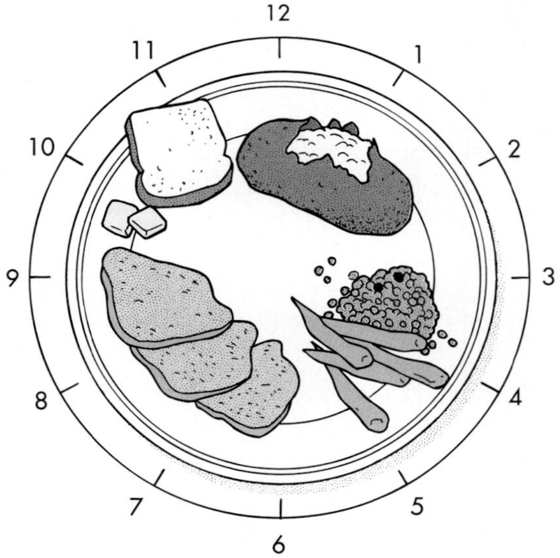

Fig. 18-15 The numbers on a clock are used to help a visually impaired person locate food on the tray.

Meals provide social contact with others. Engage the resident in pleasant conversation. However, give the resident enough time to chew and swallow food. Also, sit so that you face the resident. Sitting is more relaxing. It shows the resident that you have time to assist feeding him or her. Standing communicates nonverbally that you do not have time and that you are in a hurry. By facing the resident, you can see how well the resident is eating. You can see also if the resident has problems swallowing.

Feeding the Resident

NNAAP™ SKILL

Quality of Life

Remember to:
- ◆ *Knock before entering the resident's room*
- ◆ *Address the resident by name*
- ◆ *Introduce yourself by name and title*

Pre-Procedure

1 Explain the procedure to the resident.
2 Wash your hands.
3 Position the resident in a comfortable sitting position.
4 Bring the tray into the room or the dining room. Place it on the overbed table or dining table.

Procedure

5 Identify the resident. Check the ID bracelet against the dietary card.
6 Drape a napkin across the resident's chest and under the chin.
7 Prepare the food for eating.
8 Tell the resident what foods are on the tray.
9 Serve foods in the order the resident prefers. Alternate between solid and liquid foods. Use a spoon for safety as in Figure 18-16 on p. 434. Allow enough time for chewing. Do not rush the resident.
10 Use straws for liquids if the resident cannot drink from a glass or cup. Have one straw for each liquid. Provide a short straw for weak residents. Residents with dysphagia cannot use a straw. Give thickened liquid with a spoon.
11 Converse with the resident in a pleasant manner.
12 Encourage the resident to eat as much as possible.
13 Wipe the resident's mouth with a napkin as needed.
14 Note how much and which foods were eaten when the person is done eating (p. 434).
15 Measure and record intake if ordered.
16 Remove the tray.
17 Take the resident back to his or her room.
18 Provide oral hygiene. (Wear gloves for this step.)

Post-Procedure

19 Provide for comfort.
20 Place the signal light within reach.
21 Raise or lower bed rails if the resident is in bed. Follow the care plan.
22 Wash your hands.
23 Report your observations to the nurse
- The amount and kind of food eaten
- Complaints of nausea or dysphagia
- Signs of aspiration (see p. 438)

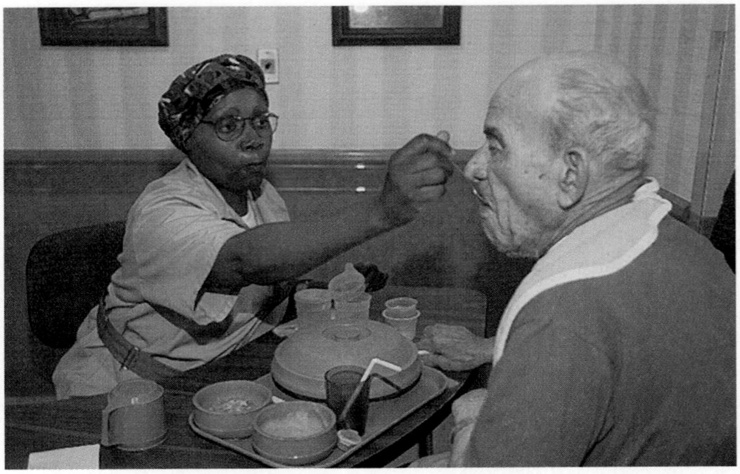

Fig. 18-16 A spoon is used to feed the person. The spoon is no more than one-third full.

Between-Meal Nourishments

Many special diets involve between-meal nourishments. Common nourishments are crackers, milk, juice, a milkshake, cake, wafers, a sandwich, gelatin, and custard. Serve nourishments as soon as they arrive on the nursing unit. Provide needed eating utensils, a straw, and a napkin. Follow the same considerations and procedures described for serving meal trays and feeding persons.

Providing Drinking Water

Residents need fresh drinking water each shift. Fresh water also is given whenever the pitcher is empty. Before providing water, ask the nurse about any special orders such as NPO or restricted fluids. Some residents are not allowed ice. Practice the rules of medical asepsis when passing drinking water. Follow center procedure for providing fresh drinking water for residents.

Calorie Counts

For some residents it is important to keep track of calorie intake. A flow sheet is used for this purpose. Your role is to note what the resident ate and how much. For example, a resident is served a chicken breast, a baked potato, beans, a roll, pudding, and two pats of butter. You note that the resident ate all the chicken, half the potato, and the roll. One pat of butter was used. The beans and pudding were not eaten. You note these on the form. A nurse or dietician then converts these portions into calories. The nurse tells you which residents require calorie counts.

OTHER METHODS OF MEETING FOOD AND FLUID NEEDS

Many residents cannot eat or drink because of illness, surgery, or injury. Other methods are used to meet their basic need for foods and fluids. The doctor orders needed methods. The nurse is responsible for carrying out the order.

Enteral Nutrition

Residents who cannot chew or swallow often require enteral nutrition. **Enteral nutrition** is giving nutrients through the gastrointestinal tract *(enteral).* Formula is given through a feeding tube inserted into the stomach or small intestine. (**Gavage** is another term for tube feeding.)

- A **nasogastric (NG) tube** is inserted through the nose *(naso)* into the stomach *(gastro)* (Fig. 18-17). A doctor or an RN performs the procedure.
- A **nasointestinal tube** is inserted through the nose into the duodenum or jejunum of the small intestine (Fig. 18-18). A doctor or a nurse performs the procedure.
- A **gastrostomy** is an opening *(stomy)* into the stomach *(gastro)* (Fig. 18-19). The opening is created surgically.
- A **jejunostomy** is an opening *(stomy)* into the middle part of the small intestine *(jejunum)* (Fig. 18-20). The opening is created surgically.

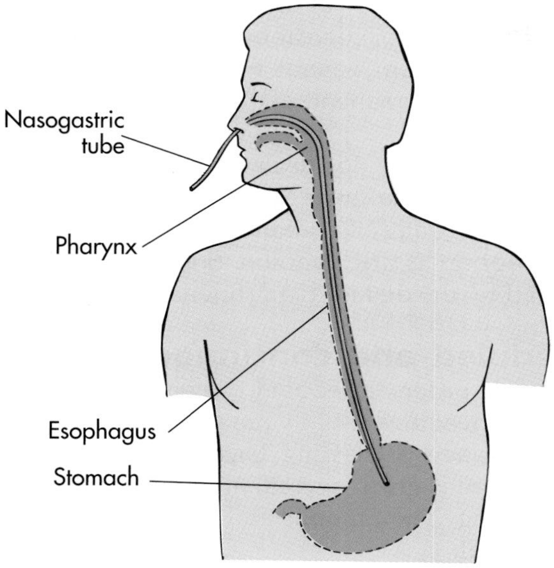

Fig. 18-17 A nasogastric tube is inserted through the nose and esophagus into the stomach.

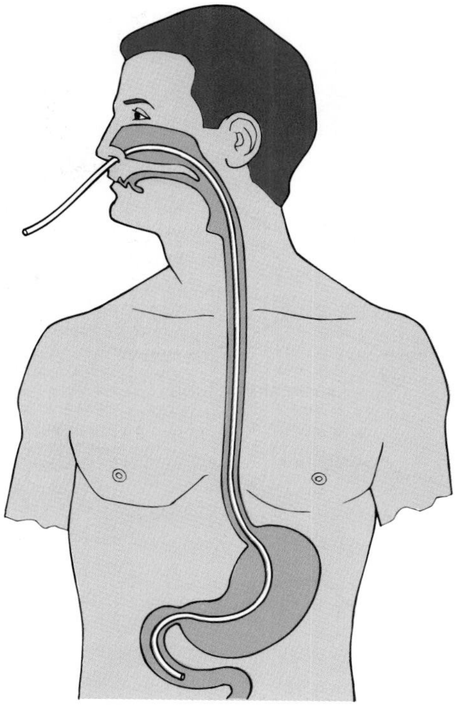

Fig. 18-18 A nasointestinal tube is inserted through the nose into the duodenum or jejunum of the small intestine.

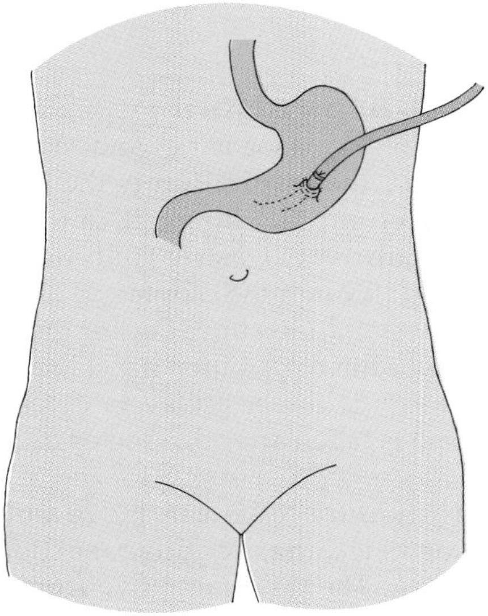

Fig. 18-19 A gastrostomy tube.

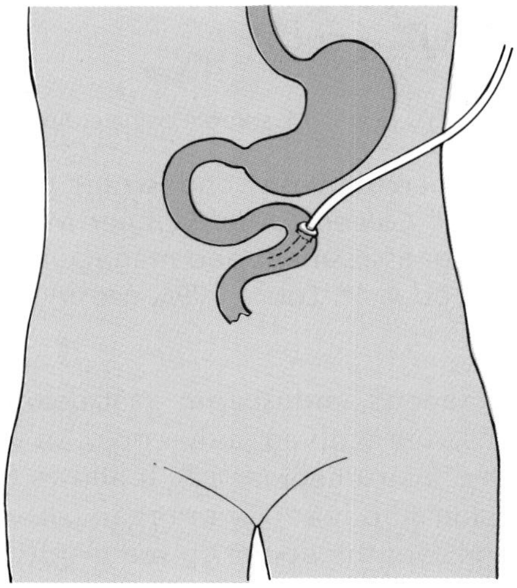

Fig. 18-20 A jejunostomy tube.

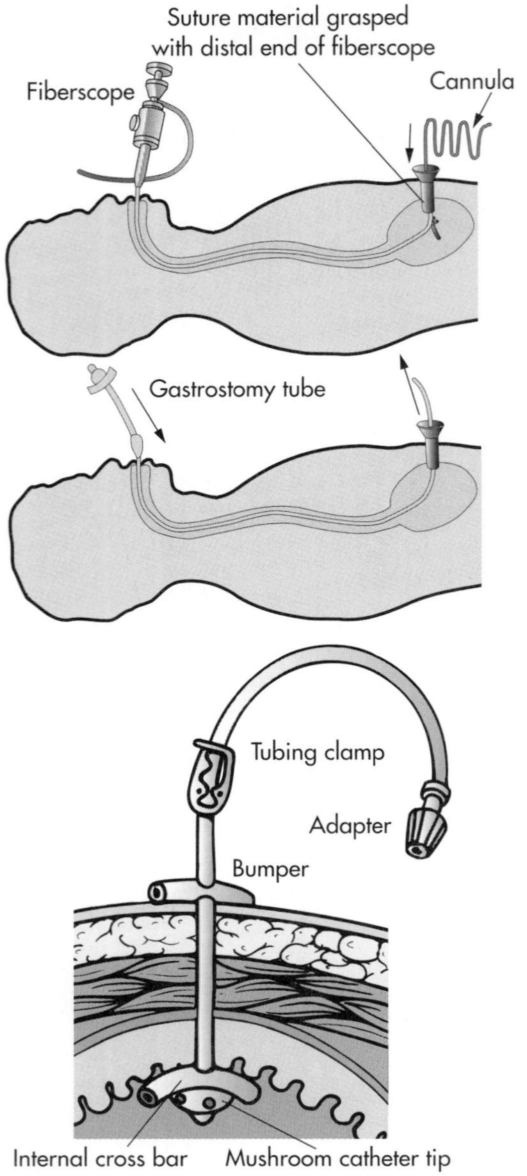

Fig. 18-21 A percutaneous endoscopic gastrostomy. *(From Lewis SH, Collier IC, Heitkemper MM:* Medical-surgical nursing: assessment and management of clinical problems, *ed 4, St. Louis, 1996, Mosby.)*

- A **percutaneous endoscopic gastrostomy (PEG) tube** is inserted with an endoscope. An endoscope is a lighted instrument *(scope)*. It allows the doctor to see inside a body cavity or organ *(endo)*. The endoscope allows the doctor to see inside the stomach. The doctor inserts the endoscope through the person's mouth and esophagus and into the stomach. A stab or puncture wound *(stomy)* is made through *(per)* the skin *(cutaneous)* and into the stomach *(gastro)*. A tube is inserted into the stomach through the stab wound (Fig. 18-21).

Feeding tubes are used when food cannot pass normally from the mouth into the esophagus and then into the stomach. Cancer of the head, neck, or esophagus is a common cause. So is trauma or surgery to the face, mouth, head, or neck. Coma is another reason for tube feedings. Some residents with dementia no longer know how to eat and may require tube feedings. Gastrostomy, jejunostomy, and PEG feedings are used for long-term enteral nutrition. The ostomy is temporary or permanent.

Formulas. The doctor orders the type of formula and the amount to give. Most formulas contain protein, carbohydrates, fat, vitamins, and minerals. Commercial formulas are common. Sometimes formula is prepared by the dietary department.

Scheduled and continuous feedings. The doctor orders scheduled or continuous feedings. Scheduled feedings usually are given four times a day with a syringe or feeding bag (Fig. 18-22). Usually about 400 ml is given over 20 minutes during a scheduled feeding. The amount and rate are like eating a regular meal.

Continuous feedings require an electronic feeding pump (Fig. 18-23). Nasointestinal and jejunostomy tube feedings are always continuous.

Formula is given at room temperature. Cold fluids can cause cramping. Sometimes continuous feedings are kept cold with ice chips around the container. Microbes grow in warm formula. The formula warms to room temperature as it drips from the bag and passes through the connecting tubing to the feeding tube. The nurse adds formula to continuous feedings every 3 to 4 hours.

Preventing aspiration. Aspiration is a major complication of nasogastric and nasointestinal tubes. Remember that **aspiration** is the breathing of fluid or an object into the lungs. It can cause pneumonia and death. Nasogastric and nasointestinal tubes are passed through the esophagus and then into the stomach or small intestine. During insertion, the tube can slip into the respiratory tract. This causes aspiration. An x-ray is the best way to determine tube placement. One is taken after the doctor or RN inserts the tube.

After insertion, the tube can move out of place from coughing, sneezing, vomiting, suctioning, and poor positioning. The tube can move from the stomach or intestines into the esophagus and then into the respiratory tract. *Therefore the RN checks tube placement before every scheduled tube feeding.* With continuous tube feedings, the RN checks tube placement every 4 to 8 hours. To assess tube placement, the RN attaches a syringe to the tube and aspirates gastrointestinal secretions. Then the RN measures the pH of the secretions.

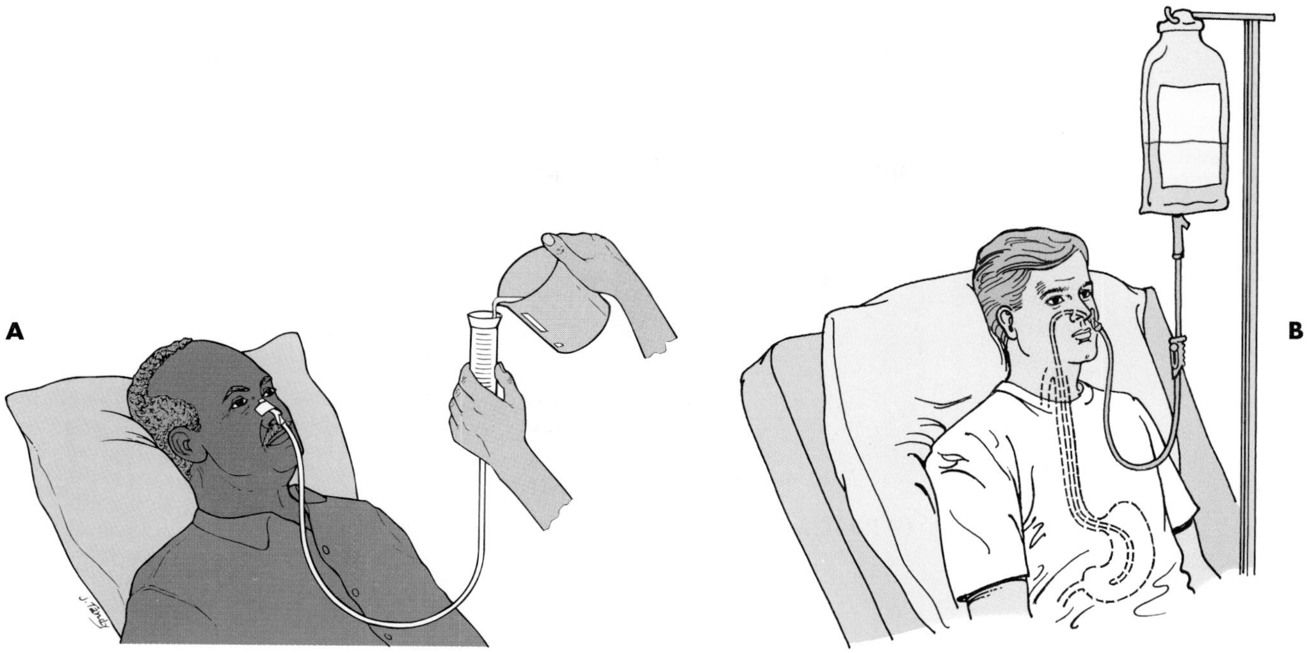

Fig. 18-22 **A,** A tube feeding is given with a syringe. **B,** Formula drips from a feeding bag into the feeding tube. *(**B** from Potter PA, Perry, AG:* Fundamentals of nursing: concepts, process, and practice, *ed 4, St Louis, 1997, Mosby.)*

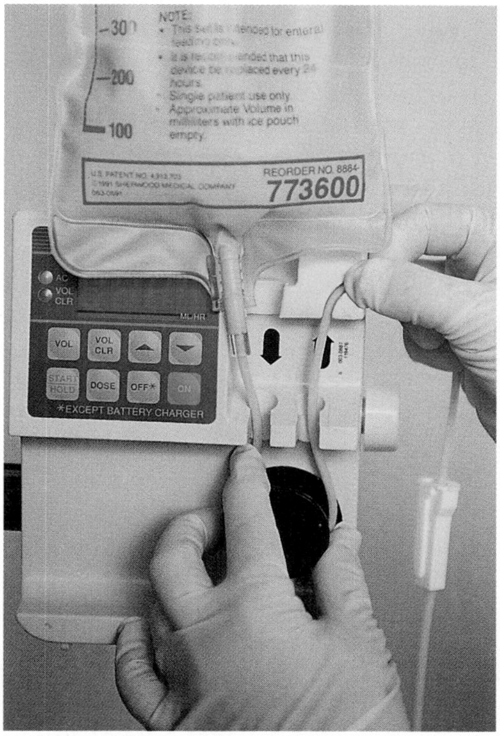

Fig. 18-23 Feeding pump. *(From Potter PA, Perry AG:* Fundamentals of nursing: concepts, process, and practice, *ed 4, St Louis, 1997, Mosby.)*

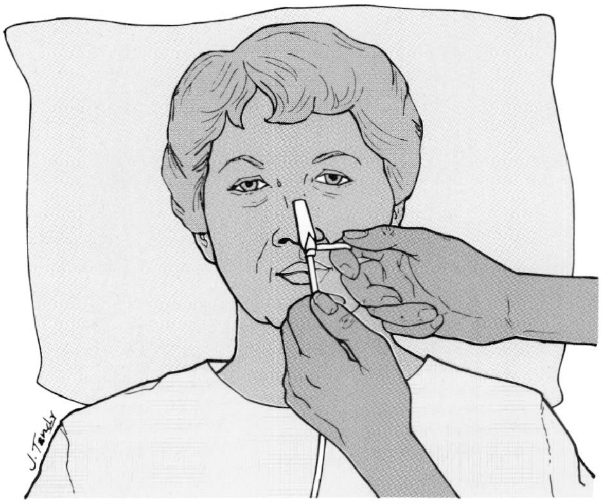

Fig. 18-24 The feeding tube is taped to the nose.

Aspiration also occurs from regurgitation. **Regurgitation** is the backward flow of food from the stomach into the mouth. This can occur with nasogastric, gastrostomy, and PEG tubes. Delayed stomach emptying and overfeeding are common causes of regurgitation. To prevent regurgitation, the resident sits or is in semi-Fowler's position for the feeding. The resident remains in this position for at least 1 hour after the feeding. This promotes movement of the formula through the gastrointestinal system and prevents aspiration. The left side-lying position is avoided. This position prevents the stomach from emptying.

The risk of regurgitation is less with nasointestinal and jejunostomy tubes. Formula passes directly into the small intestine. Also, formula is given at a slow rate. Remember that during digestion, food slowly passes from the stomach to the small intestine. The stomach handles larger amounts of food at one time than does the small intestine.

Observations. The nurse must be alert to signs and symptoms of aspiration. Other complications include diarrhea, constipation, and delayed stomach emptying. When a resident is receiving a tube feeding, you must report the following to the nurse immediately:

- Nausea
- Discomfort during the tube feeding
- Vomiting
- Diarrhea
- Distended (enlarged and swollen) abdomen
- Coughing
- Complaints of indigestion or heart burn
- Redness, swelling, drainage, odor, or pain at the ostomy site
- Elevated temperature
- Signs and symptoms of respiratory distress (see Chapter 25)
- Increased pulse rate
- Complaints of flatulence (see Chapter 17)

Comfort measures. The resident with a feeding tube is usually NPO. Dry mouth, dry lips, and sore throat are sources of discomfort. Some residents are allowed hard candy or gum. The resident's care plan will include frequent oral hygiene, lubricant for the lips, and mouth rinses. The nose and nostrils also are cleaned every 4 to 8 hours as directed by the nurse and the care plan.

Nasogastric and nasointestinal tubes can irritate and cause pressure on the nose. Sometimes they alter the shape of the nostrils. Securing the tube helps prevent these problems. Tape or a tube holder is used to secure the tube to the nose (Fig. 18-24). Tube holders have foam cushions that prevent pressure on the nose. They also eliminate the need for retaping, which irritates the nose. The tube also is secured to the person's gown. Loop a rubber band around the tube. Then pin the rubber band to the gown with a safety pin. Or tape the tube to the gown. Follow center policy for securing the tube to the gown.

Intravenous Therapy

Many residents receive fluid through a needle inserted into a vein (**intravenous therapy**). Minerals and vitamins often are given in the same manner. The terms IV and IV infusion often are used in referring to intravenous therapy. Fluid is in a plastic bag. Clear IV tubing connects the container to the needle in a vein (Fig. 18-25). The doctor orders the amount of fluid to give

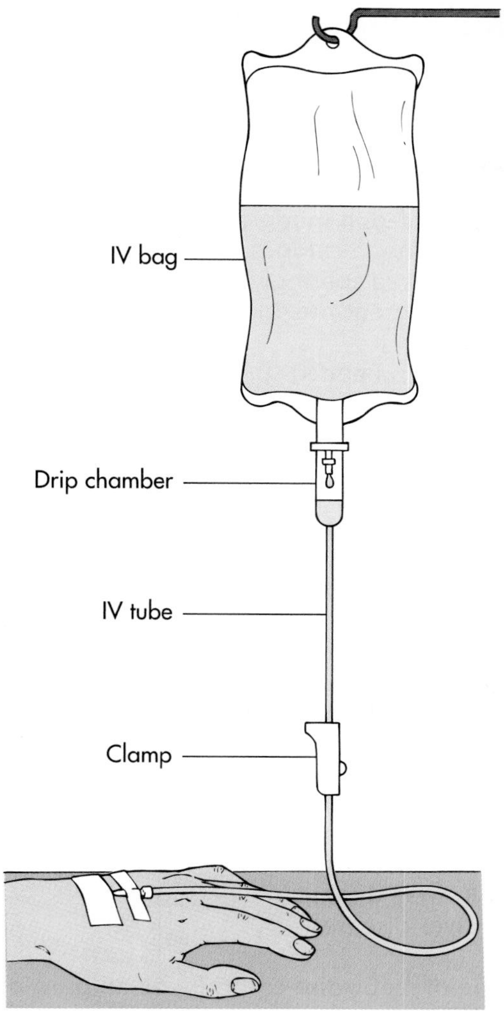

Fig. 18-25 Intravenous therapy. The needle is inserted into a vein in the arm or hand. The needle is attached to the bottle by the tubing.

(infuse) per hour. The nurse is responsible for making sure this amount is given. Special pumps control IV flow rates. These pumps have an alarm if something is wrong. Tell the nurse immediately if you hear an IV pump alarm. *You are never responsible for IV therapy or for regulating the flow rate.*

Hyperalimentation. Hyperalimentation is the intravenous administration of a highly concentrated solution of proteins, carbohydrates, vitamins, and minerals. The solution is far more nutritious than a regular IV solution. Hyperalimentation is used for seriously ill and injured residents. These residents are usually in long-term care subacute units or in hospital-based subacute care units. *You are never responsible for administering or regulating hyperalimentation solutions.*

Quality of Life

As explained in previous chapters, OBRA serves to promote the resident's quality of life. This includes the resident's health and safety. Nutrition and fluid balance are important for quality of life.

The resident's right to personal choice is important in meeting food and fluid needs. Everyone has a lifetime of food likes and dislikes. These do not change when a person enters a nursing center. Food preferences may be based on religious practices or cultural background. The dietitian works with the resident to plan healthy meals that include personal choices. Residents may tell you that they like or want certain foods. You must share this information with the nurse.

Residents with dementia may require special approaches to meet their nutritional needs. You must be patient and help to provide a quiet and calm dining experience. Remember that all residents have the right to be treated with dignity and respect.

Sometimes family and friends bring the resident food from home. This can help the resident's need for love and belonging. Sometimes it is very hard for the dietary department to provide all of the resident's food preferences. Residents usually are very pleased when family and friends bring favorite foods. Certain foods and food traditions are part of holidays. Holidays are more meaningful to residents when they can share in lifelong family traditions. Many families and friends bring residents food as holiday gifts. The nurse needs to know when food is brought to the resident. The food must not interfere with a special diet.

OBRA requires that the resident's food be served correctly. Hot food must be hot; cold food must be cold. Mashed potatoes are not very appetizing if cold. You would not eat them, and the resident should not have to. Make sure meals are served promptly. If there is an unavoidable delay in serving a tray, get a new tray of food from the dietary department. Tell the resident why the meal was delayed. Make sure the resident is given any necessary assistance in eating. This includes providing any special equipment or eating utensils.

Review Questions

Circle T if the statement is true and F if the statement is false.

1 T F Mr. Bonner is on a sodium-restricted diet. He asks for some salt for his chicken. You should bring him the salt.

2 T F Nasointestinal tube feedings are continuous.

3 T F Jejunostomy tube feedings are scheduled.

4 T F Jejunostomy tube feedings are given with a syringe.

Circle the BEST answer.

5 Nutrition is
- A Fats, proteins, carbohydrates, vitamins, and minerals
- B The many processes involved in the ingestion, digestion, absorption, and use of food and fluids by the body
- C The Food Guide Pyramid
- D The balance between calories taken in and calories used by the body

6 The Food Guide Pyramid encourages
- A A low-fat diet
- B A high-fat diet
- C A low-fiber diet
- D A low-salt diet

7 How many daily servings of breads, cereals, rice, and pasta are recommended?
- A 6 to 11
- B 3 to 5
- C 2 to 4
- D 2 to 3

8 How many daily servings of the meat group are recommended?
- A 6 to 11
- B 3 to 5
- C 2 to 4
- D 2 to 3

9 Which food groups contain the most fat?
- A Breads, cereal, rice, and pasta
- B Fruits
- C Milk, yogurt, and cheese
- D Meat, poultry, fish, dry beans, eggs, and nuts

10 Fats, oils, and sweets
- A Are used in moderate amounts
- B Are low in calories
- C Are used sparingly
- D Have great nutritional value

11 Protein is needed for
- A Tissue growth and repair
- B Energy and the fiber for bowel elimination
- C Body heat and the protection of organs from injury
- D Improving the taste of food

12 Which foods provide the *most* protein?
- A Butter and cream
- B Tomatoes and potatoes
- C Meats and fish
- D Corn and lettuce

13 Sodium-restricted diets are usually ordered for the following persons *except* those with
- A Diabetes mellitus
- B Heart disease
- C Kidney disease
- D Liver disease

14 The diabetic diet controls the amount of
- A Water
- B Sodium
- C Carbohydrates
- D Nutrients

15 Diet planning for the diabetic diet involves
- A Calculating the amount of sodium
- B A consistent amount of carbohydrate daily
- C Measuring fluid intake
- D Giving insulin with meals

16 OBRA requires that
- A Hot foods be served hot; cold foods be served cold
- B Foods smell good
- C Foods taste good
- D All of the above

17 OBRA requires
- A Two regular meals
- B Three regular meals
- C Three regular meals and a bedtime snack
- D Four regular meals

18 Adult fluid requirements for normal fluid balance are about
A 1000 to 1500 ml daily
B 1500 to 2000 ml daily
C 2000 to 2500 ml daily
D 2500 to 3000 ml daily

19 A resident is NPO. You should
A Provide a variety of fluids
B Offer fluids in small amounts and small containers
C Remove the water pitcher and glass
D Prevent the resident from having oral hygiene

20 Which are not counted as liquid foods?
A Coffee, tea, juices, and soft drinks
B Butter, sauces, and melted cheese
C Ice cream, sherbet, custard, and pudding
D Jell-O, Popsicles, and creamed cereals

21 Residents eating in a dining room serve themselves from bowls and platters on their table. This is a
A Social dining program
B Family dining program
C Low stimulation feeding program
D Serve-yourself dining program

22 You get information about a resident's diet from
A The care plan
B The diet card
C End-of-shift report
D Resident care conference

23 Residents with dysphagia should
A Use a straw for all liquids
B Get a regular diet
C Be fed using a swallow guide
D Eat alone in their room

24 Which is not a sign of a swallowing problem?
A Drooling
B Coughing while eating
C Pocketing
D Dysphagia

25 Which is *false?*
A Between-meal nourishments are served promptly.
B You are never responsible for IV therapy.
C You are never responsible for hyperalimentation.
D You can insert an NG tube and give a tube feeding.

26 Which statement about feeding a resident is *false?*
A Ask if he or she wants to pray before eating.
B A fork is used to feed the resident.
C The resident is asked the order in which to serve foods.
D Engage the resident in a pleasant conversation.

27 A resident with a feeding tube is usually
A Allowed a regular diet
B On bedrest
C NPO
D In a coma

28 To prevent regurgitation after a tube feeding, the resident is positioned
A In semi-Fowler's position for 30 minutes after the feeding
B In semi-Fowler's position for 1 hour after the feeding
C In the left side-lying position for 30 minutes after the feeding
D In the left side-lying position for 1 hour after the feeding

Answers to these questions are on p. 698.

19 Exercise and Activity

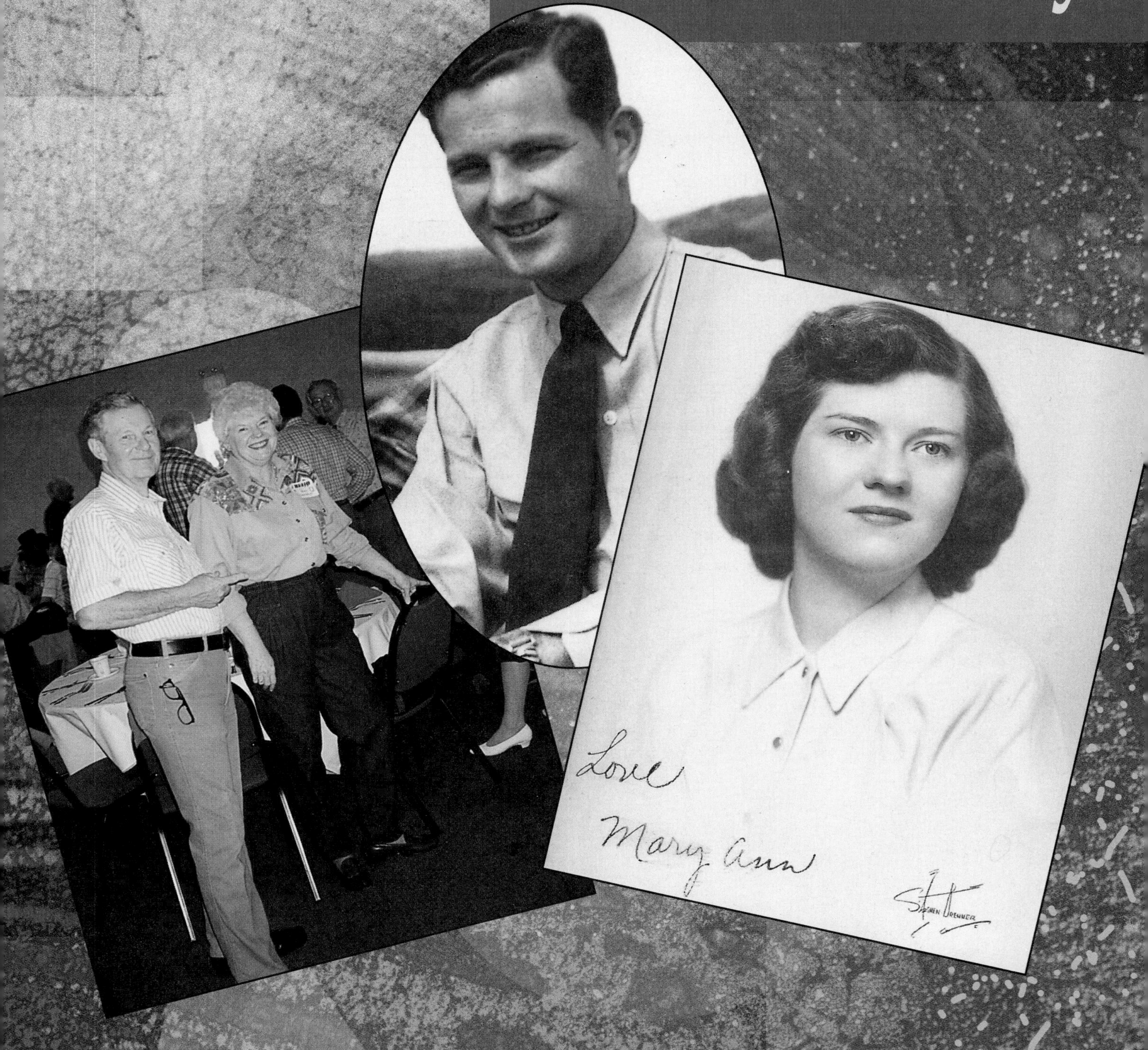

What You Will Learn

- The definition of the key terms listed in this chapter
- The purpose of bedrest
- The complications of bedrest and how to prevent them
- The devices used to support and maintain body alignment
- The purpose of a trapeze
- How to perform range-of-motion exercises
- How to help a resident walk
- The purpose of four walking aids
- How to help a falling resident
- The procedures described in this chapter

Key Terms

abduction Moving a body part away from the midline of the body

adduction Moving a body part toward the midline of the body

ambulation The act of walking

atrophy A decrease in size or a wasting away of tissue

contracture The lack of joint mobility caused by abnormal shortening of a muscle

deconditioning The loss of muscle strength as a result of inactivity

dorsiflexion A toe-up motion of the foot at the ankle

extension Straightening of a body part

external rotation Turning the joint outward

flexion Bending a body part

footdrop The foot falls down at the ankle (permanent plantar flexion)

hyperextension Excessive straightening of a body part

internal rotation Turning the joint inward

orthostatic hypotension A drop in *(hypo)* blood pressure when the person stands *(ortho* and *static)*; postural hypotension

plantar flexion The foot *(plantar)* is bent *(flexion)* down at the ankle

postural hypotension Orthostatic hypotension

pronation Turning downward

range of motion (ROM) The movement of a joint to the extent possible without causing pain

rotation Turning the joint

supination Turning upward

syncope A brief loss of consciousness; fainting

Being active is important for physical and mental well-being. Most people move about and function without help. However, aging, illnesses, surgery, injuries, and pain can cause weakness and some activity limits. Some people are weak from chronic illnesses. Others are in bed for a long time. Some have permanent paralysis. Some disorders are progressive, causing decreases in activity. Examples include multiple sclerosis, Parkinson's disease, arthritis, and nervous system and muscular disorders (see Chapter 26). Inactivity, whether mild or severe, affects the normal function of every body system. Mental well-being also is affected.

Deconditioning is the loss of muscle strength from inactivity. When inactive, older persons become deconditioned quickly. Nurses use the nursing process to promote exercise and activity in all residents to the extent possible. The health care team promotes exercise and activity for all residents. Each resident is encouraged to be as active as physically possible. The care plan tells you about each resident's activity level and what exercises to perform.

To assist in promoting exercise and activity, you need to understand:

- Bedrest
- How to prevent complications from bedrest
- How to help residents exercise

BEDREST

Bedrest is ordered by the doctor to treat a resident's health problem. Sometimes it is a nursing measure because of a change in the resident's condition. You must know what activities are allowed for each resident. The resident's care plan and your assignment sheet will have this information. Check with the nurse if you have any questions. Generally bedrest is ordered to:

- Reduce physical activity
- Reduce pain
- Encourage rest
- Regain strength
- Promote healing

The following types of bedrest are common. Always ask the nurse what bedrest means for each resident:

- *Bedrest*—the resident remains in bed but some activities of daily living (ADL) are allowed. Self-feeding, oral hygiene, bathing, shaving, and hair care often are allowed.
- *Strict bedrest*—everything is done for the resident. No ADL are allowed.
- *Bedrest with commode privileges*—the resident can use the bedside commode for elimination needs.
- *Bedrest with bathroom privileges (bedrest with BRP)*—the resident can use the bathroom for elimination needs.

Complications of Bedrest

Bedrest and lack of exercise and activity can cause serious complications. Every body system is affected. Pressure ulcers, constipation, and fecal impaction can result. Urinary tract infections, renal stones (renal calculi), blood clots (thrombi), and pneumonia (infection of the lung [see Chapter 26]) can occur.

Contractures and muscle atrophy occur in the musculoskeletal system. A **contracture** is the lack of joint mobility caused by abnormal shortening of a muscle. The contracted muscle is fixed into position, is deformed, and cannot stretch (Fig. 19-1). Common sites are the fingers, wrists, elbows, toes, ankles, knees, and hips. Contractures can occur also in the neck and spine. The person with a contracture is permanently deformed and disabled. **Atrophy** is the decrease in size or the wasting away of tissue. Muscle atrophy is a decrease in size or a wasting away of muscle (Fig. 19-2). These complications must be prevented to maintain normal body movement.

Orthostatic hypotension and blood clots (see Chapter 14) occur in the cardiovascular system. **Orthostatic hypotension** is a drop in *(hypo)* blood pressure when the person stands *(ortho* and *static)*. When a person moves from lying or sitting to a standing position, the blood pressure drops. The person experiences dizziness, weakness, and spots before the eyes. Syncope can

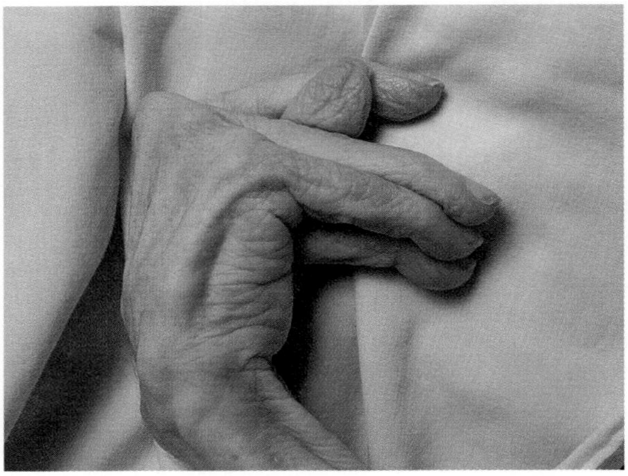

Fig. 19-1 A contracture.

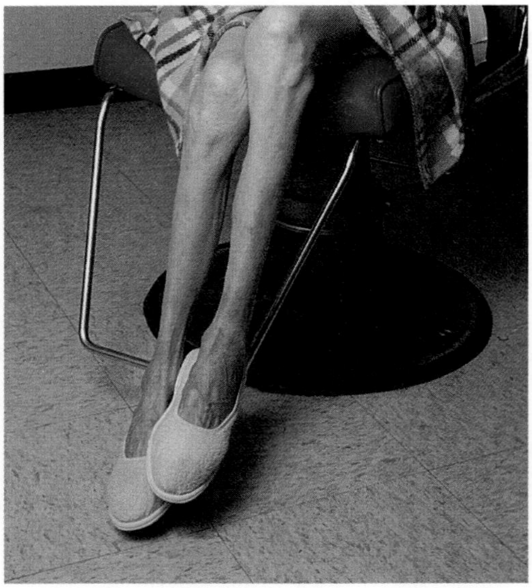

Fig. 19-2 Muscle atrophy.

Box 19-1 Preventing Orthostatic Hypotension

- Measure blood pressure when the resident is supine. Also count the resident's pulse and respirations.
- Raise the head of the bed so the resident is in Fowler's position. Raise the head of the bed slowly.
  - Ask the resident about weakness, dizziness, or spots before the eyes. Lower the head of the bed if these symptoms occur.
  - Measure blood pressure, pulse, and respirations when the resident is in Fowler's position.
  - Keep the resident in Fowler's position for a short while. Ask the resident about weakness, dizziness, or spots before the eyes.
- Assist the resident to sit on the side of the bed (see Chapter 10).
  - Ask the resident about weakness, dizziness, or spots before the eyes. Assist the resident to Fowler's position if any of these symptoms occur.
  - Measure blood pressure, pulse, and respirations when the resident is sitting on the side of the bed.
  - Have the resident continue to sit on the side of the bed for a short while.
- Assist the resident to stand.
  - Ask the resident about weakness, dizziness, or spots before the eyes. Help the resident sit on the side of the bed if any of these symptoms occur.
  - Measure blood pressure, pulse, and respirations.
- Help the resident sit in a chair or walk as directed by the nurse.
  - Ask the resident about weakness, dizziness, or spots before the eyes. If the resident is walking, help the resident to sit if symptoms occur.
  - Measure blood pressure, pulse, and respirations.
- Report blood pressure, pulse, and respirations to the nurse. Also report other symptoms.

occur. **Syncope** (fainting) is a brief loss of consciousness. (Syncope comes from the Greek word *synkoptein,* which means to cut short.) Orthostatic hypotension is also called **postural hypotension.** *(Postural* relates to posture or standing.) Box 19-1 lists the measures that prevent orthostatic hypotension. Slowly changing positions is key.

Complications from bedrest are prevented by good nursing care. Positioning in good body alignment, range-of-motion exercises, and frequent position changes are important preventive measures. These are part of the resident's care plan.

Positioning

Body alignment and positioning are discussed in Chapter 10. Supportive devices often are used to support and maintain the resident in a certain position:

- *Bed boards*—are placed under the mattress. They keep the resident in alignment by preventing the mattress from sagging (Fig. 19-3). They are usually made of plywood and are covered with canvas or other material. There are 2 sections so the head of the bed can be raised. One section is for the head of the bed and the other for the foot of the bed.

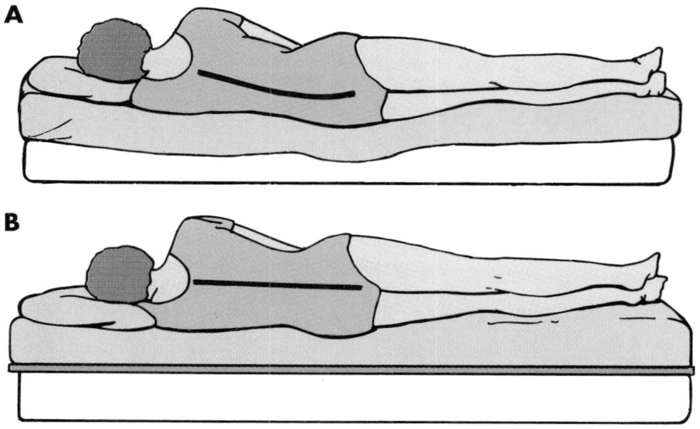

Fig. 19-3 A, Mattress sagging without bed boards. **B,** Bed boards are placed under the mattress. No sagging occurs.

- *Footboards*—are placed at the foot of the mattress (Fig. 19-4). They prevent plantar flexion that can lead to footdrop. In **plantar flexion** the foot *(plantar)* is bent *(flexion)*. **Footdrop** is when the foot falls down at the ankle (permanent plantar flexion). The footboard is placed so the soles of the feet are flush against it. The feet are in good alignment as when standing. Footboards also serve as bed cradles. They keep top linens off the feet.
- *Trochanter rolls*—prevent the hips and legs from turning outward (external rotation) (Fig. 19-5). They are made from bath blankets. A blanket is folded to the desired length and rolled up. The loose end is placed under the resident from the hip to the knee. Then the roll is tucked alongside the body. Pillows or sandbags also are used to keep the hips and knees in alignment.
- *Hip abduction wedges*—keep the hips abducted (Fig. 19-6). The wedge is positioned between the resident's legs. These are common after hip replacement surgery.

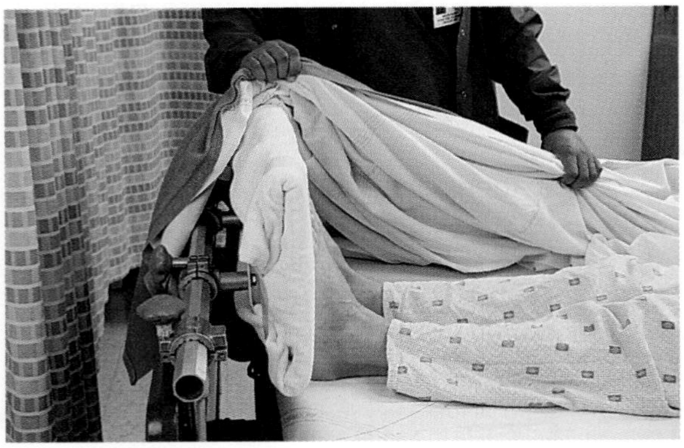

Fig. 19-4 Footboard. Feet are flush with the board to keep them in normal alignment.

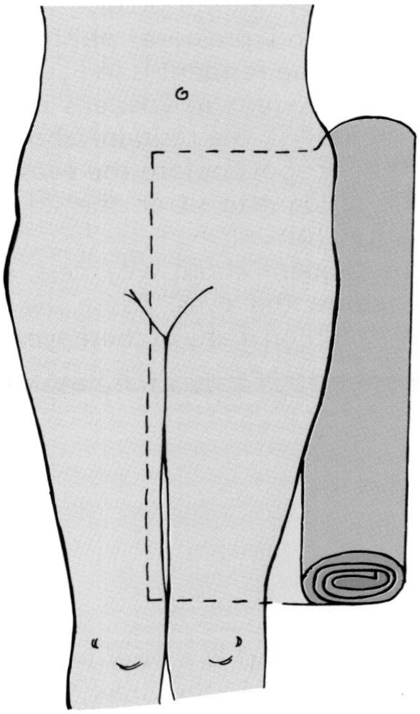

Fig. 19-5 Trochanter roll made from a bath blanket. It extends from the hip to the knee.

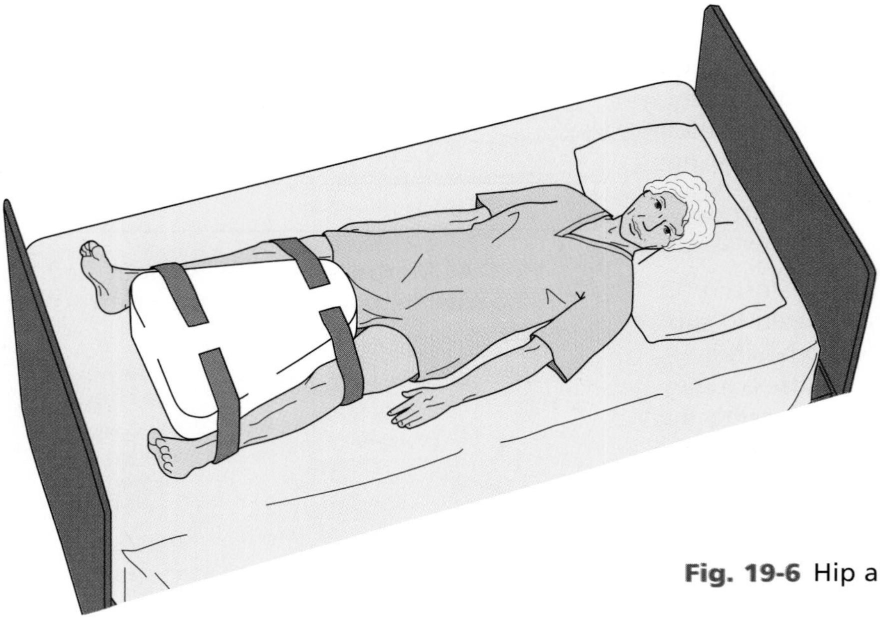

Fig. 19-6 Hip abduction wedge.

- *Hand rolls* or *hand grips*—prevent contractures of the thumb, fingers, and wrist. Commercial hand rolls are common (Fig. 19-7). Foam rubber sponges, rubber balls, and finger cushions (Fig. 19-8) also are used.
- *Splints*—keep the wrist, thumb, and fingers in normal position. They are usually secured in place with Velcro. Some have foam padding (Fig. 19-9).
- *Bed cradles*—keep the weight of top linens off the feet (see Fig. 14-6, p. 306). The weight of top linens can cause footdrop and pressure ulcers.

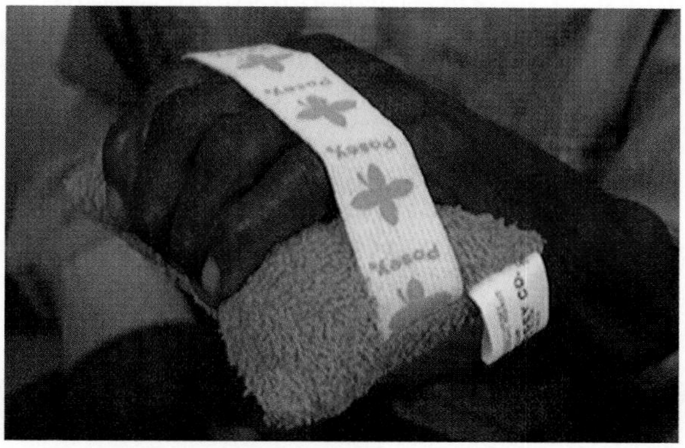

Fig. 19-7 Hand roll. *(Courtesy J.T. Posey Co., Arcadia, Calif.)*

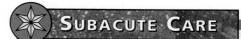

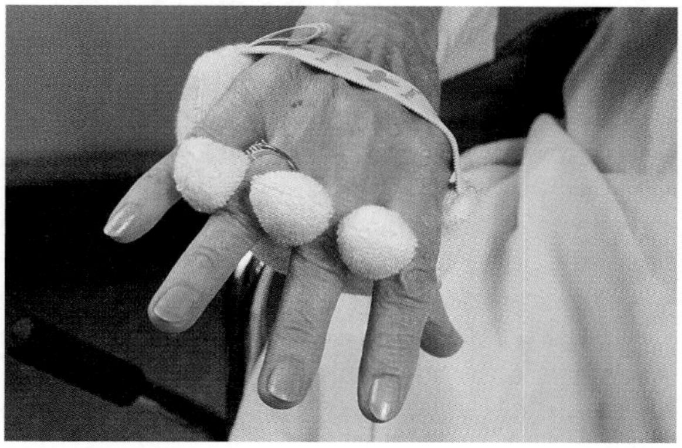

Fig. 19-8 Finger cushion. *(Courtesy J.T. Posey Co., Arcadia, Calif.)*

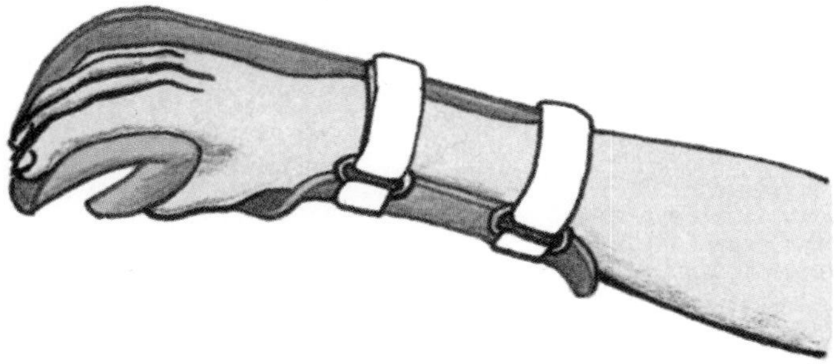

Fig. 19-9 Splint. *(From Birchenall J, Streight, E:* Mosby's textbook for the home care aide, *St Louis, 1997, Mosby.)*

Exercise

Exercise helps prevent contractures, muscle atrophy, and other complications of bedrest. (*See Subacute Care.*) Some exercise occurs with activities of daily living and when turning and moving in bed without assistance. Additional exercises are needed for muscles and joints.

A trapeze is used for exercises to strengthen arm muscles. The trapeze is suspended from an overbed frame (see Fig. 10-9, p. 203). The resident grasps the bar with both hands to lift the trunk off the bed. The trapeze is used also to move up and turn in bed.

Subacute Care

For persons who need subacute care, the exercise and activity plan is focused on rehabilitation. The persons work closely with physical therapists and occupational therapists to improve strength and endurance. Care plan goals for exercise and ambulation may change daily. The goal is to improve the person's independence so he or she can go home. The entire health care team works with the person to help meet rehabilitation goals. You must know and follow the care plan carefully.

Range-of-motion exercises.

The movement of a joint to the extent possible without causing pain is the **range of motion (ROM)** of that joint. Range-of-motion exercises involve exercising the joints through their complete range of motion. The exercises are usually done at least twice a day. Range-of-motion exercises are active, passive, or active-assistive:

- *Active* range-of-motion exercises are done by the person.
- *Passive* range-of-motion exercises involve having another person move the joints through their range of motion.
- *Active-assistive* range of motion is when the person does the exercises with some help from another person.

Range-of-motion exercises naturally occur during activities of daily living. Bathing, hair care, eating, reaching, and walking all involve joint movements. Residents on bedrest may require more frequent range-of-motion exercises. So may those who have mobility loss from a stroke or injury. Therefore the doctor or nurse may order more frequent range-of-motion exercises.

OBRA

OBRA requires that nursing centers have an assessment and care planning process that prevents any unnecessary reduction in a resident's range of motion. Preventive care may involve active, active-assistive, or passive range-of-motion exercises. Splints and braces are used if necessary (p. 462).

The nurse tells you which joints to exercise, the frequency of the exercises, and if the exercises are to be active, passive, or active-assistive. This information is also in the care plan. Box 19-2 describes the movements involved in range-of-motion exercises.

Range-of-motion exercises can cause injury if not done properly. The rules in Box 19-3 are practiced when performing or assisting with range-of-motion exercises.

Text continued on p. 454

Box 19-2 Joint Movements

Abduction—moving a body part away from the midline of the body
Adduction—moving a body part toward the midline of the body
Extension—straightening a body part
Flexion—bending a body part
Hyperextension—excessive straightening of a body part
Dorsiflexion—bending the toes and foot up at the ankle
Rotation—turning the joint
Internal rotation—turning the joint inward
External rotation—turning the joint outward
Plantar flexion—bending the foot down at the ankle
Pronation—turning downward
Supination—turning upward

Box 19-3 Rules for Performing Range-of-Motion Exercises

- Exercise only the joints the nurse tells you to exercise.
- Expose only the body part being exercised.
- Use good body mechanics.
- Support the extremity being exercised.
- Move the joint slowly, smoothly, and gently.
- Do not force a joint beyond its present range of motion or to the point of pain.
- *Perform range-of-motion exercises to the neck only if allowed by center policy.* In some centers, only physical or occupational therapists do neck exercises. This is because of the danger of neck injuries.

Performing Range-of-Motion Exercises

NNAAP™ SKILL

Quality of Life

Remember to:

- *Knock before entering the resident's room*
- *Address the resident by name*
- *Introduce yourself by name and title*

Pre-Procedure

1 Identify the resident. Check the ID bracelet against the assignment sheet.
2 Explain the procedure to the resident.
3 Wash your hands.
4 Obtain a bath blanket.
5 Provide for privacy.
6 Raise the bed to the best level for good body mechanics. Make sure bed rails are up.

Procedure

7 Lower the bed rail near you.
8 Position the resident supine and in good alignment.
9 Cover the resident with a bath blanket. Fanfold top linens to the foot of the bed.
10 Exercise the neck if allowed by the center and if the nurse instructs you to (Fig. 19-10, p. 451):
  a Place your hands over the resident's ears to support the head.
  b Flexion—bring the head forward so the chin touches the chest.
  c Extension—straighten the head.
  d Hyperextension—bring the head backward until the chin is pointing up.
  e Rotation—turn the head from side to side.
  f Lateral flexion—move the head to the right and to the left.
  g Repeat flexion, extension, hyperextension, rotation, and lateral flexion 5 times—or the number of times stated on the care plan.
11 Exercise the shoulder (Fig. 19-11, p. 451):
  a Grasp the wrist with one hand and the elbow with the other.
  b Flexion—raise the arm straight in front and over the head.
  c Extension—bring the arm down to the side.
  d Hyperextension—move the arm behind the body. (This is done if the resident sits in a straight-back chair or is standing.)
  e Abduction—move the straight arm away from the side of the body.
  f Adduction—move the straight arm to the side of the body.
  g Internal rotation—bend the elbow, and place it at the same level as the shoulder. Move the forearm down toward the body.
  h External rotation—move the forearm toward the head.
  i Repeat flexion, extension, hyperextension, abduction, adduction, and internal and external rotation 5 times—or the number of times stated on the care plan.
12 Exercise the elbow (Fig. 19-12, p. 452):
  a Grasp the resident's wrist with one hand and the elbow with the other.
  b Flexion—bend the arm so the same-side shoulder is touched.
  c Extension—straighten the arm.
  d Repeat flexion and extension 5 times—or the number of times stated on the care plan.
13 Exercise the forearm (Fig. 19-13, p. 452):
  a Pronation—turn the hand so the palm is down.
  b Supination—turn the hand so the palm is up.
  c Repeat pronation and supination 5 times—or the number of times stated on the care plan.

Continued

Performing Range-of-Motion Exercises—cont'd

NNAAP™ SKILL

Procedure—cont'd

14 Exercise the wrist (Fig. 19-14, p. 452):
   a Hold the wrist with both of your hands.
   b Flexion—bend the hand down.
   c Extension—straighten the hand.
   d Hyperextension—bend the hand back.
   e Radial flexion—turn the hand toward the thumb.
   f Ulnar flexion—turn the hand toward the little finger.
   g Repeat flexion, extension, hyperextension, and radial and ulnar flexion 5 times—or the number of times stated on the care plan.

15 Exercise the thumb (Fig. 19-15, p. 452):
   a Hold the resident's hand with one hand and the thumb with your other hand.
   b Abduction—move the thumb out from the inner part of the index finger.
   c Adduction—move the thumb back next to the index finger.
   d Opposition—touch each fingertip with the thumb.
   e Flexion—bend the thumb into the hand.
   f Extension—move the thumb out to the side of the fingers.
   g Repeat flexion, extension, abduction, adduction, and opposition 5 times—or the number of times stated on the care plan.

16 Exercise the fingers (Fig. 19-16, p. 452):
   a Abduction—spread the fingers and the thumb apart.
   b Adduction—bring the fingers and thumb together.
   c Extension—straighten the fingers so the fingers, hand, and arm are straight.
   d Flexion—make a fist.
   e Repeat abduction, adduction, extension, and flexion 5 times—or the number of times stated on the care plan.

17 Exercise the hip (Fig. 19-17, p. 452):
   a Place one hand under the knee and the other under the ankle to support the leg.
   b Flexion—raise the leg.
   c Extension—straighten the leg.
   d Abduction—move the leg away from the body.
   e Adduction—move the leg toward the other leg.
   f Internal rotation—turn the leg inward.
   g External rotation—turn the leg outward.
   h Repeat flexion, extension, abduction, adduction, and inward and outward rotation 5 times—or the number of times stated on the care plan.

18 Exercise the knee (Fig. 19-18, p. 453):
   a Place one hand under the knee and the other under the ankle to support the leg.
   b Flexion—bend the leg.
   c Extension—straighten the leg.
   d Repeat flexion and extension of the knee 5 times—or the number of times stated on the care plan.

19 Exercise the ankle (Fig. 19-19, p. 453):
   a Place one hand under the foot and the other under the ankle to support the part.
   b Dorsiflexion—pull the foot forward, and push down on the heel at the same time.
   c Plantar flexion—turn the foot down, or point the toes.
   d Repeat dorsiflexion and plantar flexion 5 times—or the number of times stated on the care plan.

20 Exercise the foot (Fig. 19-20, p. 453):
   a Pronation—turn the outside of the foot up and the inside down.
   b Supination—turn the inside of the foot up and the outside down.
   c Repeat pronation and supination 5 times—or the number of times stated on the care plan.

21 Exercise the toes (Fig. 19-21, p. 453):
   a Flexion—curl the toes.
   b Extension—straighten the toes.
   c Abduction—spread the toes apart.
   d Adduction—pull the toes together.
   e Repeat flexion, extension, abduction, and adduction 5 times—or the number of times stated on the care plan.

Performing Range-of-Motion Exercises—cont'd

NNAAP™ SKILL

Procedure—cont'd

22 Cover the leg, and raise the bed rail.

23 Go to the other side. Lower the bed rail near you.

24 Repeat steps 11 through 21.

Post-Procedure

25 Provide for comfort.

26 Cover the resident. Remove the bath blanket.

27 Raise or lower bed rails. Follow the care plan.

28 Lower the bed to its lowest level.

29 Place the signal light within reach.

30 Unscreen the resident.

31 Return the bath blanket to its proper place.

32 Wash your hands.

33 Report the following to the nurse:
- The time the exercises were performed
- The joints exercised
- The number of times the exercises were performed on each joint
- Any complaints of pain or signs of stiffness or spasm
- The degree to which the resident participated in the exercises

34 Document according to center policy.

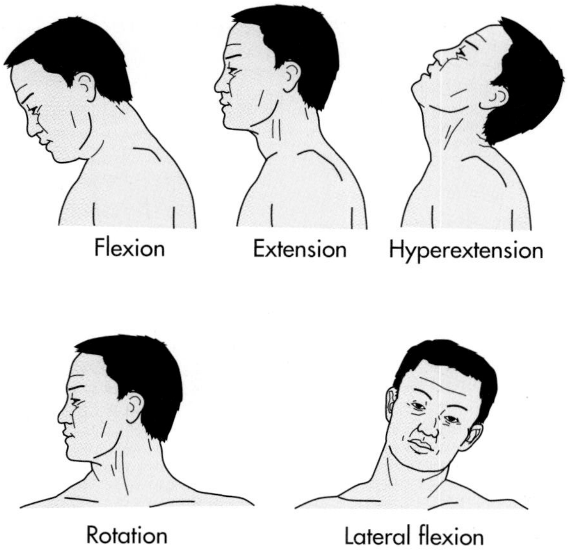

Fig. 19-10 Range-of-motion exercises for the neck.

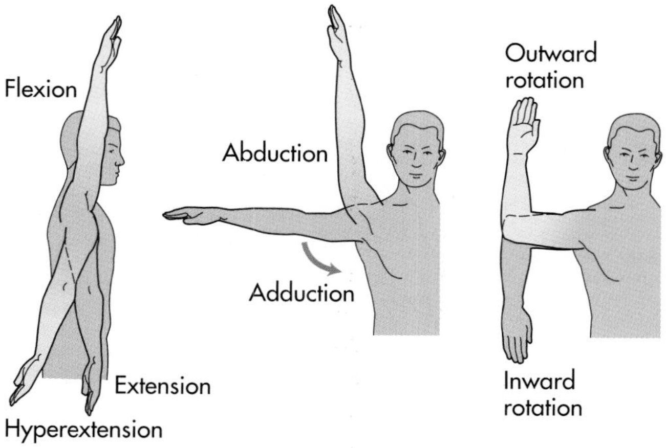

Fig. 19-11 Range-of-motion exercises for the shoulder.

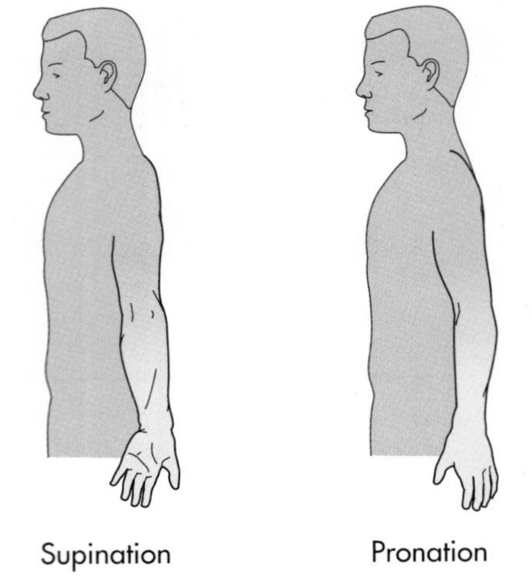

Fig. 19-12 Range-of-motion exercises for the elbow.

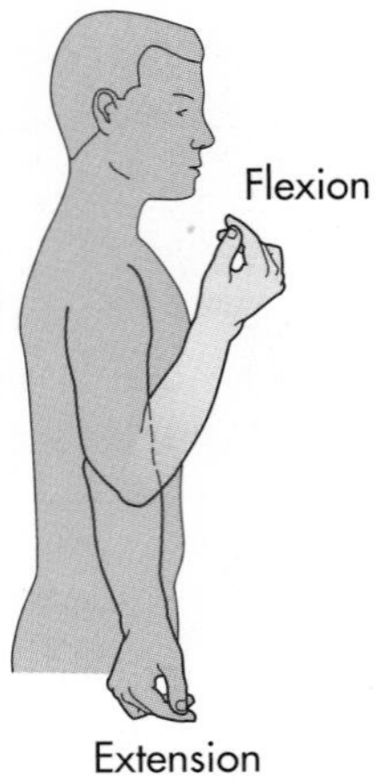

Fig. 19-13 Range-of-motion exercises for the forearm.

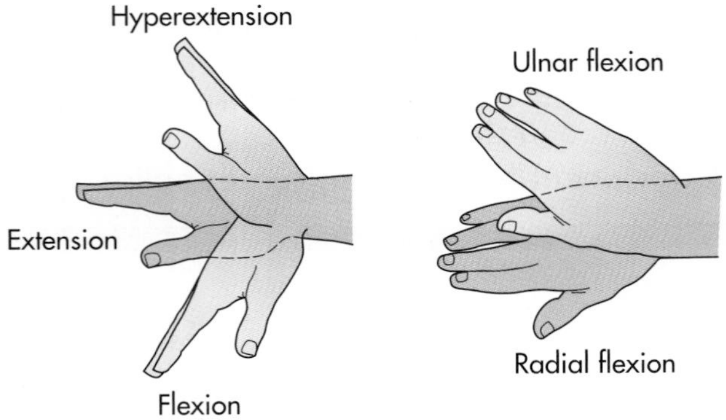

Fig. 19-14 Range-of-motion exercises for the wrist.

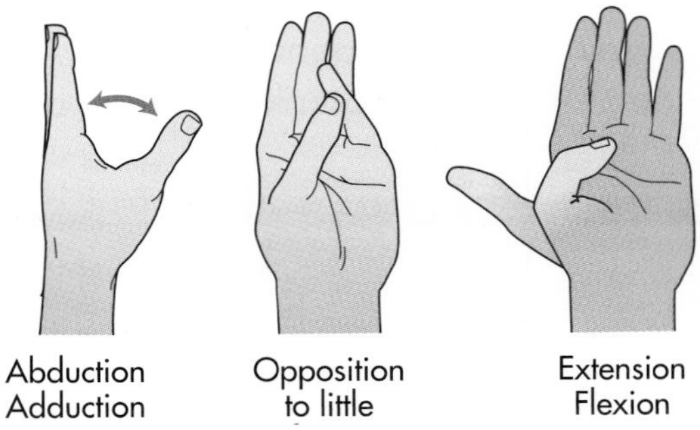

Fig. 19-15 Range-of-motion exercises for the thumb.

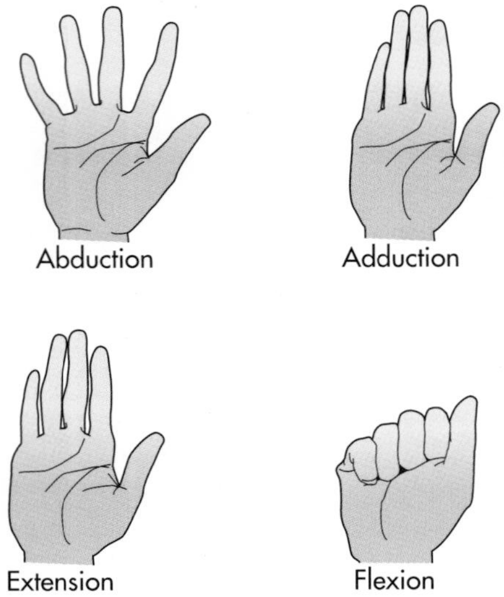

Fig. 19-16 Range-of-motion exercises for the fingers.

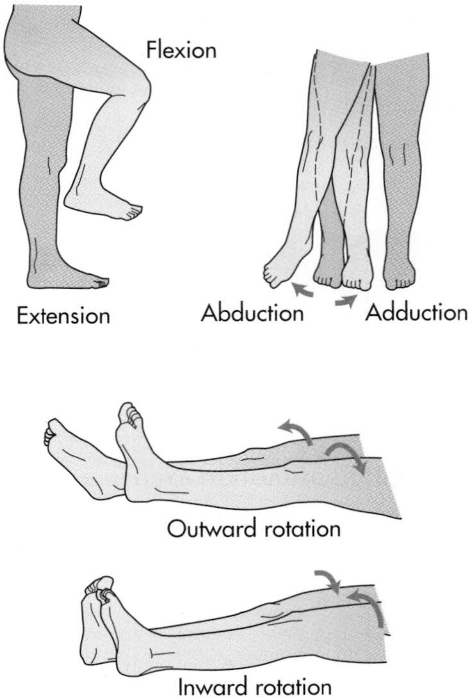

Fig. 19-17 Range-of-motion exercises for the hip.

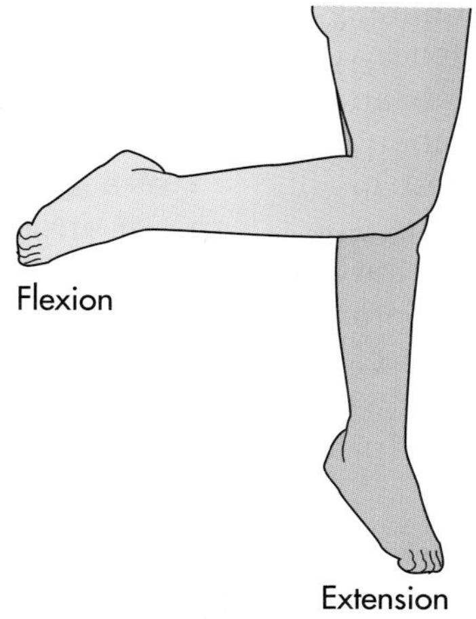

Fig. 19-18 Range-of-motion exercises for the knee.

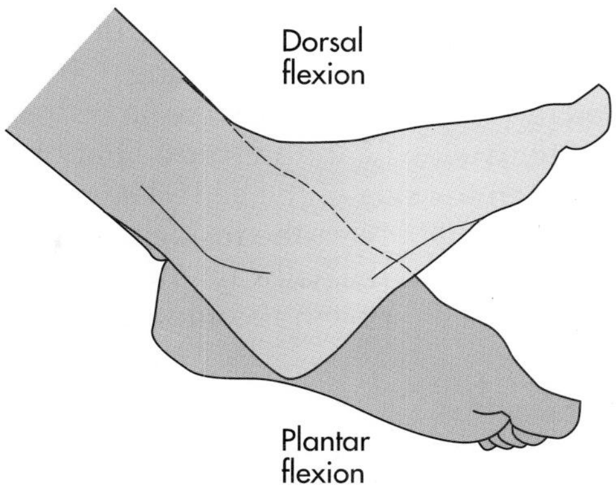

Fig. 19-19 Range-of-motion exercises for the ankle.

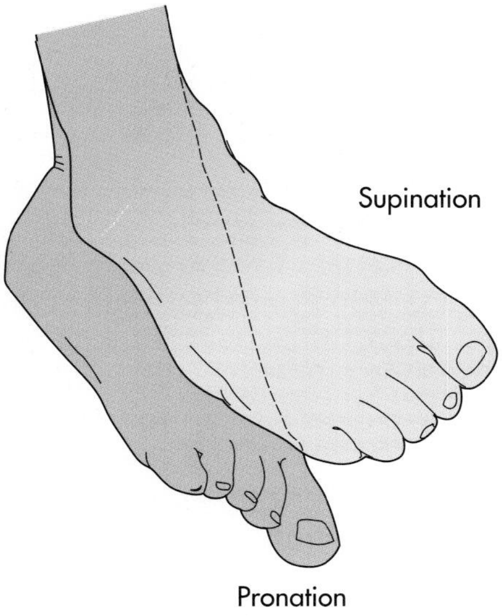

Fig. 19-20 Range-of-motion exercises for the foot.

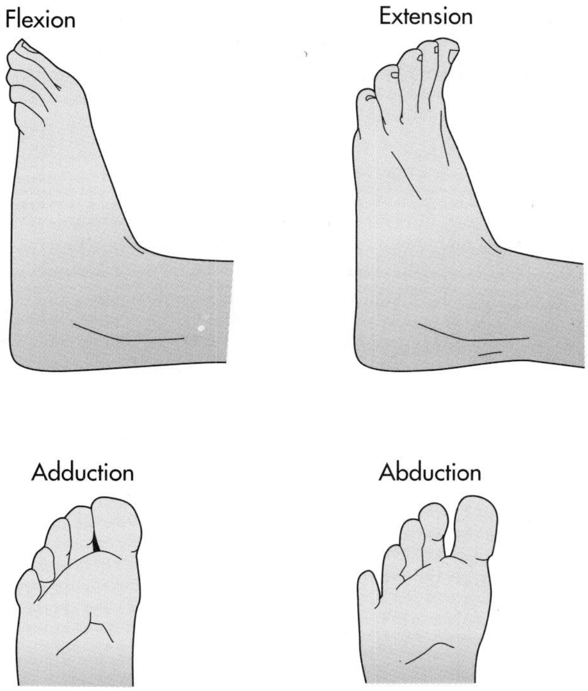

Fig. 19-21 Range-of-motion exercises for the toes.

AMBULATION

Many residents cannot walk without help. However, they must walk regularly to prevent deconditioning. Some become independent in walking. Others will always need help. Residents who were on bedrest need to increase activity slowly and in steps. First the resident dangles (sits on the side of the bed). The next step is to sit in a bedside chair. Next the resident walks about in the room and then in the hallway. **Ambulation,** the act of walking, is not a problem if complications were prevented. Deconditioning, contractures, and muscle atrophy are prevented by proper positioning and exercise.

Some residents are weak and unsteady from inactivity, illness, or injury. You need to help them begin to walk after bedrest or illness. Use a gait (transfer or safety) belt if the person is weak or unsteady. For additional support, the resident can use the handrails along the wall. Some residents in wheelchairs can walk with assistance. They should ambulate as stated in the care plan. Always check the resident for orthostatic hypotension (p. 445).

Helping the Resident to Walk

NNAAP™ SKILL

Quality of Life

Remember to:
- *Knock before entering the resident's room*
- *Address the resident by name*
- *Introduce yourself by name and title*

Pre-Procedure

1 Explain the procedure to the resident.
2 Wash your hands.
3 Collect the following:
- Robe and nonskid shoes
- Paper or sheet to protect bottom linens
- Transfer (gait or safety) belt

4 Identify the resident. Check the ID bracelet against the assignment sheet.
5 Provide for privacy.

Procedure

6 Move furniture as needed for moving space for you and the resident.
7 Lower the bed to its lowest position. Lock the bed wheels.
8 Fanfold top linens to the foot of the bed.
9 Place the paper or sheet under the resident's feet. This protects the bottom sheet from the shoes. Put the shoes on the resident.
10 Help the resident to dangle. (See *Helping the Resident to Sit on the Side of the Bed,* p. 214.)
11 Help the resident put on the robe.
12 Apply the gait belt. (See *Applying a Gait [Transfer or Safety] Belt,* p. 216.)
13 Help the resident stand:
 a Stand facing the resident.
 b Grasp the gait belt at each side.
 c Brace your knees against the resident's knees. Block his or her feet with your feet (see Fig. 10-21, p. 219).
 d Tell the resident to lean forward and stand on the count of three.
 e Assist the resident to a standing position as you straighten your knees (see Fig. 10-22, p. 219).
14 Stand at the resident's side while he or she gains balance. Do not let go of the gait belt. Grasp the belt at the side and back.
15 Encourage the resident to stand erect with the head up and back straight.
16 Assist the resident to walk. Walk at his or her side, and provide support with the gait belt (Fig. 19-22).

Helping the Resident to Walk—cont'd

NNAAP™ SKILL

Procedure

17 Encourage the resident to walk normally. The heel of the foot strikes the floor first. Discourage shuffling, sliding, or walking on tiptoes.

18 Walk the required distance if the resident can tolerate the activity. Do not rush the resident.

19 Help the resident return to bed:

a Have the resident stand at the side of the bed.

b Pivot him or her a quarter turn. The backs of the knees should touch the bed.

c Grasp the sides of the gait belt.

d Lower the resident onto the bed as you bend your knees. Remove the gait belt and robe.

e Help the resident lie down. (See *Helping the Resident to Sit on the Side of the Bed,* p. 214.)

20 Lower the head of the bed. Help the resident to the center of the bed.

21 Remove the shoes, and remove the paper or sheet over the bottom sheet.

Post-Procedure

22 Provide for comfort. Cover the resident.

23 Place the signal light within reach.

24 Raise or lower bed rails. Follow the care plan.

25 Return the robe and shoes to their proper place.

26 Return furniture to its proper location.

27 Unscreen the resident.

28 Wash your hands.

29 Report the following to the nurse:
- How well the resident tolerated the activity
- Any complaints of pain or discomfort
- The distance walked

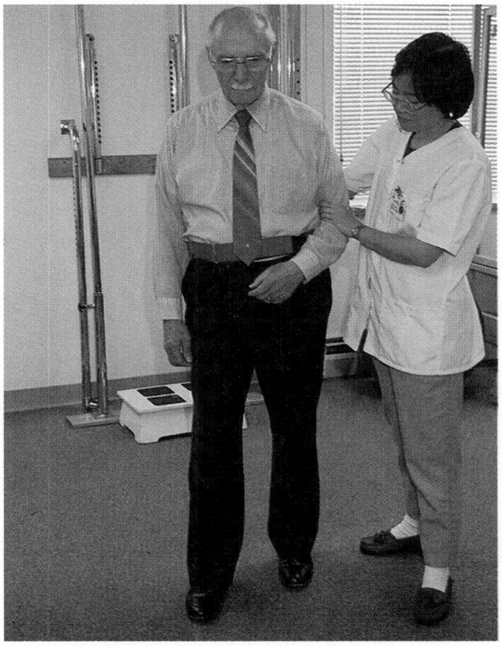

Fig. 19-22 Assist with ambulation by walking at the person's side. Use a transfer (safety) belt for the person's safety.

The Falling Resident

A resident may start to fall when standing or walking. The resident may be weak, lightheaded, or dizzy. Fainting may occur. Falling may be caused by slipping or sliding on spills, waxed floors, throw rugs, or improper shoes (see Chapter 8).

When a resident is falling, there is a tendency to try to prevent the fall. However, trying to prevent a fall could cause greater harm. You could injure yourself and the resident as you twist and strain to stop the fall. Balance is lost as a resident falls. If you try to prevent the fall, you could lose your balance. Thus both you and the resident could fall or cause the other person to fall. Head, hip, and knee injuries are common from falls.

If a resident starts to fall, ease him or her to the floor. This lets you control the direction of the fall. You can also protect the resident's head. Do not move the resident once he or she is on the floor. The nurse must check the resident before he or she is moved. Do not allow the resident to move or get up before the nurse checks for injuries. Calmly explain that a nurse must check all residents who fall to make sure there are no serious injuries such as broken bones. (*See Residents With Dementia.*) An incident report is completed after all falls. The nurse may ask you to help fill out the incident report.

Residents With Dementia

A confused resident may not understand why he or she cannot move or get up after a fall. Trying to force a confused or agitated resident not to move may injure the resident and you. You may need to let the resident move about for his or her safety and your own. Stay calm, and protect the resident from injury. Talk to the resident in a quiet and soothing voice until someone can assist you. Never use force or hold a resident down. See Chapter 27 for safe approaches to use when caring for residents with dementia.

Helping the Falling Resident

Procedure

1 Stand with your feet apart. Keep your back straight.

2 Bring the resident close to your body as quickly as possible. Use the gait belt if one is worn. If not, wrap your arms around the resident's waist. You can also hold the resident under the arms (Fig. 19-23, *A*).

3 Move your leg so the resident's buttocks rest on it (Fig. 19-23, *B*). Move the leg near the resident.

4 Lower the resident to the floor. Let him or her slide down your leg to the floor (Fig. 19-23, *C*). Bend at your hips and knees as you lower the resident.

5 Call a nurse to check the resident.

6 Help the nurse return the resident to bed. Get other workers to help if necessary.

7 Report the following to the nurse:
- How the fall occurred
- How far the resident walked
- How activity was tolerated before the fall
- Any complaints before the fall
- The amount of assistance needed by the resident while walking

8 Complete an incident report.

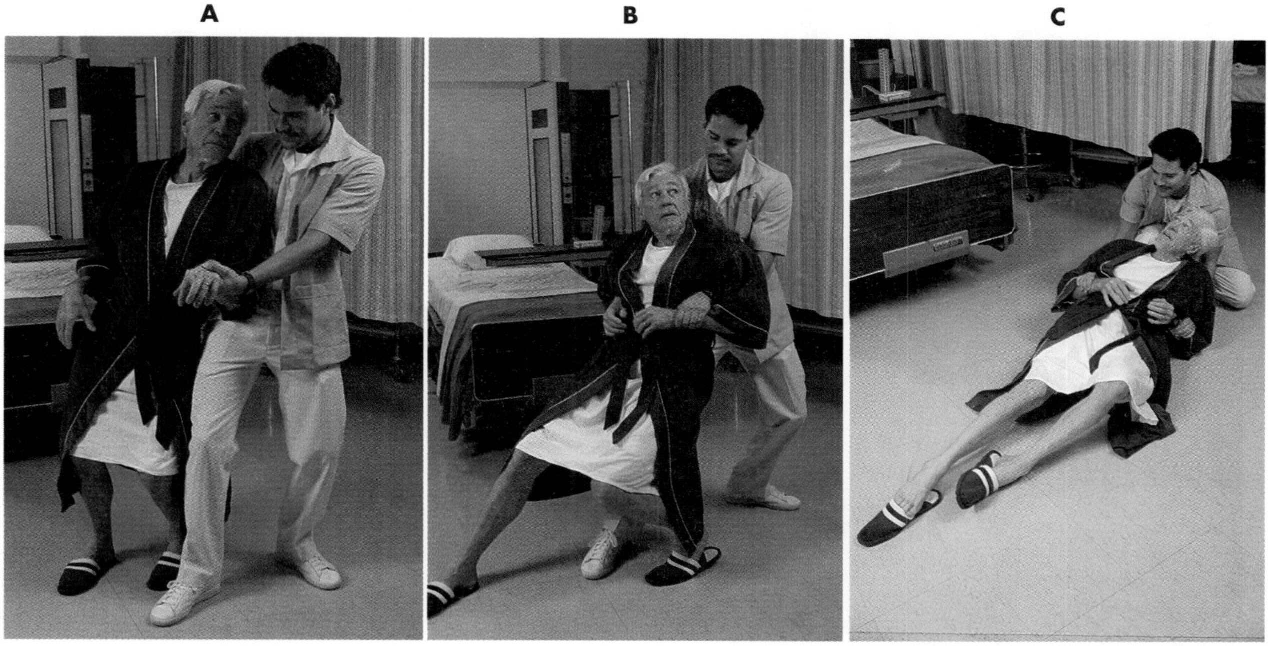

Fig. 19-23 **A,** The falling person is supported under the arms. **B,** The person's buttocks are on the nursing assistant's leg. **C,** The person is eased to the floor on the nursing assistant's leg.

Walking Aids

Walking aids support the body. Older residents often need a walker or cane for safety while they walk. Walking aids are ordered by the doctor, physical therapist, or nurse. The need is temporary or permanent. The type ordered depends on the resident's physical condition, the amount of support needed, and the type of disability. The physical therapist or nurse teaches the resident to use the walking aid.

Crutches. Crutches are used when the resident cannot use one leg or when one or both legs need to gain strength. Some residents with permanent leg weakness can use crutches. They usually use Lofstrand crutches (Fig. 19-24, p. 458). These crutches are made of metal. A metal band fits around the forearm. Axillary crutches extend from the underarm (axilla) to the ground (Fig. 19-25, p. 458). They are made of wood or metal.

The resident learns to crutch walk, climb up and down stairs, and sit and stand. Safety is important. The resident using crutches is at risk of falling. The following safety measures are followed:

- The crutches must fit. A physical therapist or a nurse measures and fits the resident with crutches. An improper fit increases the risk of falling and further injury. Back pain, nerve damage, and injuries to the underarms and palms are other risks.
- Crutch tips must be attached to the crutches. They must not be worn down or wet. Replace worn crutch tips. Dry wet tips with a towel or paper towels.
- Crutches are checked for flaws. Check wooden crutches for cracks and metal crutches for bends. All bolts on both types must be tight.
- Street shoes are worn. They must be flat and have nonskid soles.
- Clothes must fit well. Loose clothing may get caught between the crutches and underarms. Loose clothing can also hang forward and block the resident's view of the feet and crutch tips.
- Safety rules to prevent falls are followed (see Chapter 8).
- Crutches are kept where the resident can reach them. Place them next to the resident's chair or against a wall.
- Know which crutch gait the resident uses:
  - Four-point alternating gait (Fig. 19-26, p. 458)
  - Three-point alternating gait (Fig. 19-27, p. 459)
  - Two-point alternating gait (Fig. 19-28, p. 459)
  - Swing-to gait (Fig. 19-29, p. 459)
  - Swing-through gait (Fig. 19-30, p. 460)

Text continued on p. 460

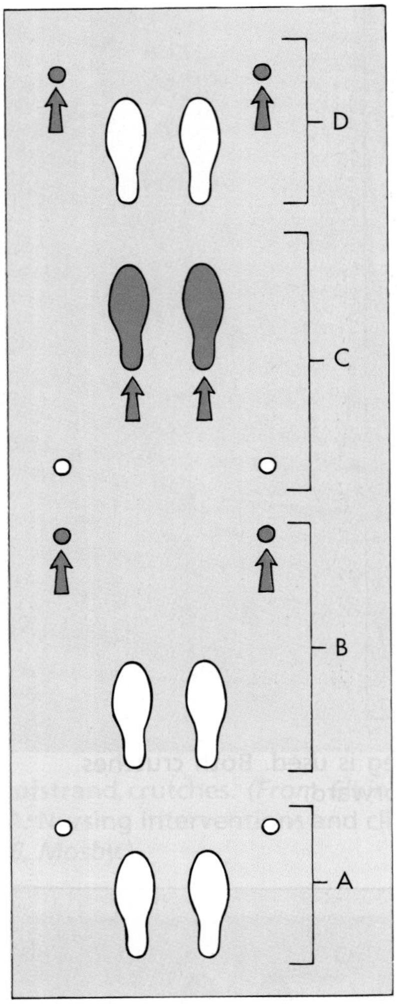

Fig. 19-30 Swing-through gait. The person bears some weight on each leg. Both crutches are moved forward. Then the person lifts both legs and swings *through* the crutches.

Canes. Canes are used for weakness on one side of the body. They help provide balance and support. There are single-tip, three-point (tripod), and four-point (quad) canes (Fig. 19-31). A cane is held on the *strong side* of the body. (If the left leg is weak, the cane is held in the right hand.) Three-point and four-point canes give more support than single-tip canes. However, they are harder to move.

The cane tip is about 6 to 10 inches to the side of the foot and about 6 to 10 inches in front of the foot on the strong side. The grip is level with the hip. The resident walks as follows:

Step A: The cane is moved forward 6 to 10 inches (Fig. 19-32, *A*).
Step B: The weak leg (opposite the cane) is moved forward even with the cane (Fig. 19-32, *B*).
Step C: The strong leg is brought forward and ahead of the cane and the weak leg (Fig. 19-32, *C*).

Walkers. A walker is a four-point walking aid (Fig. 19-33, p. 462). It gives more support than a cane. Many people feel safer and more secure with a walker than with a cane. There are many kinds of walkers. The standard walker is picked up and moved about 6 to 8 inches in front of the resident. The resident then moves the right foot and then the left foot up to the walker (Fig. 19-34, p. 462).

You may see older persons using wheeled walkers (Fig. 19-35, p. 462). Residents who cannot use a standard walker use them. A wheeled walker has wheels on the front legs and rubber tips on the back legs. The resident pushes the walker ahead about 6 to 8 inches and then walks up to it. The rubber tips on the back legs prevent the walker from moving while the resident is walking.

Baskets, pouches, and trays can be attached to the walker (see Fig. 19-33). These attachments allow residents to carry needed items rather than relying on others to do so. This allows them greater independence. The attachment also keeps the hands free to grip the walker.

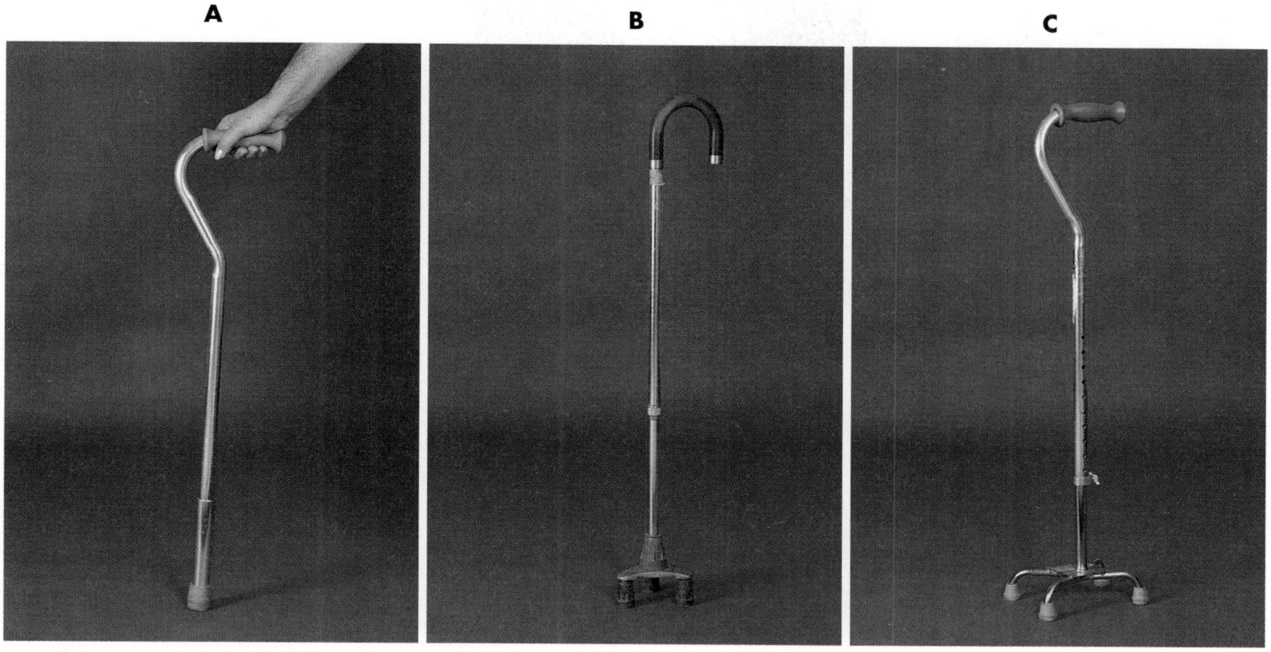

Fig. 19-31 **A,** Single-tip cane. **B,** Three-point (tripod) cane. **C,** Four-point (quad) cane.

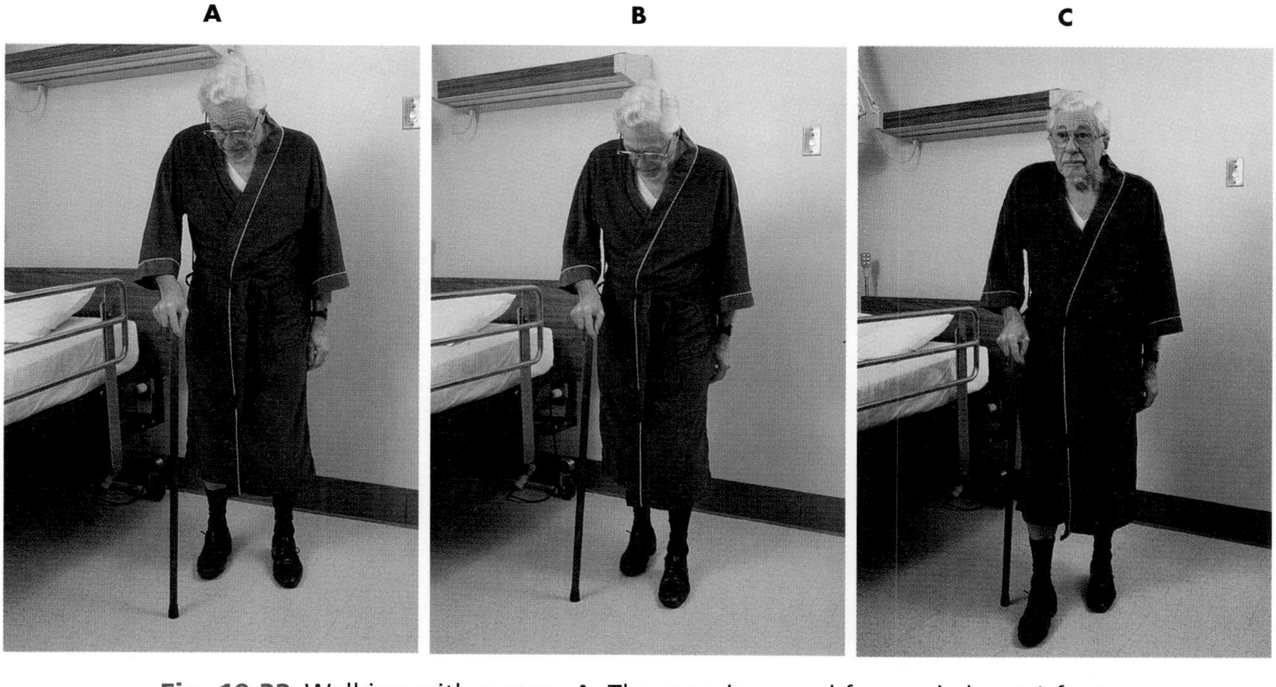

Fig. 19-32 Walking with a cane. **A,** The cane is moved forward about 1 foot. **B,** The leg opposite the cane (weak leg) is brought forward even with the cane. **C,** The leg on the cane side (strong leg) is moved ahead of the cane and the weak leg.

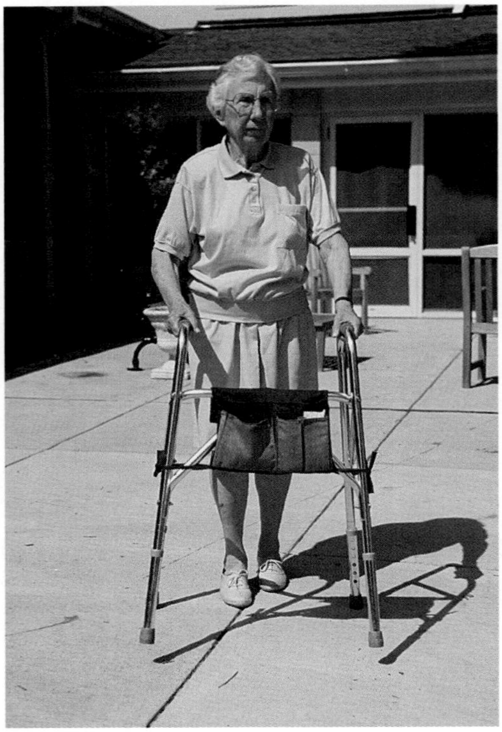

Fig. 19-33 A walker.

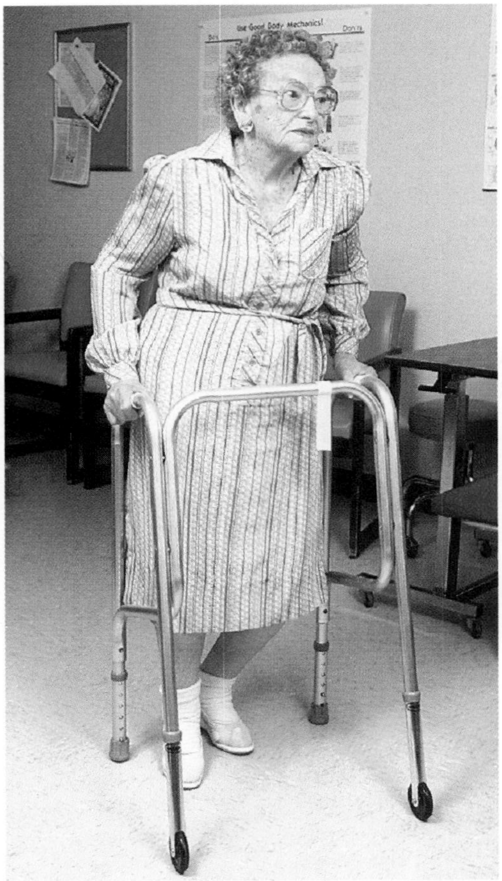

Fig. 19-35 An older woman using a wheeled walker.

A

B

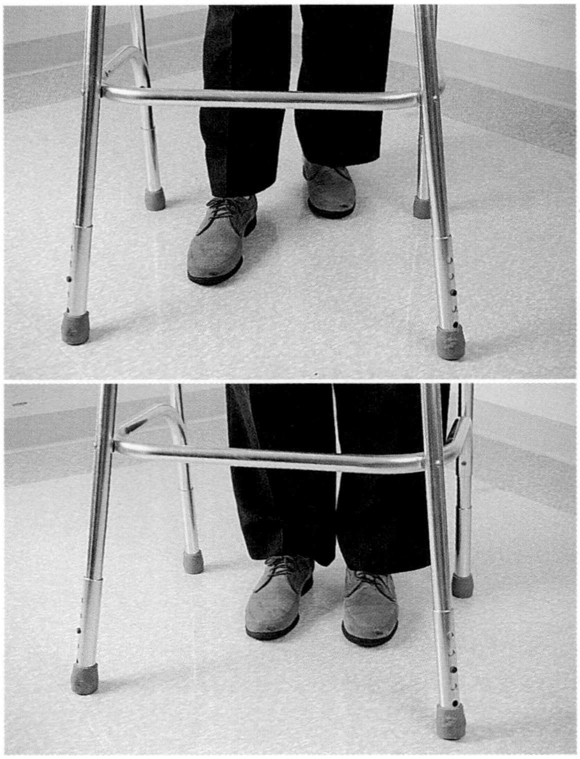

Fig. 19-34 Walking with a walker. **A,** The walker is moved about 6 inches in front of the person. **B,** The right foot and then the left foot are moved up to the walker.

Braces. Braces support weak body parts. They also prevent or correct deformities or prevent movement of a joint. Metal, plastic, or leather is used for braces. A brace is applied over the ankle, knee, or back (Fig. 19-36). An ankle-foot orthosis (AFO) is positioned in the shoe (Fig. 19-37). Then the foot is inserted. The device is secured in place with Velcro. This type of brace is commonly used after a stroke.

Skin under braces is kept clean and dry to prevent skin breakdown. When you apply or remove a brace, report any redness or signs of skin breakdown to the nurse immediately. Also report complaints of pain or discomfort. The nurse assesses the skin under braces every shift. The care plan tells you the schedule for applying and removing braces.

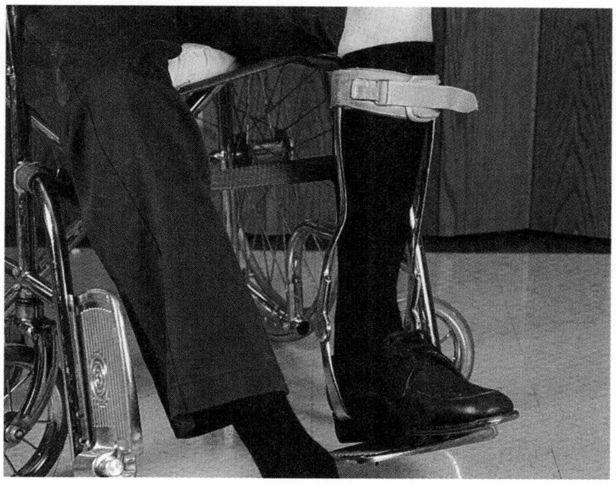

Fig. 19-36 Leg brace.

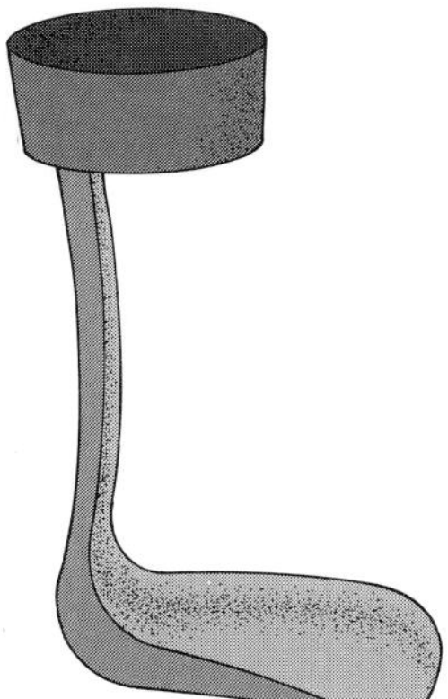

Fig. 19-37 Ankle-foot orthosis (AFO).

RECREATIONAL ACTIVITIES

OBRA OBRA requires activity programs for residents. Recreational activities are important for the physical and mental well-being of older persons. Joints and muscles are exercised, and circulation is stimulated. Recreational activities also provide social opportunities and are mentally stimulating. A good activity program helps to increase a resident's quality of life.

OBRA According to OBRA, activities must meet the interests and physical, mental, and psychosocial needs of each resident. Bingo, movies, dances, exercise groups, shopping trips, museum trips, concerts, and guest speakers are often arranged. Some centers have gardening activities.

OBRA The right to personal choice is protected. The resident chooses which activities to take part in. OBRA requires that activities promote physical, intellectual, social, and emotional well-being. Well-being is promoted when the resident attends activities of personal choice. The resident must not be forced to take part in an activity that has no interest to him or her. OBRA

Residents may need help getting to an activity. Some also need help in participating. You must provide assistance as necessary.

New ideas for activities always are welcome. Residents may share ideas with you or tell you about favorite pastimes. Or you may have ideas of your own. Be sure to share these with the health care team. They can be passed on to the resident group responsible for planning activities. Remember that OBRA also requires that residents be allowed to participate in resident group activities. OBRA

QUALITY OF LIFE

The rights to privacy and personal choice are protected when exercising residents. Make sure the resident's privacy is protected when performing range-of-motion exercises. Also make sure that residents are properly clothed when walking in hallways. The resident's body must not be exposed.

Personal choice in ambulating is encouraged. The person may want to walk outside. The person may prefer to walk in the morning, afternoon, or evening. The resident may want to wait until a family member arrives or leaves. The resident is allowed to make such decisions whenever safe and possible. Be sure to get the nurse's approval.

On subacute care units, it is important to help the person gain strength and independence as quickly as possible. You must know and follow the care plan. This helps the person meet goals and return home if possible.

OBRA requires activity programs for residents. As explained in Chapter 1, activities must meet the interests and physical, mental, and psychosocial needs of each resident. The resident's right to personal choice is protected. The resident is allowed to choose which activities to take part in. The resident must not be forced to take part in an activity that is of no interest to him or her. Remember that OBRA requires that activities promote physical, intellectual, social, and emotional well-being. Well-being is promoted when the resident attends activities of personal choice.

REVIEW QUESTIONS

Circle the BEST answer.

1 Mr. Parker is on bedrest. Which statement is *false?*
- A He has orthostatic hypotension.
- B Bedrest helps reduce pain and promote healing.
- C Complications of bedrest include pressure ulcers, constipation, and blood clots.
- D Contractures and muscle atrophy can occur.

2 Which helps to prevent plantar flexion?
- A Bed boards
- B A footboard
- C Trochanter rolls
- D Hand rolls

3 Which prevents the hip from turning outward?
- A Bed boards
- B A footboard
- C Trochanter roll
- D All of the above

4 A contracture is
- A The loss of muscle strength as a result of inactivity
- B The lack of joint mobility caused by shortening of a muscle
- C A decrease in the size of a muscle
- D All of the above

5 A trapeze is used to
- A Lift the trunk off the bed
- B Move up or turn in bed
- C Strengthen arm muscles
- D All of the above

6 Passive range-of-motion exercises are performed by
- A The resident
- B A health team member
- C The resident with the assistance of another
- D The resident with the use of a trapeze

7 ROM exercises are ordered for Mr. Parker. You should do the following *except*
- A Support the extremity being exercised
- B Move the joint slowly, smoothly, and gently
- C Force the joint through full range of motion
- D Exercise only the joints indicated by the nurse

8 Flexion involves
- A Bending the body part
- B Straightening the body part
- C Moving the body part toward the body
- D Moving the body part away from the body

9 Which statement about ambulation is *false?*
- A A transfer belt is used if the resident is weak or unsteady.
- B The resident is allowed to shuffle or slide when beginning to walk after bedrest.
- C Walking aids may be needed permanently or temporarily.
- D Crutches, canes, walkers, and braces are common walking aids.

10 You are getting a resident ready to crutch walk. You should do the following *except*
- A Check the crutch tips
- B Have the resident wear street shoes
- C Get any pair of crutches from physical therapy
- D Make sure bolts on the crutches are tight

11 A single-tip cane is used
- A At waist level
- B On the strong side
- C On the weak side
- D On either side

Circle T if the statement is true and F if the statement is false.

12 T F A single-tip cane and a four-point cane give equal support.

13 T F When using a cane, the feet are moved first.

14 T F Mr. Parker uses a walker. First he moves the walker in front of him. Then he moves his right foot and left foot forward.

15 T F Mr. Parker starts to fall. You should try to prevent the fall.

16 T F A resident has a brace. Bony areas need protection from skin breakdown.

Answers to these questions are on p. 698.

20 Comfort, Rest, and Sleep

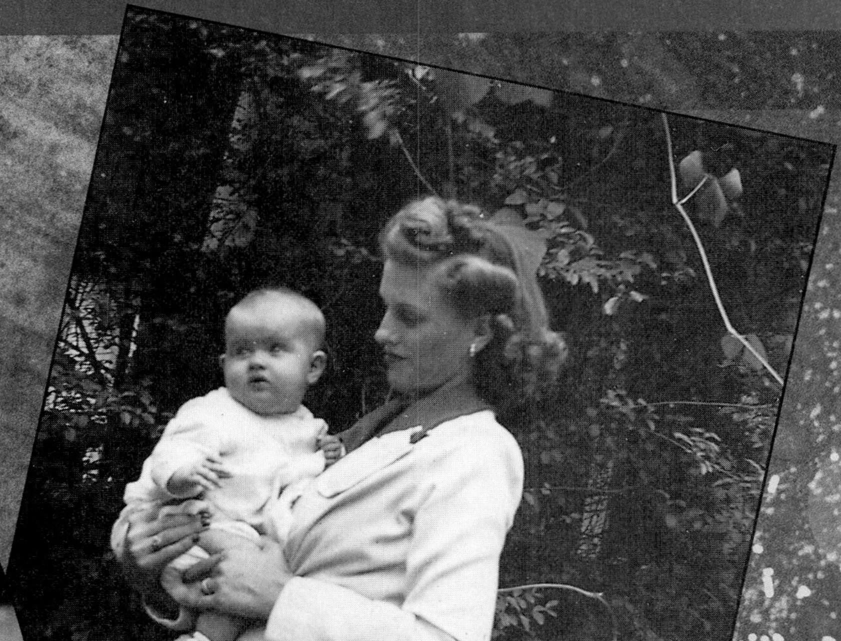

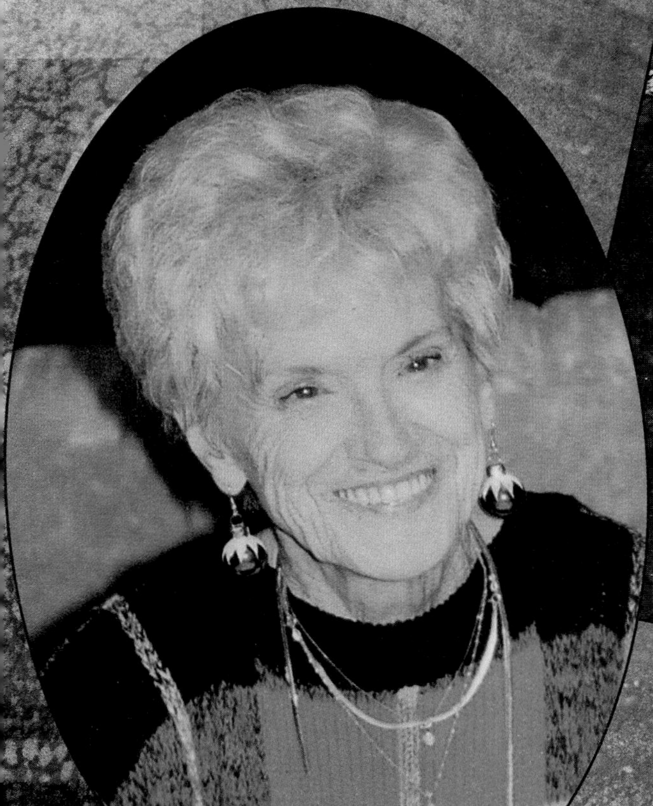

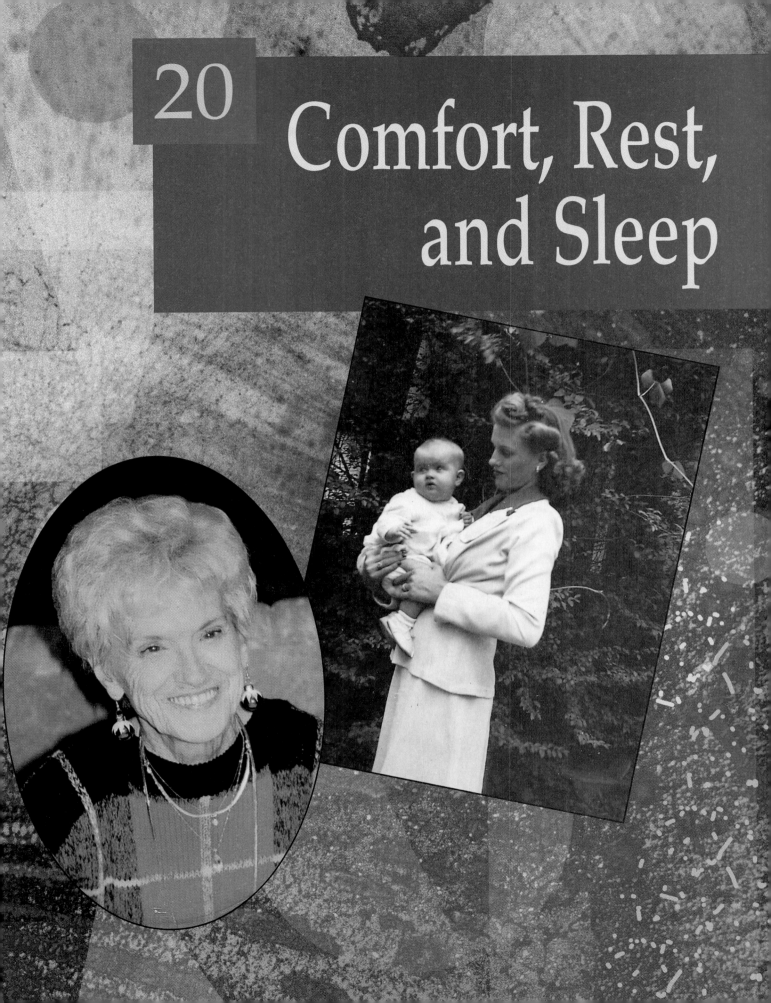

What You Will Learn

- The definition of the key terms listed in this chapter
- Why comfort, rest, and sleep are important
- Four types of pain
- Why pain is a personal experience
- The factors that affect pain
- The signs and symptoms of pain
- The nursing measures that relieve pain
- Why meeting basic needs is important for rest
- The nursing measures that promote rest
- When rest is needed
- The factors that affect sleep
- The common sleep disorders
- Circadian rhythm and how it affects sleep
- The stages of sleep
- The sleep requirements for each age-group
- How dementia affects sleep
- The nursing measures that promote sleep
- The OBRA requirements for comfort, rest, and sleep

Key Terms

acute pain Pain that is felt suddenly from injury, disease, trauma, or surgery; it generally lasts less than 6 months

chronic pain Pain lasting longer than 6 months; it may be constant or occur off and on

circadian rhythm is daily rhythm based on a 24-hour cycle; the day-night cycle or body rhythm

comfort A state of well-being; the person has no physical or emotional pain and is calm and at peace

discomfort To ache, hurt, or be sore; pain

distraction To change a person's center of attention

enuresis Urinary incontinence in bed at night

guided imagery Creating and focusing on an image

insomnia A chronic condition in which the person cannot sleep or stay asleep throughout the night

NREM sleep The stage of sleep when there is no rapid eye movement; nonREM sleep

pain Discomfort

phantom pain Pain felt in a body part that is no longer there

radiating pain Pain felt at the site of tissue damage and in nearby areas

relaxation To be free from mental or physical stress

REM sleep The stage of sleep when there is rapid eye movement

rest To be calm, at ease, and relaxed; to be free of anxiety and stress

sleep A state of unconsciousness, reduced voluntary muscle activity, and lowered metabolism

Comfort, rest, and sleep are needed for well-being. The total person—the physical, emotional, social, and spiritual—is affected by comfort, rest, and sleep problems. Discomfort and pain can be physical or emotional. Whatever the cause, discomfort and pain affect rest and sleep. They also decrease the resident's function and quality of life.

Rest and sleep restore energy and well-being. Illness and injury increase the need for rest and sleep. The body needs more energy for healing and repair. When a resident is ill or injured, he or she needs more energy than normal to perform daily activities. The health care team plays a major role in promoting the resident's comfort, rest, and sleep.

COMFORT

Comfort is a state of well-being. There is no physical or emotional pain. The person is calm and at peace. Age, illness, and activity affect comfort. So do factors like temperature, ventilation, noise, odors, and lighting. The health care team controls these factors to meet the resident's needs.

Temperature and Ventilation

Heating, air conditioning, and ventilation systems maintain comfortable temperatures and provide fresh air. A temperature range of 68° F to 74° F is usually comfortable for most healthy people. A comfortable temperature for one person may be too hot or too cold for another.

Aging results in the loss of the fatty tissue layer. This increases the older person's sensitivity to cold. Higher room temperatures often are necessary (p. 468). Sweaters, lap blankets, socks, and extra blankets often are needed for warmth. Older persons need protection from drafts and extreme cold.

Stale room air and lingering odors affect comfort and rest. A good ventilation system provides fresh air and moves room air. Drafts can occur as air moves. Some residents are sensitive to drafts. Adequate clothing is necessary. Move residents away from drafty areas when possible.

Odors

Many odors are pleasant, like food aromas and flower scents. Others are unpleasant. Wound drainage, vomitus, and bowel movements have unpleasant smells. These odors can embarrass the resident. Body, breath, and smoking odors may offend residents, visitors, and staff. Ill and older persons often have a reduced sense of smell. They may not notice odors. Good nursing care, good ventilation, and good housekeeping practices help eliminate odors. Odors are reduced by:

- Emptying and washing bedpans and kidney basins promptly
- Changing soiled linens promptly
- Cleaning incontinent residents promptly
- Providing good personal hygiene to prevent body and breath odors
- Using room deodorizers when necessary and if allowed by the center
- Emptying waste baskets promptly

Smoke odors cause special problems. Most centers ban smoking. Staff and visitors cannot smoke anywhere in the building. If you smoke, follow the center's policy. Wash your hands after handling smoking materials and before giving care. Smoke odors cling to your uniform, hair, and breath. Your own personal hygiene is important.

OBRA provides for residents who smoke. This is done to provide a homelike setting. The center must allow residents to smoke in an area that maintains their quality of life. Nursing centers often let residents smoke in certain areas. This can be in an outside area if weather permits. The resident and family are informed about the center's smoking policy when the person is admitted to the center.

OBRA

Noise

Ill people are sensitive to noises and sounds around them. They often are disturbed by common health care sounds. The clanging of metal bedpans, urinals, and wash basins is annoying. So is the clatter of dishes and trays. Loud talking and laughing in hallways and at the nurses' station, loud televisions and radios, ringing telephones, signal lights, and buzzing intercoms often are irritating. So is noise from equipment needing repair or oil.

When in a strange place, people want to know the cause and meaning of new sounds. This is part of the basic need for safety and security. Residents may find some sounds dangerous, frightening, or irritating. They may become upset, anxious, and uncomfortable. Remember that noise to one person may not be noise to another. For example, loud stereo music may please a teenager but disturb parents.

Nursing centers are designed to reduce noise. Drapes, carpeting, and acoustical tiles help absorb noise. Plastic items make less noise than metal equipment. Reduce noise by controlling the loudness of your voice. Also handle equipment carefully. Keeping equipment working properly and promptly answering telephones, signal lights, and intercoms also decrease noise.

Lighting

Good lighting is needed for the safety and comfort of residents and staff. Glares, shadows, and dull lighting can cause falls, headaches, and eyestrain. People usually relax and rest better in dim light. However, a bright room is more cheerful and stimulating.

Adjust lighting to meet the resident's changing needs. Pull shades or draw drapes to control natural light. Adjust the overbed light to provide soft, medium, and bright lighting. Some centers have ceiling lights over beds. These provide low to very bright light. Bright lighting is helpful when giving care. Light controls should be within the resident's reach.

OBRA Requirements

OBRA requires that residents receive care that promotes well-being. Comfort, rest, and sleep are necessary for physical, emotional, and mental well-being. OBRA requires that resident rooms be designed and equipped to provide for comfort.

The following OBRA room requirements promote comfort:

OBRA

- No more than four residents in a room
- Suspended curtain that extends around the bed for privacy
- A bed of proper height and size for the resident
- Clean, comfortable mattress
- Linens appropriate to the weather and climate
- Clean and orderly room
- Odor-free room
- Room temperature between 71°F and 81°F
- Acceptable noise level
- Adequate ventilation and room humidity
- Appropriate lighting

PAIN

Discomfort or **pain** means to ache, hurt, or be sore. Discomfort is unpleasant. Comfort and discomfort are subjective (see Chapter 4). That is, you cannot see, hear, touch, or smell the resident's comfort or discomfort. You must rely on what the resident tells you. You must report complaints to the nurse. The information is used for the nursing process. The nurse uses the nursing process to help the health care team plan the resident's care.

Pain is personal. It differs for each person. What *hurts* to one person may *ache* to another. What one person calls *sore*, another may call *aching*. Pain is subjective. If a resident complains of pain or discomfort, the resident *has* pain or discomfort. You must believe the resident. Remember that you cannot see, hear, feel, or smell the pain.

Pain is a warning from the body. It means there is damage to body tissues. Pain often causes the person to seek health care.

Types of Pain

There are different types of pain. The doctor uses the type of pain when diagnosing. The type of pain also is used in the nursing process:

- **Acute pain** is felt suddenly from injury, disease, trauma, or surgery. There is tissue damage. Acute pain lasts a short time—usually less than 6 months. It decreases with healing.
- **Chronic pain** lasts longer than 6 months. Pain is constant or occurs off and on. There is no longer tissue damage. Chronic pain remains long after healing. Arthritis and cancer are common causes of chronic pain.
- **Radiating pain** is felt at the site of tissue damage and in nearby areas. Pain from a heart attack is often felt in the left side of the chest, left jaw, left shoulder, and left arm. A diseased gallbladder can cause pain in the right upper abdomen, the back, and the right shoulder (Fig. 20-1).
- **Phantom pain** is felt in a body part that is no longer there. A person with an amputated leg may still sense leg pain (see Chapter 26).

Factors Affecting Pain

A resident may handle pain well one time and poorly the next time. Many factors can affect reactions to pain.

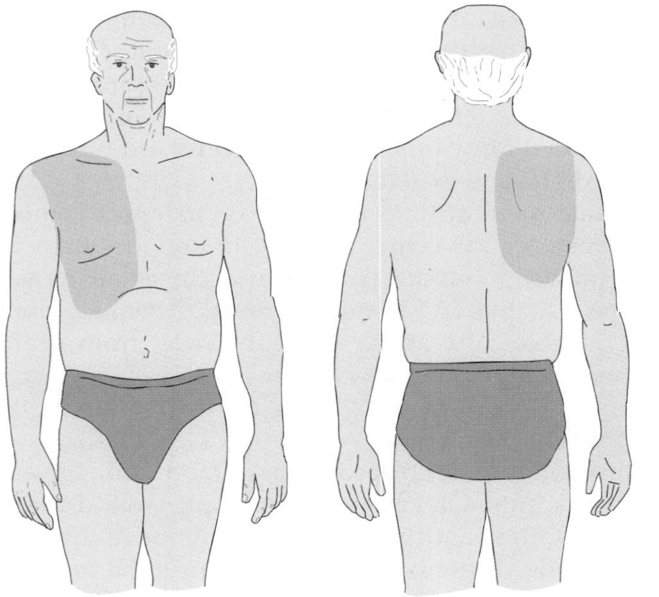

Fig. 20-1 Gallbladder pain radiates to the right upper abdomen, the back, and the right shoulder.

Past experience. We learn from past experiences. They help us know what to do or what to expect. Whether its going to school, driving a car, taking a test, shopping, having a baby, or caring for children, the past prepares us for similar events at another time. We also learn from the past experiences shared by family and friends.

A person may have had pain before. The severity of pain, its cause, how long it lasted, and if relief occurred all affect the person's current response to pain. Knowing what to expect can help or hinder how the person handles pain.

Some people have not had pain. When pain is felt, the person may be very afraid and anxious. Fear and anxiety affect pain.

Anxiety. Anxiety relates to feelings of fear, dread, worry, and concern. The person feels uneasy and tense. The person may feel troubled or threatened or sense danger. Something is wrong but the person does not know what or why.

Pain and anxiety are related. Pain can cause anxiety. Anxiety increases the amount of pain the person feels. Lessening anxiety helps reduce pain. For example, the nurse explains to Mr. Smith that he will have pain after surgery. The nurse also explains that he will receive drugs for pain relief. Mr. Smith knows the cause of the pain and what to expect. This helps reduce his anxiety and therefore the amount of pain felt.

Rest and sleep. Rest and sleep restore energy. They reduce body demands, and the body repairs itself. Lack of needed rest and sleep affects how a person thinks and copes with daily life. Ill and injured persons need more sleep than usual. Many also have pain. Lack of rest and sleep affects how the person deals with pain. Pain seems worse when the person is tired or restless. Also, the person usually pays more attention to pain when tired and unable to rest or sleep.

Attention. The more a person thinks about the pain, the worse it can seem. Sometimes pain is so severe that it is all the person thinks about. However, even mild pain can seem worse if the person thinks about it all the time. Pain often seems worse at night. Activity is less; it is quiet; there are no visitors; the radio or television is off; others are asleep. When unable to sleep the person has time to think about the pain.

Personal and family duties. How a person deals with pain often relates to personal and family obligations. Often pain is ignored if children must be cared for. Some people go to work when having pain. Others deny pain because they fear a serious illness. The illness can interfere with earning money, going to school, or caring for children, a partner, or ill parents.

The value or meaning of pain. Some people view pain as a sign of weakness. It also may mean a serious illness and the need for painful tests and treatments. Therefore pain is ignored or denied. Sometimes pain results in pleasure. The pain of childbirth is one example.

For some persons, pain means not having to work or assume daily routines. Pain is used to avoid certain people or things. Pain is useful for the person. Some people like doting and pampering by others. The person values and wants such attention.

Support from others. Pain is often easier to deal with when family and friends offer comfort and support. The pain of childbirth is easier when a loving father gives support and encouragement. A child bears pain much better when comforted by a caring mother, father, or family member. The use of touch by a valued person is very comforting. Just being nearby also helps.

Some people do not have caring family or friends. They must deal with pain alone. Being alone can increase anxiety. It also gives the person more time to think about the pain. Facing pain alone is hard for everyone, especially children and older persons.

Culture. Culture affects how a person responds to pain. In some cultures the person in pain is *stoic*. To be stoic means to show no reaction to joy, sorrow, pleasure, or pain. Strong verbal and nonverbal reactions to pain are seen in other cultures. (*See Caring About Culture, p. 470.*)

OBRA and JCAHO require the health care team to consider a resident's culture in the care-planning process. Non–English speaking residents may have problems telling the care team about pain. The center must know who these residents are. They must have someone available who can interpret the resident's needs to the care team. All residents have the right to be comfortable and as pain-free as possible. **OBRA**

Age/Illness. Persons with certain diseases may have decreased pain sensations. They do not feel pain, or it may not feel severe. This places them at greater risk for undetected disease or injury. Remember that pain occurs with tissue damage. Therefore pain alerts the person to illness or injury. If pain is not felt, the person does not know to seek health care.

Some older persons have many health problems that cause pain. Chronic pain may mask new pain. Older persons may also ignore or deny new pain. They may think it is related to an existing health problem.

Caring About Culture

Pain Reactions

People of Mexico and the Philippines may appear stoic in reaction to pain. In the Philippines, pain is viewed as the will of God and that God will give strength to bear the pain.

In Vietnam, pain may be severe before pain relief measures are requested. The people of India accept pain quietly and will accept some relief measures. In China, showing emotion is considered a weakness of character. Therefore pain is often suppressed. Pain relief measures must be offered more than once before they are accepted. The people of China find it impolite to accept something the first time it is offered.

Modified from Geissler EM: *Pocket guide to cultural assessment,* ed 2, St Louis, 1998, Mosby.

Residents With Dementia

Residents with dementia may not be able to tell you about their pain. Changes in a resident's usual behavior may mean that the person has pain. A resident who normally moans and groans may become quiet and withdrawn. A resident who is friendly and outgoing may become agitated and aggressive. One who is nonverbal and quiet may become restless and cry easily. Loss of appetite is also a sign of pain. You must report any changes in a resident's usual behavior to the nurse. All residents have the right to have their pain managed correctly.

OBRA: OBRA requires that the nurse do a pain assessment when there is a change in the resident's behavior.

Like other adults, older persons often deny or ignore pain because of what it may mean.

Thinking and reasoning are affected in some older persons. Some cannot verbally communicate pain. Nursing staff must be alert for the signs of pain. (*See Residents With Dementia.)*

Signs and Symptoms

You cannot see, hear, feel, or smell the resident's pain. You must rely on what the resident tells you. Promptly report to the nurse any information you collect about pain. Use the resident's exact words when you report and record. The nurse needs the following information when assessing the resident's pain:

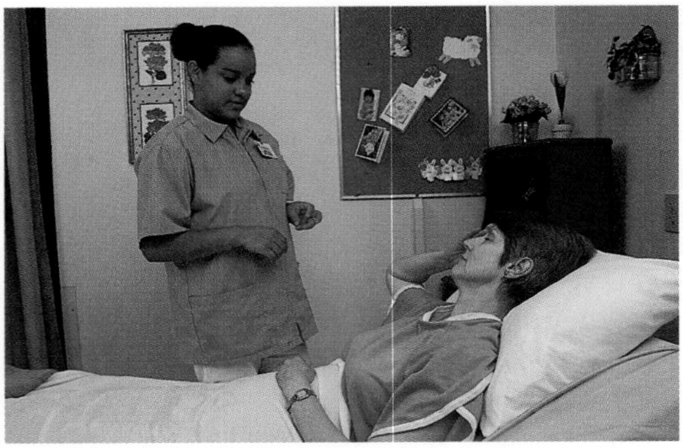

Fig. 20-2 The person points to the area of pain.

Box 20-1 Words Used to Describe Pain

- Aching
- Burning
- Cramping
- Crushing
- Dull
- Gnawing
- Knifelike
- Piercing
- Pressure
- Sharp
- Sore
- Squeezing
- Stabbing
- Throbbing
- Viselike

- ***Location.*** Where is the pain? Ask the resident to point to the area of pain (Fig. 20-2). Remember that pain can radiate. Ask the resident if the pain is anywhere else and to point to those areas.
- ***Onset and duration.*** When did the pain start? How long has the pain lasted?
- ***Intensity.*** Does the resident complain of mild, moderate, or severe pain? Ask the resident to rate the pain on a scale of 1 to 10, with 10 being the most severe.
- ***Description.*** Ask the resident to describe the pain. Box 20-1 lists some words used to describe pain. Write down what the resident says. Use the resident's words when reporting to the nurse.
- ***Factors causing pain.*** These are called *precipitating* factors. To precipitate means to cause. Such factors include moving or turning in bed, coughing or deep breathing, and exercise. Ask what the resident was doing before the pain started and when it started.
- ***Vital signs.*** What are the resident's pulse, respirations, and blood pressure? Increases in these vital signs often occur with pain.
- ***Other signs and symptoms.*** Does the resident have other symptoms: dizziness, nausea, vomiting, weakness, numbness or tingling, or others? Box 20-2 lists the signs and symptoms that often occur with pain.

Nursing Measures

The nurse uses the nursing process to promote comfort and relieve pain. Box 20-3 lists the nursing measures that are often part of care plans. You learned how to perform most of the measures in earlier chapters (Fig. 20-3, p. 472). You also learned why they are important for comfort.

Other measures often are needed to control pain. These include distraction, relaxation, and guided imagery. Nurses, physical therapists, occupational therapists, and recreational therapists may assist residents with these measures. The nurse or therapist may ask you to assist with these measures. The nurse or therapist instructs you on how to properly perform them.

Distraction means to change the resident's center of attention. The resident's attention is moved away from the pain. Listening to music, playing games, singing, praying, watching television, and needlework are some ways to distract attention (Fig. 20-4, p. 472).

Relaxation means to be free from mental and physical stress. This state reduces pain and anxiety. The nurse or therapist teaches the resident relaxation techniques. The resident is taught to breathe deeply and slowly and to contract and relax muscle groups. A comfortable position and a quiet room are important.

Box 20-2 Signs and Symptoms of Pain

Body Responses
- Increased pulse, respirations, and blood pressure
- Sweating (diaphoresis)
- Nausea
- Vomiting
- Pale skin (pallor)

Behaviors
- Changes in speech: slow or rapid; loud or quiet
- Crying
- Gasping
- Grimacing

Behaviors—cont'd
- Groaning
- Grunting
- Holding the affected body part (splinting)
- Irritability
- Maintaining one position; refusing to move
- Moaning
- Quietness
- Restlessness
- Rubbing
- Screaming

Box 20-3 Nursing Measures to Promote Comfort and Relieve Pain

- Position the resident in good body alignment; use pillows for support.
- Keep bed linens tight and wrinkle free.
- Make sure the resident is not lying on drainage tubes.
- Assist the resident to the bathroom or commode, or offer the bedpan or urinal.
- Provide blankets for warmth and to prevent chilling.
- Use correct lifting, moving, and turning procedures.
- Wait one-half hour after pain medication was given before performing procedures.
- Give a back massage.
- Provide soft music to distract the resident.
- Use touch to provide comfort.
- Allow family members and friends at the bedside as requested by the resident.
- Avoid sudden or jarring movements of the bed.
- Handle the resident gently.
- Practice safety measures if the resident is receiving strong pain medication or sedatives:
  - Keep the bed in the low position.
  - Raise bed rails as directed. Follow the care plan.
  - Check on the resident every 10 to 15 minutes.
  - Provide assistance when the resident is up.
- Apply warm or cold applications as directed by the nurse (see Chapter 24).
- Provide a calm, quiet, darkened environment.

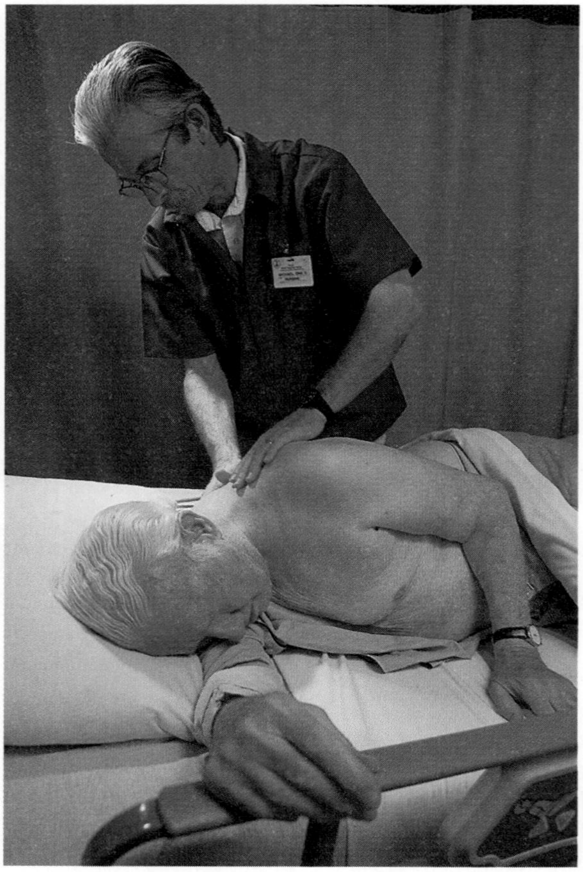

Fig. 20-3 Measures are implemented to relieve pain. The person is positioned in good body alignment with pillows used for support. The room is darkened. Blankets provide warmth. A back massage provides touch and promotes relaxation.

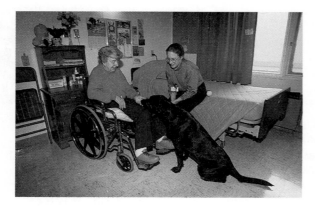

Fig. 20-4 A comforting pet can provide needed distraction from pain.

Guided imagery is creating and focusing on an image. The resident is asked to create a pleasant scene. This is noted on the care plan so all staff use the same image with the resident. The nurse or therapist uses a calm, soft voice when helping the resident focus on the image. Soft music, a blanket for warmth, and a darkened room may help. The nurse or therapist coaches the resident to focus on the image and then to practice relaxation exercises.

Doctors often order drugs to control or relieve pain. Nurses give these drugs. Such drugs can cause orthostatic hypotension, drowsiness, dizziness, and coordination problems. Therefore the resident is protected from injury, falls, and fractures. The nurse alerts you to any needed safety measures. Specific safety measures for the resident are found in the care plan.

REST

Rest means being calm, at ease, and relaxed. The resident is free of anxiety and stress. Rest may involve physical inactivity. Or the resident may do things that he or she finds calming and relaxing. Examples include reading, music, television, needlework, prayer, gardening, baking, golf, walking, and carpentry (Fig. 20-5).

Basic needs must be met for a resident to rest. Thirst, hunger, elimination needs, and pain or discomfort can affect rest. You can promote rest by meeting physical needs. A comfortable position and good body alignment also are important. A quiet environment promotes rest. So does a clean, dry, and wrinkle-free bed. Some residents rest easier in a clean, neat, and uncluttered room.

Safety and security needs must be met. The resident must feel safe from falling or other injuries. The resident is secure with the signal light within reach. Understanding the reasons for treatments also helps the resident feel safe. So does knowing how procedures are done. That is why you always explain the procedure before it is performed.

Many residents have rituals or routines before resting. These may include going to the bathroom, brushing teeth, washing the face and hands, praying, having a snack or beverage, locking doors, or making sure children or loved ones are safe at home. The resident may want a favorite blanket or afghan. Follow routines and rituals whenever possible.

Love and belonging are important for rest. Visits or telephone calls from family and friends may help the resident relax. The resident knows that others care and are concerned. Reading cards and letters may also help the resident relax and rest (Fig. 20-6).

Esteem needs relate to feeling good about oneself. A resident may find hospital gowns embarrassing. Others fear exposure. Many residents rest better wearing their own gown or pajamas. Personal appearance also affects esteem. Hair care, being clean and free of body odors, and other hygiene and grooming measures all help people feel good about themselves. If esteem needs are met, the resident may rest easier.

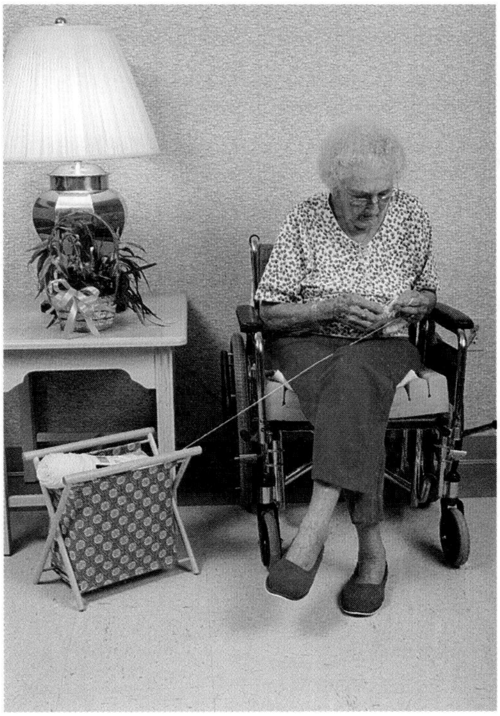

Fig. 20-5 Needlework is relaxing for this lady.

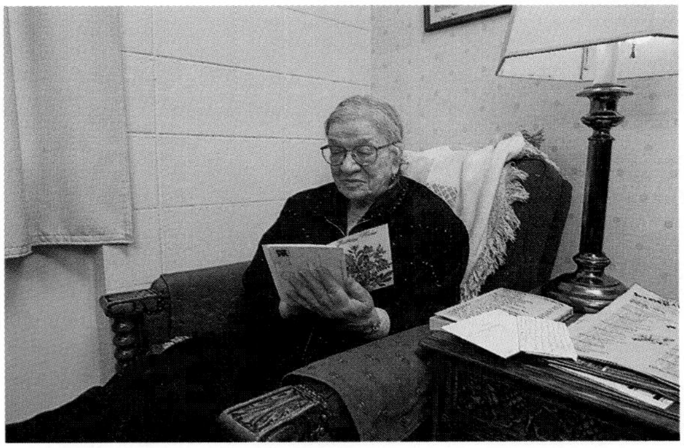

Fig. 20-6 The resident reads cards and letters from family and friends.

Some people are refreshed after resting for 15 or 20 minutes. Others need more time. Health care routines usually allow time for afternoon rest.

Ill or injured residents need to rest more often. Some need to rest during or after a procedure. For example, a bath tires Mr. Smith. So does getting dressed. You need to let him rest before making the bed. Some people need a few hours to complete oral hygiene, bathing, grooming, and dressing. Others need to rest after meals. Do not push the resident beyond his or her limits. Allow rest periods as they are needed. Do not rush the resident.

Distraction, relaxation, and guided imagery also promote rest. So does a back massage. You must plan and organize care so that the resident can rest without interruptions.

The doctor may order bedrest for a resident. Bedrest, its complications, and how to prevent complications are presented in Chapter 19.

SLEEP

Sleep is a state of unconsciousness, reduced voluntary muscle activity, and lowered metabolism. An unconscious person is unaware of the environment and cannot respond to people and things in the environment. The unconsciousness is temporary. People awake from sleep. Alarm clocks, voices, and crying babies easily awaken sleeping persons. Voluntary muscles are skeletal muscles. During sleep, there are no voluntary arm or leg movements. Metabolism is the burning of food and energy for use by the body. Less energy is needed during sleep. Thus metabolism is reduced during sleep.

Sleep is a basic need. It lets the mind and body rest. The body saves energy. Body functions slow. Vital signs fall. That is, blood pressure, temperature, and pulse and respiration rates are lower than when awake. Tissue healing and repair occur during sleep. Sleep lowers stress, tension, and anxiety. It refreshes and renews the person. That is, the person regains energy and mental alertness. The person thinks and functions better after needed sleep.

Circadian Rhythm

Sleep occurs regularly. It is part of circadian rhythm. Circadian comes from the Latin words *circa* meaning *about* and *dies* meaning *day*. **Circadian rhythm** is a pattern based on a 24-hour cycle. It is a daily rhythm called the *day-night cycle* or *body rhythm*. Functioning is affected by circadian rhythm. Some people function better in the morning. They are more alert and active; they think and react better. Others do better in the evening.

Circadian rhythm includes a sleep-wake cycle. The person's *biological clock* signals the time for sleep and the time to wake up. You have usual times for going to sleep and waking up. You may awaken before the alarm clock goes off. That is all part of your biological clock. Health care centers often interfere with a person's circadian rhythm and the sleep-wake cycle. Sleep problems easily occur.

Many people work evening and night shifts. They include health care workers, police officers, fire fighters, fast food workers, and factory workers. Their bodies must adjust to changes in the sleep-wake cycle.

Sleep Cycle

There are two phases of sleep. Nonrapid eye movement is **NREM sleep** *or nonREM sleep.* NREM sleep has four stages. Sleep goes from light to deep as the person moves through the four stages.

The rapid eye movement phase is called **REM sleep**. The person is hard to arouse. Mental restoration occurs during REM sleep. Events and problems of the previous day are thought to be reviewed during REM sleep. The person prepares for the next day.

Box 20-4 shows the stages of NREM and REM sleep. There are usually 4 to 6 cycles of NREM and REM sleep during the 7 to 8 hours of sleep each night. Stage 1 of NREM is usually not repeated.

Sleep Requirements

The amount of sleep needed varies for each age-group. The amount needed decreases with age (Table 20-1). Infants need more sleep than toddlers. Toddlers need more than preschool children. School-age children need more than teenagers. Older persons need less sleep than middle-age adults.

Table 20-1 Average Sleep Requirements

Age-Group	Hours Per Day
Newborns (birth to 4 weeks)	14 to 18
Infants (4 weeks to 1 year)	12 to 14
Toddlers (1 to 3 years)	11 to 12
Preschoolers (3 to 6 years)	11 to 12
Middle and late childhood (6 to 12 years)	10 to 11
Adolescents (12 to 18 years)	8 to 9
Young adults (18 to 40 years)	7 to 8
Middle-age adults (40 to 65 years)	7
Older adults (65 years and older)	5 to 7

Box 20-4 Sleep Cycle

Stage 1: NREM Sleep
- Lightest sleep level
- Lasts a few minutes
- Gradual fall in vital signs
- Gradual lowering of metabolism
- Feels drowsy and relaxed
- Easily aroused
- Daydreaming feeling after being aroused

Stage 2: NREM Sleep
- Sound sleep
- Relaxation increases
- Still easy to arouse
- Lasts 10 to 20 minutes
- Body functions continue to slow

Stage 3: NREM Sleep
- First stages of deep sleep
- Hard to arouse
- Rarely moves
- Muscles relax completely
- Vital signs fall
- Lasts 15 to 30 minutes

Stage 4: NREM Sleep
- Deepest stage of sleep
- Hard to arouse
- Body rests and is restored
- Vital signs much lower than when awake
- Lasts about 15 to 30 minutes
- Sleepwalking and enuresis (urinary incontinence in bed at night) may occur

REM Sleep
- Vivid, full-color dreaming
- Usually starts 50 to 90 minutes after sleep has begun
- Rapid eye movements
- Blood pressure, pulse, and respirations may fluctuate
- Voluntary muscles are relaxed
- Mental restoration occurs
- Hard to arouse
- Lasts about 20 minutes

Modified from Potter PA, Perry AG: *Fundamentals of nursing: concepts, process and practice*, ed 4, St Louis, 1997, Mosby.

Factors Affecting Sleep

Several factors affect the amount and quality of sleep. Quality relates to how well the person slept and if needed amounts of NREM and REM sleep were obtained:

- ***Illness.*** Illness increases the need for sleep. However, the signs and symptoms of illness can interfere with sleep. They include pain, nausea, vomiting, coughing, difficulty breathing, diarrhea, frequent voiding, and itching. Treatments and therapies also can interfere with sleep. Often residents are awakened for treatments or medications. Traction or a cast can cause uncomfortable positions. The emotional effects of illness can affect sleep. These include fear, anxiety, and worry.
- ***Nutrition.*** Weight loss or gain affects sleep. The need for sleep increases with weight gain. It decreases with weight loss. Some foods affect sleep. Those with caffeine (chocolate, coffee, tea, and colas) prevent sleep. The protein L-tryptophan tends to help sleep. It is found in milk, cheese, and beef.
- ***Exercise.*** Exercise is good for the body. It improves health and fitness. Exercise requires energy. The person usually feels good after exercising. Eventually the person tires. Being tired helps the person sleep well at night. Exercising right before bedtime interferes with sleep. Exercise causes the release of substances into the bloodstream that stimulate the body. Therefore there should be at least 2 hours between exercise and bedtime.
- ***Environment.*** People adjust to their usual sleep settings. They get used to such things as the bed, pillows, noises in the home or neighborhood, lighting, and a sleeping partner. Any change in the usual setting can affect the amount and quality of sleep.
- ***Drugs and other substances.*** Some drugs promote sleep. These are commonly called *sleeping pills.* Drugs given for anxiety, depression, and pain may cause the person to sleep. However, these drugs and sleeping pills reduce the length of REM sleep. Remember that mental restoration occurs during REM sleep. Behavior problems and sleep deprivation can occur. Alcohol is a drug. Alcohol tends to cause drowsiness and sleep. However, it interferes with REM sleep. Those under the influence of alcohol may awaken during sleep. Difficulty returning to sleep is common. Some drugs contain caffeine. As stated earlier, caffeine is a stimulant and prevents sleep. Besides in drugs, it is found in coffee, tea, chocolate, and colas. The side effects of some drugs can disrupt sleep. These include frequent voiding and nightmares.
- ***Life-style changes.*** Life-style relates to a person's daily routines and way of living. Work, school, play, and social events are all part of life-style. Life-style changes can affect sleep. Travel, vacation, and social events often affect usual bedtimes and when the person awakens. Children usually stay up later during school holidays. They may sleep later too. If work hours change, the person needs to change sleep hours. Such changes affect normal sleep-wake cycles and the circadian rhythm.
- ***Emotional problems.*** Fear, worry, depression, and anxiety affect sleep. These may be caused by work, personal, or family problems. Loss of a close family member or friend is another cause. Money problems are stressful. People may have difficulty falling asleep, or they awaken often. Difficulty getting back to sleep may occur.

Sleep Disorders

Sleep disorders involve repeated sleep problems. The amount and quality of sleep are affected. Sleep disorders affect life-style. Box 20-5 on p. 476 lists the signs and symptoms that occur.

Insomnia.

Insomnia is a chronic condition in which the person cannot sleep or stay asleep throughout the night. There are three forms of insomnia:

- Unable to fall asleep
- Unable to stay asleep
- Early awakening and unable to fall back asleep

Emotional problems are common causes of insomnia. The fear of dying during sleep is another cause. Some people are afraid of not waking up. This may occur after recent heart disease or after being told of a terminal illness. The fear of not being able to sleep is another cause. The physical and emotional discomforts of illness also can cause insomnia.

The health care team plans measures to promote sleep (p. 476). However, the emotional or physical problems causing the insomnia also are treated.

Sleep deprivation.

With sleep deprivation, the amount and quality of sleep are decreased. Sleep is interrupted. NREM and REM sleep stages are not completed. Illness, pain, and hospital care are common causes of sleep deprivation. Patients in intensive care units (ICUs) are at great risk. ICU lights are on much of the time. The many care measures and sounds from equipment interfere with sleep. Factors that affect sleep can also lead to sleep deprivation. Sleep deprivation results in many of the signs and symptoms listed in Box 20-5.

Sleepwalking.

The person who sleepwalks leaves the bed and walks about. The person is not aware of sleepwalking and has no memory of the event on awakening. Children sleepwalk more than adults. The event may last 3 to 4 minutes or longer.

Box 20-5 Signs and Symptoms of Sleep Disorders

- Hand tremors
- Slowed responses to questions, conversations, or situations
- Reduced word memory; difficulty finding the right word
- Decreased reasoning and judgment
- Irregular pulse
- Redness and puffiness around the eyes
- Dark circles under the eyes
- Moodiness; mood swings
- Disorientation
- Irritability
- Fatigue
- Sleepiness
- Agitation
- Restlessness
- Decreased attention
- Hallucinations (see Chapter 26)
- Coordination problems
- Slurred speech

Stress, fatigue, and some drugs can cause sleepwalking. A resident who sleepwalks needs protection from injury. The risk of falling is great. Intravenous infusions, catheters, nasogastric tubes, and other tubings are possible sources of injury. The tubes or catheters can be pulled out of the body when the resident gets out of bed. Guide sleepwalkers back to bed. They startle easily. Awaken them gently.

Residents With Dementia

Frequent sleep disturbances are common in residents with Alzheimer's disease and other types of dementia. Night wandering is common. Restlessness and confusion often increase at night. This increases the risk of falls. Quietly and calmly directing the resident to his or her room is often helpful. Allowing nighttime wandering in a safe and supervised setting is the best approach for some residents. Other measures listed in Box 20-6 also are tried. Specific measures for a resident are in the care plan.

Promoting Sleep

The nurse assesses the resident's sleep patterns. Your observations are important. Report any of the signs and symptoms listed in Box 20-5. The health care team plans measures to promote sleep (Box 20-6). Check the care plan so that you give the correct care. *(See Residents With Dementia.)* Also report your observations so the nurse can evaluate if the goal of a regular sleep pattern was met.

Many residents have specific rituals and routines before bedtime. They are allowed if safe. The resident may perform personal hygiene measures in a certain order. Some residents like to check on friends in the center before going to bed. Some are given the responsibility of turning off lights at bedtime. A bedtime snack may be important. Watching certain television shows in bed is a bedtime routine for some persons. Others may read religious writings, pray, or say a rosary before going to sleep. Whatever the routine or ritual, it is important to the resident.

The resident is involved in planning care. The resident is allowed to choose when to take a nap or go to sleep. The resident also has the right to choose what measures are helpful in promoting comfort, rest, and sleep. You must follow the care plan and the resident's wishes.

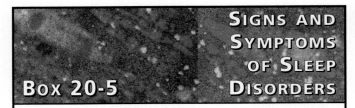

Box 20-6 Nursing Measures to Promote Sleep

- Organize care to allow for uninterrupted rest.
- Avoid physical activity before bedtime.
- Encourage the resident to avoid tending to business or family matters before bedtime.
- Allow a flexible bedtime. Bedtime is when the resident is tired and fatigued—not a certain time.
- Provide a comfortable room temperature.
- Allow the resident to take a warm bath or shower.
- Provide a bedtime snack (milk).
- Avoid caffeine (coffee, tea, colas, and chocolate).
- Avoid alcoholic beverages.
- Have the resident void before going to bed. Make sure incontinent residents are clean and dry.
- Follow bedtime rituals.
- Make sure the resident wears loose-fitting nightwear.
- Provide adequate warmth (blankets, socks) for those who tend to be cold.
- Reduce noise.
- Darken the room by closing shades, blinds, and the privacy curtain. Shut off or dim lights.
- Dim lights in hallways and the nursing unit.
- Make sure linens are clean, dry, and wrinkle free.
- Position the resident in good alignment.
- Support body parts as ordered.
- Make sure the resident is in a comfortable position.
- Give a back massage.
- Implement measures to relieve pain.
- Allow the resident to read. Read to children.
- Allow the resident to listen to music.
- Allow the resident to watch television.
- Assist with relaxation exercises as ordered.
- Sit and talk with residents.

Quality of Life

Comfort, rest, and sleep are important for quality of life and well-being. OBRA has certain requirements that promote the resident's comfort, rest, and sleep. They relate to the bed, mattress, room temperature, noise level, lighting, linens, odors, and number of residents in each room. The right to personal choice and being involved in planning care are other ways to promote the resident's comfort, rest, and sleep.

Residents have the right to have their pain assessed and managed. Untreated pain decreases the resident's quality of life. You must know the signs and symptoms of pain to help the nurse meet the resident's needs.

REVIEW QUESTIONS

Circle the BEST answer.

1 These statements are about pain. Which is *false?*
- A Pain is objective. It can be seen, heard, smelled, or felt.
- B Pain is a warning from the body. It means there is damage to tissues.
- C Pain is personal. It is different for each person.
- D Pain is used to make diagnoses.

2 A resident complains of pain in the left side of the chest, up into the left jaw, and down to the left shoulder and left arm. This is
- A Acute pain
- B Chronic pain
- C Radiating pain
- D Phantom pain

3 Mr. Smith complains of pain. You should do the following *except*
- A Ask him to point to where the pain is felt
- B Ask him when the pain started
- C Ask him to describe the pain
- D Ask to look at the pain

4 The nurse gives Mr. Smith a drug for pain. A procedure is scheduled for this time. You should
- A Perform the procedure before the drug is given
- B Perform the procedure right after the drug is given
- C Wait one-half hour to let the drug take effect
- D Omit the procedure for the day

5 Mr. Smith is protected from injury after receiving a drug for pain relief. You should do the following *except*
- A Keep the bed in the high position
- B Raise bed rails as directed
- C Check on him every 10 to 15 minutes
- D Provide assistance if he needs to get up

6 Which measure will not help relieve pain?
- A Providing blankets as needed
- B Keeping the room well lighted
- C Providing soft music
- D Giving a back massage

7 Mr. Smith's care plan has the following nursing measures. Which will *not* help him rest or sleep?
- A Have the resident urinate before rest or sleep.
- B Assist the resident to assume a comfortable position.
- C Assist the resident to ambulate before rest or sleep.
- D Allow him to choose sleep attire.

8 Mr. Smith tires very easily. His morning care includes a bath, hair care, and getting dressed. His bed is made after he is dressed. When should he rest?
- A After morning care is completed
- B After his bath and before hair care
- C After you make the bed
- D Whenever he needs to

9 These statements are about sleep. Which is *false?*
- A Tissue healing and repair occur during sleep.
- B Voluntary muscle activity increases during sleep.
- C Sleep refreshes and renews the person.
- D All of the above

10 Mr. Smith was awake several nights when he first entered the center. Which is *false?*
- A His circadian rhythm may be affected.
- B NREM and REM sleep are affected.
- C His biological clock will still tell him when to sleep and wake up.
- D His functioning is affected.

11 Mr. Smith is 70 years old. When healthy, he probably needs about
- A 12 to 14 hours of sleep per day
- B 8 to 9 hours of sleep per day
- C 7 to 8 hours of sleep per day
- D About 6 hours of sleep per day

12 Mr. Smith asks for a snack. He said a friend brought him a chocolate chip cheesecake and some beef summer sausage. He asks for milk with his snack. Which prevents sleep?
- A Chocolate
- B Cheese
- C Milk
- D Beef

REVIEW QUESTIONS—cont'd

13 Mr. Smith has difficulty sleeping, and he awakens several times during the night. He has difficulty answering your questions and seems moody. His pulse is irregular, and his eyes are red and puffy. He is showing signs of

A Insomnia
B Sleep deprivation
C Enuresis
D Distraction

14 These measures are part of Mr. Smith's care plan. Which should you question?

A Let Mr. Smith choose his bedtime.
B Provide a bedtime snack of hot tea and a cheese sandwich.
C Make sure his cast is properly supported.
D Follow his bedtime rituals.

Circle T if the statement is true and F if the statement is false.

15 T F Changes in a resident's usual behavior may be a sign of pain.

16 T F Residents with dementia usually sleep well at night.

17 T F A resident's culture may affect how he or she reacts to pain.

Answers to these questions are on p. 699.

21 Measuring Vital Signs

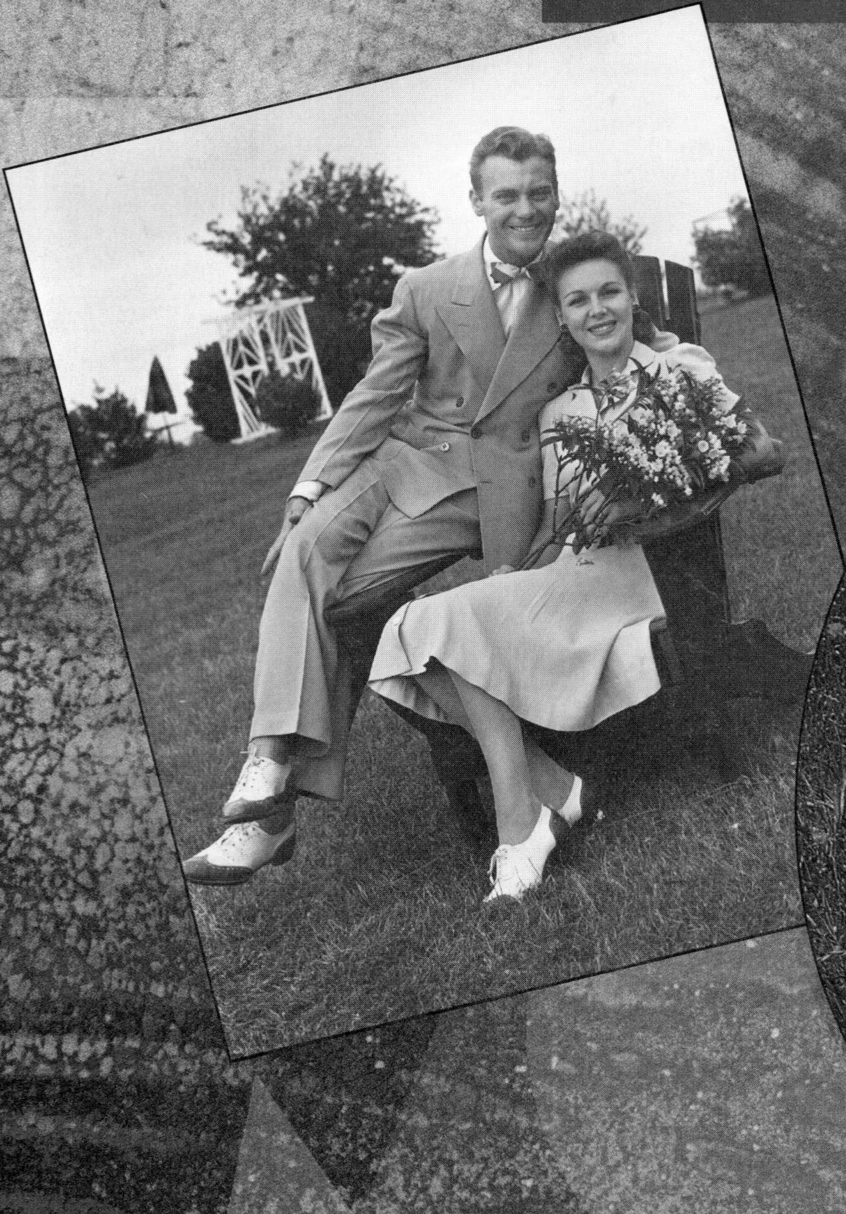

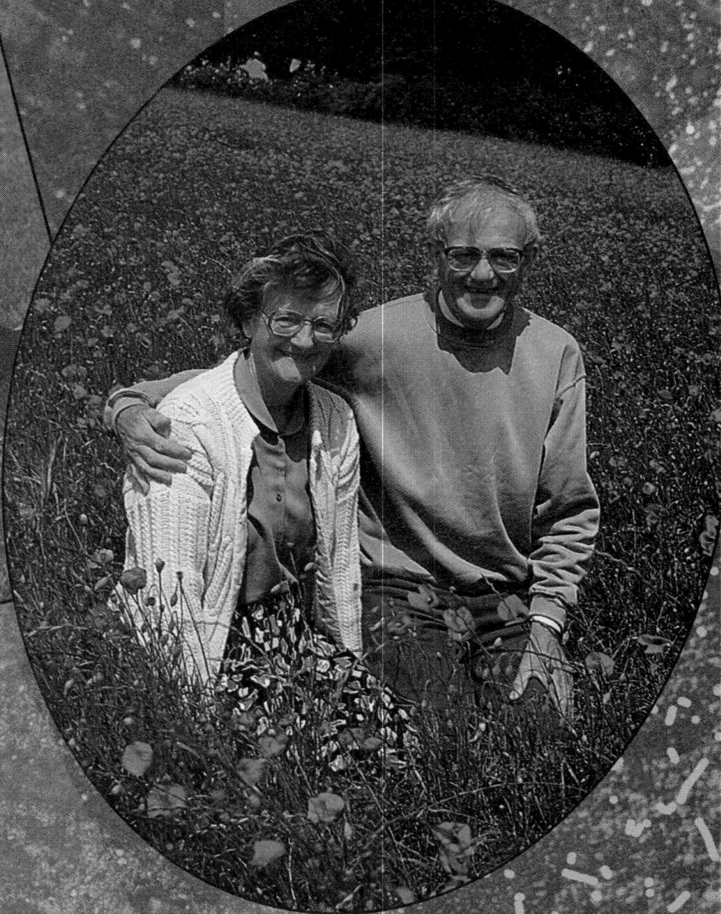

What You Will Learn

- The definition of the key terms listed in this chapter
- Why vital signs are measured
- The factors affecting vital signs
- The normal ranges of oral, rectal, axillary, and tympanic membrane temperatures
- When to take oral, rectal, axillary, and tympanic membrane temperatures
- The sites for taking a pulse
- The characteristics of normal respirations
- The factors affecting blood pressure
- The practices to follow when measuring blood pressure
- The normal pulse, respiration, and blood pressure ranges for different age-groups
- The procedures described in this chapter

Key Terms

apical-radial pulse Taking the apical and radial pulses at the same time

blood pressure The amount of force exerted against the walls of an artery by the blood

body temperature The amount of heat in the body that is a balance between the amount of heat produced and the amount lost by the body

bradycardia A slow *(brady)* heart rate *(cardia)*; the rate is less than 60 beats per minute

diastole The period of heart muscle relaxation

diastolic pressure The pressure in the arteries when the heart is at rest

hypertension Persistent blood pressure measurements above *(hyper)* the normal systolic (140 mm Hg) or diastolic (90 mm Hg) pressures

hypotension A condition in which the systolic blood pressure is below *(hypo)* 90 mm Hg and the diastolic pressure is below 60 mm Hg

pulse The beat of the heart felt at an artery as a wave of blood passes through the artery

pulse deficit The difference between the apical and radial pulse rates

pulse rate The number of heartbeats or pulses felt in 1 minute

respiration The act of breathing air into (inhalation) and out of (exhalation) the lungs

sphygmomanometer The instrument used to measure blood pressure

stethoscope An instrument used to listen to the sounds produced by the heart, lungs, and other body organs

systole The period of heart muscle contraction

systolic pressure The amount of force it takes to pump blood out of the heart into the arterial circulation

tachycardia A rapid *(tachy)* heart rate *(cardia)*; the heart rate is more than 100 beats per minute

vital signs Temperature, pulse, respirations, and blood pressure

▲ Vital signs reflect the function of three body processes essential for life: regulation of body temperature, breathing, and heart function. The four **vital signs** of body function are temperature, pulse, respirations, and blood pressure.

MEASURING AND REPORTING VITAL SIGNS

A person's vital signs vary within certain limits during any 24-hour period. Many factors affect vital signs. They include sleep, activity, eating, weather, noise, exercise, drugs, fear, anxiety, pain, and illness.

Vital signs are measured to detect changes in normal body function. They tell about a person's response to treatment. They often signal life-threatening events. Vital signs are part of the assessment step of the nursing process. Vital signs are measured:

- During physical examinations
- When a person is admitted to the nursing center
- Several times a day for persons in subacute care units
- Before and after surgery
- Before and after complex procedures or diagnostic tests
- After some nursing procedures or measures, such as ambulation
- When drugs are taken that affect the respiratory or circulatory system
- Whenever the resident complains of pain, fainting, shortness of breath, rapid heart rate, or not feeling well
- As stated on the care plan (Nursing center residents have vital signs measured daily or weekly. Follow the resident's care plan and the nurse's instructions for taking the person's vital signs.)

Vital signs show even minor changes in a resident's condition. Accuracy is essential in measuring, recording, and reporting vital signs. If unsure of your measurements, promptly ask the nurse to take them again. Unless otherwise ordered, take vital signs with the resident lying or sitting. The resident is at rest when vital signs are measured. Immediately report the following to the nurse:

- Any vital sign that is changed from a previous measurement
- Vital signs above the normal range
- Vital signs below the normal range

Many centers have *temp boards* or *TPR books.* These are divided into columns. Resident names are listed down the left side of the page. The other columns are for times (such as 0800, 1200, 1600, 2000). Vital signs are recorded on the line in the column appropriate for the resident and time. In some centers, changed or abnormal vital signs are circled in red. The nurse or doctor compares current and previous measurements.

BODY TEMPERATURE

Body temperature is the amount of heat in the body. It is a balance between the amount of heat produced and the amount lost by the body. Heat is produced as cells use food for energy. It is lost through the skin, breathing, urine, and feces. Body temperature stays fairly stable. It is lower in the morning and higher in the afternoon and evening. Factors affecting body temperature include age, weather, exercise, pregnancy, the menstrual cycle, emotions, stress, and illness.

Normal Body Temperature

Temperature is measured using the Fahrenheit (F) and Centigrade or Celsius (C) scales. Common sites for measuring body temperature are the mouth, rectum, axilla (underarm), and ear (tympanic membrane). Normal body temperature depends on the site and usually stays within a normal range (Table 21-1).

Older persons generally have a lower body temperature than younger adults. An oral temperature of 98.6° F may signal fever in an older person. Always report temperatures that are above the lower end of the normal range.

Thermometers are used to measure temperature. Glass and disposable thermometers are common in homes. So are tympanic thermometers. Electronic and tympanic thermometers are common in hospitals and nursing centers. Glass and disposable thermometers also are used for residents requiring Transmission-Based Precautions.

Glass Thermometers

The glass thermometer (clinical thermometer) is a hollow glass tube with a mercury-filled bulb (Fig. 21-1). When heated, the mercury expands and rises in the tube. The mercury contracts and moves down the tube when cooled.

Long-tip or slender-tip thermometers are used for oral and axillary temperatures. So are thermometers with stubby and pear-shaped tips. Rectal thermometers have stubby tips that are color coded in red.

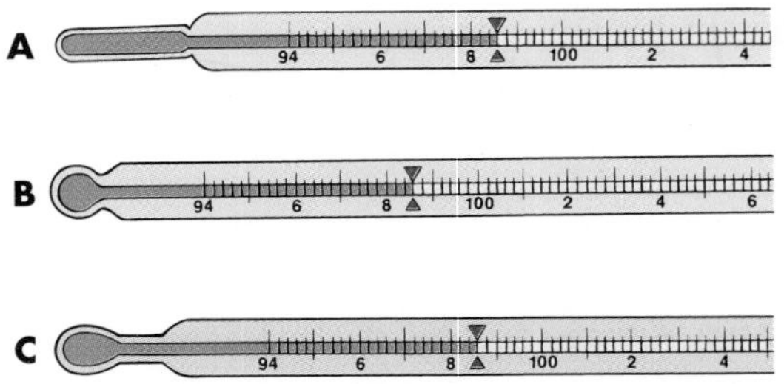

Fig. 21-1 Types of glass thermometers. **A,** The long or slender tip. **B,** The stubby tip (rectal thermometer). **C,** The pear-shaped tip.

TABLE 21-1 NORMAL BODY TEMPERATURES

Site	Baseline	Normal Range
Oral	98.6° F (37° C)	97.6° to 99.6° F (36.5 to 37.5° C)
Rectal	99.6° F (37.6° C)	98.6° to 100.6° F (37.0° to 38.1° C)
Axillary	97.6° F (36.5° C)	96.6° to 98.6° F (35.9° to 37.0° C)
Tympanic membrane	98.6° F (37° C)	98.6° F (37° C)

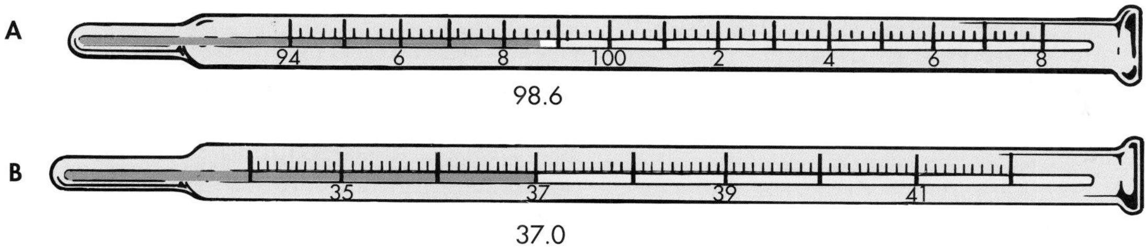

Fig. 21-2 **A,** Fahrenheit thermometer. The mercury level is at 98.6° F. **B,** Centigrade thermometer. The mercury level is at 37.0° C.

Glass thermometers are reusable. However, they have the following disadvantages:

- They take a long time to register—3 to 10 minutes depending on the site. Oral temperatures take 2 to 3 minutes, rectal temperatures take at least 2 minutes, and axillary temperatures take 5 to 10 minutes.
- They break easily. Broken rectal thermometers can injure the rectum and colon.
- The resident may bite down on an oral thermometer and cause it to break. Cuts to the oral mucous membranes are risks. Any swallowed mercury can cause mercury poisoning.

NOTE: *If a glass thermometer breaks, you must report it to the nurse immediately. Mercury is a hazardous substance and requires special disposal procedures. Do not touch the mercury, and do not let the resident do so. The center must follow special procedures for handling all hazardous materials. See Chapter 8.*

How to read a glass thermometer.

Fahrenheit thermometers have both long and short lines. Every other long line is marked in an even degree from 94° to 108° F. The short lines indicate 0.2 (two tenths) of a degree (Fig. 21-2, *A*).

Centigrade thermometers also have both long and short lines. Each long line represents 1 degree, from 34° to 42° C. Each short line represents 0.1 (one tenth) of a degree (Fig. 21-2, *B*).

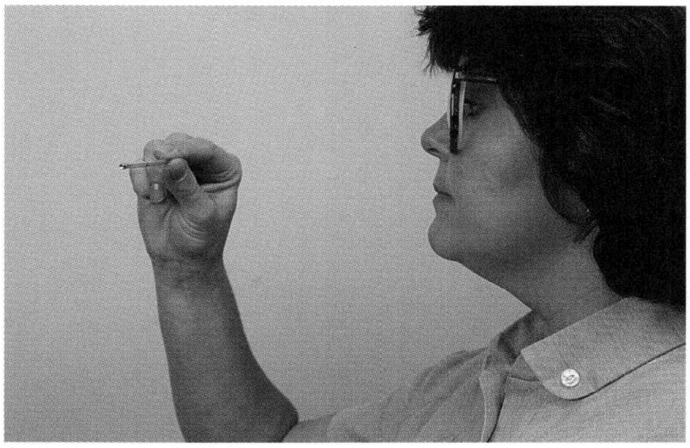

Fig. 21-3 The thermometer is read at eye level.

Do the following to read a glass thermometer:

- Hold the thermometer at the stem (Fig. 21-3).
- Bring the thermometer to eye level.
- Rotate the thermometer until you see both the numbers and the long and short lines.
- Turn the thermometer back and forth slowly until you see the silver (or red) mercury line.
- Read the thermometer to the nearest degree (long line). Read the nearest tenth of a degree (short line)—an even number if using a Fahrenheit thermometer.

Using a glass thermometer. The thermometer is inserted into the mouth, rectum, or axilla. Each area has many microbes. Therefore each resident has a thermometer. This prevents the spread of microbes and infection. The following measures are practiced when using a glass thermometer:

- Use only the resident's thermometer.
- Use a rectal thermometer only for rectal temperatures.
- Rinse the thermometer under cold running water if it was soaking in a disinfectant. Use tissues to dry it from the stem to the bulb end.
- Check the thermometer for breaks and chips.
- Shake down the thermometer so the mercury is below the lines and numbers. Hold the thermometer at the stem. Stand away from walls, tables, or other hard surfaces. Flex and snap your wrist until the mercury is shaken down (Fig. 21-4).

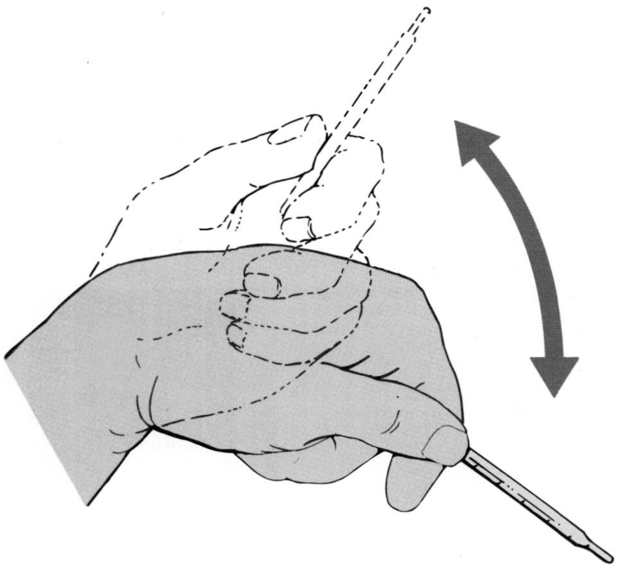

Fig. 21-4 The wrist is snapped to shake down the thermometer.

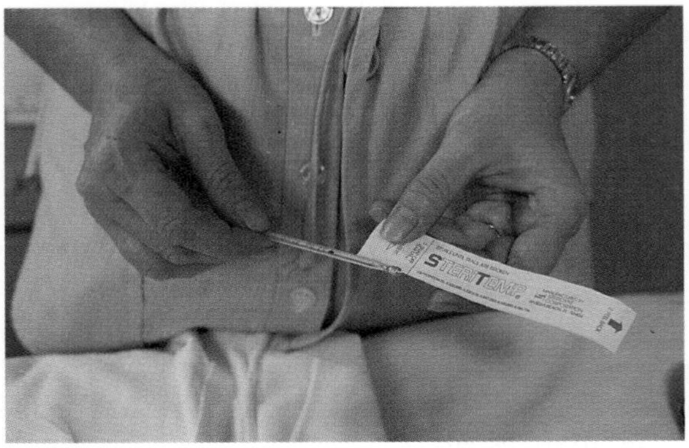

Fig. 21-5 The thermometer is inserted into a plastic cover.

- Clean and store the thermometer following center policy. Wipe it with tissues first to remove mucus or feces. Do not use hot water for cleaning. It causes the mercury to expand so much that the thermometer could break. After cleaning, rinse the thermometer under cold running water. Then store it in a case or a container filled with disinfectant solution.
- Use plastic covers following center policy (Fig. 21-5). A cover is used once and then discarded. The thermometer is inserted into a cover and the temperature taken. The cover is removed to read the thermometer. The thermometer never touches the resident.
- Practice medical asepsis, and follow Standard Precautions.

Taking oral temperatures. Oral temperatures are usually taken on adults and older children. The glass thermometer remains in place 2 to 3 minutes or as required by center policy. Temperatures are not taken orally if the person:

- Is an infant or a child younger than 4 to 5 years
- Is unconscious
- Has had surgery or an injury to the face, neck, nose, or mouth
- Is receiving oxygen
- Breathes through the mouth
- Has a nasogastric tube in place
- Is delirious, restless, confused, or disoriented
- Is paralyzed on one side of the body
- Has a sore mouth
- Has a history of convulsive disorders

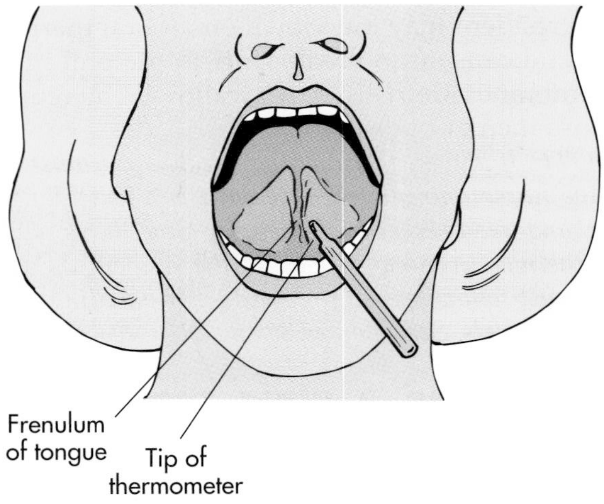

Fig. 21-6 The thermometer is positioned at the base of the tongue next to the frenulum.

Taking an Oral Temperature With a Glass Thermometer

NNAAP™ SKILL

Quality of Life

Remember to:
- *Knock before entering the resident's room*
- *Address the resident by name*
- *Introduce yourself by name and title*

Pre-Procedure

1 Explain the procedure to the resident. Ask him or her not to eat, drink, smoke, or chew gum for at least 15 minutes.

2 Collect the following:
- Oral thermometer and holder
- Tissues
- Plastic covers if used
- Gloves

3 Wash your hands.

4 Identify the resident. Check the ID bracelet against the assignment sheet.

5 Provide for privacy.

Procedure

6 Put on the gloves.

7 Rinse the thermometer in cold water if it was soaking in a disinfectant solution. Dry it with tissues.

8 Check the thermometer for breaks or chips.

9 Shake down the thermometer.

10 Place a plastic cover on the thermometer if used.

11 Ask the resident to moisten his or her lips.

12 Place the bulb end of the thermometer under the resident's tongue (Fig. 21-6).

13 Ask the resident to close his or her lips around the thermometer to hold it in place. Ask the resident not to talk while the thermometer is in place. Also remind the resident not to bite down on the thermometer.

14 Leave the thermometer in place for 2 to 3 minutes or as required by center policy.

15 Remove the thermometer by grasping the stem.

16 Use tissues to remove the plastic cover. Wipe the thermometer with a tissue from the stem to the bulb end if no cover was used.

17 Read the thermometer.

18 Record the resident's name and temperature on your note pad or assignment sheet.

19 Shake down the thermometer.

20 Clean the thermometer according to center policy.

Post-Procedure

21 Provide for comfort.

22 Place the signal light within reach.

23 Unscreen the resident.

24 Remove the gloves, and wash your hands.

25 Report any abnormal temperature to the nurse. Record the measurement in the proper place.

Taking rectal temperatures. Rectal temperatures are taken when the oral route cannot be used. Rectal temperatures are not taken if the resident has diarrhea, a rectal disorder or injury, or heart disease or has had rectal surgery.

The rectal thermometer is lubricated for easy insertion and to prevent tissue injury. The thermometer is held in place so it is not lost into the rectum or broken. A glass thermometer remains in the rectum for 2 minutes or as required by center policy.

Privacy is important when taking rectal temperatures. The buttocks and anus are exposed. Many people are embarrassed by the procedure.

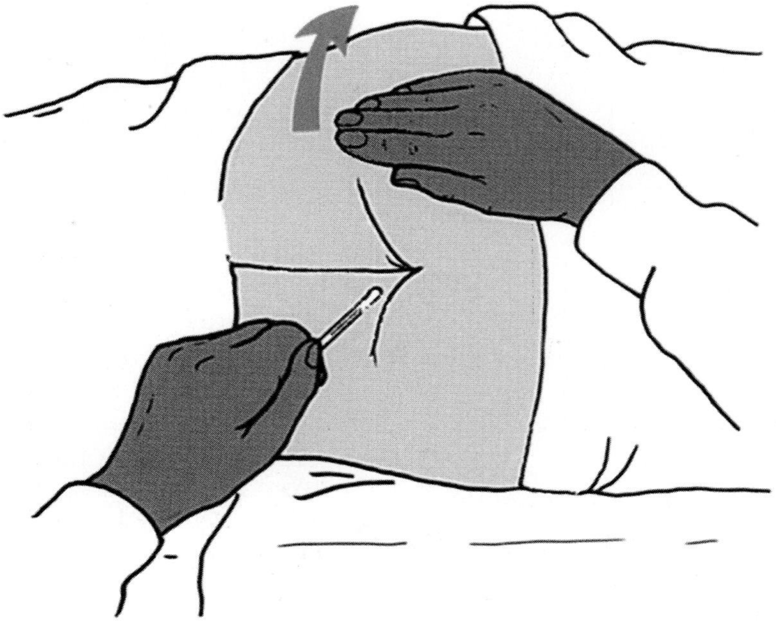

Fig. 21-7 The rectal temperature is taken with the resident in side-lying position. The buttock is raised to expose the anus.

Taking a Rectal Temperature With a Glass Thermometer

Quality of Life

Remember to:
- *Knock before entering the resident's room*
- *Address the resident by name*
- *Introduce yourself by name and title*

Pre-Procedure

1 Explain the procedure to the resident.
2 Collect the following:
   - Rectal thermometer and holder
   - Toilet tissue
   - Plastic cover if used
   - Gloves
   - Water-soluble lubricant
3 Wash your hands.
4 Identify the resident. Check the ID bracelet against the assignment sheet.
5 Provide for privacy.

Procedure

6 Rinse the thermometer in cold water if it was soaking in a disinfectant solution. Dry it with tissues.
7 Check the thermometer for breaks or chips.
8 Shake down the thermometer.
9 Place a plastic cover on the thermometer if used.
10 Position the person in side-lying position.
11 Put on the gloves.
12 Put a small amount of lubricant on a tissue. Lubricate the bulb end of the thermometer.
13 Fold back top linens to expose the anal area.
14 Raise the upper buttock to expose the anus (Fig. 21-7).
15 Insert the thermometer 1 inch into the rectum. Do not force the thermometer. Remember, glass thermometers can break.
16 Hold thermometer in place for 2 minutes or as required by center policy.
17 Remove the thermometer.
18 Remove the plastic cover. Wipe the thermometer with tissues from the stem to the bulb end if no cover was used.
19 Place used toilet tissue on a paper towel or several thicknesses of toilet tissue. Place the thermometer on clean toilet tissue.
20 Wipe the anal area to remove excess lubricant and any feces. Cover the resident.
21 Provide for comfort. Place the signal light within reach.
22 Dispose of tissue.
23 Read the thermometer. Record the resident's name and temperature on your note pad or assignment sheet. Write *R* to indicate a rectal temperature.
24 Shake down the thermometer.
25 Clean the thermometer according to center policy.
26 Remove the gloves, and wash your hands.

Post-Procedure

27 Unscreen the resident.
28 Report any abnormal temperature to the nurse. Record the measurement with an *R* in the proper place.

Taking axillary temperatures. Axillary temperatures are less reliable than oral, rectal, or tympanic membrane temperatures. They are used when the other routes cannot be used. The axilla must be dry for the measurement. This site is not used right after bathing. The thermometer is held in place to maintain proper position. A glass thermometer is held in place for 5 to 10 minutes or as required by center policy.

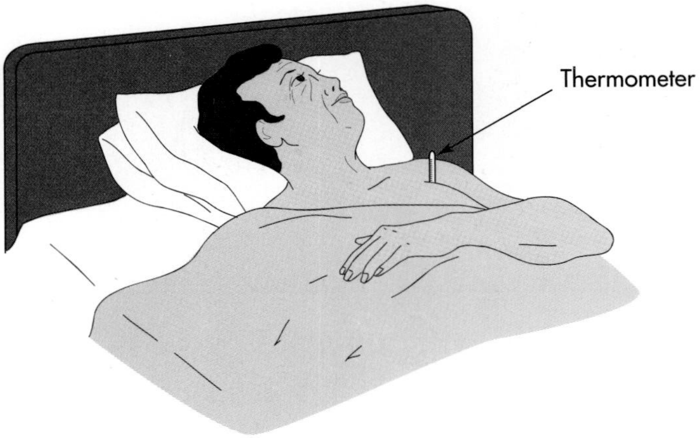

Fig. 21-8 The thermometer is held in place in the axilla by bringing the person's arm over the chest.

Taking an Axillary Temperature With a Glass Thermometer

Quality of Life

Remember to:
- Knock before entering the resident's room
- Address the resident by name
- Introduce yourself by name and title

Pre-Procedure

1 Explain the procedure to the resident.
2 Collect the following:
   - Oral glass thermometer and holder
   - Plastic cover if used
   - Tissues
   - Towel
3 Wash your hands.
4 Identify the resident. Check the ID bracelet against the assignment sheet.
5 Provide for privacy.

Procedure

6 Rinse the thermometer in cold water if it was soaking in a disinfectant solution. Dry it with tissues.
7 Check the thermometer for breaks or chips.
8 Shake down the thermometer.
9 Place a plastic cover on the thermometer if used.
10 Help the resident remove an arm from the gown. Do not expose the resident.
11 Dry the axilla with the towel.
12 Place the bulb end of the thermometer in the center of the axilla.
13 Ask the resident to place the arm over the chest to hold the thermometer in place (Fig. 21-8). Hold it and the arm in place if he or she cannot help.
14 Leave the thermometer in place for 5 to 10 minutes or as required by center policy.
15 Remove the thermometer from the plastic cover. Wipe it with tissues from the stem to the bulb end if no cover was used.
16 Read the thermometer.
17 Record the resident's name and temperature with an *A* (for axillary temperature) on your note pad or assignment sheet.
18 Help the resident put the gown back on.
19 Provide for comfort. Place the signal light within reach.
20 Shake down the thermometer.
21 Rinse and wash the thermometer. Place it in the holder with disinfectant or in a plastic cover.

Post-Procedure

22 Unscreen the resident.
23 Follow center policy for soiled linen.
24 Wash your hands.
25 Report any abnormal temperature to the nurse. Record the measurement with an *A* in the proper place.

Electronic Thermometers

Electronic thermometers are battery operated. They measure temperature in a few seconds. The temperature is displayed on the front of the instrument. The hand-held unit is kept in a battery charger when not in use.

Electronic thermometers have oral and rectal probes. A disposable cover (sheath) covers the probe. Disposable probe covers are used once and then discarded. This helps prevent the spread of infection. Medical asepsis and Standard Precautions also help prevent the spread of infection.

Taking a Temperature With an Electronic Thermometer

NNAAP™ SKILL

Quality of Life

Remember to:

- *Knock before entering the resident's room*
- *Address the resident by name*
- *Introduce yourself by name and title*

Pre-Procedure

1 Explain the procedure to the resident. Ask him or her not to eat, drink, smoke, or chew gum for at least 15 minutes if you will take an oral temperature.

2 Collect the following:
- Electronic thermometer
- Probe (blue for an oral or axillary temperature; red for a rectal temperature)
- Disposable probe cover
- Toilet tissue (for a rectal temperature)
- Water-soluble lubricant (for a rectal temperature)
- Gloves

3 Plug the probe into the thermometer.

4 Wash your hands.

5 Identify the resident. Check the ID bracelet against the assignment sheet.

Procedure

6 Provide for privacy. Position the resident for an oral, rectal, or axillary temperature.

7 Put on gloves if contact with blood, body fluids, secretions, or excretions is likely.

8 Insert the probe into a probe cover.

9 **For an *oral temperature*:**

a Ask the resident to open the mouth and raise the tongue.

b Place the covered probe at the base of the tongue on either side (Fig. 21-9).

c Ask the resident to lower the tongue and close the mouth.

For a *rectal temperature:*

a Lubricate the end of the covered probe using the lubricant on the toilet tissue.

b Fold back top linens to expose the anal area.

c Raise the upper buttock to expose the anus.

d Insert the probe ½ inch into the rectum.

For an *axillary temperature:*

a Help the resident remove an arm from the gown. Do not expose the resident.

b Dry the axilla with the towel.

c Place the covered probe in the axilla. Place the resident's arm over the chest.

Taking a Temperature With an Electronic Thermometer—cont'd

NNAAP™ SKILL

Procedure—cont'd

10 Hold the probe in place until you hear a tone or see a flashing or steady light. It means the temperature was measured.

11 Read the temperature on the display.

12 Remove the probe. Press the eject button to discard the cover.

13 Record the resident's name and temperature on your note pad or assignment sheet.

14 Return the probe to the holder.

15 Provide for comfort. Help the resident put the gown back on if an axillary temperature was taken. For a *rectal temperature*:

- a Wipe the anal area with tissue to remove lubricant.
- b Cover the resident.
- c Discard used toilet tissue.
- d Remove the gloves.

Post-Procedure

16 Place the signal light within the resident's reach.

17 Unscreen the resident.

18 Remove the gloves, and wash your hands.

19 Return the thermometer to the charging unit.

20 Wash your hands.

21 Report any abnormal temperature to the nurse. Record the measurement in the proper place. Note if an oral, rectal, or axillary temperature was taken.

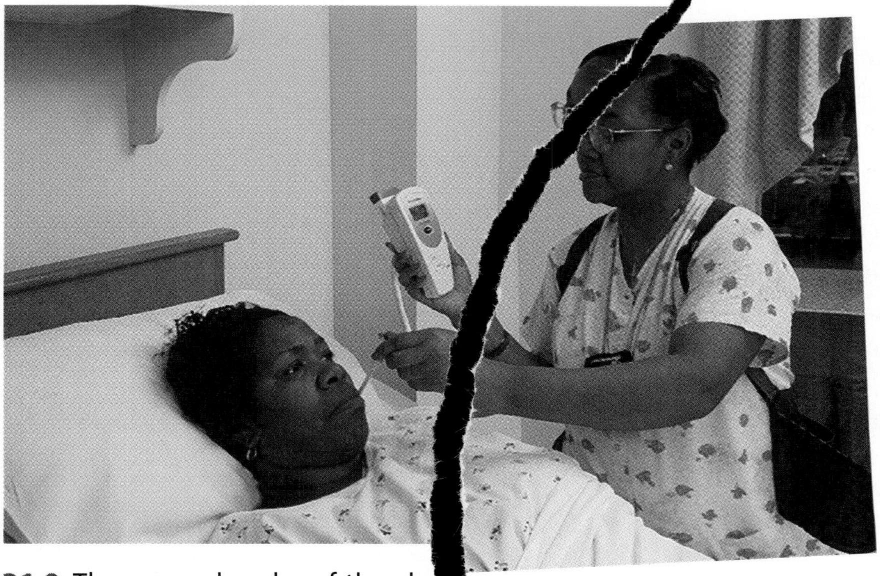

Fig. 21-9 The covered probe of the electronic thermometer is inserted under the tongue.

◈ Tympanic Membrane Thermometers

Tympanic membrane thermometers measure temperature at the tympanic membrane in the ear (Fig. 21-10). The covered probe is gently inserted into the ear. The temperature is measured in 1 to 3 seconds. These thermometers are battery operated and use a disposable probe cover. They must be kept charged.

Tympanic membrane thermometers are comfortable for the resident. They are not invasive like rectal thermometers. They are useful for confused residents because of their speed and comfort. There are fewer microbes in the ear than in the mouth or rectum. Therefore the risk of spreading infection is reduced. These thermometers are not used if there is ear drainage.

Taking a Tympanic Membrane Temperature

Quality of Life

Remember to:
- ◆ *Knock before entering the resident's room*
- ◆ *Address the resident by name*
- ◆ *Introduce yourself by name and title*

Pre-Procedure

1 Explain the procedure to the resident.
2 Get the tympanic membrane thermometer and a probe cover.
3 Wash your hands.
4 Identify the resident. Check the ID bracelet against the assignment sheet.
5 Provide for privacy.

Procedure

6 Ask the resident to turn his or her head so the ear is in front of you.
7 Insert the probe gently. Pull back on the ear to straighten the ear canal (Fig. 21-11).
8 Start the thermometer.
9 Read the measurement when you hear a tone or see a flashing light.
10 Remove the probe from the ear.
11 Record the resident's name and temperature on your note pad or assignment sheet. Note that a tympanic temperature was taken.
12 Press the eject button, and discard the probe.

Post-Procedure

13 Provide for comfort.
14 Place the signal light within reach.
15 Unscreen the resident.
16 Return the thermometer to the charging unit.
17 Wash your hands.
18 Report any abnormal temperature to the nurse. Record the measurement in the proper place. Note that a tympanic membrane temperature was taken.

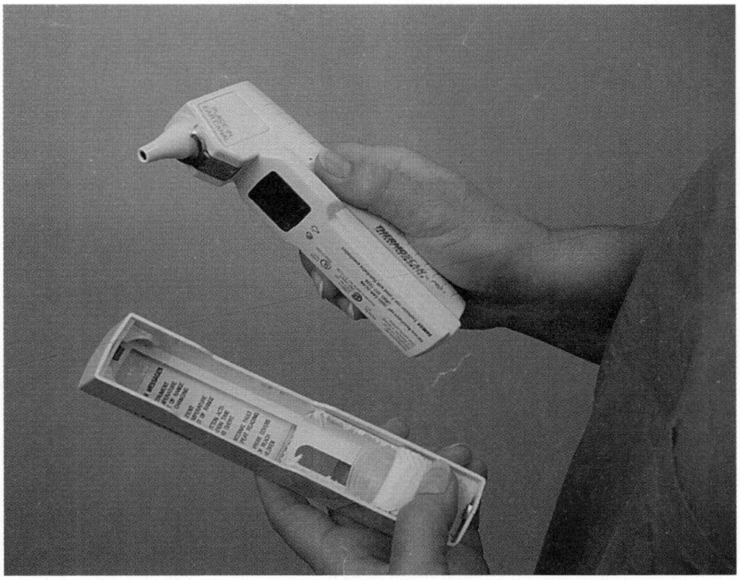

Fig. 21-10 Tympanic membrane thermometer. *(Courtesy Thermoscan, Inc, San Diego, Calif.)*

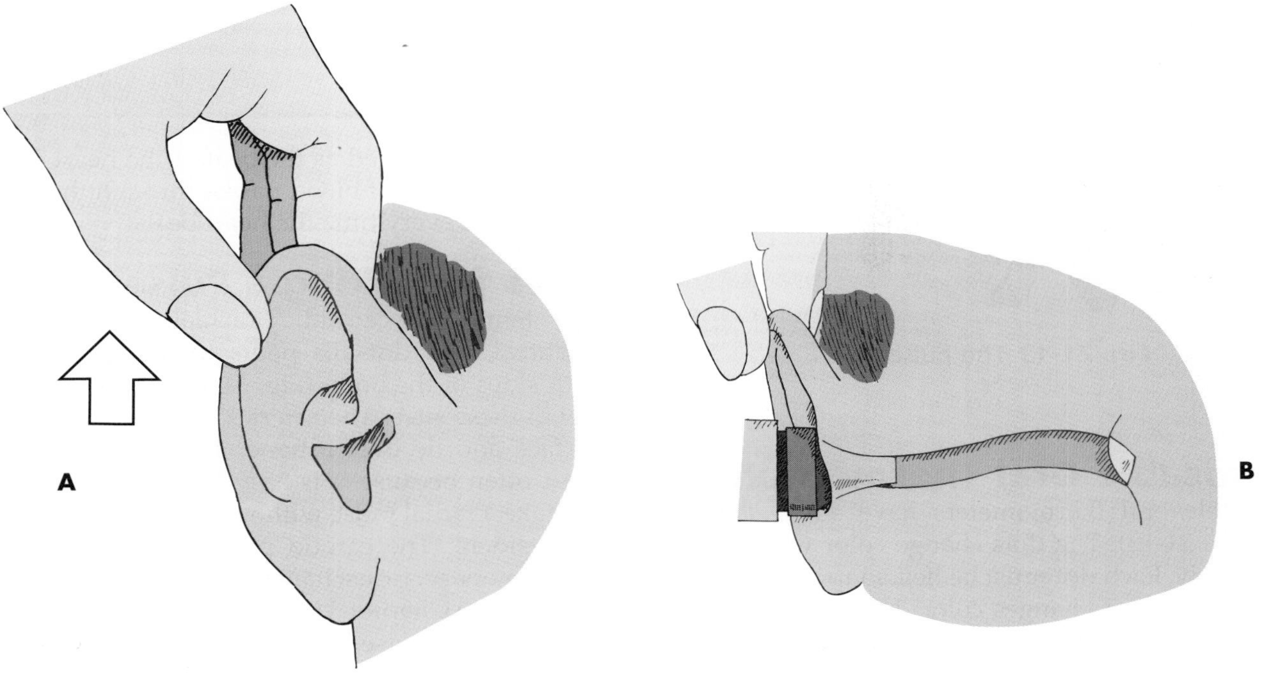

Fig. 21-11 A, The ear is pulled back and, **B,** the tympanic membrane thermometer probe is inserted into the ear canal.

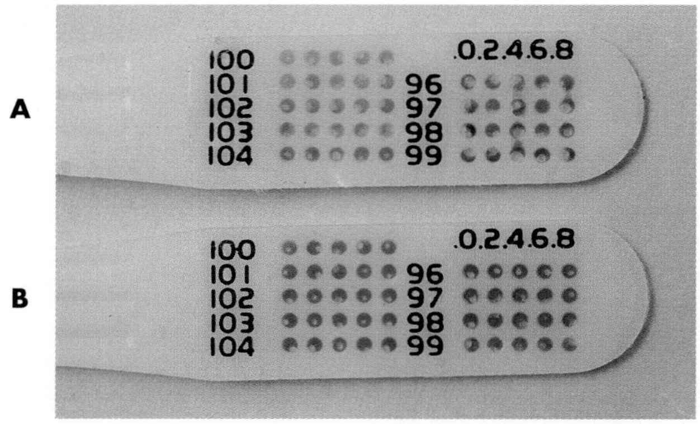

Fig. 21-12 A, Disposable oral thermometer with chemical dots. **B,** The dots change color when the temperature is taken.

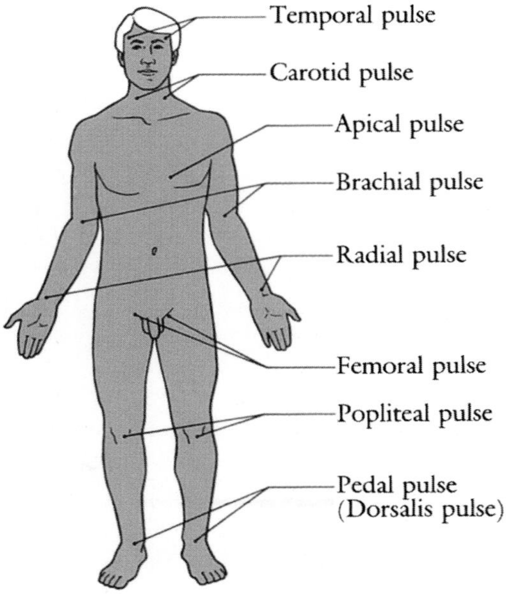

Fig. 21-13 The pulse sites.

Disposable Oral Thermometers

Disposable oral thermometers have small chemical dots (Fig. 21-12). The dots change color when heated by the body. Each dot must be heated to a certain temperature before it changes color. These thermometers are used only once. They measure temperature in 45 to 60 seconds.

Temperature-Sensitive Tape

Temperature-sensitive tape changes color in response to body heat. The tape is applied to the forehead or abdomen. It shows if the temperature is normal or above normal. Exact body temperature is not measured. The color change takes about 15 seconds.

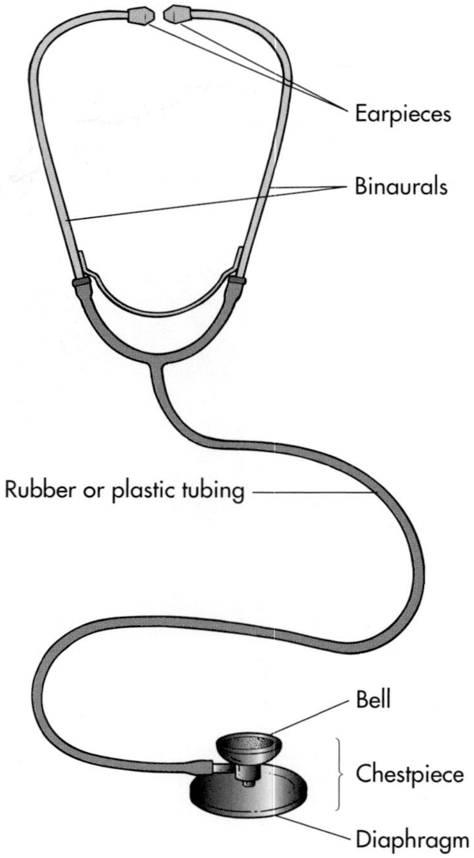

Fig. 21-14 Parts of a stethoscope.

PULSE

The **pulse** is defined as the beat of the heart felt at an artery as a wave of blood passes through the artery. A pulse is felt every time the heart beats.

Sites for Taking a Pulse

The temporal, carotid, brachial, radial, femoral, popliteal, and dorsalis pedis (pedal) pulses are on both sides of the body (Fig. 21-13). Pulses are easy to feel at these sites. The arteries are close to the body's surface and lie over a bone. The radial site is used most often because it is easy to reach and find. You can take a radial pulse without disturbing or exposing the resident. The carotid pulse is taken during cardiopulmonary resuscitation (CPR) and other emergencies (see Chapter 31).

The apical pulse is felt over the apex *(apical)* of the heart. The apex is at the tip of the heart, just below the left nipple (p. 498). The apical pulse is taken with a stethoscope.

Using a Stethoscope

A **stethoscope** is an instrument used to listen to the sounds produced by the heart, lungs, and other body organs (Fig. 21-14). It is used to take the apical pulse

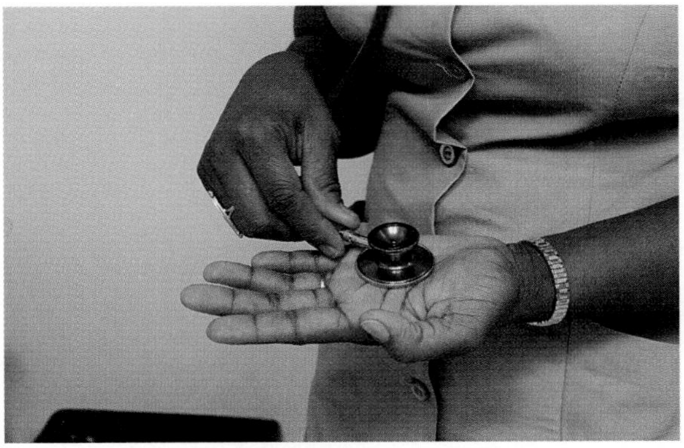

Fig. 21-15 The diaphragm of the stethoscope is warmed in the palm of the hand.

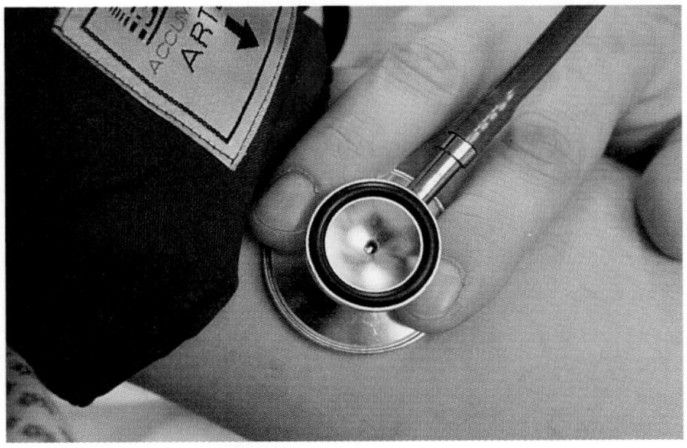

Fig. 21-16 The stethoscope is held in place with the fingertips of the index and middle fingers.

and to measure blood pressure. The stethoscope amplifies the sounds for easy hearing.

Stethoscopes are in contact with many residents and health care team members. Therefore infection control is important. The earpieces and diaphragm are cleaned before and after use. Cleaning prevents the spread of microbes.

The following measures are practiced when using a stethoscope:

- Wipe the earpieces and diaphragm with alcohol wipes.
- Warm the diaphragm in your hand (Fig. 21-15).
- Place the earpiece tips in your ears so the bend of the tips points forward. Earpieces should fit snugly to block out external noises. They should not cause pain or ear discomfort.
- Place the diaphragm over the artery. Hold it in place as in Figure 21-16.
- Prevent noise. Do not let anything touch the tubing. Ask the resident to be silent during the procedure.
- Wipe the earpiece tips and diaphragm with alcohol wipes after the procedure.

Table 21-2 Pulse Ranges for Different Ages

Age	Pulse Rates per Minute
Birth to 4 weeks	80-180
4 weeks to 1 year	80-160
1 to 2 years	80-130
2 to 6 years	80-120
6 to 12 years	70-110
12 years and older	60-100

Pulse Rate

The **pulse rate** is the number of heartbeats or pulses felt in 1 minute. The rate varies for different age-groups (Table 21-2). The pulse rate is affected by many factors. They include elevated body temperature (fever), exercise, fear, anger, anxiety, excitement, heat, position, and pain. These and other factors cause the heart to beat faster. Some drugs also increase the pulse rate. Other drugs slow down the pulse.

The adult pulse rate is between 60 and 100 beats per minute. A rate of less than 60 or more than 100 is considered abnormal. **Tachycardia** is a rapid *(tachy)* heart rate *(cardia)*. The heart rate is more than 100 beats per minute. **Bradycardia** is a slow *(brady)* heart rate *(cardia)*. The rate is less than 60 beats per minute. Report abnormal rates to the nurse immediately.

Rhythm and Force of the Pulse

The rhythm of the pulse should be regular. That is, a pulse is felt in a pattern. The same time interval should occur between beats. An irregular pulse occurs when the beats are unevenly spaced or beats are skipped (Fig. 21-17, p. 496).

The force of the pulse relates to its strength. A forceful pulse is easy to feel and is described as strong, full, or bounding. Pulses that are hard to feel are described as weak, thready, or feeble.

Electronic blood pressure equipment (p. 504) can also count pulses. The pulse rate is displayed along with the blood pressure. However, no information is given about the rhythm and force of the pulse. If electronic blood pressure equipment is used, you still need to feel the pulse to determine rhythm and force.

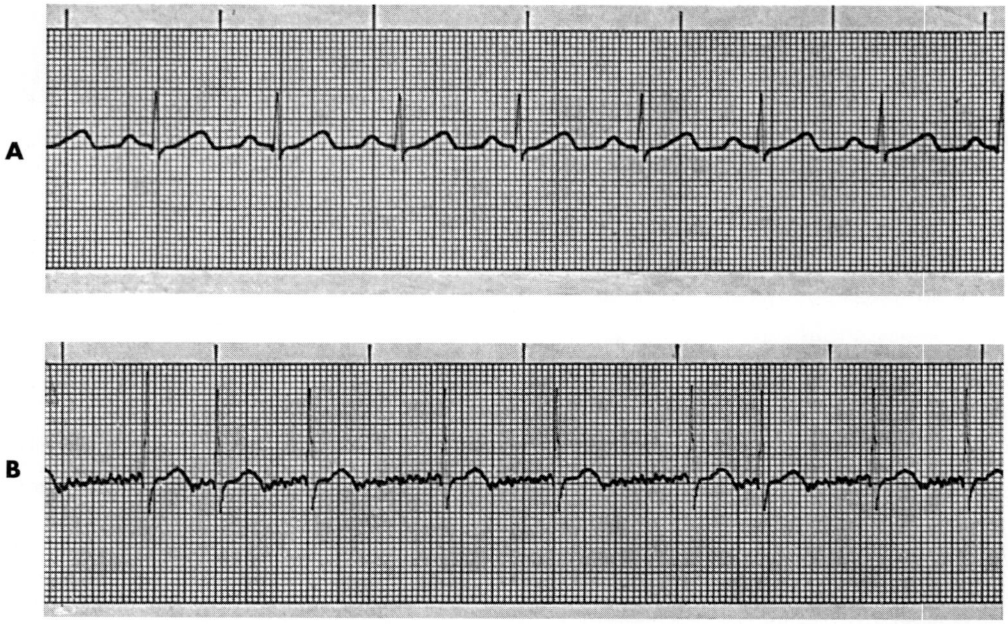

Fig. 21-17 **A,** The electrocardiogram shows a regular pulse. The beats occur at regular intervals. **B,** The beats in this electrocardiogram occur at irregular intervals. *(From Atwood S, Stanton C, Storey J:* Introduction to basic cardiac dysrhythmias, *ed 2, St Louis, 1996, Mosby.)*

◈ Taking a Radial Pulse

The radial pulse is used for routine vital signs. The pulse is felt by placing the first three fingers of one hand against the radial artery. The radial artery is on the thumb side of the wrist (Fig. 21-18). Do not use your thumb to take a pulse; it has a pulse of its own. You could mistake the pulse in your thumb for the person's pulse. Count the pulse for 30 seconds. Then multiply the number by 2 to get the number of beats per minute. If the pulse is irregular, count the pulse for 1 full minute.

In some centers, all radial pulses are taken for 1 full minute. Follow your center's policy.

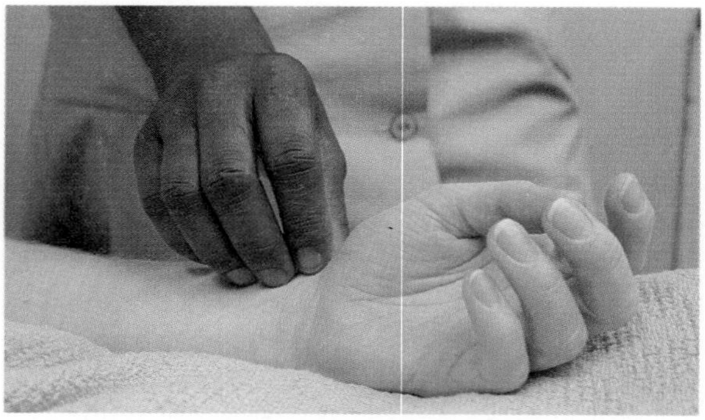

Fig. 21-18 The middle three fingers are used to locate the radial pulse on the thumb side of the wrist.

Taking a Radial Pulse

NNAAP™ SKILL

Quality of Life

Remember to:

- *Knock before entering the resident's room*
- *Address the resident by name*
- *Introduce yourself by name and title*

Pre-Procedure

1 Wash your hands.

2 Identify the resident. Check the ID bracelet against the assignment sheet.

3 Explain the procedure to the resident.

4 Provide for privacy.

Procedure

5 Have the resident sit or lie down.

6 Locate the radial pulse with your 3 middle fingers (see Fig. 21-18).

7 Note if the pulse is strong or weak, and regular or irregular.

8 Count the pulse for 30 seconds. Multiply the number of beats by 2. Or count the pulse for 1 full minute if required by center policy.

9 Count the pulse for 1 full minute if it is irregular.

10 Record the resident's name and pulse on your note pad or assignment sheet. Make a note about the strength of the pulse and if it was regular or irregular.

Post-Procedure

11 Provide for comfort.

12 Place the signal light within reach.

13 Unscreen the resident.

14 Wash your hands.

15 Report the following to the nurse:
- A pulse rate of less than 60 or more than 100 beats per minute is reported immediately
- Whether the pulse is regular or irregular
- The pulse rate
- The strength of the pulse (strong, full, or bounding; or weak, thready, or feeble)

16 Record the pulse rate in the proper place.

◈ Taking an Apical Pulse

The apical pulse is taken with a stethoscope. Apical pulses are taken on residents who have heart disease or who take drugs that affect the heart. The apical pulse is on the left side of the chest slightly below the nipple (Fig. 21-19). The apical pulse is counted for 1 full minute.

The heartbeat normally sounds like a *lub-dub*. Each *lub-dub* is counted as 1 beat. Do not count the *lub* as 1 beat and the *dub* as another.

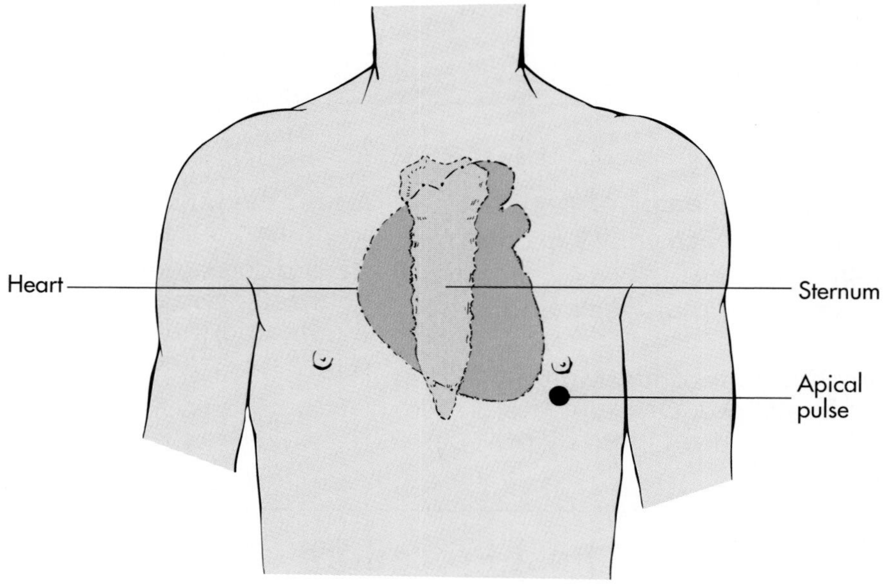

Fig. 21-19 The apical pulse is located 2 to 3 inches to the left of the sternum (breastbone) and below the left nipple.

Taking an Apical Pulse

Quality of Life

Remember to:
- ◆ *Knock before entering the resident's room*
- ◆ *Address the resident by name*
- ◆ *Introduce yourself by name and title*

Pre-Procedure

1 Collect the following:
- Stethoscope with diaphragm
- Alcohol wipes

2 Wash your hands.

3 Identify the resident. Check the ID bracelet against the assignment sheet.

4 Explain the procedure to the resident.

5 Provide for privacy.

Procedure

6 Wipe the earpieces and diaphragm with alcohol wipes.

7 Have the resident sit or lie down.

8 Expose the nipple area of the left chest.

9 Warm the diaphragm in your palm.

10 Place the earpieces in your ears.

11 Locate the apical pulse. Place the diaphragm 2 to 3 inches to the left of the breastbone and below the left nipple (see Fig. 21-19).

12 Count the pulse for 1 full minute. Note if it is regular or irregular.

13 Cover the resident. Remove the earpieces.

14 Record the resident's name and pulse on your note pad or assignment sheet. Note whether the pulse was regular or irregular.

15 Provide for comfort.

16 Place the signal light within reach.

17 Unscreen the resident.

18 Clean the earpieces and diaphragm of the stethoscope with alcohol wipes.

19 Return the stethoscope to its proper place.

Post-Procedure

20 Wash your hands.

21 Report the following to the nurse:
- A pulse rate of less than 60 or more than 100 beats per minute is reported immediately
- Whether the pulse was regular or irregular
- The pulse rate

22 Record the pulse rate in the proper place with an *Ap* for an apical pulse.

Taking an Apical-Radial Pulse

The apical and radial pulse rates should be equal. Sometimes heart contractions are not strong enough to create pulses in the radial artery. Then the radial pulse is less than the apical pulse. This may occur in people with heart disease. To see if there is a difference between the apical and radial rates, two staff members take the pulses at the same time. This is called an **apical-radial pulse.** The **pulse deficit** is the difference between the apical and radial pulse rates. To obtain the pulse deficit, subtract the radial rate from the apical rate. The apical pulse rate is never less than the radial pulse rate.

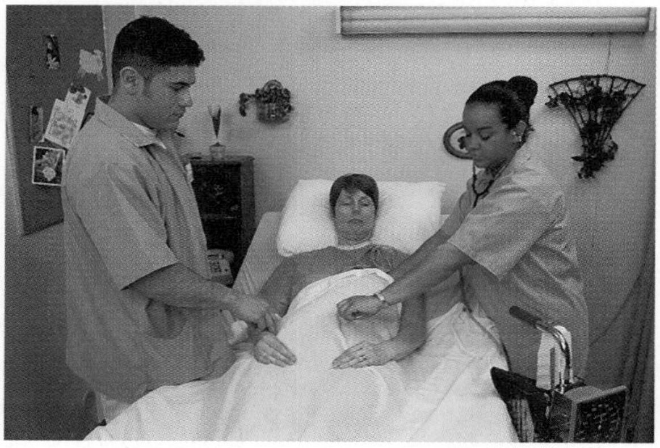

Fig. 21-20 Two workers take an apical-radial pulse. One worker takes the apical pulse, and the other takes the radial pulse.

Taking an Apical-Radial Pulse

Quality of Life

Remember to:
- *Knock before entering the resident's room*
- *Address the resident by name*
- *Introduce yourself by name and title*

Pre-Procedure

1. Ask a nurse or another nursing assistant to help you.
2. Collect a stethoscope and alcohol wipes.
3. Wash your hands.
4. Identify the resident. Check the ID bracelet against the assignment sheet.
5. Explain the procedure to the resident.
6. Provide for privacy.

Procedure

7. Wipe the earpieces and diaphragm with the alcohol wipes.
8. Have the resident sit or lie down.
9. Warm the diaphragm in your palm.
10. Expose the left nipple area of the chest.
11. Place the earpieces in your ears.
12. Find the apical pulse. Have your helper find the radial pulse (Fig. 21-20).
13. Give the signal to begin counting.
14. Count the pulse for 1 full minute.
15. Give the signal to stop counting.
16. Cover the resident. Remove the earpieces.
17. Record the resident's name and the apical and radial pulses on your note pad or assignment sheet. Subtract the radial pulse from the apical pulse for the pulse deficit. Note whether the pulse was regular or irregular.
18. Provide for comfort.
19. Place the signal light within reach.
20. Unscreen the resident.
21. Clean the earpieces and diaphragm with alcohol wipes.
22. Return the stethoscope to its proper place.

Post-Procedure

23. Wash your hands.
24. Report the following to the nurse:
    - An apical pulse rate of less than 60 or more than 100 beats per minute is reported immediately
    - The apical and radial pulse rates
    - The pulse deficit
    - Whether the pulse was regular or irregular
25. Record the pulses in the proper place. Indicate that an apical-radial pulse was taken.

RESPIRATIONS

Respiration is the act of breathing air into the lungs (inhalation) and out of the lungs (exhalation). Oxygen is taken into the lungs during inhalation. Carbon dioxide is moved out of the lungs during exhalation. Each respiration involves one inhalation and one exhalation. The chest rises during inhalation and falls during exhalation.

The healthy adult has 10 to 20 respirations per minute. The respiratory rate is affected by many of the factors that affect body temperature and pulse. Heart and respiratory diseases usually cause an increased number of respirations per minute.

Respirations are normally quiet, effortless, and regular. Both sides of the chest rise and fall equally. See Chapter 25 for abnormal respiratory patterns.

Respirations are counted when the resident is at rest. The resident is positioned so you can see the chest rise and fall. To a certain extent, a person can control the depth and rate of breathing. People tend to change breathing patterns when they know their respirations are being counted. Therefore the resident should not know that you are counting respirations.

Respirations are counted right after taking a pulse. Keep your fingers or stethoscope over the pulse site. (The resident assumes you are still taking the pulse.) Count respirations by watching the rise and fall of the chest. Count them for 30 seconds. Then multiply the number by 2 for the total number of respirations in 1 minute. If an abnormal pattern is noted, count the respirations for 1 full minute.

Counting Respirations

NNAAP™ SKILL

Procedure

1 Continue to hold the wrist after taking the radial pulse. Keep the stethoscope in place if you took an apical pulse.
2 Do not tell the resident you are counting respirations.
3 Begin counting when the chest rises. Count each rise and fall of the chest as 1 respiration.
4 Observe if respirations are regular and if both sides of the chest rise equally. Also note the depth of respirations and if the resident has any pain or difficulty in breathing.
5 Count respirations for 30 seconds. Multiply the number by 2.
6 Count respirations for 1 full minute if they are abnormal or irregular.
7 Record the resident's name, respiratory rate, and other observations on your note pad or assignment sheet.

Post-Procedure

8 Provide for comfort.
9 Place the signal light within reach.
10 Wash your hands.
11 Report the following to the nurse:
- The respiratory rate
- Equality and depth of respirations
- If the respirations were regular or irregular
- If the resident experienced pain or difficulty in breathing
- Any respiratory noises
- Any abnormal respiratory patterns (see Chapter 25)

12 Record the respiratory rate in the proper place.

BLOOD PRESSURE

Blood pressure is the amount of force exerted against the walls of an artery by the blood. Blood pressure is controlled by:

- The force of heart contractions
- The amount of blood pumped with each heartbeat
- How easily the blood flows through the blood vessels

The period of heart muscle contraction is called **systole.** The period of heart muscle relaxation is called **diastole.**

Both the systolic and diastolic pressures are measured. The **systolic pressure** is the higher pressure. It represents the amount of force needed to pump blood out of the heart into the arterial circulation. The **diastolic pressure** is the lower pressure. It reflects the pressure in the arteries when the heart is at rest. Blood pressure is measured in millimeters (mm) of mercury (Hg). The systolic pressure is recorded over the diastolic pressure. The average adult has a systolic pressure of 120 mm Hg and a diastolic pressure of 80 mm Hg. This is written as 120/80 mm Hg.

Factors Affecting Blood Pressure

Blood pressure can change from minute to minute. Such changes are related to the factors described in Box 21-1.

Because it can vary so easily, blood pressure has normal ranges. Systolic pressures between 100 and 140 mm Hg are considered normal. Normal diastolic pressures are between 60 and 90 mm Hg.

Persistent measurements above (*hyper*) the normal systolic and diastolic pressures are abnormal. This condition is known as **hypertension.** Report any systolic pressure above 140 mm Hg to the nurse immediately. A diastolic pressure above 90 mm Hg also is

Box 21-1 Factors Affecting Blood Pressure

- **Age**—blood pressure increases as a person grows older. It is lowest in infancy and childhood and highest in adulthood. Blood pressure continues to increase with aging.
- **Gender** (male or female)—women usually have lower blood pressures than men do. Blood pressures rise in women after menopause.
- **Blood volume**—is the amount of blood in the system. Severe bleeding lowers the blood volume. Therefore the blood pressure lowers. The rapid administration of IV fluids increases the blood volume. The blood pressure rises.
- **Stress**—includes anxiety, fear, and emotions. Heart rate and blood pressure increase as part of the body's response to stress.
- **Pain**—generally increases blood pressure. However, severe pain can cause shock. Blood pressure is seriously low in the state of shock (see Chapter 31).
- **Exercise**—increases heart rate and blood pressure. Blood pressure is not measured right after exercise.
- **Weight**—blood pressure is higher in overweight persons. The blood pressure lowers with weight loss.
- **Race**—black persons generally have higher blood pressures than white persons do.
- **Diet**—a high-sodium diet increases the amount of water in the body. The extra fluid volume increases blood pressure (see Chapter 18).
- **Drugs**—drugs can be given to raise or lower blood pressure. Other drugs have the side effects of high or low blood pressure.
- **Position**—blood pressure is generally lower when lying down and higher in the standing position. Sudden changes in position can cause sudden changes in blood pressure (orthostatic hypotension). A person who stands suddenly may have a sudden drop in blood pressure. Dizziness and fainting can occur. (See Chapter 19.)
- **Smoking**—increases blood pressure. Nicotine in cigarettes causes blood vessels to narrow. The heart must work harder to pump blood through narrowed vessels.
- **Alcohol**—excessive alcohol intake can raise blood pressure.

reported immediately. Likewise, systolic pressures below (*hypo*) 90 mm Hg and diastolic pressures below 60 mm Hg are reported. This is called **hypotension.** Some people normally have low blood pressures. However, hypotension may be a sign of a serious condition that can lead to death if not corrected.

Arteries narrow and lose their elasticity. The heart has to work harder to pump blood through the vessels. Therefore both the systolic and diastolic pressures are higher in older persons. A blood pressure of 160/90 mm Hg is normal for many older persons. Older persons also are at risk for orthostatic hypotension (see Chapter 19).

Residents on certain heart drugs may need their blood pressure taken and reported to the nurse before the drug is given. The nurse tells you when this is needed. The information also is in the resident's care plan.

Equipment

A stethoscope and a sphygmomanometer are used to measure blood pressure. The **sphygmomanometer** consists of a cuff and a measuring device. There are three types of sphygmomanometers: aneroid, mercury, and electronic. (*See Subacute Care.*) The aneroid type has a round dial and a needle that points to the calibrations (Fig. 21-21, *A*). The aneroid manometer is small and easy to carry. The mercury manometer is more accurate than the aneroid type. The mercury type has a column of mercury within a calibrated tube (Fig. 21-21, *B*).

Electronic sphygmomanometers display the systolic and diastolic blood pressures on the front of the instrument (Fig. 21-21, *C*). The pulse rate also is usually displayed. The cuff automatically inflates and deflates on some models. Others have automatic deflation only. If electronic blood pressure equipment is used where you work, you need to learn how to use the equipment. Follow the manufacturer's instructions. These devices are available for home use.

The blood pressure cuff is wrapped around the upper arm. Tubing connects the cuff to the manometer. Another tube connects the cuff to a small hand-held bulb. A valve on the bulb is turned so the cuff inflates as the bulb is squeezed. The inflated cuff causes pressure over the brachial artery. The valve is turned in the other way for cuff deflation. Blood pressure is measured as the cuff is deflated.

Sounds are produced as blood flows through the arteries. The stethoscope is used to listen to the sounds in the brachial artery as the cuff is deflated. Stethoscopes are not needed with electronic sphygmomanometers.

Residents with very small arms may need a pediatric blood pressure cuff. Those with very large arms may need an extra-large cuff. Using the right size cuff is necessary for accuracy. If a resident needs a special cuff, the information is found in the care plan.

Subacute Care

Centers with subacute units may have a wall-mounted mercury sphygmomanometer in the person's room.

A

B

C

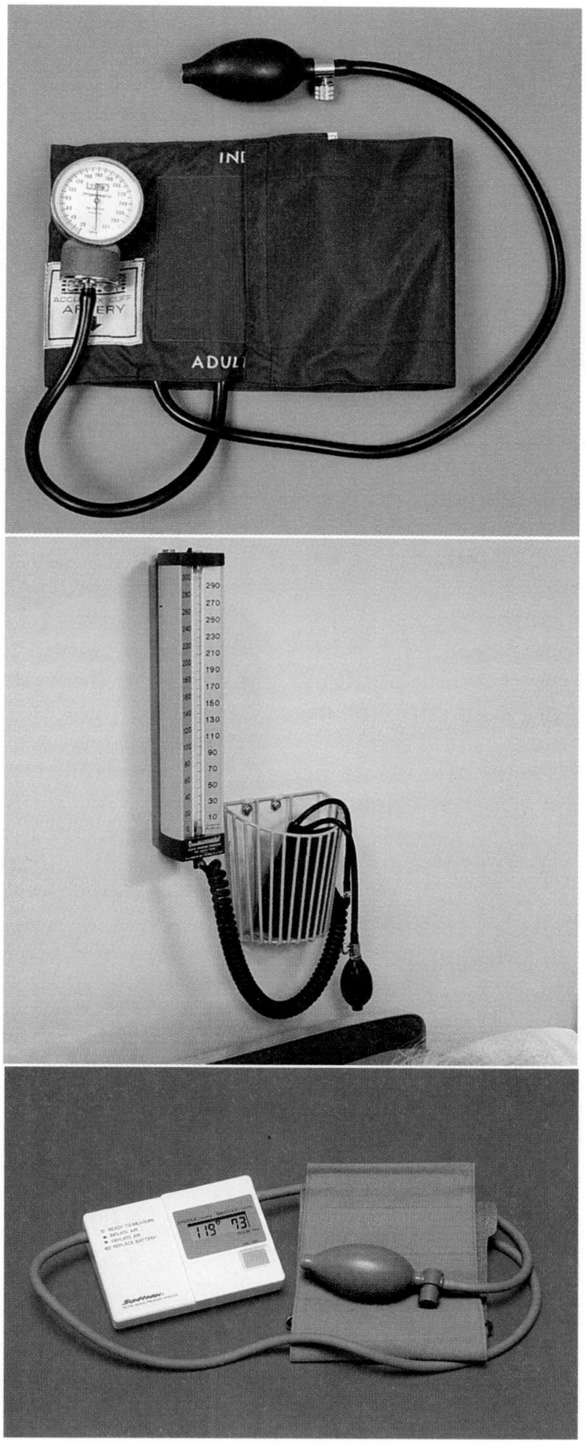

Fig. 21-21 A, Aneroid manometer and cuff. **B,** Mercury manometer and cuff. **C,** Electronic sphygmomanometer.

Measuring Blood Pressure

Blood pressure is normally measured in the brachial artery. Box 21-2 lists the guidelines for measuring blood pressure.

Box 21-2 Guidelines for Measuring Blood Pressure

- Do not take blood pressure on an arm with an IV infusion, a cast, or a dialysis access site. If a person had breast surgery, blood pressure is not taken on that side. Also avoid taking blood pressure on an injured arm.
- Let the resident rest for 10 to 20 minutes before measuring the blood pressure.
- Measure blood pressure with the person sitting or lying. Sometimes the doctor orders measurement of blood pressure in the standing position.
- Use the correct size blood pressure cuff (for example, a pediatric cuff for a very small arm).
- Apply the cuff to the bare upper arm. Clothing can affect the measurement. Do not apply the cuff over clothing.
- Make sure the cuff is snug. Loose cuffs can cause inaccurate readings.
- Place the diaphragm of the stethoscope firmly over the artery. The entire diaphragm must have contact with the skin.
- Make sure the room is quiet. Talking, television, radio, and sounds from the hallway can affect an accurate measurement.
- Have the sphygmomanometer clearly visible.
- Locate the radial artery, and then inflate the cuff. When you no longer feel the radial pulse, inflate the cuff another 30 mm Hg. This prevents cuff inflation to an unnecessarily high pressure, which is painful to the person.
- Measure the systolic and diastolic pressures. Expect to hear the first blood pressure sound at the point where you last felt the radial pulse. The first sound is the systolic pressure. The point where the sound disappears is the diastolic pressure.
- Take the blood pressure again if you are not sure of an accurate measurement. Wait 30 to 60 seconds before repeating the measurement.
- Notify the nurse immediately if you cannot hear the blood pressure.

Measuring Blood Pressure

NNAAP™ SKILL

Quality of Life

Remember to:
- *Knock before entering the resident's room*
- *Address the resident by name*
- *Introduce yourself by name and title*

Pre-Procedure

1 Collect the following:
- Sphygmomanometer (blood pressure cuff)
- Stethoscope
- Alcohol wipes

2 Wash your hands.

3 Identify the resident. Check the ID bracelet against the assignment sheet.

4 Explain the procedure to the resident.

5 Provide for privacy.

Procedure

6 Wipe the stethoscope earpieces and diaphragm with alcohol wipes.

7 Have the resident sit or lie down.

8 Position the resident's arm so it is level with the heart. The palm is up.

9 Stand no more than 3 feet away from the sphygmomanometer. A mercury model is vertical, on a flat surface, and at eye level. The aneroid type is directly in front of you.

10 Expose the upper arm.

11 Squeeze the cuff to expel any remaining air. Close the valve on the bulb.

12 Find the brachial artery at the inner aspect of the elbow.

13 Place the arrow on the cuff over the brachial artery (Fig. 21-22, *A*, p. 508). Wrap the cuff around the upper arm at least 1 inch above the elbow. It should be even and snug.

14 Place the stethoscope earpieces in your ears.

15 Locate the radial artery. Inflate the cuff until you can no longer feel the pulse. Inflate the cuff 30 mm Hg beyond the point where you last felt the pulse.

16 Position the diaphragm over the brachial artery (Fig. 21-22, *B*, p. 508).

17 Deflate the cuff at an even rate of 2 to 4 millimeters per second. Turn the valve counterclockwise to deflate the cuff.

18 Note the point on the scale where you hear the first sound. This is the systolic reading. It is near the point where the radial pulse disappeared.

19 Continue to deflate the cuff. Note the point where the sound disappears for the diastolic reading.

20 Deflate the cuff completely. Remove it from the resident's arm. Remove the stethoscope.

21 Record the resident's name and blood pressure on your note pad or assignment sheet.

22 Return the cuff to the case or wall holder.

Post-Procedure

23 Provide for comfort.

24 Place the signal light within reach.

25 Unscreen the resident.

26 Clean the earpieces and diaphragm with alcohol wipes.

27 Return the equipment to its proper place.

28 Wash your hands.

29 Report the blood pressure to the nurse. Record it in the proper place.

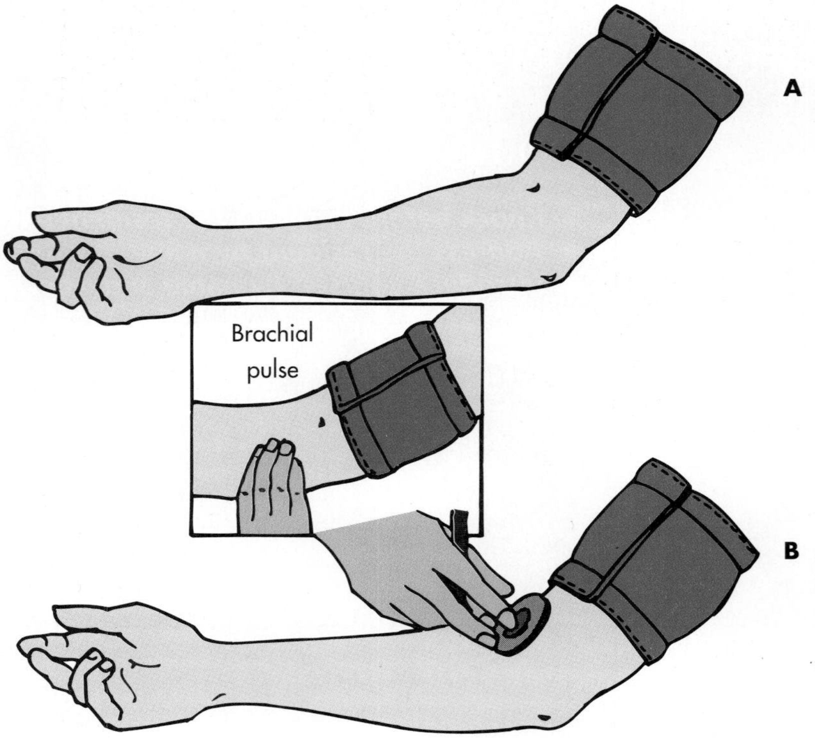

Fig. 21-22 A, The cuff is over the brachial artery. **B,** The diaphragm of the stethoscope is over the brachial artery.

QUALITY OF LIFE

You must protect the resident's right to privacy when measuring vital signs. Privacy is provided during the procedures. This is especially important if you are taking axillary or rectal temperatures and apical pulses. You must not expose the resident unnecessarily.

Always keep resident information confidential. Vital signs are just as private as other resident information. Share this information only with the nurse. Refer questions from family and visitors to the nurse.

The right to personal choice is important. Unless orders note otherwise, vital signs are measured with the resident sitting or lying down. Let the resident choose the position. The resident also may prefer that you use the right or left arm for pulses and blood pressures. Use the arm the resident prefers if it is safe to do so (see Box 21-2).

REVIEW QUESTIONS

Circle the BEST answer.

1 Which statement is *false?*
A The vital signs are temperature, pulse, respirations, and blood pressure.
B Vital signs detect changes in body function.
C Vital signs change only during illness.
D Sleep, exercise, drugs, emotions, and noise affect vital signs.

2 Which temperature should you report immediately?
A An oral temperature of 98.4° F
B A rectal temperature of 101.6° F
C An axillary temperature of 97.6° F
D An oral temperature of 99.0° F

3 You broke a glass thermometer. You must do all of the following *except*
A Notify the nurse immediately
B Immediately clean up the mercury with a paper towel
C Follow center policy for handling hazardous materials
D Protect the resident and yourself from exposure to the mercury

4 A rectal temperature is *not* taken when the resident
A Is unconscious
B Has diarrhea
C Has a nasogastric tube
D Is receiving oxygen

5 Which gives the least accurate measurement of body temperature?
A Oral temperature
B Rectal temperature
C Axillary temperature
D Tympanic temperature

6 Which is usually used to take a pulse?
A The radial pulse
B The apical-radial pulse
C The apical pulse
D The brachial pulse

7 Which is reported to the nurse immediately?
A A resident has a radial pulse of 66 beats per minute.
B A resident has an apical pulse of 40 beats per minute.
C A resident's apical-radial pulse is 80 beats per minute.
D A resident has a radial pulse of 96 beats per minute.

8 Normal respirations are
A Between 10 and 20 per minute
B Quiet and effortless
C Regular with both sides of the chest rising and falling equally
D All of the above

9 Respirations are usually counted
A After taking the temperature
B After taking the pulse
C Before taking the pulse
D After taking the blood pressure

10 Which blood pressure is normal for an adult?
A 88/54 mm Hg
B 210/100 mm Hg
C 130/82 mm Hg
D 152/96 mm Hg

11 When taking a blood pressure, you should do the following *except*
A Take the blood pressure in the arm with an IV infusion
B Apply the cuff to a bare upper arm
C Turn off the television and radio
D Locate the brachial artery

12 Which is the systolic blood pressure?
A The point at which the pulse is no longer felt
B The point where the first sound is heard
C The point where the last sound is heard
D The point 30 mm Hg above where the pulse was felt

Answers to these questions are on p. 699.

22 Admitting, Transferring, and Discharging Residents

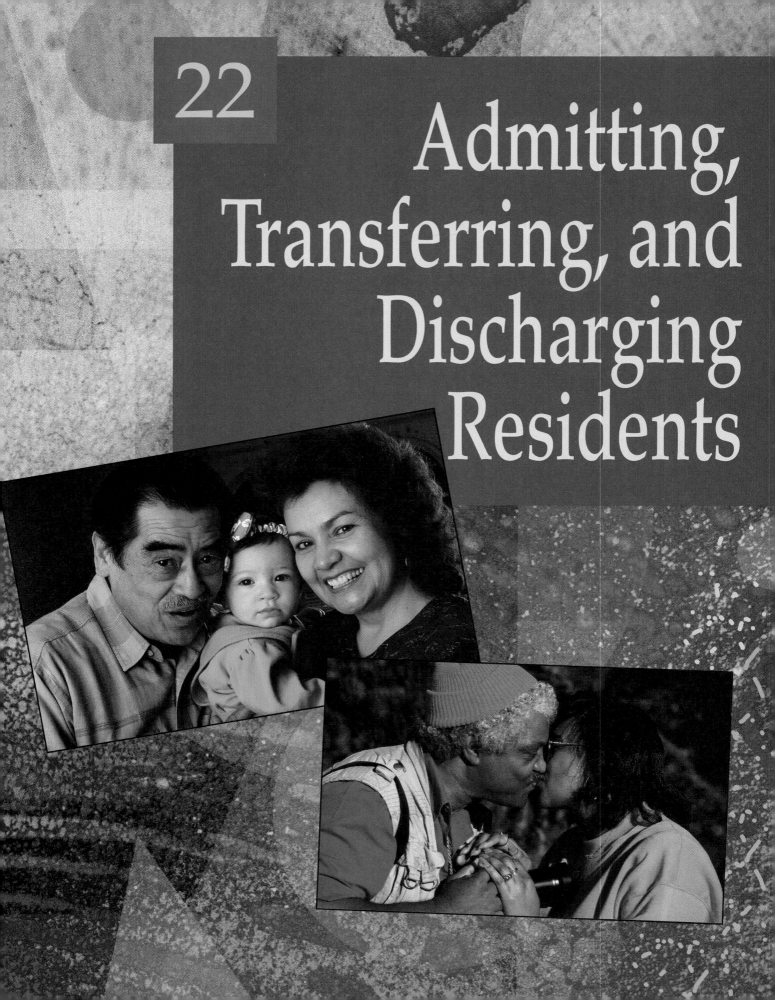

What You Will Learn

- The definition of the key terms listed in this chapter
- The admission process followed by the admissions office
- Ways to help the resident feel comfortable in the nursing center
- The family's role in the admission, transfer, and discharge processes
- How to admit a resident to the nursing unit
- How to weigh and measure a resident
- How to handle the resident's clothing and valuables
- Why residents are transferred to another nursing unit within the center
- How to prepare a resident for discharge
- The procedures described in this chapter

Key Terms

admission Official entry of a person into a nursing center or nursing unit

discharge The official departure of a person from a nursing center or nursing unit

transfer Moving a resident from one room, nursing unit, or nursing center to another

Admission to a nursing center often causes anxiety and fear. New residents and families may be unfamiliar with nursing centers. There are fears of never returning home. Some residents know they will not return home. There also are concerns about the care: who gives it, and is it given? Residents do not know what is expected of them. They worry about getting meals, finding the bathroom, and how to get help. The center's strange sights and sounds frighten some residents. They do not know the staff members or other residents. They are separated from family and friends. They leave behind their home and possessions.

Residents may have similar concerns when transferred to another nursing unit within the center. Discharge usually is a happy time. However, the resident may need to adapt to other changes. The resident may be going to another health care center or may need home care.

OBRA

The center must follow OBRA standards for the transfer and discharge of residents. Reasons for a resident's transfer and discharge are carefully documented to make sure that the resident's rights are protected. The resident and family are notified of any plans for transfer or discharge. The resident may object to a transfer or discharge. If so, the resident follows procedures that allow him or her to be heard. An ombudsman often works with the resident and family to ensure that the resident's best interests are considered.

Admission, transfer, and discharge are critical events for both residents and families. All persons involved need to feel comfortable and secure. Residents leave your unit because of a transfer or discharge. This is your last chance to leave a good impression. You want the resident to leave feeling good about you, the nursing unit, the center, and the care given.

You will use what you have learned from previous chapters when admitting, transferring, and discharging residents. This includes privacy, confidentiality, reporting and recording, communicating with the health team, communication rules, and understanding and communicating with residents. Respect for the resident and the resident's property also applies.

ADMISSIONS

The admission process begins in the admissions office. **Admission** is the official entry of a person into the center. *(See Residents With Dementia, p. 512.)* A health care team member conducts the initial admitting procedures. *(See Subacute Care, p. 512.)* Many centers now have admission coordinators. They make

Residents With Dementia

Persons with dementia and their families may need special help during the admission process. The person's confusion may increase in new surroundings. He or she may become fearful and agitated and want to leave. Family members are also fearful and often feel guilty about admitting the person to a nursing center. The health care team works together to help the resident and the family feel safe and welcome. The nurse, social worker, activities coordinator, and nursing assistant are very important members of this team.

Subacute Care

Persons admitted to subacute care units are usually very ill and need rehabilitation. They often arrive with special equipment and medical supplies. An RN usually greets the person and starts the admission process. You may need to assist the RN. The nurse may ask you to complete the admission process if the person has no serious discomfort or distress.

sure the resident's admission is as simple and easy as possible. Often admission procedures are completed 2 or 3 days before the person enters the center. Identifying information is obtained from the person or a family member. This includes the person's full name, age, date of birth, doctor's name, Social Security number, and religion. The information is recorded on the admission record.

The nursing staff is told of the admission and room assignment before the resident arrives. Some residents arrive by ambulance or wheelchair van. The attendants take them directly to their rooms. Some residents arrive by private car. A nurse or nursing assistant takes them to their rooms. Some residents want a family member with them. Then the family also goes to the room. This is a critical and emotional time for the resident and family. They are not separated until they are comfortable doing so. Remember that the center is now the person's home.

Admitting papers and a general consent for treatment are signed. The resident signs them. If the resident is not mentally competent, the responsible family member does so. This is done before or after the resident is taken to his or her room.

At some time after admission, a photograph is taken and the resident is given an ID bracelet. This is used to identify the resident (see Chapter 8).

Preparing the Room

The room needs to be ready for the new resident. This usually is your responsibility. Fig. 22-1 shows a room ready for a resident's arrival.

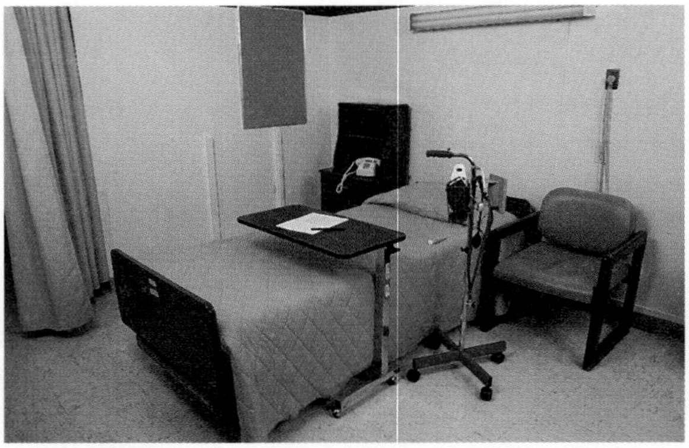

Fig. 22-1 The room is ready for a resident to be admitted.

Preparing the Resident's Room

Pre-Procedure

1 Know which room and bed to prepare. Find out if the resident will arrive by wheelchair or stretcher.

2 Wash your hands.

3 Collect the following:
- Personal-care items: bath basin, pitcher, glass, bedpan, and urinal (for a male resident)
- Admission checklist (Fig. 22-2, p. 514)
- Sphygmomanometer
- Stethoscope
- Gown or pajamas, towel, and washcloth
- IV pole if needed

Procedure

4 For the resident arriving by stretcher:
   a Open the bed as for a surgical bed (see Chapter 12).
   b Raise the bed to its highest level.

5 For the ambulatory or wheelchair resident:
   a Leave the bed closed.
   b Lower the bed to its lowest level.

6 Attach the signal light to the bed linens.

7 Place the sphygmomanometer, stethoscope, and admission checklist on the overbed table.

8 Place the gown or pajamas, towel, washcloth, and personal-care items in the bedside stand.

9 Place the water pitcher and glass on the bedside stand or overbed table. (If the resident is NPO, omit this step.)

10 Wash your hands.

BONELL NURSING UNIT ADMISSION CHECKLIST

For Nursing Assistants

_____ 1. Check the room before resident arrives to see that: _____ room is clean.
_____ bed made _____ straw & H_2O pitcher _____ washcloth & hand towel.
_____ 2. Introduce resident to yourself, other residents, and staff. Likes to be called ____________.
_____ 3. Orient resident to room and call lights _____.
_____ 4. _____ T. _____ P. _____ R. _____ BP. _____ Wt. _____ Ht.
_____ 5. Fill out Inventory of Personal Effects form _____.
_____ 6. Laundry service: _____ family to do _____ sign posted at receptacle
_____ facility to do _____ clothes marked
_____ 7. Mark comb, brush, toothbrush, denture cup, dentures, eyeglasses, etc. _____.
_____ 8. Assist in putting personal possessions away _____.

Signature ______________________ Date __________

For Medical Records Unit Assistant or Charge Nurse

_____ 1. Alert CNA of new admission _____.
_____ 2. Copy Face Sheet and sent to medical records _____ Kitchen (also sent written request).
_____ 3. Order lab work: _____ X-ray _____ Other
_____ 4. Complete chart: _____.
_____ 5. Place name in the following places: _____ bath schedule _____ room door
_____ medicine cabinet _____ closet door _____ bed _____ dresser
_____ daily census _____ daily report _____ wheelchair _____ towel rack
_____ 6. Place name tag on resident.

Signature ______________________ Date __________

Continued

For Social Services

_____ 1. Take 2 pictures.
_____ 2. _____ Desire beauty shop _____ Barber shop
_____ 3. Placement of door badge.

Signature ______________________ Date __________

For Admitting Nurse

_____ 1. Talked with resident of Philosophy of Independence and of going to dining room for meals.
_____ 2. Complete Nursing Assessment, Pain Assessment, Braden, Bladder Assessment, and Safety Assessment. Send communique to P.T. for a Rehab Assessment one week prior to Care Conference.
_____ 3. Determine allergies.
_____ 4. Remove all medication from room.
_____ 5. Make out nursing care plan and aide assignment sheet.
_____ 6. Chart admission remarks—(date, time, admitted from, with whom, mode of transportation, mobility, (V.S., etc.).
_____ 7. Check Physicians Orders: clarify orders, obtain missing Dx (i.e.: catheter, psych Dx), write treatment on treatment profile sheet.
_____ 8. Call Pharmacy, inform them of Pay Status, order medication if needed. Write medication on medication profile sheet.
_____ 9. Obtain V.S. × each shift × 3 days.
_____ 10. Chart each shift × 3 days.
_____ 11. Schedule Glucose monitoring next AM.
_____ 12. Obtain order for 2-step TB test.
_____ 13. Place name on daily census and 24 hour report. Place name on resident roster along with pertinent data.
_____ 14. Supply Care Enrollment form.
_____ 15. Write name in lab book.

Signature ______________________ Date __________

Discharge Check List

_____ 1. Physician order received _____.
_____ 2. Responsible party notified _____, who ______________.
_____ 3. Update MDS for discharge; make 2 copies _____.
 a. _____ one for resident
 b. _____ one for Medical Records
_____ 4. Complete Discharge Summary and Post Discharge Plan GSS #227.
_____ 5. If discharge to hospital or other health care facility, transfer form filled out _____.
_____ 6. If discharged to home, a discharge form filled out_____. Was a home health care agency ordered and contracted? _____.
_____ 7. Discharge instructions: Medications (for home) special instructions _____; other written instructions _____ (retain a copy).
 a. _____ equipment ______________.
 b. _____ dietary instructions ______________.
_____ 8. Document on Nurses Notes the time of discharge, on the above information, document dispensation of all medications, and on the physical, mental, and psychosocial assessment of resident.
_____ 9. Place name on daily census for discharge _____ and on daily report _____, and remove from Resident Roster.
_____ 10. Remove name from bath list _____.
_____ 11. Notify kitchen _____.
_____ 12. Notify housekeeping _____.
_____ 13. Confirm forwarding address _____ and notify finance of discharge and address.
_____ 14. Send chart to Medical Records _____.
_____ 15. Place Schedule II, III, IV, and V count sheets and unused medications in locked Narcotic cupboard in medication room. Inform Nurse Manager.
_____ 16. Notify Pharmacy _____ Date _____ Time _____.
_____ 17. Inventory of personal effects reviewed, and disposition noted on Inventory of Personal Effects form.
_____ 18. Place discharge information in OPUS Book and Lab Book.

Signature ______________________ Date __________

Fig. 22-2 Admission checklist. *(Courtesy Bonell Good Samaritan Center, Greeley, Colo.)*

Admitting the Resident

The resident usually is greeted and escorted to the room by the nurse. However, the nurse may ask you to do so if the resident is in no apparent discomfort or distress. The admission record will give you the resident's name.

The resident needs to feel physically and mentally comfortable, safe, and secure. Avoid rushing into admission procedures. Rather, treat the resident and family as if they are guests in your home. Offer them a cup of coffee, tea, or other beverage. Visit with them, and tell them some of the many good things about the center. This is a good time to introduce the person's roommate. You also can introduce the person to other residents in nearby rooms. You might write down their names for the new resident. Remembering names given during introductions is hard for many people. It is important that when the family leaves, the resident will know others. He or she will not be left in the awkward position of not knowing anyone. Other residents are a source of great comfort and support to the new resident. They understand, better than any health care team member, what it is like to enter a nursing center.

Remember that this is the resident's home. You need to help the resident make the room as homelike as possible. You can help the resident unpack. Perhaps the resident needs help hanging clothes and putting things in drawers. Maybe the resident wants to hang a picture or display photographs. This is a time to show caring and compassion. Do all that you can to help the person feel safe, comfortable, and secure.

When the resident is comfortable, an admission checklist is completed. The resident's vital signs, weight, and height are measured. The resident is oriented to the room and told about the nursing unit and the center.

The nurse or social worker explains the resident's rights to the resident and family. They also are given a booklet explaining these rights. This is required by OBRA. OBRA

The following will promote positive communication during the admission process:

- Greet the resident by name. Use the admission record to find out the resident's name. Ask if he or she prefers a certain name.
- Introduce yourself to the resident and family or friends present. Give your title, and explain that you assist the nurses in giving care.
- Introduce the roommate.
- Provide for privacy. Ask family members or friends to leave the room. Tell them how much time you need and where they can wait comfortably. (Allow a family member or friend to stay if the resident prefers.)
- Complete a clothing and valuables list (see Chapter 8). Help the resident hang clothes in the closet and put personal items in the drawers and bedside stand. (The resident's family may wish to help with this.)
- Measure vital signs (see Chapter 21).
- Weigh and measure the resident (p. 516). (If the resident is fully dressed, this is done at bedtime.)
- Orient the resident to furniture and equipment in the room. Also, explain meal times and the location of the nurses' station, lounge, chapel, and dining room.
- Fill the water pitcher if oral fluids are allowed (see Chapter 18).
- Place the signal light within reach (see Chapter 8). Place other controls and needed items within reach.
- Keep the bed in its lowest position (see Chapter 8).
- Raise or lower bed rails as instructed by the nurse (see Chapter 8).

Measuring height and weight. Height and weight are measured on admission. The resident wears only a gown or pajamas. Shoes or slippers add weight. They also cause inaccurate height measurement. Residents who are fully dressed on admission are weighed and measured at bedtime. The resident should urinate before being weighed. A full bladder can affect the weight measurement.

There are standing, chair, and lift scales (Fig. 22-3, p. 518). Chair and lift scales are used for residents who cannot stand. Some centers use electronic digital chair and lift scales. You must follow the manufacturer's instructions and center procedures when using chair or lift scales.

Text continued on p. 519

Measuring Height and Weight

NNAAP™ SKILL

Quality of Life

Remember to:
- ***Knock before entering the resident's room***
- ***Address the resident by name***
- ***Introduce yourself by name and title***

Pre-Procedure

1 Explain the procedure to the resident.
2 Ask the resident to urinate (see Chapter 16).
3 Wash your hands.
4 Collect the following:
   a Scale (standing, chair, wheelchair, or lift scale)
   b Paper towels
5 Identify the resident. Check the ID bracelet against the assignment sheet.
6 Provide for privacy.

Procedure

7 Standing scale:
   a Place the paper towels on the scale platform.
   b Raise the height-measurement rod.
   c Ask the resident to remove the robe and slippers. Assist if necessary.
   d Help the resident stand on the scale platform with the arms to the sides.
   e Move the weights until the balance pointer is in the middle (Fig. 22-4, p. 518).

Measuring Height and Weight—cont'd

NNAAP™ SKILL

Procedure—cont'd

- f Record the name and weight on your notepad or assignment sheet.
- g Ask the resident to stand as straight as possible.
- h Lower the height measurement rod until it rests on the resident's head.
- i Record the height on your notepad or assignment sheet.

8 Chair scale:

- a Help the resident transfer from the wheelchair to the chair scale (see *Transferring the Resident to a Chair or Wheelchair,* p. 217).
- b Place the resident's feet on the foot platform (Fig. 22-3, *B,* p. 518).
- c Move the weights until the balance pointer is in the middle.
- d Record the weight on your notepad or assignment sheet.

9 Lift scale:

- a Attach the sling and chains to the lift.
- b Place both weights on zero.
- c Level and balance the scale according to the manufacturer's instructions.
- d Remove the sling from the scale.
- e Place the resident on the sling, and attach it to the lift. Raise the resident about 4 inches off the bed (see *Using a Mechanical Lift,* p. 223).
- f Move the weights until the balance pointer is in the middle.
- g Record the weight on your notepad or assignment sheet.
- h Lower the resident to the bed.
- i Remove the sling.

Post-Procedure

10 Help the resident put on robe and slippers or clothing if he or she will be up. Or help him or her back to bed.

11 Provide for comfort.

12 Place the signal light within reach.

13 Raise or lower bed rails. Follow the care plan.

14 Unscreen the resident.

15 Return the scale to its proper place.

16 Wash your hands.

17 Report the height and weight to the nurse. Record the measurements in the proper place.

A **B** **C**

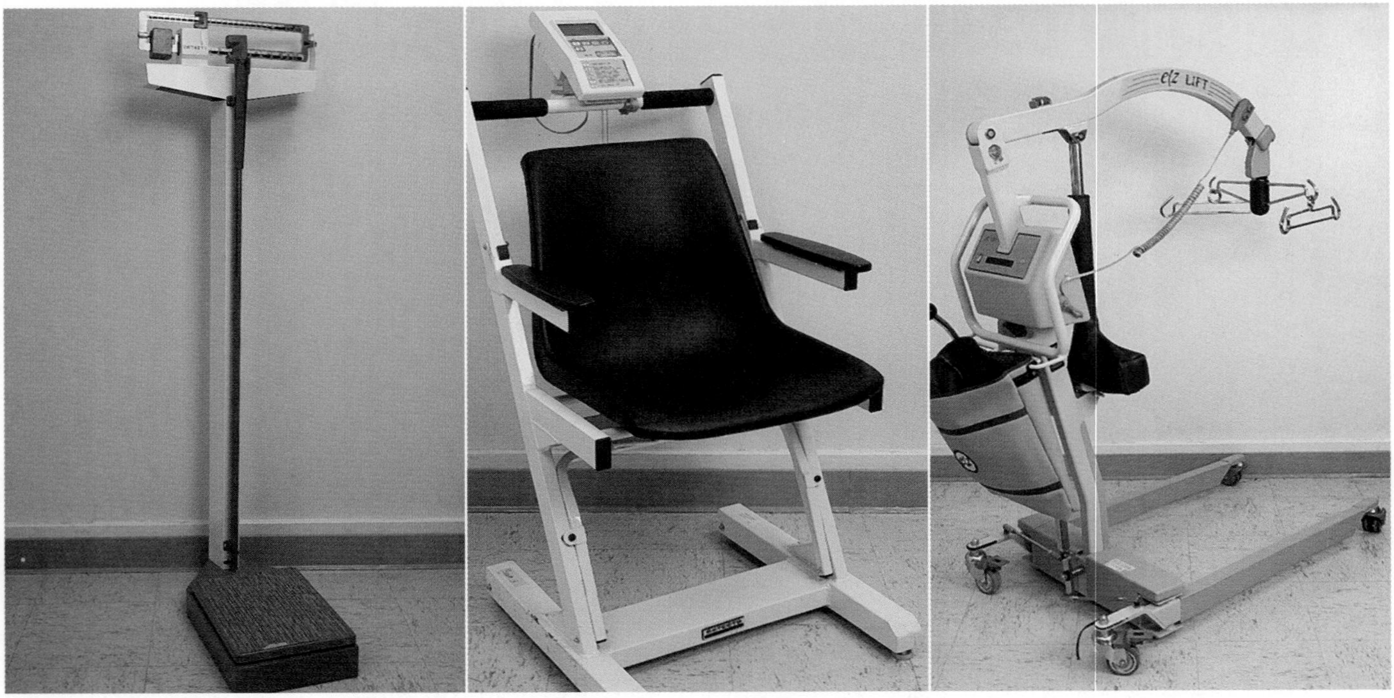

Fig. 22-3 **A,** Standing scale. **B,** Chair scale. **C,** Lift scale.

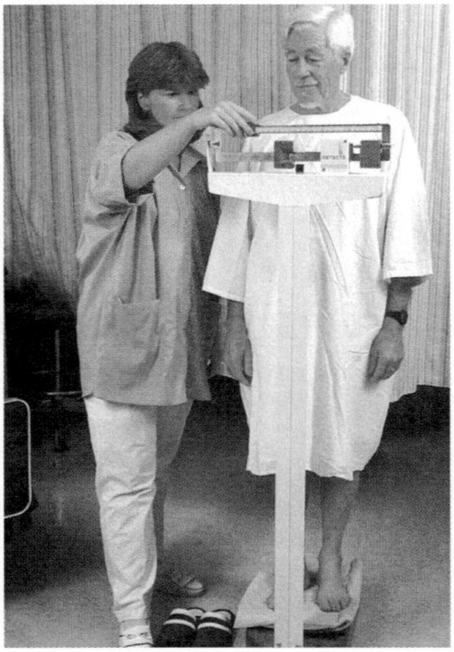

Fig. 22-4 The resident is weighed and measured. The weight is read when the balance pointer is in the middle.

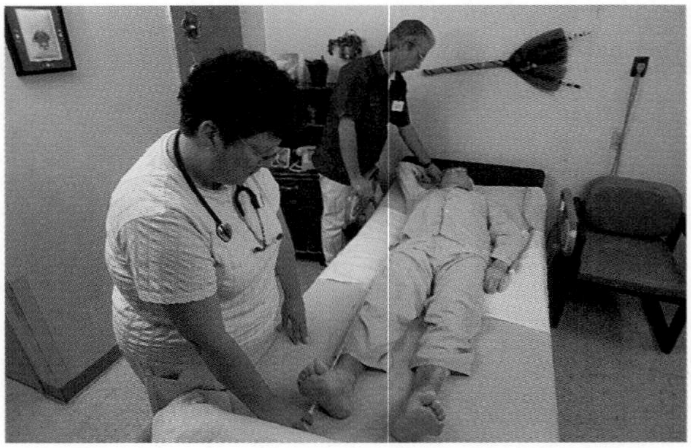

Fig. 22-5 The resident is measured in bed. The ruler extends from the top of his head to his heel.

Measuring Height: the Wheelchair or Bed Resident

Quality of Life

Remember to:
- *Knock before entering the resident's room*
- *Address the resident by name*
- *Introduce yourself by name and title*

Pre-Procedure

1 Explain the procedure to the resident.
2 Wash your hands.
3 Collect a measuring tape and ruler.
4 Get a helper.
5 Provide for privacy.

Procedure

6 Position the resident supine if this position is allowed.
7 Have your helper hold the end of the measuring tape at the resident's heel.
8 Pull the measuring tape alongside the resident's body until it extends past the head.
9 Place the ruler flat across the top of the head. It should extend from the resident's head to the measuring tape. Make sure the ruler is level (Fig. 22-5).
10 Record the height on your notepad or assignment sheet.

Post-Procedure

11 Provide for comfort. Assist the resident back to the wheelchair if appropriate.
12 Raise or lower bed rails if the resident stays in bed. Follow the care plan.
13 Place the signal light within reach. Unscreen the resident.
14 Return equipment to its proper location.
15 Wash your hands.
16 Report the height to the nurse. Record the measurement in the proper place.

Clothing and valuables. A list is made of the resident's clothing and valuables (see Chapter 8). Valuables, including money and jewelry, are kept in a safe place. If the resident wishes, they are sent home with a family member. The staff member admitting the resident completes a clothing list. Each item is identified and described on the list. The staff member and resident both sign the completed list. If the resident cannot sign, a family member does so.

A valuables envelope is used for money and jewelry. Each jewelry piece is listed and described on the envelope. It is placed in the envelope while the resident watches. Money is counted with the resident before being put in the envelope. The envelope is sealed and signed like the clothing checklist. The envelope is given to the nurse. The nurse or social worker takes the envelope to the safe or sends it home with the family.

Some valuables are kept at the bedside. These include dentures, eyeglasses, contact lenses, hearing aids, watches, electric shavers, clocks, and radios. Valuables kept at the bedside are listed in the resident's record. Also, include wheelchairs, walkers, canes, crutches, or other special equipment brought from home. Most centers do safety checks of any medical equipment brought from home. Follow center policy for handling such equipment. Some residents keep money for newspapers, telephone calls, and vending machines. The amount of money kept by the resident is noted in the resident's record.

TRANSFERS

Sometimes a resident is transferred to another room or nursing unit. A **transfer** is moving a resident from one room, nursing unit, or nursing center to another. Transfers usually are related to a change in condition. Some residents are transferred to a hospital. Others may transfer to a hospice unit. A resident may request a room change. Room changes may be necessary if roommates do not get along.

The doctor, nurse, or social worker explains the reasons for the transfer. The family and business office are notified. You may assist in the transfer or carry out the entire procedure. The resident usually is transported by wheelchair or stretcher. Sometimes the bed is used.

The resident needs support and reassurance during a transfer. The resident is going to a new unit or agency and does not know the staff. Use good communication skills at this time. Avoid pat answers such as "everything will be OK." Touch is often comforting at this time. Also help the resident by introducing him or her to new health care team members. Wish the resident well as you leave him or her.

Transferring the Resident to Another Nursing Unit

Quality of Life

Remember to:
- *Knock before entering the resident's room*
- *Address the resident by name*
- *Introduce yourself by name and title*

Pre-Procedure

1 Find out where the resident is going. Find out if you need to use the bed, a wheelchair, or stretcher.

2 Explain the procedure to the resident.

3 Get a stretcher or wheelchair, bath blanket, and a utility cart if needed.

Procedure

4 Wash your hands.

5 Identify the resident. Check the ID bracelet against the transfer slip. Call the resident by name.

6 Put the resident's personal belongings and bedside equipment on the utility cart.

7 Assist the resident to the wheelchair or stretcher (see *Transferring the Resident to a Chair or Wheelchair,* pp. 217-218, or *Transferring the Resident to a Stretcher,* p. 225). Cover the resident with a bath blanket.

8 Transport the resident to the assigned place.

9 Introduce the resident to the receiving nurse.

10 Help the nurse transfer the resident from the wheelchair or stretcher into bed. Help position the resident. (If the resident does not wish to go to bed, make sure he or she is comfortable in the wheelchair or assist the resident to a comfortable chair.)

11 Bring the resident's personal belongings and equipment to the new room. Help put them away.

12 Report the following to the receiving nurse:
- How the resident tolerated the transfer
- That a nurse will bring the resident's chart, care plan, and medications

Post-Procedure

13 Return the wheelchair or stretcher and utility cart to the storage area.

14 Wash your hands.

15 Strip the bed, clean the unit, and make a closed bed. (In some centers, the housekeeping department does this.) Follow center policy.

DISCHARGES

Discharges usually are planned in advance. **Discharge** is the official departure of the resident from the center. This is usually a happy time if the resident is going home. Some residents are discharged to a hospital or to another nursing center. Others need home care. These residents may have fears and concerns. The doctor, nurse, dietitian, social worker, and other health care team members plan the resident's discharge. They teach the resident and family about diet, exercise, and drugs. They also teach the resident and family how to perform care procedures or give treatments. They arrange for special home care and therapy. *(See Subacute Care.)* A doctor's appointment may be given.

The resident or family needs to make arrangements for payment at the business office. Sometimes financial arrangements are made on admission or before discharge.

You will help the resident dress and pack belongings. You also may transport the resident out of the center. The nurse tells you when to start the discharge procedure. The doctor must write a discharge order before the resident can leave. The nurse tells you when the resident may leave and how to transport him or her. Usually a wheelchair is used. Some centers allow the resident to walk if able. Occasionally a resident leaves by ambulance. Ambulance staff bring the stretcher to the room. They are responsible for transport.

SUBACUTE CARE

Persons discharged from a subacute care unit need teaching about their rehabilitation program. The physical therapist, occupational therapist, speech/language pathologist, respiratory therapist, nurse, social worker, and dietician are involved in discharge teaching. Special equipment also is obtained. Therapists often make a home visit with the person before discharge to assure that the person will be safe in the home setting. Follow-up visits by the therapist, nurse, and social worker may be needed. Some centers have a case manager who makes sure that the person has all needed services, equipment, and supplies for returning home.

Always use good communication skills when assisting with a resident's discharge. Wish the resident and family well as they leave the center.

A resident may wish to leave the center without the doctor's permission. You must notify the nurse immediately if the resident expresses the wish or intent to leave. The nurse or social worker handles the situation.

Discharging the Resident

QUALITY OF LIFE

Remember to:
- *Knock before entering the resident's room*
- *Address the resident by name*
- *Introduce yourself by name and title*

Procedure

1. Make sure the resident is to be discharged. Find out if transportation arrangements were made.
2. Explain the procedure to the resident.
3. Wash your hands.
4. Identify the resident. Check the ID bracelet against the discharge slip. Call the resident by name.
5. Provide for privacy.
6. Help the resident dress if assistance is needed (see *Dressing the Resident,* p. 341).
7. Help the resident pack. Check all drawers and closets to make sure all items are collected.
8. Check off the clothing list. Ask the resident or responsible party to sign the form indicating that all clothing was returned.

Continued

Discharging the Resident—cont'd

Procedure—cont'd

9 Tell the nurse that the resident is ready for the final visit. The nurse:
 a Gives prescriptions written by the doctor
 b Provides discharge instructions
 c Secures valuables from the safe

10 Get a wheelchair and a utility cart for the resident's belongings. Ask a co-worker to help you.

11 Assist the resident into the wheelchair (see *Transferring the Resident to a Wheelchair,* p. 217).

12 Take the resident to the exit area. Lock the wheels of the wheelchair. Help the resident out of the wheelchair and into the car (Fig. 22-6).

13 Help put the belongings into the car.

14 Return the wheelchair and utility cart to the storage area.

15 Wash your hands.

16 Report the following to the nurse:
 a The time of discharge
 b How the resident was transported
 c Who accompanied the resident
 d The resident's destination
 e Any other observations

17 Strip the bed, clean the resident unit, and make a closed bed. (In some centers, the housekeeping department does this.) Follow center policy.

18 Wash your hands.

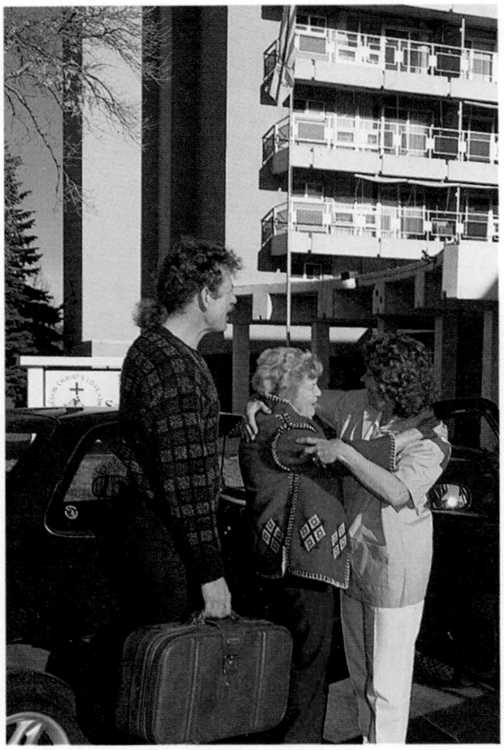

Fig. 22-6 The resident is being discharged.

Quality of Life

Admission to a nursing center usually is a difficult time for the resident and family. Transfers also can cause fear and apprehension. Discharge usually is a happy and pleasant event. However, it may cause worries and concerns if more care and treatment are needed. You can help the resident and family cope with these events. Be courteous, caring, efficient, and competent. You must be sensitive to the resident's and the family's fears and concerns. The person's property and valuables are handled carefully and with respect. They are kept in a safe place and protected from loss or damage. Always treat the resident and family the way you would like your loved ones treated.

The first hours and days in the center are often very lonely and difficult. It is important to check on new residents often. Introduce them to other residents. Encourage them to take part in activities. Remember to explain all procedures and what the various sounds mean. You may need to repeat the same information often. Remember that the new resident is in a new place and is receiving all kinds of new information. It may take a while to remember things. The resident will feel safer and more secure if he or she knows what is happening and why. Remember to always protect the resident's rights and to promote quality of life for the resident.

Review Questions

Circle T if the statement is true and F if the statement is false.

1 T F Identifying information is obtained when the resident arrives on the nursing unit.

2 T F Residents who arrive by ambulance are taken to their room by the ambulance staff.

3 T F The resident should be greeted by name during the admission process.

4 T F The admission checklist is completed when the resident arrives in his or her room.

5 T F You are responsible for explaining the resident's rights to the resident and family.

6 T F A resident complains of pain. You should report the complaint after completing the admission checklist.

7 T F You help orient the resident to the new environment.

8 T F A robe and slippers are worn when the resident is weighed and measured.

9 T F A tape measure is used to measure the height of ambulatory residents.

10 T F A list is made of clothing and valuables during the admission process.

11 T F The resident's condition may require a transfer to another nursing unit within the center.

12 T F A doctor's order is required for discharge from the nursing center.

13 T F You are responsible for instructing the resident about diet and drugs.

14 T F Starting with admission, the resident's rights are protected.

15 T F A confused person may become more confused in a new environment.

Circle the BEST answer.

16 You are admitting a person to the nursing unit. Your first action is to
- A Greet the person by name
- B Ask the person his or her name
- C Tell the person that everything will be OK
- D Introduce the roommate

17 A resident is discharged. You should
- A Tell the resident that everything will be OK
- B Tell the resident not to worry
- C Wish the resident well
- D Introduce the resident to new nursing staff

18 Mr. Jones objects to a transfer. Which is *false?*
- A You report the information to the nurse.
- B You tell Mr. Jones not to worry.
- C Mr. Jones has the right to be heard.
- D The ombudsman will help Mr. Jones to ensure his rights are respected.

Answers to these questions are on p. 699.

23 Assisting With the Physical Examination

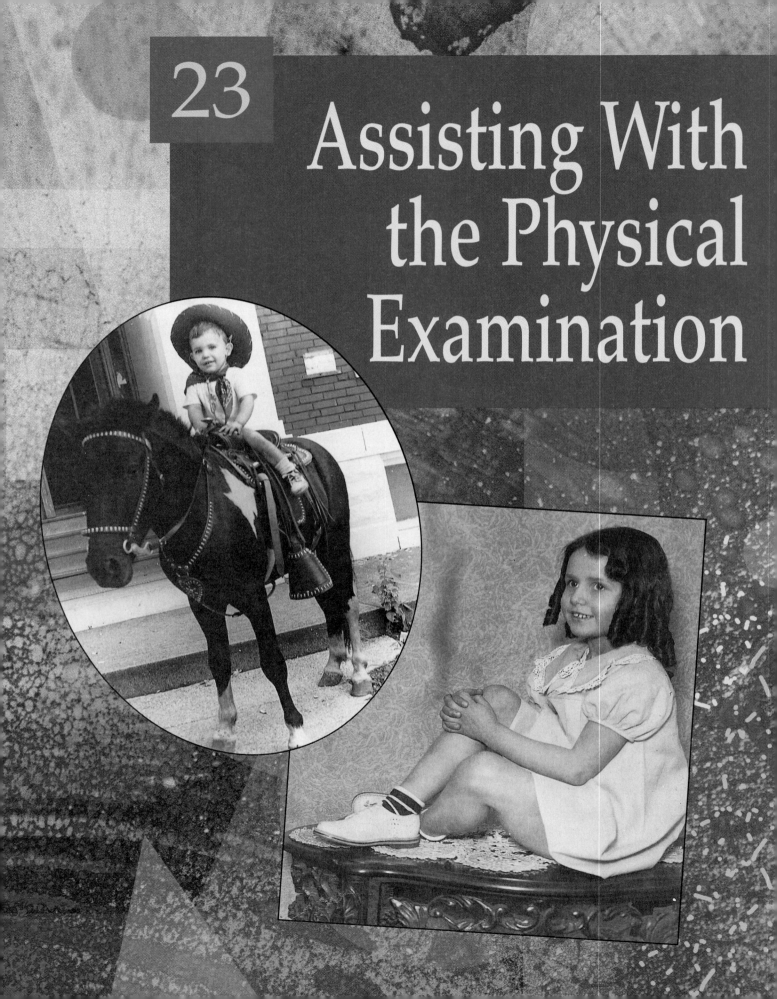

What You Will Learn

- The definition of the key terms listed in this chapter
- What to do before, after, and during a physical examination
- The equipment used during a physical examination
- How to prepare a resident for an examination
- Four examination positions and how to drape the resident for each position
- How to promote quality of life for the resident having an examination
- The rules for assisting with a physical examination
- The procedure described in this chapter

Key Terms

dorsal recumbent position The supine or back-lying examination position; the legs are together

horizontal recumbent position The dorsal recumbent position

knee-chest position The person kneels and rests the body on the knees and chest; the head is turned to one side, the arms are above the head or flexed at the elbows, the back is straight, and the body is flexed about 90 degrees at the hips

laryngeal mirror An instrument used to examine the mouth, teeth, and throat

lithotomy position The person is in a back-lying position, the hips are brought down to the edge of the examination table, the knees are flexed, the hips are externally rotated, and the feet are supported in stirrups

nasal speculum An instrument used to examine the inside of the nose

ophthalmoscope A lighted instrument used to examine the internal structures of the eye

otoscope A lighted instrument used to examine the external ear and the eardrum (tympanic membrane)

percussion hammer An instrument used to tap body parts to test reflexes

tuning fork An instrument used to test hearing

vaginal speculum An instrument used to open the vagina so that it and the cervix can be examined

Doctors usually perform physical examinations. Many RNs also perform them. They are done for many reasons. Routine health examinations are done to promote health. Pre-employment physicals are done to determine fitness for work. Physical examinations are used also to diagnose and treat disease. In nursing centers, each resident has a physical examination at least once a year. You may be asked to assist a doctor or RN with a physical examination.

NURSING ASSISTANT RESPONSIBILITIES

Your responsibilities depend on the center's policies and procedures. The examiner's preferences also affect what you are expected to do. You may do some or all of the following:

- Collect linens for draping the resident and for the procedure.
- Collect equipment used for the examination.
- Prepare the examination room or the resident unit for the examination.
- Provide enough lighting.
- Transport the resident to and from the examination room.
- Measure vital signs, height, and weight.
- Position and drape the resident for the examination.
- Hand equipment and instruments to the examiner.
- Label specimen containers.
- Dispose of soiled linen, and discard used disposable supplies.
- Clean reusable equipment after the examination.
- Help the resident dress or assume a comfortable position after the examination.

EQUIPMENT

Some equipment and supplies used in a physical examination are used for resident care. You may recognize some of the instruments. You need to know the instruments shown in Figure 23-1.

- **Ophthalmoscope**—is a lighted instrument used to examine the internal structures of the eye.
- **Otoscope**—is a lighted instrument used to examine the external ear and the eardrum (tympanic membrane). Some scopes have interchangeable parts. They are changed into an ophthalmoscope or otoscope.
- **Percussion hammer**—is used to tap body parts to test reflexes.
- **Vaginal speculum**—is used to open the vagina so that it and the cervix can be examined.
- **Nasal speculum**—is used to examine the inside of the nose.
- **Tuning fork**—is vibrated to test hearing.
- **Laryngeal mirror**—is used to examine the mouth, teeth, and throat.

Some centers have examination trays in the central supply department. If not, collect needed items. Items listed in *Preparing the Resident for an Examination* (p. 527) usually are used for an examination. They are arranged on a tray or table for the examiner.

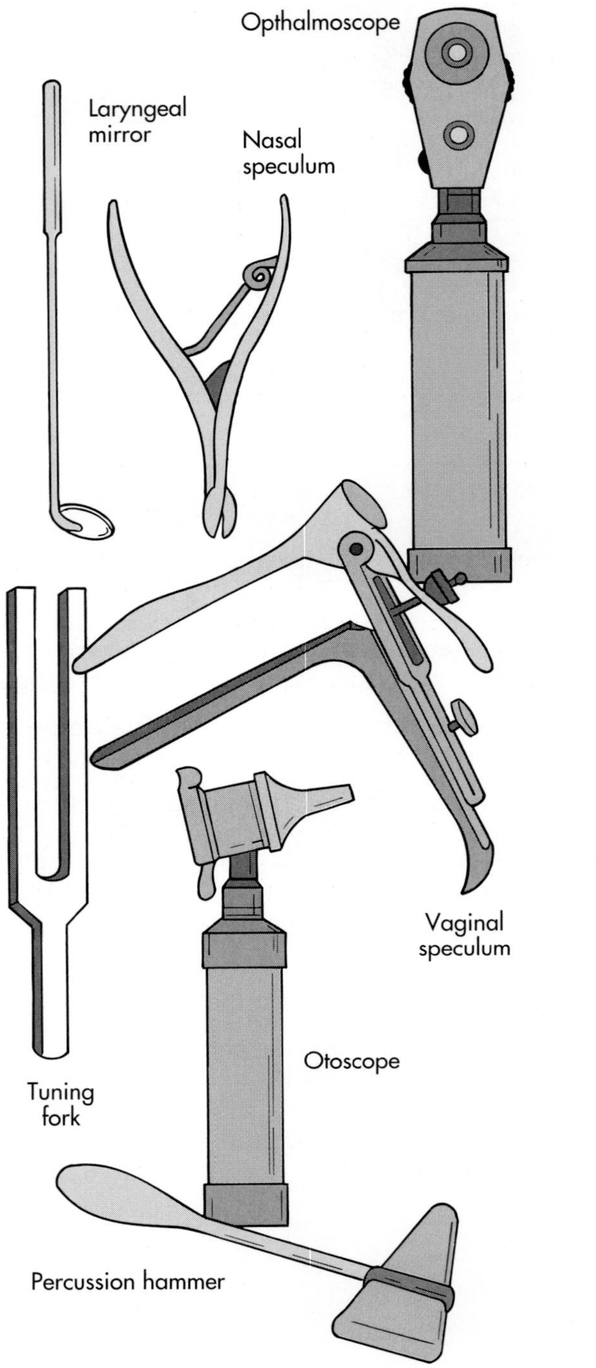

Fig. 23-1 Instrument used for a physical examination.

◈ PREPARING THE RESIDENT

The physical examination causes anxiety for many people. They are concerned about possible findings. Often residents are confused or fearful about what the examiner is going to do. Other factors can add to their anxiety. These include discomfort, embarrassment, the fear of exposure, and not knowing the procedure. You need to be sensitive to the resident's feelings and concerns. The resident is prepared physically and psychologically for the examination. Under OBRA, the resident has the right to know who will do the examination, why it is being done, and what to expect. The doctor or nurse explains these things to the resident.

OBRA

The resident's quality of life is promoted. The resident has the right to personal choice. The doctor or nurse is responsible for informing the resident about the examination. Reasons for the examination are given. The resident is told who will do the examination and when it will be done. The procedure is explained. The resident must give consent. The resident may want a different examiner. Or, the resident may want a family member present. Some residents want the examination results explained with a family member present. All of these are part of the resident's right to personal choice.

Usually all clothes are removed for a complete physical examination. The resident is covered with a drape. A disposable paper drape, a bath blanket, a sheet, or a drawsheet is used. Usually a hospital gown is worn. It reduces the feeling of nakedness and the fear of exposure. Explain to the resident that little exposure occurs during the examination. The resident needs to understand that some exposure is necessary to examine the body. However, only the body part being examined is exposed. You must screen the resident and close the door to the room. This further protects the resident's right to privacy.

The resident urinates before the examination. An empty bladder is necessary for the examiner to feel the abdominal organs. A full bladder can change the normal position and shape of organs. It can also cause discomfort, especially when the abdominal organs are felt. If a urine specimen is needed, obtain it at this time. Explain how to collect the specimen, and label the container properly (see Chapter 16).

Warmth is a major concern during the examination. The resident is protected from chilling. Have an extra bath blanket nearby. Also, take measures to prevent drafts.

The examiner may want height, weight (see Chapter 22), and vital signs (see Chapter 21) measured. These are obtained before the examination starts. They are recorded on the examination form. The resident is then positioned and draped for the examination.

Preparing the Resident for an Examination

Quality of Life

Remember to:
- ***Knock before entering the resident's room***
- ***Address the resident by name***
- ***Introduce yourself by name and title***

Procedure

1. Explain the procedure to the resident.
2. Wash your hands.
3. Assemble the following items on a tray at the bedside or in the examination room:
   - Flashlight
   - Sphygmomanometer
   - Stethoscope
   - Thermometer
   - Tongue depressors (blades)
   - Laryngeal mirror
   - Ophthalmoscope
   - Otoscope
   - Nasal speculum
   - Percussion (reflex) hammer
   - Tuning fork
   - Tape measure
   - Gloves
   - Water-soluble lubricant
   - Vaginal speculum (female resident)
   - Cotton-tipped applicators

Continued

Preparing the Resident for an Examination—cont'd

Procedure—cont'd

- Specimen containers and labels
- Disposable bag
- Emesis basin
- Towel
- Bath blanket
- Tissues
- Drape (sheet, bath blanket, drawsheet, or disposable drape)
- Paper towels
- Cotton balls
- Waterproof bed protector
- Eye chart (Snellen chart)
- Slides
- Gown
- Alcohol wipes
- Wastebasket
- Container for soiled instruments
- Marking pencils or pens

4 Identify the resident. Check the ID bracelet against the assignment sheet.

5 Provide for privacy.

6 Ask the resident to put on the gown. Instruct him or her to remove all clothes. Assist as necessary.

7 Ask the resident to urinate. If the resident is not ambulatory, offer the bedpan or urinal. Provide for privacy.

8 Transport the resident to the examination room.

9 Weigh and measure the resident (see Chapter 22).

10 Help the resident get on the examination table. Have him or her use a stool if necessary. Omit this step if the examination is done in the resident's room.

11 Position the resident as directed. Raise the bed to its highest level. Raise the bed rails if the resident is in bed.

12 Drape the resident.

13 Place a bed protector under the buttocks.

14 Arrange for adequate lighting.

15 Put the signal light on for the nurse or examiner. Do not leave the resident unattended.

POSITIONING AND DRAPING

The resident may have to assume a special position for the examination. Some examination positions (Fig. 23-2) are uncomfortable and embarrassing. The examiner tells you how to position the resident. Help the resident assume and maintain the position. But first explain the following to the resident:

- The need for the position
- How the position is assumed
- How the body is draped
- How long the resident can expect to stay in the position

The **dorsal recumbent (horizontal recumbent)** or supine (back-lying) position is used to examine the abdomen, anterior chest, and breasts. The resident is supine with the legs together. If the perineal area is examined, the knees are flexed and hips externally rotated (see Fig. 23-2, *A*). The resident is draped as for perineal care (see *Female Perineal Care,* p. 292).

The **lithotomy position** (Fig. 23-2, *B*) is used to examine the vagina. The resident lies on her back, and her hips are brought to the edge of the examination table. The knees are flexed, and the hips are externally rotated. The feet are supported in stirrups. The resident is draped as for the dorsal recumbent position. Some centers provide socks to cover the feet and calves. Some residents cannot assume this position. The examiner tells you how to position the resident.

The **knee-chest position** (Fig. 23-2, *C*) is used to examine the rectum. Sometimes it is used to examine the vagina. The resident kneels on the bed or examination table. Then the resident rests his or her body on the knees and chest. The head is turned to one side, and the arms are above the head or flexed at the elbows. The back is straight, and the body is flexed about 90 degrees at the hips. The resident wears a gown and sometimes socks. The drape is applied in a diamond shape to cover the back, buttocks, and thighs. This position is rarely used for older persons. They usually assume the side-lying position.

The *Sims' position* (Fig. 23-2, *D*) is sometimes used to examine the rectum or vagina. The drape is applied in a diamond shape. The corner near the examiner is folded back to expose the rectum or vagina.

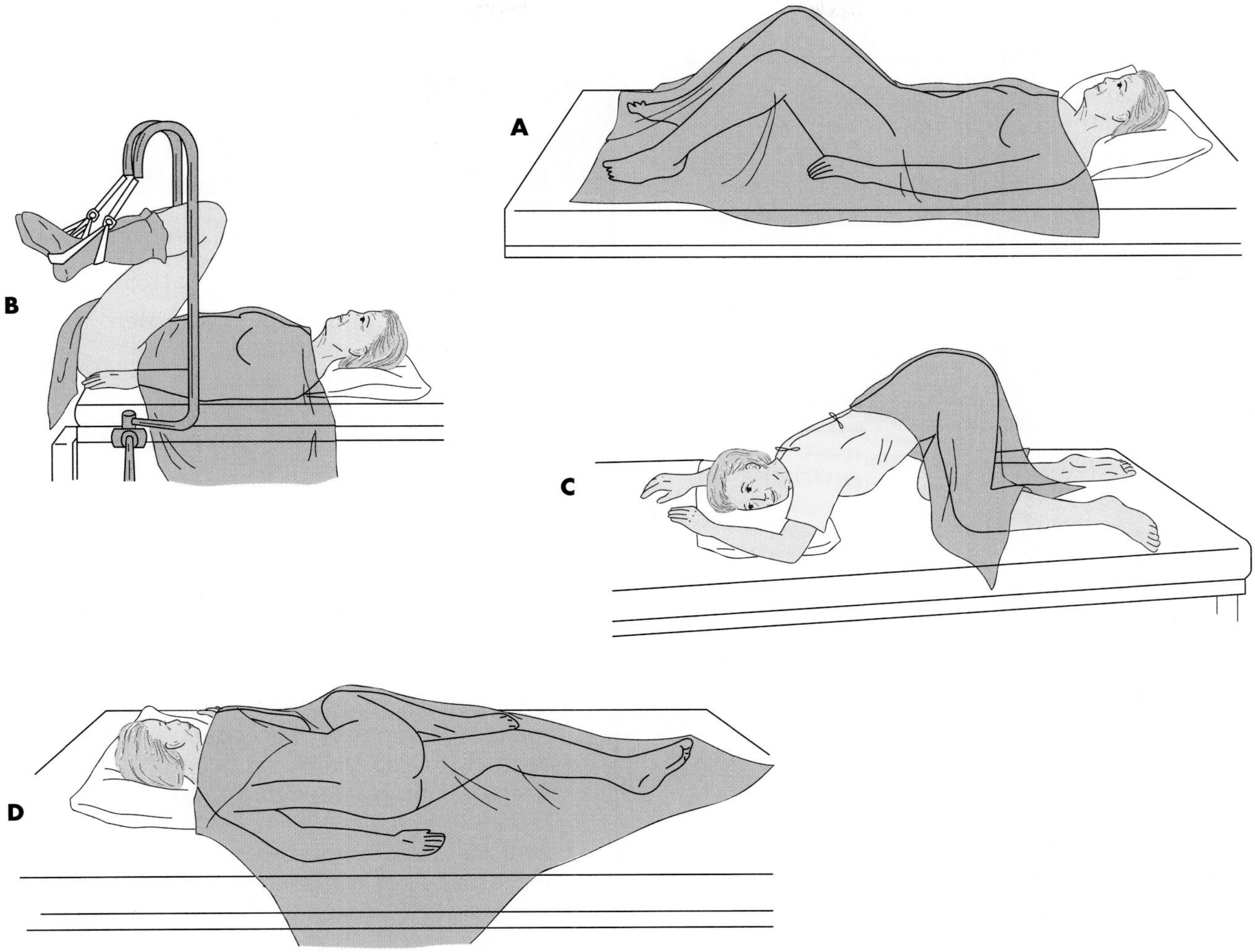

Fig. 23-2 Positioning and draping for the physical examination. **A,** Dorsal recumbent position. **B,** Lithotomy position. **C,** Knee-chest position. **D,** Sims' position.

Residents With Dementia

Residents with dementia may resist the examiner's efforts. The resident may be agitated and physically aggressive because of confusion and fear. A resident who refuses or actively resists an examination is not restrained or forced into allowing an examination. The health care team may need to try at another time. Having a family member present may help calm the resident. Sometimes the doctor orders medication to help the resident relax. The residents' rights are always respected.

ASSISTING WITH THE EXAMINATION

You may be asked to prepare, position, and drape the resident. You also might assist the doctor or RN during the examination. (*See Residents With Dementia.*) When assisting with the examination, follow the rules in Box 23-1.

After the Examination

After the examination the resident is taken back to the room. If the resident will be out of bed, help him or her to dress. Lubricant is used for the vaginal or rectal examination. The area is wiped or cleaned before the resident dresses or returns to the room.

Used disposable items are put in a waste container. Examples are bed protectors, paper drapes, tongue blades, applicators, and cotton balls. These supplies are replaced so the tray is ready for the next examination. Reusable items are cleaned according to center policy and returned to the tray or storage place. This includes the otoscope and ophthalmoscope tips, speculum, and stethoscope. The examination table is covered with a clean drawsheet or paper. All specimens are labeled and taken to the designated area with a requisition slip. The resident's unit or examination room should be neat and orderly after the examination. Follow center policy for soiled linens. Follow Standard Precautions and the Bloodborne Pathogen Standard.

Box 23-1 Rules for Assisting With the Physical Examination

- Wash your hands before and after the examination.
- Provide for privacy. This is done by screening, closing doors, and draping. Expose only the body part being examined.
- Assist the resident in assuming positions as directed by the examiner.
- Place instruments and equipment in a handy location for the examiner.
- Stay in the room when a female is examined (unless you are a male). When a man examines a woman, another female is in the room. This is for the legal protection of the woman and the male examiner. A female attendant also adds to the psychological comfort of the woman. A female examiner may want a male attendant present when she examines a male. This also is for her legal protection.
- Protect the resident from falling.
- Reassure the resident throughout the examination.
- Anticipate the examiner's need for equipment.
- Place paper or paper towels on the floor if the resident is asked to stand.
- Practice medical asepsis and Standard Precautions. Also follow the Bloodborne Pathogen Standard.

QUALITY OF LIFE

OBRA requires that residents be cared for in a way that promotes dignity, self-esteem, and physical, mental, and social well-being. The resident wears only a gown for the examination. An uncomfortable position may be required. Private body parts (breasts, vagina, penis, and rectum) may be examined. The resident may have fears about who will perform the examination and how it will be done. There may also be fears about why the examination is needed. Is the person dying? Will cancer be found? Will surgery be needed? Will more medicine be needed? Will an illness or a disorder be found? All these factors affect the resident's dignity, self-esteem, and well-being.

The resident's quality of life is promoted. The resident has the right to personal choice (see p. 527). The right to privacy and confidentiality is also very important. The resident is protected from exposure. Only those involved in the examination have the right to see the resident's body. They are the examiner and the examiner's assistant. The resident must give consent for others to be present. Proper draping and screening are important during the examination. Only the body part being examined is exposed. If assisting with the examination, you must help keep the resident covered.

Confidentiality also is important. Only staff members involved in the resident's care need to know the reason for the examination and the results. To give good care, the health care team needs to know. The doctor or nurse shares the results with those who need to know. Family members are told only if the resident consents. Other residents and visitors do not need to know. The resident can share the information if he or she wants to.

The examination environment is important for the resident's quality of life. The resident needs to feel safe and secure. The resident is protected from falls and other injuries. Remember that the resident wears only a hospital gown. The resident is kept warm and free from chills and drafts. The resident also must feel covered and protected from exposure.

Safety and security also relate to mental well-being. Knowing why the examination is needed and how it will be done helps the resident feel safe and secure. The presence of a friendly staff member is important. The person assisting with the examination should be someone with whom the resident feels comfortable. Touch and reassuring words also help the resident feel safe and secure.

REVIEW QUESTIONS

Circle the BEST answer.

1 The otoscope is used to
- A Examine the internal structures of the eye
- B Examine the external ear and the eardrum
- C Test reflexes
- D Open the vagina

2 You are preparing Mrs. Porter for an examination. You should do the following *except*
- A Have her urinate
- B Ask her to undress
- C Drape her
- D Go tell the nurse when Mrs. Porter is ready

3 Which part of Mrs. Porter's examination can you do?
- A Examine her eyes and ears
- B Inspect her mouth, teeth, and throat
- C Measure her height, weight, and vital signs
- D Observe her perineum and rectum

4 Mrs. Porter is supine. Her hips are flexed and externally rotated. Her feet are supported in stirrups. She is in the
- A Dorsal recumbent position
- B Lithotomy position
- C Knee-chest position
- D Sims' position

5 You will assist with Mrs. Porter's examination. Which is *false?*
- A Handwashing is done before and after the examination.
- B Instruments are placed near the examiner.
- C You leave the room when Mrs. Porter is examined.
- D Provide for privacy by screening, closing the door, and proper draping.

6 Which statement is *true?*
- A You can explain the reason for the examination to the resident.
- B The resident must be safe from injury during the examination.
- C You can tell the family the results of the examination.
- D All of the above

7 Proper screening and draping are important for
- A The right to privacy
- B Quality of life
- C Safety and security
- D All of the above

Answers to these questions are on p. 699.

24 Heat and Cold Applications

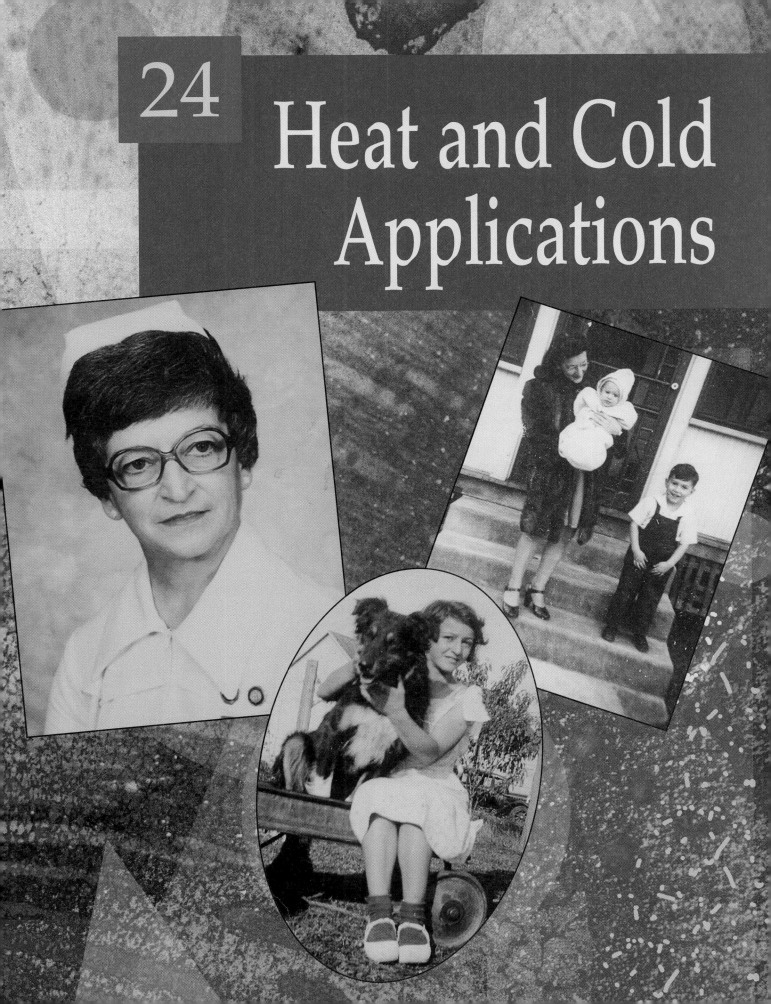

What You Will Learn

- The definition of the key terms listed in this chapter
- The purposes, effects, and complications of heat and cold applications
- The residents at risk for complications from heat and cold applications
- The differences between moist and dry heat and cold applications
- The rules for the application of heat and cold
- How cooling and warming blankets are used
- The procedures described in this chapter

Key Terms

constrict To narrow

dilate To expand or open wider

hyperthermia A body temperature *(thermia)* that is much higher *(hyper)* than the person's normal range

hypothermia A very low *(hypo)* body temperature *(thermia);* body temperature is below 95° F (35° C)

Doctors order heat and cold applications to promote healing and comfort. These applications also reduce tissue swelling. Heat and cold have opposite effects on body function. Severe injuries and changes in body function can occur. The risks are great. You must thoroughly understand the purposes, effects, and complications of heat and cold applications.

In some centers, only nurses apply heat and cold. Other centers let nursing assistants apply heat and cold. Before you perform these procedures, make sure that:

- Your state allows you to perform the procedure
- The procedure is in your job description
- You have the necessary training
- You are familiar with the equipment
- You review the procedure with a nurse
- A nurse is available to answer questions and to supervise you

HEAT APPLICATIONS

Heat applications can be applied to almost any body part. They are often used for musculoskeletal injuries or problems (sprains, arthritis). Heat applications are used to:

- Relieve pain
- Relax muscles
- Promote healing
- Reduce tissue swelling
- Decrease joint stiffness

Effects

When heat is applied to the skin, blood vessels in the area dilate. **Dilate** means to expand or open wider (Fig. 24-1). More blood flows through the vessels. The tissues have more oxygen and nutrients for healing. Excess fluid is removed from the area faster. The skin is reddened and feels warm.

Complications

High temperatures can cause burns. Pain, excessive redness, and blisters are danger signs. Report these signs immediately. Also observe for pale skin. When heat is applied too long, blood vessels **constrict** (narrow) (see Fig. 24-1). Blood flow decreases when vessels constrict. This reduces the amount of blood for the tissues. Tissue damage occurs, and the skin is pale.

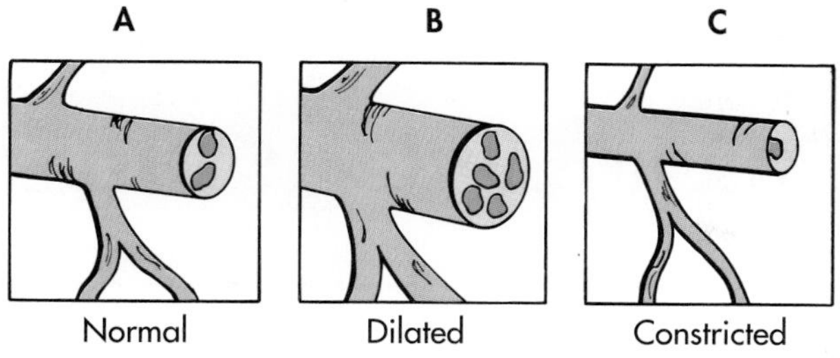

Fig. 24-1 A, Blood vessel under normal conditions. **B,** Dilated blood vessel. **C,** Constricted blood vessel.

Residents With Dementia

Confused persons and those with dementia may not recognize pain. Look for changes in the resident's behavior. Behavior changes can signal pain.

Older and fair-skinned people are at great risk for complications. Their delicate and fragile skin is easily burned. Residents with difficulty sensing heat or pain also are at risk. *(See Residents With Dementia.)* Nervous system damage, loss of consciousness, circulatory disorders, and some drugs interfere with sensation.

Persons with metal implants are at risk. Metal conducts heat. Deep tissues can be burned. Pacemakers and joint replacements are made of metal. Heat is not applied in the area of the implant.

Moist and Dry Applications

A *moist heat application* means that water is in contact with the skin. Water conducts heat. The effects from moist heat are greater and occur faster than from dry heat applications. Heat penetrates deeper with a moist application. To prevent injury, moist heat applications have lower (cooler) temperatures than dry heat applications.

Water is not in contact with the skin with *dry heat applications.* Dry heat has advantages:

- The application stays at the desired temperature longer.
- Dry heat does not penetrate as deeply as moist heat.

Because water is not used, dry heat needs higher (hotter) temperatures to achieve the desired effect. Therefore burns are still a risk.

The resident is protected from injury during local heat applications. Practice the rules in Box 24-1 to prevent burns and other complications.

Box 24-1 Rules for Applying Heat and Cold

- Know how to operate equipment used in the procedure.
- Measure the temperature of moist applications. Use a bath thermometer.
- Follow center policies for safe temperature ranges. See Table 24-1 on p. 536 for guidelines.
- Do not apply *very hot* (above 106° to 115° F, or 41° to 46° C) applications. Tissue damage can occur. A nurse applies *very hot* applications.
- Ask the nurse what the temperature of the application should be:
  - Heat—cooler temperatures are used for persons at risk.
  - Cold—warmer temperatures are used for persons at risk.
- Know the precise site of the heat application. Ask the nurse to show you the site.
- Cover dry heat or cold applications before applying them. Use a flannel cover, towel, or pillowcase according to center policy.
- Observe the skin for signs of complications. Immediately report the following to the nurse:
  - Complaints of pain, numbness, or burning
  - Excessive redness
  - Blisters
  - Pale, white, or gray skin
  - Cyanosis
  - Shivering
- Do not let the resident change the temperature of the application.
- Ask the nurse how long to leave the application in place. Carefully watch the time. Heat and cold are applied for no longer than 20 minutes.
- Follow the rules of electrical safety when using electrical appliances to apply heat (see Chapter 8).
- Expose only the body part where you will apply heat or cold. Provide for privacy through proper draping and screening.
- Place the signal light within the resident's reach.

Table 24-1 Heat and Cold Temperature Ranges

Temperature	Fahrenheit Range	Centigrade Range
Very hot	106° to 115° F	41.1° to 46.1° C
Hot	98° to 106° F	36.6° to 41.1° C
Warm	93° to 98° F	33.8° to 36.6° C
Tepid	80° to 93° F	26.6° to 33.8° C
Cool	65° to 80° F	18.3° to 26.6° C
Cold	50° to 65° F	10.0° to 18.3° C

From Perry AG, Potter PA: *Clinical nursing skills and techniques*, ed 4, St Louis, 1997, Mosby.

Hot Compresses and Packs

Hot compresses and packs are moist heat applications. They consist of a washcloth, small towel, or gauze dressing. A compress is applied to a small area. Packs are applied to large areas.

The application is left in place for 20 minutes. Sometimes an aquathermia pad (p. 542) is applied over the compress or pack. This maintains the temperature of the compress or pack.

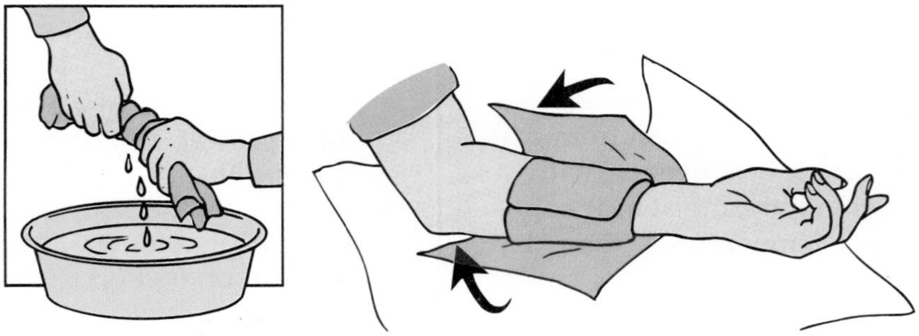

Fig. 24-2 A hot compress is covered with plastic and a bath towel. These keep the compress warm.

Applying Hot Compresses

Quality of Life

Remember to:
- *Knock before entering the resident's room*
- *Address the resident by name*
- *Introduce yourself by name and title*

Pre-Procedure

1 Explain the procedure to the resident.
2 Wash your hands.
3 Collect the following:
- Basin
- Bath thermometer
- Small towel, washcloth, or gauze squares
- Plastic wrap or aquathermia pad
- Ties, tape, or rolled gauze
- Bath towel
- Waterproof bed protector

4 Identify the resident. Check the ID bracelet against the assignment sheet.
5 Provide for privacy.

Procedure

6 Place the protector under the body part.
7 Fill the basin one-half to two-thirds full with hot water as directed by the nurse. Measure water temperature with a bath thermometer.
8 Place the compress in the water.
9 Wring out the compress.
10 Apply the compress to the area. Note the time.
11 Cover the compress quickly. Do one of the following as directed by the nurse:
  a Cover it with plastic wrap and then with a bath towel (Fig 24-2). Secure the towel in place with ties, tape, or rolled gauze.
  b Cover it with an aquathermia pad (p. 542).
12 Place the signal light within reach. Raise or lower bed rails. Follow the care plan.
13 Check the area every 5 minutes. Check for redness and complaints of pain, discomfort, or numbness. Remove the compress if any occur. Tell the nurse immediately.
14 Change the compress if cooling occurs.
15 Remove the compress after 20 minutes or as directed by the nurse. Pat the area dry with a towel. (If the bed rail is up, lower it for this step.)

Post-Procedure

16 Provide for comfort.
17 Unscreen the resident.
18 Raise or lower bed rails. Follow the care plan.
19 Place the signal light within reach.
20 Clean equipment. Discard disposable items.
21 Follow center policy for soiled linen.
22 Wash your hands.
23 Report the following to the nurse:
- Time, site, and length of the application
- Observations of the skin
- The resident's response

Commercial compresses. Commercial compresses are premoistened and packaged in foil. An infrared lamp is used to heat the wrapped compress as instructed by the manufacturer. The lamp is kept in the clean utility room, treatment room, medication room, or the resident's room.

Commercial compresses are sterile. Sometimes doctors order them for nonsterile compresses. Nurses may decide they are needed in certain situations. Commercial compresses are costly and are used only when necessary.

Applying a Commercial Compress

Quality of Life

Remember to:
- ***Knock before entering the resident's room***
- ***Address the resident by name***
- ***Introduce yourself by name and title***

Pre-Procedure

1 Explain the procedure to the resident.
2 Wash your hands.
3 Collect the following:
- Commercial compress
- Infrared lamp
- Towel
- Ties, tape, or rolled gauze
- Waterproof bed protector
- Aquathermia pad (if ordered)

4 Heat the compress following the manufacturer's instructions.
5 Identify the resident. Check the ID bracelet against the assignment sheet.
6 Provide for privacy.

Procedure

7 Place the bed protector under the body part.
8 Open the foil-wrapped compress.
9 Apply the compress quickly. Use the outside of the foil to pick up and apply the compress.
10 Cover the compress with a towel.
11 Secure the towel in place with ties, tape, or rolled gauze.
12 Apply the aquathermia pad (if ordered). See *Applying an Aquathermia Pad*, p. 543.
13 Place the signal light within reach. Raise or lower bed rails. Follow the care plan.
14 Check the area every 5 minutes. Check for redness and complaints of pain, discomfort, or numbness. Remove the compress if any occur. Tell the nurse immediately.
15 Change the compress if cooling occurs.
16 Remove the compress after 20 minutes or as directed by the nurse. Pat the area dry with the towel. (If the bed rail is up, lower it for this step.)

Post-Procedure

17 Follow steps 16 through 23 in *Applying Hot Compresses.*

Hot Soaks

A hot soak involves putting the body part into water. This usually is used for smaller parts, such as a hand, lower arm, foot, or lower leg (Fig. 24-3). Sometimes larger areas are soaked (arm, leg, or torso). Then a tub is used. The soak lasts 15 to 20 minutes. The resident's comfort and body alignment are maintained during the hot soak.

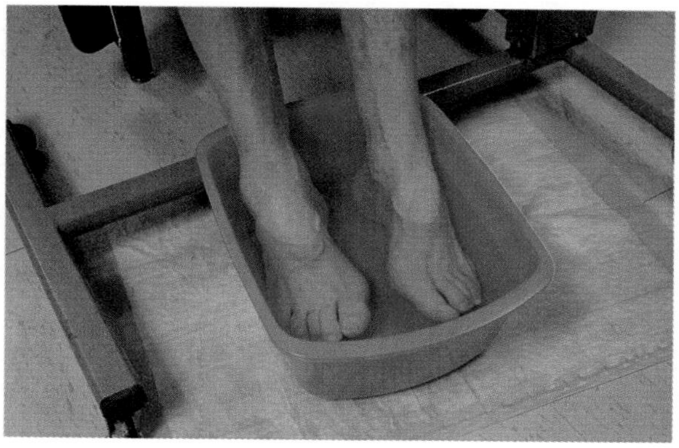

Fig. 24-3 The hot soak.

The Hot Soak

Quality of Life

Remember to:
- *Knock before entering the resident's room*
- *Address the resident by name*
- *Introduce yourself by name and title*

Pre-Procedure

1 Explain the procedure to the resident.
2 Wash your hands.
3 Collect the following:
- Water basin or an arm or foot bath
- Bath thermometer
- Bath blanket
- Waterproof pads

4 Identify the resident. Check the ID bracelet against the assignment sheet.
5 Provide for privacy.

Procedure

6 Position the resident for the treatment. Place the signal light within reach.
7 Place a waterproof pad under the area.
8 Fill the container one-half full with hot water as directed by the nurse. Measure water temperature.
9 Expose the area. Avoid unnecessary exposure.
10 Place the part into the water. Pad the edge of the container with a towel. Note the time.
11 Cover the resident with a bath blanket for extra warmth.
12 Check the area every 5 minutes. Check for redness and complaints of pain, numbness, or discomfort. Remove the part from the soak if any of these complications occur. Wrap the part in a towel, and tell the nurse immediately.
13 Check water temperature every 5 minutes. Change water as necessary. Wrap the part in a towel while changing the water.
14 Remove the part from the water in 15 to 20 minutes. Pat dry with a towel.

Post-Procedure

15 Follow steps 16 through 23 in *Applying Hot Compresses.*

◈ The Sitz Bath

The sitz bath involves immersing the perineal and rectal areas in warm or hot water for 20 minutes. (*Sitz* means *seat* in German.) Sitz baths are used to clean perineal and anal wounds. They are used also to promote healing, relieve pain and soreness, increase circulation, and stimulate voiding. They are common after rectal and female pelvic surgery, for hemorrhoids, and after childbirth.

The disposable plastic sitz bath fits onto the toilet seat (Fig. 24-4). A sitz tub is a built-in fixture with a deep seat. The resident sits in a seat filled with water (Fig. 24-5).

Blood flow to the perineal and rectal areas increases. Therefore less blood flows to other body parts. The resident may become weak or feel faint. Drowsiness can occur from the treatment's relaxing effect. Observe the resident for signs of weakness, faintness, or fatigue. Also protect the resident from injury. Check the resident often, keep the signal light within reach, and prevent chills and burns.

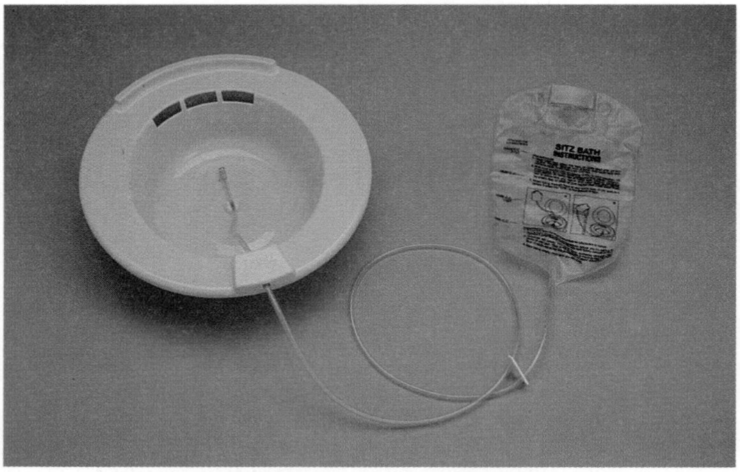

Fig. 24-4 The disposable sitz bath.

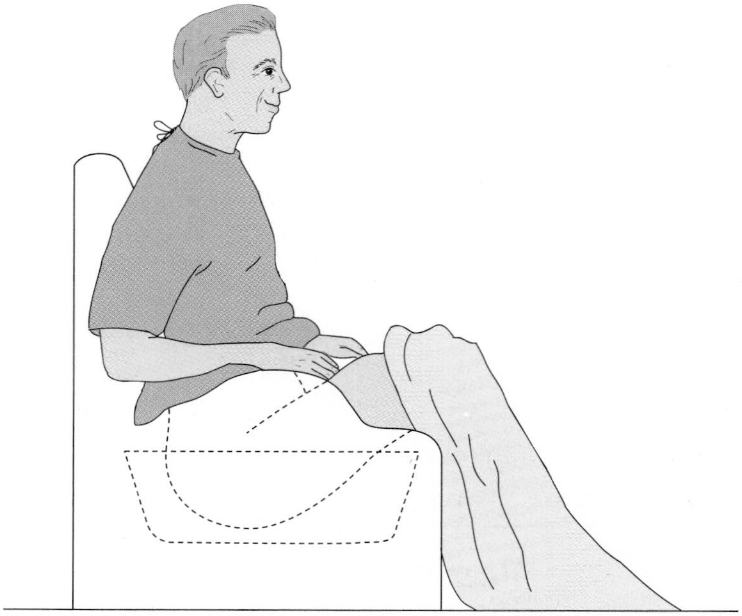

Fig. 24-5 The built-in sitz bath.

Assisting the Resident to Take a Sitz Bath

Quality of Life

Remember to:
- *Knock before entering the resident's room*
- *Address the resident by name*
- *Introduce yourself by name and title*

Pre-Procedure

1 Explain the procedure to the resident.
2 Wash your hands.
3 Collect the following:
- Disposable sitz bath or wheelchair if the built-in sitz bath is used
- Bath thermometer
- Large water container
- Two bath blankets, bath towels, and a clean gown
- Footstool if the resident is short
- Disinfectant solution
- Utility gloves

4 Identify the resident. Check the ID bracelet against the assignment sheet.
5 Provide for privacy.

Procedure

6 Do one of the following:
  a Place the disposable sitz bath on the toilet seat.
  b Transport the resident by wheelchair to the sitz bath room.
7 Fill the sitz bath two-thirds full with water as directed by the nurse. Measure water temperature.
8 Use bath towels to pad the metal parts that will have contact with the resident.
9 Raise the gown, and secure it above the waist.
10 Help the resident sit in the sitz bath.
11 Place a bath blanket around the shoulders. Place another over the legs for warmth.
12 Provide a footstool if the edge of the sitz bath causes pressure under the knees.
13 Place the signal light within reach, and provide for comfort.
14 Stay with a resident who is weak or unsteady.
15 Check the resident every 5 minutes for complaints of weakness, faintness, and drowsiness. Check for a rapid pulse. If any occur, get assistance to help the resident back to bed.
16 Help the resident out of the sitz bath after 20 minutes or as directed by the nurse.
17 Assist the resident with drying and dressing.
18 Assist the resident back to bed.

Post-Procedure

19 Provide for comfort.
20 Unscreen the resident.
21 Place the signal light within reach.
22 Raise or lower bed rails. Follow the care plan.
23 Clean the sitz bath with disinfectant solution. Wear utility gloves for this step.
24 Return reusable items to their proper place. Follow center policy for soiled linen.
25 Wash your hands.
26 Report your observations to the nurse.

◈ The Aquathermia Pad

The aquathermia pad (Aqua-K, K-Pad) is an electric device used for dry heat. Tubes inside the pad are filled with distilled water. A bedside heating unit is also filled with distilled water. The heated water flows to the pad through a connecting hose (Fig. 24-6). Another hose returns water to the heating unit. The water is reheated and returned back to the pad.

The heating unit is kept level with the pad and connecting hoses. Water must flow freely. Hoses must not have kinks and air bubbles. The temperature usually is set at 105° F (40.5° C) with a key. Then the key is removed. This prevents anyone from changing the temperature. The temperature is often set in the central supply department. The key is kept in that department.

The following safety measures are practiced:

- Follow electrical safety precautions (see Chapter 8).
- Place the heating unit on an even, uncluttered surface. This prevents it from being knocked over or knocked off of the surface.
- Use a flannel cover to insulate the pad. It also absorbs perspiration at the application site. (Some centers use a towel or pillowcase).
- Secure the pad in place with ties, tape, or rolled gauze. Do not use pins. They can puncture the pad and cause leaks.
- Do not place the pad under the resident or under a body part. This prevents the escape of heat. Burns can result if heat cannot escape.

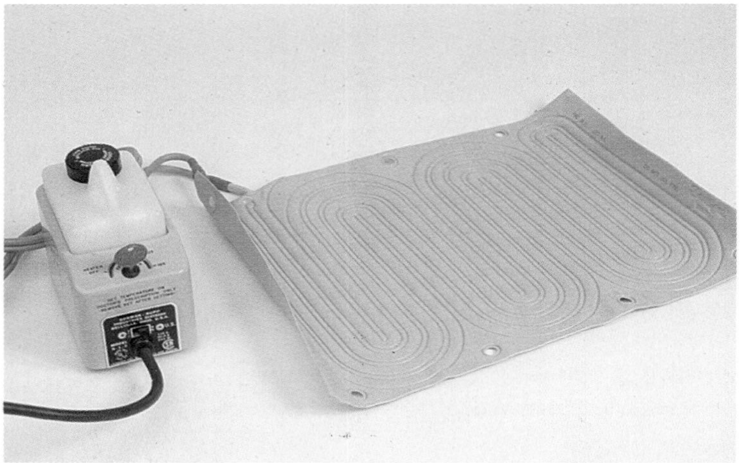

Fig. 24-6 The aquathermia pad and heating unit.

Applying an Aquathermia Pad

Quality of Life

Remember to:
- *Knock before entering the resident's room*
- *Address the resident by name*
- *Introduce yourself by name and title*

Pre-Procedure

1 Explain the procedure to the resident.
2 Wash your hands.
3 Collect the following:
- Aquathermia pad and heating unit
- Distilled water
- Flannel cover, pillowcase, or towel
- Ties, tape, or rolled gauze

4 Identify the resident. Check the ID bracelet against the assignment sheet.
5 Provide for privacy.

Procedure

6 Fill the heating unit to the fill line with distilled water.
7 Remove air bubbles. Place the pad and tubing below the heating unit. Tilt the unit from side to side.
8 Set the temperature as instructed by the nurse (usually 105° F, or 40.5° C). Remove the key. (Give the key to the nurse when you complete the procedure).
9 Place the pad in the cover.
10 Plug in the unit. Let water warm to the desired temperature.
11 Set the heating unit on the bedside stand. Keep the pad and connecting hoses level with the unit. Hoses must not have kinks.
12 Apply the pad to the part. Note the time.
13 Secure the pad in place with ties, tape, or rolled gauze. Do not use pins.
14 Unscreen the resident. Place the signal light within reach.
15 Raise or lower bed rails. Follow the care plan.
16 Check the skin for redness, swelling, and blisters. Ask about pain, discomfort, or decreased sensation. Remove the pad if any occur. Tell the nurse immediately.
17 Remove the pad at the specified time. (If the bed rail is up, lower it for this step.)

Post-Procedure

18 Follow steps 16 through 23 in *Applying Hot Compresses.*

COLD APPLICATIONS

Cold applications are often used to treat sprains and fractures. They reduce pain, prevent swelling, and decrease circulation and bleeding. Cold cools the body when fever is present.

Effects

Cold has the opposite effect of heat. When cold is applied to the skin, blood vessels constrict (see Fig. 24-1). Decreased blood flow results. Less oxygen and nutrients are carried to the tissues. Cold applications are useful right after injury. The decreased circulation reduces the amount of bleeding. The amount of fluid collecting in tissues also is reduced. Cold has a numbing effect on the skin. This helps reduce or relieve pain in the part.

Complications

Complications include pain, burns and blisters, and *cyanosis* (bluish skin color). Burns and blisters tend to occur from intense cold. They also occur when dry cold applications are in direct contact with the skin. When cold is applied for a long time, blood vessels dilate. Blood flow increases. The prolonged application of cold has the same effects as local heat applications.

Fair-skinned residents have fragile skin. They are at great risk for complications. So are residents with mental or sensory impairments. Check the resident often.

Moist and Dry Applications

Cold applications are moist or dry. The ice bag and ice collar are dry cold applications. The cold compress is a moist application. Moist cold applications penetrate deeper than dry ones. Therefore temperatures of moist applications are not as cold as dry applications.

Injuries from cold applications are prevented. See the rules listed in Box 24-1.

◈ Ice Bags, Ice Collars, and Disposable Cold Packs

Ice bags and ice collars are dry cold applications. Ice collars are applied to the neck. The bag or collar is filled with crushed ice. Then it is placed in a cover. If the cover becomes moist, it is removed and a dry one applied.

Commercial ice bags are kept frozen until needed. They are refrozen for reuse. Covers are also needed with ice collars or commercial ice bags.

Disposable cold packs are used once and discarded. They come in many sizes. Some have an outer covering allowing direct application to the skin. Otherwise a cover is used.

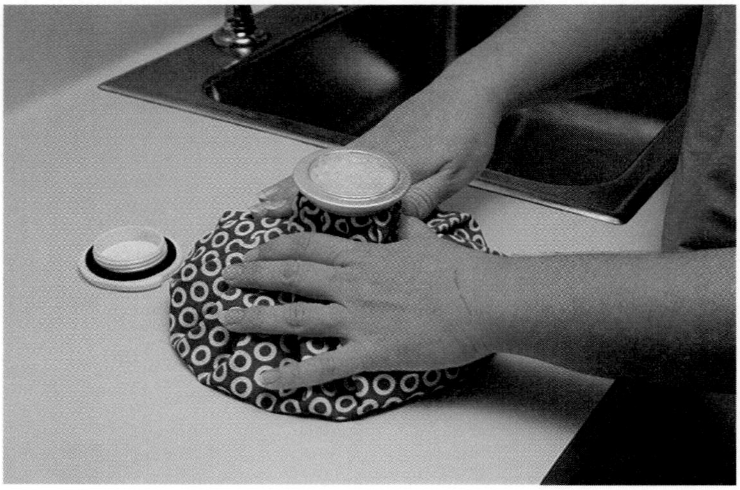

Fig. 24-7 The ice bag is filled one-half to two-thirds full with ice.

Applying an Ice Bag, Ice Collar, or Disposable Cold Pack

Quality of Life

Remember to:
- ◆ *Knock before entering the resident's room*
- ◆ *Address the resident by name*
- ◆ *Introduce yourself by name and title*

Pre-Procedure

1 Explain the procedure to the resident.
2 Wash your hands.
3 Collect a disposable cold pack or the following:
   - Ice bag or collar
   - Crushed ice
   - Flannel cover, towel, or pillowcase
   - Paper towels
4 Apply an ice bag or collar:
   a Fill the ice bag with water. Put in the stopper. Turn the bag upside down to check for leaks.
   b Empty the bag.
   c Fill the bag one-half to two-thirds full with crushed ice or ice chips (Fig. 24-7).
   d Remove excess air. Bend, twist, or squeeze the bag; or press it against a firm surface.
   e Place the cap or stopper on securely.
   f Dry the bag with the paper towels.
   g Place the bag in the cover.
5 Apply a disposable cold pack:
   a Squeeze, knead, or strike the cold pack as directed by the manufacturer. This releases cold.
   b Place the bag in the cover.
6 Identify the resident. Check the ID bracelet against the assignment sheet.
7 Provide for privacy.

Procedure

8 Apply the ice bag. Secure it in place with ties, tape, or rolled gauze. Note the time.
9 Place the signal light within reach. Raise or lower bed rails. Follow the care plan.
10 Check the skin every 10 minutes. Check for blisters; pale, white, or gray skin; cyanosis; and shivering. Ask about numbness, pain, or burning. Remove the bag if any occur. Tell the nurse immediately.
11 Remove the bag after 20 minutes or as directed by the nurse.

Post-Procedure

12 Follow steps 16 through 23 in *Applying Hot Compresses.*

Cold Compresses

Applying a cold compress is like applying a hot compress. The cold compress is a moist application. Moist cold compresses are left in place no longer than 20 minutes.

Applying Cold Compresses

Quality of Life

Remember to:
- *Knock before entering the resident's room*
- *Address the resident by name*
- *Introduce yourself by name and title*

Pre-Procedure

1 Explain the procedure to the resident.
2 Wash your hands.
3 Collect the following:
- Large basin with ice
- Small basin with cold water
- Gauze squares, washcloths, or small towels
- Waterproof pad
- Bath towel

4 Identify the resident. Check the ID bracelet against the assignment sheet.
5 Provide for privacy.

Procedure

6 Place the small basin with cold water into the large basin with ice.
7 Place the compresses into the cold water.
8 Place a bed protector under the affected body part. Expose the area.
9 Wring out a compress so water is not dripping.
10 Apply the compress to the part. Note the time.
11 Place the signal light within reach. Raise or lower bed rails. Follow the care plan.
12 Check the area every 5 minutes. Check for blisters; pale, white, or gray skin; cyanosis; or shivering. Ask about numbness, pain, or burning. Remove the compress if any occur. Tell the nurse immediately.
13 Change the compress when it warms. Usually compresses are changed every 5 minutes.
14 Remove the compress after 20 minutes or as directed by the nurse.
15 Pat dry the area with the bath towel.

Post-Procedure

16 Follow steps 16 through 23 in *Applying Hot Compresses.*

COOLING AND WARMING BLANKETS

Hyperthermia is a body temperature *(thermia)* that is much higher *(hyper)* than the person's normal range. Generally, body temperature is greater than 103° F (39.4° C). It is often called *heat stroke* when caused by hot weather temperatures. Other causes include illness, dehydration, and not being able to perspire. Lowering the resident's body temperature is necessary. Otherwise death can occur. The doctor orders ice packs applied to the resident's head, neck, underarms, and groin. Sometimes a cooling blanket is used alone or with ice packs.

A cooling blanket is an electric device. Made of rubber or plastic, the device has tubes filled with distilled water or other fluid. The fluid circulates through the tubes. The blanket is placed on the resident's bed and covered with a sheet. The blanket is turned on to the cool setting and allowed to cool. The resident lies on the blanket. The resident's vital signs are measured often. Rapid and excess cooling are prevented.

Hypothermia is a very low *(hypo)* body temperature *(thermia)*. Body temperature is less than 95° F (35° C). Cold weather temperatures are a common cause. The resident is warmed to prevent death. The resident's treatment may include a warming blanket. A warming blanket is the same as a cooling blanket except that the temperature is turned to warm. Vital signs are checked often to prevent rapid or excess warming.

When used to cool the body, the device is called a *hypothermia blanket*. When used to warm the body, it is called a *hyperthermia blanket*. The device has warm and cool settings.

QUALITY OF LIFE

Heat and cold applications are ordered to promote healing and comfort and to reduce tissue swelling. Residents who need these applications have some injury or disorder. A resident may worry about why the heat or cold application is needed. You can promote the resident's quality of life by trying to understand the resident's concern. Be kind, caring, and patient. Refer any questions about the need for the application to the nurse. Remember that the resident has the right to personal choice. This means that the resident has the right to be involved in planning care. To do so, the resident must know why the application is needed.

Also remember to explain procedures to residents. What is familiar to you may not be so to them. Also, residents can plan if they know what will happen. A resident may want to make a phone call or finish an activity before the treatment. Or a resident may want the treatment done by a certain time—for example, before visitors arrive, before a favorite TV program, or before a scheduled activity. Having residents help plan when treatments are done protects their right to personal choice.

The right to privacy is protected. Protecting privacy shows respect for the resident. It also protects the resident's dignity. Only the body part involved in the procedure is exposed. Unnecessary exposure violates the resident's right to privacy. It also can affect comfort if there is unnecessary chilling.

You can promote quality of life by making sure the resident's environment is safe and comfortable. Heat and cold applications take between 20 and 30 minutes. The resident is not free to move about during this time. Encourage the resident to use the toilet, commode, urinal, or bedpan before the procedure. Make sure the room is free of unpleasant equipment or odors. Place needed items within the resident's reach. These include the signal light, water, books or magazines, needlework, telephone, and other items requested by the resident. Check the resident often. You are responsible for the resident's safety.

Review Questions

Circle the BEST answer.

1 Local heat has the following effects *except*
A Pain relief
B Muscle relaxation
C Healing
D Decreased blood flow

2 Which is the greatest threat from heat applications?
A Infection
B Burns
C Chilling
D Pressure ulcers

3 Who has the greatest risk of complications from local heat applications?
A A 10-year-old boy
B A teenager
C A 40-year-old woman
D An older person

4 These statements are about moist heat applications. Which is *false?*
A Water is in contact with the skin.
B The effects of moist heat are less than with a dry heat application.
C Moist heat penetrates deeper than dry heat.
D The temperature of a moist heat application is lower than a dry heat application.

5 The temperature of a hot application is usually between
A 80° and 93° F
B 93° and 98° F
C 98° and 106° F
D 106° and 115° F

6 These statements are about the sitz bath. Which is *false?*
A The perineal and rectal areas are immersed in warm or hot water for 20 minutes.
B The sitz bath lasts 25 to 30 minutes.
C The sitz bath cleans the perineum, relieves pain, increases circulation, or stimulates voiding.
D Weakness and fainting can occur.

7 Mrs. Parks is using an aquathermia pad. Which is *false?*
A The aquathermia pad is a dry heat application.
B The temperature of an aquathermia pad is usually set at 105° F.
C Electrical safety precautions are practiced.
D Pins secure the pad in place.

8 Local cold applications
A Reduce pain, prevent swelling, and decrease circulation
B Dilate blood vessels
C Prevent the spread of microbes
D All of the above

9 Which is *not* a complication of local cold applications?
A Pain
B Burns and blisters
C Cyanosis
D Infection

10 Before applying an ice bag
A Place the bag in a freezer
B Measure the temperature of the bag
C Place the bag in a cover
D Ask the resident to void

11 Moist cold compresses are left in place no longer than
A 20 minutes
B 30 minutes
C 45 minutes
D 60 minutes

12 A cooling blanket is used for
A Hypothermia
B Hyperthermia
C Cyanosis
D Shivering

Answers to these questions are on p. 699.

25 Oxygen Needs

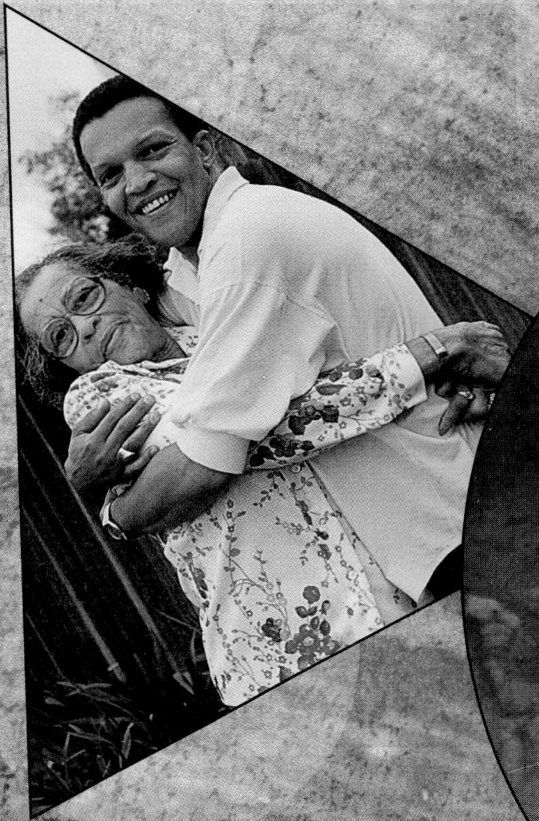

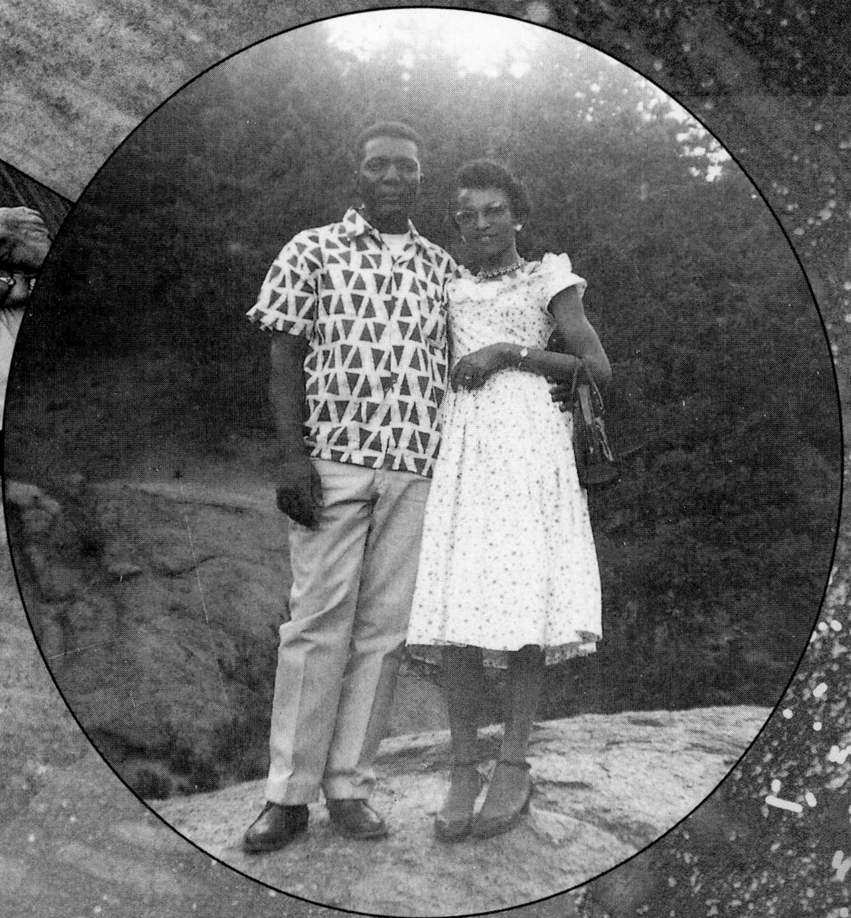

What You Will Learn

- The definition of the key terms listed in this chapter
- The factors affecting oxygen needs
- The signs and symptoms of hypoxia and altered respiratory function
- The tests used to diagnose respiratory problems
- How positioning, coughing and deep breathing, and incentive spirometry promote oxygenation
- The devices used to administer oxygen
- How to safely assist with oxygen therapy
- How to assist in the care of persons with an artificial airway
- The safety measures for oral suctioning
- How to assist in the care of persons on mechanical ventilation
- How to assist in the care of persons with chest tubes
- The procedures described in this chapter

Key Terms

allergy A sensitivity to a substance that causes the body to react with signs and symptoms

apnea The lack or absence *(a)* of breathing *(pnea)*

Biot's respirations Irregular breathing with periods of apnea; respirations may be slow and deep or rapid and shallow

bradypnea Slow *(brady)* breathing *(pnea)*; respirations are fewer than 10 per minute

Cheyne-Stokes Respirations gradually increase in rate and depth and then become shallow and slow; breathing may stop (*apnea*) for 10 to 20 seconds

dyspnea Difficult, labored, or painful *(dys)* breathing *(pnea)*

hemoptysis Bloody *(hemo)* sputum (*ptysis* meaning "to spit")

hemothorax The collection of blood *(hemo)* in the pleural space *(thorax)*

hyperventilation Respirations that are rapid *(hyper)* and deeper than normal

hypoventilation Respirations that are slow *(hypo)*, shallow, and sometimes irregular

hypoxemia A reduced amount *(hypo)* of oxygen *(ox)* in the blood *(emia)*

hypoxia A deficiency *(hypo)* of oxygen *(oxia)* in the cells

intubation The process of inserting an artificial airway

Kussmaul's respirations Very deep and rapid respirations; a sign of diabetic coma

mechanical ventilation Using a machine to move air into and out of the lungs

orthopnea Being able to breathe *(pnea)* deeply and comfortably only while sitting or standing *(ortho)*

orthopneic position Sitting up in bed *(ortho)* and leaning forward over the bedside table

oxygen concentration The amount of hemoglobin that contains oxygen (O_2)

pleural effusion The escape and collection of fluid *(effusion)* in the pleural space *(thorax)*

pneumothorax The collection of air *(pneumo)* in the pleural space *(thorax)*

pollutant A harmful chemical or substance in the air or water

respiratory arrest Breathing stops

respiratory depression Slow, weak respirations that occur at a rate of less than 12 per minute; respirations are not deep enough to bring enough air into the lungs

sputum Expectorated (expelled) mucus

suction The process of withdrawing or sucking up fluid (secretions)

tachypnea Rapid *(tachy)* breathing *(pnea)*; respirations are usually more than 24 per minute

Oxygen is a tasteless, odorless, and colorless gas. It is a basic need and is necessary for survival. Death occurs within minutes if a person stops breathing. Serious illnesses occur without enough oxygen. Illness, surgery, and injuries affect the amount of oxygen in the blood and cells. You need to know how to give safe and effective care to residents with oxygen needs. *(See Subacute Care.)*

Before giving any care described in this chapter, you must make sure that:

- Your state allows nursing assistants to perform the procedure
- The procedure is in your job description
- You have the necessary training
- You are familiar with the equipment
- You review the procedure with the nurse
- A nurse is available to supervise you

SUBACUTE CARE

Centers with a subacute care unit often have a respiratory rehabilitation program. These programs are managed by a *pulmonologist* (a doctor with special education and training in the care of persons with respiratory problems). Persons needing respiratory rehabilitation are often very ill. Complex procedures and special equipment often are needed. The health care team must have the necessary education and training to provide effective and safe care. JCAHO requires centers to provide educational programs to ensure that all staff members caring for these persons have the knowledge and skills to do so.

Many of the procedures described in this chapter are done or supervised by an RN or a respiratory therapist. Subacute care units must always have an RN on duty.

Persons admitted to subacute respiratory care programs often get better and go home. The goal is to help the person reach his or her highest level of function and live as independently as possible.

FACTORS AFFECTING OXYGEN NEEDS

The respiratory and cardiovascular systems must function properly for cells to get enough oxygen. Any disease, injury, or surgery involving these systems affects the body's ability to take in oxygen and deliver it to the cells. Each body system depends on the other. Altered function of any system (e.g., the nervous, musculoskeletal, or urinary system) affects the body's ability to meet its oxygen needs. Major factors affecting oxygen needs are:

- ***Respiratory system status***—Structures must be intact and functioning. The airway must be open (patent). Alveoli must exchange oxygen (O_2) and carbon dioxide (CO_2).
- ***Cardiovascular system function***—Blood flow must flow freely to and from the heart. Narrowed vessels affect the delivery of oxygen-rich blood to the cells and blood return to the heart. Capillaries and cells must exchange O_2 and CO_2.
- ***Red blood cell count***—The blood must have enough red blood cells (RBCs). RBCs contain hemoglobin that picks up oxygen in the lungs and carries it to the cells. The bone marrow must produce enough RBCs. Poor diet, chemotherapy, and leukemia affect bone marrow function. Blood loss also reduces the number of RBCs.
- ***Intact nervous system***—Nervous system diseases and injuries can affect respiratory muscle function. Breathing may be difficult or impossible. Brain damage affects respiratory rate, rhythm, and depth. Narcotics and depressant drugs are chemicals that affect the brain. They slow respirations. The amount of O_2 and CO_2 in the blood also affects brain function. Respiratory rate increases when O_2 is lacking. The body tries to bring in more oxygen. It also increases when CO_2 increases. The body tries to get rid of CO_2.
- ***Aging***—Respiratory muscles weaken, and lung tissue becomes less elastic. Strength for coughing decreases. Coughing and removing secretions from the upper airway are important. Otherwise, upper respiratory tract infections can lead to *pneumonia* (inflammation of the lung). Older persons are at a higher risk for respiratory complications after surgery.
- ***Exercise***—Oxygen needs increase with exercise. Normally, respiratory rate and depth increase to bring enough O_2 into the lungs. Residents with heart and respiratory diseases may have enough oxygen at rest. However, even slight activity can increase their oxygen needs. Their bodies may not be able to bring in oxygen and to deliver it to cells.
- ***Fever***—Oxygen needs increase. As with exercise, respiratory rate and depth must increase to meet the body's needs.
- ***Pain***—Pain increases the need for oxygen. Respiratory rate increases to meet this need. However, chest and abdominal injuries and surgeries often involve the respiratory muscles. This interferes with breathing in and out.
- ***Medications***—Some drugs depress the respiratory center in the brain. **Respiratory depression** is slow, weak respirations at a rate of fewer than

12 per minute. Respirations are too shallow to bring enough air into the lungs. **Respiratory arrest** is when breathing stops. Narcotics such as morphine and Demerol can have these effects. (The word narcotic comes from the Greek word *narkoun.* It means stupor or to be numb.) These drugs are given in safe amounts for severe pain. Substance abusers are at risk for respiratory depression and respiratory arrest from overdoses from narcotics and depressants. Narcotics include opium, heroin, and methadone. Depressant drugs include barbiturates (Nembutal, phenobarbital, secobarbital, Tuinal, and others) and the benzodiazepines (Dalmane, diazepam, Halcion, Librium, Tranxene, Valium, Xanax, and others).

- *Smoking*—Smoking causes lung cancer and chronic obstructive pulmonary disease (COPD). It is a risk factor for coronary artery disease.
- *Allergies*—An **allergy** is a sensitivity to a substance that causes the body to react with signs and symptoms. Respiratory signs and symptoms include runny nose, wheezing, and congestion. Mucous membranes in the upper airway swell. With severe swelling, the airway closes. Shock and death are risks. Pollens, dust, foods, drugs, and cigarette smoke often cause allergies. Residents with allergies are at risk for chronic bronchitis and asthma.
- *Pollutant exposure*—A **pollutant** is a harmful chemical or substance in the air or water. Dust, fumes, toxins, asbestos, coal dust, and sawdust are some air pollutants. They damage the lungs. Pollutant exposure occurs in home, work, and community settings.
- *Nutrition*—Good nutrition is needed for red blood cell production. RBCs live about 3 to 4 months. New ones must replace those that die off. The body needs iron and vitamins (vitamin B12, vitamin C, and folic acid) to produce RBCs.
- *Substance abuse*—Alcohol depresses the brain. Excessive amounts reduce the cough reflex and increase the risk of aspiration. Obstructed airway and pneumonia are risks from aspiration. Respiratory depression and respiratory arrest are risks when narcotics and depressant drugs are abused.

ALTERED RESPIRATORY FUNCTION

Respiratory system function involves three processes. Air moves in and out of the lungs. Oxygen and carbon dioxide are exchanged at the alveoli. The blood transports O_2 to the cells and removes CO_2 from them. Respiratory function is altered if even one process is affected.

Box 25-1 Signs and Symptoms of Hypoxia

- Restlessness
- Dizziness
- Disorientation
- Confusion
- Behavior and personality changes
- Difficulty concentrating and following directions
- Apprehension
- Anxiety
- Fatigue
- Agitation
- Increased pulse rate
- Increased rate and depth of respirations
- Sitting position, often leaning forward
- Cyanosis (bluish color to the skin, lips, mucous membranes, and nail beds)
- Dyspnea

Hypoxia

Hypoxia is a deficiency *(hypo)* of oxygen *(oxia)* in the cells. Cells do not receive enough oxygen. Therefore they do not function properly. Any illness, disease, injury, or surgery affecting respiratory function can cause hypoxia. The brain is very sensitive to inadequate oxygen. Restlessness is an early sign of hypoxia. So are dizziness and disorientation. Report signs and symptoms of hypoxia to the nurse immediately (Box 25-1).

Hypoxia is life threatening. The heart, brain, and other organs must receive enough oxygen to function. Oxygen is given, and treatment is directed at the cause of the hypoxia.

Abnormal Respirations

Normal respirations occur between 12 and 20 times per minute in the adult. Infants and children have faster rates. Respirations are normally quiet, effortless, and regular. Both sides of the chest rise and fall equally. The following breathing patterns are abnormal:

- **Tachypnea**—rapid *(tachy)* breathing *(pnea).* Respirations are usually more than 24 per minute. Fever, exercise, pain, pregnancy, airway obstruction, and hypoxemia are common causes. **Hypoxemia** is a reduced amount *(hypo)* of oxygen *(ox)* in the blood *(emia).*

Box 25-2 Signs and Symptoms of Altered Respiratory Function

- Signs and symptoms of hypoxia (see Box 25-1)
- Any abnormal breathing pattern
- Complaints of shortness of breath or being "winded" or "short-winded"
- Cough (note frequency and time of day)
  - Dry and hacking
  - Harsh and barking
  - Productive (produces sputum) or nonproductive
- Sputum
  - Color—clear, white, yellow, green, brown, or red
  - Odor—none or foul odor
  - Consistency—thick, watery, or frothy (with bubbles or foam)
  - **Hemoptysis**—bloody *(hemo)* sputum (*ptysis* meaning "to spit"); note if the sputum is bright red, dark red, blood-tinged, or streaked with blood
- Noisy respirations
  - Wheezing
  - Wet-sounding respirations
  - Crowing sounds
- Chest pain (note location)
  - Constant
  - Person's description (stabbing, knifelike, aching)
  - What makes it worse (movement, coughing, yawning, sneezing, sighing, deep breathing)
- Cyanosis
  - Skin
  - Mucous membranes
  - Lips
  - Nail beds
- Changes in vital signs
- Body position
  - Sitting upright
  - Leaning forward or hunched over a table

- **Bradypnea**—slow *(brady)* breathing *(pnea)*. Respirations are fewer than 10 per minute. Bradypnea is seen with drug overdoses and central nervous system disorders.
- **Apnea**—the lack or absence *(a)* of breathing *(pnea)*. It occurs in cardiac arrest and respiratory arrest. Sleep apnea and periodic apnea of newborns are other types of apnea.
- **Hypoventilation**—respirations that are slow *(hypo)*, shallow, and sometimes irregular. Lung disorders affecting the alveoli are common causes. Pneumonia is an example. Other causes include obesity, airway obstruction, drug side effects, and nervous system and musculoskeletal disorders affecting the respiratory muscles.
- **Hyperventilation**—respirations that are rapid *(hyper)* and deeper than normal. Its many causes include asthma, emphysema, infection, fever, central nervous system disorders, hypoxia, anxiety, pain, and some drugs.
- **Dyspnea**—difficult, labored, or painful *(dys)* breathing *(pnea)*. Heart disease, exercise, and anxiety are common causes.
- **Cheyne-Stokes**—respirations gradually increase in rate and depth and then become shallow and slow. Breathing may stop (apnea) for 10 to 20 seconds. Drug overdose, heart failure, renal failure, and brain disorders are common causes. These respirations are common when death is near.
- **Orthopnea**—breathing *(pnea)* deeply and comfortably only while sitting or standing *(ortho)*. Common causes include emphysema, asthma, pneumonia, angina pectoris, and other heart and respiratory disorders.
- **Biot's respirations**—irregular breathing with periods of apnea. Respirations are slow and deep or rapid and shallow. They occur with central nervous system disorders.
- **Kussmaul's respirations**—very deep and rapid respirations. They are a sign of diabetic coma.

Assisting With Assessment and Diagnostic Testing

Altered respiratory function may be an acute or chronic problem. Doctors, nurses, and respiratory therapists are always alert for altered respiratory function. When caring for residents with acute or chronic respiratory problems, you must report your observations to the nurse promptly and accurately (Box 25-2). Quick action is necessary to meet the resident's oxygen needs. Measures are taken to correct the situation and prevent the problem from getting worse.

The doctor orders tests to determine the cause of altered respiratory function. Residents go to the hospital or other diagnostic center for some tests. Others are done at the nursing center. The following tests are common. You are likely to assist with pulse oximetry and in collecting sputum specimens.

- *Chest x-ray (CXR)*—An x-ray is taken of the chest. It is used to evaluate changes in the lungs. All clothing and jewelry from the waist to the neck are removed. The resident wears a hospital gown. Chest x-rays are often done at the center. A portable x-ray machine is used in the resident's room.
- *Lung scan*—The lungs are scanned to see what areas are not getting air or blood. The resident inhales radioactive gas and is injected with a radioisotope. *Radioactive* means to give off radiation. A *radioisotope* is an element that gives off radiation. Lung tissue getting air and blood flow "take up" the radioactive substances. A scanner senses areas with radioactive substances. The resident goes to the hospital or a diagnostic center for this procedure.
- *Bronchoscopy*—A scope *(scopy)* is passed into the trachea and bronchi *(broncho)*. The doctor inspects the larynx, trachea, and bronchi for bleeding and tumors. The doctor can take tissue samples (biopsy) or remove mucous plugs and foreign objects. The resident is NPO 6 to 8 hours before the procedure. This reduces the danger of vomiting and aspiration. A local or general anesthetic is given. After the procedure, the resident is NPO and watched carefully until the gag and swallow reflexes return. The resident goes to the hospital or a diagnostic center for this procedure. Preoperative and postoperative care are given as directed by the nurse.
- *Thoracentesis*—The pleura *(thora)* is punctured, air or fluid is aspirated *(centesis)* from it. The doctor inserts a needle through the chest wall into the pleural sac. Injury or disease can cause the pleural sac to fill with air, blood, or fluid. This affects respiratory function. The procedure also is done to remove fluid for laboratory study or to inject anticancer drugs into the pleural sac. The procedure takes a few minutes. Vital signs are taken before a local anesthetic is given. The resident sits up or leans forward and is asked not to talk, cough, or move suddenly (Fig. 25-1). Postprocedure care involves applying a dressing to the puncture site and taking vital signs. A chest x-ray is taken to check for lung damage. The resident is checked often for shortness of breath, dyspnea, cough, sputum, chest pain, cyanosis, vital sign changes, and other respiratory signs and symptoms. The resident usually goes to the hospital or a diagnostic center for this procedure. Some centers do this procedure in a subacute unit.
- *Pulmonary function tests*—Tests measure the amount of air moving in and out of the lungs (volume) and how much air the lungs can hold (capacity). The resident takes as deep a breath as possible. Using a mouthpiece, the resident blows into a machine (Fig. 25-2). The tests are used to evaluate residents at risk for lung diseases or postoperative pulmonary complications. They are used also to measure the progress of lung disease and its treatment. Fatigue is common after the tests. The resident should rest after the procedure.

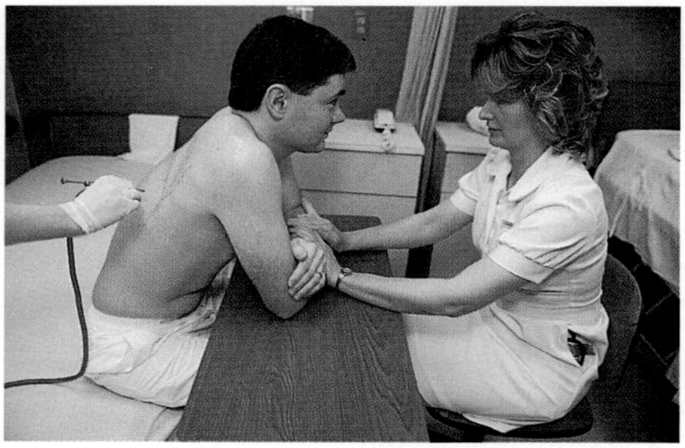

Fig. 25-1 The person is positioned for a thoracentesis. *(From Elkin MK, Perry AG, Potter PA:* Nursing interventions and clinical skills, *St Louis, 1996, Mosby.)*

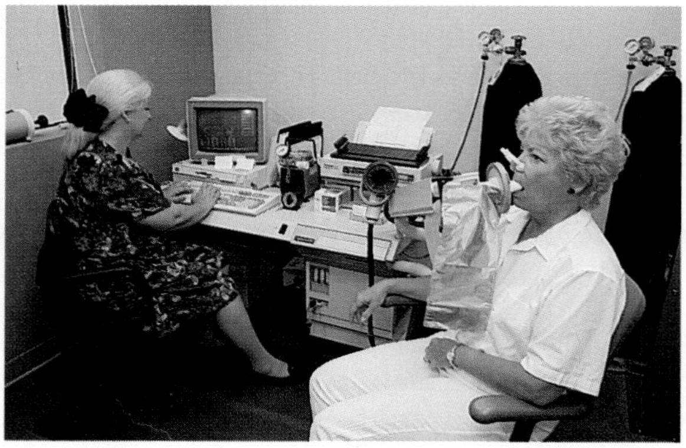

Fig. 25-2 Pulmonary function testing.

- *Arterial blood gases (ABGs)*—A radial or femoral artery is punctured to obtain arterial blood. Laboratory tests measure the amount of oxygen in the blood. Hemorrhage from the artery is prevented. Pressure is applied to the artery for at least 5 minutes after the procedure. Pressure is applied longer if the resident has blood clotting problems. A specially trained RN or a respiratory therapist draws blood for this procedure.

Pulse oximetry. Pulse oximetry measures *(metry)* oxygen *(oxi)* concentration in arterial blood. **Oxygen concentration** is the amount (percent) of hemoglobin that contains oxygen. The normal range is 95% to 100%. For example if 97% of all the hemoglobin (100%) carries O_2, tissues get enough oxygen. If only 90% of the hemoglobin contains O_2, tissues do not get enough oxygen to function. Measurements are used to prevent hypoxia and to evaluate treatment.

A sensor (or probe) is attached to the resident's finger, toe, earlobe, nose, or forehead (Fig. 25-3). Two light beams on one side of the sensor pass through the tissues. A detector on the other side measures the amount of light passing through the tissues. The oximeter receives this information and measures the oxygen concentration. The value and the resident's pulse rate are displayed on the monitor. Oximeters have alarms. The alarms sound if oxygen concentration is low, the pulse is too fast or slow, or other problems occur.

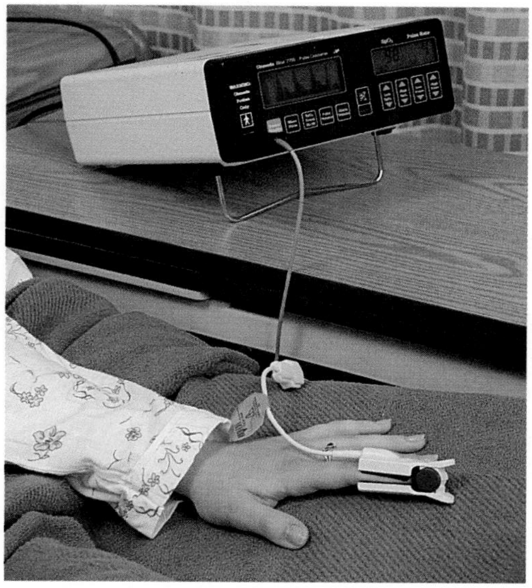

Fig. 25-3 A pulse oximetry sensor is attached to a person's finger.

A good sensor site is needed. The nurse tells you what site to use based on the resident's condition. Swollen sites are avoided. So are sites with breaks in the skin. Older persons often have poor circulation from aging or vascular disease. Blood flow to the toe or finger site may be poor. If so, the ear, nose, or forehead site is used.

Bright light, dark nail polish, and movements affect measurements. Place a towel over the sensor to block bright light. Remove nail polish, or use another site. Movements from shivering, seizures, or tremors affect finger sensors. The earlobe is a better site for these problems. Blood pressure cuffs affect blood flow. If using a finger site, do not measure blood pressure on that side.

Report and record measurements accurately. Use the abbreviation SpO_2 when recording the oxygen concentration value (S=saturation, p=pulse, O_2= oxygen). Also, report and record:

- The date and time
- What the resident was doing at the time of the measurement
- Oxygen flow rate and the device used (pp. 563-564)
- Reason for the measurement (routine or change in the resident's condition)
- Other observations

Pulse oximetry does not lessen the need for good observations. The resident's condition can change rapidly. You assist the nurse and respiratory therapist in observing for signs and symptoms of hypoxia.

Using a Pulse Oximeter

Quality of Life

Remember to:
- ◆ ***Knock before entering the resident's room***
- ◆ ***Address the resident by name***
- ◆ ***Introduce yourself by name and title***

Pre-Procedure

1 Review the procedure with the nurse.
2 Ask the nurse what site to use.
3 Explain the procedure to the resident.
4 Wash your hands.
5 Collect the following:
   - Oximeter and sensor
   - Nail polish remover
   - Cotton balls
   - SpO_2 flow sheet
   - Tape
   - Towel

6 Identify the resident. Check the ID bracelet against the assignment sheet.
7 Provide for privacy.

Continued

Using a Pulse Oximeter—cont'd

Procedure

8 Provide for comfort.
9 Remove nail polish with a cotton ball. (Some women put nail polish on their toes. If a toe site is used, remove any nail polish.)
10 Dry the site with a towel.
11 Clip or tape the sensor to the site.
12 Turn on the oximeter.
13 Check the resident's pulse (apical or radial) with the pulse on the display. The pulses should be equal. Tell the nurse if the pulses are not equal.
14 Read the SpO_2 on the display. Note the value on the flow sheet.
15 Leave the sensor in place for continuous monitoring. Otherwise, turn off the oximeter and remove the sensor.

Post-Procedure

16 Provide for comfort.
17 Place the signal light within the resident's reach.
18 Raise or lower bed rails. Follow the care plan.
19 Unscreen the resident.
20 Return the pulse oximeter to its proper place if continuous monitoring is not ordered.
21 Wash your hands.
22 Report the SpO_2 and your other observations to the nurse.

◈ Collecting sputum specimens. Respiratory disorders cause the lungs, bronchi, and trachea to secrete mucus. The mucus is called **sputum** when expectorated (expelled) through the mouth. Sputum is different from saliva. Saliva is a thin, clear liquid produced by the salivary glands in the mouth. Saliva is often called "spit."

Sputum specimens are studied for blood, microbes, and abnormal cells. The resident coughs up sputum from the bronchi and trachea. This is often painful and difficult. Specimen collection is easier in the early morning when secretions are coughed up upon awakening. The resident rinses the mouth with water. Rinsing decreases saliva and removes food particles. Mouthwash is not used before the procedure. It destroys some of the microbes in the mouth.

Collecting a sputum specimen can embarrass the resident. Coughing and expectorating sounds can upset or nauseate other residents nearby. Also, sputum is unpleasant to look at. For these reasons, privacy is important. The specimen container is covered and placed in a bag. Some centers use sputum containers that conceal the contents. Always follow Standard Precautions and the Bloodborne Pathogen Standard when collecting a sputum specimen.

Older persons may not have the strength to cough up sputum. Coughing is easier after postural drainage. Postural drainage involves draining secretions by gravity. Gravity causes fluids to flow down. Therefore the resident is positioned so a lung part is lower than the airway (Fig. 25-4, p. 558). Different positions are used depending on what part of the lungs need draining. The nurse or respiratory therapist is responsible for postural drainage.

Collecting a Sputum Specimen

Quality of Life

Remember to:
- ◆ *Knock before entering the resident's room*
- ◆ *Address the resident by name*
- ◆ *Introduce yourself by name and title*

Pre-Procedure

1 Explain the procedure to the resident.

2 Wash your hands.

3 Collect the following:
- Sputum specimen container
- Tissues
- Label
- Laboratory requisition
- Disposable bag
- Gloves

Procedure

4 Label the container.

5 Identify the resident. Check the ID bracelet against the requisition slip.

6 Provide for privacy. If able, the resident goes into the bathroom to obtain the specimen.

7 Ask the resident to rinse the mouth with clear water.

8 Put on the gloves.

9 Have the resident hold the container. Only the outside of the container is touched.

10 Ask the resident to cover the mouth and nose with tissues when coughing.

11 Ask him or her to take 2 or 3 deep breaths and cough up the sputum.

12 Have the resident expectorate directly into the container (Fig. 25-5, p. 558). Sputum should not touch the outside of the container.

13 Collect 1 to 2 tablespoons of sputum unless told to collect more.

14 Put the lid on the container immediately.

15 Place the container in the bag. Attach the requisition to the bag.

16 Remove the gloves.

Post-Procedure

17 Provide for comfort.

18 Place the signal light within reach.

19 Unscreen the resident.

20 Wash your hands.

21 Take the bag to the laboratory.

22 Wash your hands.

23 Report the following to the nurse:
- The time the specimen was collected and taken to the laboratory
- The amount of sputum collected
- How easily the resident raised the sputum
- The consistency and appearance of sputum (see Box 25-2)
- Any other observations

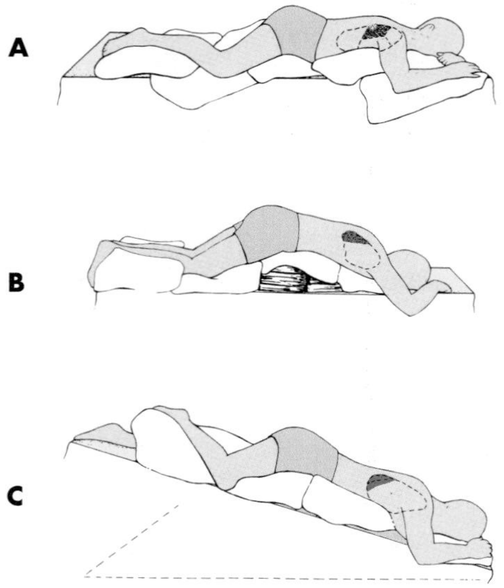

Fig. 25-4 Some positions used for postural drainage. **A,** Draining the right upper lobe. **B,** Draining the right middle lobe. **C,** Draining the right lower lobe. *(From Potter PA, Perry AG:* Fundamentals of nursing: concepts, process, and practice, *ed 4, St Louis, 1997, Mosby.)*

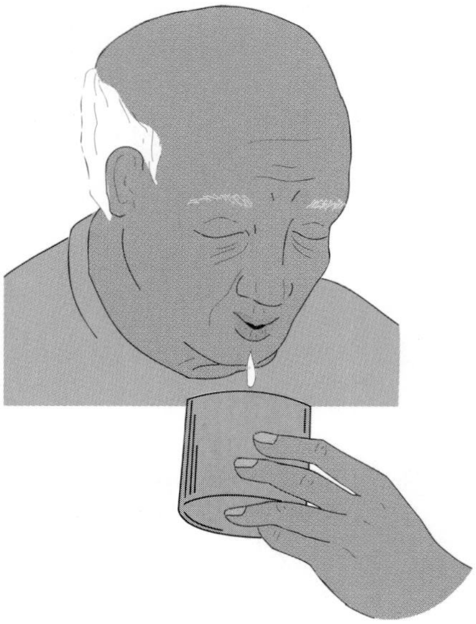

Fig. 25-5 The person expectorates into the center of the specimen container.

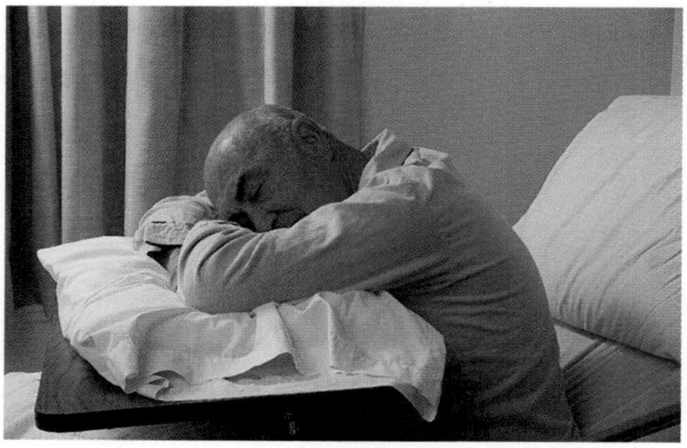

Fig. 25-6 The person is in the orthopneic position. Note that a pillow is on the overbed table for the person's comfort.

PROMOTING OXYGENATION

For the body to get enough oxygen, air must move deeply into the lungs. Air must reach the alveoli for the exchange of oxygen and carbon dioxide with the blood. Disease and injury can prevent air from reaching the alveoli. Secretions can congest lung tissue and the airway. Pain, immobility, and narcotics interfere with deep breathing and coughing up secretions. Therefore secretions collect in the respiratory system. They interfere with air movement and alveolar function in the affected part of the lung. Secretions also provide an environment for microbes. Infection is a threat.

The health care team plans measures to meet the resident's oxygen needs. The following measures often are included in resident care plans.

Positioning

Breathing is usually easier in semi-Fowler's and Fowler's position. Residents with difficulty breathing often prefer to sit up in bed and lean forward over the overbed table. This is called the **orthopneic position.** *Ortho* means sitting or standing; *pnea* means breathing. You can increase the resident's comfort by placing a pillow on the overbed table (Fig. 25-6).

Frequent position changes are important. Unless the doctor limits positioning, the resident must not lie on one side for a long time. This prevents lung expansion on that side and allows secretions to pool. Position changes are usually done at least every 2 hours. You must follow the resident's care plan.

◈ Coughing and Deep Breathing

Mucus is removed by coughing. Deep breathing promotes air movement into most parts of the lungs. Coughing and deep breathing exercises are helpful for residents with respiratory disorders. They are routinely done after surgery and are important for residents on bedrest. The exercises are painful after injury or surgery. The resident may be afraid of breaking open an incision while coughing.

Coughing and deep breathing help prevent pneumonia and atelectasis. *Atelectasis* is the collapse of a portion of the lung. It occurs when mucus collects in the airway. Air cannot get to a part of the lung, and the lung collapses.

The frequency of coughing and deep breathing varies. Some doctors order the exercises every 1 or 2 hours while the resident is awake. Others want them done 4 times a day. The nurse tells you when coughing and deep breathing are done. You are told how many deep breaths and coughs the resident should do. Remember to follow the resident's care plan.

Assisting the Resident With Coughing and Deep Breathing Exercises

Quality of Life

Remember to:

- ***Knock before entering the resident's room***
- ***Address the resident by name***
- ***Introduce yourself by name and title***

Pre-Procedure

1 Explain the procedure to the resident.
2 Identify the resident. Check the ID bracelet against the assignment sheet.
3 Wash your hands.
4 Provide for privacy.

Procedure

5 Help the resident to a comfortable sitting position: dangling, semi-Fowler's, or Fowler's.
6 Have the resident deep breathe:
  a Have the resident place the hands over the rib cage (Fig. 25-7, p. 560).
  b Ask the resident to exhale. Explain that when exhaling, the ribs should move as far down as possible.
  c Have the resident take a deep breath. It should be as deep as possible. Remind the resident to inhale through the nose.
  d Ask the resident to hold the breath for 3 seconds.
  e Ask the resident to exhale slowly through pursed lips (Fig. 25-8, p. 560). The resi-dent should exhale until the ribs move as far down as possible.
  f Repeat this step 4 more times.
7 Ask the resident to cough:
  a Have the resident interlace the fingers over the incision (Fig. 25-9, *A*, p. 560). The resident can also hold a small pillow or folded towel over the incision (Fig. 25-9, *B*, p. 560).
  b Have the resident take in a deep breath as in step 6.
  c Ask the resident to cough strongly twice with the mouth open.

Post-Procedure

8 Provide for comfort.
9 Raise or lower bed rails. Follow the care plan.
10 Place the signal light within reach.
11 Unscreen the resident.
12 Report your observations to the nurse:
- The number of times the resident coughed and deep breathed
- How the resident tolerated the procedure

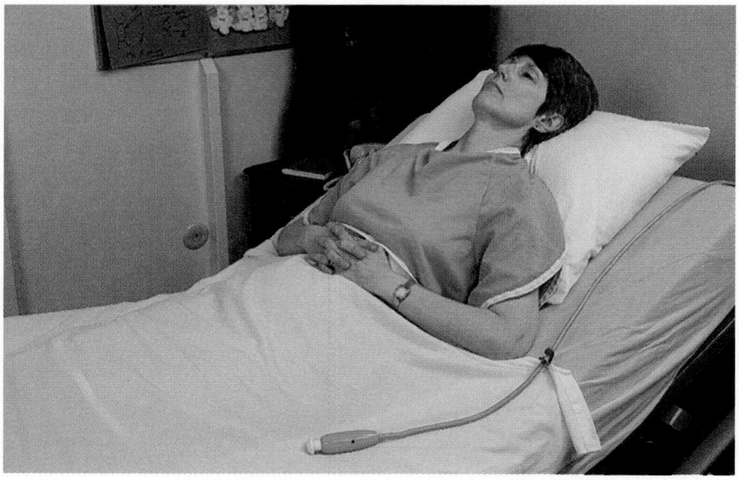

Fig. 25-7 The hands are over the rib cage for deep breathing.

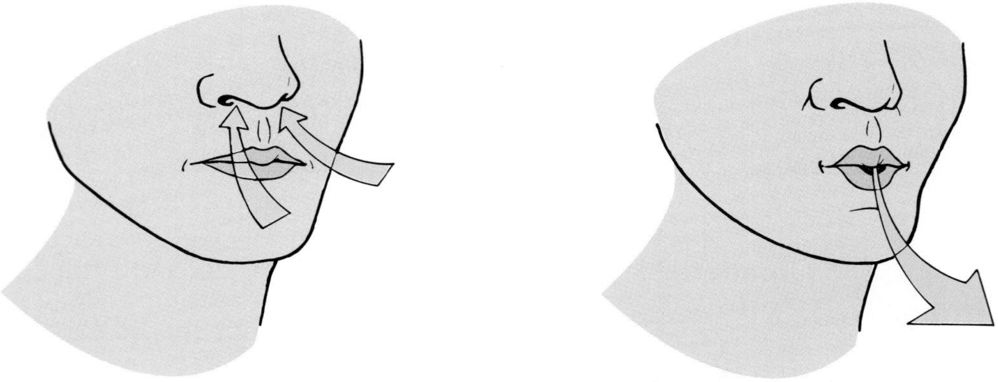

Fig. 25-8 The person inhales through the nose and exhales through pursed lips during the deep-breathing exercise.

A

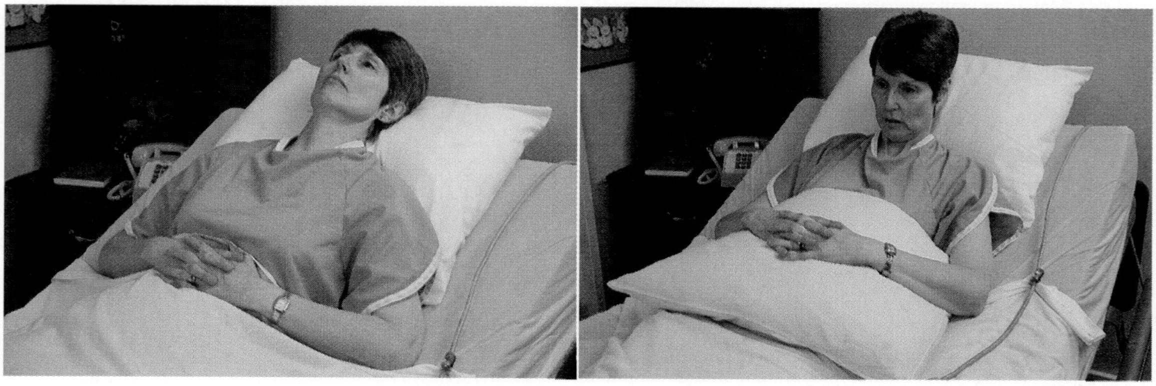

B

Fig. 25-9 The person supports an incision for the coughing exercise. **A,** Fingers are interlaced over the incision. **B,** A small pillow is held over the incision.

Incentive Spirometry

Incentive means to give encouragement. A *spirometer* is a machine that measures and records the amount (volume) of air inhaled. Thus incentive spirometry involves encouraging the resident to inhale until reaching a preset volume of air. Balls or bars in the spirometer allow the resident to see the movement of air when inhaling (Fig. 25-10).

The spirometer is placed upright. The resident exhales normally and then seals the lips around a mouthpiece. The resident takes in a slow, deep breath until the balls rise to the desired height. The breath is held for 2 to 6 seconds to keep the balls floating. Then the resident removes the mouthpiece and exhales slowly. The resident may cough at this time. The nurse tells you how often the resident needs incentive spirometry and how many breaths the resident needs to take. This information is also found in the care plan. Follow center policy for cleaning and replacing disposable mouthpieces.

ASSISTING WITH OXYGEN THERAPY

Disease, injury, and surgery often interfere with breathing. The amount of oxygen in the blood may be less than normal (hypoxemia). If so, the doctor orders supplemental oxygen.

Oxygen is treated as a drug. The doctor orders the amount of oxygen to give and the device to use. The order also states if oxygen is given continuously or intermittently (periodically). *Continuous oxygen therapy* means that the oxygen is never stopped. That is, the administration of oxygen is not interrupted for any reason. *Intermittent oxygen therapy* is for symptom relief. Chest pain and exercise are common reasons for intermittent oxygen. The oxygen helps relieve chest pain. Residents with a chronic respiratory disease may have enough oxygen at rest. With mild exercise or activities of daily living, they become short of breath. Oxygen helps to relieve the shortness of breath.

You are not responsible for administering oxygen. The nurse and respiratory therapist start and maintain oxygen therapy. You assist the nurse in providing safe care to residents receiving oxygen.

Oxygen Sources

Oxygen is supplied through wall outlets, oxygen tanks, oxygen concentrators, and liquid oxygen systems. With the wall outlet (Fig. 25-11), O_2 is piped into each resident unit. Each unit is connected to a centrally located oxygen supply. *(See Subacute Care.)*

The oxygen tank is portable. It is brought to the resident's unit when the doctor orders oxygen therapy. A small tank is used during emergencies and transfers. Some ambulatory residents need continuous oxygen. A portable tank is used when walking (Fig. 25-12, p. 562). The gauge on the tank tells how much oxygen is left in the tank (Fig. 25-13, p. 562). Tell the nurse if the tank is low.

Oxygen concentrators (Fig. 25-14, p. 562) do not need an oxygen source (wall outlet or tank). The concentrator

SUBACUTE CARE

Centers with a subacute care unit often supply oxygen through wall outlets.

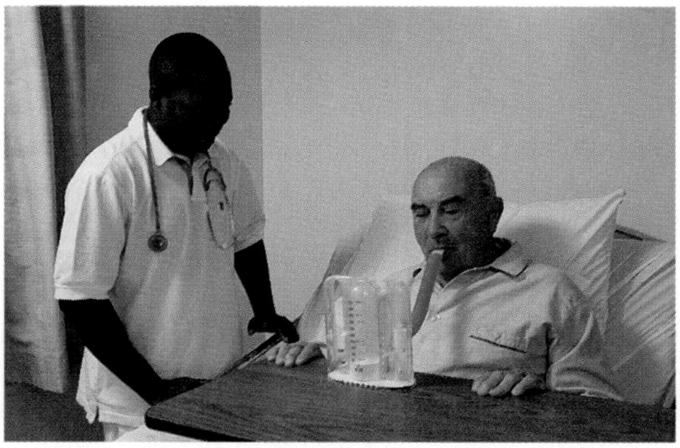

Fig. 25-10 The person uses a spirometer.

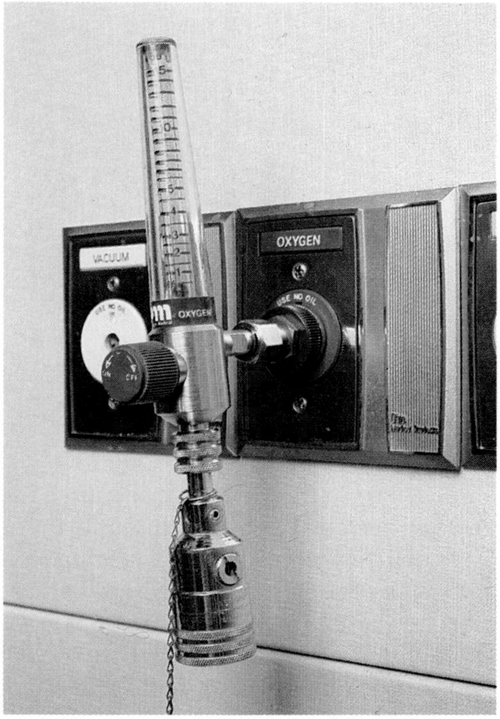

Fig. 25-11 Wall oxygen outlet.

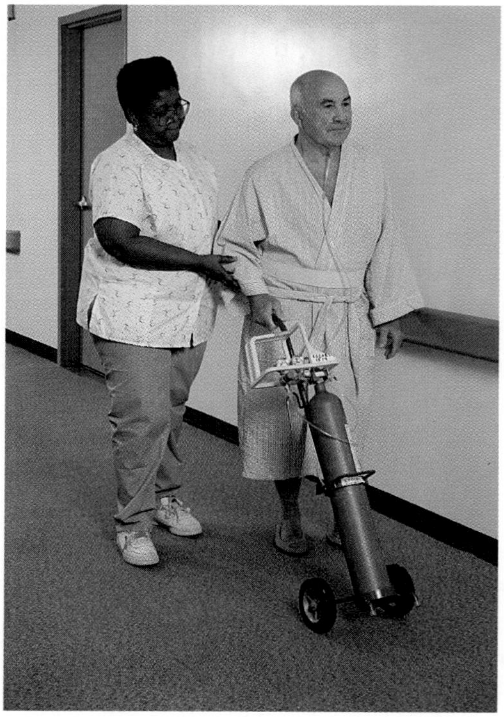

Fig. 25-12 The person uses a portable oxygen tank during ambulation.

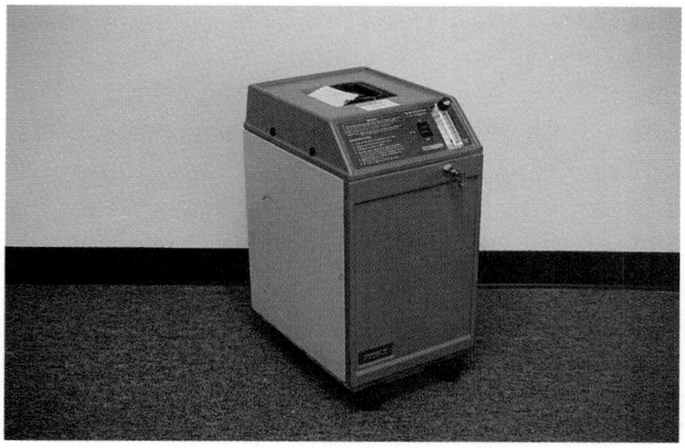

Fig. 25-14 Oxygen concentrator.

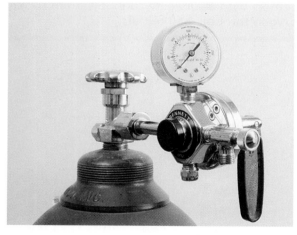

Fig. 25-13 The gauge shows the amount of oxygen remaining in the tank.

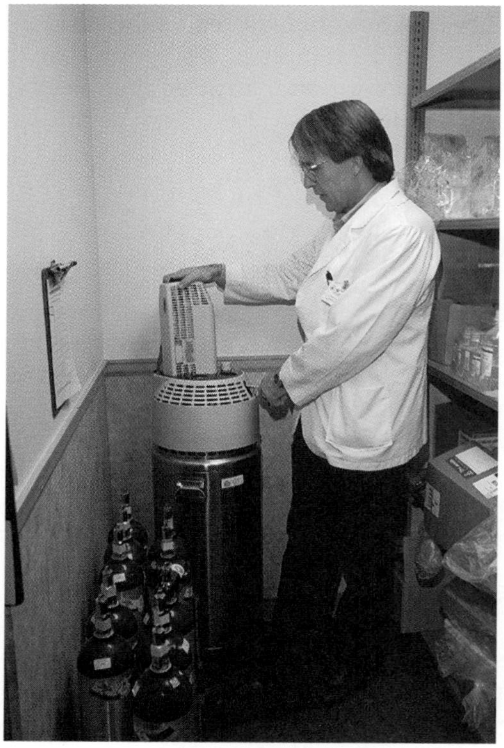

Fig. 25-15 Liquid oxygen system.

removes oxygen from the air. A power source is needed. If the concentrator is not portable, moving about is limited. The resident stays close to the machine. A portable oxygen tank is needed in case of a power failure and for mobility.

Liquid oxygen systems are used in some centers (Fig. 25-15). A portable unit is filled from a stationary unit. The portable unit will last as long as 8 hours. A liquid content indicator tells you when the unit needs refilling. Tell the nurse if the tank is low. The portable unit may be worn over the shoulder. This allows the resident to be mobile. Liquid oxygen is very cold. If touched, it can cause the skin to freeze. Never tamper with the equipment. Doing so is unsafe and could damage the equipment. Follow center policies and procedures and the manufacturer's instructions when working with liquid oxygen.

Some residents will use a liquid oxygen system at home after discharge from the center. The nurse and the respiratory therapist teach the resident and family about how to safely use the liquid oxygen system before discharge.

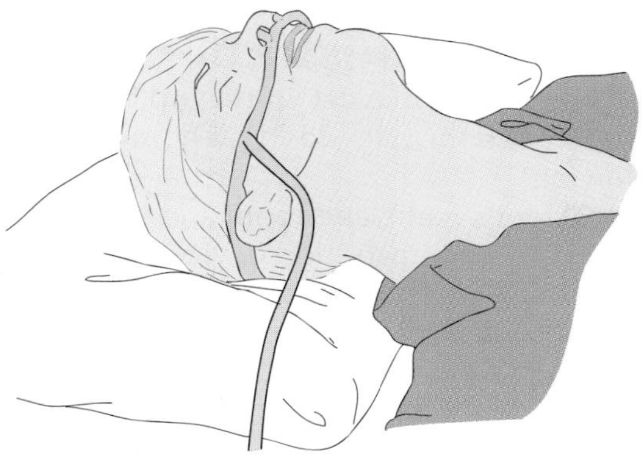

Fig. 25-16 Nasal cannula.

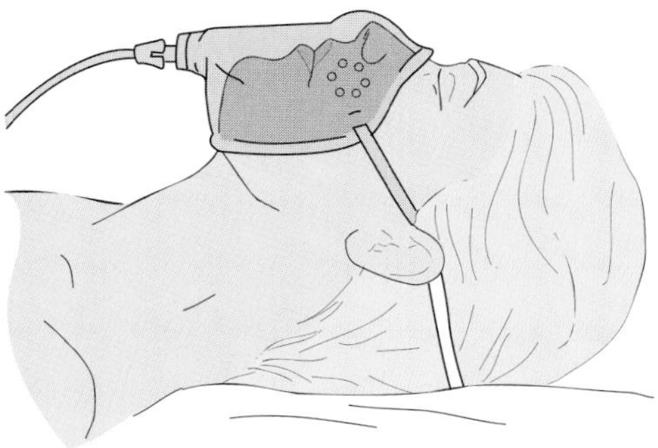

Fig. 25-17 Simple face mask.

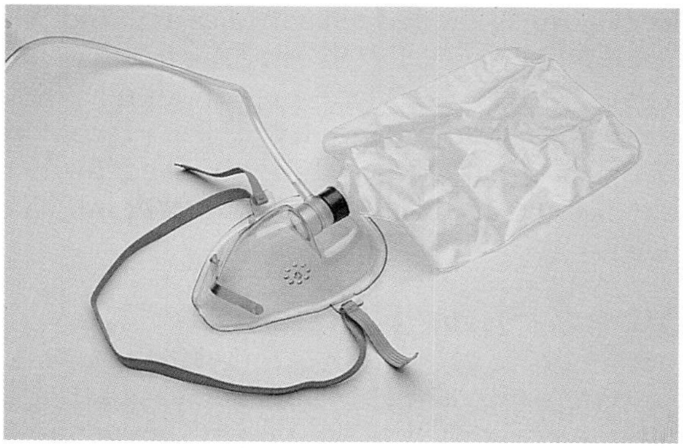

Fig. 25-18 Partial-rebreathing face mask.

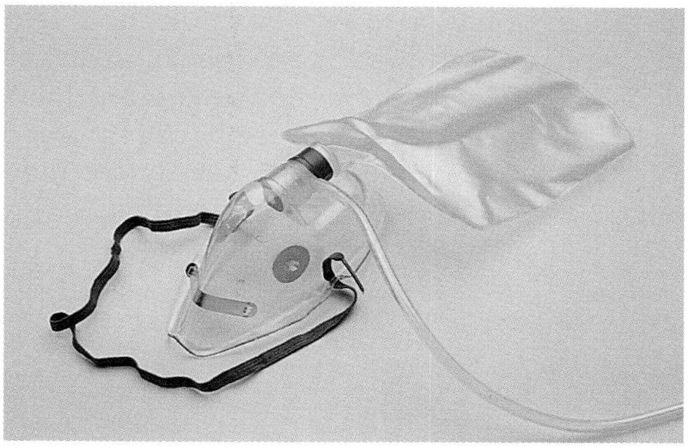

Fig. 25-19 Nonrebreathing face mask.

Devices Used to Administer Oxygen

The doctor orders the device used to administer oxygen. These devices are common:

- **Nasal cannula** (Fig. 25-16)—two prongs project from the tubing. The prongs are inserted a short distance into the nostrils. The prongs point downward. This prevents drying of the sinuses. An elastic headband or tubing brought behind the ears keeps the cannula in place. The resident can eat and talk with a cannula in place. Nasal irritation occurs with tight prongs. Pressure on the ears is possible.
- **Simple face mask** (Fig. 25-17)—covers the nose and mouth. The mask has small holes in the sides. Carbon dioxide escapes during exhalation. Room air enters during inhalation.
- **Partial-rebreathing mask** (Fig. 25-18)—a reservoir bag is added to the simple face mask. The bag is for exhaled air. With inhalation, the resident inhales oxygen and some of the exhaled air. Some room air also is inhaled. The bag should not totally deflate when the resident inhales.

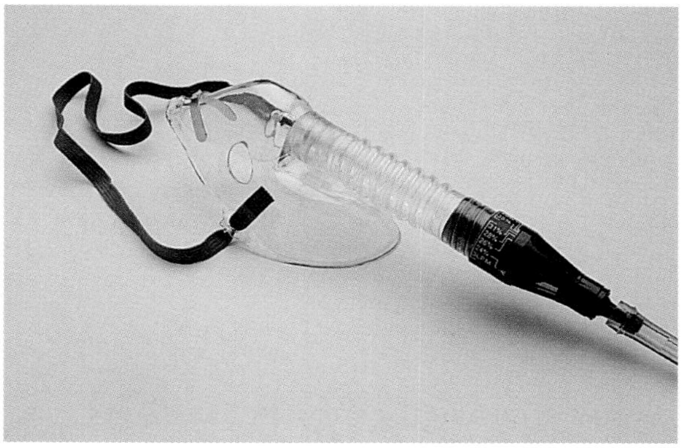

Fig. 25-20 Venturi mask.

- **Nonrebreathing mask** (Fig. 25-19)—prevents exhaled air from entering the reservoir bag. Exhaled air leaves through holes in the mask. When the resident inhales, oxygen from the reservoir bag is inhaled. The bag must totally collapse during exhalation.
- **Venturi mask** (Fig. 25-20)—allows precise amounts of oxygen to be given. Color-coded adapters indicate the amount of oxygen being delivered.

Special care is needed when masks are used. Masks make talking difficult. Listen carefully to what the resident says. Moisture can build up under masks. Keep the resident's face clean and dry to help prevent irritation from the mask. Masks are removed for eating. Usually oxygen is administered by nasal cannula during meals.

Oxygen Flow Rates

The amount of oxygen given is called the *flow rate.* The doctor orders this. The flow rate is measured in liters per minute (L/min). The flow rate is anywhere from 2 to 15 liters of oxygen per minute. The flowmeter (see Fig. 25-11) is set for the desired rate. The nurse or respiratory therapist does this.

The nurse tells you what the flow rate is for the resident. This information is also found in the care plan. When giving care and checking residents, always check the flow rate. Tell the nurse immediately if the flow rate is too high or too low. A nurse or respiratory therapist adjusts the flow rate. Some states and centers let nursing assistants adjust oxygen flow rates.

◈ Preparing for Oxygen Administration

Your job description may let you set up the oxygen administration system (Fig. 25-21). The nurse tells you the following:

- The resident's name and room and bed number
- The oxygen administration device ordered
- If humidification is ordered

Oxygen is a dry gas. If not humidified (made moist), oxygen dries the airway's mucous membranes. Distilled water is added to the humidifier to create water vapor. Oxygen tubing is attached to the humidifier. Oxygen picks up water vapor as it flows into the system. Bubbling in the humidifier means water vapor is being produced. If humidification is not ordered, distilled water and the humidifier are not used.

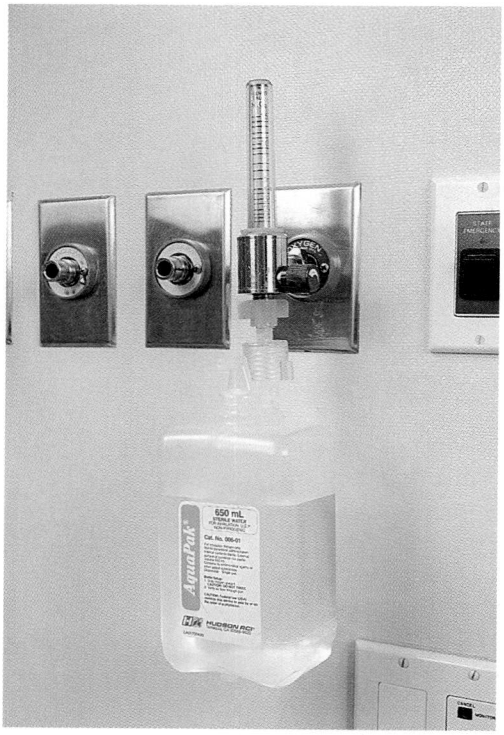

Fig. 25-21 Oxygen administration system with humidifier.

Setting Up for Oxygen Administration

Quality of Life

Remember to:
- ***Knock before entering the resident's room***
- ***Address the resident by name***
- ***Introduce yourself by name and title***

Pre-Procedure

1 Review the doctor's orders with the nurse.
2 Wash your hands.
3 Collect the following:
- Oxygen administration device with connecting tubing
- Oxygen tank
- Flowmeter
- Humidifier (if ordered)
- Distilled water (if using a humidifier)

Procedure

4 Identify the resident. Check the ID bracelet against the assignment sheet.
5 Explain to the resident what you are going to do.
6 Make sure the flowmeter is in the *OFF* position.
7 Attach the flowmeter to the wall outlet or oxygen tank.
8 Fill the humidifier with distilled water.
9 Attach the humidifier to the bottom of the flowmeter.
10 Attach the oxygen administration device and connecting tubing to the humidifier. *Do not set the flowmeter or apply the oxygen administration device on the resident.*

Post-Procedure

11 Discard packaging.
12 Make sure the cap is securely on the distilled water. Store it according to center policy.
13 Provide for comfort.
14 Place the signal light within reach.
15 Tell the nurse that you completed the procedure. *The nurse will:*
- *Turn on the oxygen and set the flow rate*
- *Apply the oxygen administration device on the resident*

16 Wash your hands.

Oxygen Safety

Remember that you assist the nurse with oxygen therapy. You are not responsible for administering oxygen. You do not adjust the flow rate unless allowed by your state and center. However, you must give safe care to residents receiving oxygen. Box 25-3 lists the rules for assisting with oxygen therapy. Also, follow the rules for fire and use of oxygen (see Chapter 8).

ASSISTING WITH RESPIRATORY THERAPY

Persons in a subacute care unit may require an artificial airway, suctioning, mechanical ventilation, and chest tubes. Often these persons are recovering from an illness or injury that affects the airway and lungs. The nurse may ask you to assist in their care. *(See Subacute Care, p. 567.)*

Box 25-3 Safety Rules for Oxygen Therapy

- Never remove the device (cannula, mask) used to administer oxygen.
- Make sure the oxygen administration device is secure but not tight.
- Check for signs of irritation from the device. Check behind the ears, under the nose (cannula), and around the face (mask).
- Never shut off oxygen flow from the wall outlet, tank, or oxygen concentrator.
- Do not adjust the flow rate unless allowed by your state and center.
- Notify the nurse immediately if the flow rate is too high or too low.
- Make sure the humidifier is bubbling. Notify the nurse immediately if the humidifier is not bubbling.
- Tape or pin connecting tubing to the person's gown. Tubing must be secured in place.
- Make sure there are no kinks in the tubing.
- Make sure the resident is not lying on any part of the tubing.
- Report signs and symptoms of hypoxia, respiratory distress, or abnormal breathing patterns to the nurse immediately (see Boxes 25-1 and 25-2).
- Give oral hygiene as directed by the nurse. Follow the care plan.
- Make sure the device is clean and free of mucus.
- Maintain an adequate water level in the humidifier.

SUBACUTE CARE

Artificial Airways

Artificial airways keep the airway patent (open). They are used when the airway is obstructed from disease, injury, secretions, or aspiration. Persons needing mechanical ventilation require an artificial airway (p. 569). So do some persons who are semiconscious or unconscious.

Intubation is the process of inserting an artificial airway. Usually plastic, disposable airways are used. They come in adult, pediatric, and infant sizes. The *oropharyngeal airway* is inserted through the mouth and into the pharynx (Fig. 25-22, *A,* p. 571). An RN or respiratory therapist can insert the airway. The *nasopharyngeal airway* is inserted through a nostril and into the pharynx (Fig. 25-22, *B,* p. 571). An RN or respiratory therapist can insert the airway. An *endotracheal tube* is inserted through the mouth or nose and into the trachea (Fig. 25-22, *C,* p. 571). A doctor, RN, or respiratory therapist with special training intubates using a lighted scope. A balloon (called a *cuff*) at the end of the tube is inflated to keep the airway in place. A *tracheostomy tube* is inserted through a surgical incision *(ostomy)* into the trachea *(tracheo)* (Fig. 25-22, *D,* p. 571). Some tracheostomy tubes have cuffs. The cuff is inflated to keep the tube in place. The tracheostomy is done by a doctor.

You assist the nurse in caring for persons with artificial airways. The person's vital signs are checked often. The person is observed for hypoxia and other respiratory signs and symptoms. If an airway comes out or is dislodged, tell the nurse immediately. The person needs frequent oral hygiene. The nurse tells you when and how to perform oral hygiene. This information is also found in the care plan.

Gagging and choking sensations are common with artificial airways. Imagine something in your mouth, nose, or throat. The person needs comforting and reassurance. Remind the person that the airway helps breathing. Use touch to show you care.

Persons with an endotracheal tube cannot speak. Some tracheostomy tubes allow the resident to speak. Paper and pencils, Magic Slates, communication boards, and hand signals are ways to communicate.

Tracheostomies

Tracheostomies are temporary or permanent. They are temporary when the person requires mechanical ventilation (p. 569). They are permanent when airway structures are surgically removed. Some cancers require removing airway structures. Sometimes a permanent tracheostomy is required when severe trauma injures the airway or a closed head injury damages the breathing center in the brain.

Tracheostomy tubes are made of plastic or metal. A tracheostomy tube has three parts (Fig. 25-23, p. 571): the outer tube, the inner tube, and obturator. *Cannula* is another word for tube. The inner and outer tubes are often called the inner and outer cannulas. The obturator has a rounded end. It is used to insert the outer cannula. After the outer cannula is inserted, the obturator is removed. (The obturator is placed within easy reach in case the tracheostomy tube falls out and needs to be reinserted. It is taped to the wall or bedside stand.) The inner cannula is inserted and locked in place. The outer cannula is secured in place with ties around the person's neck or a Velcro collar. The inner cannula is removed for cleaning and mucus removal. This keeps the airway patent. The outer cannula is not removed.

Some plastic tracheostomy tubes do not have an inner cannula. These are used for persons who are suctioned often. With frequent suctioning, mucus does not stick to the cannula.

The cuffed tracheostomy tube provides a seal between the cannula and the trachea (see Fig. 25-22, *D,* p. 571). This type is used with mechanical ventilation. The cuff prevents air from leaking around the tube. It also prevents aspiration. The RN or respiratory therapist inflates and deflates the cuff.

Securing tracheostomy tubes in place is important. The tube must not come out (extubation). If not secured properly, the tube could come out with coughing or if pulled on. Damage to the airway is possible if the tube is loose and moves up and down in the trachea.

The tracheostomy tube must remain patent (open). Some persons can cough secretions up and out of the tracheostomy. Others require suctioning (p. 568). *Call for the RN if the person shows signs and symptoms of hypoxia or respiratory distress. Also, call the RN if the outer cannula comes out.*

Measures are needed to prevent aspiration. Nothing can enter the stoma. Otherwise, the patient can aspirate. Some patients go home with a tracheostomy. The RN and respiratory therapist teach the patient and family the following:

- Make sure dressings do not have loose gauze or lint.
- Keep the stoma or tube covered when outside. Wear a stoma cover, scarf, or shirt or blouse that buttons at the neck. The cover prevents dust, insects, and other small particles from entering the stoma.

Continued

Subacute Care—cont'd

- Take tub baths instead of showers. If showers are taken, wear a shower guard and use a hand-held nozzle. Direct water away from the stoma.
- Be careful when shampooing. Ask another person to help you.
- Cover the stoma when shaving.
- Do not swim. Water will enter the tube or stoma.
- Wear a medical alert bracelet. Also, carry a medical alert ID card.

Tracheostomy care involves cleaning the inner cannula, cleaning the stoma, and applying clean ties or Velcro collar. Cleaning the inner cannula removes mucus. This keeps the airway patent. A clean stoma and clean ties or collar help prevent infection at the tracheostomy site. Cleaning the stoma also helps prevent skin breakdown.

The nurse may ask you to assist with tracheostomy care. It may be done daily or every 8 to 12 hours. Tracheostomy care is done when there are excess secretions, the ties or collar are soiled, or the dressing is soiled or moist. When the ties are removed, you must hold the outer cannula in place. Ties or collar must be secure but not tight. A finger should slide under the ties or collar (Fig. 25-24, p. 571). Standard Precautions and the Bloodborne Pathogen Standard are followed when assisting the nurse.

Suctioning the Airway

Injury and illness often cause secretions to collect in the upper airway. Removing the secretions is necessary so air can flow into and out of the airway. Retained secretions obstruct the airway. They provide an environment for microbes and interfere with oxygen and carbon dioxide exchange. Hypoxia occurs if secretions are not removed. Usually coughing removes the secretions. Sometimes the person cannot cough or the cough is too weak to remove secretions. Then suctioning is necessary.

Suction is the process of withdrawing or sucking up fluid (secretions). A tube is connected to a suction source (wall outlet or suction machine) at one end and to a suction catheter at the other end. The catheter is inserted into the airway. Secretions are withdrawn through the catheter.

Suction routes involve the upper airway and the lower airway. The nose, mouth, and pharynx make up the upper airway. The trachea and bronchi are the lower parts of the airway.

The *oropharyngeal* route involves suctioning the mouth *(oral)* and pharynx *(pharyngeal).* The nurse passes the suction catheter through the mouth and into the pharynx. The *nasopharyngeal* route involves suctioning the nose *(nasal)* and pharynx *(pharyngeal).* The suction catheter is passed through the nose and into the pharynx. These routes are used for persons who cannot expectorate or swallow secretions after coughing. Lower airway suctioning is done through an endotracheal tube or a tracheostomy tube (p. 567).

If not done correctly, suctioning can seriously harm the person. Suctioning removes oxygen from the airway. Therefore the person does not get a fresh supply of oxygen during suctioning. Hypoxia and life-threatening complications can arise from the respiratory, cardiovascular, and nervous systems. Cardiac arrest can occur. Infection and injury to the airway's mucous membranes also are possible. The nurse may ask you to assist with suctioning. Therefore you need to understand the principles and safety measures involved in safe suctioning. These are described in Box 25-4, p. 572.

Always make sure needed suction equipment and supplies are at the bedside. When the person needs suctioning, you do not have time to collect supplies from the supply area.

For oropharyngeal suctioning, one complete cycle involves inserting the catheter, suctioning, and removing the catheter. A suction cycle takes no more than 10 to 15 seconds to complete. (Hold your breath during the suction cycle. This helps you experience what the patient feels during suctioning.)

Some persons have large amounts of thick secretions. The Yankauer suction catheter often is used for these persons (Fig. 25-25, p. 572). It is larger and stiffer than other suction catheters.

Hypoxia is a risk during suctioning. Remember that the person does not receive oxygen when the suction catheter is inserted. Also, suction removes air out of the airway. Therefore the person's lungs are hyperventilated before suctioning a tracheostomy. To *hyperventilate* means to give extra (hyper) breaths (ventilate). This is done with a manual resuscitation or Ambu bag (Fig. 25-26, p. 572). The Ambu bag is attached to an oxygen source. Then the oxygen delivery device is removed from the tracheostomy tube. The Ambu bag is attached to the tracheostomy tube. The bag is compressed (squeezed) with both hands as the person inhales. The RN or respiratory therapist gives 3 to 5 breaths.

Remember that an oxygen source is attached to the Ambu bag. Oxygen is treated like a drug. Nursing assistants are not allowed to administer drugs. Therefore you need to check if your state and center allow you to use an Ambu bag attached to an oxygen source.

SUBACUTE CARE—CONT'D

Some centers limit suctioning to 10 seconds. Others allow 10 to 15 seconds for the suction cycle (inserting the catheter, applying suction, and removing the catheter).

Mechanical Ventilation

Weak muscle effort, airway obstruction, and damaged lung tissue cause hypoxia. Central nervous system diseases and injuries can affect the respiratory center in the brain. Nerve damage can interfere with sending messages between the lungs and the brain. Drug overdose can depress the brain. These and other respiratory problems are so severe that some people cannot breathe on their own. Or they cannot maintain enough oxygen in the blood. These persons often need mechanical ventilation. **Mechanical ventilation** is using a machine to move air into and out of the lungs (Fig. 25-27, p. 572). Oxygen enters the lungs, and carbon dioxide leaves the lungs. Mechanical ventilation is started in the hospital.

Often persons are taken off the ventilator within hours or days of needing the device. However, some persons need the ventilator for longer periods of time. These persons may require subacute care. Often the person needs weaning from the ventilator. That is, the person needs to breathe without the ventilator. It may take several weeks to get the person off the ventilator. The doctor, respiratory therapist, and RN plan the weaning process.

Persons on mechanical ventilation have an artificial airway. Depending on the person's problems, an endotracheal tube or tracheostomy tube is used. You assist the RN with the care described on p. 567.

Ventilators have alarms that warn when something is wrong. One alarm is for when the person gets disconnected from the ventilator. *When any alarm sounds, first check to see if the person's endotracheal tube or tracheostomy tube is attached to the ventilator. If it is disconnected, attach the tube to the ventilator.* Then notify the RN immediately about the alarm. Do not reset alarms. Remember that the person is on a ventilator because of respiratory difficulties. *The person can die if not connected to the ventilator.*

Persons needing mechanical ventilation are seriously ill. They often have other problems and injuries. Their reactions to mechanical ventilation are many. Some are confused, disoriented, or unable to think clearly. Many are frightened by the machine and fear dying. Some feel relief when their bodies get enough oxygen. Many fear staying on the machine for life. Mechanical ventilation can be painful for those with a chest injury or chest surgery. Tubes and hoses restrict movement, adding to the person's discomfort.

The RN may ask you to assist with the person's care. The following are important aspects of the person's care:

- Keep the signal light within the person's reach.
- Make sure there is enough slack on hoses and connecting tubing. They should not pull on the endotracheal or tracheostomy tube.
- Answer signal lights promptly. Remember that the person depends on others for basic needs.
- Explain who you are and what you are going to do whenever you enter the room.
- Orient the person to day, date, and time.
- Tell the RN immediately if the person shows signs of respiratory distress or discomfort.
- Do not change any settings on the ventilator or reset alarms.
- Provide a means of communication. Remember that the person on mechanical ventilation cannot talk.
- Use established hand or eye signals for "yes" and "no." All health team members (nursing staff, doctors, respiratory therapists, and others) and the family must use the same signals. Otherwise, communication does not occur.
- Ask questions that have simple answers. The person may not have the strength to write out long responses.
- Watch what you say when within the person's hearing distance. The person may pay close attention to what you are saying. Do not say anything that could upset the person.
- Watch your nonverbal communication. Although seriously ill and unable to speak, the person may be very aware of nonverbal messages. Avoid communicating worry and concern to the person.
- Take time to comfort and reassure the person. Tell the person what you are going to do and why. Also, tell the person about such things as the weather, pleasant news events, and gifts and cards.
- Meet the person's basic needs for personal and oral hygiene, elimination, and activity (repositioning, range-of-motion exercises, sitting in a chair) as directed by the RN. Follow the person's care plan.
- Apply a moist washcloth or lubricant to the person's lips as directed by the RN. This helps prevent the lips from drying and cracking.
- Use touch to reassure and comfort the person.
- Tell the person when you are leaving the room and when you will return.

Continued

SUBACUTE CARE—CONT'D

Chest Tubes

When the chest is entered, air, blood, or fluid can collect in the pleural space (sac or cavity). Chest entry occurs with chest surgery or injury. **Pneumothorax** is the collection of air *(pneumo)* in the pleural space *(thorax)*. **Hemothorax** is the collection of blood *(hemo)* in the pleural space *(thorax)*. **Pleural effusion** is the collection of fluid *(effusion)* in the plueral space (thorax).

Pressure caused by the collection of air, blood, or fluid collapses the lung. Air cannot reach the affected aveoli. O_2 and CO_2 are not exchanged at the alveoli. Respiratory distress and hypoxia result. Sometimes there is pressure on the heart. This affects the heart's ability to pump blood and is a life-threatening problem.

The doctor inserts chest tubes to remove the air, fluid, or blood (Fig. 25-28, p. 573). The sterile procedure is done in surgery, in the emergency room, or at the bedside in the hospital. An RN assists with the procedure. The person may transfer to a subacute care unit when his or her condition is stable.

The chest tubes are attached to a drainage system (Fig. 25-29, p. 573). The system must be airtight so that air does not enter the pleural space. Water-seal drainage is used to keep the system airtight (Fig. 25-30, p. 573). This is done as follows:

- A chest tube is attached to connecting tubing.
- Connecting tubing is then attached to a tube in the drainage container.
- The tube in the drainage container extends under water. The water prevents air from entering the chest tube and then the pleural space.

A 1- , 2- , or 3-bottle system or a disposable system is used (see Fig. 25-30). Disposable systems are common. Bottles are shown in Figure 25-30 to give you a clearer understanding of how the system works. Sometimes suction is applied to the drainage system.

When caring for persons with chest tubes, you need to:

- Keep the drainage system below the level of the person's chest.
- Measure the person's vital signs as directed by the RN. Report any changes in vital signs immediately.
- Report signs and symptoms of hypoxia and respiratory distress to the RN immediately. Also, report patient complaints of pain or difficulty breathing.
- Keep connecting tubing coiled on the bed. Allow enough slack so the chest tubes are not dislodged when the person moves. If tubing hangs in loops, drainage collects in the loop.
- Make sure the tubing is not kinked. Kinking obstructs the chest tube causing air, blood, or fluid to collect in the pleural space.
- Observe chest drainage. Immediately report to the RN any change in chest drainage. This includes increases in drainage or the appearance of bright red drainage.
- Record chest drainage according to center policy.
- Turn and position the person as directed by the RN. The person is turned carefully and gently to prevent the chest tubes from dislodging.
- Assist the person with coughing and deep breathing as directed by the RN. Also, assist with incentive spirometry as directed.
- Note bubbling activity in the drainage system. Tell the RN immediately if the bubbling increases, decreases, or stops.
- Tell the RN immediately if any part of the system is loose or disconnected.
- Make sure petrolatum gauze is at the bedside in case a chest tube comes out.
- Call for help immediately if a chest tube comes out. Cover the insertion site with sterile petrolatum gauze. Stay with the person until an RN arrives. Follow the RN's directions.

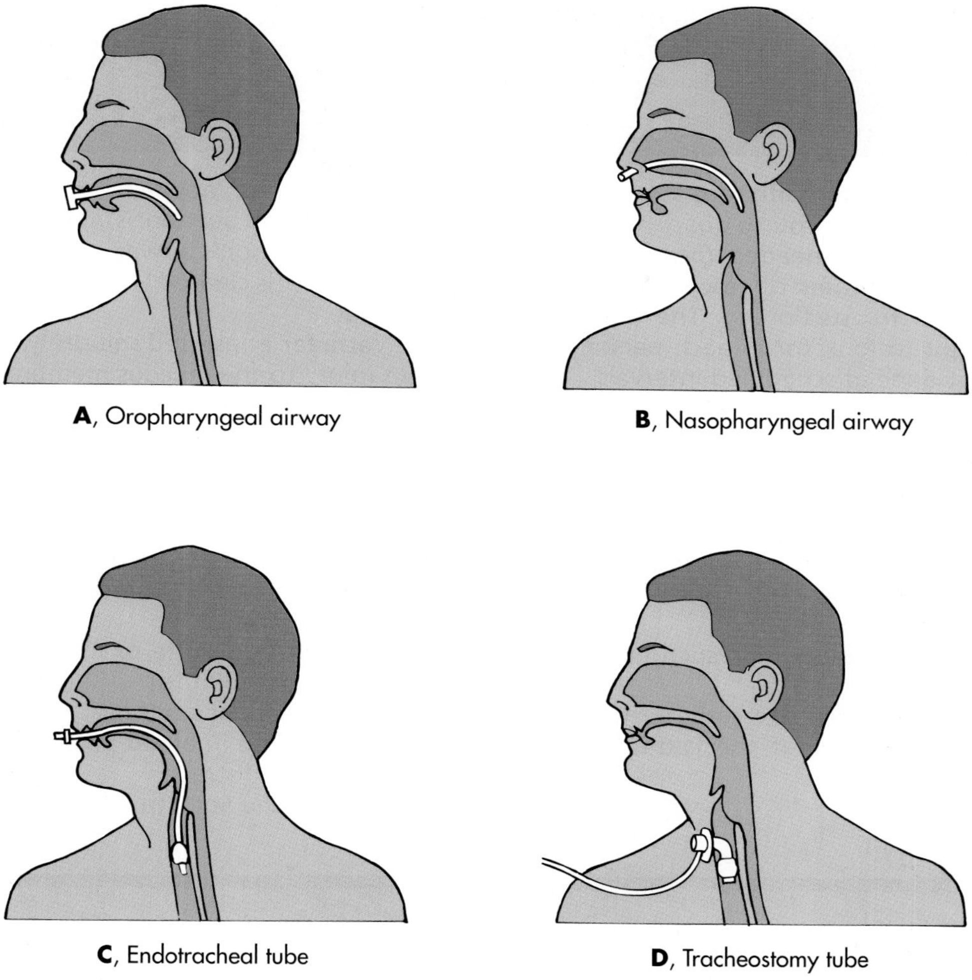

Fig. 25-22 Artificial airways. **A,** Oropharyngeal airway. **B,** Nasopharyngeal airway. **C,** Endotracheal tube. **D,** Tracheostomy tube.

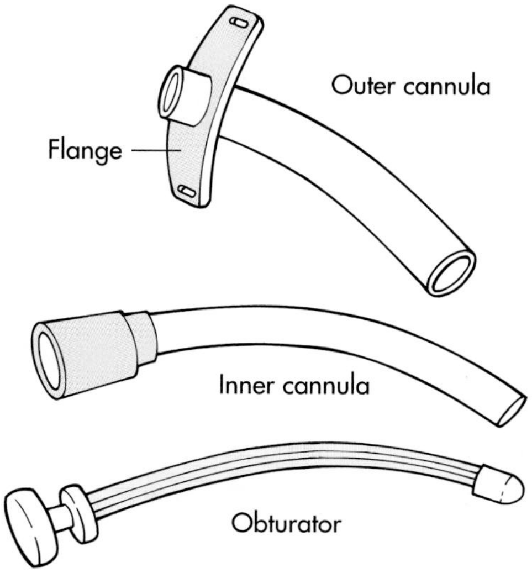

Fig. 25-23 Parts of a tracheostomy tube.

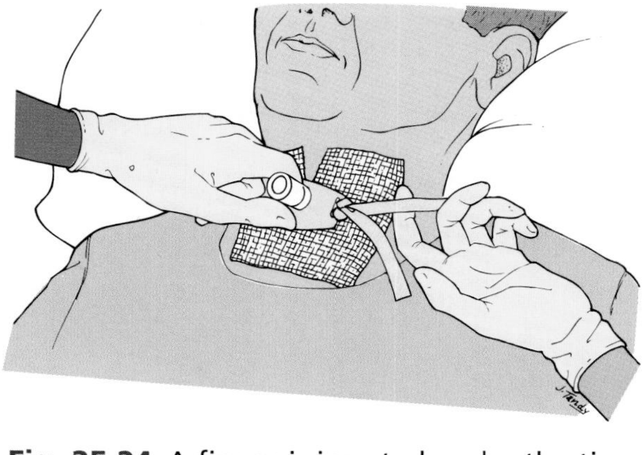

Fig. 25-24 A finger is inserted under the ties.

Box 25-4 Principles and Safety Measures for Suctioning

- Review the procedure with the nurse. Know what the nurse expects you to do.
- Suctioning is done as needed *(prn)*. Coughing and signs and symptoms of respiratory distress signal the need for suctioning. The nurse tells you what signs to look for in each person. Suctioning is not done at scheduled intervals.
- Standard Precautions and the Bloodborne Pathogen Standard are followed. Remember, secretions can contain blood and are potentially infectious.
- The mouth is clean, not sterile. Microbes enter the mouth through breathing, eating, and drinking. Oropharyngeal suctioning does not require sterile technique.
- Sterile technique is used when suctioning a tracheostomy (see Chapter 9).
- The nurse tells you what size catheter to collect. Airway injury can occur if the catheter is too large.
- Suction is not applied while inserting the catheter. When suction is applied, air is sucked out of the person's airway.
- The catheter is cleared with water or saline after removal.
- The catheter is inserted smoothly. This helps prevent injury to the mucous membranes.
- The suction catheter is passed no more than 3 times. The risk of injury increases each time the suction catheter is passed.
- Check the person's pulse, respirations, and pulse oximeter before, during, and after the procedure. Also observe the person's level of consciousness. Tell the RN immediately if any of the following occur:
  - A drop in pulse rate or a pulse rate less than 60 beats per minute
  - Irregular cardiac rhythms
  - A drop or rise in blood pressure
  - Respiratory distress
  - A drop in the SpO_2 (p. 554)

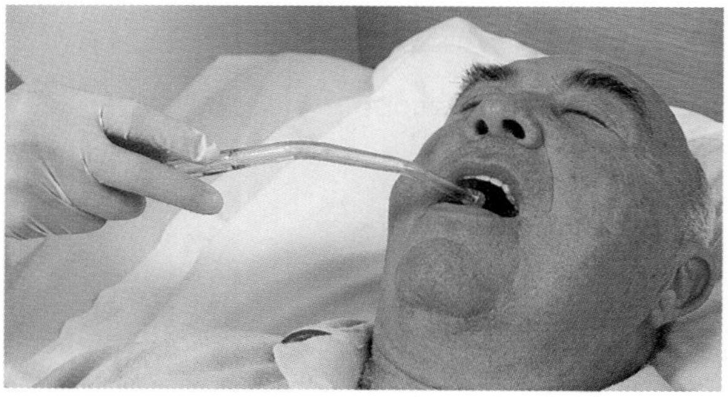

Fig. 25-25 The Yankauer suction catheter.

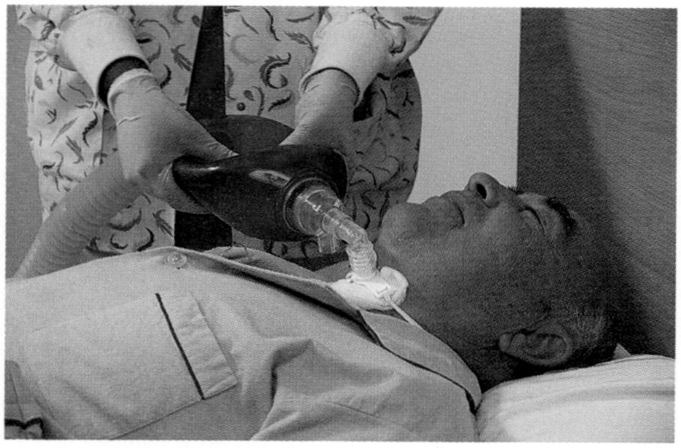

Fig. 25-26 The Ambu bag. Two hands are used to compress the bag.

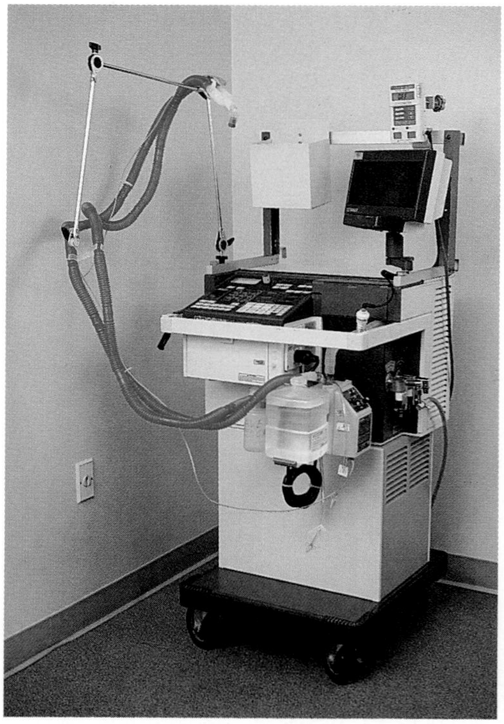

Fig. 25-27 A mechanical ventilator.

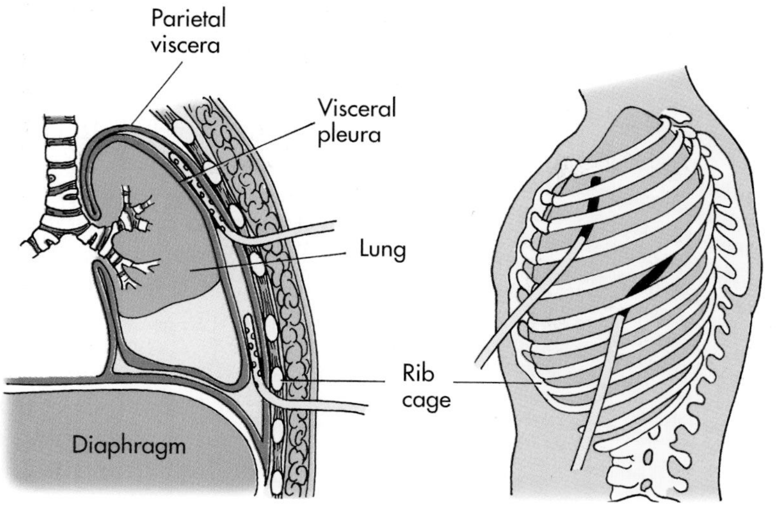

Fig. 25-28 Chest tubes inserted into the pleural space. *(From Elkin MK, Perry AG, Potter PA:* Nursing interventions and clinical skills, *St Louis, 1996, Mosby.)*

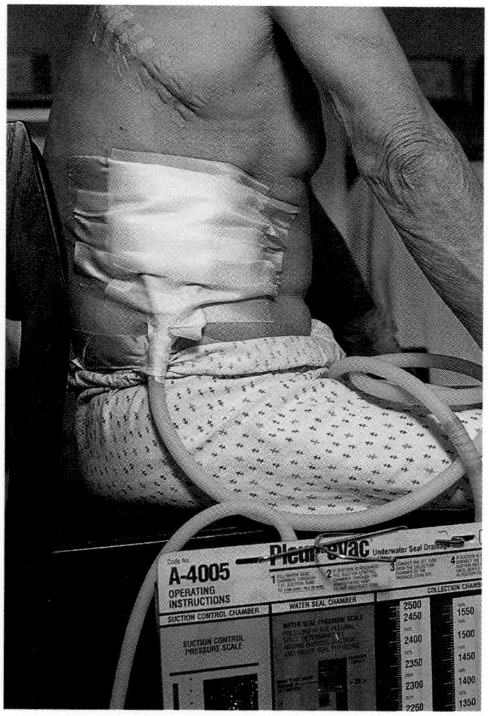

Fig. 25-29 Chest tubes attached to a disposable water-seal drainage system. *(From Elkin MK, Perry AG, Potter PA:* Nursing interventions and clinical skills, *St Louis, 1996, Mosby.)*

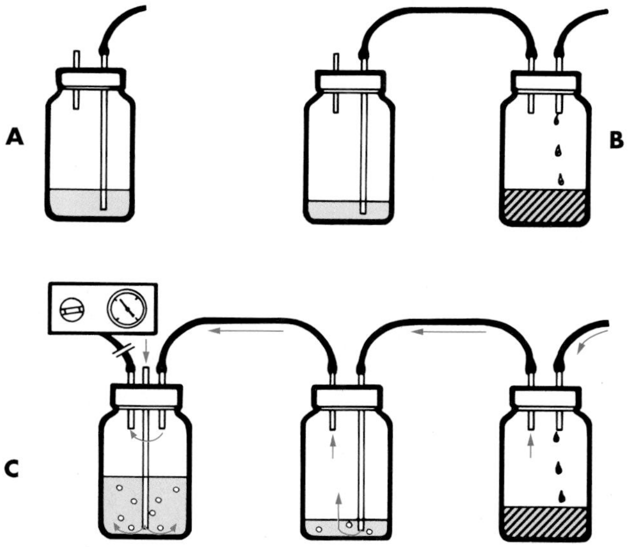

Fig. 25-30 Water-seal drainage system. *(From Potter PA, Perry AG:* Fundamentals of nursing: concepts, process, and practice, *ed 4, St Louis, 1997, Mosby.)*

QUALITY OF LIFE

Residents have the right to safe and effective care. Do not perform or assist with procedures in this chapter unless you have received the necessary training. The procedures in this chapter are complex. Many require an RN's supervision. Serious complications can occur if incorrect care is given. You may be assigned to care for residents who need suctioning or oxygen therapy. You must provide safe care. A safe environment promotes quality of life for the resident. Always follow the safety measures and the rules for suctioning and oxygen therapy.

The right to privacy is very important when diagnostic procedures are performed. Do all you can to provide privacy. Merely pulling the privacy curtain is not enough. If possible, schedule the procedure when the roommate is out of the room. Close doors and window shades, blinds, or curtains. The resident raising a sputum specimen is allowed to do so in private if able.

You will work with the health care team to help meet the resident's oxygen needs. You are not responsible for administering oxygen. You will assist in providing safe care to residents receiving oxygen. You need to have a sound, basic understanding of oxygen therapy and general safety rules. Resident safety is never overlooked. Careful observation of the resident is necessary. You must promptly report observations and resident complaints. The side effects and complications of some treatments and procedures can be severe. *Every sign, symptom, or resident complaint is important.*

Finally, you need to know your own limits. Do not perform any procedure that you do not understand or with which you are unfamiliar. Remember your legal and ethical responsibilities. *You have the right to say no.* You should not do anything that is beyond your legal scope, preparation, and skill level.

REVIEW QUESTIONS

Circle the BEST answer.

1 Alcohol and narcotics affect oxygen needs because they
- A Depress the brain
- B Are pollutants
- C Cause allergies
- D Cause a pneumothorax

2 Hypoxia is
- A A deficiency of oxygen in the blood
- B The amount of hemoglobin that contains oxygen
- C A deficiency of oxygen in the cells
- D The lack of oxygen

3 One of the earliest signs of hypoxia is
- A Cyanosis
- B Increased pulse and respiratory rates
- C Restlessness
- D Dyspnea

4 A resident can breathe deeply and comfortably only while sitting or standing. This is called
- A Biot's respirations
- B Orthopnea
- C Bradypnea
- D Kussmaul's respirations

5 The resident will probably need to rest after
- A A chest x-ray
- B A lung scan
- C Arterial blood gases
- D Pulmonary function tests

6 A resident has pulse oximetry. The resident's $Sp0_2$ is 98%. Which is *true?*
- A The machine is not accurate.
- B The resident's pulse is 98 beats per minute.
- C The measurement is within normal range.
- D The resident needs suctioning.

7 Which is not a site for a pulse oximetry sensor?
- A Toe
- B Finger
- C Ear lobe
- D Upper arm

8 The best time to collect a sputum specimen is
- A On awakening
- B After meals
- C At bedtime
- D After suctioning

9 Before collecting a sputum specimen, you should
- A Ask the resident to use mouthwash
- B Ask the resident to rinse the mouth with clear water
- C Ask the resident to brush the teeth
- D Apply lubricant to the resident's lips

10 You are assisting a resident with coughing and deep breathing. Which is *false?*
- A The resident inhales through pursed lips.
- B The resident needs to be in a comfortable sitting position.
- C The resident inhales deeply through the nose.
- D The resident holds a small pillow over an incision.

11 Which is useful for deep breathing?
- A Pulse oximeter
- B Incentive spirometry
- C Chest tubes
- D Partial-rebreathing mask

12 You are assisting with oxygen therapy. You can
- A Turn the oxygen on and off
- B Start the oxygen
- C Decide what device to use
- D Make sure the connecting tubing is secure and free of kinks

13 A person has a tracheostomy. Which is *false?*
- A A nondisposable inner cannula is removed for cleaning.
- B The obturator is inserted after the outer cannula.
- C The outer cannula must be secured in place.
- D The person must be protected from aspiration.

14 A person has a tracheostomy. The resident can do the following *except*
- A Shampoo
- B Shave
- C Shower with a hand-held nozzle
- D Swim

15 These statements are about oral pharyngeal suctioning. Which is *true?*
- A Suction is applied while inserting the catheter.
- B Suctioning is done every 2 hours.
- C A suction cycle is no more than 10 to 15 seconds.
- D The mouth is considered sterile.

16 Oral pharyngeal suctioning requires
- A Following Standard Precautions and the Bloodborne Pathogen Standard
- B Sterile technique
- C An artificial airway
- D All of the above

17 Which is used to hyperventilate the lungs?
- A Incentive spirometer
- B Pulse oximeter
- C Ambu bag
- D Partial-rebreathing mask

18 Mr. Long requires mechanical ventilation. Which is *false?*
- A He has an endotracheal tube or a tracheostomy tube.
- B His signal light must always be within his reach.
- C You should use touch to provide comfort and reassurance.
- D You can reset alarms on the ventilator.

19 An alarm sounds on Mr. Long's ventilator. What should you do first?
- A Reset the alarm.
- B Check to see if his airway is attached to the ventilator.
- C Call the nurse immediately.
- D Ask him what is wrong.

20 Chest tubes are attached to water-seal drainage. You should do the following *except*
- A Notify the RN if bubbling increases, decreases, or stops
- B Make sure the tubing is not kinked
- C Keep the drainage system below the resident's chest
- D Hang tubing in loops

Answers to these questions are on p. 699.

26 Common Health Problems

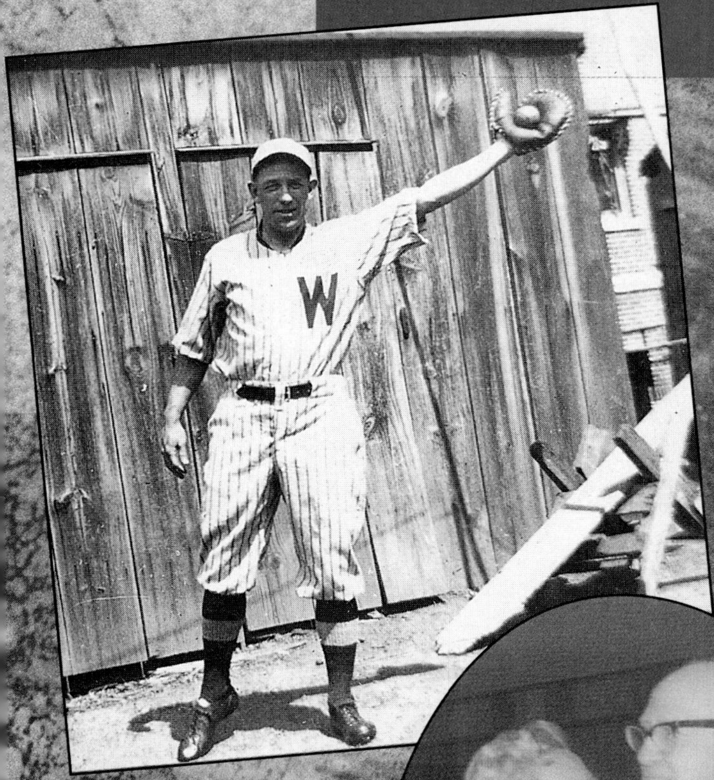

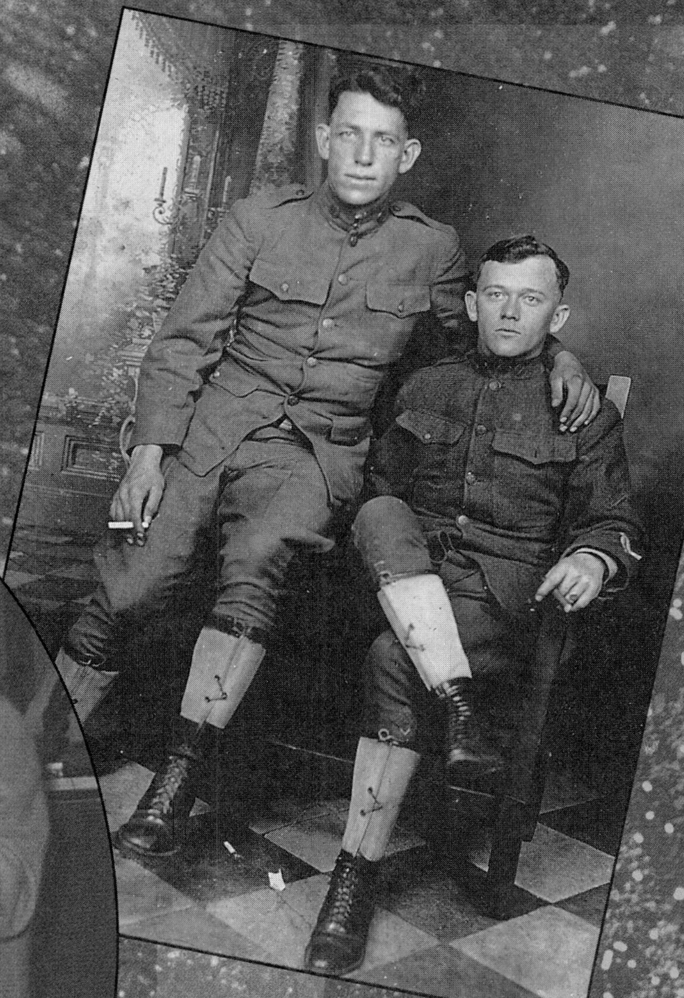

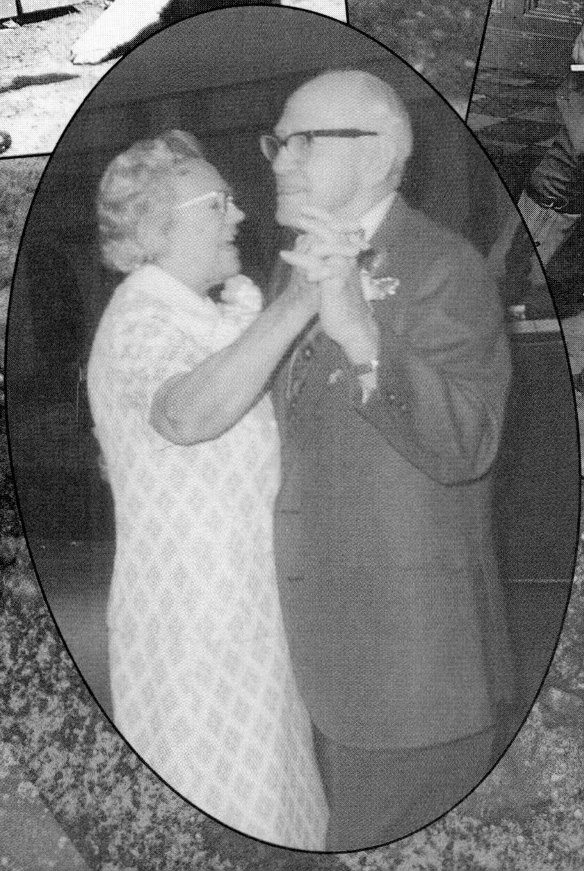

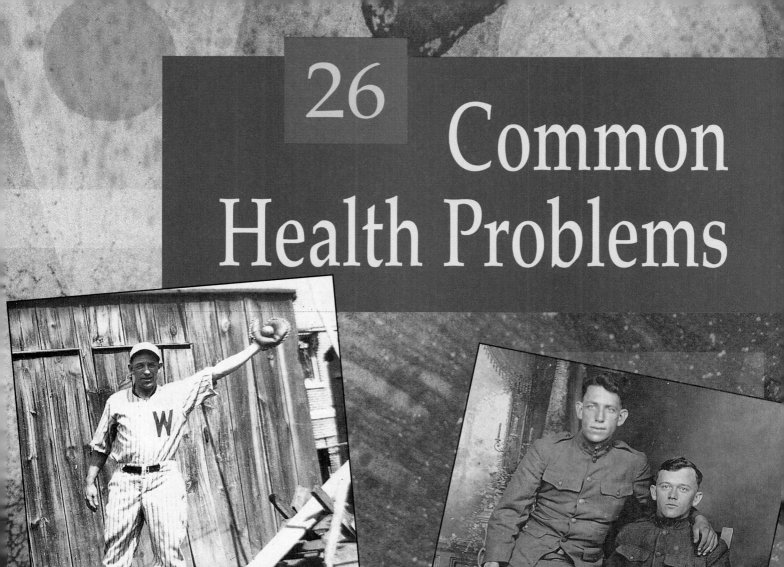

What You Will Learn

- The definition of the key terms listed in this chapter
- The seven warning signs of cancer
- How to maintain joint function in persons with arthritis
- How to care for residents in casts, in traction, and with hip pinnings
- The care required for residents with osteoporosis
- The effects of amputation
- The signs and symptoms of stroke, and the care required by residents after a stroke
- The signs and symptoms of Parkinson's disease and multiple sclerosis
- How to care for residents with hearing and vision impairments
- The causes and effects of head and spinal cord injuries and the care required
- Common respiratory disorders and the care required
- The signs, symptoms, and treatment of hypertension
- The risk factors for coronary artery disease
- The care required for residents with angina pectoris, myocardial infarction, and heart failure
- The care required by residents with urinary system disorders
- The signs, symptoms, and complications of diabetes
- How to help the resident who is vomiting
- The signs and symptoms of hepatitis, AIDS, and sexually transmitted diseases, and the necessary precautions when caring for residents with these disorders
- The different types of mental health disorders

Key Terms

affect Feelings and emotions

amputation The removal of all or part of an extremity

anxiety A vague, uneasy feeling that occurs in response to stress

aphasia The inability *(a)* to speak *(phasia)*

arthritis Joint *(arthr)* inflammation *(itis)*

arthroplasty The surgical replacement *(plasty)* of a joint *(arthro)*

benign tumor A tumor that grows slowly and within a localized area

braille A method of writing that uses raised dots; raised dots are arranged to represent each letter of the alphabet; the first 10 letters represent the numbers 0 through 9

cancer Malignant tumor

closed fracture The bone is broken but the skin is intact; simple fracture

compound fracture The bone is broken and has come through the skin; open fracture

compulsion The uncontrolled performance of an act

defense mechanism An unconscious reaction that blocks unpleasant or threatening feelings

delusion A false belief

delusion of grandeur An exaggerated belief about one's own importance, wealth, power, or talents

delusion of persecution A false belief that one is being mistreated, abused, or harassed

dialysis The process of removing waste products from the blood

dysphagia Difficulty *(dys)* swallowing *(phagia)*

emotional illness Mental illness, mental disorder, psychiatric disorder

expressive aphasia Difficulty expressing or sending out thoughts

expressive-receptive aphasia Difficulty expressing or sending out thoughts and difficulty receiving information

fracture A broken bone

KEY TERMS—cont'd

gangrene A condition in which there is death of tissue; tissues become black, cold, and shriveled

hallucination Seeing, hearing, or feeling something that is not real

hemiplegia Paralysis on one side of the body

hyperglycemia High *(hyper)* sugar *(glyc)* in the blood *(emia)*

hypoglycemia Low *(hypo)* sugar *(glyc)* in the blood *(emia)*

malignant tumor A tumor that grows rapidly and invades other tissues; cancer

mental Relating to the mind; something that exists in the mind or is performed by the mind

mental disorder Mental illness, emotional illness, psychiatric disorder

mental health A state of mind in which the person copes with and adjusts to the stresses of everyday living in ways acceptable to society

mental illness A disturbance in the person's ability to cope or adjust to stress; behavior and functioning are impaired; mental disorder, emotional illness, psychiatric disorder

metastasis The spread of cancer to other parts of the body

obsession A persistent thought or idea

open fracture Compound fracture

panic An intense and sudden feeling of fear, anxiety, terror, or dread

paranoia A disorder *(para)* of the mind *(noia)*; false beliefs (delusions) and suspicion about a person or situation

paraplegia Paralysis of the legs

phobia Fear, panic, or dread

psychiatric disorder Mental illness, mental disorder, emotional illness

psychosis A serious mental disorder; the person does not view or interpret reality correctly

quadriplegia Paralysis of the arms, legs, and trunk

receptive aphasia Difficulty receiving information

schizophrenia Split *(schizo)* mind *(phrenia)*

simple fracture Closed fracture

stomatitis Inflammation *(itis)* of the mouth *(stomat)*

stress The response or change in the body caused by any emotional, physical, social, or economic factor

stressor Any emotional, physical, social, or economic factor that causes stress

tinnitus Ringing in the ears

tumor A new growth of abnormal cells; tumors are benign or malignant

vertigo Dizziness

This chapter gives basic information about common health problems. The nurse uses the nursing process to help the health care team meet the needs of residents with these and other health problems. Understanding a disorder makes the required care meaningful. The nurse gives you more information as needed.

A review of Chapter 6 (Body Structure and Function) will help you study this chapter.

CANCER

A **tumor** is a new growth of abnormal cells. Tumors are benign or malignant (Fig. 26-1, p. 580). **Benign** tumors grow slowly and within a localized area. They usually do not cause death. A malignant tumor is cancerous. A **malignant** tumor **(cancer)** grows rapidly and invades healthy tissues (Fig. 26-2, p. 580). Death occurs if the cancer is not treated and controlled. **Metastasis** is the spread of cancer to other body parts (Fig. 26-3, p. 580). It occurs if the cancer is not treated and controlled. Cancer can occur in almost any body part. The most common sites are the lung, colon and rectum, breast, prostate, uterus, and urinary tract. Cancer is the second leading cause of death in the United States. It occurs in people of all ages.

The exact causes of cancer are unknown. However, certain factors contribute to its development. They include:

- A family history of cancer
- Exposure to radiation (including the sun)
- Exposure to certain chemicals

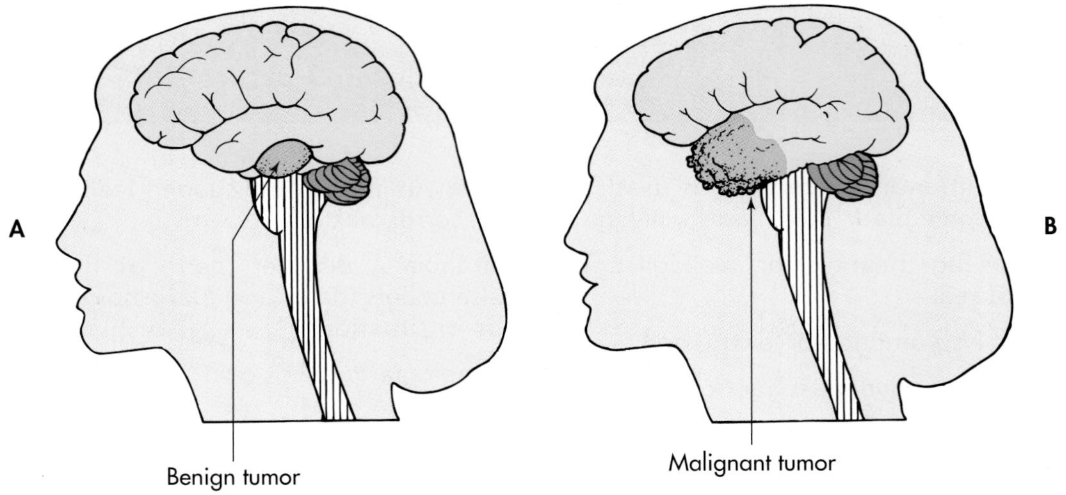

Fig. 26-1 A, Benign tumors grow within a localized area. **B,** Malignant tumors invade other tissues.

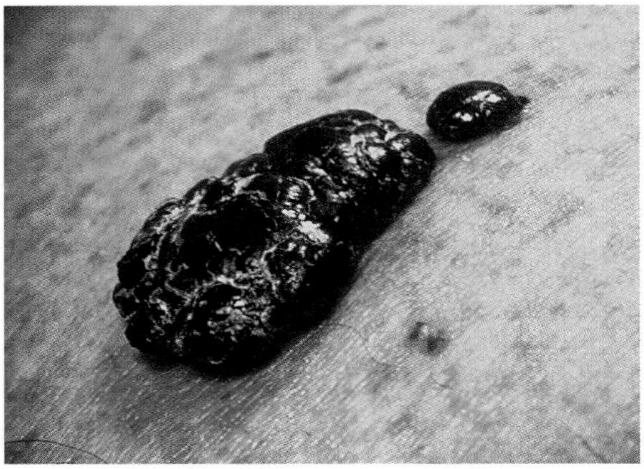

Fig. 26-2 A malignant tumor on the skin. *(From Belcher AE:* Cancer nursing, *St Louis, 1992, Mosby.)*

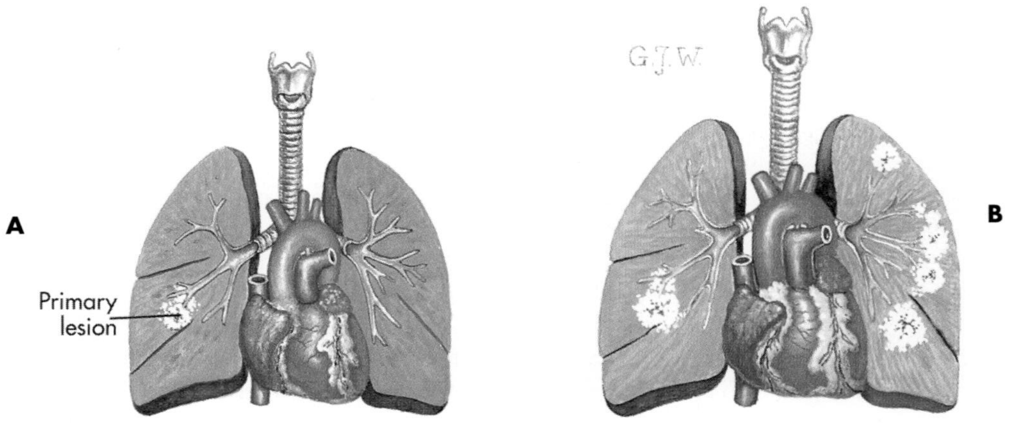

Fig. 26-3 A, A tumor in the lung. **B,** The tumor has metastasized to the other lung. *(From Belcher AE:* Cancer nursing, *St Louis, 1992, Mosby).*

Box 26-1 Seven Warning Signs of Cancer

- Change in bowel or bladder habits
- A sore that does not heal
- Unusual bleeding or discharge from a body opening
- Thickening or lump in the breast or elsewhere in the body
- Indigestion or difficulty swallowing
- Obvious change in a wart or mole
- Nagging cough or hoarseness

- Smoking
- Alcohol
- High-fat, high-calorie diet
- Food additives
- Viruses
- Hormones

Cancer can be treated and controlled with early detection. The seven warning signs identified by the American Cancer Society (ACS) are listed in Box 26-1.

Treatment depends on the type of tumor, its site and size, and if it has spread. One or a combination of treatments is used. The three major cancer treatments are surgery, radiation therapy, and chemotherapy.

Surgery involves removing malignant tissue. Surgery is done to cure or control cancer. It is also done to relieve pain from advanced cancer. Some surgeries are very disfiguring. The person's self-esteem and body image are affected.

Radiation therapy destroys living cells. X-rays are directed at the tumor. Cancer cells and normal cells are exposed to radiation. Both are destroyed. Radiation therapy is used to cure certain cancers or to control the growth of cancer cells. Pain is relieved or prevented by controlling cell growth. Radiation therapy has side effects. Discomfort, nausea and vomiting, fatigue (tiredness), anorexia (loss of appetite), and diarrhea are common. Skin breakdown can occur in the exposed area. The doctor may order special skin care procedures.

Chemotherapy involves drugs that kill cells. Like radiation, chemotherapy affects normal cells and cancer cells. It is used to cure cancer or control the growth rate of cancer cells. Side effects can be severe. They are caused by the destruction of normal cells. The gastrointestinal tract is irritated. Nausea, vomiting, and diarrhea result. **Stomatitis,** an inflammation *(itis)* of the mouth *(stomat)*, may also develop. Hair loss (alopecia) may occur. Decreased production of blood cells occurs. As a result, the person is at risk for bleeding and infection. Other organs may also be affected.

Residents with cancer have many needs. They include:

- Pain relief or control
- Adequate rest and exercise
- Fluids and nutrition
- Preventing skin breakdown
- Preventing bowel elimination problems (constipation occurs from pain relief drugs; diarrhea occurs from chemotherapy)
- Dealing with the side effects of radiation therapy and chemotherapy
- Psychological and social needs
- Spiritual needs

The resident's psychological and social needs are great. Anger, fear, and depression are common. Disfigurement from surgery may cause the resident to feel unwhole, unattractive, or unclean. The resident and family need much emotional support. Talk to the resident. Do not avoid the resident because you are uncomfortable. Use touch to communicate that you care. Listen to the resident. Often the resident needs to talk and have someone listen. Being there when needed is important. You may not have to say anything. Just be there to listen.

The resident's spiritual needs also are important. Some residents get much comfort by talking to a spiritual leader. To many people, meeting spiritual needs is as important as meeting their physical needs.

Residents with cancer often are referred to a hospice program (see Chapter 32). Hospice staff provide added support to the residents and their families. They are also a source of education and support for center staff caring for residents with cancer.

MUSCULOSKELETAL DISORDERS

Musculoskeletal disorders affect the ability to move about. Some are caused by injury. Others result from age-related changes.

Arthritis

Arthritis means joint *(arthr)* inflammation *(itis)*. It is the most common joint disease. Pain and decreased mobility occur in the affected joints. There are two basic types of arthritis.

Osteoarthritis (degenerative joint disease). This type of arthritis occurs with aging. Joint injury and obesity are other causes. The hips, knees, and spine are commonly affected. These joints bear the body's weight. Joints in the fingers and thumbs can also be affected. Symptoms are joint stiffness and pain. Joint stiffness occurs with rest and lack of motion. Pain occurs with weight-bearing and joint motion. Severe pain can interfere with rest and sleep. Cold weather and dampness seem to increase the

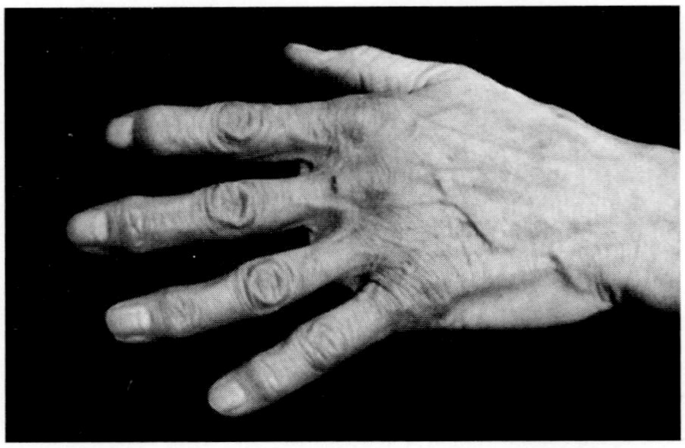

Fig. 26-4 Heberden's nodes occur in the finger joints. *(From Lewis SM, Collier IC, Heitkemper MM:* Medical-surgical nursing: assessment and management of clinical problems, *ed 4, St Louis, 1996, Mosby.)*

symptoms. Bony growths called *Heberden's nodes* (Fig. 26-4) are common in the fingers.

Osteoarthritis has no cure. Treatment involves relieving pain and stiffness. Doctors often order aspirin for pain. Local heat or local cold applications may be ordered. For obese persons, weight loss is stressed. A low-fat, low-calorie diet often is ordered. When the condition is advanced, the person may need a cane or walker. Measures to prevent falls are important. Assistance with activities of daily living (ADL) is given as needed. Elevated toilet seats are helpful when there is limited range of motion in the hips and knees. Sometimes joint replacement surgery is necessary (p. 583).

Rheumatoid arthritis. Rheumatoid arthritis (RA) is a chronic disease. It occurs at any age and is more common in women. Connective tissue throughout the body is affected. The disease affects the heart, lungs, eyes, kidneys, and skin. However, mainly the joints are affected. Smaller joints in the fingers, hands, and feet are affected first (Fig. 26-5). Eventually, larger joints are involved (wrists, elbows, and shoulders; ankles, knees, and hips). Joint inflammation usually occurs on both sides of the body. For example, if the right wrist is involved, so is the left wrist.

Severe inflammation causes very painful and swollen joints. The person restricts movement with severe pain. As the disease progresses, more and more joints become involved. Changes in other organs eventually occur.

Signs and symptoms of RA include:

- Pain, redness, warmth, and swelling in the joint area
- Joint stiffness upon awakening and after inactivity
- Limitation of joint motion
- Fever
- Fatigue
- Loss of appetite

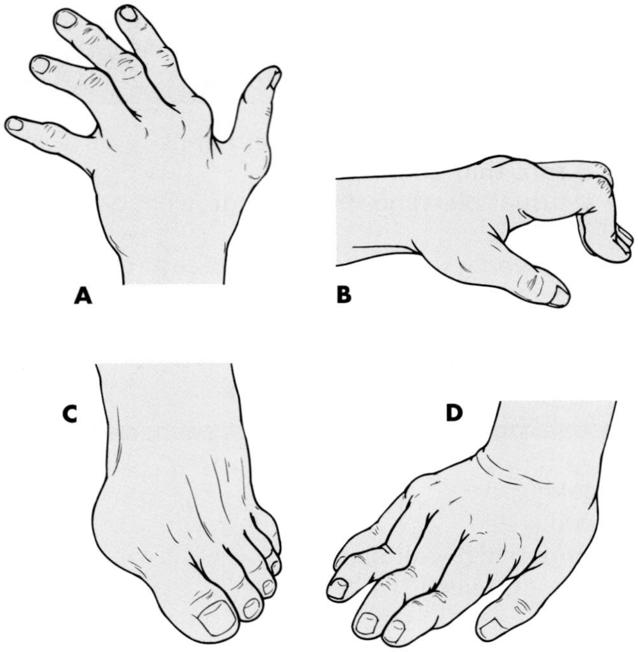

Fig. 26-5 Finger deformities caused by rheumatoid arthritis. *(From Lewis SM, Collier IC, Heitkemper, MM:* Medical-surgical nursing: assessment and management of clinical problems, *ed 4, St Louis, 1996, Mosby.)*

- Weight loss
- Muscle aches

Treatment goals are to maintain joint motion, control pain, and prevent deformities. Rest is balanced with exercise. Bedrest is needed if several joints are involved and when fever is present. Turning and repositioning are done every 2 hours. Good body alignment is essential. Positioning to prevent contractures and deformities promotes comfort. Bed boards, a bed cradle, trochanter rolls, and pillows are used for alignment and positioning. Adequate sleep—8 to 10 hours—is needed each night. Morning and afternoon rest periods also are necessary.

Range-of-motion exercises are done. Walking aids may be needed. Splints may be applied to the affected body parts. Safety measures to prevent falls are practiced.

The doctor orders drugs for pain. Local heat or local cold applications may be ordered (see Chapter 24). Back massages are relaxing. Joint replacement surgery may be indicated.

Emotional support and reassurance are needed. The disease is chronic. Death from other organ involvement is always possible. A good attitude is important. Being active is important. The health care team focuses on helping the residents stay as active as possible. The more residents can do for themselves, the better off they are. You can help by providing encouragement and praise. You must be a good listener when the resident needs to talk.

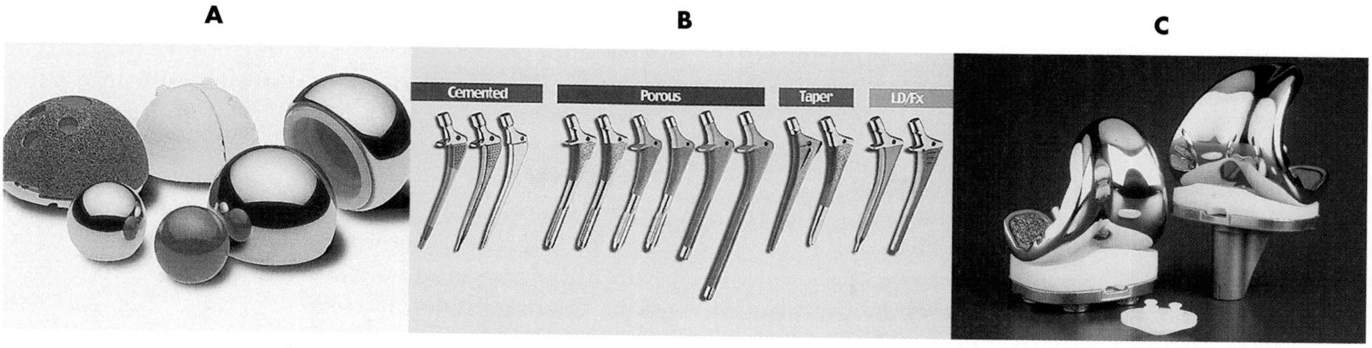

Fig. 26-6 A, Hip replacement prosthesis. **B,** Hip replacement prosthesis stems. **C,** Knee replacement prosthesis. *(From Lewis SM, Collier IC, Heitkemper MM:* Medical-surgical nursing: assessment and management of clinical problems, *ed 4, St Louis, 1996, Mosby.)*

Total joint replacement.

Arthroplasty is the surgical replacement *(plasty)* of a joint *(arthro)*. Ankle, knee, hip, shoulder, wrist, finger, and toe joints can be replaced. The diseased joint is removed and replaced with a prosthesis (Fig. 26-6). The surgery relieves pain and restores joint motion.

Osteoporosis

Osteoporosis is a bone *(osteo)* disorder in which the bone becomes porous and brittle *(porosis)*. Bones are fragile and break easily. Bones of the spine, hips, and wrists are affected most often. It is common in older persons and in women after menopause. The ovaries do not produce the hormone *estrogen* after menopause. The lack of estrogen results in bone changes. Lack of dietary calcium is also a major cause of osteoporosis. Smoking, high alcohol intake, and lack of exercise also are risk factors. Bedrest and immobility are other causes. Immobility does not allow for proper bone use. For bone to form properly, it must bear weight. If not, calcium is absorbed and the bone becomes porous and brittle.

Signs and symptoms of osteoporosis include low back pain, gradual loss of height, and stooped posture. Fractures are a major threat. Sometimes bones are so brittle that the slightest stress can cause a fracture. Turning in bed or getting up from a chair can cause a fracture. Fractures are a great risk if the resident falls or has an accident.

Prevention is important. Calcium, estrogen replacement therapy, and exercise are key. The diet must contain enough calcium. Often doctors order calcium and vitamin supplements. Estrogen is often ordered for women after menopause. Exercise that involves weight bearing is best. Walking, jogging, dancing, and stair climbing are examples. Good posture is also important. Some people wear a back brace or corset or need walking aids. Protect the resident from falls and accidents (see Chapter 8). Always turn and reposition the resident gently.

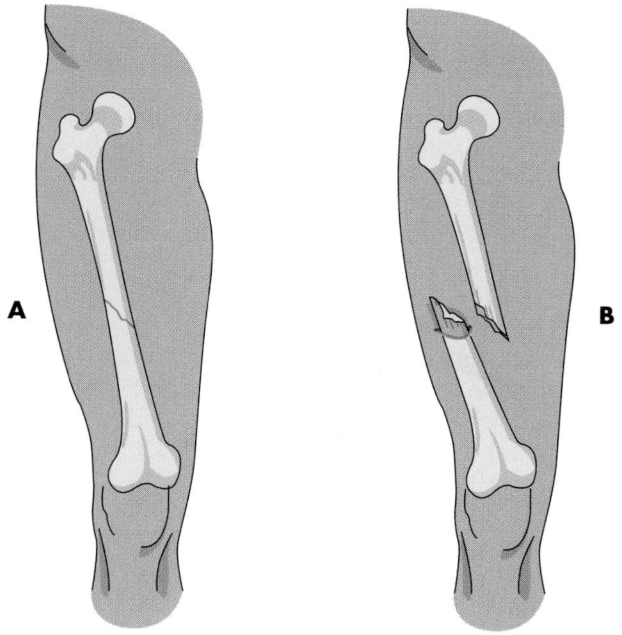

Fig. 26-7 A, Closed fracture. **B,** Open fracture. *(From Beare PG, Myers JL:* Principles and practice of adult health nursing, *ed 3, St Louis, 1998, Mosby.)*

Fractures

A **fracture** is a broken bone. Tissues around the fracture (muscles, blood vessels, nerves, and tendons) are usually injured. Fractures are open or closed (Fig. 26-7). A **closed fracture (simple fracture)** means the bone is broken but the skin is intact. An **open fracture (compound fracture)** means the broken bone has come through the skin.

Fractures are caused by falls and accidents. Bone tumors, metastatic cancer, and osteoporosis are other causes. Signs and symptoms of a fracture are:

- Pain
- Swelling
- Limited movement and loss of function
- Bruising and color changes in the skin at the fracture site
- Bleeding (internal or external)

The bone has to heal. The bone ends are brought into normal position. This is called *reduction*. *Closed reduction* involves moving the bone back into place. The skin is not opened. *Open reduction* involves surgery. The bone is exposed and brought back into alignment. Nails, rods, pins, screws, plates, or wires keep the bone in place (Fig. 26-8). After reduction, the fracture is immobilized. That is, movement of the bone ends is prevented. This is done with a cast or traction. Residents in traction are usually in a subacute care unit.

Cast care. Casts are made of plaster of paris, plastic, or fiberglass. The cast covers all or part of an extremity (Fig. 26-9). Before the doctor applies a cast, the extremity is covered with stockinette. This protects the skin. Casting material comes in rolls. The rolls are moistened and wrapped around the part. Plastic and fiberglass casts dry quickly. A plaster of paris cast needs 24 to 48 hours to dry. It is odorless, white, and shiny when dry. When wet, it is gray and cool and has a musty smell. The rules listed in Box 26-2 are for cast care.

Box 26-2 Rules for Cast Care

- Do not cover the cast with blankets, plastic, or other material. A plaster cast gives off heat as it dries. Covers prevent the escape of heat. Burns can occur if the heat cannot escape.
- Turn the resident as directed by the nurse. All cast surfaces are exposed to the air at one time or another. Turning promotes even drying.
- Do not place a wet cast on a hard surface. A hard surface flattens the cast. The cast must maintain its shape. Use pillows to support the entire length of the cast (Fig. 26-10, p. 586).
- Support a wet cast with your palms when turning and positioning the resident (Fig. 26-11, p. 586). Fingers can dent the cast. The dents can cause pressure areas that can lead to skin breakdown.
- Protect the resident from rough edges of the cast. Petaling involves covering the cast edges with tape (Fig. 26-12, p. 587). If stockinette is used, the doctor pulls it up over the cast. The stockinette is secured in place with a roll of cast material.
- Keep a plaster cast dry. A wet plaster cast loses its shape. It is protected from moisture from the perineal area. The nurse may apply a waterproof material around the perineal area once the cast is dry.
- Do not let the resident insert anything into the cast. Itching often occurs under the cast and causes an intense desire to scratch. Items used for scratching (pencils, coat hangers, knitting needles, back scratchers) can open the skin. An infection can develop. Items used for scratching can also wrinkle the stockinette. The object can be lost into the cast. Both can cause pressure and lead to skin breakdown.
- Elevate a casted arm or leg on pillows. This reduces swelling.
- Have enough help when turning and repositioning the resident. Plaster casts are heavy and awkward. Balance is lost easily.
- Position the person as directed by the nurse. This information is also in the care plan.
- Report these signs and symptoms to the nurse immediately:
  - Pain—warns of a pressure ulcer, poor circulation, or nerve damage
  - Swelling and a tight cast—a sign of reduced blood flow to the part
  - Pale skin—a sign of reduced blood flow to the part
  - Cyanosis—a sign of reduced blood flow to the part
  - Odor—a sign of infection
  - Inability to move the fingers or toes—a sign of pressure on a nerve
  - Numbness—a sign of pressure on a nerve or reduced blood flow to the part
  - Temperature changes—cool skin means poor circulation; hot skin means inflammation
  - Drainage on or under the cast—a sign of infection under the cast
  - Chills, fever, nausea, and vomiting—may signal an infection under the cast

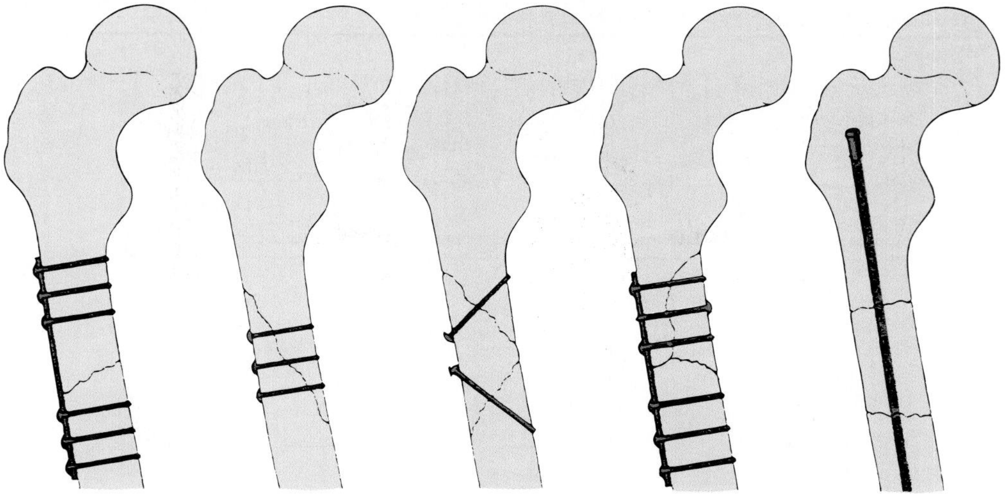

Fig. 26-8 Devices used to reduce a fracture. *(From Beare PG, Myers JL:* Principles and practice of adult health nursing, *ed 3, St Louis, 1998, Mosby.)*

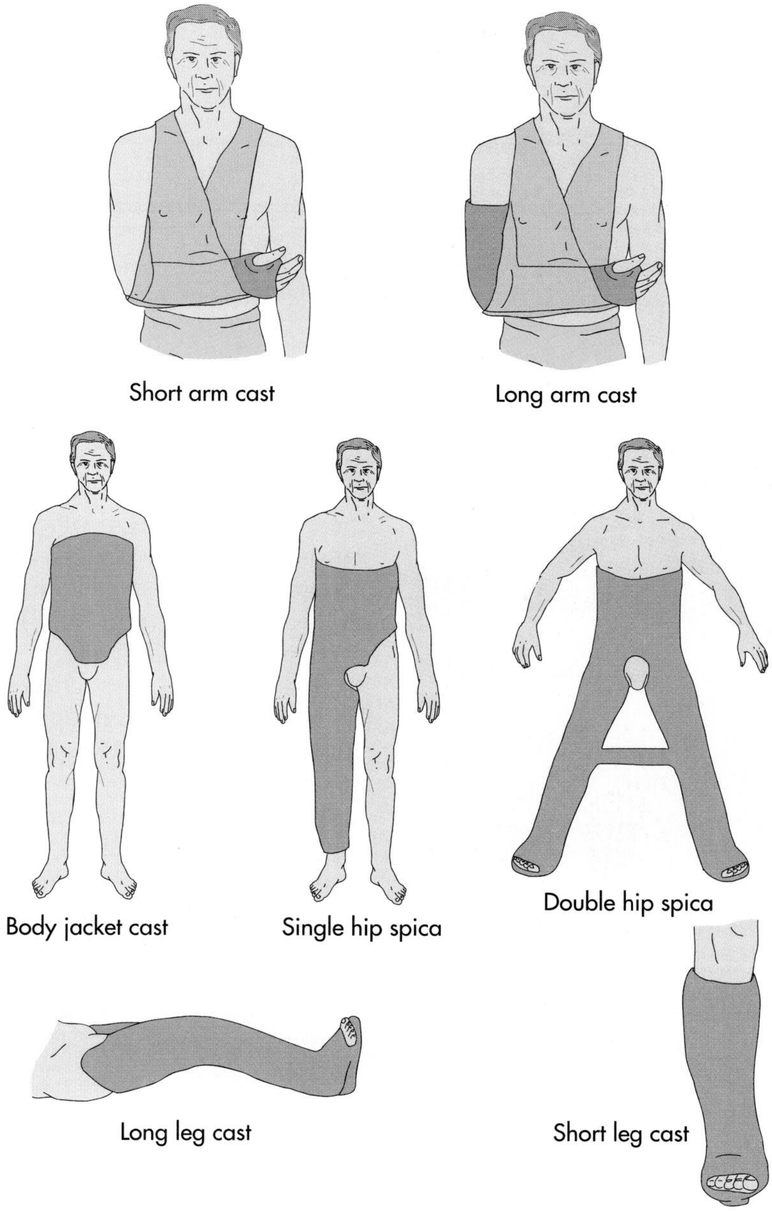

Fig. 26-9 Common casts.

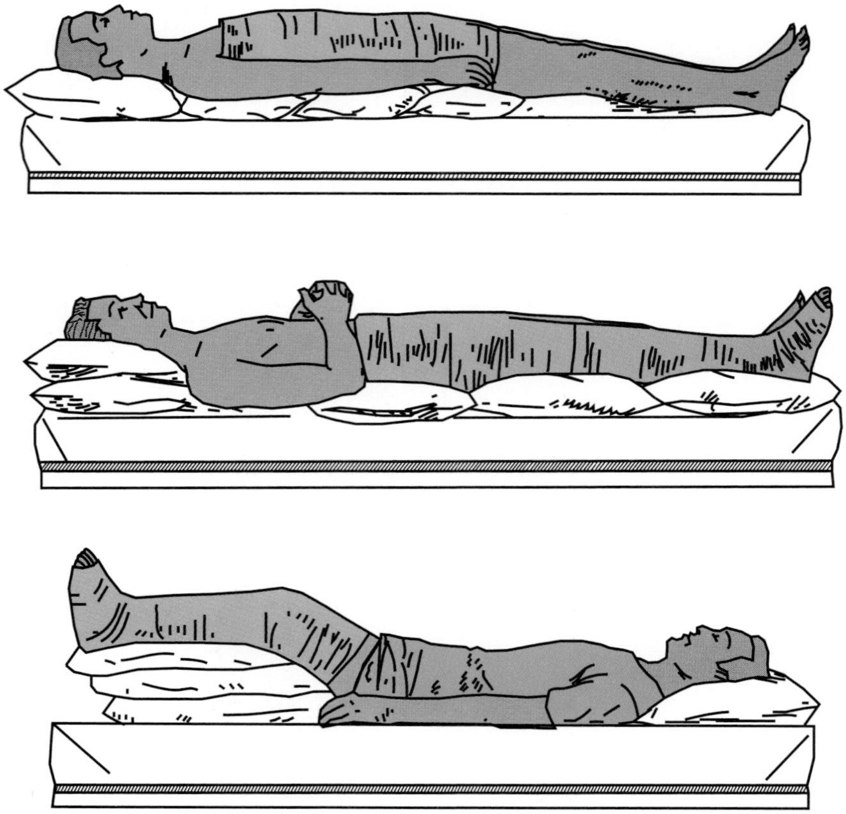

Fig. 26-10 Pillows support the entire length of the wet cast. *(From Harkness GH, Dincher JR:* Medical-surgical nursing: total patient care, *ed 9, St Louis, 1996, Mosby.)*

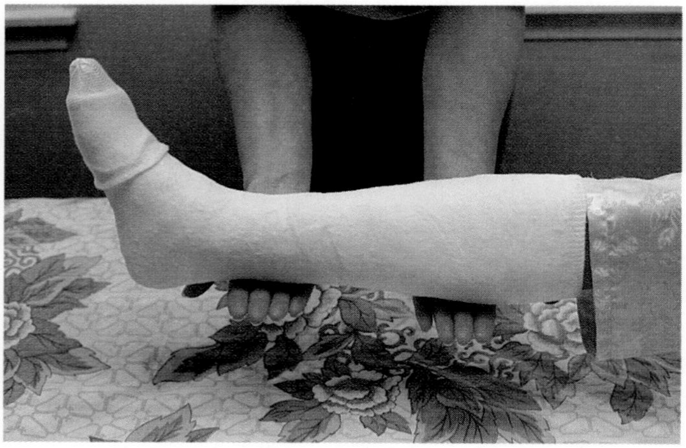

Fig. 26-11 The cast is supported with the palms during lifting.

Traction. Traction is used to reduce and immobilize fractures. A steady pull from two directions keeps the fractured bone in place. Traction is also used for muscle spasms, to correct or prevent deformities, and for other musculoskeletal injuries. Weights, ropes, and pulleys are used (Fig. 26-13). Traction is applied to the neck, arms, legs, or pelvis.

A doctor applies traction to the skin or to the bone. With *skin traction,* bandages and strips of material are applied to the skin. Weights are attached to the material or bandage (see Fig. 26-13). Traction applied directly to the bone is called *skeletal traction.* It is used for some arm and leg fractures. A pin, nail, or wire is inserted through the bone (Fig. 26-14, p. 588). For traction to the cervical spine, tongs are applied to the skull (Fig. 26-15). Weights are attached to the device.

The rules listed in Box 26-3 on p. 588 apply when caring for a person in traction.

A

B

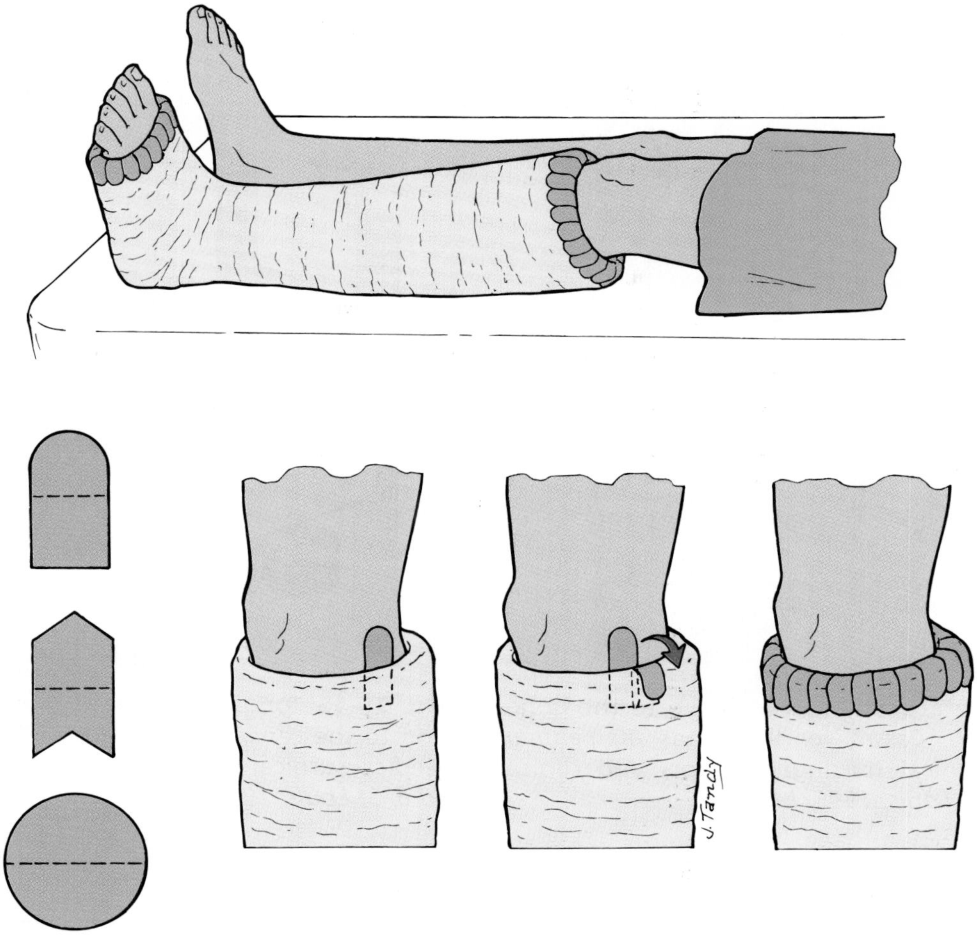

Fig. 26-12 **A,** The edges of the cast are petaled. **B,** Pieces of tape are used to make petals. The petal is placed inside the cast and then brought over the edge.

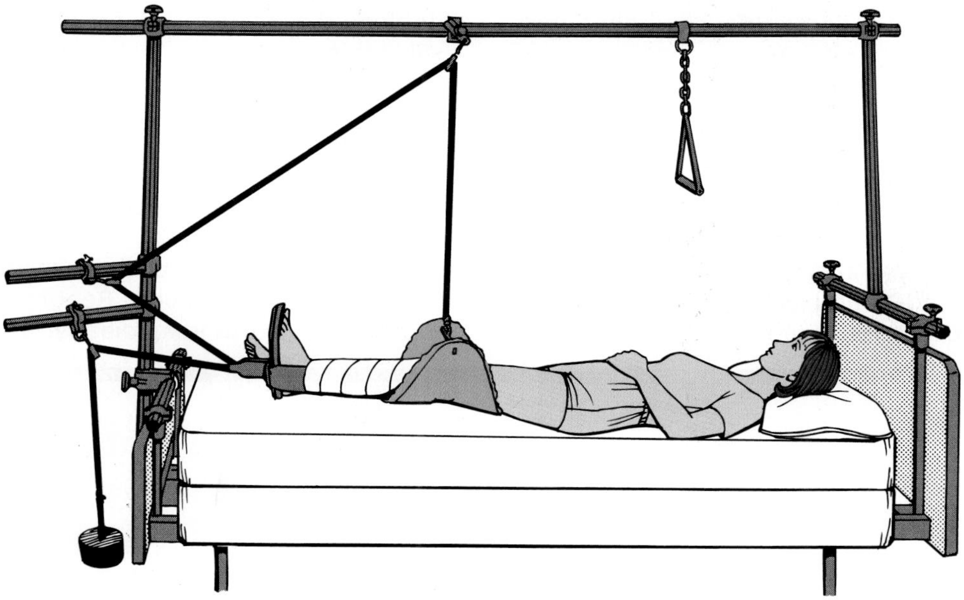

Fig. 26-13 Traction setup. Note the weights, pulleys, and ropes. *(From Phipps WJ, Cassmeyer VL, Sands JK, Lehman MK:* Medical-surgical nursing: concepts and clinical practice, *ed 5, St Louis, 1995, Mosby.)*

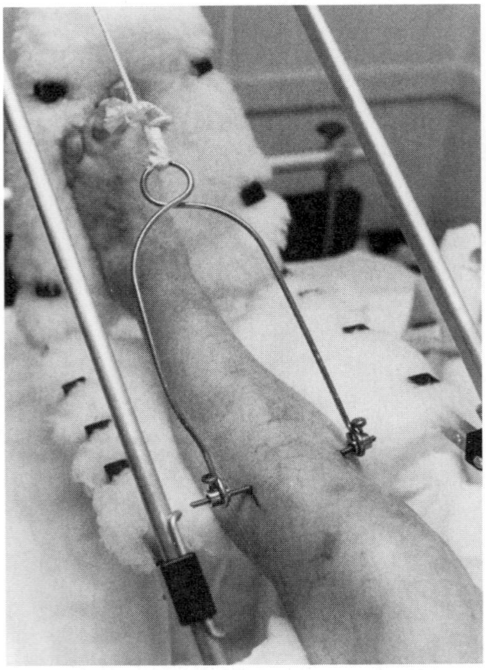

Fig. 26-14 Skeletal traction is attached to the bone. *(From Phipps WJ, Cassmeyer VL, Sands JK, Lehman MK:* Medical-surgical nursing: concepts and clinical practice, *ed 5, St Louis, 1995, Mosby.)*

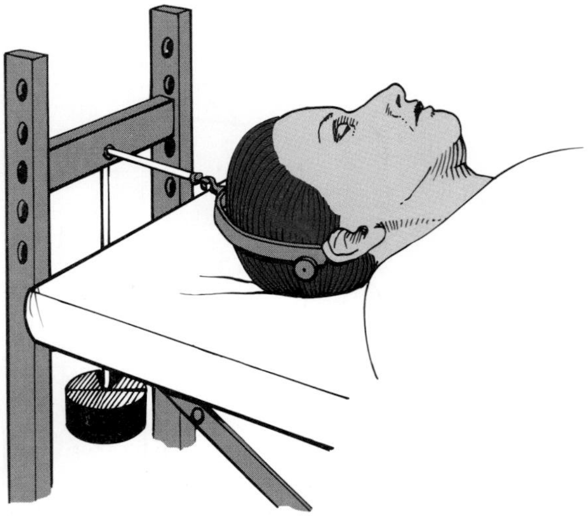

Fig. 26-15 Tongs are inserted into the skull for traction to the cervical spine. *(From Phipps WJ, Sands JK:* Medical-surgical nursing: concepts and clinical practice, *ed 6, St Louis, 1999, Mosby.)*

Box 26-3 Care of the Resident in Traction

- Keep the resident in good body alignment.
- Do not remove the traction.
- Keep weights off the floor. Weights must hang freely from the traction setup (see Fig. 26-13).
- Do not remove weights from the traction setup.
- Do not add weights to the traction setup.
- Perform range-of-motion exercises for the uninvolved body parts as directed by the nurse.
- Position the resident as directed by the nurse. Usually only the back-lying position is allowed. Slight turning is allowed with some types of traction.
- Provide the fracture pan for elimination.
- Give skin care. Follow the care plan.
- Put bottom linens on the bed from the top down. The resident uses the trapeze to raise the body off the bed.
- Check pin, nail, wire, or tong sites for redness, drainage, or odors. Report any observations to the nurse immediately.
- Observe for the signs and symptoms listed under cast care (see Box 26-2). Report these observations to the nurse immediately.

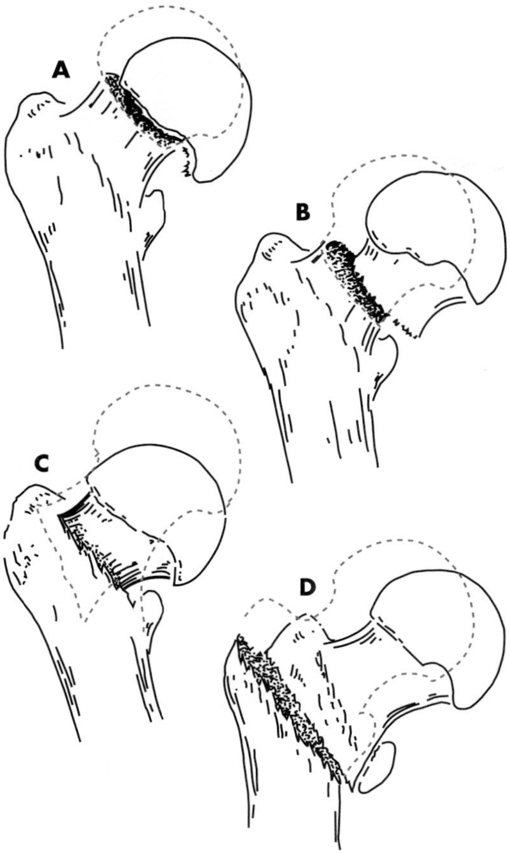

Fig. 26-16 Hip fractures. *(From Phipps WJ, Cassmeyer VL, Sands JK, Lehman MK:* Medical-surgical nursing: concepts and clinical practice, *ed 5, St Louis, 1995, Mosby.)*

A

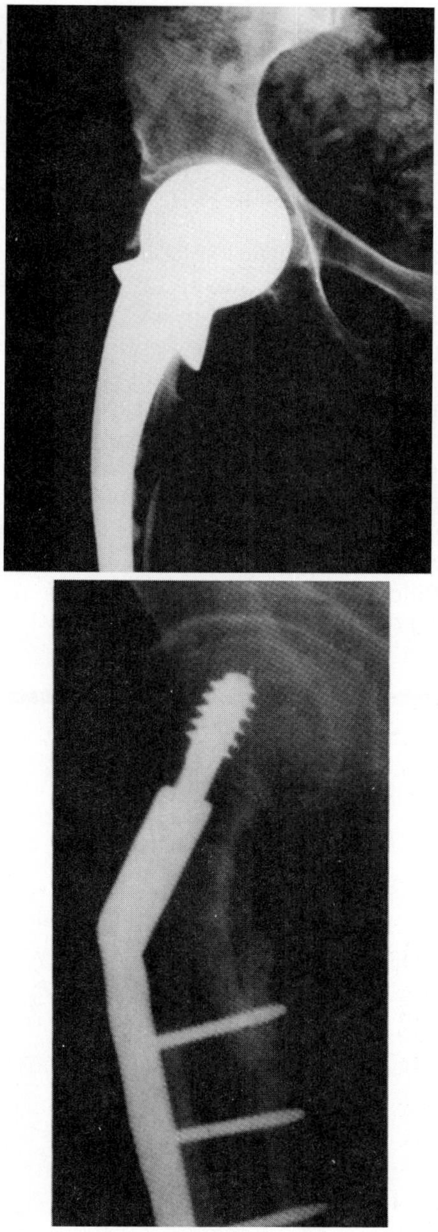

B

Fig. 26-17 A, Hip fracture repaired with a prosthesis. **B,** Hip fracture repaired with a hip nail. *(From Lewis SM, Collier IC, Heitkemper MM:* Medical-surgical nursing: assessment and management of clinical problems, *ed 4, St Louis, 1996, Mosby.)*

Hip fractures. Fractured hips are common in older persons, especially older women (Fig. 26-16). They are especially serious because healing is slower in older people. The resident may have other disorders. These disorders and slow healing may complicate the resident's condition and care. The resident is also at great risk for postoperative complications. These include pneumonia, atelectasis, urinary tract infections, and thrombi in the leg veins. The resident can die from these complications. The resident is also at risk for pressure ulcers, constipation, and confusion.

Open reduction is usually required. The fracture is fixed in position with a pin, nail, plate, screw, or prosthesis (Fig. 26-17). This procedure requires hospital care. Often the person requires rehabilitation in a nursing center after surgery. Some centers admit the person to a subacute unit. The person requires the care described in Box 26-4 on p. 590.

Box 26-4 Care of the Resident With a Hip Fracture

- Give good skin care. Skin breakdown can occur rapidly.
- Encourage incentive spirometry and coughing and deep breathing exercises as directed by the nurse (see Chapter 25).
- Turn and reposition the resident as directed by the nurse. The doctor's orders for turning and positioning depend on the type of fracture and the surgery performed. Usually the resident is not positioned on the operative side.
- Keep the operated leg abducted at all times. The leg is abducted when the resident is supine, being turned, or in a side-lying position (Fig. 26-18, *A*). Pillows or abductor splints are used as directed (Fig. 26-18, *B*).
- Prevent external rotation of the hip (turning outward). Use trochanter rolls or abduction splints as directed.
- Perform range-of-motion exercises as directed (see Chapter 19). Do not exercise the affected leg.
- Provide a straight-back chair with armrests when the resident is to be up. The resident needs a high, firm seat. A low, soft chair is not used.
- Place the chair on the unaffected side.
- Assist the nurse in transferring the resident from the bed to the chair as directed.
- Do not let the resident stand on the operated leg unless allowed by the doctor.
- Support and elevate the leg as directed when the resident is in the chair.
- Apply elastic stockings as directed (see Chapter 14).

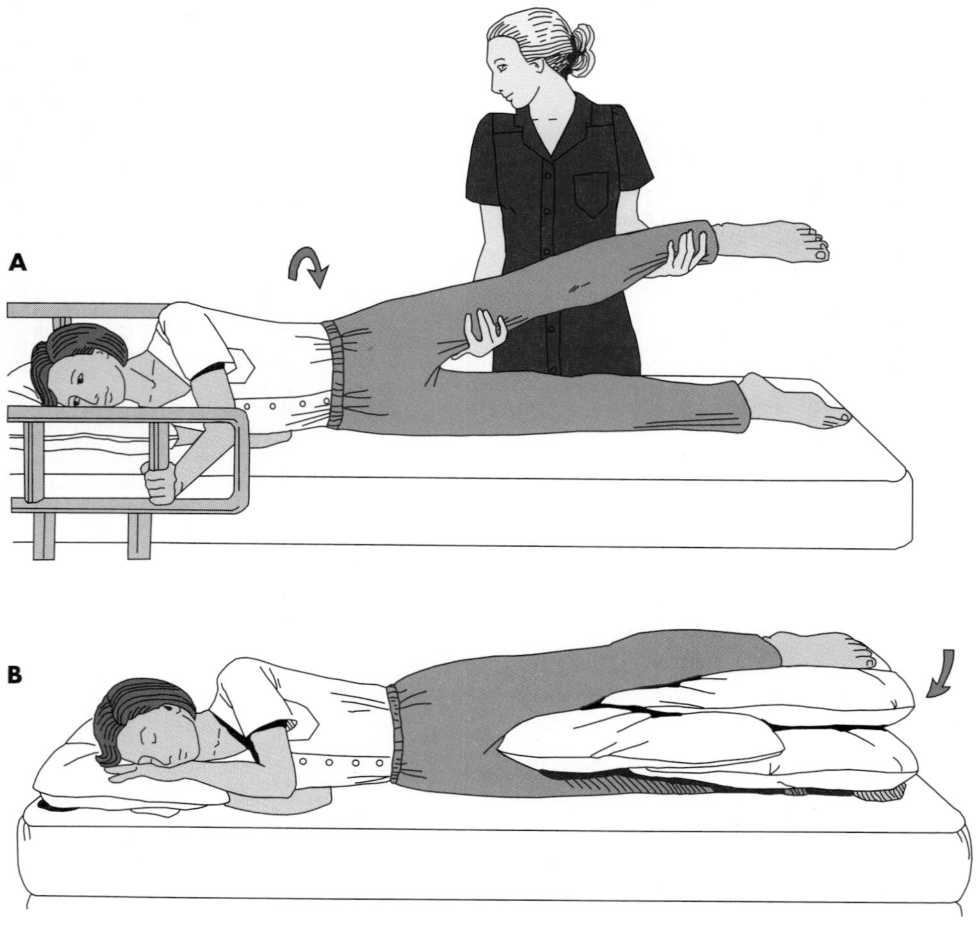

Fig. 26-18 **A,** The hip is abducted when the person is turned. **B,** Pillows are used to maintain the hip in abduction. *(From Lewis SM, Collier IC, Heitkemper MM:* Medical-surgical nursing: assessment and management of clinical problems, *ed 4, St Louis, 1996, Mosby.)*

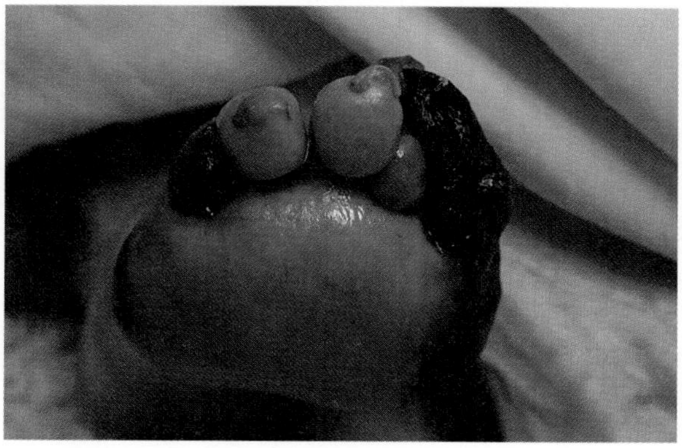

Fig. 26-19 Gangrene.

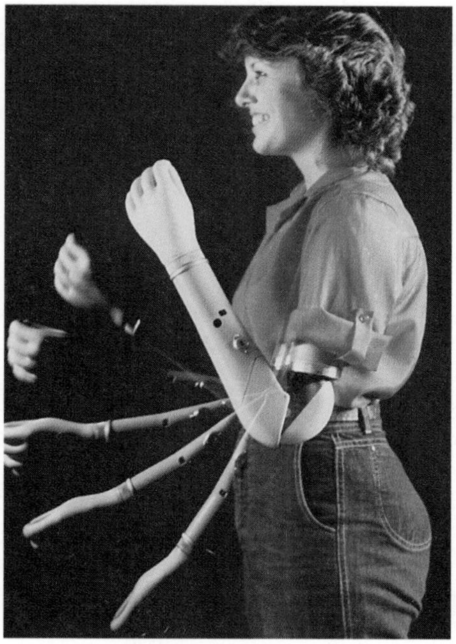

Fig. 26-20 Arm prosthesis. *(Courtesy Motion Control, Division of IOMED Inc., Salt Lake City, Utah.)*

Loss of a Limb

An **amputation** is the removal of all or part of an extremity. Usually the part is removed surgically. Traumatic amputations can occur from vehicle and workplace accidents. Severe injuries, bone tumors, severe infections, and circulatory disorders may require amputations.

Gangrene is a condition in which there is death of tissue. It can result from infection, injuries, and circulatory disorders. These conditions interfere with blood supply to the tissues. The tissues do not get enough oxygen and nutrients. Poisonous substances and waste products build up in the affected tissues. Tissue death results. The tissue becomes black, cold, and shriveled (Fig. 26-19) and eventually falls off. If untreated, gangrene spreads through the body and causes death.

All or part of an extremity may be amputated. Fingers, the hand, forearm, or entire arm may be removed. Toes, the foot, lower leg, upper leg, or entire leg may be amputated.

Much support is needed. A major psychological adjustment is necessary. The resident's life is affected by the amputation. Appearance, activities of daily living, moving about, and work are some areas affected.

At some point most persons with an amputation are fitted with a prosthesis. A prosthesis is an artificial replacement for a missing body part (Fig. 26-20). The stump is conditioned so the prosthesis fits. Stump conditioning involves shrinking and shaping the stump into a cone shape. An elastic stocking or bandage is used to shrink and shape the stump (Fig. 26-21). Exercises are ordered to strengthen the other limbs. Physical therapists help the resident use the prosthesis. Occupational therapy is necessary if the stump or prosthesis is used for activities of daily living.

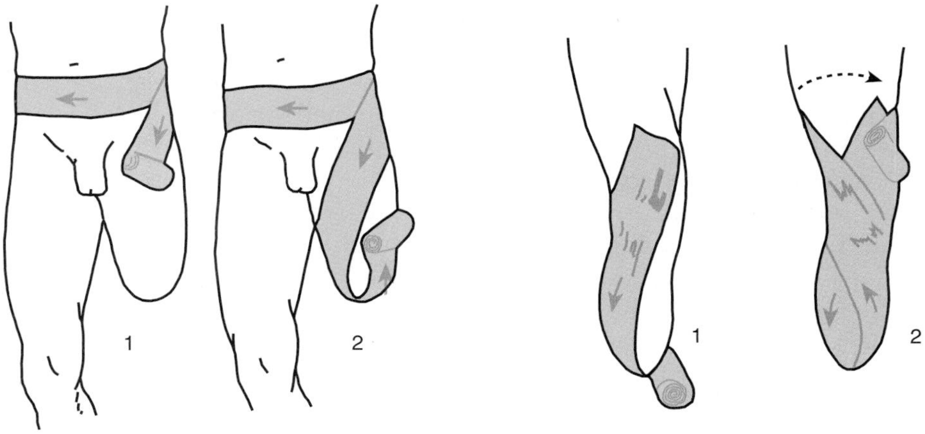

Fig. 26-21 A midthigh amputation is bandaged to shrink and shape the stump. *(From Phipps WJ, Cassmeyer VL, Sands JK, Lehman MK:* Medical-surgical nursing: concepts and clinical practice, *ed 5, St Louis, 1995, Mosby.)*

The resident may feel that the limb is still there or may complain of pain in the amputated part. This is called *phantom limb pain.* The exact cause is unknown. However, it is a normal reaction. The sensation may occur only for a short time after surgery, but some persons have phantom limb pain for many years.

NERVOUS SYSTEM DISORDERS

Nervous system disorders can affect mental and physical functions. They can affect the ability to speak, understand, feel, see, hear, touch, think, control bowels and bladder, or move.

Stroke

The American Heart Association (AHA) defines stroke as a cardiovascular disease affecting the blood vessels that supply blood to the brain. Blood supply to a part of the brain is suddenly interrupted. Brain cells in the area affected do not get oxygen and nutrients. Brain damage occurs. Functions controlled by that part of the brain are lost or impaired. A ruptured blood vessel is one cause of stroke. This causes hemorrhage (excessive bleeding) into the brain. Blood clots are another cause. A blood clot obstructs blood flow to the brain. A stroke is also called a *cerebrovascular accident (CVA)* or *brain attack.*

Stroke is the third leading cause of death in the United States. It is the leading cause of disability in adults. Stroke is a medical emergency. The person needs immediate medical attention. (See Chapter 31 for emergency care.) Box 26-5 lists the warning signs of stroke. Sometimes the warning signs last a few minutes. This is called a *transient ischemic attack (TIA). (Transient* means temporary or short term. *Ischemic* means to hold back *[ischein]* blood *[hemic].*) Blood supply to the brain is interrupted for a short time. Sometimes a TIA occurs before a stroke. The person having a TIA needs medical attention. The TIA warns of a stroke.

Stroke is more common among persons over 65 years of age. However, it does occur in young and middle-age adults. A common cause of stroke is hypertension (high blood pressure). Other risk factors include diabetes, family history of stroke, hardening of the arteries, smoking, heart disease, and stress. Lack of exercise and high alcohol intake also are risk factors. So is race. Black men and women are at greater risk than white persons.

Box 26-5 Warning Signs of Stroke (CVA, Brain Attack)

- Sudden weakness or numbness of the face, arm, or leg on one side of the body
- Sudden dimness or loss of vision, particularly in one eye
- Loss of speech or trouble talking or understanding speech
- Sudden, severe headaches with no known cause
- Unexplained dizziness, unsteadiness, or sudden falls (especially with any of the other signs)

From American Heart Association, 1997.

Signs and symptoms vary. Warning signs may occur (see Box 26-5). Dizziness, ringing in the ears, headache, nausea and vomiting, and memory loss also can occur. The stroke may occur suddenly. Unconsciousness, noisy breathing, high blood pressure, slow pulse, redness of the face, seizures, and paralysis on one side of the body **(hemiplegia)** may occur. The person may lose bowel and bladder control and the ability to speak. **Aphasia** is the inability *(a)* to speak *(phasia).*

If the person survives, some brain damage is likely. The functions lost depend on the area of brain damage (Fig. 26-22). The effects of a stroke include:

- Loss of hand, arm, leg, or body control
- Loss of face control
- Hemiplegia
- Changing emotions (the person can cry easily—sometimes for no reason)
- Difficulty swallowing (**dysphagia** means difficulty *[dys]* swallowing *[phagia]*)
- Dimmed vision
- Aphasia
- Slow or slurred speech
- Changes in perception (sight, touch, movement, and thought)
- Impaired memory
- Urinary frequency, urgency, or incontinence
- Depression
- Frustration

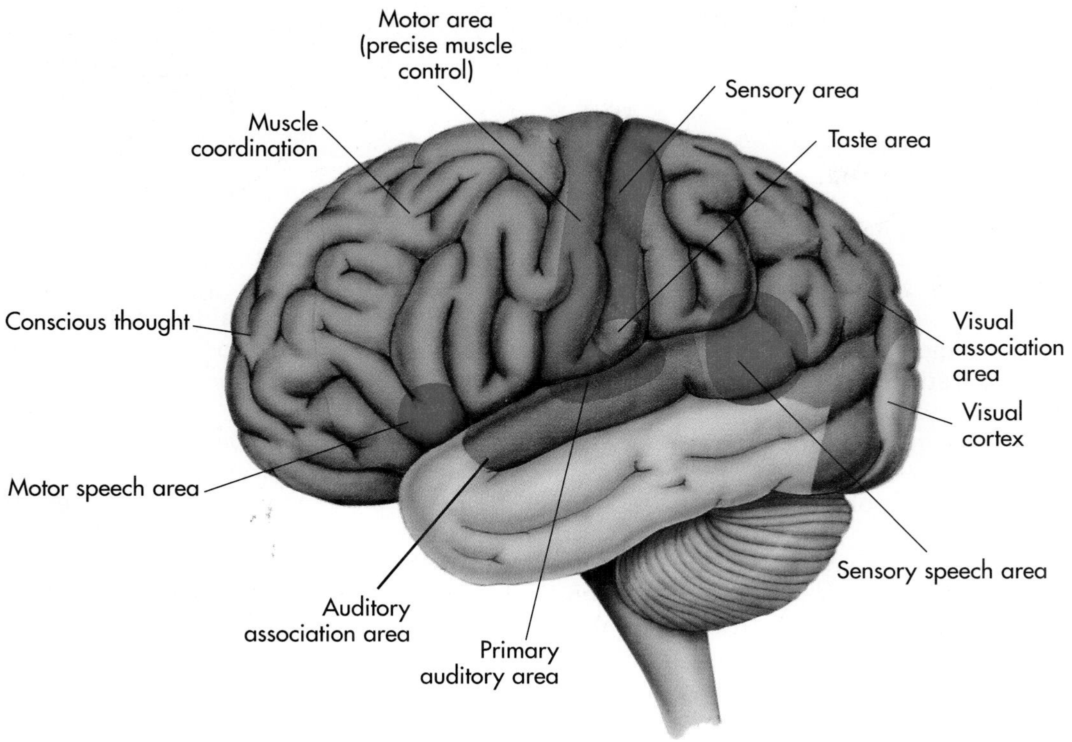

Fig. 26-22 Functions lost from a stroke depend on the area of brain damage. *(Modified from Thibodeau GA, Patton KT:* The human body in health & disease, *ed 2, St Louis, 1997, Mosby.)*

These effects change the person's behavior. The person may forget about or ignore the weaker side. This is from loss of movement and feeling on that side. If vision is affected, the person may not see that side of the body. The person may not recognize or know how to use familiar items. Activities of daily living and other tasks are difficult. The person may forget what to do and how to do it. If the person does know, the body may not respond.

Rehabilitation starts immediately. The resident may depend partially or totally on others for care. The nurse uses the nursing process to help the health care team meet the resident's needs. The entire team works together to help the resident regain the highest possible level of function. Common care measures are listed in Box 26-6 on p. 594.

Aphasia. There are two basic types of aphasia. **Expressive aphasia** involves difficulty expressing or sending out thoughts. There are problems with speaking, spelling, counting, gesturing, or writing. The person thinks one thing but says another. For example, the person thinks about food but asks for a newspaper. People are called the wrong names even when correct names are known. The person thinks clearly but cannot speak. Some produce only sounds and no words. The person may cry or swear for no apparent reason.

Receptive aphasia relates to receiving information. The person has trouble understanding what is said or read. Everyday objects are not recognized. The person may not know how to use a fork, toilet, water glass, TV, telephone, or other items. The person may not recognize people.

Remember that for communication to occur, the message sent must be received and correctly interpreted. The person with *receptive* aphasia simply cannot interpret the message received. The person with *expressive* aphasia cannot send messages. Some people have both expressive and receptive aphasia. This is called **expressive-receptive aphasia.**

Residents with aphasia have many emotional needs. Frustration, depression, and anger are common. Communication is important for functioning and relationships with others. Remember that the resident wants to communicate but cannot. You need to be patient and kind.

Box 26-6 Care of the Resident With a Stroke (CVA, Brain Attack)

- The lateral position is used to prevent aspiration.
- Coughing and deep breathing are encouraged.
- The bed is kept in semi-Fowler's position.
- Turning and repositioning are done at least every 2 hours.
- Food and fluid needs are met.
- Elastic stockings are ordered to prevent thrombi (blood clots) in the legs.
- Range-of-motion exercises are performed to prevent contractures.
- A catheter may be inserted or a bladder training program started.
- A bowel training program may be necessary.
- Safety precautions are practiced. Check with the nurse and follow the care plan about the use of bed rails.
- Assistance is given for self-care activities. The resident should do as much as possible.
- Communication methods are established. Magic Slates, pencil and paper, a picture board, or other methods are used. Questions are limited to those that have "yes" or "no" answers. Speak slowly. Allow the resident time to respond (see Chapter 5).
- Good skin care is given to prevent pressure ulcers.
- Speech therapy, physical therapy, and occupational therapy are ordered. Assistive devices are used as necessary (see Chapter 29).
- Emotional support and encouragement are given. Praise is given for even the slightest accomplishment.

Parkinson's Disease

Parkinson's disease is a slow, progressive disorder with no cure. Degeneration of a part of the brain occurs. The disease is usually seen in persons over 50 years of age. Signs and symptoms are a mask-like expression, tremors, pill-rolling movements of the fingers, a shuffling gait, stooped posture, impaired balance, stiff muscles (rigidity), slow movements, and drooling. Difficulty swallowing and chewing, bowel and bladder problems, sleep problems, and depression can occur. Some persons have memory loss, slow thinking, and emotional changes (fear and insecurity). Speech changes include slurred, monotone, and soft speech. Some persons talk too fast or repeat what they said.

The doctor orders drugs specific for Parkinson's disease. Exercise and physical therapy are ordered. These help the resident improve strength, posture, balance, and mobility. The resident may need help with eating and other self-care activities. Measures to promote normal elimination are practiced. Safety practices are followed to prevent injury. Remember that mental function may not be affected. Talk to and treat the resident as an adult with dignity and respect.

Multiple Sclerosis

Multiple sclerosis (MS) is a progressive disease. The myelin sheath (which covers the nerves), the spinal cord, and the white matter in the brain are destroyed. Nerve impulses are not sent to and from the brain in a normal manner. Functions are impaired or lost.

Symptoms start between the ages of 20 and 40. Women are affected more often than men. The onset is gradual. Blurred or double vision occurs first. Muscle weakness and difficulty with balance and walking occur. Tremors, numbness and tingling, loss of feeling, speech impairment, dizziness, and poor coordination eventually occur. So do urinary incontinence, anal incontinence or constipation, and behavior changes. The person's condition worsens over many years. As care needs increase, the person may need long-term care. Blindness, contractures, paralysis of all extremities (quadriplegia), loss of bowel and bladder control, and respiratory muscle weakness are among the person's many problems. The person becomes totally dependent on others for care. Anger and depression are common.

There is no known cure. Residents are kept active as long as possible. They need to do as much for themselves as possible. Nursing care depends on the resident's needs and condition. Skin care, hygiene, and range-of-motion exercises are important. Measures are taken to prevent injury and to promote bowel and bladder elimination. Turning, positioning, coughing, and deep breathing also are important. Complications from bedrest are prevented.

The care plan reflects the resident's changing needs. Occupational and physical therapists and the speech/language pathologist are often involved in the resident's care. The National Multiple Sclerosis Society can provide resources for the resident and family.

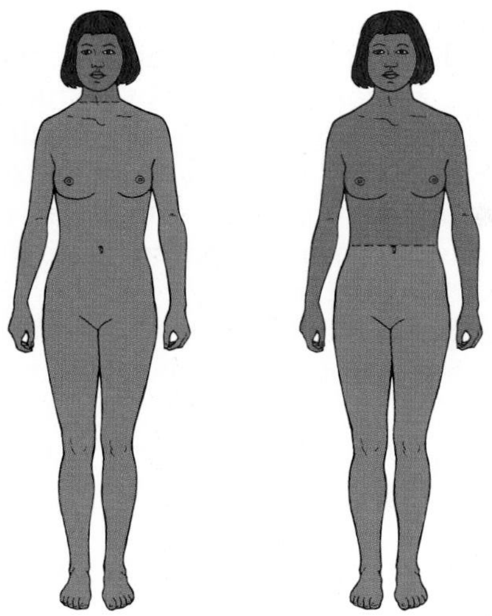

Fig. 26-23 The shaded areas indicate the areas of paralysis.

Head Injuries

Injuries can occur to the scalp, skull, and brain tissue. Some injuries are minor. They cause only temporary loss of consciousness. Others are more serious. Brain tissue is bruised or torn. Bleeding can occur in the brain or surrounding structures. Permanent brain damage or death may result.

Head injuries are caused by falls, vehicle accidents, workplace accidents, and sports injuries. Other body parts often are injured. Spinal cord injuries are likely. Hospital care is required. If the person survives a severe head injury, some permanent damage is likely. Paralysis, mental retardation, personality changes, speech problems, breathing difficulties, and loss of bowel and bladder control may be permanent. Rehabilitation is required. Some persons are admitted to nursing centers for rehabilitation or for permanent placement. Nursing care depends on the resident's needs and remaining abilities. The care plan outlines the resident's care.

Spinal Cord Injuries

Spinal cord injuries can permanently damage the nervous system. Common causes are stab or bullet wounds, motor vehicle accidents, workplace accidents, falls, or sports injuries. Hospital care is required. Cervical traction often is necessary (see Fig. 26-15). The person in cervical traction is placed on a device (Stryker frame, rotation bed) that keeps the spine straight while the person is turned.

The type of damage depends on the level of injury. The higher the level of injury, the greater the loss of function (Fig. 26-23). With lumbar injuries, muscle function in the legs is lost. Injuries at the thoracic level cause loss of muscle function below the chest. Persons with an injury at the lumbar or thoracic level are paraplegics. **Paraplegia** is paralysis of the legs. Cervical injuries cause loss of function to the arms, chest, and all muscles below the chest. Persons with these injuries are quadriplegics. **Quadriplegia** is paralysis of the arms, legs, and trunk.

If the person survives, rehabilitation is necessary. Transfer to a rehabilitation or nursing center may be necessary. Some subacute care units have special rehabilitation programs for persons with a spinal cord injury. The person learns to function at his or her highest possible level. The resident learns to use self-help and assistive devices and other special equipment. Paralyzed residents generally need the care listed in Box 26-7. The resident's needs and the rehabilitation program depend on the functions lost and remaining abilities. Attention is given to emotional needs. These residents have severe emotional reactions to paralysis and the loss of function.

Some residents require permanent placement in the nursing center. Others return home and live independently. Some may require home care or assisted-living housing.

Box 26-7 Care of the Resident With Paralysis

- Prevent falls. Keep bed rails up, the bed in low position, and the signal light within reach. Check the resident often if he or she cannot use the signal light.
- Prevent burns. Check bath water, heat applications, and food for the proper temperature.
- Turn and reposition the person at least every 2 hours.
- Give skin care and other measures to prevent pressure ulcers.
- Maintain good body alignment at all times. Use pillows, trochanter rolls, footboards, and other devices as needed.
- Carry out bowel and bladder training programs.
- Perform range-of-motion exercises to maintain muscle function and prevent contractures. Assist with other exercises as ordered.
- Assist with food and fluids as needed. Provide self-help devices as ordered. Feed the resident if necessary.
- Give emotional and psychological support. The resident's care may involve a psychiatrist or psychologist.
- Physical therapy, occupational therapy, speech therapy, and vocational rehabilitation are ordered. They help the resident regain independent functioning to the extent possible.

EAR DISORDERS

The ear is important for hearing and balance. Middle ear infections, Meniere's disease, and hearing loss are presented in this section.

Otitis Media

Otitis media is infection *(itis)* of the middle *(media)* ear *(ot)*. The infection is acute or chronic. Chronic otitis media can damage the tympanic membrane (eardrum) or the ossicles (see Fig. 6-13, p. 103). The eardrum and ossicles are needed for hearing. Permanent hearing loss can occur from chronic otitis media.

Fluid buildup occurs in the ear. It causes pain and hearing loss. Other signs and symptoms include fever and ringing in the ears **(tinnitus).** Antibiotics usually are ordered by the doctor.

Meniere's Disease

Meniere's disease involves increased fluid in the inner ear. The increased fluid causes pressure in the middle ear. There are three symptoms. Vertigo is the major symptom. **Vertigo** means dizziness. The resident feels whirling and spinning sensations. The resident must lie down. Severe dizziness can cause nausea and vomiting. The other main symptoms are ringing in the ears (tinnitus) and hearing loss.

The doctor can order drugs for the resident. Sometimes a low-salt diet decreases the amount of fluid in the ear. Safety is important during vertigo. The resident must lie down. Falls are prevented. Bed rails usually are ordered. The head is kept still, and the resident avoids turning the head. To talk to the resident, stand directly in front of him or her. When movement is necessary, the resident moves slowly. Bright or glaring lights are avoided. Assistance is given with ambulation. The resident should not walk alone in case vertigo occurs.

Hearing Problems

Hearing losses range from slight hearing impairments to complete deafness. Clear speech, responding to others, safety, and awareness of surroundings all require hearing. Many people deny having difficulty hearing. This is because hearing loss often is associated with aging. However, temporary hearing loss can occur when the ear canal is blocked with ear wax (cerumen). Hearing improves when the ear wax is removed. Wax is removed by a doctor or nurse.

Effects on the person. A person may be unaware of gradual difficulty in hearing. Others may see changes in the person's behavior or attitude. They may not know that the changes are the result of hearing problems. Symptoms and effects of hearing loss vary. They are not always obvious to the person or to others. Obvious signs of hearing impairment include:

- Speaking too loudly
- Leaning forward to hear
- Turning and cupping the better ear toward the speaker
- Answering questions or responding inappropriately
- Asking for words to be repeated

Psychological and social effects are less obvious. Residents may give wrong answers or responses. Therefore they tend to avoid social situations. This is to avoid embarrassment. Loneliness, boredom, and feeling left out often result. Only parts of conversations are heard. People with hearing loss may become suspicious. They think they are being talked about or that others are talking softly on purpose. There is the fear of being labeled "senile" because of inappropriate responses. Some control conversations to avoid answering questions. Straining and working to hear can cause fatigue, frustration, and irritability.

Hearing loss may cause speech problems. How you pronounce words and voice volume depend on how you hear yourself. Hearing loss may result in slurred speech and improper pronunciation. Monotone speech and dropping word endings also may occur. It may be hard to understand what the resident is saying. Do not assume that you understand what the resident says. Do not pretend to understand to avoid embarrassing the resident. Serious problems can result if you assume or pretend to understand. Follow the guidelines in Box 26-8 to communicate with the speech-impaired resident.

Communicating with the resident. Hearing-impaired residents may wear a hearing aid or read lips. They also watch facial expressions, gestures, and body language. Some residents learn sign language (Figs. 26-24 and 26-25 on pp. 598-599). Some hearing-impaired residents have a *hearing* dog. The dog alerts the resident to such things as ringing phones, doorbells, sirens, or oncoming cars. Certain measures are needed when communicating with the resident. The measures listed in Box 26-9 can help the resident hear or speech-read (lip-read).

Box 26-8 Communicating With the Speech-Impaired Resident

- Listen, and give the resident your full attention.
- Ask the resident questions to which you know the answer. This helps you become familiar with the resident's speech.
- Determine the subject being discussed. This helps you understand main points.
- Ask the resident to repeat or rephrase statements if necessary.
- Repeat what the resident has said. Ask if you have understood correctly.
- Ask the resident to write down key words or the message.
- Watch the resident 's lip movements.
- Watch facial expressions, gestures, and body language for clues about what is being said.

Box 26-9 Communicating With the Hearing-Impaired Resident

- Gain attention, and alert the resident to your presence. Raise an arm or hand, or lightly touch the resident's arm. Do not startle or approach the resident from behind.
- Face the resident directly when speaking. Do not turn or walk away while you are talking.
- Stand or sit in good light. Shadows and glares affect the resident's ability to see your face clearly.
- Speak clearly, distinctly, and slowly.
- Speak in a normal tone of voice. Do not shout.
- Do not cover your mouth, smoke, eat, or chew gum while talking. These things affect mouth movements.
- Stand or sit on the side of the better ear.
- State the topic of conversation first.
- Use short sentences and simple words.
- Write out important names and words.
- Say things in a different way if the resident does not seem to understand.
- Keep conversations and discussions short to avoid tiring the resident.
- Repeat and rephrase statements as needed.
- Be alert to the messages sent by your facial expressions, gestures, and body language.
- Reduce or eliminate background noises.

Hearing aids. A *hearing aid* makes sounds louder (Fig. 26-26, p. 599). It does not correct or cure the hearing problem. Hearing ability does not improve. However, the person hears better because the hearing aid makes sounds louder. Both background noise and speech are louder. The measures for communicating with hearing-impaired persons apply to those with hearing aids.

Hearing aids operate on batteries. There is an *on* and *off* switch. Sometimes hearing aids do not seem to work properly. Often only simple measures are needed to get them to work:

- Check if the hearing aid is *on.*
- Check the battery position.
- Insert a new battery if needed.
- Clean the earmold if necessary.

Hearing aids are expensive. You must handle and care for them properly. Report lost or damaged hearing aids to the nurse immediately. *Check with the nurse before washing or cleaning a hearing aid. Also follow the manufacturer's instructions for proper care and use.* Only the earmold is washed. It is usually washed daily with soap and water. The battery is removed at night. When not in use, the hearing aid is turned off.

Text continued on p. 600

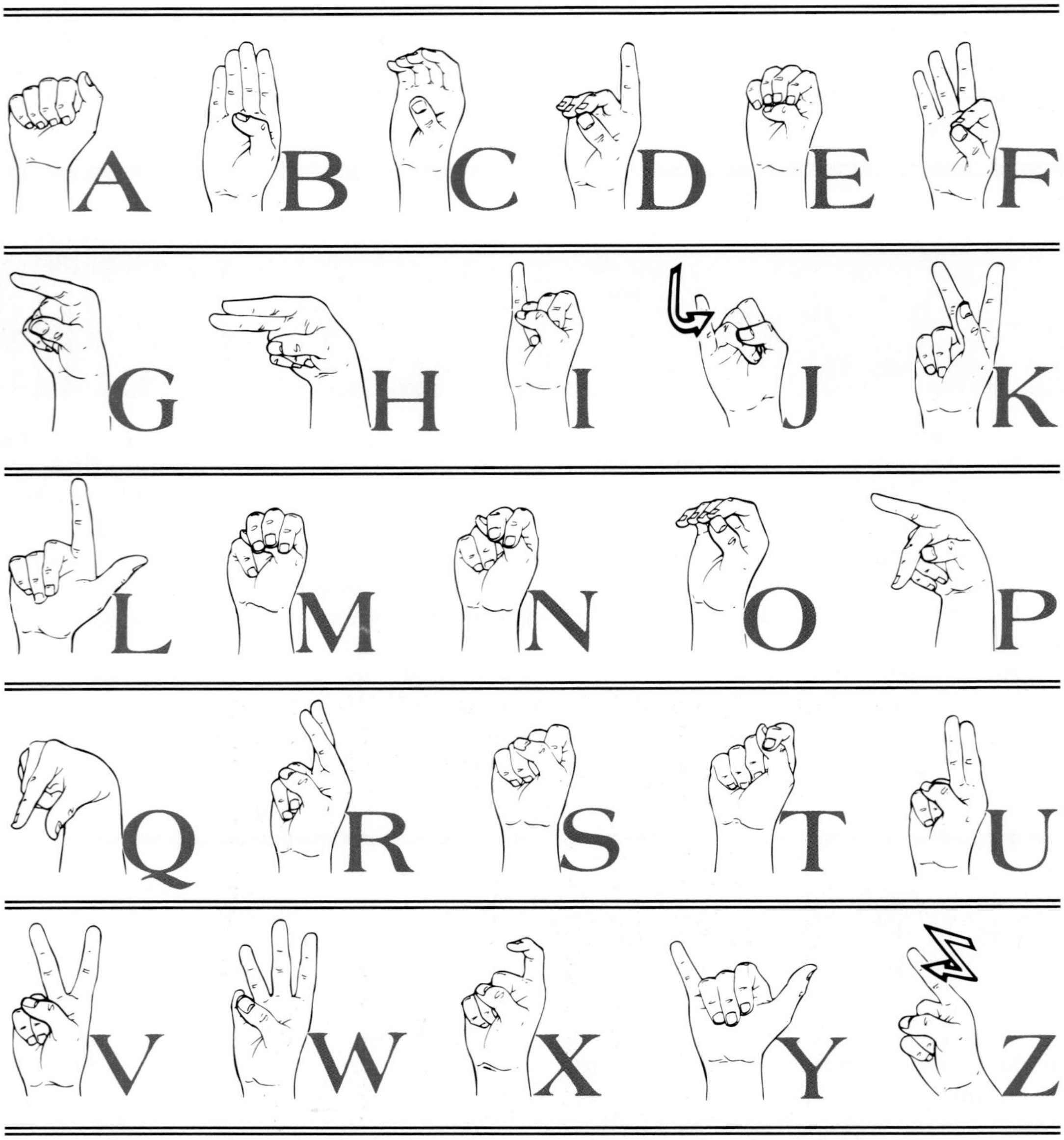

Fig. 26-24 Manual alphabet. *(Courtesy National Association of the Deaf, Silver Springs, Md.)*

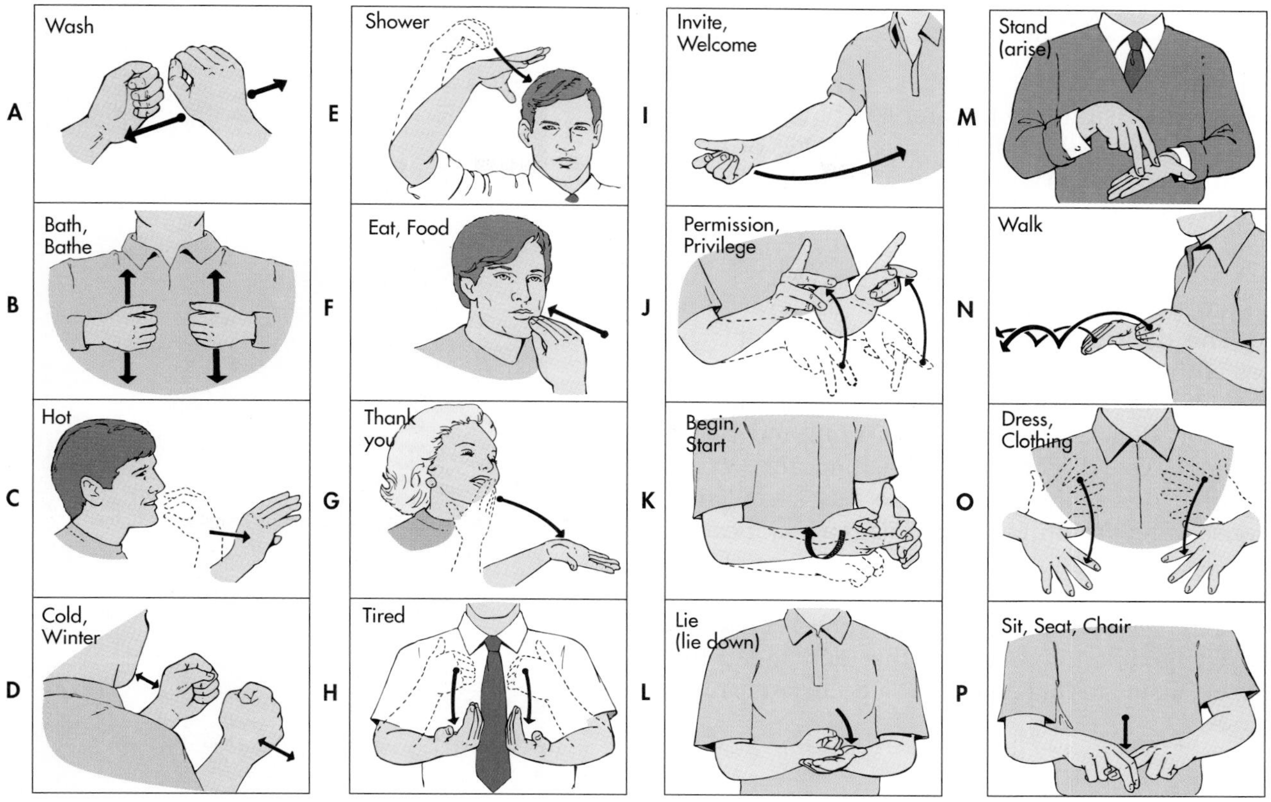

Fig. 26-25 Sign language.

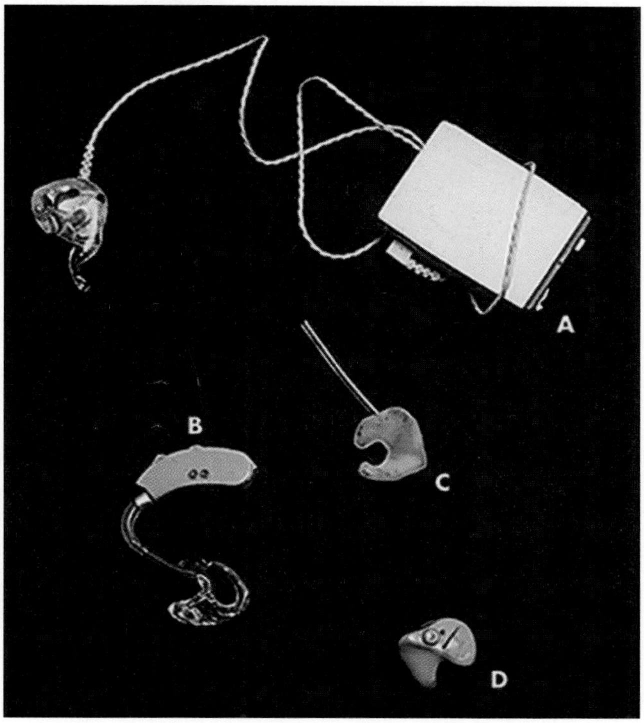

Fig. 26-26 Types of hearing aids. *(Courtesy CLG Photographics, St. Louis.)*

EYE DISORDERS

Vision problems occur at all ages. Problems range from very mild vision loss to complete blindness. Vision loss is sudden or gradual in onset. One or both eyes are affected. Surgery, eyeglasses, or contact lenses are often necessary.

Glaucoma

With glaucoma, fluid pressure within the eye is increased. This damages the optic nerve. The result is vision loss with eventual blindness. The disease is gradual or sudden in onset. Signs and symptoms include tunnel vision (Fig. 26-27), blurred vision, and halos around lights. Eye discomfort and aching also occur. With sudden onset, the person also has severe eye pain, nausea, and vomiting. Glaucoma is a major cause of blindness. Blacks and persons over 40 years of age are at risk.

Treatment involves drug therapy and possibly surgery. The goal is to prevent further damage to the optic nerve. Damage that has already occurred cannot be reversed.

Cataract

Cataract is an eye disorder in which the lens becomes cloudy (opaque). The cloudiness prevents light from entering the eye (Fig. 26-28). Cataract comes from the Greek word that means *waterfall*. Trying to see is like looking through a waterfall. Gradual blurring and dimming of vision occur. The person is sensitive to light and glares. A cataract can occur in one or both eyes. Aging is the most common cause. Persons age 60 and older are at risk.

Surgery is the only treatment. A tiny incision is made into the eye. The cloudy lens is removed. A plastic lens is implanted into the eye. Vision returns to near normal.

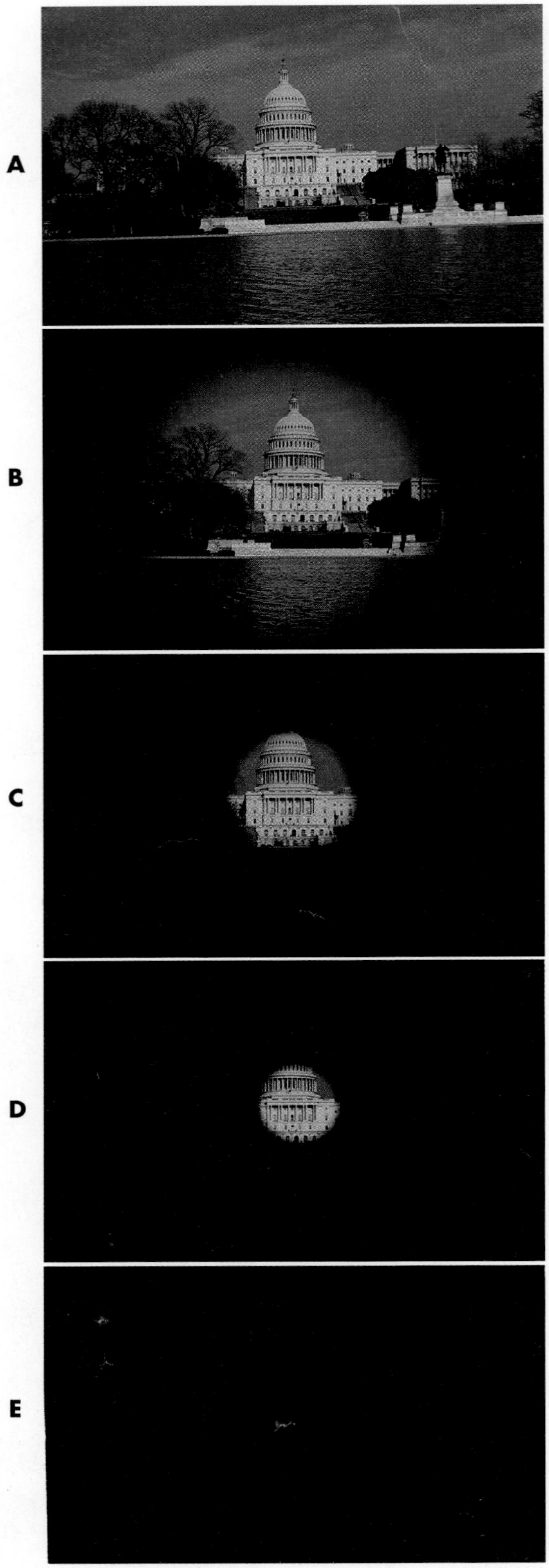

Fig. 26-27 **A,** Normal vision. **B,** Tunnel vision. **C, D, E,** Vision loss continues with eventual blindness.

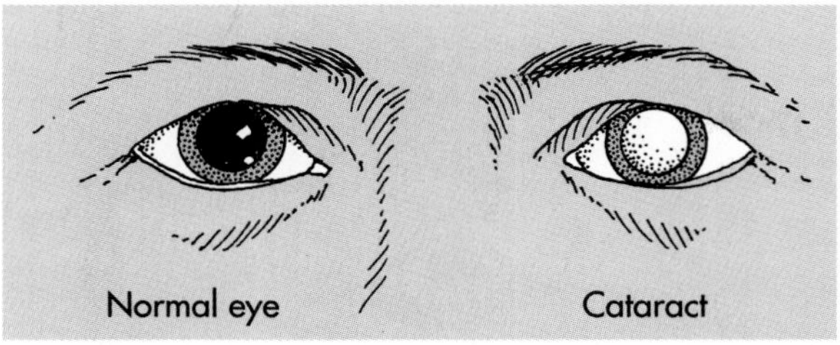

Fig. 26-28 The left eye has a cataract. *(From Phipps WJ, Cassmeyer VL, Sands JK, Lehman MK:* Medical-surgical nursing: concepts and clinical practice, *ed 5, St Louis, 1995, Mosby.)*

The person may have to wear an eye shield or patch for a day or two after surgery. The shield protects the eye from injury. The following rules are important in caring for a resident with a new lens implant:

- Keep the eye shield in place as directed. Some doctors allow the shield to be left off during the day if the resident wears eyeglasses. The shield is worn for sleep, including napping.
- Do not shampoo or shower the resident without a doctor's order.
- Take care not to bump the eye.
- Report the following to the nurse immediately:
  - Increasing pain after the first 24 hours following surgery
  - Drainage from the eye
- Remind the resident not to rub the eye.

Measures for the blind person are practiced when an eye shield is worn (see p. 602). The person may have vision loss in the other eye from a cataract or other causes.

Corrective Lenses

Eyeglasses and contact lenses are prescribed to correct vision problems. Often eyeglasses are worn only for certain activities, such as reading or seeing at a distance. Some residents wear them all the time while awake. Contact lenses are usually worn continuously while awake.

Eyeglasses. Lenses are made of hardened glass or plastic. They are made to prevent shattering. Glass lenses are washed with warm water and dried with soft tissue. Plastic lenses are easily scratched. Special cleaning solutions, tissues, and cloths are used to clean and dry them.

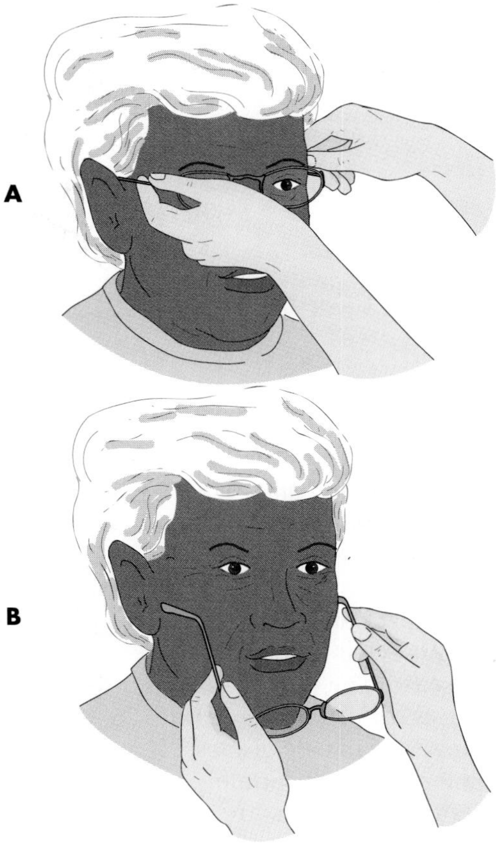

Fig. 26-29 A, Remove eyeglasses by holding the frames in front of both ears. **B,** Lift the frames from the ears, and bring the glasses down away from the face.

Glasses are costly. They are protected from breakage or other damage (Fig. 26-29). When not worn, they are put in their case. The case is put in the drawer of the bedside stand to prevent loss or damage to the glasses. To prevent loss, most centers mark eyeglasses with the resident's name.

Contact lenses. Contact lenses fit directly on the eye. Many people like contacts because they cannot be seen. However, contacts are easily lost. Depending on the type of lens, contacts can be worn for 12 to 24 hours or for 1 week. Contact lenses are removed and cleaned following manufacturer's instructions and center procedures.

Report any redness or drainage from the eyes to the nurse right away. Also report resident complaints of eye pain or blurred vision.

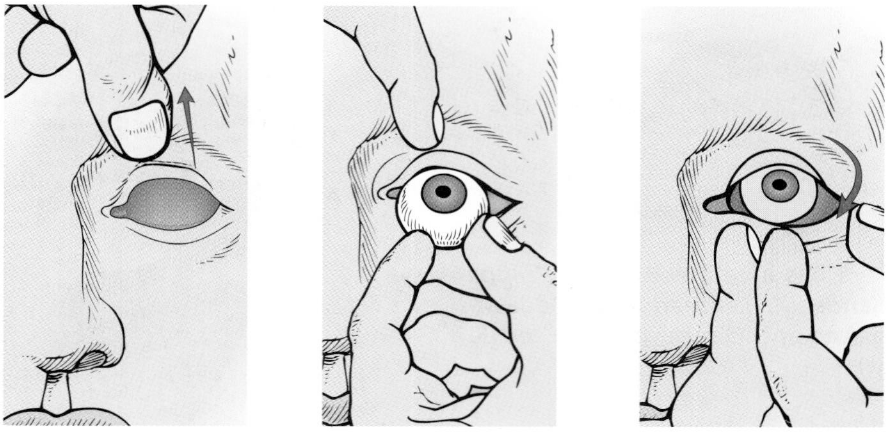

Fig. 26-30 Inserting an artificial eye. *(From Lewis SM, Collier IC, Heitkemper MM:* Medical-surgical nursing: assessment and management of clinical problems, *ed 4, St Louis, 1996, Mosby.)*

Artificial Eyes

Removal of an eye is sometimes necessary because of injury or disease. The person is then fitted with an ocular prosthesis, or artificial eye (Fig. 26-30). The artificial eye is made of plastic or glass. It matches the other eye in color and shape. Some prostheses are permanent implants, and others are removable. If the prosthesis is removable, the person is taught to remove, clean, and insert it. The person performs routine care of the prosthesis.

An artificial eye is the resident's property. Like dentures, eyeglasses, and other valuables, it is protected from loss or damage. The following measures are practiced if the eye is removed and will not be reinserted:

- Wash the eye with a mild soap and warm water. Then rinse it well.
- Line a container with a soft cloth or 4 × 4 gauze. This prevents scratches and damage to the eye.
- Fill the container with water or a saline (salt) solution.
- Place the eye in the container. Close the container.
- Label the container with the person's name and room number.
- Place the labeled container in the drawer in the bedside stand.
- Wash the eye socket with warm water or saline. Use a washcloth or gauze square to clean the eye socket. Use a gauze square to remove excess moisture.
- Wash the eyelid with mild soap and warm water. Clean from the inner to the outer aspect of the eyelid (see Chapter 13). Dry the eyelid.

The resident is blind on the side of the artificial eye. Vision in the other eye may be normal or impaired.

Blindness

Birth defects, accidents, and eye diseases are among the many causes of blindness. It is also a complication of some diseases. The level of blindness varies. Some blind persons cannot sense light and have no usable vision. They are totally blind. Others sense some light but have no usable vision. Still others have some usable vision but cannot read newsprint. The legally blind person sees at 20 feet what a person with normal vision sees at 200 feet.

A person's life is seriously affected by the loss of sight. Physical and psychological adjustments are hard and long. Special education and training are needed. Moving about, activities of daily living, reading braille, and using a guide dog all require training.

Braille is a method of writing that uses raised dots. Dots are arranged to represent each letter of the alphabet. The first ten letters also represent the numbers 0 through 9 (Fig. 26-31). The person feels the arrangement of dots with the fingers (Fig. 26-32). Many books, magazines, and newspapers are available in braille. So are typewriters and computer keyboards.

Braille is hard to learn, especially for many older persons. Entire books and articles are available on compact disks and tapes. They are bought in bookstores or borrowed from libraries.

The blind person is taught to move about using a white cane with a red tip or a guide dog. Both are recognized worldwide as signs that the person is blind. The dog serves as the eyes of the blind person. The dog recognizes danger and guides the person through traffic. Assist the person with ambulating, if necessary (Fig. 26-33).

Treat the blind resident with respect and dignity—not with pity. Most blind people adjust well. They lead independent lives. Some were blind for a long time and others for a short time. The practices in Box 26-10 on p. 604 are necessary for all blind persons.

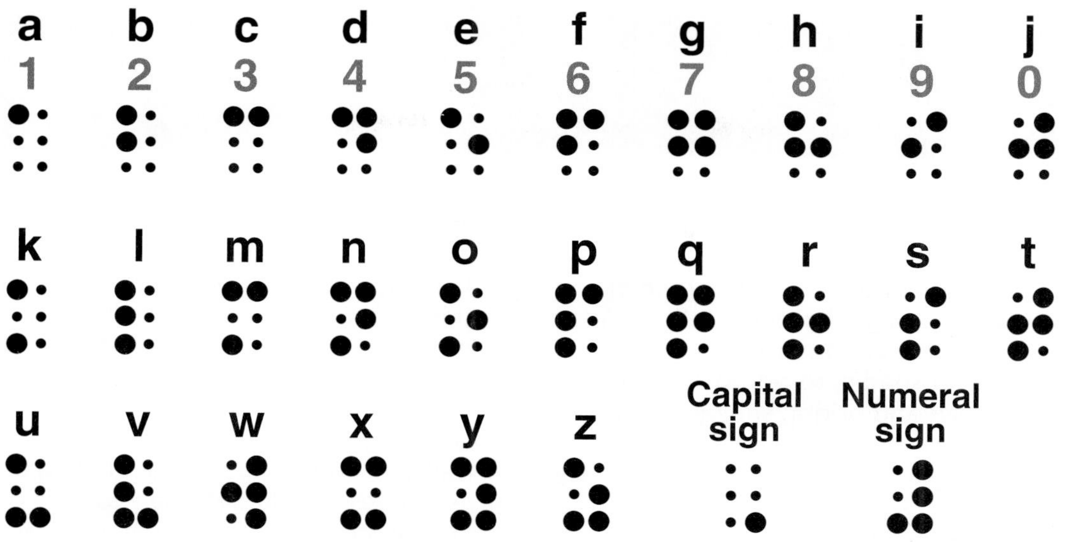

Fig. 26-31 Braille.

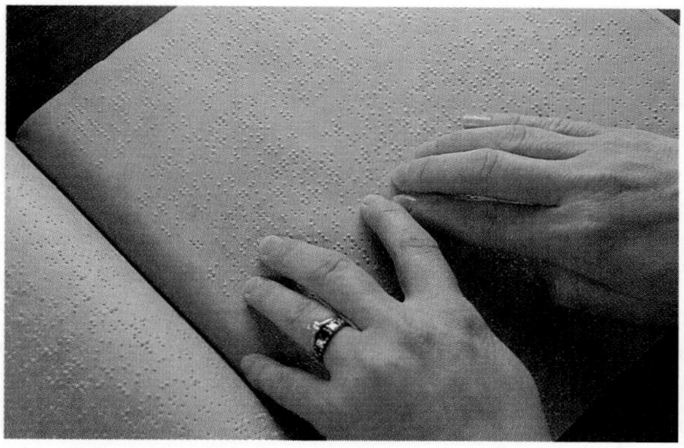

Fig. 26-32 Braille is "read" with the fingers.

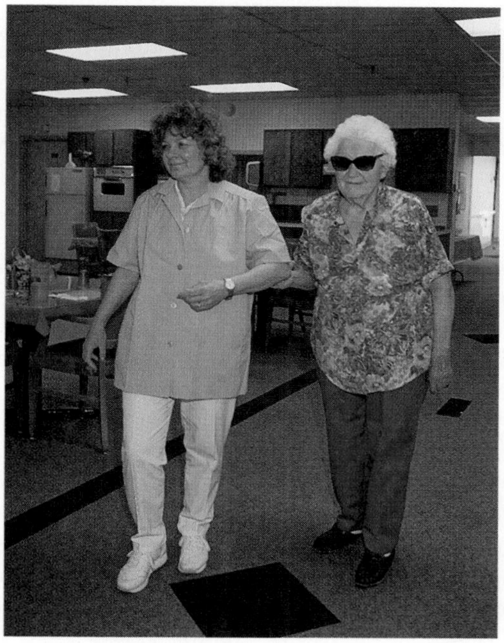

Fig. 26-33 The blind person walks slightly behind the nursing assistant. She takes the assistant's arm.

Box 26-10 Caring for the Blind Resident

- Ask the resident how much he or she can see. Do not assume the resident is totally blind or that the resident has some vision.
- Ask the resident what type of lighting he or she prefers. Provide enough lighting. Tell the resident when the lights are on or off.
- Adjust blinds and shades to adjust lighting for glares. Sunny days and bright, snowy days cause glares.
- Face the resident when speaking. Speak slowly and clearly.
- Use a normal tone of voice. Do not shout or speak loudly. Blindness does not mean the resident is hearing impaired.
- Identify yourself when you enter the room. Give your name, title, and reason for being there. Do not touch the resident until you have indicated your presence in the room.
- Identify others in the room. Explain where each person is located and what the person is doing.
- Address the resident by name. This lets the resident know that you are directing a comment or question to him or her.
- Do not avoid using the words "see," "look," or "read."
- Orient the resident to the room. Describe the layout. Also identify the location and purpose of furniture and equipment.
- Let the resident move about and touch and locate furniture and equipment if able.
- Do not let the resident alone in the middle of a room. Make sure the resident can reach a wall, chair, table, or sofa.
- Do not rearrange furniture and equipment.
- Keep doors open or shut (never partially open).
- Give step-by-step explanations of procedures as you perform them. Indicate when the procedure is over.
- Offer assistance. Simply say, "May I help you?" Respect the resident's answer.
- Tell the resident when you are leaving the room.
- Assist the resident in ambulating by walking slightly ahead of him or her (see Fig. 26-33). Offer your right or left arm. Tell the resident which arm you are offering so he or she can take your arm. Never push, pull, or guide the resident in front of you.
- Walk at a normal pace when guiding the resident.
- Let the resident know when you are coming to a curb or steps. Let the resident know if you will step up or down.
- Inform the resident of doors, turns, furniture, and other obstructions when assisting with ambulation.
- Give specific directions. For example, say "right behind you," "on your left," or "in front of you." Avoid phrases like "over here" or "over there."
- Keep hallways and walkways free of carts, equipment, and other items.
- Assist in food selection by reading the menu to the resident.
- Avoid plates, napkins, place mats, and tablecloths with patterns and designs. These items should be solid colors and provide contrast. For example, a white plate is placed on a dark place mat or tablecloth.
- Explain the location of food and beverages on the tray. Use the face of a clock (see Chapter 18), or guide the resident's hand to each item on the tray.
- Cut meat, open containers, butter bread, and perform other similar activities if needed.
- Keep the signal light within the resident 's reach.
- Provide a radio, compact disks or audiotapes, television, and braille books for entertainment.
- Let the resident perform self-care if able.

RESPIRATORY DISORDERS

The respiratory system brings oxygen (O_2) into the lungs and removes carbon dioxide (CO_2) from the body. Respiratory disorders interfere with this function and threaten life.

Chronic Obstructive Pulmonary Disease (COPD)

Three disorders are grouped under chronic obstructive pulmonary disease (COPD). They are chronic bronchitis, emphysema, and asthma. These disorders interfere with the exchange of O_2 and CO_2 in the lungs. They obstruct air flow.

Chronic bronchitis. Chronic bronchitis occurs after repeated episodes of bronchitis (inflammation of the bronchi). Cigarette smoking is the major cause. Air pollution and industrial dusts are other causes. *Smoker's cough* in the morning is usually the first symptom. At first the cough is dry. Eventually the person coughs up mucus, which may contain pus. The cough becomes more frequent as the disease progresses. The person has difficulty breathing and tires easily. The mucus and inflamed breathing passages *obstruct* airflow into the lungs. Therefore the body cannot get normal amounts of oxygen.

The person must stop smoking. Oxygen therapy and breathing exercises are often ordered. Respiratory tract infections are prevented. If one occurs, prompt treatment is essential.

Emphysema. In emphysema, the alveoli enlarge. Walls of the alveoli are less elastic. They do not expand and shrink normally with inspiration and expiration. As a result, some air is trapped in the alveoli during expiration. Trapped air is not exhaled. As the disease progresses, more alveoli are involved. Therefore more air is trapped. The normal exchange of O_2 and CO_2 cannot occur in affected alveoli. Chronic bronchitis and emphysema often occur together.

Cigarette smoking is the most common cause. Signs and symptoms include shortness of breath and smoker's cough. At first, shortness of breath occurs with exertion. As the disease progresses, it occurs at rest. Sputum may contain pus. As more air is trapped in the lungs, the person develops a *barrel chest* (Fig. 26-34). These residents usually prefer to sit upright and slightly forward. Breathing is easier in this position. You may need to assist the resident in assuming such a position. To do so, place the overbed table at chest height in front of the resident. Then place a pillow on the table. Have the resident lean forward slightly and rest the arms and head on the pillow.

Respiratory therapy, breathing exercises, oxygen, and drug therapy are ordered. For successful therapy, the person must stop smoking.

Asthma. Air passages narrow with asthma. Dyspnea results. Allergies and emotional stress are common causes. Episodes occur suddenly and are called *asthma attacks*. The person also has shortness of breath, wheezing, coughing, rapid pulse, perspiration, and cyanosis. The person is very frightened during the attack. Fear causes the attack to become worse.

Drugs are used to treat asthma. Emergency room treatment may be necessary for severe attacks. The person and family are taught how to prevent asthma attacks. Repeated attacks can damage the respiratory system.

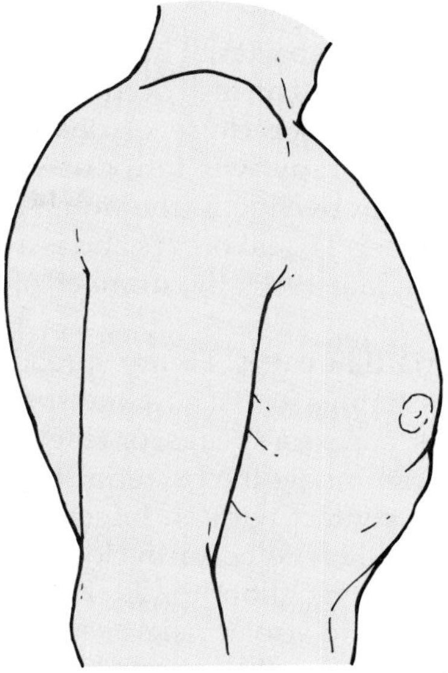

Fig. 26-34 Barrel chest from emphysema.

Pneumonia

Pneumonia is an inflammation of lung tissue. Alveoli in the affected area fill with fluid. Because of fluid in the alveoli, O_2 and CO_2 are not exchanged normally.

Pneumonia is caused by bacteria, viruses, aspiration, or immobility. The resident is very ill. Fever, chills, painful cough, chest pain on breathing, and a rapid pulse occur. Cyanosis may be present. Sputum is clear, green, yellow, or rust colored. The color depends on the cause.

Drugs are ordered for infection and pain. Fluids are encouraged because of fever. Fluids also help to thin mucous secretions. Thin secretions are easier to cough up. IV fluids and oxygen may be ordered. Most residents prefer semi-Fowler's position for breathing. Frequent position changes help prevent pooling of secretions in dependent areas of the lungs. Standard Precautions are followed. Transmission-Based Precautions may be necessary, depending on the cause. Mouth care is important. Frequent linen changes are needed because of fever.

The older person is at high risk for pneumonia. Changes from aging, other diseases, and decreased mobility increase the risk of pneumonia. Other diseases and the drugs taken for them can mask the signs and symptoms of pneumonia. Pneumonia can lead to death.

Aspiration pneumonia is common in older persons. Dysphagia, decreased cough and gag reflexes, and nervous system disorders increase the risk of aspiration. So do drugs that depress the brain. Such drugs include narcotics and sedatives. Alcohol also depresses the brain.

Tuberculosis

Tuberculosis (TB) is a bacterial infection. The lungs are affected. However, TB can also occur in the kidney and bones. TB was a major cause of death in the early 1900s. TB drug therapy was introduced in the 1940s and 1950s. A great decline in the number of TB cases resulted. However, TB still occurs and is a major health problem. In the late 1980s the number of cases began to increase.

The bacteria that cause TB are spread by airborne droplets (see Chapter 9). Bacteria are spread when the person coughs, sneezes, speaks, or sings. Others in the environment can inhale the bacteria. Those who have close, frequent contact with an infected person are at risk. TB is more likely to occur in close, crowded areas such as inner-city neighborhoods. Persons with HIV infection (p. 614) are also at risk.

Sometimes bacteria do not cause an infection until many years later. The person may not have symptoms at first. The disease is found when a routine chest x-ray is done or when a TB skin test is required for a job. Early signs and symptoms are tiredness, loss of appetite, weight loss, fever, and night sweats. Coughing occurs. The cough is more frequent as the disease progresses. Sputum production also increases. Chest pain occurs.

Treatment involves drugs for TB. Usually, hospital care is not necessary. Persons with TB need to cover their nose and mouth with tissues when coughing or sneezing. Tissues are flushed down the toilet or placed in a paper bag and burned. In health care centers, tissues are placed in a biohazard bag and disposed of following center policy. Handwashing after contact with sputum is essential. Standard Precautions and Airborne Precautions are practiced. Most nursing centers do not admit persons with active TB.

CARDIOVASCULAR DISORDERS

Cardiovascular disorders are the leading causes of death in the United States. Problems occur in the heart or in the blood vessels.

Hypertension

Hypertension *(high blood pressure)* is a condition in which the blood pressure is abnormally high. The systolic pressure is 140 mm Hg or higher. Or the diastolic pressure is 90 mm Hg or higher. Elevated measurements must occur on two different occasions. Risk factors are listed in Box 26-11. Narrowed blood vessels are a common cause. When vessels narrow, the heart pumps with more force to move blood through the vessels. Kidney disorders, head injuries, some complications of pregnancy, and adrenal gland tumors also cause hypertension.

Box 26-11 Risk Factors for Hypertension

- Age—the risk increases with aging beginning at about age 35
- Sex—younger men are at greater risk than younger women; the risk increases for women after menopause
- Race—blacks are at greater risk than whites
- Family history—tends to run in families
- Obesity—related to lack of exercise and atherosclerosis
- Stress—increased sympathetic nervous system activity
- Cigarette smoking—nicotine narrows blood vessels
- High-salt diet—sodium causes fluid retention; increased fluid raises the blood volume
- Alcohol—increases chemical substances in the body that increase blood pressure
- Lack of exercise—leads to obesity
- Atherosclerosis—arteries narrow because of fatty buildup in the vessels

Hypertension can damage other body organs. The heart may enlarge so it can pump with more force. Blood vessels in the brain may burst and cause a stroke. Blood vessels in the eyes and kidneys may be damaged.

At first, hypertension may not cause signs or symptoms. Usually it is discovered when blood pressure is measured. Signs and symptoms develop as the disorder progresses. Headache, blurred vision, and dizziness may be reported. Complications of hypertension include TIAs, stroke, heart attack, kidney (renal) failure, and blindness.

Certain drugs can lower blood pressure. The person needs to exercise, get enough rest, and quit smoking. A sodium-restricted diet may also be ordered. If the person is overweight, a low-calorie diet is ordered.

Coronary Artery Disease

The coronary arteries are in the heart. They supply the heart with blood. In coronary artery disease (CAD), the coronary arteries narrow. One or all of the arteries may be affected. Because of narrowed vessels, the heart muscle gets less blood. The most common cause is atherosclerosis. In atherosclerosis, fatty material collects on the arterial walls (Fig. 26-35). The arteries narrow and obstruct blood flow. Blood flow through an artery may be totally blocked. Permanent damage occurs in the part of the heart receiving its blood supply from that artery.

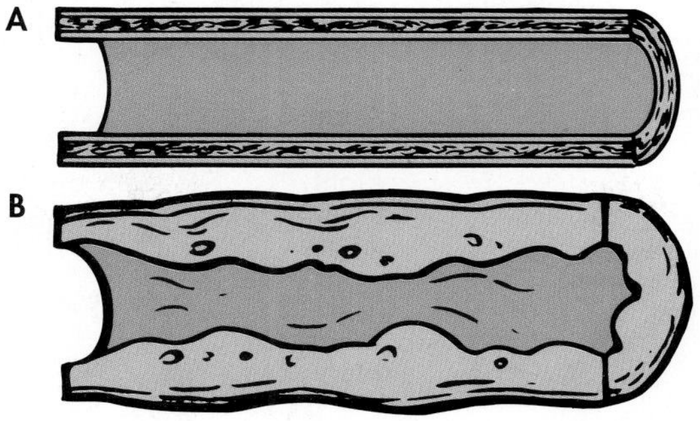

Fig. 26-35 **A,** Normal artery. **B,** Fatty deposits collect on the walls of arteries in atherosclerosis.

CAD is the leading cause of death in the United States. Risk factors include:

- Sex (male gender)
- Age (more common in older persons)
- Obesity
- Cigarette smoking
- Lack of exercise
- A diet high in fat and cholesterol
- Hypertension
- Family history of CAD
- Uncontrolled diabetes (p. 611)

The major complications of CAD are angina pectoris and myocardial infarction (heart attack). Treatment involves reducing risk factors. Nothing can be done about the person's sex, age, and family history. However, efforts are directed at losing weight, regular exercise, no smoking, and eating a healthy diet. Controlling blood pressure and diabetes also is important.

Angina pectoris. Angina *(pain)* pectoris *(chest)* means chest pain. The chest pain is from reduced blood flow to a part of the heart muscle (myocardium). Commonly called *angina,* it occurs when the heart needs more oxygen. Normally, blood flow to the heart increases when the heart's need for oxygen increases. Physical exertion, a heavy meal, emotional stress, and excitement increase the heart's need for oxygen. In CAD, narrowed vessels prevent increased blood flow.

Signs and symptoms include chest pain. The pain may be described as a tightness or discomfort in the left side of the chest. Pain may radiate to other sites (Fig. 26-36). Pain in the left jaw and down the inner aspect of the left arm is common. The person may be pale, feel faint, and perspire. Dyspnea is common. These signs and symptoms cause the person to stop activity and rest. Rest often relieves the symptoms in 3 to 15 minutes. Rest reduces the heart's need for oxygen. Therefore normal blood flow is achieved and heart damage prevented.

Besides rest, a drug called *nitroglycerin* is taken to relieve angina. A nitroglycerin tablet is taken when an angina attack occurs. The tablet is put under the tongue.

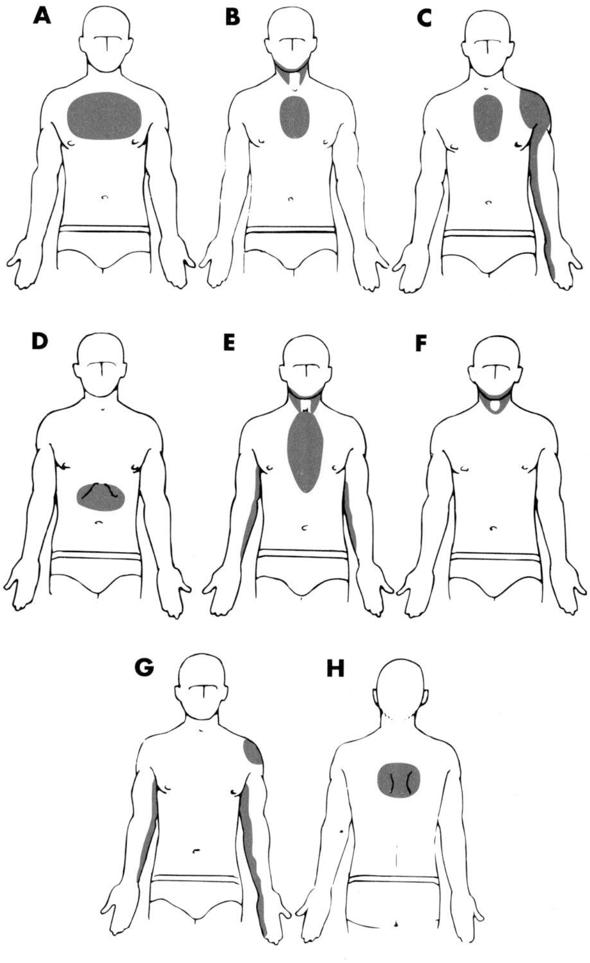

Fig. 26-36 Shaded areas show where the pain of angina pectoris is located. *(From Phipps WJ, Cassmeyer VL, Sands JK, Lehman MK:* Medical-surgical nursing: concepts and clinical practice, *ed 5, St Louis, 1995, Mosby.)*

It dissolves under the tongue and is rapidly absorbed into the bloodstream. Most doctors want the tablets kept at the bedside. The resident takes a tablet when one is needed and then tells the nurse. The resident

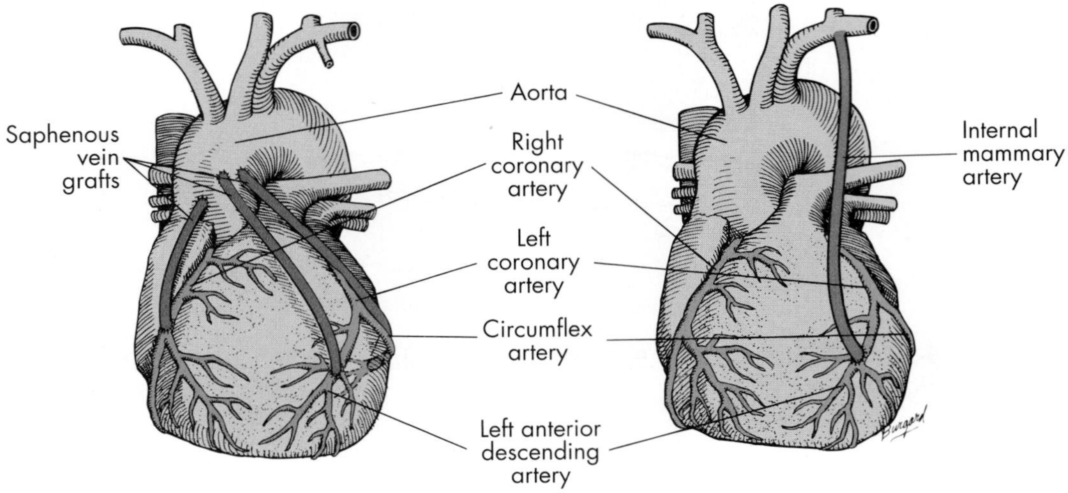

Fig. 26-37 Coronary artery bypass surgery. *(From Phipps WJ, Cassmeyer VL, Sands JK, Lehman MK:* Medical-surgical nursing: concepts and clinical practice, *ed 5, St Louis, 1995, Mosby.)*

does not wait for someone to answer the signal light and then for a nurse to get the tablet. The resident needs the tablets nearby at all times. This includes when the resident goes to physical therapy, occupational therapy, the dining room, lounge, or other areas.

Persons are taught to avoid things likely to cause angina pectoris. These include overexertion, heavy meals and overeating, and emotional times. They need to stay indoors during cold weather or during hot, humid weather. Exercise programs supervised by doctors are helpful.

Some people need coronary artery bypass surgery. The surgery bypasses the diseased part of the artery (Fig. 26-37) and increases blood flow to the heart. Many persons with angina pectoris eventually have heart attacks. Chest pain that is not relieved by rest and nitroglycerin may have a more serious cause.

Myocardial infarction. A myocardial infarction (MI) is caused by lack of blood supply to the heart muscle (myocardium). Tissue death occurs (infarction). Common terms for MI are *heart attack, coronary, coronary thrombosis,* and *coronary occlusion.* Blood flow to the myocardium is suddenly interrupted. Atherosclerosis or a thrombus (blood clot) obstructs blood flow through an artery. The area of damage may be small or large (Fig. 26-38). Sudden cardiac death *(cardiac arrest)* can occur (see Chapter 31).

The person suffering from myocardial infarction has one or more of the signs and symptoms listed in Box 26-12. Myocardial infarction is an emergency. Efforts are directed at relieving pain, stabilizing vital signs, giving oxygen, and calming the person. Many drugs are given. The person is treated in a coronary care unit (CCU). The unit has the equipment and drugs needed during cardiac arrest. Measures are taken to prevent life-threatening complications.

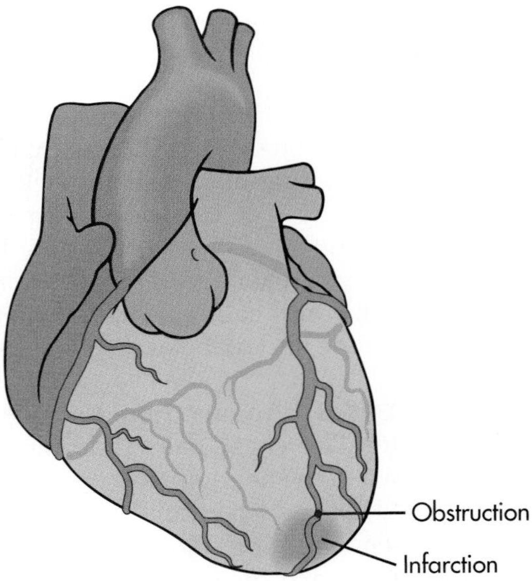

Fig. 26-38 Myocardial infarction. *(From Lewis SM, Collier IC, Heitkemper, MM:* Medical-surgical nursing: assessment and management of clinical problems, *ed 4, St Louis, 1996, Mosby.)*

The person is in the CCU for 2 to 3 days. When stable, the person is transferred. Activity is increased gradually. Drug therapy and measures to prevent complications are continued. Cardiac rehabilitation is planned. The goal is to prevent another heart attack. The program includes exercise; teaching about drugs, dietary changes, and sexual activity; and life-style changes. *(See Subacute Care, p. 609.)*

Box 26-12 Signs and Symptoms of Myocardial Infarction

- Sudden, severe chest pain
- Pain is usually on the left side
- Pain is described as crushing, stabbing, or squeezing; some describe pain in terms of someone sitting on the chest
- Pain may radiate to the neck and jaw, and down the arm or to other sites
- Pain is more severe and lasts longer than angina pectoris
- Pain is not relieved by rest and nitroglycerin
- Indigestion
- Dyspnea
- Nausea
- Dizziness
- Perspiration
- Pallor
- Cyanosis
- Cold and clammy skin
- Low blood pressure
- Weak and irregular pulse
- Fear and apprehension
- A feeling of doom

Subacute Care

Some subacute care units have cardiac rehabilitation programs. The program is managed by a cardiologist. This is a doctor with special education and training in caring for persons with a cardiovascular disorder.

Heart Failure

Heart failure, or congestive heart failure (CHF), occurs when the heart cannot pump blood normally. Blood backs up and causes tissue congestion. Left-sided heart failure, right-sided heart failure, or both can occur.

When the heart's left side fails to pump efficiently, blood backs up into the lungs. Signs and symptoms of respiratory congestion occur. These include dyspnea, increased sputum, cough, and gurgling sounds in the lungs. Also, blood is not pumped out of the heart to the rest of the body in adequate amounts. Organs do not get enough blood. Signs and symptoms occur from effects on the organs. Poor blood flow to the brain causes confusion, dizziness, and fainting. Poor blood flow to the kidneys causes reduced kidney function and decreased urinary output. The skin becomes pale or cyanotic. Blood pressure falls. A very severe form of left-sided failure is *pulmonary edema* (fluid in the lungs). Pulmonary edema is an emergency. Death can occur.

With right-sided failure, blood backs up into the venae cavae and into the venous system. Feet and ankles swell. Neck veins bulge. Liver congestion causes decreased liver function. The abdomen becomes congested with fluid. The right side of the heart cannot pump blood to the lungs efficiently. Normal blood flow does not occur from the lungs to the left side of the heart. Less blood than normal is pumped from the left side of the heart to the rest of the body. As with left-sided heart failure, the body's organs have a reduced blood supply. The signs and symptoms described in the previous paragraph eventually occur.

Heart failure is usually caused by a weakened heart. Myocardial infarction and hypertension are common causes. Damaged heart valves are another cause.

Heart failure can be treated and controlled. Drugs strengthen the heart and reduce the amount of fluid in the body. A sodium-restricted diet is ordered. Oxygen is given. Most residents prefer semi-Fowler's or Fowler's position for breathing. If acutely ill, the resident is transferred to the hospital for treatment. You may be involved in these aspects of the resident's care:

- Maintaining bedrest or a limited activity program
- Measuring intake and output
- Measuring weight daily
- Restricting fluids as ordered by the doctor
- Giving good skin care to prevent skin breakdown
- Performing range-of-motion exercises
- Assisting with transfers or ambulation
- Assisting with self-care activities
- Maintaining good body alignment
- Applying elastic stockings

The older person is at risk for skin breakdown. Tissue swelling, poor circulation, and fragile skin combine to increase the risk of pressure ulcers. Good skin care and regular position changes are essential.

URINARY SYSTEM DISORDERS

The kidneys, ureters, bladder, and urethra are the major urinary system structures. Disorders can occur in one or more of these structures.

Urinary Tract Infections

Urinary tract infections (UTIs) are common. They can occur in the bladder or in a kidney. Infection in one area can lead to infection of the entire system. Normally the urinary system is sterile. It has no pathogens or nonpathogens. Microbes can enter the urinary system through the urethra. Catheterization, urological examinations, sexual intercourse, poor perineal hygiene, and poor fluid intake are common causes. UTI is a common nosocomial infection (see Chapter 9).

Women are at greater risk for UTIs than men. Women have a shorter urethra, which microbes can easily enter. In men, prostate gland secretions offer protection from UTIs. An enlarged prostate increases the risk of a UTI. Therefore older men are at risk.

Cystitis. Cystitis is inflammation *(itis)* of the bladder *(cyst)*. It is caused by bacteria. The person may have one or more of the following:

- Urinary frequency
- Urgency
- Dysuria—difficult or painful *(dys)* urination *(uria)*
- Pain
- Foul-smelling urine
- Hematuria—blood *(hemat)* in the urine *(uria)*
- Pyuria—pus *(py)* in the urine *(uria)*

Antibiotics are the treatment of choice. Persons also are encouraged to drink at least 2000 ml of fluids per day.

Pyelonephritis. Pyelonephritis is inflammation *(itis)* of the kidney *(nephr)* pelvis *(pyelo)*. Infection is the most common cause. Chills, fever, back pain, and nausea and vomiting occur. So do the signs and symptoms of cystitis. Treatment consists of antibiotics and fluids.

Renal Calculi

Renal calculi are kidney *(renal)* stones *(calculi)*. White men between the ages of 20 and 40 have the greatest risk. Bedrest and immobility also are risk factors. Stones vary in size. Signs and symptoms include:

- Severe, cramping pain in the back and side; pain can occur also in the abdomen, thigh, and urethra
- Nausea and vomiting
- Fever and chills
- Dysuria—difficult or painful *(dys)* urination *(uria)*
- Urinary frequency and urgency
- Oliguria—scant *(olig)* urine *(uria)*
- Hematuria—blood *(hemat)* in the urine *(uria)*

Treatment involves pain relief and encouraging fluids. The resident needs to drink about 4000 ml of fluid a day. Encouraging fluids helps promote passage of the stone through the urine. All urine is strained (see Chapter 16). Surgical removal of the stone may be necessary.

Renal Failure

In renal failure (kidney failure) the kidneys do not function or are severely impaired. Waste products are not removed from the blood. Fluids are retained in the body. Heart failure and hypertension easily result. Renal failure may be acute or chronic. The resident is very ill.

Acute renal failure. Acute renal failure occurs suddenly. Severe decreased blood flow to the kidneys is a common cause. The many causes of decreased blood flow to the kidneys include postoperative bleeding, bleeding from trauma, myocardial infarction (heart attack), severe congestive heart failure, burns, and severe allergic reactions. Persons with acute renal failure need hospital care.

At first the person has *oliguria* (scant amount of urine). Urine output is less than 400 ml in 24 hours. This is followed by *anuria* (absence of urine). It can last a few days to 2 weeks. Then diuresis occurs. *Diuresis* means the process *(esis)* of passing *(di)* the urine *(ur)*. Large amounts of urine are produced. Urine output ranges from 1000 to 5000 ml a day. Kidney function improves and returns to normal during the recovery phase. This phase can take anywhere from 1 month to 1 year. Some persons develop chronic renal failure.

Every system is affected by the buildup of waste products in the blood. Death can occur.

The doctor orders drug therapy, restricted fluids, and diet therapy. The person's diet is low in protein, high in carbohydrates, and low in potassium. The health care team plans for the person's physical and psychological needs. The person's care plan is likely to include:

- Measuring and recording urine output every hour; an output of less than 30 ml per hour is reported to the nurse immediately
- Measuring and recording intake and output every shift
- Restricting fluid intake
- Daily weight measurements using the same scale
- Turning and repositioning at least every 2 hours
- Measures to prevent pressure ulcers
- Frequent oral hygiene
- Measures to prevent infection
- Coughing and deep breathing exercises
- Measures to meet the person's emotional needs

Chronic renal failure. In chronic renal failure the kidneys cannot meet the body's needs. Nephrons of the kidney are slowly destroyed over many years. Hypertension and diabetes are the most common causes. Infections, urinary tract obstructions, and tumors are other causes.

Signs and symptoms appear when 80% to 90% of kidney function is lost. Every body system is affected by the buildup of waste products in the blood. Box 26-13 lists some of the signs and symptoms that occur.

Treatment includes fluid restriction, diet therapy, drugs, and dialysis. **Dialysis** is the process of removing waste products from the blood (see Chapter 16). It is a complex process. Specially trained nurses perform the procedure. Some residents have a kidney transplant.

Nursing measures for the resident in chronic renal failure are listed in Box 26-14.

ENDOCRINE SYSTEM DISORDERS

The endocrine system is made up of glands. The endocrine glands secrete hormones that affect other organs and glands. The most common endocrine disorder is diabetes mellitus.

Diabetes Mellitus

In diabetes mellitus the body cannot use sugar properly. Insulin is needed for the proper use of sugar. Insulin is secreted by the pancreas. In this disorder the pancreas does not secrete enough insulin. Sugar builds up in the blood. Cells do not have enough sugar for energy. Therefore cells cannot perform their functions.

Diabetes mellitus occurs in children and adults. Risk factors include obesity and a family history of diabetes. The risk increases after age 40.

Box 26-13 Signs and Symptoms of Chronic Renal Failure

- Yellow, tan, or dusky skin
- Dry, itchy skin
- Thin, brittle skin
- Bruises
- Bad breath (halitosis)
- Stomatitis (inflammation of the mouth)
- Nausea and vomiting
- Loss of appetite
- Diarrhea or constipation
- Bleeding tendencies
- Susceptibility to infection
- Hypertension
- Heart failure
- Gastric ulcers
- Irregular pulse
- Abnormal breathing patterns
- Burning sensation in the legs and feet
- Muscle twitching
- Leg cramps at night
- Fatigue
- Headache
- Convulsions
- Confusion
- Coma

Box 26-14 Care of the Resident in Chronic Renal Failure

- A diet low in protein, potassium, and sodium
- Fluid restriction
- Measuring blood pressure in the supine, sitting, and standing positions
- Measuring weight daily (with the same scale)
- Measuring and recording intake and output
- Turning and repositioning
- Measures to prevent pressure ulcers
- Range-of-motion exercises
- Measures to prevent itching (bath oils, lotions, and creams)
- Measures to prevent injury and bleeding
- Frequent oral hygiene
- Measures to prevent infection
- Measures to prevent diarrhea or constipation
- Measures to meet the resident's emotional needs
- Measures to promote rest

There are three types of diabetes mellitus:

- *Insulin-dependent diabetes (IDDM, or type 1)*—occurs most often in children and young adults. The pancreas does not secrete insulin. The person needs daily insulin injections. Onset is rapid.
- *Non-insulin-dependent diabetes (NIDDM, or type 2)*—occurs in adults over 40 years of age. The pancreas secretes insulin. However, the body cannot use it effectively. Onset is slow.
- *Gestational diabetes mellitus (GDM)*—develops during pregnancy. (Gestation comes from the Latin word *gestare, which* means to *bear.*) It usually disappears after the baby is born. However, the woman is at risk for NIDDM.

Signs and symptoms include increased urine production, increased thirst, hunger, weight loss, and extreme tiredness. Blurred vision is common. Frequent infections and slow healing of sores are common in persons with NIDDM. In both types, blood tests show increased sugar levels.

If diabetes is not controlled, complications occur. These include blindness, renal failure, nerve damage, hypertension, and circulatory disorders. Circulatory disorders can lead to stroke, heart attack, and slow wound healing. Foot and leg wounds are very serious (see Chapter 14). Infection and gangrene can occur and require amputation of the part.

Risk factors include a family history of the disease. Obesity is also a risk factor. Blacks, Hispanics, and Native Americans are at risk. So are older persons.

Insulin-dependent diabetes is treated with daily insulin therapy, diet, and exercise. The amount of sugar in the diet is limited (see Chapter 18). Meals are served on time to balance insulin needs. The doctor may order between-meal nourishments (see Chapter 18). Remember, food raises the blood sugar, and insulin lowers blood sugar. The person needs to eat all foods served.

Non-insulin-dependent diabetes is treated with diet and exercise. Calories and sugar in the diet are restricted. Overweight persons need to lose weight. Oral medications may be ordered. Some persons need insulin.

Both types require blood glucose monitoring. Good foot care is very important. Corns, blisters, and calluses on the feet can lead to an infection and amputation.

Hypoglycemia (insulin shock) occurs with too much insulin. **Hypoglycemia** means low *(hypo)* sugar *(glyc)* in the blood *(emia).* Hyperglycemia (diabetic coma) develops if a person does not get enough insulin. **Hyperglycemia** means high *(hyper)* sugar *(glyc)* in the blood *(emia).* Table 26-1 lists the causes, signs, and symptoms of hypoglycemia and hyperglycemia. Both can lead to death if not corrected.

DIGESTIVE DISORDERS

The digestive system breaks down food for absorption by the body. It also eliminates solid wastes. Some digestive disorders are discussed in Chapter 17: diarrhea, constipation, flatulence, fecal incontinence, and care of residents with colostomies and ileostomies.

Vomiting

Vomiting is the act of expelling stomach contents through the mouth. It is a sign of illness or injury. It can be life threatening. The vomitus (material vomited) can be aspirated and obstruct the airway. Shock also can occur if large amounts of blood are vomited. The following measures are practiced:

- Use Standard Precautions, and follow the Bloodborne Pathogen Standard.
- Turn the resident's head well to one side. This prevents aspiration.
- Place a kidney basin under the resident's chin.
- Remove the vomitus from the resident's immediate environment.
- Provide for oral hygiene. This helps eliminate the taste of vomitus.
- Eliminate odors.
- Change linens as necessary.
- Observe vomitus for color, odor, and undigested food. Vomitus that looks like coffee grounds contains digested blood. This indicates bleeding.
- Measure the amount of vomitus. Report the amount to the nurse. Note the amount on the I&O record.
- Save a specimen for laboratory study.
- Do not discard vomitus until it is observed by the nurse.

COMMUNICABLE DISEASES

Communicable diseases (contagious or infectious diseases) can be transmitted from one person to another. They are transmitted in the following ways:

- Direct—from the infected person
- Indirect—from dressings, linens, or surfaces
- Airborne—from the person through sneezing or coughing
- Vehicle—through ingestion of contaminated food, water, drugs, blood, or fluids
- Vector—from animals, fleas, and ticks

This section discusses hepatitis, AIDS, and sexually transmitted diseases. Standard Precautions and Transmission-Based Precautions are followed.

TABLE 26-1 HYPOGLYCEMIA AND HYPERGLYCEMIA

	Causes	Signs and Symptoms
Hypoglycemia (insulin shock)	Too much insulin Omitting a meal Eating too little food Increased exercise Vomiting	Hunger Weakness Trembling Perspiration Headache Dizziness Rapid pulse Low blood pressure Confusion Cold, clammy skin Convulsions Unconsciousness
Hyperglycemia (diabetic coma)	Undiagnosed diabetes Not enough insulin Eating too much food Too little exercise Stress (e.g., from surgery, illness, emotional upset)	Weakness Drowsiness Thirst Hunger Frequent urination Flushed face Sweet breath odor Slow, deep, and labored respirations Rapid, weak pulse Low blood pressure Dry skin Headache Nausea and vomiting Coma

Hepatitis

Hepatitis is an inflammation of the liver. The major types of hepatitis are:

- *Hepatitis A*—is spread by the fecal-oral route. Food, water, or drinking or eating vessels can be contaminated with feces. The virus is ingested when eating or drinking contaminated food or water. It is ingested also when eating or drinking from a contaminated vessel. Causes include poor sanitation, crowded living conditions, poor nutrition, and poor hygiene. Handle bedpans, feces, and rectal thermometers carefully. Good handwashing is essential for everyone.
- *Heptatitis B*—is caused by the hepatitis B virus (HBV). The virus is present in blood and body fluids (saliva, semen, vaginal secretions) of infected persons. It is transmitted by needle sharing among IV drug users. The virus is spread also by sexual contact, especially anal sex. (The HBV vaccine is discussed in Chapter 9.)
- *Hepatitis C*—is caused by a virus spread through needle sharing and sexual contact.
- *Hepatitis D*—occurs in persons infected with HBV. Persons who receive frequent blood transfusions are at risk.
- *Hepatitis E*—occurs in countries with poor sanitation. It is spread by the fecal-oral route.

Hepatitis can be mild or can cause death. The signs and symptoms of hepatitis are listed in Box 26-15 on p. 614. Treatment involves bedrest and a healthy diet. The person is not allowed to drink alcohol. Full recovery takes about 8 weeks.

You must protect yourself and others from the hepatitis virus. Standard Precautions and the Bloodborne Pathogen Standard are followed. Transmission-Based Precautions are ordered as necessary (see Chapter 9).

Box 26-15 Signs and Symptoms of Hepatitis

- Loss of appetite
- Weakness, fatigue, exhaustion
- Nausea and vomiting
- Fever
- Skin rash
- Dark urine
- Jaundice (yellowish color to the skin and whites of the eyes)
- Light-colored stools
- Headache
- Chills
- Abdominal pain
- Muscle aches

Acquired Immunodeficiency Syndrome

Acquired immunodeficiency syndrome (AIDS) is caused by a virus. The virus is called the human immunodeficiency virus (HIV). The virus attacks the immune system. The person's ability to fight other diseases is affected. AIDS has no cure at present. It eventually leads to death.

The virus is spread through certain body fluids—blood, semen, vaginal secretions, and breast milk. HIV is not spread by saliva, tears, sweat, sneezing, coughing, insects, or casual contact. AIDS is transmitted mainly by:

- Unprotected anal, vaginal, or oral sex with an infected person ("unprotected" is without a latex condom)
- Needle-sharing among IV drug users
- HIV-infected mothers before or during childbirth
- HIV-infected mothers through breast feeding

The virus enters the bloodstream through the rectum, vagina, penis, or mouth. Small breaks in the mucous membrane of the vagina or rectum may occur when the penis, finger, or other objects are inserted. Gum disease can cause breaks in the mucous membrane of the gums. The breaks in the mucous membranes of the mouth, vagina, or rectum provide a route for the virus to enter their bloodstreams.

Intravenous drug users transmit AIDS through the use of contaminated needles and syringes. The virus is carried in the contaminated blood left in needles or syringes. When needles and syringes are used by others, contaminated blood enters their bloodstream.

Infection can occur also when infected body fluids come in contact with open areas on the skin. Babies can become infected during pregnancy, shortly after birth, or from breast feeding.

The virus is very fragile. It cannot live outside the body. Therefore HIV is not spread by casual, everyday contact. Such contact includes using public telephones, restrooms, or water fountains. Other forms of casual contact include talking to, hugging, or dancing with an infected person. HIV is not transmitted by food prepared by the infected person.

Signs and symptoms of AIDS are listed in Box 26-16. Some persons infected with HIV do not develop AIDS for as long as 10 to 15 years. They may not show signs or symptoms of the disease. However, they are carriers of the virus. They can spread the disease to others.

Persons with AIDS develop other diseases. Their bodies do not have the ability to fight disease. Their immune systems, which fights diseases, are damaged. The person is at risk for pneumonia, tuberculosis, Kaposi's sarcoma (a type of cancer), and central nervous system damage. The person with central nervous system damage may show memory loss, loss of coordination, paralysis, mental health disorders, and dementia.

You may care for residents with AIDS or who are HIV carriers (Box 26-17). You may have contact with the resident's blood and body fluids. Mouth-to-mouth contact is possible during CPR. Certain precautions are necessary to protect yourself and others from the AIDS virus. Standard Precautions and the Bloodborne Pathogen Standard are followed. *These precautions apply when caring for all residents.* Remember that you may care for a resident who has the HIV virus but shows no symptoms. You may also care for a resident who has not yet been diagnosed as having AIDS.

AIDS is often viewed as a young person's disease. People often think that older persons do not use IV drugs and that they are not sexually active. Therefore older people are not considered to be at risk for AIDS. Also many older persons do not consider themselves to be at risk. They do not practice safe sex. Except for childbirth and breast feeding, older persons do get and spread AIDS in the same ways as younger persons.

In older persons, the disease is often missed during diagnosis. Aging and other diseases can mask the signs and symptoms of AIDS. Often the person dies without the disease being diagnosed.

Box 26-16 Signs and Symptoms of Acquired Immunodeficiency Syndrome (AIDS)

- Loss of appetite
- Weight loss
- Fever
- Night sweats
- Diarrhea
- Painful or difficulty swallowing
- Tiredness, extreme or constant
- Skin rashes
- Swollen glands in the neck, underarms, and groin
- Cough
- Sores or white patches in the mouth or on the tongue
- Purple blotches or bumps on the skin that look like bruises but do not disappear
- Confusion
- Forgetfulness
- Dementia (see Chapter 27)

Box 26-17 Caring for the Resident With AIDS

- Practice Standard Precautions.
- Follow the Bloodborne Pathogen Standard.
- Provide daily hygiene. Avoid harsh soaps that irritate the skin.
- Provide oral hygiene before meals and at bedtime. Make sure the resident uses a toothbrush with soft bristles.
- Provide oral fluids as ordered.
- Measure and record intake and output.
- Measure weight daily.
- Have the resident perform deep breathing and coughing exercises as ordered.
- Practice measures to prevent pressure ulcers.
- Assist with range-of-motion exercises and ambulation as ordered.
- Encourage the resident to perform self-care as able. The resident may need assistive devices (walker, commode, eating devices).
- Encourage the resident to be as active as possible.
- Change linens, gowns, or pajamas as often as needed when fever is present.
- Be a good listener, and provide emotional support.

Sexually Transmitted Diseases

Sexually transmitted diseases (STDs) are spread by sexual contact (Table 26-2, p. 616). Some people are not aware of being infected. Others know but do not seek treatment. Embarrassment is a common reason for not seeking treatment.

The genital area is usually associated with STDs. However, other areas may be involved. These areas include the rectum, ears, mouth, nipples, throat, tongue, eyes, and nose. Most STDs are spread by sexual contact. The use of condoms helps prevent the spread of STDs. The use of condoms is very important for preventing the spread of HIV and AIDS. Some STDs are spread also through a break in the skin, by contact with infected body fluids (blood, sperm, saliva), or by contaminated blood or needles.

Standard Precautions are necessary. The Bloodborne Pathogen Standard also is followed.

MENTAL HEALTH DISORDERS

The whole person has physical, social, psychological, and spiritual parts. Each part affects the other. A physical problem has social, mental, and spiritual effects. Likewise, mental health problems affect the person physically, socially, and spiritually. A social problem can have physical, mental health, and spiritual effects.

Mental relates to the mind. It is something that exists in the mind or is done by the mind. Therefore mental health involves the mind. Definitions of mental

Table 26-2 Sexually Transmitted Diseases

Disease	Signs and Symptoms	Treatment
Genital herpes	Painful, fluid-filled sores on or near the genitalia (Fig. 26-39) The sores may have a watery discharge Itching, burning, and tingling in the genital area Fever Swollen glands	No known cure Medications can be given to control discomfort
Venereal warts	Male—Warts appear on the penis, anus, or genitalia Female—Warts appear near the vagina, cervix, and labia	Application of special ointment that causes the warts to dry up and fall off Surgical removal may be necessary if the ointment is not effective
AIDS (acquired immunodeficiency syndrome)	See pp. 614-615	See pp. 614-615
Gonorrhea	Burning on urination Urinary frequency and urgency Vaginal discharge in the female Urethral discharge in the male	Antibiotic medications
Syphilis	*Stage 1*—10 to 90 days after exposure Painless chancre on the penis, in the vagina, or on genitalia; the chancre may also be on the lips or inside the mouth or anywhere else on the body *Stage 2*—About 2 months after the chancre General fatigue, loss of appetite, nausea, fever, headache, rash, sore throat, bone and joint pain, hair loss, lesions on the lips and genitalia *Stage 3*—3 to 15 years after infection Damage to the cardiovascular system and central nervous system, blindness	Antibiotic medications

A

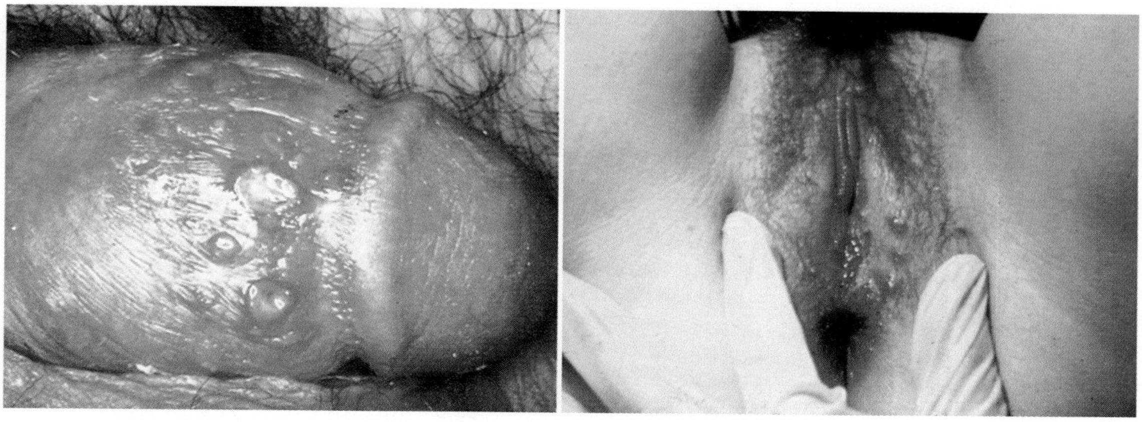

B

Fig. 26-39 Genital herpes. **A,** Sores on the penis. **B,** Sores on the perineum. *(Courtesy USPHS, Washington, D.C.)*

health and mental illness vary among textbooks and cultures. Most definitions include the concept of stress. In this textbook, these definitions are used:

- **Stress**—the response or change in the body caused by any emotional, physical, social, or economic factor.
- **Mental health**—a state of mind in which the person copes with and adjusts to the stresses of everyday living in ways acceptable to society.
- **Mental illness**—a disturbance in the person's ability to cope or adjust to stress. The person's behavior and functioning are impaired. **Mental disorder, emotional illness**, and **psychiatric disorder** also mean mental illness.

Mental health disorders have many causes. Some result when the person cannot cope or adjust to stress. Others are caused by chemical imbalances in the body. Some are genetic in origin. (Genes are found in chromosomes. Characteristics from parents are passed onto children through genes contained in the chromosomes.) Other causes include drug or substance abuse. Social and cultural factors also can lead to mental illness.

Anxiety Disorders

Anxiety is a vague, uneasy feeling. It is a response to stress. The person may not know the source or cause of the uneasy feeling. The person has a sense of danger or harm. Danger or harm is real or imagined. Anxiety is usually a normal emotion. The person acts to relieve the unpleasant feeling. Anxiety generally occurs when the person's needs are not met. Anxiety is seen in all mental health disorders.

The many signs and symptoms of anxiety are listed in Box 26-18, p. 618. They depend on the degree of anxiety. Persons with mental health disorders have higher levels of anxiety.

Anxiety level depends on the stressor. A **stressor** is any emotional, physical, social, or economic factor that causes stress. Past experiences with the same or a similar stressor affect how a person reacts. The number of stressors also affects the person's reaction. A stressor at one time in a person's life may produce only mild anxiety. The same stressor may produce a higher level of anxiety at another time.

Coping and defense mechanisms are used to relieve anxiety. Common coping mechanisms include eating, drinking, smoking, exercising, talking about the problem, and fighting. Some people play music, go for a walk, take a hot bath, or want to be alone. Some coping mechanisms are healthier than others.

Defense mechanisms are unconscious reactions that block unpleasant or threatening feelings. Defense mechanisms protect the ego. They are used by everyone. Some use of defense mechanisms is normal. They relieve anxiety. Persons with mental health disorders use defense mechanisms poorly. Box 26-19, p. 618 describes the common defense mechanisms.

Panic disorder.

Panic is the highest level of anxiety. **Panic** is an intense and sudden feeling of fear, anxiety, terror, or dread. It occurs suddenly with no obvious reason. The person cannot function and has severe signs and symptoms of anxiety. *Panic attacks* can last for a few minutes or for hours. They can occur several times a week.

Phobic disorders.

Phobia means fear, panic, or dread. The person with a phobia has an intense fear of an object or situation. Common phobias are described in Box 26-20, p. 619.

Box 26-18 Signs and Symptoms of Anxiety

- A "lump" in the throat
- "Butterflies" in the stomach
- Rapid pulse
- Rapid respirations
- Increased blood pressure
- Rapid speech
- Voice changes
- Dry mouth
- Perspiration
- Nausea
- Diarrhea
- Urinary frequency
- Urinary urgency
- Poor attention span
- Difficulty following directions
- Difficulty sleeping
- Loss of appetite

Box 26-19 Defense Mechanisms

Compensation—to compensate means to make up for, replace, or substitute. Compensation means to make up for or substitute a strength for a weakness.

Example: A boy is not good in sports. But he learns to play the guitar well.

Conversion—to convert means to change. Conversion is when an emotion is expressed or changed into a physical symptom.

Example: A girl knows she will have to read out loud in school today. She does not want to go to school. She complains of a stomachache.

Denial—to deny means to refuse to accept or believe something that is true or correct. Denial is when the person refuses to face or accept something that is unpleasant or threatening.

Example: A man had a heart attack. He is told to quit smoking and to eat a low-fat diet. He continues to smoke and eat fatty foods.

Displacement—to displace means to move or take the place of. Displacement is when an individual moves behaviors or emotions from one person, place, or thing to another person, place, or thing. The behavior or emotion is directed at a safe person, place, or thing.

Example: You are angry with your supervisor. Instead of yelling at your supervisor, you yell at a friend.

Identification—to identify means to relate or recognize. Identification is when a person assumes the ideas, behaviors, and traits of another person.

Example: A little girl admires her neighbor who is a high school cheerleader. The little girl practices cheerleading in her back yard.

Projection—to project means to blame or assign responsibility to another. Projection is blaming another person or object for one's own unacceptable behavior, emotions, ideas, or wishes.

Example: Two girls are in the same class. One fails a test. She blames the other girl for not helping her study.

Rationalization—to rationalize means to give some acceptable reason or excuse for one's behavior or actions. The real reason is not given. Rational means sensible, reasonable, or logical.

Example: A student does not study for a test and gets a poor grade. She says that the teacher is too hard and does not like her.

Reaction formation—a person acts in a way that is opposite to what he or she truly feels.

Example: A man does not like his boss. He buys the boss an expensive gift for Christmas.

Regression—to regress means to move back or to retreat. Regression means to retreat or move back to an earlier time or condition.

Example: A 3-year-old wants to drink from a baby bottle when a new baby comes into the family.

Repression—to repress means to hold down or keep back. Repression is keeping unpleasant or painful thoughts or experiences from the conscious mind. Such thoughts and experiences are in the unconscious mind and cannot be recalled or remembered.

Example: A little girl was sexually abused by her father. She is now 33 years old and has no memory of the event.

Box 26-20 Common Phobias

Agoraphobia—*agora* means marketplace. *Fear of being in an open, crowded, or public place.*

Algophobia—*algo* means pain. *Fear of being in pain or seeing others in pain.*

Aquaphobia—*aqua* means water. *Fear of water.*

Claustrophobia—*claustro* means closing. *Fear of being in or being trapped in an enclosed or narrow space.*

Gynephobia—*gyne* means woman. *Fear of women.*

Laliophobia—*lalio* means to talk or babble. *Fear of talking because of the fear of stuttering.*

Mysophobia—*myso* means anything that is disgusting. *Fear of the slightest uncleanliness; fear of dirt or contamination.*

Nyctophobia—*nycto* means night or darkness. *Fear of night or darkness.*

Photophobia—*photo* pertains to light. *Fear of light with the need to avoid light places.*

Pyrophobia—*pyro* means fire. *Fear of fire.*

Xenophobia—*xeno* means strange. *Fear of strangers.*

Obsessive-compulsive disorder. An **obsession** is a persistent thought or idea. The thought or idea may be violent. **Compulsion** is the uncontrolled performance of an act. The person knows the act is wrong but has much anxiety if the act is not done. Some eating disorders are obsessive-compulsive. The person is obsessed with thoughts of food and eats constantly. Constant handwashing because of mysophobia (fear of dirt or contamination) is another. Some obsessive-compulsive disorders involve violent acts.

Schizophrenia

Schizophrenia means split *(schizo)* mind *(phrenia)*. You need to know the following terms to understand schizophrenia:

- **Psychosis** means a serious mental disorder. The person does not view or interpret reality correctly.
- **Delusion** is a false belief. A person believes he or she is God, a movie star, or some other person.
- **Hallucination** is seeing, hearing, or feeling something that is not real. A person may see animals, insects, or people that are not present.
- **Paranoia** means a disorder *(para)* of the mind *(noia)*. The person has false beliefs (delusions) and is suspicious about a person or situation. For example, a person believes his or her food and drinks are poisoned.
- **Delusion of grandeur** is an exaggerated belief about one's own importance, wealth, power, or talents. For example, a man believes he is Superman or a woman believes she is the Queen of England.
- **Delusion of persecution** is the false belief that one is mistreated, abused, or harassed. For example, a person believes that someone is "out to get" him or her.

The person with schizophrenia has a disorder of the mind (psychosis). Thinking and behavior are disturbed. The person has delusions (false beliefs) and hallucinations (seeing, hearing, or feeling things that are not real). The person has difficulty relating to others and may be paranoid (suspicion about a person or situation). The person's responses are inappropriate. Communication is disturbed. The person may ramble or repeat what another says. Sometimes speech is not understood. The person may withdraw from others and the world. That is, the person lacks interest in others and is not involved with people or society. The person may sit for hours alone without moving, speaking, or responding. Some persons *regress*. To regress means to retreat or move back to an earlier time or condition. For example, it is normal for a 5-year-old to regress back to bedwetting when a new baby comes into the family. It is not normal for an adult to have the behaviors of an infant or child. However, that is often seen in schizophrenia.

Affective Disorders

Affect relates to feelings and emotions. Affective disorders involve feelings, emotions, and moods. There are two major affective disorders.

Bipolar disorder. *Bipolar* means two *(bi)* poles or ends *(polar)*. The person with bipolar disorder has extreme mood swings. Depression is at one extreme. Mania (elation) is at the other extreme. The person may:

- Be more depressed than manic
- Be more manic than depressed
- Alternate between depression and mania

When depressed, the person is very sad and feels lonely, worthless, empty, and hopeless. Self-esteem is low. The person may think about suicide.

In the manic phase, the person is excited, has much energy, and is very busy. The person cannot sleep and does not take time to eat or tend to self-care needs. Delusions of grandeur are common.

Major depression. The person is very unhappy, lacks motivation, and feels unwanted. These feelings are extreme. Problems with concentration occur. Body functions are depressed. Sleeping problems and inactivity are common. Constipation can occur.

Personality Disorders

The individual with a personality disorder has rigid, inflexible, and maladaptive behaviors. To *adapt* means to change or adjust. *Mal* means bad, wrong, or ill. *Maladaptive* means to change or adjust in the wrong way. Because of their behaviors, individuals with a personality disorder cannot function well in society. Personality disorders include:

- ***Abusive personality***—the person copes with anxiety by abusing others. Behavior may be violent.
- ***Paranoid personality***—the person is very suspicious. There is distrust of others.
- ***Antisocial personality***—the person has poor judgment, lacks responsibility, and is hostile. The person has no loyalty to any person or group. Morals and ethics are lacking. The person blames others for actions and behaviors. The rights of others are not considered. The person has no guilt and does not learn from past experiences or punishment. The person is often in trouble with law enforcement authorities.

Care of Persons With Mental Health Disorders

Treatment of mental health disorders involves having the person explore his or her thoughts and feelings. This is done through psychotherapy, group therapy, occupational therapy, art therapy, and family therapy. Often drugs are ordered for anxiety or depression.

The nurse uses the nursing process to meet the person's needs. The needs of the total person must be met. This includes the person's physical, safety and security, and emotional needs.

Communication is important. Be alert to nonverbal communication. This includes the person's nonverbal communication and your own.

Quality of Life

A resident may have one or many disorders described in this chapter. For example, a resident may have arthritis, diabetes, heart disease, and osteoporosis. Problems increase if a fracture occurs. The resident is then at risk for infection, pneumonia, and the complications of bedrest. The amount of care required depends on the nature of the problem and the number of problems a resident has.

Only very basic information is given about each disorder. Entire textbooks are written on many of these disorders. You are not expected to have an in-depth understanding of your residents' diagnoses. However, the information in this chapter will help you better understand your resident's physical, psychological, and social needs.

The care you give affects the quality of life for persons with the health problems described in this chapter. The care you give them was presented in previous chapters. Safety, good alignment, turning and repositioning, preventing infection, skin care, urinary and bowel elimination, and nutrition are some examples. Quality-of-life issues discussed for such care also apply to the care of residents with these common health problems.

Respecting the resident's right to privacy and confidentiality is very important. Remember to discuss the resident's problems only with the nurse and health care team members involved in the resident's care. You are not responsible for giving information to families and visitors. You must not discuss your residents outside the center. Your own family and friends should not hear about the residents.

The right to personal choice is protected. Always explain what you are going to do. The resident's consent is necessary. Also involve the resident in deciding when to begin care or procedures.

Always protect the resident's right to be free from abuse, mistreatment, and neglect. This is very important for residents with a communicable disease. Health care team members may tend to avoid the resident because they fear getting the disease themselves. Following Standard Precautions and the Bloodborne Pathogen Standard protects others from contamination. You must treat all residents with dignity and respect.

REVIEW QUESTIONS

Circle the BEST answer.

1 Which is *not* a warning sign of cancer?
A Painful, swollen joints
B A sore that does not heal
C Unusual bleeding or discharge from a body opening
D Nagging cough or hoarseness

2 Martha Powers has arthritis. Care includes the following *except*
A Measures to prevent contractures
B Range-of-motion exercises
C A cast or traction
D Assistance with activities of daily living

3 A cast needs to dry. Which is *false?*
A The cast is covered with blankets or plastic.
B The resident is turned as directed so the cast dries evenly.
C The entire length of the cast is supported with pillows.
D The cast is supported by the palms when lifted.

4 A resident has a cast. Which are reported immediately?
A Pain, numbness, or inability to move the fingers or toes
B Chills, fever, or nausea and vomiting
C Odor, cyanosis, or temperature changes of the skin
D All of the above

5 A resident is in traction. You should do the following *except*
A Perform range-of-motion exercises as directed
B Keep the weights off the floor
C Remove the weights if the resident is uncomfortable
D Give skin care at frequent intervals

6 Mr. Doe had an amputation. Why will he have a psychological adjustment?
A Activities of daily living are affected.
B Appearance is affected.
C His life-style is affected.
D All of the above

7 After a hip pinning, the operated leg is
A Abducted at all times
B Adducted at all times
C Externally rotated at all times
D Flexed at all times

8 Martha Powers has osteoporosis. She is at risk for
A Fractures
B An amputation
C Phantom limb pain
D All of the above

9 A resident had a stroke. The nurse tells you to do the following. Which should you question?
A Elevate the head of the bed to a semi-Fowler's position.
B Do range-of-motion exercises every 2 hours.
C Turn, reposition, and give skin care every 2 hours.
D Keep the bed in the highest horizontal position.

10 Receptive aphasia means that the person
A Cannot talk
B Cannot write
C Has trouble understanding messages
D All of the above

11 A resident has Parkinson's disease. Which is *false?*
A Parkinson's disease affects part of the brain.
B The person's mental function is affected first.
C Signs and symptoms include stiff muscles, slow movements, and a shuffling gait.
D The person is protected from injury.

12 A resident has multiple sclerosis. Which is *false?*
A Nerve impulses are sent to and from the brain in a normal manner.
B Symptoms begin in young adulthood.
C There is no cure.
D The person is eventually paralyzed and totally dependent on others for care.

13 Residents with head or spinal cord injuries require
A Rehabilitation
B Speech therapy
C Long-term care
D Psychiatric care

14 Mr. Young has Meniere's disease. It is important to prevent
A Infection
B Falls
C Constipation
D All of the above

15 Mr. Young has hearing loss. You can do the following *except*
A State the topic of discussion
B Chew gum while talking
C Use short sentences and simple words
D Write out important names and words

16 A resident has a speech problem. You should
A Pretend to understand so the person is not embarrassed
B Have the person write out all messages
C Ask the person to repeat or rephrase statements when necessary
D All of the above

17 Mr. Young's hearing aid does not seem to work. First, you should
A See if it is turned on
B Wash the entire instrument with soap and water
C Have it repaired
D Remove the batteries

18 Mr. Young has a cataract. Which is *true?*
A Surgery is the only treatment.
B There is no cure.
C He will become blind.
D There is pressure in the eye.

19 Mr. Young is not wearing his eyeglasses. They should be
A Soaked in a cleansing solution
B Kept within his reach
C Put in the case and in the top drawer of the bedside stand
D Placed on the overbed table

20 Mr. Goldman is blind. You should do the following *except*
A Identify yourself when you enter the room
B Move equipment and furniture to provide variety
C Explain procedures step by step
D Have him walk behind you

21 You can provide for Mr. Goldman's safety by
A Keeping doors partially open
B Informing him of steps and curbs
C Rearranging furniture
D All of the above

22 A resident has emphysema. Which is *false?*
A The person has dyspnea only with activity.
B Cigarette smoking is the most common cause.
C The resident will probably breathe easier sitting upright and slightly forward.
D Sputum may contain pus.

23 A resident has hypertension. Which complication can occur?
A Stroke
B Heart attack
C Renal failure
D All of the above

24 A resident has hypertension. Treatment will probably include the following *except*
A No smoking and regular exercise
B A high-sodium diet
C A low-calorie diet if the person is obese
D Medications to lower the blood pressure

25 A resident has angina pectoris. Which is *true?*
A Damage to the heart muscle occurs.
B The pain is described as crushing, stabbing, or squeezing.
C The pain is relieved with rest and nitroglycerin.
D All of the above

26 A resident is having a myocardial infarction. You know that
A The resident is having a heart attack
B This is an emergency situation
C The resident may have a cardiac arrest
D All of the above

27 A resident has heart failure. The following measures are ordered. Which should you question?
A Encourage fluids
B Measure intake and output
C Measure weight daily
D Perform range-of-motion exercises

28 A resident has cystitis. This is
A A kidney infection
B Kidney stones
C A urinary tract infection
D An inflammation of the bladder

29 A resident has chronic renal failure. Care will include all of the following *except*
A A diet low in protein, potassium, and sodium
B Measuring urinary output every hour
C Measures to prevent pressure ulcers
D Measuring weight daily

30 Which is *not* a sign of diabetes mellitus?
A Increased urine production
B Weight gain
C Hunger
D Increased thirst

31 Martha Powers has diabetes. She needs all of the following *except*
A Her meals served on time
B Good foot care
C Oral insulin
D Diet therapy

32 Vomiting is dangerous. It can result in
A Aspiration
B Cardiac arrest
C Hypertension
D Stroke

33 AIDS and hepatitis require
A Airborne Precautions
B Droplet Precautions
C Standard Precautions
D Contact Precautions

34 AIDS is usually spread by contact with infected
A Blood
B Urine
C Tears
D Saliva

35 These statements are about HIV and AIDS. Which is *false?*
A Standard Precautions are practiced, and the Blood Pathogen Standard is followed.
B There may be signs and symptoms of central nervous system damage.
C The person is at risk for infection.
D The person always shows some signs and symptoms.

36 Which statement is *false?*
A STDs are usually spread by sexual contact.
B STDs can affect the genital area and other parts of the body.
C Signs and symptoms of STDs are always obvious.
D Some STDs result in death.

37 A person has a mental health problem. The doctor says that she is under stress. Stress is
A The way she copes with and adjusts to everyday living
B A response or change in the body caused by some factor
C A mental or emotional disorder
D A thought or idea

38 A person uses defense mechanisms. Defense mechanisms are used to
A Blame others
B Make excuses for behavior
C Return to an earlier time
D Block unpleasant feelings

39 A person has phobias. A phobia is
A A serious mental disorder
B A false belief
C An intense fear of an object or situation
D Feelings and emotions

40 A woman believes she is married to a rock singer. This is called a
A Fantasy
B Delusion of grandeur
C Delusion of persecution
D Hallucination

41 A person has bipolar disorder. This means that the person
A Is very suspicious
B Has poor judgment, lacks responsibility, and is hostile
C Is very unhappy and feels unwanted
D Has severe mood swings

42 A person has an abusive personality. You know that the person
A Abuses drugs or alcohol
B Has an eating disorder
C Has bulimia
D May have violent behavior

Answers to these questions are on pp. 699-700.

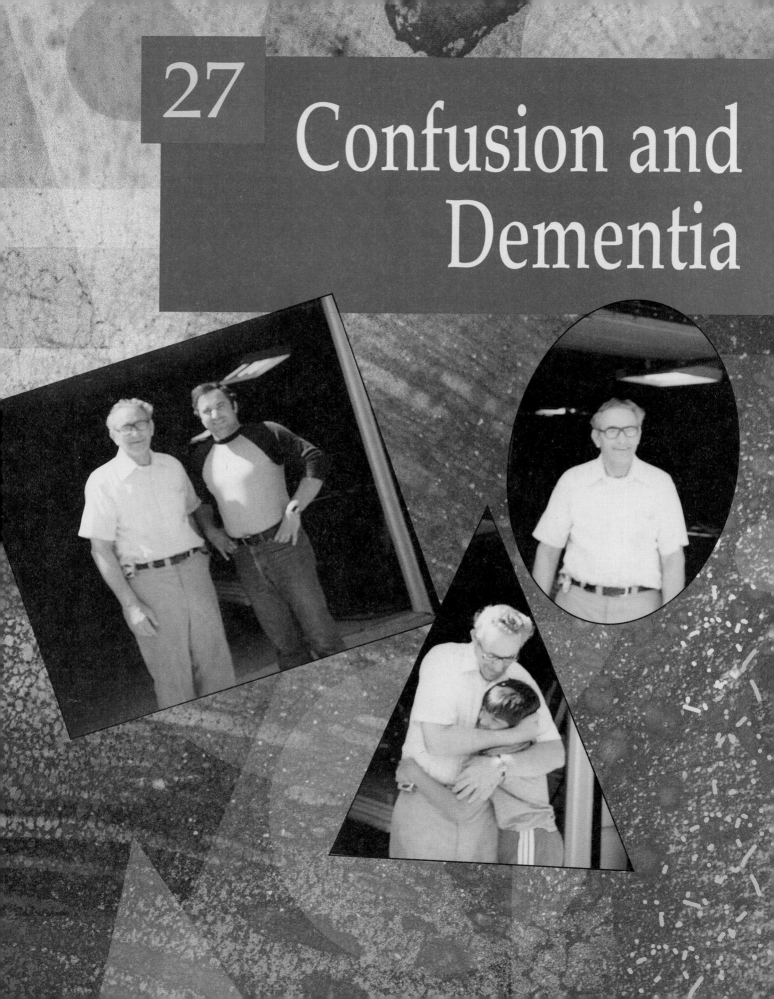

27

Confusion and Dementia

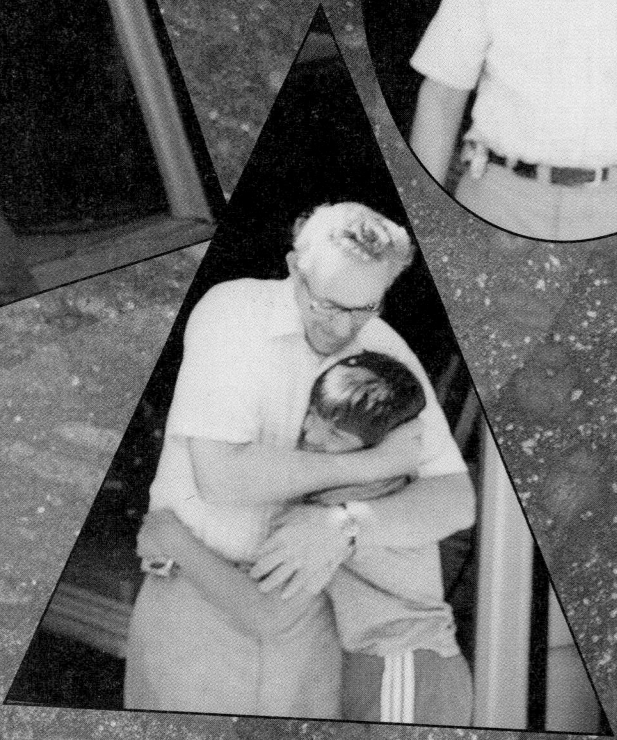

What You Will Learn

- The definition of the key terms listed in this chapter
- The definition of confusion and its causes
- The measures that help confused persons
- The difference between delirium, depression, and dementia
- How to describe Alzheimer's disease
- The signs, symptoms, and behaviors associated with Alzheimer's disease
- The care required by the resident with Alzheimer's disease and other dementia disorders
- The effects of Alzheimer's disease and other dementias on the family

Key Terms

delirium A state of temporary but acute mental confusion that comes on suddenly

delusion A false belief

dementia The term used to describe the loss of cognitive function (thinking, remembering, and reasoning) caused by changes in the brain

hallucination Seeing, hearing, or feeling something that is not real

pseudodementia False *(pseudo)* disorder of the mind *(dementia)*

sundowning Increased signs, symptoms, and behaviors of Alzheimer's disease during hours of darkness

Some changes in the brain and nervous system occur normally with aging (Box 27-1). Certain diseases can also cause changes in the brain. No matter the cause, changes in the brain can affect a person's cognitive function. (*Cognitive* relates to knowledge.) Cognitive functioning relates to memory, thinking, reasoning, ability to understand, judgment, and behavior. Quality of life is affected by a person's cognitive functioning. Many residents in nursing centers have a decrease in cognitive function.

Box 27-1 Changes in the Nervous System From Aging

- Loss of brain cells
- Slower nerve conduction
- Slower response and reaction times
- Slower reflexes
- Decreased vision and hearing
- Decreased senses of taste and smell
- Reduced sense of touch and sensitivity to pain
- Reduced blood flow to the brain
- Changes in sleep patterns
- Shorter memory
- Forgetfulness
- Confusion
- Dizziness

CONFUSION

Confusion has many causes. Diseases, infections, losses of hearing and sight, and reactions to medications are some major causes. Brain injury and physical changes from aging are other causes. With aging, there is reduced blood supply to the brain and progressive loss of brain cells. Sometimes personality and mental changes result. Memory and the ability to make good judgments are lost. A person may not know people, the time, or the place. There also may be gradual loss in the ability to perform activities of daily living.

Box 27-2 Caring for the Confused Resident

- Follow the resident's care plan to meet basic needs.
- Provide for the resident's safety.
- Call the resident by name every time you are in contact with him or her.
- State your name, and show your name tag.
- Tell the resident the date and time each morning. Repeat the information as often as necessary during the day or evening.
- Explain what you are going to do and why.
- Give clear and simple answers to questions.
- Ask clear and simple questions. Allow enough time for the resident to respond.
- Give short, simple instructions.
- Keep a calendar and a clock with large numbers in the resident's room and in nursing areas (Fig. 27-1).
- Encourage the resident to wear glasses and a hearing aid if needed.
- Use touch to communicate (see Chapter 5).
- Allow the resident to place familiar objects and pictures within view.
- Provide newspapers and magazines. Read to the resident if appropriate.
- Discuss current events with the resident.
- Provide access to television and radios.
- Maintain the day-night cycle. Open curtains, shades, and drapes during the day, and close them at night. Use a night-light at night. Encourage the resident to wear regular clothes during the day rather than a gown or pajamas.
- Maintain a calm, relaxed, and peaceful atmosphere. Prevent loud noises, rushing, and congested hallways and dining rooms.
- Maintain the resident's routine. Meals, bathing, exercise, television programs, and other activities are on a schedule. This promotes a sense of order and anticipation of what to expect.
- Do not rearrange furniture or the resident's belongings.
- Encourage the resident to participate in self-care activities.
- Be consistent.
- Remind the resident of holidays, birthdays, and other special events.

Behavior changes are common. Anger, restlessness, depression, and irritability may occur.

Acute confusion (delirium) occurs suddenly. Acute confusion is usually caused by infection, illness, injury, or drugs. It can occur after surgery. Treatment is aimed at the cause of the confusion. Usually acute confusion is temporary.

Confusion caused by physical changes cannot be cured. Some measures help to improve the person's functioning (Box 27-2). The person's physical and safety needs must be met.

DEMENTIA

Dementia is the term used to describe the loss of cognitive function (thinking, remembering, and reasoning) caused by changes in the brain. The prefix *de* means opposite, away, off of, to remove, down, or from. *Mentia* comes from the Latin word for mind. Alzheimer's disease is the most common type of dementia. Other types and causes of dementia are listed in Box 27-3.

Dementia is not a normal part of aging. Most people over age 60 never show signs of cognitive decline.

Box 27-3 Types and Causes of Dementia

- Alcohol-related dementia and Korsakoff's disease—alcohol has a toxic effect on brain cells
- AIDS-related dementia—see Chapter 26
- Brain tumors—see Chapter 26
- Cerebrovascular disease—diseased blood vessels *(vascular)* in the brain *(cerebro)*
- Delirium—a temporary state of acute confusion
- Depression—see p. 627
- Drugs—some drugs affect how the brain functions
- Huntington's disease—a nervous system disease
- Infection—see Chapter 9
- Multi-infarct dementia—many *(multi)* strokes leave areas of damage *(infarct)*
- Multiple sclerosis—see Chapter 26
- Parkinson's disease—see Chapter 26
- Pick's disease—a rare brain disorder
- Stroke—see Chapter 26
- Syphilis—see Chapter 26
- Trauma and head injury—see Chapter 26

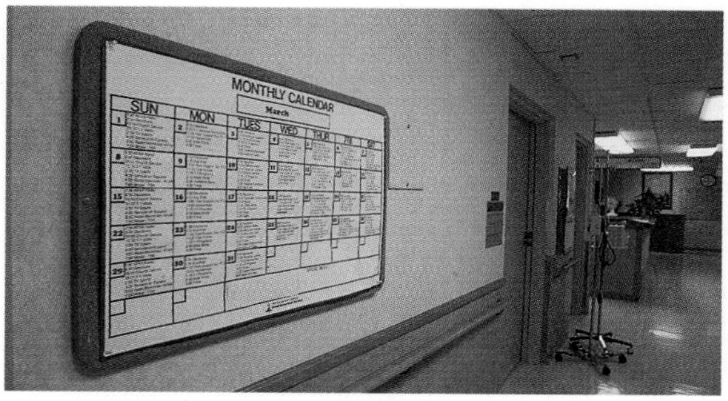

Fig. 27-1 A large calendar can help confused residents.

Dementia affects only a small number of older people. Some early warning signs of dementia are:
- Recent memory loss that affects job skills
- Difficulty with familiar tasks (e.g., dressing, cooking, driving)
- Problems with language; forgetting simple words
- Getting lost in familiar places
- Misplacing things and putting things in unusual places (e.g., putting a watch in the refrigerator)
- Changes in personality
- Poor or decreased judgement (e.g., going outdoors in the snow without shoes)
- Loss of interest in life

Persons with signs and symptoms of dementia need to see a doctor. To determine the cause and type of problem, the doctor orders many tests. Treatment depends on the cause and problem. Some dementias can be reversed. When the cause is removed, so are the signs and symptoms of dementia. Treatable causes include:
- Drugs
- Alcohol
- Delirium
- Depression
- Tumors
- Heart, lung, and blood vessel problems
- Head injuries
- Infection
- Vision and hearing problems

Permanent dementias result from changes in the brain. Parkinson's disease and cerebrovascular disease cause permanent changes in the brain. Multi-infarct dementia (MID) is caused by many *(multi)* strokes. The stroke leaves an area of damage called an *infarct.* Alzheimer's disease is the most common type of permanent dementia.

Permanent dementias have no cure. The loss of cognitive function becomes progressively worse. The rate at which it progresses varies.

Pseudodementia means false *(pseudo)* dementia. The person has the signs and symptoms of dementia. However, changes in the brain do not occur. This can occur with depression. Depression can be treated. It is very important that the correct diagnosis is made.

Delirium and Depression

Delirium and depression can be mistaken for dementia. They can occur alone or with dementia. Or the person with dementia can also suffer from delirium and depression.

Delirium.

Delirium is a state of temporary but acute mental confusion. It comes on suddenly. Delirium is common in older persons with an acute or chronic illness. Infections, heart and lung diseases, poor nutrition, and hormone disorders are common causes. Hypoglycemia is also a cause (see Chapter 26). Alcohol can cause delirium. So can many types of drugs. Delirium is an emergency. The cause must be identified and treated. Signs and symptoms of delirium include:
- Anxiety
- Disorientation
- Tremors
- Hallucinations (p. 628)
- Delusions (p. 628)
- Disturbances in attention
- Decline in level of consciousness

Depression.

Depression is the most common mental health problem in older persons. It is often overlooked when the person has physical problems. A correct diagnosis is important. Otherwise the person does not receive proper treatment. The person and family both experience unnecessary emotional, physical, social, and financial discomfort.

Some signs and symptoms of depression are also signs of aging. They also are the side effects of some drugs. Signs and symptoms of depression include:
- Sadness
- Inactivity
- Difficulty thinking
- Problems concentrating
- Feelings of despair
- Problems sleeping
- Changes in appetite
- Fatigue
- Agitation
- Withdrawal

ALZHEIMER'S DISEASE

Alzheimer's disease (AD) is a brain disease. Brain cells that control intellectual function are damaged. Memory, thinking, judgment, and behavior are affected. Mood and personality changes are seen. The person has difficulty with work and everyday functions. The person also has problems with family and social relationships.

Gradual in onset, the disease progresses over 3 to 20 years. It gets worse and worse. AD occurs in both men and women. Though more common in older persons, it also occurs in younger people. Some people in their 40s and 50s have AD. The risk increases after the age of 65. The cause is unknown. However, a family history of AD and Down syndrome are risk factors. (Down syndrome is a congenital disease [*congenital* means to be born with]. The child has mental retardation and many physical defects. See Chapter 28.)

Signs of AD

According to the Agency for Health Care Policy and Research, the classic sign of AD is gradual loss of short-term memory. Other early signs include:

- Problems finding or speaking the right word
- Not recognizing objects
- Forgetting how to use simple, everyday things (like using a pencil)
- Forgetting to turn off the stove, close windows, or lock doors
- Mood and personality changes
- Agitation
- Poor judgment

AD affects the person's ability to perform complex and simple tasks. Problems with complex tasks appear first. The person has problems using the telephone, driving a car, managing money, planning meals, and working. As the disease progresses, problems occur with simple tasks. The person has problems with bathing, dressing, eating, using the toilet, and walking.

Stages of Alzheimer's Disease

There are three stages of Alzheimer's disease (Box 27-4). Signs and symptoms become more severe with each stage. The disease ends in death. The following behaviors are common.

Wandering. Persons with Alzheimer's disease are disoriented to person, time, and place. They may wander from home or the center and not find their way back. They may be with caregivers one moment and gone the next. Judgment is poor. They cannot tell what is safe or dangerous. They are in danger of accidents. A person may walk into traffic or into a nearby river, lake, or forest. If not properly dressed, overexposure to heat and cold is a risk.

Sundowning. **Sundowning** occurs in the late afternoon and evening hours. As daylight ends and darkness occurs, confusion, restlessness, and other symptoms increase. The person's behavior is worse after the sun goes down. Sundowning may relate to being tired or hungry. Inadequate light may cause the person to see things that are not there. Persons with Alzheimer's disease may be afraid of the dark.

Hallucinations. A **hallucination** is seeing, hearing, or feeling something that is not really there. Senses are dulled. Affected persons see animals, insects, or people that are not present. Some hear voices. They may feel bugs crawling on their bodies or feel that they are being touched.

Delusions. **Delusions** are false beliefs. People with Alzheimer's disease may think they are God, a movie star, or some other person. Some believe they are in jail, are going to be murdered, or are being attacked. A person may believe that the caregiver is actually someone else. Many other false beliefs can occur.

Catastrophic reactions. Catastrophic reactions are extreme responses. The person reacts as if a disaster or tragedy has occurred. The person may scream or cry or be agitated or combative. These reactions often occur when the person has too many stimuli at one time. Eating, music or television playing, and being asked questions all at one time can overwhelm the person.

Agitation and restlessness. The agitated and restless person may pace, hit, or yell. Such behaviors may be caused by pain or discomfort, anxiety, lack of sleep, too much or too little stimulation, hunger, or the need to eliminate. A calm, quiet setting and meeting basic needs help calm the person.

Caregivers can cause agitation and restlessness. A caregiver may rush the person or be impatient. Or a caregiver's communication may be giving mixed verbal and nonverbal messages. Caregivers always need to look at how their behaviors affect other persons.

Aggression and combativeness. Aggressive and combative behaviors occur in some persons. They may result from agitation and restlessness. Examples include hitting, pinching, grabbing, biting, and swearing. Such behaviors are frightening to caregivers, other residents, and visitors. Sometimes aggressive and combative behaviors are part of the person's personality. Care approaches are found in the care plan. Also see Chapter 5 for dealing with the angry person and Chapter 8 for workplace violence.

Screaming. Persons with AD have communication problems. At first the person has difficulty finding the right words. As the AD progresses, the person may speak only short sentences or one word. Often the person's speech is not understandable.

The person may scream to communicate. Screaming is seen in persons who are very confused and have poor communication skills. The person may scream a word or a name. Or the person may just make screaming sounds.

Box 27-4 Stages of Alzheimer's Disease

Stage 1
- Memory loss—forgetfulness; forgets recent events
- Difficulty finding words, finishing thoughts, following directions, and remembering names
- Poor judgment; bad decisions (including when driving a motor vehicle)
- Disoriented to time and place
- Lack of spontaneity—less outgoing or interested in things
- Blames others for mistakes, forgetfulness, and other problems
- Moodiness
- Difficulty performing everyday tasks

Stage 2
- Restlessness; increases during the evening hours
- Sleep disturbances
- Memory loss increases—may not know family and friends
- Dulled senses—cannot tell the difference between hot and cold; cannot recognize dangers
- Bowel and bladder incontinence
- Needs assistance with activities of daily living—problems with bathing, feeding, and dressing self; afraid of bathing; will not change clothes
- Loses impulse control—may use foul language, have poor table manners, be sexually aggressive, or be rude
- Movement and gait disturbances—walks slowly, has a shuffling gait
- Communication problems—cannot follow directions; has problems with reading, writing, and math; speaks in short sentences or single words; statements may not make sense
- Repeats motions and statements—may move things back and forth constantly; may say the same thing over and over
- Agitation—behavior may be violent

Stage 3
- Seizures (see Chapter 31)
- Cannot communicate—may groan, grunt, or scream
- Does not recognize self or family members
- Depends totally on others for all activities of daily living
- Disoriented to person, time, and place
- Totally incontinent of urine and feces
- Cannot swallow—choking and aspiration are risks
- Sleep disturbances increase
- Becomes bed bound—cannot sit or walk
- Coma
- Death

Screaming has many causes. Possible causes include hearing and vision problems, pain or discomfort, fear, and fatigue. Too much or not enough stimulation can cause the person to scream. Sometimes the person reacts to a caregiver or family member by screaming.

A calm, quiet setting is helpful. Soft music can calm the person. If it is safe for the person to have them, make sure hearing aids and eyeglasses are worn. Sometimes a family member can comfort the person. Many residents have favorite caregivers. They may have a calming effect on the person. If the person responds to touch, use touch to calm him or her.

Abnormal sexual behaviors. Sexual behaviors are labeled abnormal because of how and when they occur. Remember, persons with AD are disoriented to person, time, and place. Therefore sexual behaviors may involve the wrong person, the wrong place, and the wrong time. They also have lost the ability to control behavior. Normally they would know not to undress or expose themselves in front of others. They would know not to masturbate or engage in sexual pleasures in public. Normally they would know their sexual partners. Persons with AD often mistake a sexual partner for someone else. The person kisses and hugs the other person.

Sexual behaviors may mean that the person's sexual needs are not being met. Touching, scratching, and rubbing the genitals can signal infection, pain, or discomfort involving the urinary or reproductive system. Poor hygiene is another cause. So is being wet or soiled from urine or feces.

The nurse encourages the person's sexual partner to show affection. The couple's normal practices are encouraged. Examples include hand holding, hugging, kissing, and touching. When a person masturbates in public, lead the person to his or her room. Provide privacy, and make sure the person is safe. Good hygiene is important to prevent itching. If the person urinates or has a bowel movement, make sure the person is cleaned quickly and thoroughly. Do not let the person stay wet or soiled.

The nurse needs to assess the person for urinary or reproductive system problems. The doctor is contacted as necessary.

Repetitive behaviors. Repetitive means to repeat over and over. Persons with AD repeat the same motions over and over. For example, the person folds the same napkin over and over. Or the person says the same words or asks the same question over and over. Such behaviors are usually harmless. They do not hurt the person. However, they can annoy the caregivers and the family.

The person is allowed to continue harmless acts. Music and TV can distract the person. Taking the person for a walk can help. Such measures also are useful when the person repeats words or questions.

Care of Residents With Alzheimer's Disease and Other Dementias

Alzheimer's disease and other dementias are frustrating to the person, family, and caregivers. Usually the person is cared for at home until symptoms are severe. Adult day care may help. Care in a nursing center is often required. The person may develop other illnesses and need hospital care. Thus you may care for a person with AD or other dementias in an adult day care setting or in a hospital, nursing center, or private home. The person needs your support and understanding. So does the family.

People with AD do not choose to be forgetful, incontinent, agitated, or rude. Nor do they choose to have all of the other behaviors, signs, and symptoms of the disease. They have no control over what is happening to them. The disease causes the behaviors. The resident may do something that a healthy person would not do. When this happens, remember that the disease is responsible, not the person.

There is no effective treatment for AD. The symptoms worsen over several years. The disease progresses at different rates from person to person. Eventually persons with Alzheimer's disease depend on others for all care. They develop bowel and bladder incontinence. They need to be fed, bathed, groomed, and dressed. Residents in the third stage of the disease (see Box 27-4) cannot ask for help or tell what they need.

The nurse uses the nursing process to help the health care team plan measures to meet the resident's specific needs. The resident's safety, personal hygiene, nutrition and fluids, elimination, and activity needs must be met. So must the need for comfort and sleep. Many of the measures listed in Box 27-5 will be part of the resident's care plan.

You must keep residents with AD and other dementias comfortable and safe. Good skin care and proper body alignment are needed to prevent skin breakdown and contractures. You must take special care to treat these residents with dignity and respect. They have the same rights as residents who are alert and mobile. You must talk to these residents in a calm voice and always explain what you are going to do. Massage, soothing touch, music, and aroma therapy can provide comfort and help residents relax. Many centers provide hospice care as the resident nears death (see Chapter 32).

Your observations are important. The resident can develop other health problems or be injured. However, the resident may not know there is pain, fever, constipation, incontinence, or other signs and symptoms. You need to carefully observe the resident. Any change in the resident's usual behavior must be reported to the nurse.

Infection is a major risk. Remember that the resident's ability to give full attention to activities of daily living is greatly reduced. Infection can occur from poor hygiene. This includes skin care, oral hygiene, and perineal care after bowel and bladder elimination. Inactivity and immobility can lead to pneumonia and pressure ulcers.

Besides the measures listed in Box 27-5 on p. 631, other activities and therapies are ordered. These are intended to make the resident feel useful, worthwhile, and active. They help the resident's self-esteem. The therapist may work with one person, a small group, or a large group. Therapies and activities focus on the resident's strengths and past successes. For example:

- A resident used to cook. The resident is given the task of cleaning vegetables.
- Another resident was a good dancer. Activities are planned so the resident can dance.
- A person likes to clean. The person helps dust furniture.

Crafts, exercise, gardening activities, and listening and moving to music are among the activities planned for residents. All activities are supervised. Activities are planned to meet the resident's needs based on his or her cognitive abilities. The resident's likes and dislikes are also considered. Sing-alongs, reminiscing, and board games are appropriate for some residents. Others respond better to repeated tasks like stringing beads, folding towels, or rolling dough. Massage, range-of-motion exercises, and touch also are important activities.

Box 27-5 Care of Residents With Alzheimer's Disease and Other Dementias

Environment
- Follow established routines.
- Avoid changing rooms or roommates.
- Place picture signs on rooms, bathrooms, dining rooms, and other areas (Fig. 27-2, p. 632). Keep personal items where the resident can see them.
- Stay within the resident's sight to the extent possible.
- Place memory aids (large clocks and calendars) where the resident can see them.
- Keep noise levels low.
- Play music and show movies from the resident's past.
- Select tasks and activities specific to the resident's cognitive abilities.

Communication
- Approach the resident in a calm, quiet manner.
- Follow the rules of communication described in Chapter 5.
- Practice measures to promote communication (see Chapter 5).
- Provide simple explanations of all procedures and activities.
- Give consistent responses.

Safety
- Remove harmful, sharp, and breakable objects from the environment. This includes knives, scissors, glass, dishes, razors, and tools.
- Provide plastic eating and drinking utensils when needed. This helps prevent breakage and cuts.
- Place safety plugs in electrical outlets.
- Keep cords and electrical equipment out of reach.
- Store personal care items (e.g., shampoo, deodorant, lotion) in a safe place.
- Store household cleaners and medicines in locked storage areas.
- Store dangerous equipment and tools in a safe place.
- Supervise the resident who smokes.
- Store cigarettes, cigars, pipes, matches, and other smoking materials in a safe place.
- Practice safety measures to prevent falls (see Chapter 8).
- Practice safety measures to prevent fires (see Chapter 8).
- Practice safety measures to prevent burns (see Chapter 8).
- Practice safety measures to prevent poisoning (see Chapter 8).
- Keep all doors to kitchens, utility rooms, and housekeeping closets locked.

Wandering
- Make sure doors and windows are securely locked. Locks are often placed at the top and bottom of doors (Fig. 27-3, p. 632). The resident is not likely to look for a lock at the top or bottom of the door.
- Make sure door alarms are turned on. The alarm goes off when the door is opened. These are common in nursing centers.
- Make sure the resident wears an ID bracelet at all times.
- Exercise the resident as ordered. Adequate exercise often reduces wandering.
- Do not restrain the resident. Restraints require a doctor's order. They also tend to increase confusion and disorientation.
- Do not argue with the resident who wants to leave. Remember that the resident does not understand what you are saying.
- Go with the resident who insists on going outside. Make sure he or she is properly dressed. Guide the resident inside after a few minutes (Fig. 27-4, p. 633).
- Let the resident wander in enclosed areas if provided. Many nursing centers have enclosed areas where residents can walk about (Fig. 27-5, p. 633). These areas provide a safe place for the resident to wander.

Sundowning
- Provide a calm, quiet setting late in the day. Treatments and activities are done early in the day.
- Do not restrain the resident.
- Encourage exercise and activity early in the day.
- Make sure the resident has eaten. Hunger can increase restlessness.
- Promote urinary and bowel elimination. A full bladder or constipation can increase restlessness.
- Do not try to reason with the resident. Remember, he or she cannot understand what you are saying.

Continued

Box 27-5 Care of Residents With Alzheimer's Disease and Other Dementias cont'd

- Do not ask the resident to tell you what is bothering him or her. The resident's ability to communicate is impaired. He or she does not understand what you are asking. The resident cannot think or speak clearly.
- Dim lights and soft music may help to calm residents.

Hallucinations and Delusions

- Do not argue with the resident. He or she does not understand what you are saying.
- Reassure the resident. Tell him or her that you will provide protection from harm.
- Distract the resident with some item or activity.
- Use touch to calm and reassure the resident (Fig. 27-6).

Basic Needs

- Provide for the resident's food and fluid needs (see Chapter 18). Provide finger foods. Cut food and pour liquids as needed.
- Provide good skin care (see Chapters 13 and 14). Keep the resident's skin free of urine and feces.
- Promote urinary and bowel elimination (see Chapters 16 and 17).
- Promote exercise and activity during the day (see Chapter 19). This helps reduce wandering and sundowning behaviors. The resident may also sleep better.
- Reduce the resident's intake of coffee, tea, and cola drinks. These contain caffeine. Caffeine is a stimulant. It can increase the resident's restlessness, confusion, and agitation.
- Provide a quiet, restful setting (see Chapter 20). Soft music is better in the evening than loud television programs. Play music during care activities such as bathing and during meals.
- Promote personal hygiene (see Chapter 13). Do not force the resident into a shower or tub. People with AD are often afraid of bathing. Try bathing the resident when he or she is calm. Use the bathing method preferred by the resident (tub bath, shower, bed bath). Provide for privacy, and keep the resident warm. Do not rush the resident.
- Provide oral hygiene (see Chapter 13).
- Have equipment ready for any procedure ahead of time. This reduces the amount of time the resident is involved in care measures.
- Observe for signs and symptoms of other disorders or diseases (see Chapter 26).
- Protect the resident from infection (see Chapter 9).

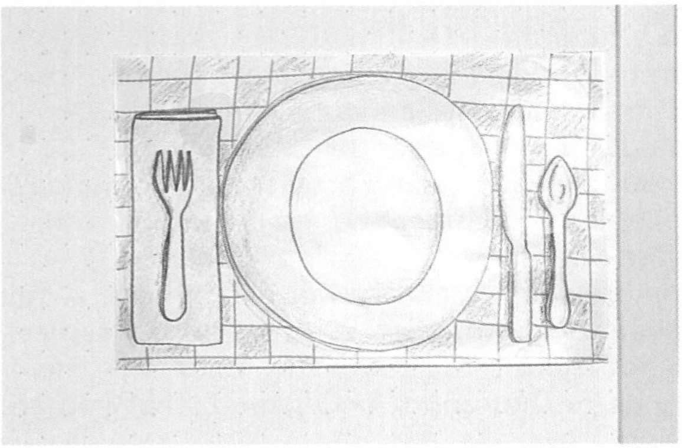

Fig. 27-2 Signs provide cues to the person with dementia.

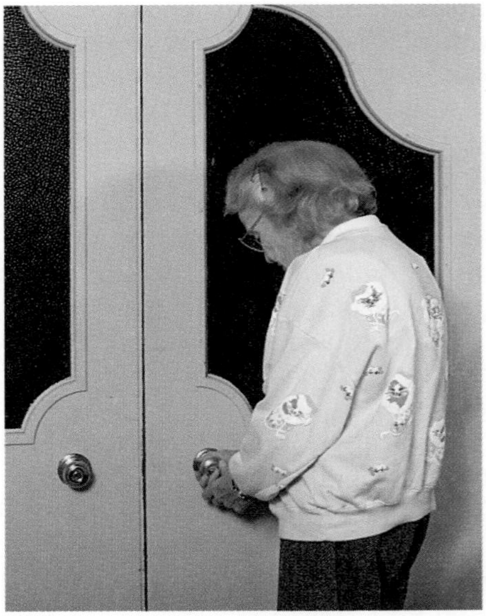

Fig. 27-3 A slide lock is at the top of the door. The person tries to open the lock on the knob.

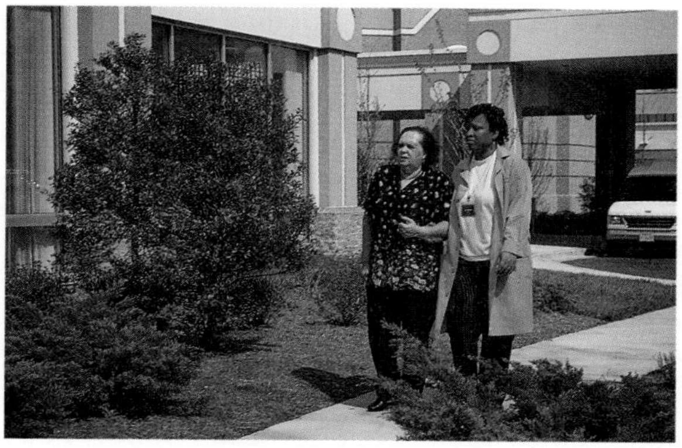

Fig. 27-4 Walk outside with the person who wanders. Then guide him back inside.

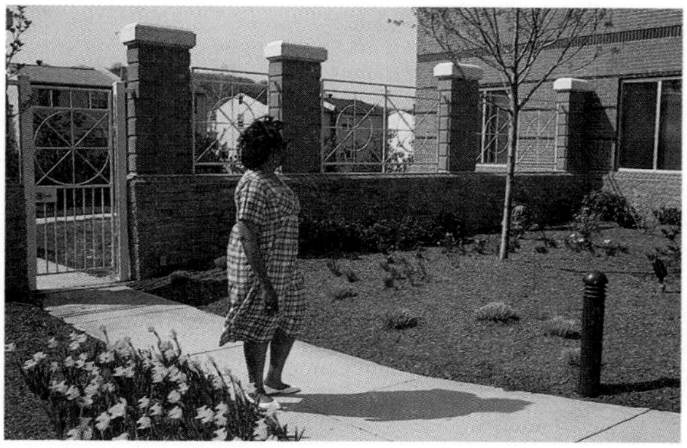

Fig. 27-5 An enclosed garden allows persons with AD to wander in a safe setting.

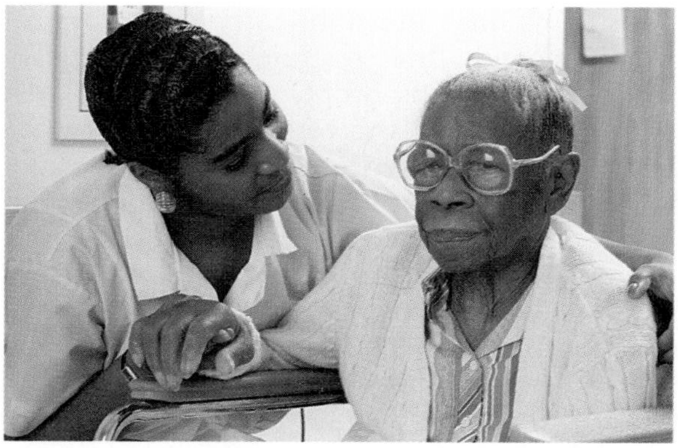

Fig. 27-6 Use touch to calm a person with Alzheimer's disease.

Special Care Units

Many centers have special care units for residents with Alzheimer's disease and other dementias. Some units are secured. Entrances and exits to the unit are locked. This prevents confused residents from wandering away. Some residents have aggressive behaviors that are disruptive or unsafe to others. They also may live on a secured unit.

According to OBRA, secured units are physical restraints. The center must follow OBRA rules and use the least restrictive approach to care. A dementia diagnosis and a doctor's order are needed before placing a person on a secured unit. The health care team meets at least every 90 days to assure that the secured unit is the best way to meet the resident's needs. The resident's rights are always protected. OBRA

The resident is transferred to another nursing unit in the center when a secured unit is no longer needed to provide safe care. For example, the person's condition progresses from stage 2 to stage 3. The person cannot sit or walk and is in bed. Wandering is no longer a concern.

JCAHO can accredit special care units. Certain standards of care must be met. All staff must receive special training in the care of residents with dementia. The unit must have programs that preserve the resident's dignity, personal freedom, and safety.

The Family

Persons with Alzheimer's disease or other dementias may live at home or with children or other family members. Family members in the household give care. Or arrangements are made for a family member or someone else to stay with the person. Help is sought from health professionals when family members can no longer deal with the situation or meet the person's needs. Home health care may help for awhile. Adult day care is another option (see Chapter 7). The decision for long-term care is usually made when:

- Family members can no longer meet the person's needs
- The person no longer knows the caregiver
- Family members have health problems
- Financial problems occur
- The person has behaviors that are dangerous to self or others

Medical care is very expensive. Diagnostic tests, doctor's visits, medicines, and home care are costly. So is long-term care. The person's medical care can drain family finances.

The family has special needs. Care of the person at home or in a nursing center is stressful. There are physical, emotional, social, and financial stresses. Children find themselves in the *sandwich generation.* They are in the middle between their own children who need attention and an ill parent who needs care. The stress of caring for two families is great. Often caregiving children have jobs too.

Caring for loved ones can be exhausting. Caregivers need much support and encouragement. Many join Alzheimer's disease support groups. Hospitals, nursing centers, and the Alzheimer's Association sponsor these groups. The Alzheimer's Association has chapters in cities and towns across the country. Support groups offer encouragement, advice, and ideas about care. People in similar situations share their feelings, anger, frustration, guilt, and other emotions. They also may share coping and care-giving ideas.

The family often feels helpless. No matter what is done for the loved one, the person only gets worse. Much time, money, energy, and emotion are required to care for the person. Anger and resentment may result. The family may then feel guilty because of their anger and resentment. They know that the person did not choose to develop the disease. The family also knows that the person does not choose to have the signs, symptoms, and behaviors of the disease. They may be frustrated and angry that the loved one can no longer show love or affection. How would you feel if your mother, father, husband, or wife did not know you? Sometimes the person's behavior is embarrassing.

The family is an important part of the health care team. The family helps plan the resident's care whenever possible. Many families are involved in unit activities. For many residents, family members provide comfort. Family members also need support and understanding from the health care team.

QUALITY OF LIFE

Quality of life is important for all persons with confusion and dementia. Those in nursing centers have the same rights under OBRA as other residents. Residents with confusion and dementia may not know or be able to exercise their rights. However, the family is aware of the resident's rights. They need to know that their loved one's rights are protected. The family also needs to know that the loved one is treated with respect and dignity.

Residents with confusion and dementia have the right to privacy and confidentiality. You must protect the resident from exposure. Only those involved in the resident's care are present for care and procedures. The resident is allowed to visit with others in private. When family and friends visit, they are given a space where they can visit privately. Confidentiality is also important. The resident's care and condition are not shared with others.

Personal choice is important. Some residents with confusion and dementia can still make simple choices. For example, a resident can choose between wearing a dress or slacks. Choosing to watch or not watch television may be a simple choice. Others cannot make choices themselves. The family may do so. The family chooses bath times, menus, clothing, activities, and other aspects of care.

The resident has the right to keep and use personal possessions. Some items comfort the resident. A pillow, blanket, afghan, or sweater may be important to the resident. The resident may not be able to tell you why or even recognize the item. Still, it is important. The resident's personal items are kept safe. You must also protect the resident's property from loss or damage.

Residents must be kept free from abuse, mistreatment, and neglect. Caring for residents with confusion and dementia is often very frustrating. The resident's behaviors may be difficult to deal with. Family and staff can become short tempered and angry. The resident is protected from abuse (see Chapter 2). Report any signs of abuse to the nurse right away. You need to be patient and calm when caring for these residents. Talk with the nurse if you find yourself becoming frustrated. Sometimes an assignment change is needed for a while.

All residents have the right to be free from restraints. Remember that restraints require a doctor's order. They are used only when it is the best method of protecting the resident. They are not used for staff convenience. Restraints can make confusion and demented behaviors worse. The nurse tells you when restraints are to be used.

Activity and a safe environment promote quality of life. Box 27-5 identifies safety measures for residents with confusion and dementia. These residents also need activities that are safe, calm, and quiet. The recreation therapist and other health team members will find activities that are best for each confused or demented resident. These are part of the resident's care plan.

REVIEW QUESTIONS

Circle the BEST answer.

1 Cognitive impairment
A Is expected in older people
B Refers to a decrease in intellectual functioning
C Refers only to memory loss
D Is a permanent condition

2 A resident is confused after surgery. The confusion is likely to be
A Permanent
B Temporary
C Caused by an infection
D Caused by brain injury

3 The confused resident is
A Restrained in bed at night
B Given many tasks to keep busy
C Easily distracted
D Never a danger to self or others

4 Joe Dunn has dementia. Dementia describes
A A false belief
B Mental disorders caused by changes in the brain
C Seeing, hearing, or feeling something that is not real
D Alzheimer's disease

5 Joe Dunn was diagnosed with Alzheimer's disease. Which is *true?*
A Alzheimer's disease occurs only in older persons.
B Diet and medications can control the disease.
C Alzheimer's disease and confusion are the same.
D Alzheimer's disease ends in death.

6 Persons with Alzheimer's disease
A Have memory loss, poor judgment, and sleep disturbances
B Lose impulse control and the ability to communicate
C May wander or have delusions and hallucinations
D All of the above

7 Sundowning means that
A The resident becomes sleepy when the sun sets
B Behaviors become worse in the late afternoon and evening hours
C Behavior improves at night
D The resident is in the third stage of the disease

8 Alzheimer's disease support groups do the following *except*
A Provide care
B Offer encouragement and care ideas
C Provide support for the family
D Promote the sharing of feelings and frustrations

9 Joe Dunn tends to wander. You should
A Make sure doors and windows are locked
B Make sure he wears an ID bracelet
C Help him with exercise as ordered
D All of the above

10 Safety is important for Joe Dunn. Which is *false?*
A Safety plugs are placed in electrical outlets.
B Cleaners and drugs are kept locked up.
C He can keep smoking materials.
D Sharp and breakable objects are removed from his environment.

11 You are caring for Joe Dunn. Which is *false?*
A It is possible to reason with him.
B Touch can calm and reassure him.
C A calm, quiet setting is important.
D Assistance is needed with ADL.

12 Joe Dunn cannot exercise his rights. Which is *true?*
A He no longer has rights.
B The nursing staff exercises his rights.
C OBRA staff protect his rights.
D The family exercises his rights.

Answers to these questions are on p. 700.

28 Developmental Disabilities

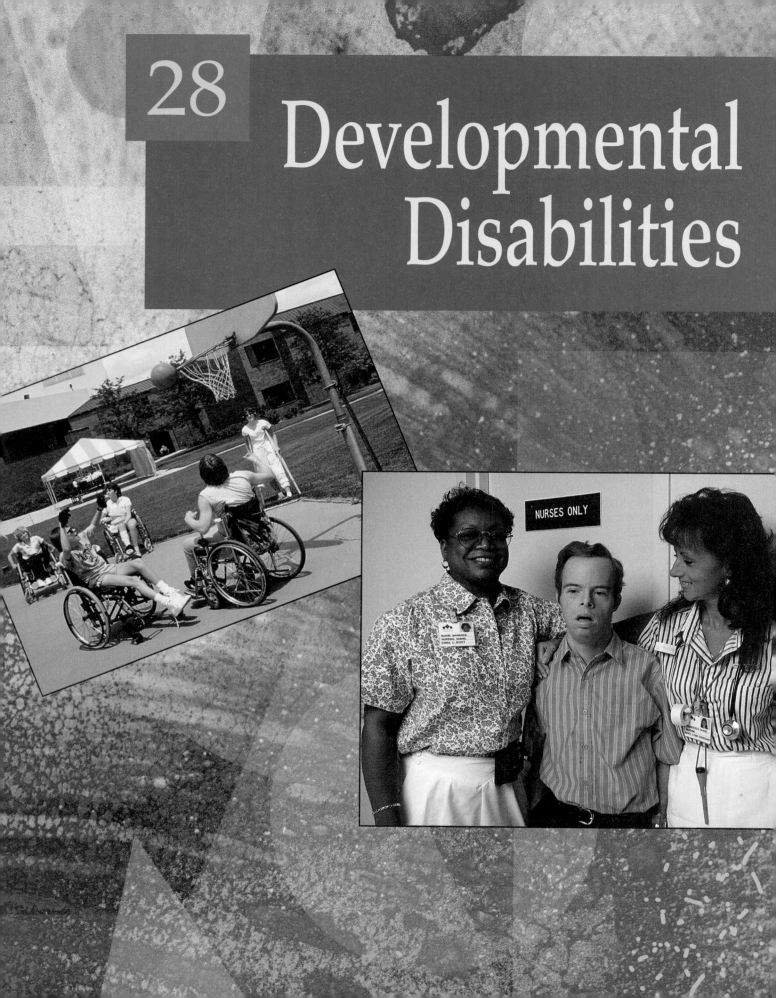

What You Will Learn

- The definition of the key terms listed in this chapter
- Areas of function limited by a developmental disability
- How a developmental disability affects the child and family across the life span
- When developmental disabilities occur
- The causes of developmental disabilities
- How mental retardation, Down syndrome, cerebral palsy, autism, epilepsy, spinal bifida, and hydrocephalus affect a person's functioning

Key Terms

cerebral palsy (CP) A term applied to a group of disorders characterized by paralysis *(palsy)* that is caused by a defect in the motor region of the brain *(cerebral)*

convulsion A seizure

developmental disability A severe, permanent physical or mental disability that occurs before 22 years of age

diplegia Similar body parts are affected on both sides of the body; paralysis of both arms or both legs

epilepsy A condition that produces brief disturbances in the brain's normal electrical functions

seizure The violent and sudden contractions or tremors of muscles; convulsion

spastic Uncontrolled contractions of skeletal muscles

Many diseases, illnesses, and injuries that cause permanent disability occur in adulthood. However, some infants are born with defects that result in disabilities. Childhood illnesses and injuries also can result in disabilities. If a disability occurs before 22 years of age, it is called a **developmental disability.** The disability is severe and permanent. It may be physical impairment, intellectual impairment, or both. The disability limits the person's ability to function in at least three of the following areas:

- Self-care
- Understanding or expressing language
- Learning
- Mobility
- Self-direction
- The ability to live independently
- Economic self-sufficiency (supporting oneself financially)

Developmentally disabled children become developmentally disabled adults. They do not remain children forever. The person needs lifelong assistance, support, and special services. The interdisciplinary health care team is involved in the person's care.

Some parents care for the child at home. Family and community agencies often provide needed support and services. However, as the child and parents grow older, caring for the child often is more difficult. The parent may not be able to lift or move an adolescent or adult child. A parent may become ill, injured, or disabled. A parent may die. Yet the person with a developmental disability still needs care.

Some severely disabled children require long-term care in a special center for those who are developmentally disabled. Some nursing centers admit developmentally disabled children and adults. OBRA and JCAHO require that centers provide age-appropriate activities for these residents. Staff must also receive special training to prepare them to meet the special care needs of developmentally disabled persons. OBRA

The causes of developmental disabilities occur before, during, and after birth. Conditions that commonly involve developmental disabilities include:

- Mental retardation
- Down syndrome
- Cerebral palsy
- Autism
- Epilepsy
- Spina bifida

MENTAL RETARDATION

Mental retardation is a disorder involving low intellectual functioning and impaired adaptive behavior. (*Intellectual function* relates to learning, thinking, and reasoning. *Adapt* means to change or adjust.) According to the American Association on Mental Retardation (AAMR), the person with mental retardation:

- *Has an IQ score below 70 to 75.* The person learns at a slower rate than normal. The ability to learn also is less than normal.
- *Is limited in 2 or more adaptive skills.* Adaptive skills are those skills needed to live, work, and play. They involve communication, self-care, home living, social skills, leisure, health and safety, self-direction, basic academics, community use, and work. The person has difficulty with activities of daily living. Understanding the behavior of others is limited. So is the person's ability to respond in socially appropriate ways.
- *Shows signs of the disorder before 18 years of age.*

In mental retardation, brain development is impaired. It can occur before birth, during birth, or before the age of 18. The many causes of mental retardation are listed in Box 28-1.

Mental retardation ranges from mild to severe. Mildly affected persons are slow to learn in school. As adults, they can function in society with some support. For example, the person needs help finding a job. However, the person does not need support every day. Some persons need extensive support every day at home or at work. Still others need constant support in all adaptive skill areas.

The Arc of the United States is a national organization on mental retardation. (It was formerly called the Association of Retarded Citizens of the United States.) The Arc believes that children with mental retardation should live in a family. They should also learn and play with children who do and do not have disabilities. Adults with mental retardation should control their life to the extent possible. That is, they should speak, make choices, and act for themselves. They should live in a home, have friends, work, and enjoy adult activities. Some have life partners. Others marry and have children.

The Arc also recognizes the sexuality of persons with mental retardation. This includes their physical, emotional, and social needs and desires. Reproductive organs develop in persons with mental retardation. Remember, adaptive skills vary from mild to severe. Some persons cannot control their sexual urges. The type and location of their sexual responses may be inappropriate. Also, some adults sexually abuse persons with mental retardation. The Arc believes that persons with mental retardation have the right to privacy and to love and be loved. The Arc also believes that persons with mental retardation should learn about sex, sexual abuse, safe sex, and other sex and sexuality issues.

DOWN SYNDROME

Down syndrome (DS) is named for a British doctor who first identified the syndrome. Down syndrome is most commonly caused by an extra 21st chromosome. Remember, at fertilization, a male sex cell (sperm) unites with a female sex cell (ovum). The sperm and the ovum each have 23 chromosomes. When they unite, the fertilized cell has 46 chromosomes. In Down syn-

BOX 28-1 CAUSES OF MENTAL RETARDATION

- **Genetic conditions**
  - Abnormal genes from one or both parents
  - Down syndrome
  - Fragile X syndrome
- **During pregnancy**
  - Alcohol use (fetal alcohol syndrome)
  - Drug use
  - Poor nutrition
  - Rubella (German measles)
  - Diabetes mellitus
  - HIV infection
  - Lack of oxygen to the brain
- **During birth**
  - Head injury
  - Prematurity
  - Low birth weight
  - Lack of oxygen to the brain
- **After birth**
  - Childhood diseases (whooping cough, chicken pox, measles)
  - Head injuries
  - Near drowning
  - Mercury poisoning
  - Lead poisoning
  - Poor nutrition
  - Child abuse (including shaken baby syndrome)

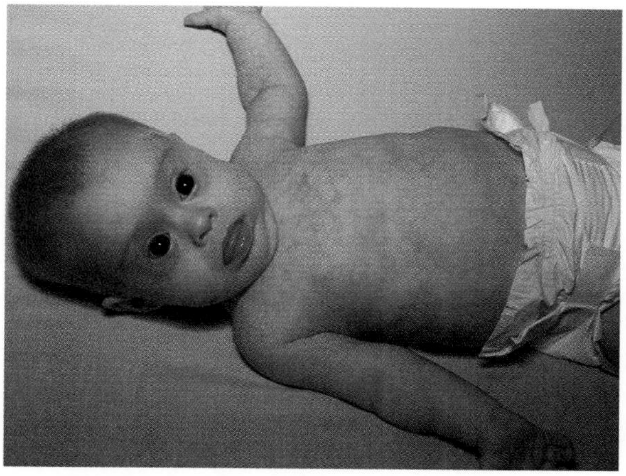

Fig. 28-1 An infant with Down syndrome. *(From Wong DL:* Whaley and Wong's nursing care of infants and children, *ed 5, St Louis, 1995, Mosby.)*

drome, an extra chromosome is present. Thus Down syndrome occurs at fertilization.

Down syndrome causes some degree of mental retardation. The child also has certain physical characteristics caused by the extra chromosome (Fig. 28-1):

- Oval-shaped eyes
- Short, wide neck
- Large tongue
- Wide, flat nose
- Small ears
- Short stature
- Short, wide hands with stubby fingers

Many children with Down syndrome are born with heart defects. They tend to have vision and hearing problems. They also are at risk for ear infections, respiratory infections, and thyroid gland problems.

Children and adults with DS need speech/language, physical, and occupational therapies. Most can learn self-care skills. They also need health and sex education. Because weight gain and constipation are problems, they need a well-balanced diet and regular exercise.

CEREBRAL PALSY

Cerebral palsy (CP) is a term applied to a group of disorders characterized by paralysis *(palsy)*. It is caused by a defect in the motor region of the brain *(cerebral)*. The defect results from brain damage that occurs before, during, or shortly after birth. Lack of oxygen to the brain is the usual cause. Congenital brain defects also can result in cerebral palsy.

Infants at risk for cerebral palsy include:

- Premature infants
- Low–birth-weight infants
- Infants who do not cry in the first 5 minutes after delivery
- Infants who require mechanical ventilation
- Infants who have bleeding in the brain
- Infants with congenital heart, kidney, or spinal cord defects
- Infants with seizure activity
- Infants with fetal alcohol syndrome

Brain damage in early childhood also can result in cerebral palsy. Lack of oxygen to the brain can occur from:

- Choking (see Chapter 31)
- Poisoning
- Near drowning
- Head injuries from accidents or child abuse (including shaken baby syndrome)
- Meningitis (inflammation of the covering around the brain and spinal cord)
- Encephalitis (inflammation of the brain)

Cerebral palsy affects body movements and body parts. Two types of CP affect body movements: spastic and athetoid. *Spastic* comes from the Greek word *spastikos*, which means to draw in. **Spastic** means uncontrolled contractions of skeletal muscles. That is, the muscles contract or shorten. The muscles cannot relax. One or both sides of the body may be involved. Posture, balance, and movement are affected. So are hand skills. Therefore eating, writing, dressing, and other activities of daily living are affected.

In athetoid cerebral palsy, the person cannot control muscle movements. *Athetoid* comes from the Greek word *athetos*, which means not fixed. The person has continuous slow weaving or writhing motions of the trunk, arms, and legs. The tongue and face and neck muscles also may be involved.

Hemiplegia, diplegia, and quadriplegia are used to describe the body parts involved:

- *Hemiplegia*—the arm and leg on one side of the body are affected.
- *Diplegia*—*di* comes from the Greek word meaning twice. Therefore **diplegia** means that similar body parts are affected on both sides of the body. The person has paralysis of both arms or both legs. The legs are commonly involved.
- *Quadriplegia*—both arms and both legs are paralyzed. So are the trunk and neck muscles. The person with CP can have many other impairments. They include:
  - Mental retardation
  - Learning disabilities
  - Hearing impairments
  - Vision impairments
  - Drooling
  - Constipation
  - Epilepsy (p. 640)
  - Difficulty swallowing (dysphagia)
  - Attention deficit hyperactivity disorder (short attention span, poor concentration, and increased activity)

AUTISM

Autism begins in early childhood. This mental disorder comes from the Greek word *autos*, which means self. Brain function is affected. Reasoning, social interaction, verbal and nonverbal communication skills, and play activities are impaired. The child has difficulty relating to people.

Children are severely to mildly affected. The following behaviors are common:

- Slow language development
- Repeats words or phrases
- Uses gestures to communicate
- Short attention span
- Spends time alone
- Little or no eye contact
- Overly reacts to touch; does not like to cuddle
- Little reaction to pain
- Frequent tantrums for no apparent reason
- Strong attachment to a single item
- Needs routines; does not like change
- No fear of danger
- Does not respond to others; may act deaf
- Very active or very quiet
- Aggressive or violent behavior; may injure self

Autism has no cure. With appropriate therapy, the person can learn to change or control behaviors. Many therapies are used to help the person. They include behavior modification, speech and language therapy, music therapy, auditory training, sensory therapies, physical therapy, occupational therapy, drugs, and diet therapy. Communication therapy and developing social and work skills also are very important.

Children with autism become adults. Some adults work and live independently. Others continue to need support and assistance from family and other services. Some live in a group home or a residential care center.

Persons with autism may have other disorders and disabilities. Mental retardation and epilepsy are common.

EPILEPSY

The Epilepsy Foundation of America describes **epilepsy** as a condition that produces brief disturbances in the brain's normal electrical functions. These disturbances occur from time to time. They involve bursts of electrical energy that cause seizures. (Epilepsy comes from the Greek word *epilepsia*, which means seizure.)

A **seizure** (or **convulsion**) involves violent and sudden contractions or tremors of muscles. The person has uncontrolled body movements and may lose consciousness. Seizures can occur in one part of the brain. These are called *partial seizures*. Some seizures involve the whole brain. They are called *generalized seizures*.

Illnesses that cause high fever or lack of oxygen to the brain can cause seizures. So can head injuries. However, having a single seizure does not mean the person has epilepsy. In epilepsy, seizures recur. The person with epilepsy has a permanent brain injury or defect. Often there are no known causes. The known causes of epilepsy include:

- Brain injury before, during, or after birth
- Maternal injury or infection during pregnancy
- Lack of oxygen during birth
- Head trauma (vehicle accident, gunshot wound, sports accident, fall, blow to the head)
- Chemical imbalance
- Poor nutrition
- Brain tumor
- Childhood fevers
- Poisons—such as lead and alcohol poisoning
- Infections—such as meningitis and encephalitis
- Stroke

Children and young adults are commonly affected. However, epilepsy can develop at any time. It also occurs with other problems affecting the brain. Such problems include cerebral palsy, mental retardation, autism, Alzheimer's disease, and traumatic brain injury.

Epilepsy has no known cure at this time. Many drugs are available to prevent seizures. However, some persons do not have complete seizure control with drugs. For other persons, drug therapy does not work.

When controlled, epilepsy usually does not interfere with learning and activities of daily living. In severe cases, persons may have activity and job limits. For example, because seizures can occur at any time, the person may not be allowed to drive a vehicle. Not being able to drive may limit job choices.

Persons with epilepsy have an increased risk of death. Prolonged seizures can result in brain damage. The Epilepsy Foundation of America reports that persons with epilepsy have higher rates for suicide and sudden unexplained death syndrome. They also have higher rates of accidental death, especially drowning.

See Chapter 31 for the emergency care of persons having a seizure.

SPINA BIFIDA

Spina bifida is a congenital defect of the spinal column. (It comes from the Latin words *spina*, which means backbone, and *bifid*, which means split in two parts.) The defect occurs during the first 29 days of pregnancy. Hydrocephalus often occurs with spina bifida (p. 641).

Bones of the spinal column are called *vertebrae*. The vertebrae protect the spinal cord. In spina bifida, bones of the vertebrae do not form properly. This leaves a split in the vertebrae. The split leaves the spinal cord

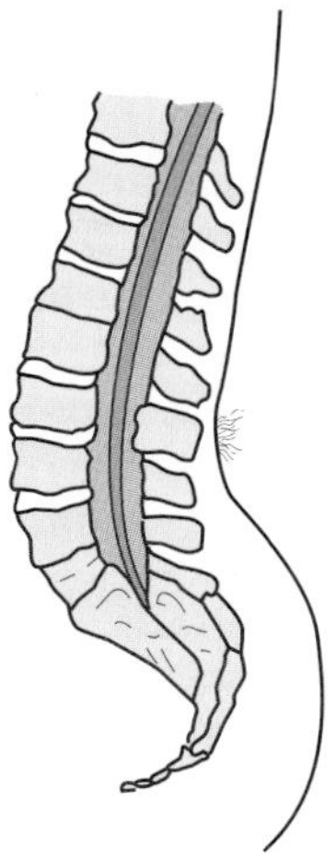

Fig. 28-2 Spina bifida occulta.

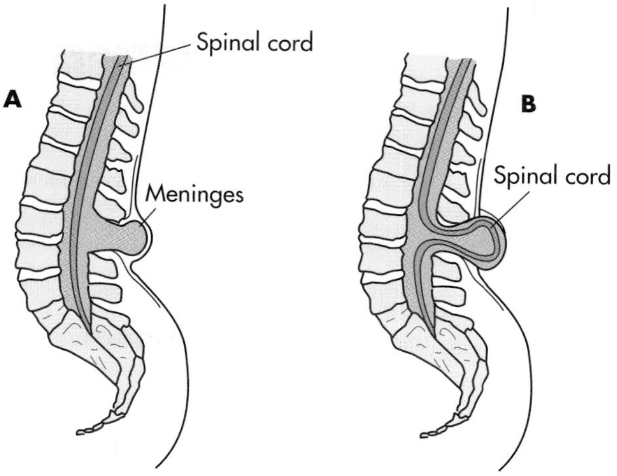

Fig. 28-3 A, Meningocele. B, Myelomeningocele.

unprotected. Only a membrane covers the spinal cord. Remember, the spinal cord contains nerves that send messages to and from the brain. If the spinal cord is unprotected, nerve damage occurs. Affected body parts do not function properly. Paralysis may occur. Bowel and bladder problems are common. Infection also is a threat.

Spina bifida can occur anywhere in the spine. However, the lower back is the most common site. The different types of spina bifida include:

- *Spina bifida occulta*—occult means hidden. The vertebrae are closed, but there is a defect in the vertebrae closure. The spinal cord and nerves are normal. The person has a dimple or tuft of hair on the back (Fig. 28-2). Often the person has no symptoms. Foot weaknesses and bowel and bladder problems can occur.
- *Spina bifida cystica*—*cystica* comes from the Greek word meaning bag, pouch, or sac. Part of the spinal column is contained in the pouch or sac. A membrane or a thin layer of skin covers the sac. It looks like a large blister on the person's back. The pouch is easily injured. Infection is a threat. There are two types of spina bifida cystica (Fig. 28-3):
    - *Meningocele*—meningo comes from the Greek word *meninx*, which means membrane, and the suffix *cele*, which means hernia or swelling. Remember, meninges is the connective tissue that covers and protects the brain and spinal cord. Cerebrospinal fluid also protects the brain and spinal cord (see Chapter 6). In meningocele the sac contains meninges and cerebrospinal fluid (see Fig. 28-3, *A* and Fig. 28-4). The sac does not contain nerve tissue. The spinal cord and nerves usually are normal. Therefore nerve damage usually is not a problem. The defect is corrected with surgery.

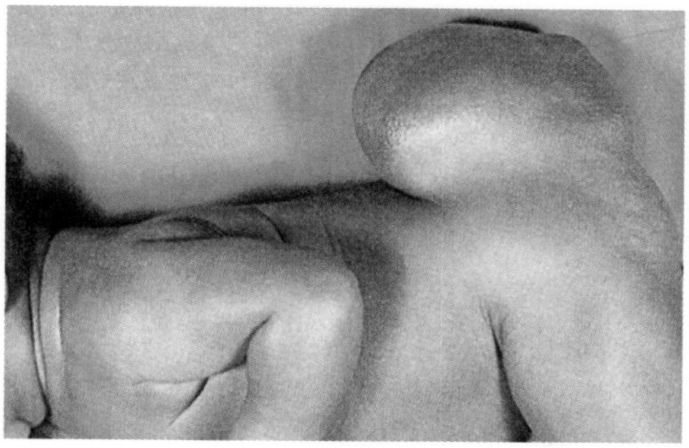

Fig. 28-4 Meningocele. *(From Zitelli BJ, Davis HW:* Atlas of pediatric physical diagnosis, *ed 1, St Louis, 1987, Gower Medical Publishing.)*

    - *Myelomeningocele (or meningomyelocele)*—*myelo* comes from the prefix meaning spinal cord. In myelomeningocele, the pouch contains nerves and spinal cord, meninges, and cerebrospinal fluid (see Fig. 28-3, *B*). Nerve damage occurs. Loss of function occurs below the level of damage. Leg paralysis, lack of sensation, and lack of bowel and bladder control are common problems. The defect is closed with surgery. Some children learn to walk using braces or crutches. Others use a wheelchair.

HYDROCEPHALUS

Hydrocephalus is a condition in which cerebrospinal fluid collects in and around the brain. (It comes from the Greek words *hydro,* meaning water, and root *cephalo,* meaning head.) A spinal defect prevents the cerebrospinal fluid from draining properly. Therefore the head enlarges (Fig. 28-5). Pressure inside the head increases. Mental retardation and neurological damage occur without treatment.

To allow draining of the cerebrospinal fluid, a shunt is placed in the brain. The shunt is a long, flexible tube that goes from the brain to a body cavity (Fig. 28-6). Fluid drains from the brain through the tube. Usually it drains into the abdominal cavity or a heart chamber. The shunt must remain patent (open). If blockage occurs, the cerebrospinal fluid cannot drain from the brain.

The person with hydrocephalus can have various problems. Visual impairment, seizures, and learning disabilities can occur.

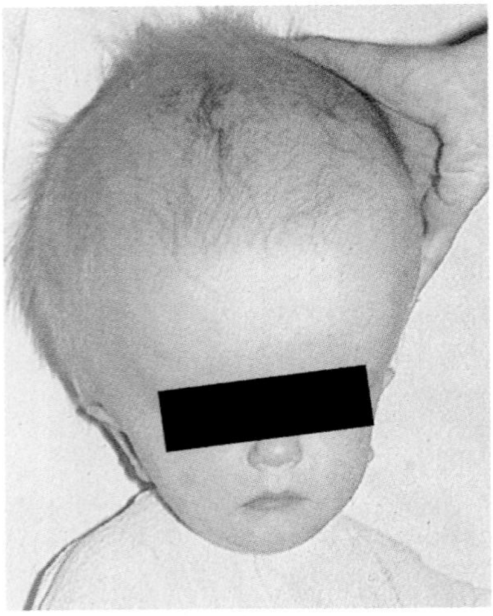

Fig. 28-5 Hydrocephalus. *(From Hart CA, Broadhead RL:* Color atlas of pediatric infectious diseases, *London, 1992, Mosby-Wolfe.)*

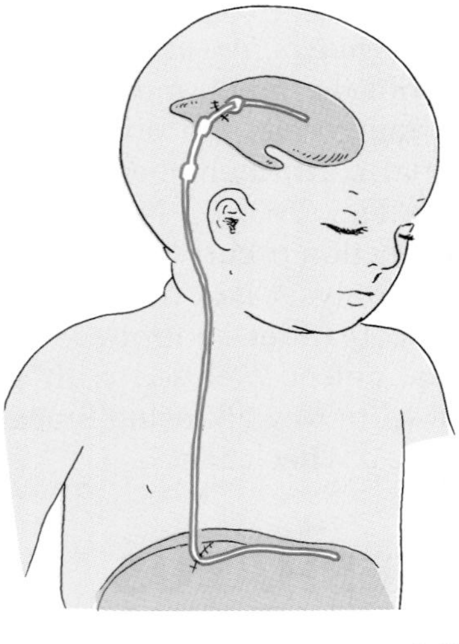

Fig. 28-6 A shunt drains cerebrospinal fluid from the brain. *(From Wong DL:* Whaley and Wong's nursing care of infants and children, *ed 5, St Louis, Mosby 1995.)*

Quality of Life

Persons with developmental disabilities have the same rights as every citizen in the United States. They have the right to live, learn, work, and enjoy life. The Americans with Disabilities Act of 1990 (ADA) further protects their rights. For those requiring care in a nursing center, the Omnibus Budget Reconciliation Act of 1987 (OBRA) offers additional protection.

Independence to the extent possible is the goal for persons with developmental disabilities. This includes having a job and living in the community. A variety of federal, state, and community resources are available to assist the person and family. Such support includes needed assistive devices, education, job training, personal assistance services, home and vehicle changes, financial assistance, and therapy services. Therapy services include physical, occupational, speech and language, respiratory, hearing, and vision therapies.

The disability affects the child and the family throughout the life span. Remember, the person with a developmental disability does not remain an infant or a child. The person grows older, becoming an adolescent, young adult, middle-age adult, and older adult. Changes from aging occur (see Chapter 7). However, the onset of such changes may occur earlier than normal in persons with severe developmental disabilities. Older parents may not have the energy or means to care for the aging child. Then long-term care may be required.

Review Questions

Circle the BEST answer.

1 All developmental disabilities occur
- A At birth
- B From trauma
- C During pregnancy
- D Before 22 years of age

2 These statements are about developmental disabilities. Which is *true?*
- A Self-care, learning, and mobility are always affected.
- B The disability is severe and permanent.
- C Physical and intellectual impairment occur together.
- D The person cannot live independently or hold a job.

3 The person with mental retardation
- A Has delayed development of sexual organs
- B Does not have the skills to live, work, and play
- C Requires care in a special setting
- D Learns at a slower rate than normal

4 Mental retardation
- A Is always severe
- B Can occur before, during, or after birth
- C Is caused by an extra chromosome
- D Affects the motor region in the brain

5 Down syndrome occurs
- A At fertilization
- B During the first 29 days of pregnancy
- C Any time before, during, or after birth
- D From trauma

6 The person with Down syndrome always has some degree of
- A Cerebral palsy
- B Autism
- C Impaired mobility
- D Mental retardation

7 Cerebral palsy is usually caused by
- A An extra chromosome
- B High fever
- C Lack of oxygen to the brain
- D Infection during pregnancy

8 The person with the spastic type of cerebral palsy has problems with
- A Learning
- B Drooling
- C Posture, balance, and movement
- D Weaving motions of the trunk, arms, and legs

9 Autism begins
- A At fertilization
- B During pregnancy
- C At birth
- D In early childhood

10 The person with autism has
- A Impaired movement
- B Difficulty relating to people
- C Diplegia
- D Mental retardation

11 The person with epilepsy has
- A Seizures
- B Diplegia
- C Athetoid cerebral palsy
- D Spastic movements

12 Which is used to control epilepsy
- A Physical therapy
- B Occupational therapy
- C Drugs
- D A shunt

13 Spina bifida involves
- A Nerve damage
- B Cerebrospinal fluid collecting in the head
- C Seizures
- D Mental retardation

14 Which is common in spina bifida?
- A Short attention span
- B Hearing and vision problems
- C Learning problems
- D Bowel and bladder problems

15 Hydrocephalus often occurs with
- A Down syndrome
- B Mental retardation
- C Spina bifida
- D Autism

Answers to these questions are on p. 700.

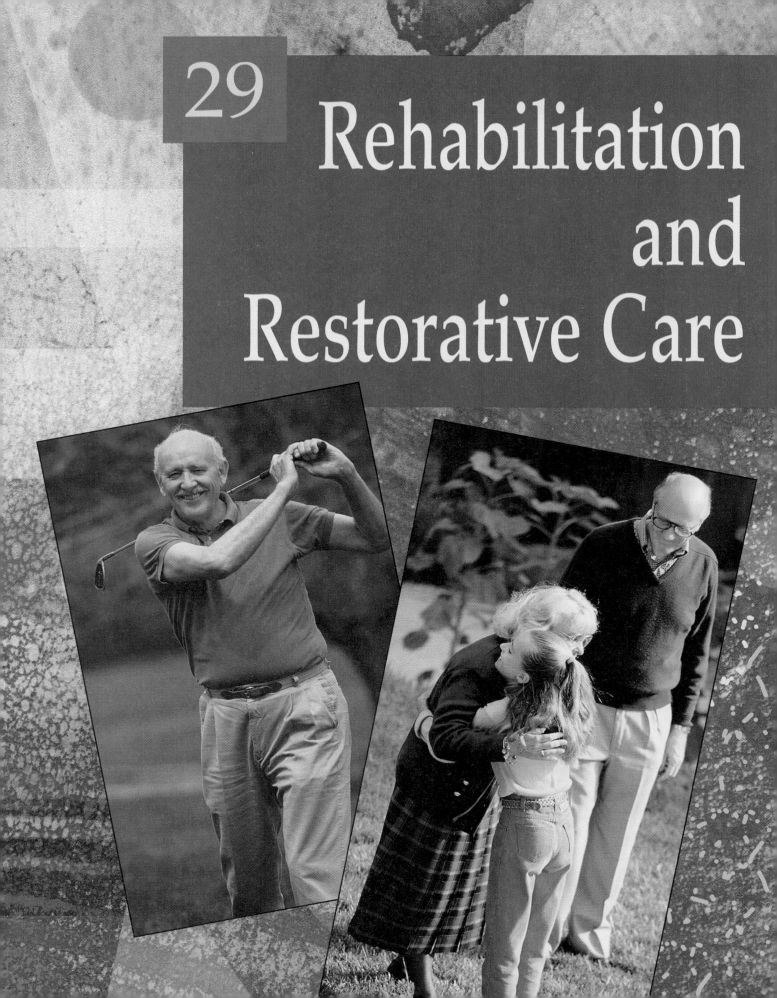

29 Rehabilitation and Restorative Care

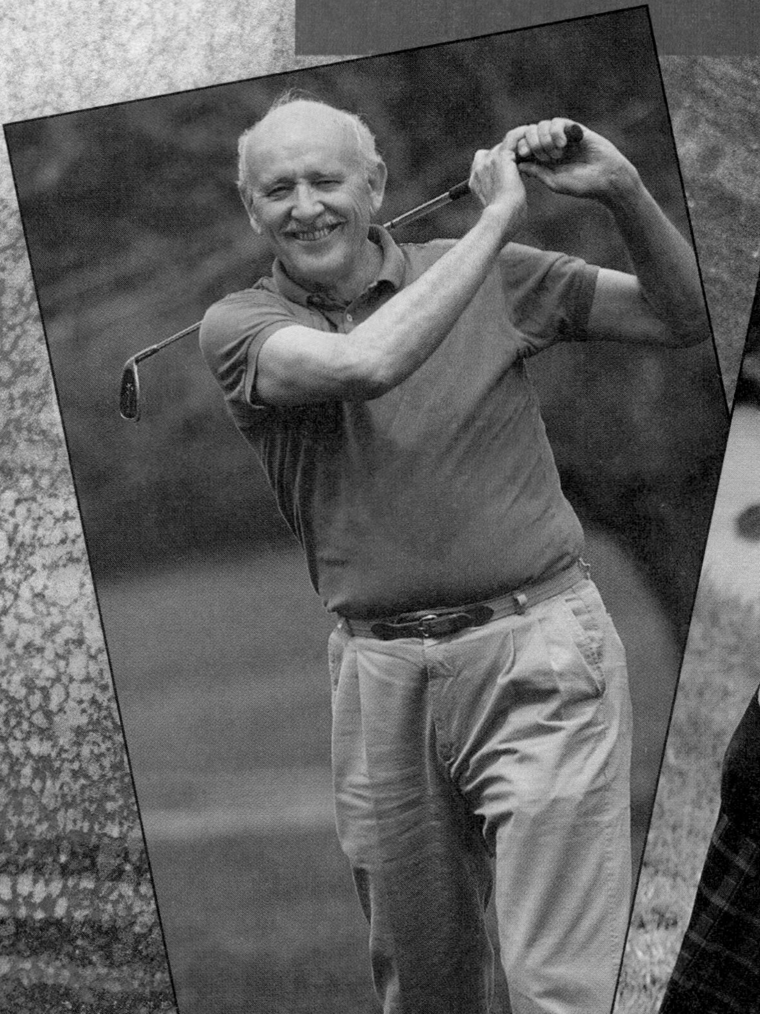

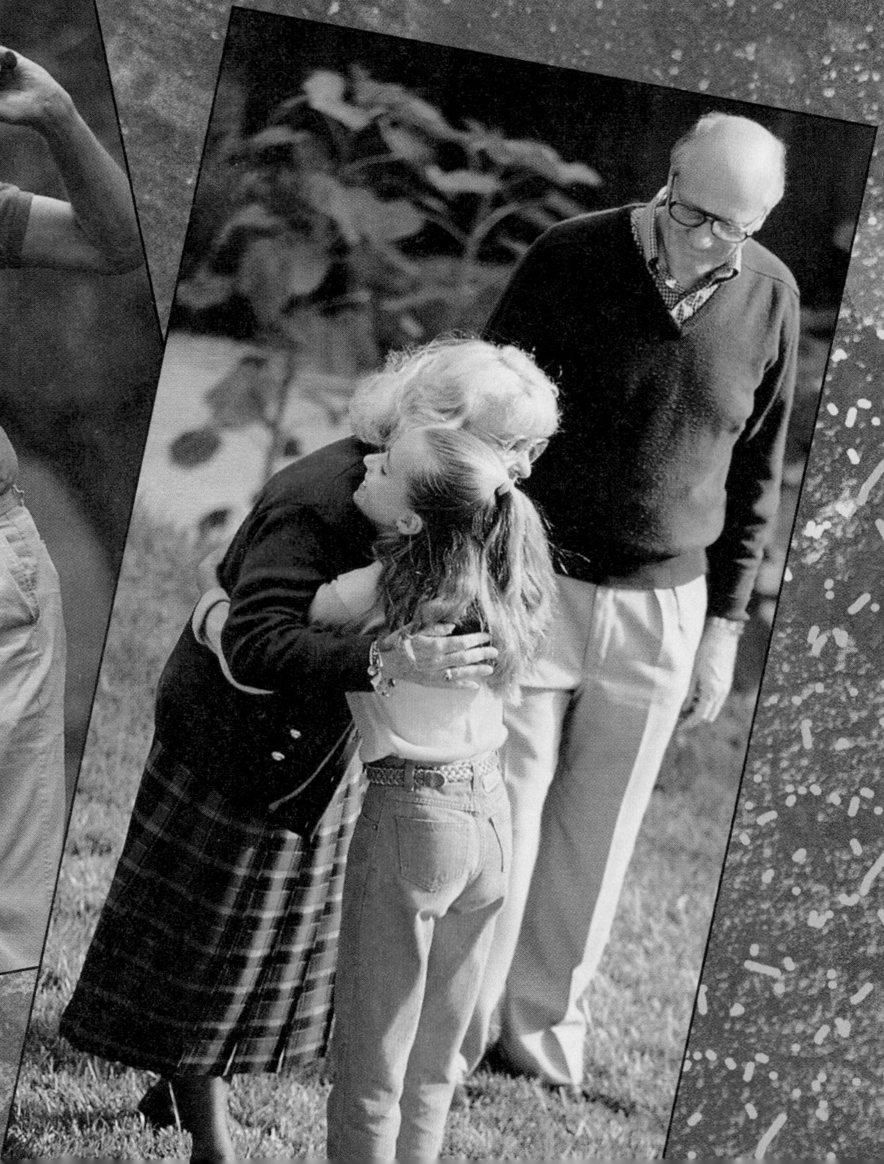

What You Will Learn

- The definition of the key terms listed in this chapter
- What rehabilitation means in terms of the whole person
- The complications that are prevented for successful rehabilitation
- Ways to help disabled residents perform activities of daily living
- The psychological reactions that are common during rehabilitation
- The members of the rehabilitation team
- The role of subacute care units in rehabilitation
- Common rehabilitation services
- Your responsibilities in rehabilitation
- How to promote quality of life during rehabilitation

Key Terms

activities of daily living (ADL) Those self-care activities a person performs daily to remain independent and to function in society

disability Any lost, absent, or impaired physical or mental function

prosthesis An artificial replacement for a missing body part

rehabilitation The process of restoring the disabled person to the highest possible level of physical, psychological, social, and economic functioning

Disease, injury, and surgery can cause decrease or loss of body function or loss of a body part. Birth injuries and birth defects also can affect a person's ability to function (see Chapter 28). Often there is loss of more than one function. The loss may be temporary or permanent. Daily activities such as eating, bathing, dressing, and walking are difficult or seem impossible. Some persons cannot work. Others cannot care for children or family.

Disability is any lost, absent, or impaired physical or mental function. It is caused by an acute or chronic illness or problem. An acute problem has a short course. Recovery is complete. A fracture is an acute problem. A chronic problem has a long course. The problem is controlled—not cured—with treatment. Diabetes mellitus and coronary artery disease are chronic health problems. Disabilities are short term or long term. The disabled person may totally or partially depend on others to meet basic needs. The degree of disability affects how much function is possible.

Health care is increasingly concerned with preventing and reducing the degree of disability. Helping the person to adjust to the disability is also important. **Rehabilitation** is the process of restoring the disabled person to the highest possible level of physical, psychological, social, and economic functioning. The health care team focuses on improving the person's abilities to function at his or her highest level of independence. Sometimes improvement in function is not possible. Then the focus is on preventing further loss of function and helping the person maintain the best possible quality of life.

Persons admitted to a nursing center often have physical disabilities. Some needed hospital care or were restricted to bedrest with an acute illness. They are weak and cannot perform activities of daily living. Restorative care helps them regain their strength and independence. Others have a progressive illness—they become more and more disabled. Rehabilitation and restorative nursing programs help these residents maintain their highest level of functioning and prevent unnecessary decline in function. Some residents have suffered strokes, fractures, amputations, or other injuries. Rehabilitation programs help them regain their former level of functioning or adjust to a long-term disability. Often these residents go home or to another level of care. You will work with different types of rehabilitation programs.

REHABILITATION AND THE WHOLE PERSON

Rehabilitation involves the whole person. A physical illness or injury always has some physical, psychological, and social effects. So does a disability. Suppose you wake up one morning and cannot move one side of your body. Would you be afraid, angry, or depressed? How would you get around in your home and care for yourself? How would you care for your family? How would you shop or visit friends or family? How would you support yourself? What work could you do?

Rehabilitation helps a person adjust physically, psychologically, socially, and economically. Abilities—what the person can do—are stressed. Complications that can cause further disability are prevented. Therefore rehabilitation begins when the person first enters the health care system. Rehabilitation usually starts at a hospital. Transfer to a nursing center for further rehabilitation may be required. This is especially true of older persons. Rehabilitation often takes longer in older persons than in other age-groups. Therefore their rehabilitation programs usually proceed at a slower pace. Older people have decreased tolerance for long and fast-paced rehabilitation programs. They often have many chronic health problems that can slow and complicate recovery. They also are at higher risk for injuries.

Physical Aspects

Rehabilitation begins when the person seeks health care. It starts with preventing complications. Complications can occur from bedrest, prolonged illness, or recovery from injury. Bowel and bladder problems are prevented. Contractures and pressure ulcers are prevented with good alignment, frequent turning and repositioning, range-of-motion exercises, and supportive devices (see Chapters 10 and 19). Good skin care is very important in preventing pressure ulcers (see Chapters 13 and 14).

Bladder training is described in Chapter 16. The method used depends on the person's physical problems, abilities, and needs. Bowel training is described in Chapter 17. It involves gaining control of bowel movements and developing a regular pattern of elimination. Fecal impaction, constipation, and anal incontinence are prevented. Follow the resident's care plan and center procedures for bladder-training and bowel-training programs.

Self-care is a major goal. **Activities of daily living (ADL)** refer to self-care activities. The person performs these activities daily to remain independent and to function in society. ADL include bathing, dressing, oral hygiene, eating, bowel and bladder elimination, and moving about. A person's ability to perform ADL and the need for self-help devices are evaluated by the rehabilitation team (p. 651).

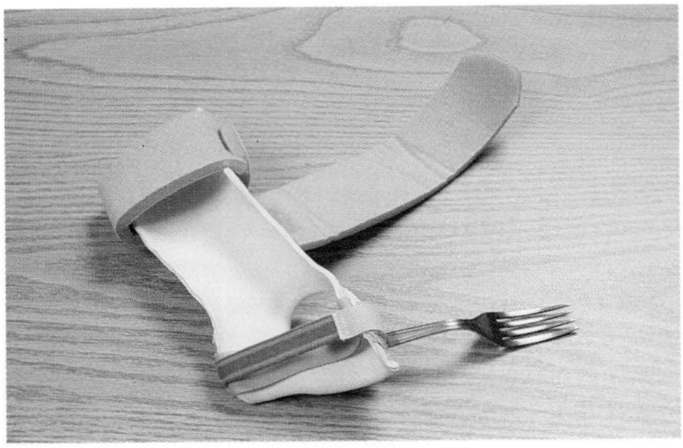

Fig. 29-1 Self-help device attached to a splint.

Disease, injury, and birth defects can affect the hands, wrists, and arms. Self-help devices often are needed. Equipment usually can be changed or made to meet the person's needs. Special eating devices include glass holders, plate guards, and silverware with curved handles or cuffs (see Fig. 18-8, p. 417) are available. Some devices are attached to special splints (Fig. 29-1). Electric toothbrushes are helpful if the resident cannot perform back-and-forth motions needed for brushing teeth. Longer handles can be attached to combs, brushes, and sponges (Fig. 29-2). There also are self-help devices for cooking, dressing, writing, dialing telephones, and many other activities (Fig. 29-3).

Some residents have lower extremity involvement. They may have to learn how to walk with a supportive device or learn how to use a wheelchair. If walking is possible, the resident may be taught to use crutches or a walker, cane, or brace (Fig. 29-4, p. 648). Both legs may be paralyzed or amputated. If so, a wheelchair is used. Residents paralyzed on one side of the body also may need a wheelchair and special positioning devices. If possible, the resident learns how to transfer from the bed to the wheelchair without help. Other transfers are taught. These include transfers to and from the toilet, bathtub, sofa, and chair and in and out of a car (Figs. 29-5 and 29-6, pp. 648-650).

Prostheses are helpful for persons with missing body parts. A **prosthesis** is an artificial replacement for the missing part. A person usually can be fitted with an artificial arm or leg and taught how to use the prosthesis (see Chapter 26). Artificial eyes are available. Technology advances will provide even better prostheses. The goal is to have a prosthesis that closely resembles the missing part in function and appearance.

Text continued on p. 651

A B C

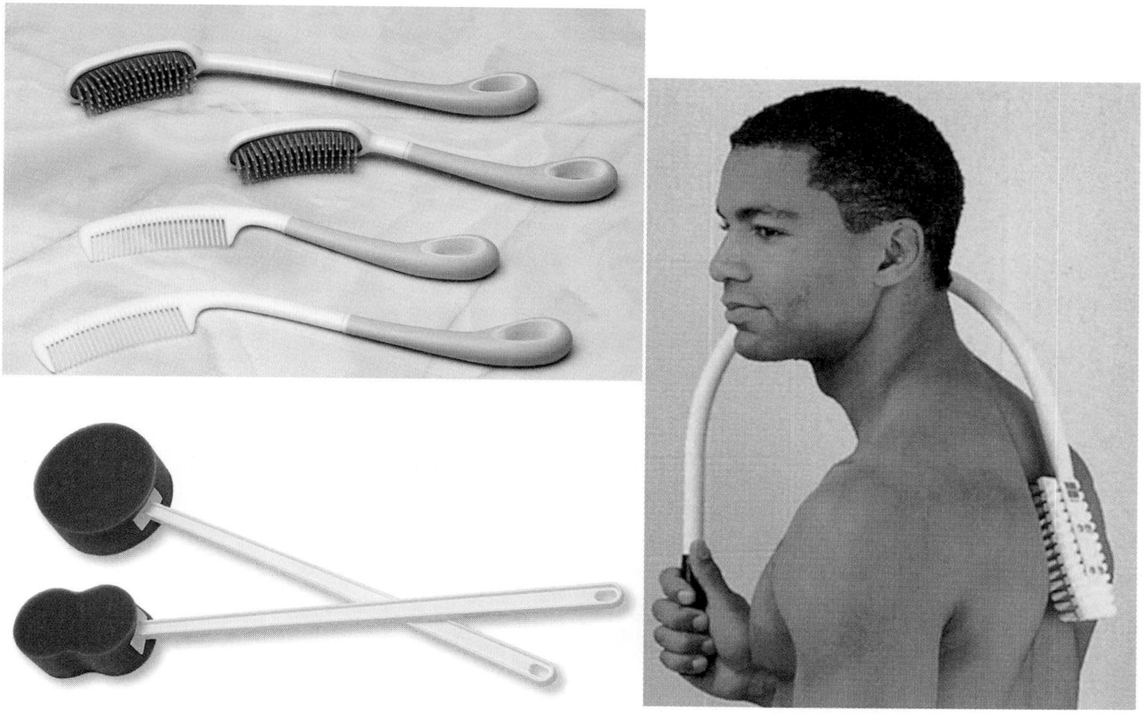

Fig. 29-2 A, A long-handled comb for hair care. **B,** The brush has a long handle for bathing. **C,** This brush has a curved handle. *(**A** and **B**, Courtesy North Coast Medical, Inc, Morgan Hill, Calif. **C**, Courtesy Sammons Preston, An AbilityOne Company, Bolingbrook, Ill.)*

A

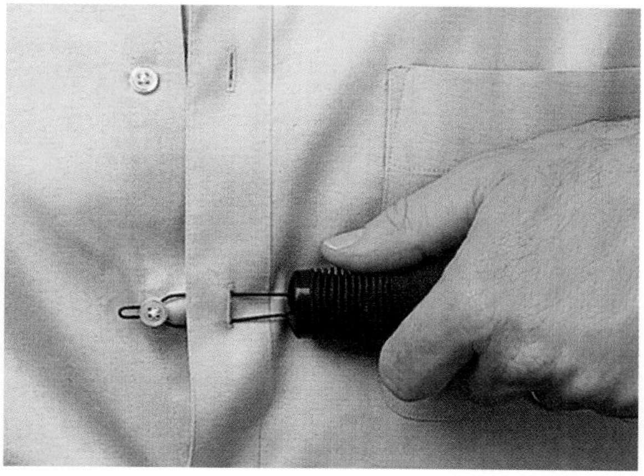

B

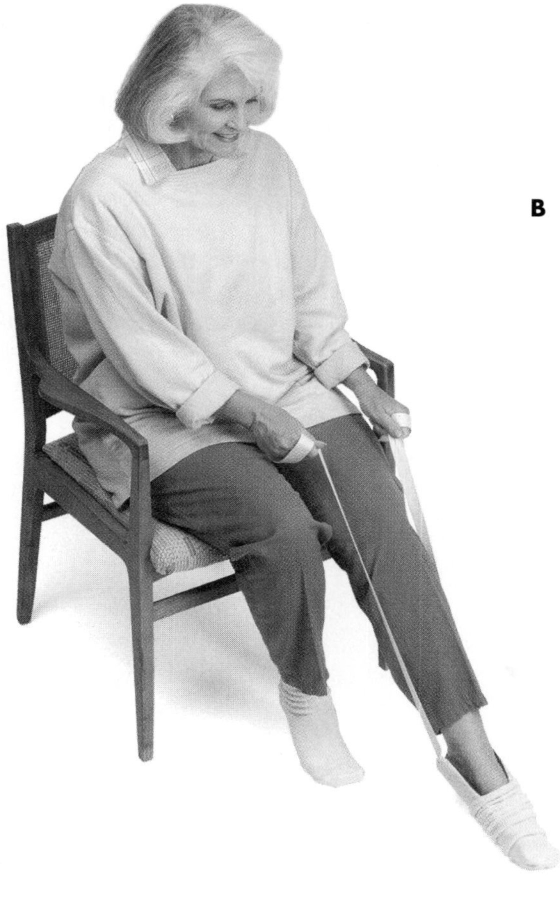

Fig. 29-3 A, A button hook is used to button and zip clothing. **B,** A sock puller is used to put on socks and stockings. *(**A** and **B**, Courtesy North Coast Medical, Inc., Morgan Hill, Calif.)*

Continued

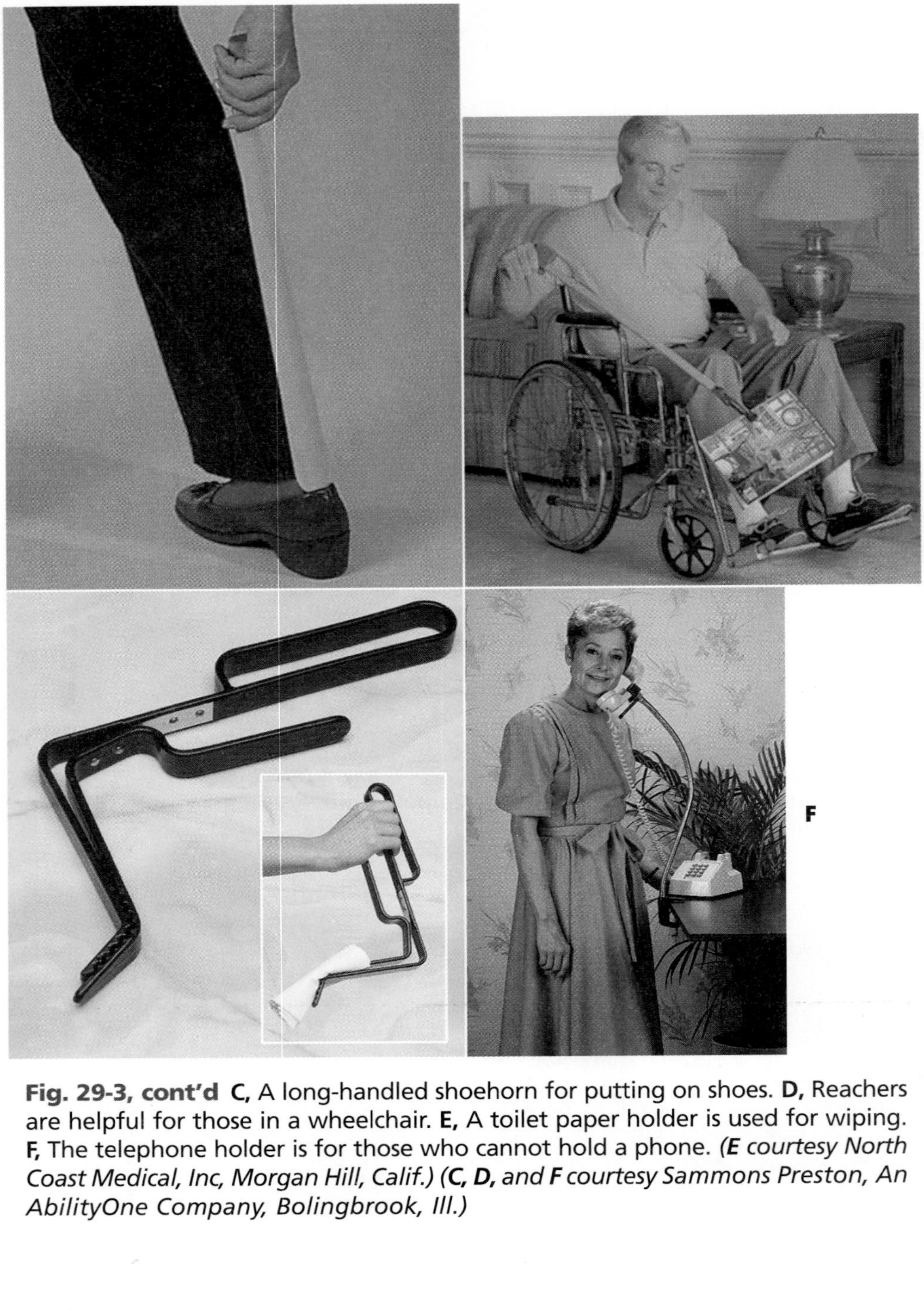

Fig. 29-3, cont'd C, A long-handled shoehorn for putting on shoes. **D,** Reachers are helpful for those in a wheelchair. **E,** A toilet paper holder is used for wiping. **F,** The telephone holder is for those who cannot hold a phone. *(**E** courtesy North Coast Medical, Inc, Morgan Hill, Calif.) (**C, D,** and **F** courtesy Sammons Preston, An AbilityOne Company, Bolingbrook, Ill.)*

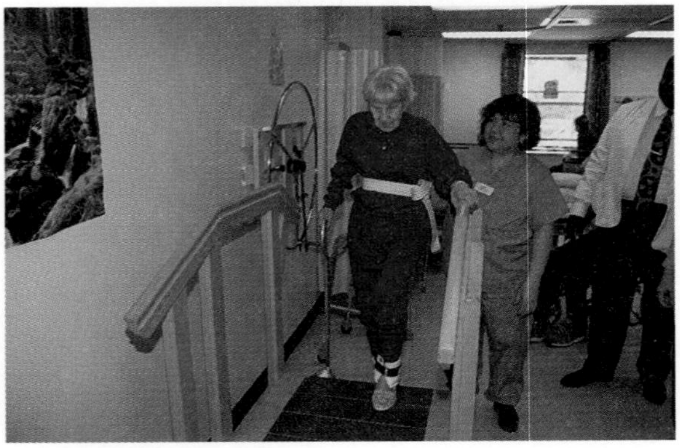

Fig. 29-4 The resident learns to walk in physical therapy.

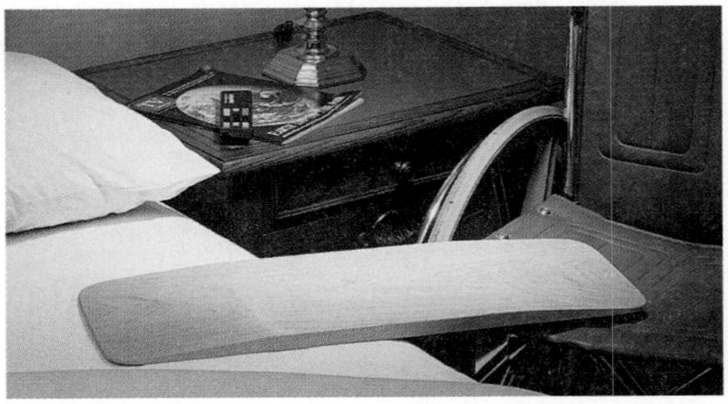

Fig. 29-5 A transfer board is used to transfer from one seat to another. *(Courtesy Northcoast Medical, Inc, Morgan Hill, Calif.)*

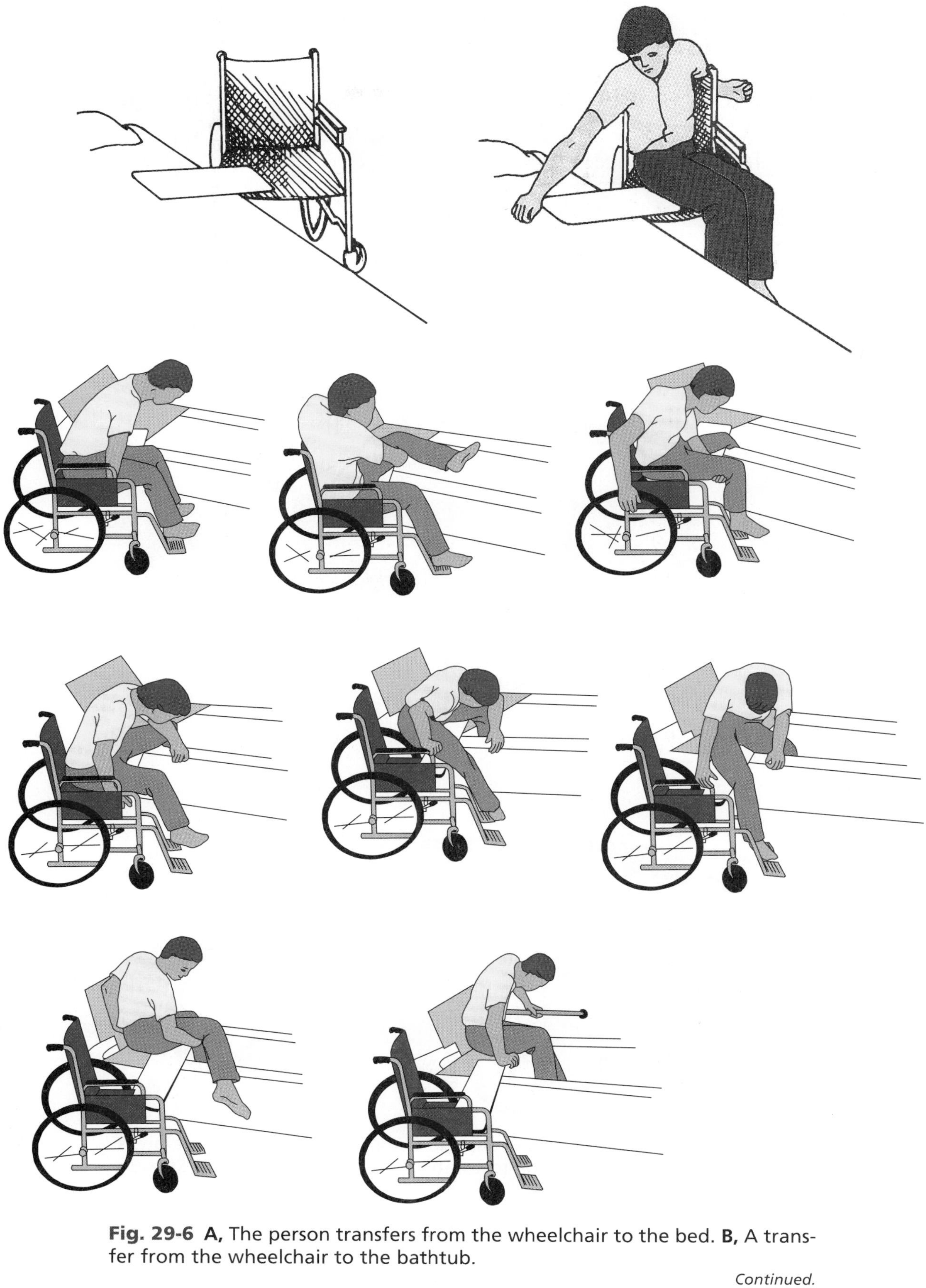

Fig. 29-6 **A,** The person transfers from the wheelchair to the bed. **B,** A transfer from the wheelchair to the bathtub.

Continued.

C

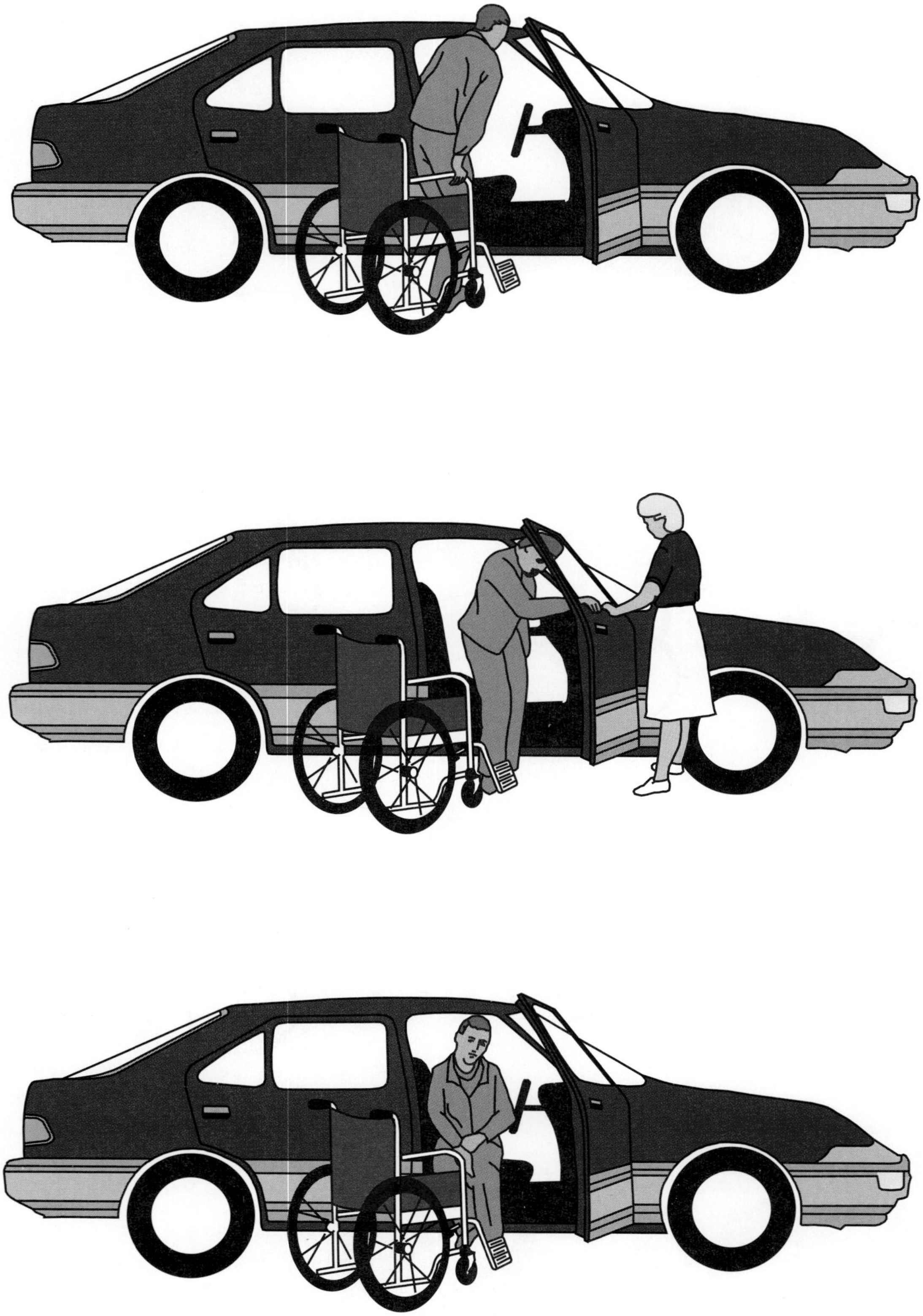

Fig. 29-6, cont'd C, A transfer to the car. The person has left-side paralysis. *(From Hoeman SP:* Rehabilitation/restorative care in the community, *St Louis, 1990, Mosby).*

Difficulty swallowing (*dysphagia*) may occur after a stroke. When possible, these residents are taught special exercises to improve swallowing. Some may never swallow again. These residents are fed through a gastrostomy tube (see Chapter 18). Difficulty speaking (*aphasia*) may occur from a stroke. Speech therapy and special devices (see Chapter 5) can help the person communicate.

Some persons need mechanical ventilation (see Chapter 25). These residents need a special respiratory rehabilitation program. Some are weaned from mechanical ventilation. Others must learn how to adapt to permanent mechanical ventilation. Special respiratory rehabilitation teams work with the residents and their families. Centers with subacute care units often have a respiratory rehabilitation program. *(See Subacute Care.)*

The center has policies and procedures for each program. The staff must be qualified to meet the needs of the residents in each program.

Subacute care units with rehabilitation programs often are accredited by JCAHO. This means that the center has met additional standards for staff education and training. The center also has specific goals for each rehabilitation program. There is a process to effectively evaluate the quality of each program. Improvements are made as needed. Resident and family education are an important part of all rehabilitation programs.

Persons admitted to subacute care rehabilitation programs usually stay for only a short time and then return home. Some may need home health care or assisted-living housing. Others will require long-term care in a nursing center.

SUBACUTE CARE

Some centers have a subacute care unit with special rehabilitation programs. These programs often focus on:

- Cardiac rehabilitation—dealing with disorders of the heart (see Chapter 26)
- Neurological rehabilitation—dealing with disorders of the nervous system (see Chapter 26)
- Respiratory rehabilitation—dealing with disorders of the respiratory system (see Chapters 25 and 26)
- Rehabilitation of complex medical/surgical conditions, such as postoperative wound care (see Chapter 14) and unstable diabetes (see Chapter 26)

Psychological and Social Aspects

A disability often affects self-esteem and relationships. Appearance and function changes may cause a person to feel unwhole, useless, unattractive, unclean, or undesirable to others. In the early stages of rehabilitation, the person may refuse to acknowledge the disability. The person also may expect therapy to correct the disability. He or she may be depressed, angry, and hostile.

Successful rehabilitation depends on the person's attitude, acceptance of limits, and motivation. The person must focus on remaining abilities. Discouragement and frustration are common feelings. Progress may be slow or efforts unsuccessful. Older persons may have greater difficulty with rehabilitation than do younger people. They often are weak and tire easily. Their progress may be slower, with fewer successes. Each new task to be learned is a reminder of the disability. Old fears and emotions may recur. Remind residents of the *progress* they have made. They need help in accepting their disabilities and limitations. Support, reassurance, encouragement, and sensitivity from the health care team are necessary. Meeting residents' psychological and social needs is an important part of the rehabilitation plan. A spiritual leader may be helpful for some residents.

THE REHABILITATION TEAM

Rehabilitation is a team effort. The team consists of the resident, the doctor, the nursing team, other health care team members (see Fig. 1-3, p. 9), and the family. All can help the disabled person regain function and independence.

The team meets regularly to discuss and evaluate the resident's progress. Goals are set for the resident. Changes in the rehabilitation plan are made when needed. The resident is included in the care plan meetings whenever possible. The family also is included if the resident wishes. Families are often a valuable part of the rehabilitation team. They provide support and encouragement. Families may also help with the person's care when he or she returns home.

REHABILITATION SERVICES

Rehabilitation begins when the person first requires health care. This usually involves hospital care. Depending on the person's needs and problems, the process may continue. The person may need more care in a nursing center. Some persons are transferred to a rehabilitation center, which has many special services. There are centers for persons who are blind, deaf, mentally retarded, and physically disabled, who have speech problems, and who are mentally ill. Home care agencies and adult day care centers also provide rehabilitation services.

OBRA Requirements

OBRA requires that nursing centers provide rehabilitation services. The services are provided by center staff members. If not, the center obtains the service from another source. For example, a center may not employ a physical therapist. Instead, the center obtains the service from a local hospital. OBRA rules state that rehabilitation services required by a resident's comprehensive care plan must be provided. If a resident requires physical therapy, it must be provided. If a resident requires occupational therapy, it must be provided. If a resident requires speech therapy, it must be provided. Such rehabilitation services require a doctor's order.

YOUR RESPONSIBILITIES

Rehabilitation and restorative nursing programs must involve the entire health care team. You are a key member of the rehabilitation team. The procedures and care measures already learned are part of the person's care. Safety, communication, legal, and ethical aspects apply in rehabilitation. Every part of your job as a nursing assistant is focused on helping residents stay as independent as possible. Good skin care, proper body alignment, range of motion, using safe transfer techniques, preventing falls, providing for the resident's spiritual needs, and treating residents with respect can increase independence and decrease the risk for decline in function. The many rules described throughout this book apply regardless of the type of disability. Box 29-1 lists your responsibilities as a member of the rehabilitation team.

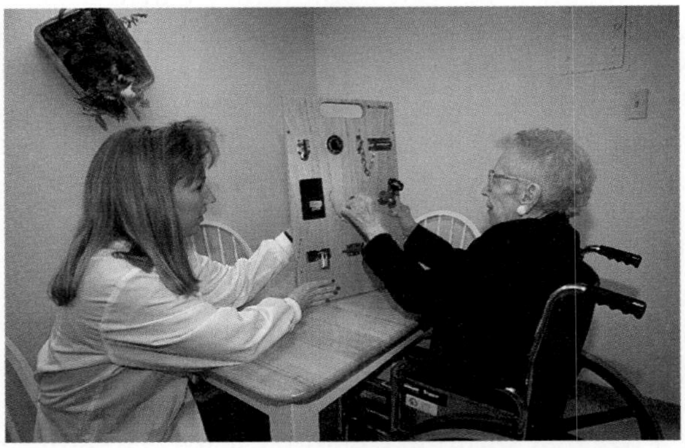

Fig. 29-7 The resident has privacy during a rehabilitation session.

Box 29-1 Nursing Assistant Responsibilities in Rehabilitation

- Follow the instructions and directions given by the nurse very carefully.
- Know and follow the resident's care plan.
- Report early signs and symptoms of complications such as pressure ulcers, contractures, and bowel and bladder problems.
- Keep the resident in good alignment at all times (see Chapter 10).
- Practice measures to prevent pressure ulcers (see Chapter 14).
- Turn and reposition the resident as directed.
- Perform range-of-motion exercises as instructed. Do them as often as stated by the nurse or resident's care plan.
- Encourage the resident to perform as many ADL as possible and to the extent possible. Allow time for the resident to complete the tasks.
- Give praise when even a little progress is made.
- Provide emotional support and reassurance.
- Practice the techniques developed by other members of the rehabilitation team when assisting the resident.
- Know how to apply self-care devices used by the resident.
- Try to understand and appreciate the resident's situation, feelings, and concerns.
- Do not pity or give the resident sympathy.
- Concentrate on the resident's abilities (not the disabilities).
- Remember that muscles will atrophy if not used.
- Practice the task that the resident must perform. This will help you guide and direct the individual.
- Know how to use and operate any special equipment that is part of the resident's rehabilitation program.
- Convey an attitude of hopefulness to the person.

Quality of Life

Successful rehabilitation will improve the resident's quality of life. A hopeful and winning attitude helps to motivate the resident. Rehabilitation, however, can be slow and frustrating. You can help the resident have the right attitude by taking measures to promote quality of life.

The resident's rights are protected. The right to privacy is important. You know why privacy is important during care. Privacy also is important during rehabilitation. Residents relearn old skills or practice new skills in private (Fig. 29-7). They do not need other residents watching them. Others do not need to see mistakes, falls, spills, or clumsiness. Nor do they need to see the person's anger or tears. Privacy protects the resident's dignity and promotes self-respect.

The right to personal choice gives the resident control. Being unable to control body movements or functions is very frustrating. Residents are allowed and encouraged to control the other aspects of their lives to the extent possible. Personal choice was discussed throughout this book. You must allow personal choice whenever possible. Residents who are sad and depressed may not want to make choices. You need to encourage them to do so. Making personal choices will help residents feel in control of those things that affect them.

The resident is part of the rehabilitation team. This allows the resident personal choice in planning care. The team plans and evaluates the resident's rehabilitation program.

The resident has the right to be free from abuse and mistreatment. Rehabilitation is often a very slow process. Sometimes improvement is not seen for weeks. Learning how to use an assistive device takes time. Learning to speak again after a stroke can take a long time. So can learning how to dress when there is paralysis on one side. These are just a few examples of the skills that may be part of rehabilitation. What seems so simple to you can be very hard for the resident. Repeated explanations and demonstrations may have no or little results. You may become impatient and short tempered with the resident. Or you may see such behavior from other team members or the family. You must protect the resident from physical and mental abuse and mistreatment. No one can shout, scream, or yell at the resident. Nor can they hit or strike the resident. The resident cannot be called names. Unkind remarks must not be made. You must report signs of abuse or mistreatment to the nurse.

You must learn to deal with your own anger and frustration. Remember that the resident wants to have function and control of body movements. The person does not choose loss of function. If the process is frustrating to you, just think how the resident must feel. Discuss your feelings with the nurse. The nurse can suggest ways to help you control your feelings. Perhaps you can be reassigned to other residents for a while.

Taking part in resident activities promotes quality of life. The resident is encouraged to join in activities. Often persons are concerned about how others view the disability. Provide support and reassurance. Remind the person that other residents have disabilities. They can be very supportive and understanding because of their own disabilities. Allow personal choice in activities. Residents usually choose those of interest and those that are the least threatening.

The environment is important for quality of life. It must be safe and must meet the resident's needs. Needed changes are made because of disabilities. Location of the overbed table or the bedside stand may need changing. The resident may need a special chair. If the signal light cannot be used, another way is needed to communicate with the staff. These and other adjustments are recommended by nurses, occupational and physical therapists, and other team members. They explain the need and purpose to the resident and family.

Rehabilitation is part of your job as a nursing assistant. It can be challenging and rewarding for all members of the health care team. Patience, understanding, and sensitivity are needed when working with the disabled person. Progress may be slow and hard to see. The resident may be frustrated and discouraged. You must give support, encouragement, and praise when needed. The disabled person does not need pity or sympathy.

Emphasizing abilities is important. So is preventing disabling complications. Contractures, pressure ulcers, and bowel and bladder problems must be prevented. Therefore good nursing care is necessary. Along with helping to prevent complications, you need to observe the techniques taught to the disabled resident. This lets you guide the resident more effectively during care. If the resident has to perform tasks in different ways for different staff members, frustration takes the place of progress. Finally, remember that the more the resident can do alone, the better the resident's quality of life.

Review Questions

Circle the BEST answer.

1 Rehabilitation is concerned with
- A Physical disabilities
- B Physical capabilities
- C The whole person
- D Psychological and social functioning

2 Physical rehabilitation begins with the prevention of
- A Anger, frustration, and depression
- B Contractures, pressure ulcers, and bowel and bladder problems
- C Illness and injury
- D Loss of self-esteem

3 Mr. Williams has paralysis of both legs. Activities of daily living are
- A Done by Mr. Williams to the extent possible
- B Done by the nursing assistant
- C Postponed until he regains use of his legs
- D Supervised by the physical therapist

4 Which reaction may be experienced by the person with a disability?
- A Feelings of being undesirable or unattractive
- B Anger and hostility
- C Depression
- D All of the above

5 The nursing assistant
- A Plans the rehabilitation program
- B Supplies prostheses
- C Gives praise when even slight progress is made
- D Does as much as possible for the disabled person

6 Which statement is *false?*
- A Sympathy and pity help the person adjust to the disability.
- B You should know how to apply self-care devices.
- C You should know how to use equipment used in the person's care.
- D Hopefulness needs to be conveyed to the person.

7 Mr. Lund is in physical therapy to learn how to use a walker. He asks to have music played. You should
- A Tell him music is not allowed
- B Choose some music
- C Let the resident choose some music
- D Ask the resident group in charge of activities to choose some music

8 Mr. Lund does not want to attend a concert scheduled at the center. This is his right to
- A Personal choice
- B Privacy
- C Be free from abuse and neglect
- D All of the above

9 Mrs. Angelo is paralyzed on the right side. The signal light is placed on the right side. You move it to the left side. You have promoted her quality of life by
- A Protecting her from abuse and mistreatment
- B Allowing personal choice
- C Providing a safe environment
- D All of the above

Circle T if the statement is true and F if the statement is false.

10 T F A resident's speech therapy should be provided in private.

11 T F You tell Mr. Lund that he cannot have dessert unless he does his exercises. This is abuse and mistreatment of the resident.

12 T F Rehabilitation programs for older persons usually proceed at a slower pace than those for the young.

13 T F The rehabilitation team includes only the doctor and the physical therapist.

14 T F The nursing assistant is involved in the resident's rehabilitation program.

15 T F Giving pity and sympathy is helpful to residents with disabilities.

Answers to these questions are on p. 700.

30 Sexuality

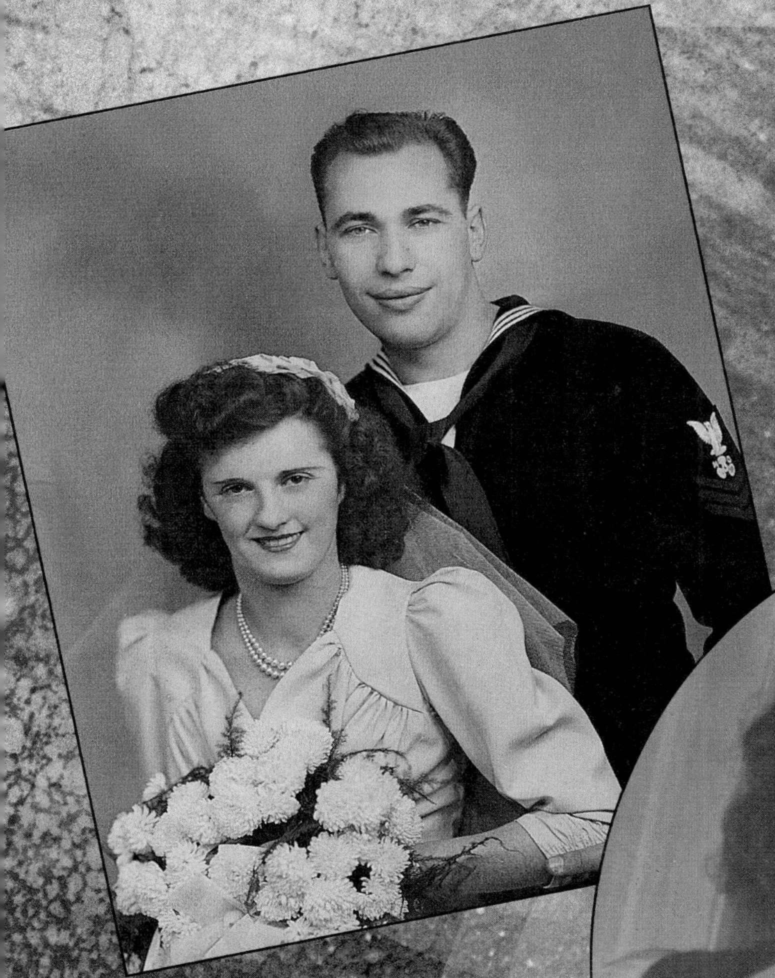

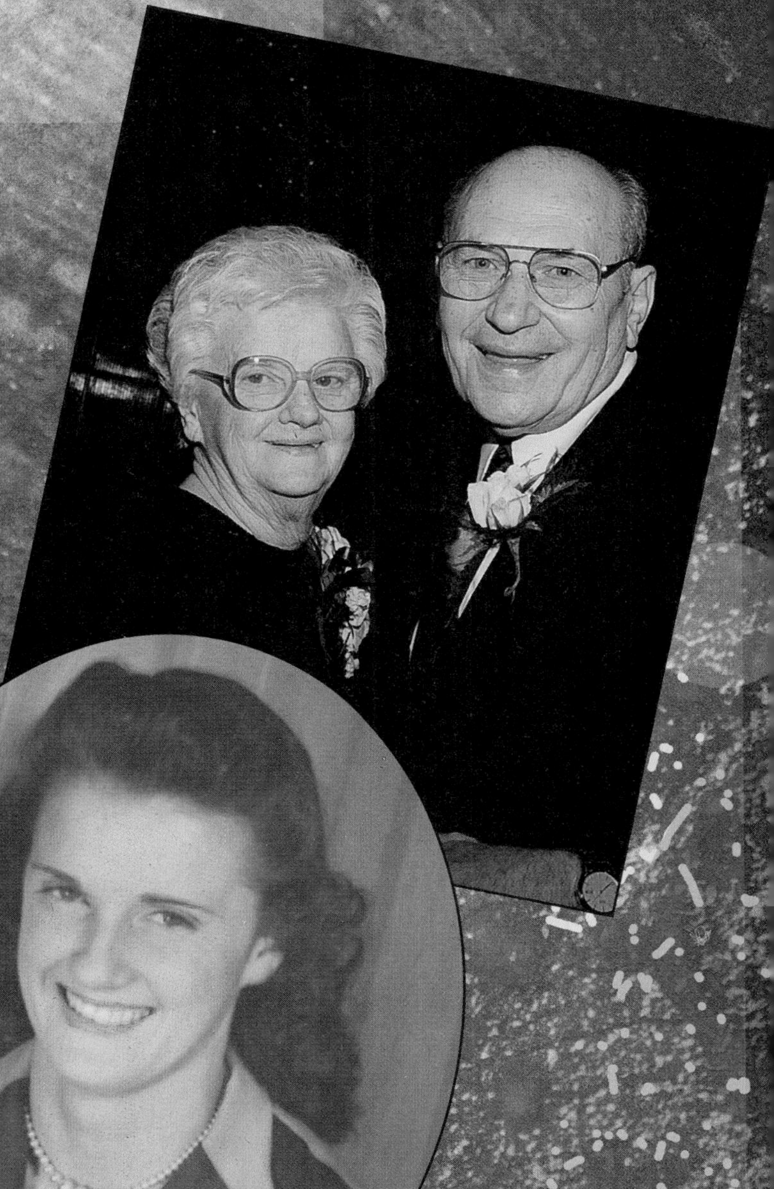

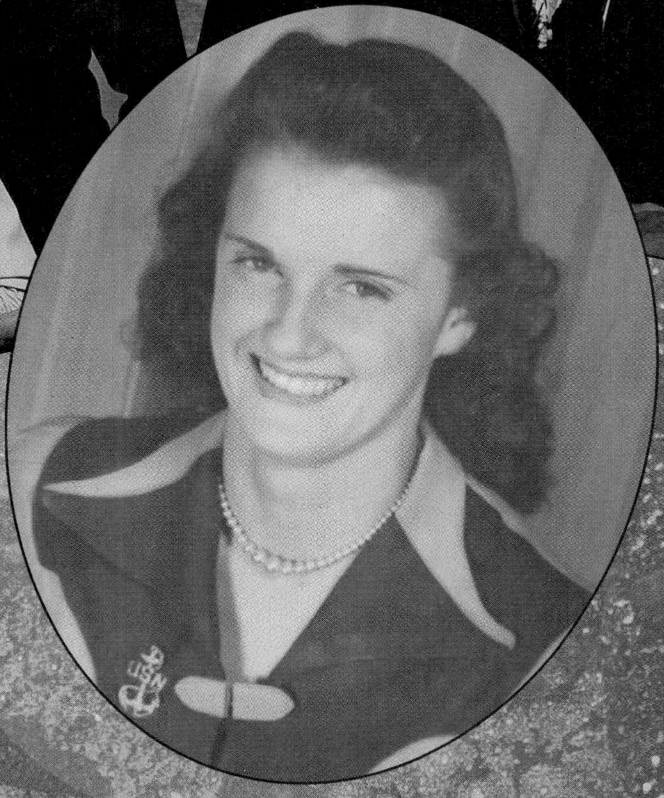

What You Will Learn

- The definition of the key terms listed in this chapter
- The differences between sex and sexuality
- The importance of sexuality throughout life
- Five types of sexual relationships
- How injury and illness can affect sexuality
- How aging affects sexuality in older persons
- How the nursing team can promote a resident's sexuality
- Why some residents become sexually aggressive
- How to deal with sexually aggressive residents

Key Terms

bisexual A person who is attracted to both sexes

heterosexual A person who is attracted to people of the other sex

homosexual A person who is attracted to members of the same sex

impotence The inability of the male to have an erection

menopause The time when menstruation stops; it marks the end of the woman's reproductive years

sex The physical activities involving the organs of reproduction; the activities are done for pleasure or to produce children

sexuality The physical, psychological, social, cultural, and spiritual factors that affect a person's feelings and attitudes about his or her sex

transsexual A person who believes that he or she is really a member of the other sex

transvestite A person who becomes sexually excited by dressing in the clothes of the other sex

▲ Nursing center residents were once viewed as having only physical problems. The resident's physical needs were the first and often the only concern. Little attention was given to the psychological or social effects of the resident's disorder. The needs for love and belonging, self-esteem, and self-actualization often were overlooked. Now attention is given to the total person. Physical, psychological, social, and spiritual needs of the resident are considered.

Sexuality is a part of the whole person. It involves the physical, psychological, social, and spiritual parts. Illness and injury can affect a person's sexuality. This chapter describes the effects of illness, injury, and aging on sexuality. You must view residents as total persons. Total persons have sexuality.

SEX AND SEXUALITY

Sex and sexuality are different. **Sex** is the physical activities involving the reproductive organs. The activities are done for pleasure or to produce children. **Sexuality** involves the personality and the body. A person's attitudes and feelings are involved. Physical, psychological, social, cultural, and spiritual factors influence sexuality. It affects how a person behaves, thinks, dresses, and responds to others.

Sexuality is present when a baby's sex is known. Names, colors, and toys reflect sexuality. Blue is used for boys and pink for girls. Dolls are for girls. Trains are for boys. By the age of 2, children know their own sex. Three-year-olds know the sex of other children. Children learn male and female roles from their parents (Fig. 30-1). Children learn early that there are certain behaviors for boys and certain ones for girls.

As children grow older, interest increases about the human body and how it works. Body changes during adolescence bring more interest about sex and the body. Their bodies respond to stimulation. Teenagers engage in sexual behaviors. They kiss, embrace, pet, or have intercourse. Pregnancy and sexually transmitted diseases (p. 660) are great risks for sexually active teenagers.

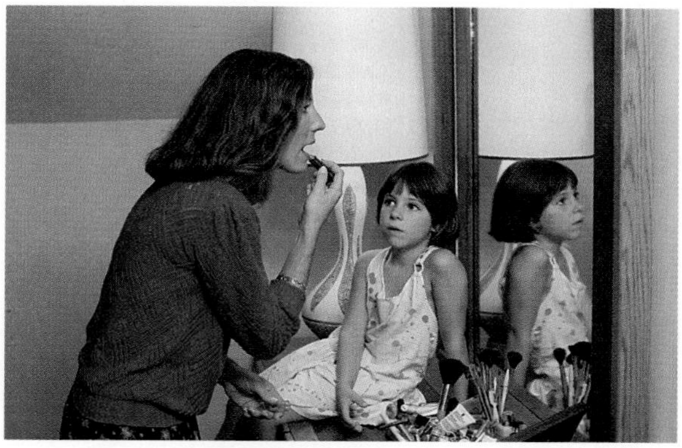

Fig. 30-1 This little girl is learning female roles from her mother.

Sex has more meaning as young adults mature. Attitudes and feelings are important. Sexual partners are selected. Sex before marriage and birth control are other decisions.

Sexuality is important into adulthood and old age. Attitudes and sex needs change as a person grows older. Life circumstances change. These include divorce, death of a partner, injury, and illness.

SEXUAL RELATIONSHIPS

Sex and sexuality usually involve a partner. A **heterosexual** is a person who is attracted to people of the other sex. Men are attracted to women, and women are attracted to men. Sexual behavior is male–female.

A **homosexual** is attracted to members of the same sex. Men are attracted to men, and women are attracted to women. *Gay* refers to homosexuality. Homosexual men are referred to as *gay men. Lesbian* refers to a female homosexual.

Homosexuality has existed for centuries. Before the 1960s and 1970s, many gay persons were secret about their sexual orientation. Now many gay men and lesbians are more open about their sexual preference and relationships.

Bisexuals are attracted to both sexes. Some alternate between same-gender and male-female behaviors. Bisexuals often are married and have children. They may seek a same-gender relationship or experience outside of marriage.

Some people believe that they are really members of the other sex. These people are **transsexuals**. A male believes he is really a female in a man's body. A female believes she is really a male in a woman's body. Transsexual persons often describe feeling "trapped" in the wrong body. Most have had these feelings for as long as they can remember. As children they usually show behaviors of the other sex. Many seek psychiatric treatment. Some have sex-change operations.

Transvestites become sexually excited by dressing in clothes of the other sex. Most are male. They usually are married and heterosexual. They dress normally as men most of the time. Dressing as a woman is usually done in private. Some dress completely as a woman. Others focus on bras and panties. The sex partner may not know about the practice. Some partners take part in transvestite activities. Some transvestites have same-gender friends with similar interests.

INJURY AND ILLNESS

Sexuality and sex involve the mind and body. Injury and illness can affect sexual function. A person may feel unclean, unwhole, unattractive, or mutilated after surgery or injury. Attitudes about sex may change. The person may feel unfit for closeness and love. Therefore the person may develop sexual problems that are psychological. Time, understanding, and a caring partner are very helpful. Counseling or psychiatric help may be needed.

Many illnesses, injuries, and surgeries affect the nervous, circulatory, and reproductive systems. If one or more of these systems are involved, the person's sexual ability may change. Most chronic illnesses affect sexual function.

Impotence is the inability of the male to have an erection. Diabetes mellitus, spinal cord injuries, multiple sclerosis, and alcoholism are common causes. Circulatory disorders and medications can interfere with achieving an erection. Impotence is a side effect of some medications that control high blood pressure. Today new drugs are available for impotence.

Heart disease, stroke, chronic obstructive pulmonary disease, and nervous system disorders can affect sexual ability. Some reproductive system surgeries have physical and psychological effects. Prostate or testes removal affects erections. Removal of the uterus, ovaries, or a breast may affect a woman psychologically.

You will care for residents with disorders that can affect sexual functioning. Changes in sexual functioning greatly impact the resident. Fear, anger, worry, and depression are common. You see these in the resident's behavior and comments. The resident's feelings are very normal and expected. The health care team must be sensitive to the resident's feelings. Helping the resident deal with these feelings is part of the care plan.

SEXUALITY AND OLDER PERSONS

Sexual relationships are important to older persons (Fig. 30-2, p. 658). They fall in love, hold hands, embrace, and have sex. They need sex, love, and affection. Many have sexual intercourse.

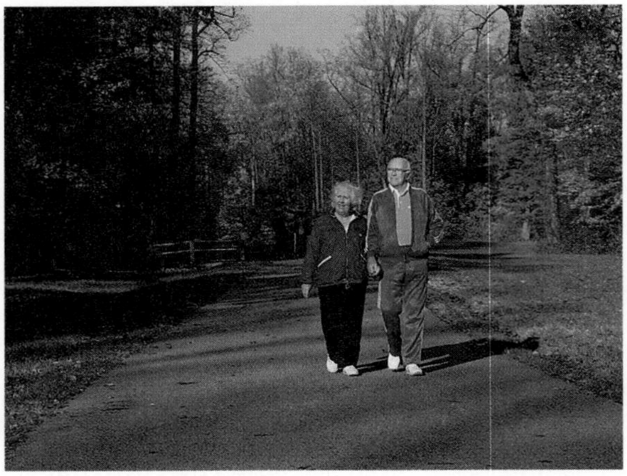

Fig. 30-2 Love and affection are important to older persons.

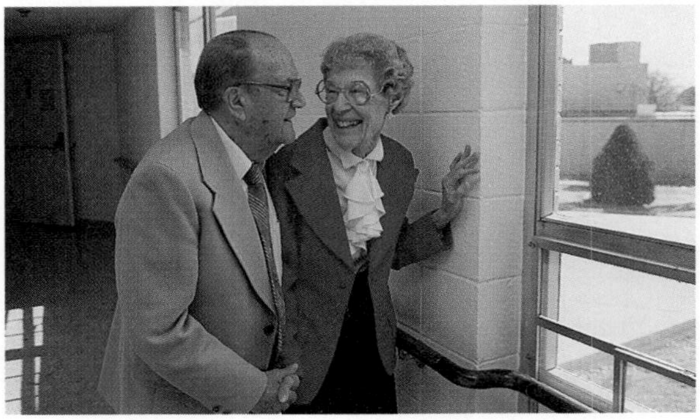

Fig. 30-3 Relationships occur in nursing centers.

Love, affection, and intimacy are needed throughout life. As other losses occur, feeling close to another person is more important. Children leave home. Friends and relatives die. People retire. Health problems may develop. Decreasing strength and a changing appearance add to these losses.

Reproductive organs change with aging (see Chapter 7). In men, the hormone *testosterone* decreases. The hormone affects strength, sperm production, and reproductive tissues. These changes affect sexual activity. It takes longer for an erection to occur. The phase between erection and orgasm is also longer. Orgasm is less forceful than in the younger years. After orgasm, the erection is lost quickly. The time between erections is also longer. Older men may need the penis stimulated for sexual arousal. These changes result in decreased frequency of sexual activity.

Mental and physical fatigue, overeating, and excessive drinking affect erections. Some men fear performance problems. Therefore they may avoid sexual activity.

Physical changes occur in women (see Chapter 7). Menopause occurs around 50 years of age. **Menopause** is when a woman stops menstruating. Her reproductive years end. Female hormones (*estrogen* and *progesterone*) decrease. Reduced hormone levels affect reproductive tissues. The uterus, vagina, and external genitalia atrophy (shrink). Intercourse may be uncomfortable or painful. This is from thin vaginal walls and vaginal dryness. Older women also have changes in sexual excitement. Arousal takes longer. The time between excitement and orgasm is longer. Orgasm is less intense. The pre-excitement state returns more quickly.

Frequency of sexual activity decreases for many men and women. Reasons relate to weakness, mental and physical fatigue, pain, and reduced mobility. The normal aging process or chronic illnesses are common causes. Pain and reduced mobility from illness and aging can affect frequency. One or both partners may have a chronic illness. It may lead to decreased frequency or no sexual activity.

Some older people do not have sexual intercourse. This does not mean sexual needs or desires are lost. They can express their needs in other ways. Handholding, touching, caressing, and embracing bring closeness and intimacy.

Having a sexual partner is also important. Death and divorce result in loss of a sexual partner. The partner may also be in a hospital or nursing center. These situations occur in adults of all ages.

MEETING THE RESIDENT'S SEXUAL NEEDS

Sexuality is part of the total person. Some residents are so ill that sexual activity is impossible. Others want and are capable of sexual activity. Sexual activity does not always mean intercourse. It may be expressed in other ways. The nursing team has an important role in sexuality. They allow and promote the meeting of sexual needs. Residents appreciate the measures listed in Box 30-1. They are carried out in cooperation with the nurse supervising your work.

Married couples in nursing centers are allowed to share the same room. This is an OBRA requirement. The couple have lived together for many years. Long-term care is no reason to keep them apart in male and female rooms. They can share the same bed if their conditions permit. OBRA

Sexual partners are lost through death and divorce. A single resident may develop a relationship with another single resident. Instead of keeping them apart, they are allowed time together (Fig. 30-3).

Box 30-1 PROMOTING SEXUALITY

- Let the resident practice grooming routines. This includes applying makeup, nail polish, and body lotion and wearing cologne. Hair care is important. Women may want to shave their legs and underarms and pluck eyebrows. Men may use after-shave lotion. Residents need help with these activities.
- Let the resident choose clothing. Hospital gowns embarrass both men and women. Street clothes are worn if the resident's condition permits.
- Protect the right to privacy. Avoid exposing the resident. Drape and screen the resident appropriately.
- Accept the resident's sexual relationships. The resident may not share your sexual attitudes, values, or practices. Do not expect the resident to follow your standards. The resident may have a homosexual, premarital, or extramarital relationship. Do not judge or gossip about relationships.
- Allow privacy. You can usually tell when two people want to be alone. If the resident has a private room, close the door for privacy. Some centers have *Do Not Disturb* signs for doors. Let the resident and partner know how much time they have alone. For example, remind them about meal times, medications, or treatments. Tell other staff members that the resident wants time alone.
- Knock before you enter any room. This is a simple courtesy that shows respect for privacy.
- Consider the resident's roommate. Privacy curtains provide little privacy. Arrange for privacy when the roommate is out of the room. Sometimes roommates volunteer to leave for a while. If the roommate cannot leave, other areas on the nursing unit are used for privacy.
- Allow privacy for masturbation. It is a normal form of sexual expression and release. Close the privacy curtain and the door. Knock before you enter any room to save you and the resident embarrassment. Sometimes confused residents masturbate in public areas. Lead the resident to a private area, or engage his or her interest in some other activity.

THE SEXUALLY AGGRESSIVE RESIDENT

Some residents want their sexual needs met by the health care team. They flirt, make sexual advances or comments, expose themselves, masturbate, or touch staff. The staff member is usually angry or embarrassed when this happens. These reactions are normal. Often there are reasons for the resident's behavior. Understanding this helps you deal with the situation.

Illness, injury, surgery, or aging often threatens a male's sense of manhood. He tries to prove to himself that he is still attractive and able to perform sexually. Therefore he may behave sexually toward a staff member.

Some sexually aggressive behaviors are caused by confusion or disorientation. Common causes are nervous system disorders, medications, fever, dementia (see Chapter 27), and poor vision. The person may confuse a staff member or another resident with his or her partner. Or the person cannot control behavior because of changes in mental function. The healthy person is able to control sexual urges. However, changes in the brain can make control difficult. Sexual behavior in these cases is usually innocent on the resident's part.

Some residents do touch workers inappropriately. Their purpose is sexual. However, sometimes touch is the only way to get someone's attention. For example, Mr. Green had a stroke. His right side is paralyzed, and he cannot speak. Your back is to him, and you are bending over. Your buttocks are the closest part of your body to him. To get your attention, he touches your buttocks. You should not consider his behavior as sexual.

Often masturbation is viewed as a sexually aggressive behavior. It could indeed be touching and manipulating the genitals for sexual pleasure. However, urinary or reproductive system disorders can cause genital soreness or itching. Poor hygiene is another cause of itching. So is being wet or soiled from urine or a bowel movement. The health care team must remember that touching the genitals could be a sign of a health problem.

Sexual advances may be intentional. You need to be professional about the matter. These suggestions may help:

- Ask the resident not to touch you. State the places where you were touched.
- Tell the resident that you will not do what he or she wants.

- Tell the resident that those behaviors make you uncomfortable. Politely ask the resident not to act in that way.
- Allow privacy if the resident is becoming sexually aroused. Provide for safety; for example, raise bed rails if ordered for the resident, place the signal light within reach (see Chapter 8). Tell the resident when you will return.
- Discuss the situation with the nurse. The nurse can help you understand the resident 's behavior.

The health care team develops approaches to deal with sexually aggressive behaviors. These approaches are based on the cause of the behavior. They are specific to each resident and are part of the resident's care plan. Many centers have special classes to help staff deal with sexually aggressive behavior. You must always stay calm and professional. If you feel that you cannot deal with a situation, talk to the nurse.

SEXUALLY TRANSMITTED DISEASES

Some diseases are spread by sexual contact. They are grouped under the heading of sexually transmitted diseases (STDs). STDs are presented in Chapter 26.

QUALITY OF LIFE

Sexuality is part of the total person. Illness or injury does not mean that sexuality is unimportant. Some residents are so ill that sexual activity is impossible. Others, however, want to be and can be sexually active. Sexual activity does not always mean intercourse. It may be expressed in other ways. The health care team plays an important role in allowing residents to meet their sexual needs. The measures listed in Box 30-1 are appreciated by residents. They are carried out in cooperation with the nurse supervising your work.

Do not make judgments or gossip about a resident's sexuality. Positive, pleasurable sexual relationships and intimacy enhance the quality of life for many persons of all ages.

REVIEW QUESTIONS

Circle the BEST answer.

1 Sex involves
- A The organs of reproduction
- B Attitudes and feelings
- C Cultural and spiritual factors
- D All of the above

2 Sexuality is important to
- A Small children
- B Teenagers and young adults
- C Middle-age adults
- D Persons of all ages

3 Impotence is
- A When menstruation stops
- B A psychological reaction to disfigurement
- C The inability of the male to achieve an erection
- D The complete absence of sexual activity

4 Reproductive organs change with aging.
- A True
- B False

5 Mr. and Mrs. Green live in the same nursing center. Which will *not* promote their sexuality?
- A Allowing their normal grooming routines
- B Having them wear hospital gowns
- C Allowing them privacy
- D Accepting their relationship

6 An older lady and an older gentleman live in a nursing center. They are holding hands. Nursing staff should keep them apart.
- A True
- B False

7 Mr. Green wants time alone with his wife. The nurse tells you this is okay. You should
- A Close the door to the room
- B Put a *Do Not Disturb* sign on the door
- C Tell other staff that Mr. and Mrs. Green want some time alone
- D All of the above

8 Mr. and Mrs. Green should be assigned to separate rooms.
- A True
- B False

9 Mr. Smith is masturbating in the dining room. You should do all of the following, *except*
- A Cover him and quietly take him to his room
- B Scold him for his bad behavior
- C Provide privacy and respect his rights
- D Report the behavior to the nurse

10 A resident makes sexual advances to you. You should do the following *except*
- A Discuss the situation with the nurse
- B Do what the resident asks
- C Explain to the resident that the behaviors make you uncomfortable
- D Ask the resident not to touch you in places where you were touched

Answers to these questions are on p. 700.

31 Basic Emergency Care

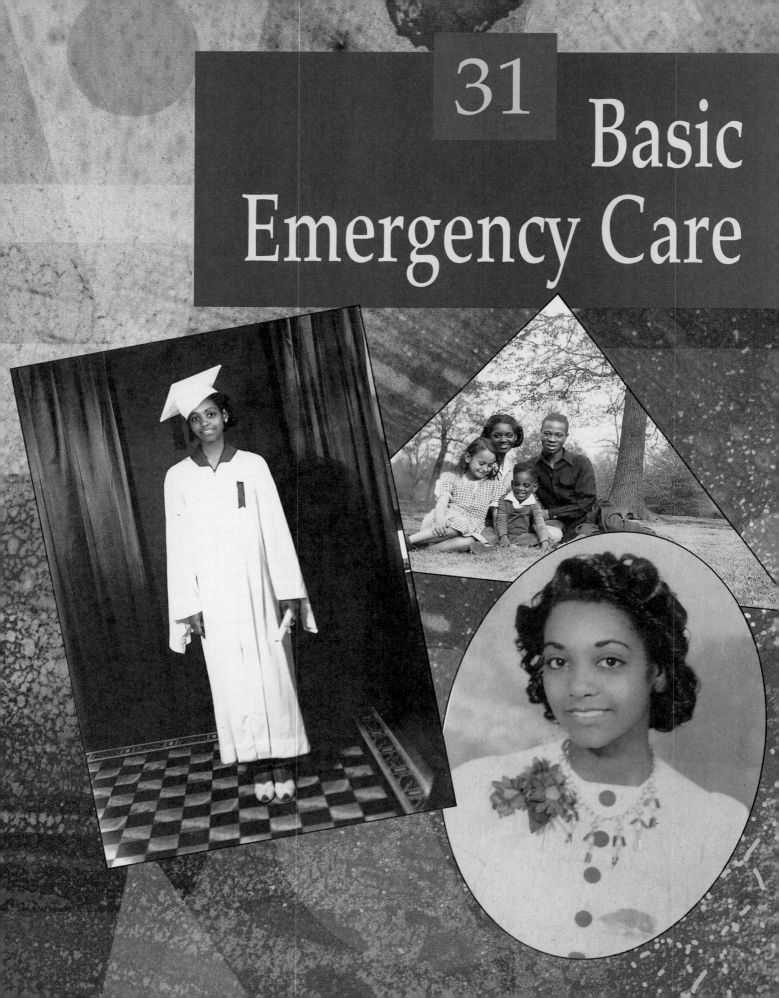

What You Will Learn

- The definition of the key terms listed in this chapter
- The general rules of emergency care
- The signs of cardiac arrest and obstructed airway
- How to perform cardiopulmoary resuscitation and relieve an obstructed airway
- The difference between internal and external hemorrhage
- The difference between arterial and venous bleeding
- How to control hemorrhage
- The different types of seizures and how to care for a person during a seizure
- Common causes of and emergency care for fainting
- Signs of stroke and emergency care for a person with stroke
- How to promote quality of life in emergency situations
- The procedures described in this chapter

Key Terms

cardiac arrest The sudden stoppage of breathing and heart action

convulsion Violent and sudden contractions or tremors of muscles; seizure

fainting The sudden loss of consciousness as a result of an inadequate blood supply to the brain

first aid Emergency care given to an ill or injured person before medical help arrives

hemorrhage The excessive loss of blood from a blood vessel

respiratory arrest Breathing stops but the heart continues to pump for several minutes

seizure A convulsion

shock A condition that results when there is an inadequate blood supply to organs and tissues

Emergency situations can occur in nursing centers, homes, public places, and on the highway. Knowing what to do may mean the difference between life and death. This chapter describes some common emergencies and the basic care that is given. You are encouraged to take a first aid course offered by the National Safety Council or the American Red Cross. A basic life support course offered by the American Heart Association, National Safety Council, or the American Red Cross also is recommended. These courses prepare you to give care in emergency situations.

GENERAL RULES OF EMERGENCY CARE

First aid is the emergency care given to an ill or injured person before medical help arrives. The goals of first aid are to prevent death and to prevent injuries from becoming worse.

When an emergency occurs, the local emergency medical service (EMS) system is activated. The system involves emergency personnel (paramedics, emergency medical technicians) who have had education and training in emergency care. They have learned how to treat, stabilize, and transport persons who are experiencing life-threatening conditions. Their emergency vehicles have the equipment, supplies, and drugs used in emergencies. Emergency personnel communicate by two-way radio with a doctor based in a hospital emergency room. The doctor tells them what to do. In many areas, dialing 911 can activate the EMS system. Calling the local fire or police department or the telephone operator also can activate the system.

In nursing centers, a nurse decides when to activate the EMS system. The nurse tells you what to do to help in the situation. If the resident has stopped breathing or is having a cardiac arrest, the nurse may start cardiopulmonary resuscitation (CPR) (p. 664). Center policies vary about nursing assistants starting CPR. Some allow nursing assistants to start CPR, and others do not. You need to know your center's policy about CPR.

Some residents are not resuscitated. The resident, family, and doctor have decided that the resident should be allowed to die with peace and dignity. If so, the doctor writes a "Do not resuscitate" (DNR) order (see Chapter 32). You need to know your center's policy about DNR orders. The nurse tells you which residents have DNR orders. This information is also in the care plan.

Each emergency is different. However, the rules in Box 31-1 apply to any emergency.

BASIC LIFE SUPPORT

When the heart and breathing stop, the person is clinically dead. Blood and oxygen are not circulated through the body. Permanent brain damage and other organ damage occur within minutes. Death may be expected. Death is expected in persons suffering from long illnesses for which there is no hope of recovery. However, the heart and breathing can stop suddenly and without warning. This is a state of **cardiac arrest.**

Cardiac arrest is a sudden, unexpected, and dramatic event. People have had a cardiac arrest while driving, shoveling snow, playing golf or tennis, watching television, eating, and sleeping. Cardiac arrest can occur anywhere and at any time. Common causes include heart disease, drowning, electrical shock, severe injury, obstruction of the air passages, and drug overdose. The person suffers permanent brain damage unless breathing and circulation are restored.

Respiratory arrest is when breathing stops but the heart continues to pump blood for several minutes. If breathing is not restored, cardiac arrest occurs. Causes of respiratory arrest include drowning, stroke, obstructed airway, drug overdose, electrocution, smoke inhalation, suffocation, injury from lightning, myocardial infarction (heart attack), coma, and other injuries.

Basic life support (BLS) involves preventing or promptly recognizing cardiac arrest or respiratory arrest. BLS procedures support breathing and circulation. These life-saving measures require speed, skill, and efficiency. Prompt activation of the EMS system is also part of BLS.

NOTE: *The American Heart Association, National Safety Council, and American Red Cross certify individuals to perform basic life support procedures. The basic life support procedures that follow are presented as information. They do not replace certification training. You are encouraged to take a basic life support course offered by one of these organizations.*

Box 31-1 General Rules of Emergency Care

- Know your limits. Do not try to do more than you are able. Do not perform a procedure with which you are unfamiliar. Do what you can under the circumstances.
- Stay calm. This helps the person feel more secure.
- Practice Standard Precautions, and follow the Bloodborne Pathogen Standard to the extent possible.
- Check for signs of life-threatening problems. Check for breathing, pulse, and bleeding.
- Keep the person lying down or in the position in which he or she was found. Moving the person could make an injury worse.
- Perform necessary emergency measures.
- Call for help, or have someone activate the EMS system. An operator sends emergency vehicles and personnel to the scene. Do not hang up until the operator has hung up. Give the operator the following information:
  - Your location—with the street address and the city or town you are in, as well as the names of cross streets or roads and landmarks if possible
  - Telephone number you are calling from
  - What happened (e.g., heart attack, accident)—police, fire equipment, and ambulances may be needed
  - How many people need help
  - Conditions of persons, any obvious injuries, and any life-threatening situations
  - What aid is being given
- Do not remove clothes unless you have to. If clothing must be removed, tear the garment along the seams.
- Keep the person warm. Cover the person with a blanket. Or use coats and sweaters.
- Reassure the conscious person. Explain what is happening and that help was called.
- Do not give the person any food or fluids.
- Do not move the person. Emergency personnel are trained to do so.
- Keep bystanders away from the person. They tend to stare, offer advice, and make comments about the person's condition. The person may think the situation is worse than it really is. Also, onlookers invade privacy.

Cardiopulmonary Resuscitation

There are three major signs of cardiac arrest—no pulse, no breathing, and unconsciousness. The person's skin is cool, pale, and gray. The person has no blood pressure.

Cardiopulmonary resuscitation (CPR) must be started as soon as cardiac arrest occurs. CPR provides oxygen to the brain, heart, kidneys, and other organs until more advanced emergency care can be given. CPR has three basic parts (the ABCs of CPR):

- **A**irway
- **B**reathing
- **C**irculation

Airway. The respiratory passages (airway) must be open to restore breathing. The airway often is blocked or obstructed during cardiac arrest. The person's tongue falls toward the back of the throat and blocks the airway. The *head-tilt/chin-lift maneuver* is used to open the airway (Fig. 31-1):

- Place one hand on the person's forehead.
- Apply pressure on the forehead with the palm to tilt the head back.
- Place the fingers of the other hand under the bony part of the chin.
- Lift the chin forward as the head is tilted backward with the other hand.

When the airway is open, check for vomitus, loose dentures, or other foreign bodies. These can obstruct the airway during rescue breathing. Remove dentures, and wipe vomitus away with your index and middle fingers. Wear disposable gloves, or cover your fingers with a cloth. Although you must not waste time, try to protect the dentures from loss or damage.

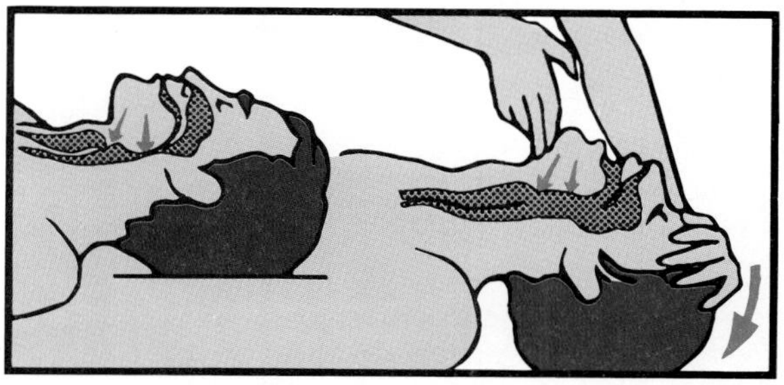

Fig. 31-1 The head-tilt/chin-lift maneuver is used to open the airway. One hand is on the person's forehead, and pressure is applied to tilt the head back. The fingers of the other hand are placed under the chin. The chin is lifted forward with the fingers.

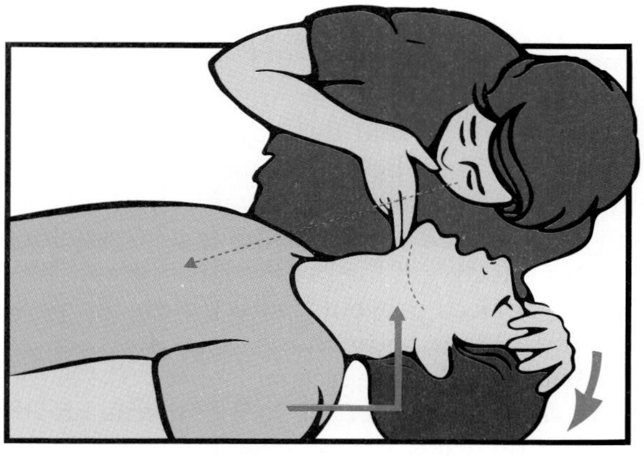

Fig. 31-2 Determine breathlessness by *looking* to see if the chest rises and falls, *listening* for the escape of air, and *feeling* for the flow of air.

Breathing. Air is not inhaled when breathing stops. The person must get oxygen. Otherwise, permanent brain and organ damage occur. Breathing is done for the person. This is called *rescue breathing*.

Before you start rescue breathing, determine breathlessness (Fig. 31-2). It should take 3 to 5 seconds to do the following:

- Maintain an open airway.
- Place your ear over the person's mouth and nose.
- Observe the person's chest.
- *Look* to see if the person's chest rises and falls.
- *Listen* for the escape of air.
- *Feel* for the flow of air.

Mouth-to-mouth resuscitation (Fig. 31-3) is the most common method of rescue breathing. The airway is kept open to give mouth-to-mouth resuscitation. The person's nostrils are pinched shut with the thumb and index finger of the hand on the forehead. Shutting the nostrils prevents air from escaping through the nose. After taking a deep breath, place your mouth tightly over the person's mouth. Blow air into the person's mouth slowly. You should see the person's chest rise as the lungs fill with air. You should also hear the escape of air when the person exhales. After you give a breath, remove your mouth from the person's mouth. Then take in a quick, deep breath.

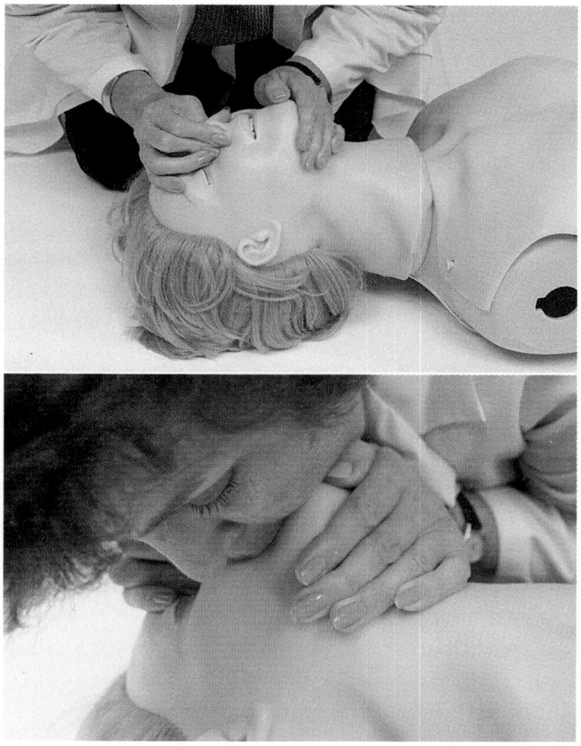

A

B

Fig. 31-3 Mouth-to-mouth resuscitation. **A,** The person's airway is opened, and the nostrils are pinched shut. **B,** The person's mouth is sealed by the rescuer's mouth.

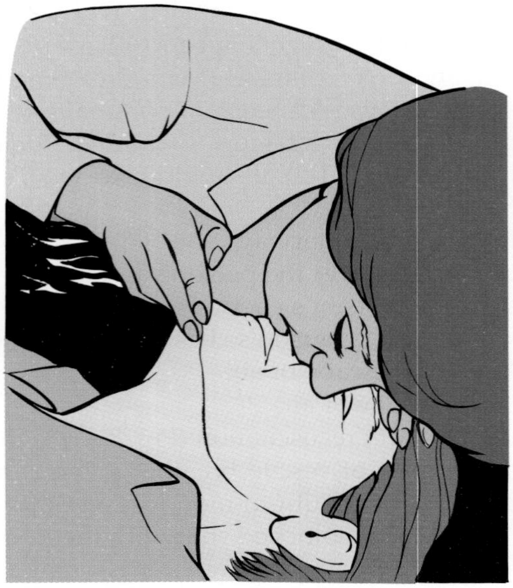

Fig. 31-4 Mouth-to-nose resuscitation.

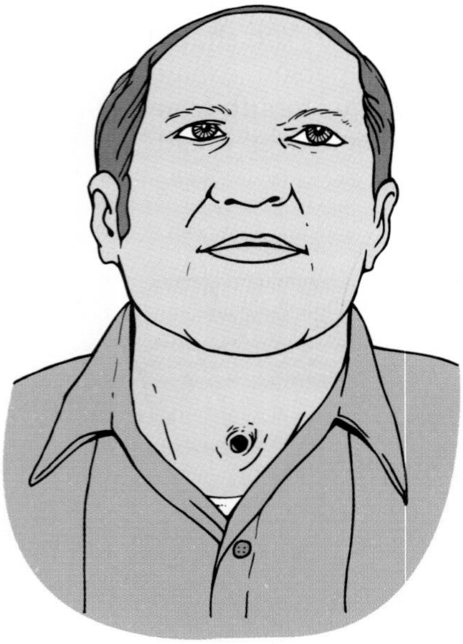

Fig. 31-5 A stoma in the neck. The person breathes air into and out of the stoma.

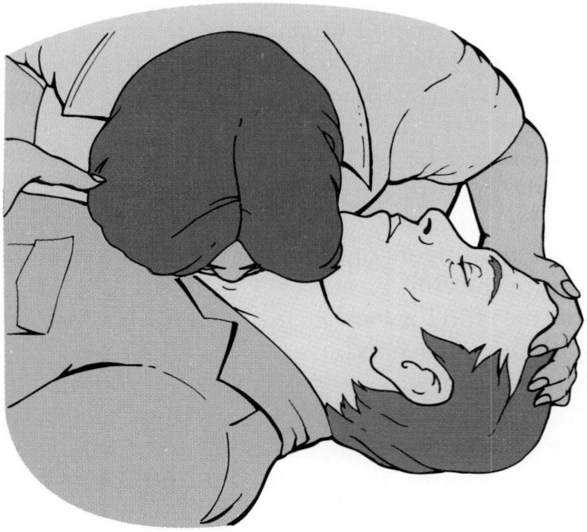

Fig. 31-6 Mouth-to-stoma resuscitation.

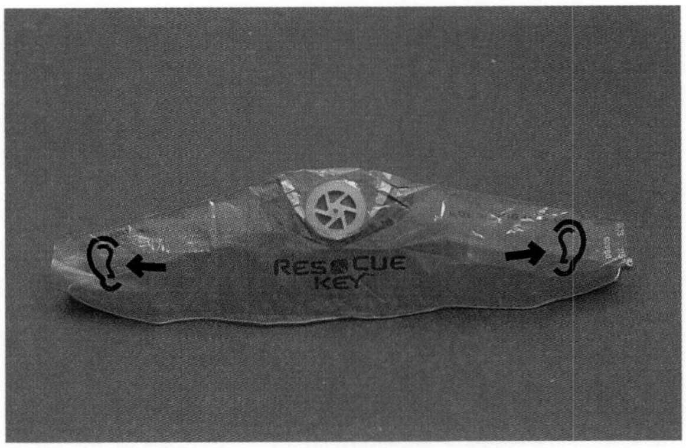

Fig. 31-7 Mask device.

Mouth-to-mouth resuscitation is not always indicated or possible. The *mouth-to-nose* technique may be necessary. The mouth-to-nose technique is used when:

- You cannot ventilate the person's mouth.
- You cannot open the mouth.
- You cannot make a tight seal for mouth-to-mouth resuscitation.
- The mouth is severely injured.

The mouth is closed for mouth-to-nose resuscitation. The head-tilt/chin-lift method is used to open the airway. Pressure is placed on the chin to close the mouth. To give a breath, place your mouth over the person's nose and blow air into the nose (Fig. 31-4). After giving a breath, remove your mouth from the person's nose.

Some people breathe through an opening *(stoma)* in their neck (Fig. 31-5). They need *mouth-to-stoma* ventilation during cardiac or respiratory arrest. You will seal your mouth around the stoma and blow air into the stoma (Fig. 31-6). Before giving mouth-to-mouth or mouth-to-nose resuscitation, always check to see if a person has a stoma. Other methods of rescue breathing are not effective if the person has a stoma.

Barrier devices prevent contact with the person's mouth and blood, body fluids, secretions, or excretions. Mask devices are available (Fig. 31-7). *Mouth-to-barrier device* is another method of rescue breathing. The barrier device is placed over the person's mouth and nose. There must be a tight seal. You breathe into the barrier device.

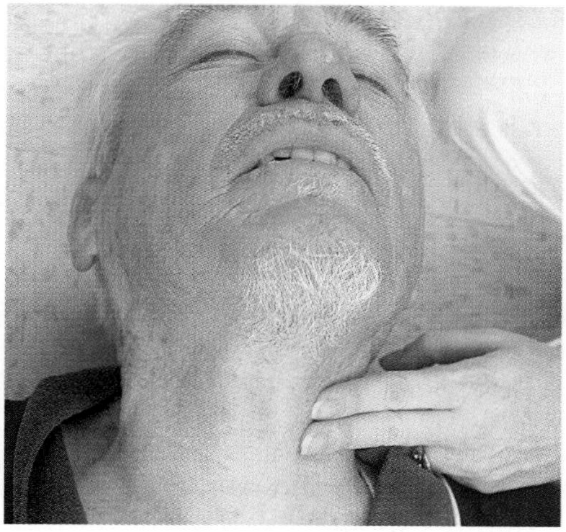

Fig. 31-8 Locating the carotid pulse. Index and middle fingers are placed on the trachea. The fingers are moved down into the groove of the neck where the carotid pulse is located.

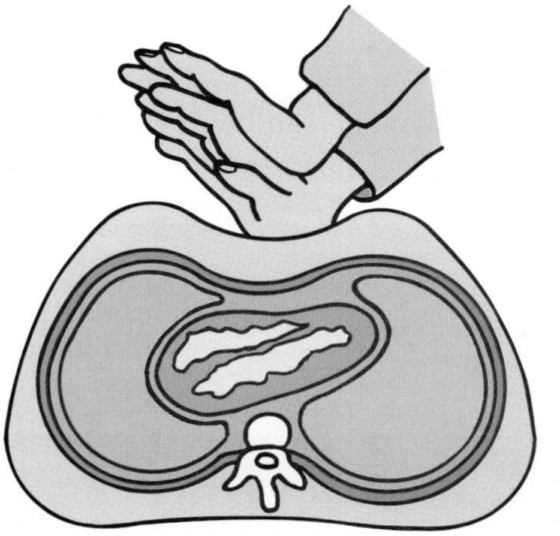

Fig. 31-9 The heart lies between the sternum and spinal cord. The heart is compressed when pressure is applied to the sternum. *(From Rosen P, Barkin RM, Brain GR, Dailey RH, Levy RC:* Emergency medicine: concepts and clinical practice, *ed 3, St Louis, 1992, Mosby.)*

When CPR is started, 2 breaths are given at first. Exhalation is allowed after each breath. Then breaths are given at a rate of 10 to 12 breaths per minute. During one-rescuer CPR, 2 breaths are given after every 15 chest compressions. During two-rescuer CPR, a breath is given after every 5 chest compressions.

Circulation. Blood flow to the brain and other organs must be maintained. Otherwise permanent damage results. In cardiac arrest the heart has stopped beating. Therefore blood must be pumped through the body in some other way. Artificial circulation is accomplished by chest compression. Each chest compression forces blood through the circulatory system.

Before starting chest compressions, pulselessness is determined. Use the carotid artery on the side near you to check for pulselessness. To find the carotid pulse, place the tips of your index and middle fingers on the person's trachea (windpipe). Then slide your finger tips down off the trachea to the groove of the neck (Fig. 31-8).

The heart lies between the sternum (breastbone) and the spinal column. When pressure is applied to the sternum, the sternum is depressed. This compresses the heart between the sternum and spinal column (Fig. 31-9). For effective chest compressions, the person must be supine and on a hard, flat surface.

Proper hand position is important for external chest compressions. The process of locating hand position for adults is shown in Fig. 31-10:

- Use your index and middle fingers to locate the lower part of the person's rib cage on the side nearest you.
- Then run your fingers up along the rib cage to the notch at the center of the chest. The notch is where the ribs and sternum meet.
- Place the heel of your other hand on the lower half of the sternum next to your index finger.

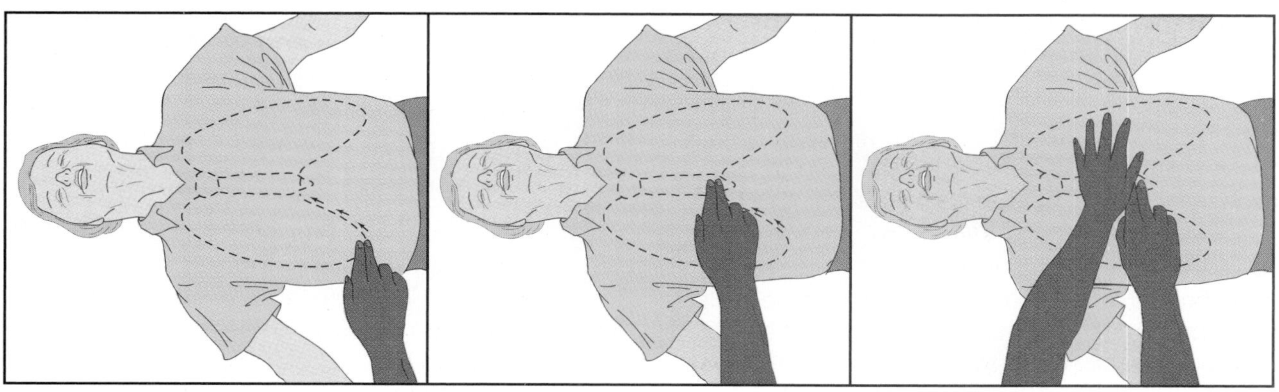

Fig. 31-10 Proper hand position for CPR. **A,** Locate the rib cage. **B,** Run the fingers along the rib cage to the notch. **C,** Place the heel of your other hand next to your index finger.

- Remove your index finger and middle finger from the notch.
- Place that hand on the hand already on the sternum.
- Extend or interlace your fingers. Keep them off the chest.

You must be positioned properly for chest compressions. Your elbows are straight. Your shoulders are directly over the person's chest (Fig. 31-11). Firm, downward pressure is exerted to depress the sternum about $1\frac{1}{2}$ to 2 inches. Then release pressure without removing your hands from the chest. Give compressions in a regular rhythm.

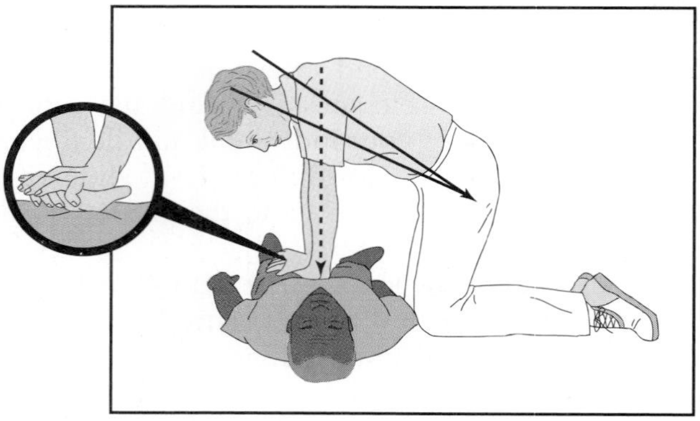

Fig. 31-11 Position of the shoulders for CPR.

Performing CPR. CPR is done only for cardiac arrest. You must determine if cardiac arrest or fainting has occurred. CPR is done when there is unresponsiveness, breathlessness, and pulselessness. That is, the person does not respond, is not breathing, and has no pulse. Basic life support involves the following sequence:

1. Determine unresponsiveness. Tap or gently shake the person, and shout, "Are you OK?" If there is no response, the person is unconscious.
2. *Activate the EMS system immediately if the person is unresponsive.*
3. Determine breathlessness. *Look* at the person's chest to see if it rises and falls. *Listen* for the escape of air during expiration. *Feel* for the flow of air. To feel for air, place your cheek near the person's nose.
4. Open the airway, and give 2 breaths if the person is not breathing.
5. Determine pulselessness.
6. Start chest compressions if the person has no pulse.

Cardiopulmonary resuscitation is done alone or with another person. *CPR is never practiced on another person.* Serious damage can be done. Mannequins are used to learn CPR.

Adult CPR—One Rescuer

Procedure

1. Check for unresponsiveness.
2. Call for help. Activate the EMS system.
3. Position the person supine. Logroll the person so there is no twisting of the spine. The person must be on a hard, flat surface. Place the person's arms alongside the body.
4. Open the airway. Use the head-tilt/chin-lift maneuver.
5. Check for breathlessness.
6. Give 2 breaths. Each should be $1\frac{1}{2}$ to 2 seconds long. Let the person's chest deflate between breaths.
7. Check for pulselessness. Check the pulse for 5 to 10 seconds. Use your other hand to keep the airway open with the head-tilt maneuver.
8. Give chest compressions at a rate of 80 to 100 per minute. Give 15 compressions and then 2 breaths:
   a. Establish a rhythm, and count out loud (try: "1 and, 2 and, 3 and, 4 and, 5 and, 6 and, 7 and, 8 and, 9 and, 10 and, 11 and, 12 and, 13 and, 14 and, 15").
   b. Open the airway, and give 2 breaths.
   c. Repeat this step until 4 cycles of 15 compressions and 2 breaths are given.
9. Check for a carotid pulse (3 to 5 seconds).
10. Continue CPR if the person has no pulse. Begin with chest compressions.
11. Continue the cycle of 15 compressions and 2 breaths. Check for a pulse every few minutes.
12. Repeat steps 10 and 11 as long as necessary.

Adult CPR—Two Rescuers

Procedure

1 Perform one-person CPR until a helper arrives.
2 Continue chest compressions. The helper says, "I know CPR. Can I help?"
3 Indicate that you want help. Ask that the EMS system be activated, if not already done.
4 Do not stop the chest compressions. The helper kneels on the other side of the person. The two-rescuer procedure begins after you complete a cycle of 15 compressions and 2 breaths.
5 Stop compressions for 3 to 5 seconds. The helper kneels on the other side of the person and checks for carotid pulse. The two-rescuer procedure starts after you complete a cycle of 15 compressions and 2 breaths.
6 Perform two-person CPR (Fig. 31-12) as follows:
   a The helper gives 2 breaths.
   b Give chest compressions at a rate of 80 to 100 per minute. Count out loud in a rhythm (try: "1 and, 2 and, 3 and, 4 and, 5").
   c The helper gives a breath immediately after the fifth compression. Pause for the breath. Continue chest compressions after the breath.
   d A breath is given after every fifth compression.
7 Stop compressions after 1 minute. Your helper checks for a carotid pulse. After the first minute, compressions are stopped every few minutes to check for breathing and circulation. Compressions are stopped for only 5 seconds.
8 Call for a switch in positions when you are tired.
9 Change positions quickly as follows:
   a Helper gives a breath after you give the fifth compression.
   b Helper moves down to kneel at the person's shoulder and finds the proper hand position.
   c You move to the person's head after giving the fifth compression.
   d Check for a pulse (3 to 5 seconds).
   e Say, "No pulse."
   f Give 1 breath before your helper starts chest compressions.
10 Give 1 breath after every fifth compression.
11 Switch positions when the person giving the compressions is tired. Check for a pulse and breathing at every position change.

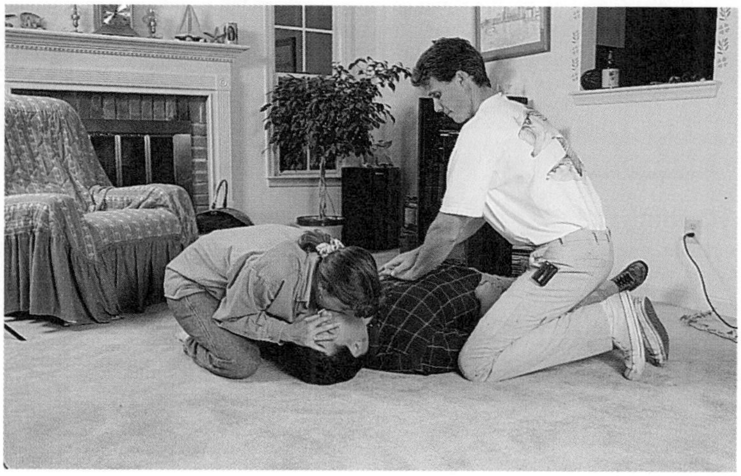

Fig. 31-12 Two people performing CPR.

Obstructed Airway

Airway obstruction *(choking)* can lead to cardiac arrest. Air cannot pass through the air passages to the lungs. The body does not get oxygen.

Foreign bodies can cause airway obstruction. This often occurs during eating. Meat is the most common food to cause airway obstruction. Choking often occurs on large, poorly chewed pieces of meat. Laughing and talking while eating also are common causes. Older persons are at risk for choking. Weakness, poorly fitting dentures, poor swallowing reflexes, and chronic illnesses can lead to choking in these persons. They also can choke on hard candy, apples, or pieces of hot dog.

Airway obstruction can occur in the unconscious person. Common causes are aspiration of vomitus and the tongue falling back into the airway. These occur during cardiac arrest.

Foreign bodies can cause partial or complete airway obstruction. With *partial obstruction,* the person can move some air into and out of the lungs. The person is conscious. Forceful coughing often can remove the object. The EMS system is activated if the partial obstruction is not relieved.

When *complete airway obstruction* occurs, the conscious person clutches at the throat (Fig. 31-13). The person cannot breathe, speak, or cough. The person appears pale and cyanotic. Air does not move into and out of the lungs. The conscious person is very apprehensive. The obstruction must be removed immediately before cardiac arrest occurs. Obstructed airway is an emergency. The EMS system must be activated.

The *Heimlich maneuver* is used to relieve an obstructed airway caused by a foreign body. It involves abdominal thrusts. The maneuver is performed with the person standing, sitting, or lying. The finger sweep is used with the Heimlich maneuver when an adult becomes unconscious.

The Heimlich maneuver is not effective in extremely obese persons or pregnant women. Chest thrusts are used. They are described in Box 31-2.

Call for help when a person has an obstructed airway. Have someone activate the EMS system.

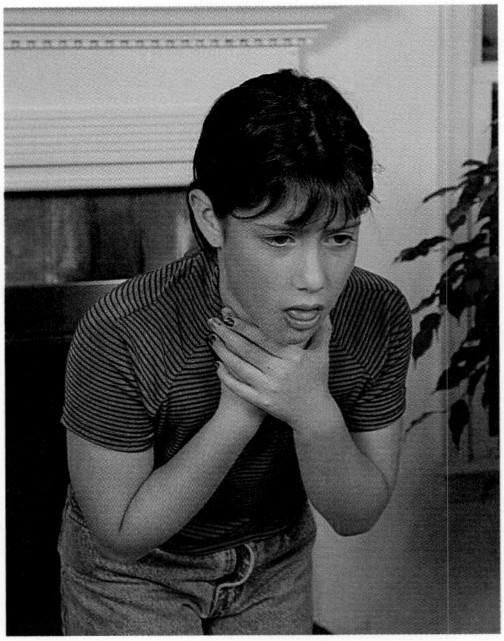

Fig. 31-13 A choking person will usually clutch the throat.

Box 31-2 Obstructed Airway: Chest Thrusts for Obese or Pregnant Persons

The person is sitting or standing:
1. Stand behind the person.
2. Place your arms under the person's arms. Wrap your arms around the person's chest.
3. Make a fist. Place the thumb side of the fist on the middle of the sternum.
4. Grasp the fist with your other hand.
5. Give backward chest thrusts until the object is expelled or the person becomes unconscious.

The person is lying down or unconscious:
1. Position the person supine.
2. Kneel next to the person's body.
3. Position your hands as for external chest compression.
4. Give chest thrusts until the object is expelled or the person becomes unconscious.

Clearing the Obstructed Airway—The Person Is Standing or Sitting

Procedure

1 Ask the person if he or she is choking.

2 Determine if the person can cough or speak.

3 Perform the Heimlich maneuver (abdominal thrusts) if the person is standing or sitting (Fig. 31-14):
   - a Stand behind the person.
   - b Wrap your arms around the person's waist.
   - c Make a fist with one hand.
   - d Place the thumb side of the fist against the abdomen. The fist is in the middle above the navel and below the end of the sternum (breastbone).
   - e Grasp your fist with your other hand.
   - f Press your fist and hand into the person's abdomen with a quick, upward thrust.
   - g Repeat the abdominal thrust until the object is expelled or the person loses consciousness.

4 Lower the unconscious person to the floor or ground.

5 Activate the EMS system.

6 Do the finger sweep maneuver to check for a foreign object:
   - a Open the person's mouth. Use the tongue-jaw lift maneuver (Fig. 31-15, *A*, p. 672):
     - Grasp the tongue and lower jaw with your thumb and fingers.
     - Lift the lower jaw upward.
   - b Insert your other index finger into the mouth along the side of the cheek and deep into the throat (Fig. 31-15, *B*, p. 672). Your finger should be at the base of the tongue.
   - c Form a hook with your index finger.
   - d Try to dislodge and remove the object. Do not push it deeper into the throat.
   - e Grasp and remove the object if it is within reach.

7 Open the airway with the head-tilt/chin-lift maneuver.

8 Give 2 breaths.

9 Reposition the person's head if you could not ventilate the person. Give 2 breaths.

10 Give up to 5 abdominal thrusts. (See *Clearing the Obstructed Airway—The Person is Lying Down*, p. 672).

11 Repeat steps 6 through 10 (finger sweeps, rescue breathing, and abdominal thrusts) until the object is expelled or emergency medical personnel arrive.

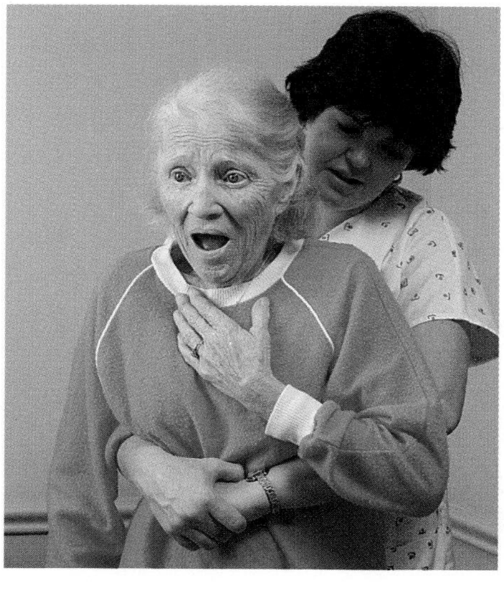

Fig. 31-14 Abdominal thrusts with the person standing.

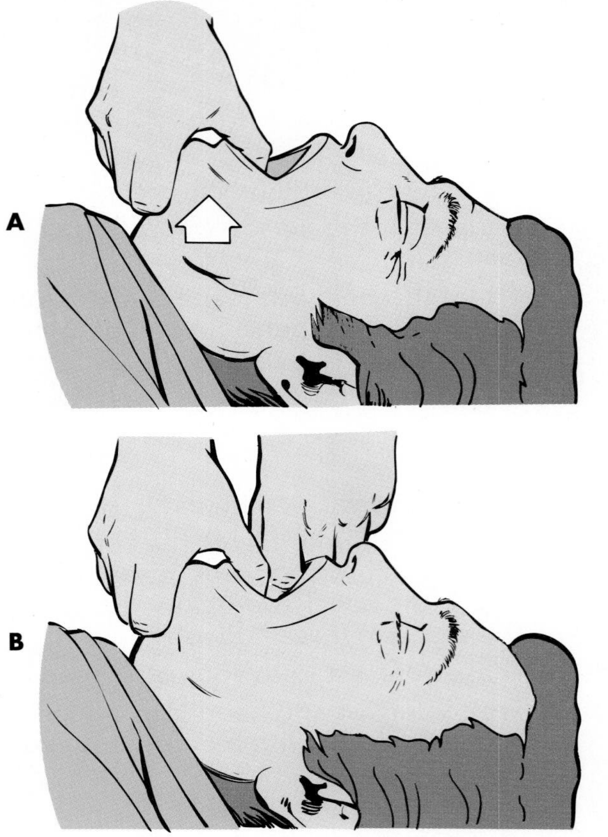

Fig. 31-15 Tongue-jaw lift maneuver. **A,** The person's tongue is grasped, and the jaw is lifted forward with one hand. **B,** The index finger of the other hand is used to check for a foreign object.

Clearing the Obstructed Airway—The Person Is Lying Down

Procedure

1 Ask the person if he or she is choking.
2 Determine if the person can cough or speak.
3 Perform the Heimlich maneuver if the person is choking (Fig. 31-16):
   a Position the person supine.
   b Kneel next to the person's thighs.
   c Place the heel of one hand against the abdomen. It should be in the middle above the navel and below the end of the sternum (breastbone).
   d Place your second hand on top of your first hand.
   e Press your fist and hand into the abdomen with a quick, upward thrust.
   f Repeat abdominal thrusts until the object is expelled or the person loses consciousness.
4 Activate the EMS system if the person becomes unconscious.
5 Do the finger sweep maneuver to check for a foreign object. See step 6 in *Clearing the Obstructed Airway—The Person Is Standing or Sitting.*
6 Open the airway with the head-tilt/chin-lift maneuver.
7 Give 2 breaths.
8 Reposition the person's head if you could not ventilate the person. Give 2 breaths.
9 Give up to 5 abdominal thrusts.
10 Repeat steps 5 though 9 (finger sweeps, rescue breathing, abdominal thrusts) until the object is expelled or emergency medical personnel arrive.

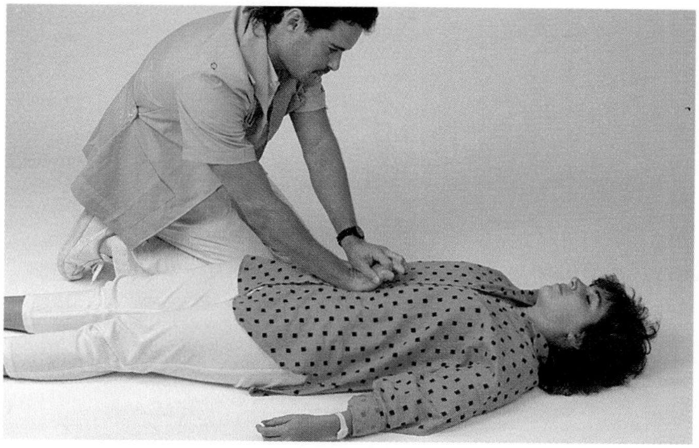

Fig. 31-16 Abdominal thrusts with the victim lying down.

◈ **Finding an unconscious adult.** You may find an adult unconscious. You did not see the person lose consciousness, and you do not know the cause. You cannot assume the cause is choking. Therefore you need to establish unresponsiveness and attempt rescue breathing. Abdominal thrusts are done if you cannot ventilate the person. Then the finger sweep maneuver is used.

Clearing the Obstructed Airway—The Unconscious Adult

Procedure

1. Check for unresponsiveness.
2. Call for help. Have someone activate the EMS system.
3. Logroll the person to the supine position with his or her face up. The person's arms should be at the sides.
4. Open the airway. Use the head-tilt/chin-lift maneuver.
5. Give 2 breaths. Reposition the person's head, and open the airway if you could not ventilate. Give 2 breaths.
6. Do the Heimlich maneuver if you cannot ventilate the person. See *Clearing the Obstructed Airway—The Person Is Lying Down.*
7. Do the finger sweep maneuver to check for a foreign object. See Step 6 in *Clearing the Obstructed Airway—The Person is Standing or Sitting.*
8. Repeat steps 4 through 7 until the object is expelled or emergency personnel arrive.

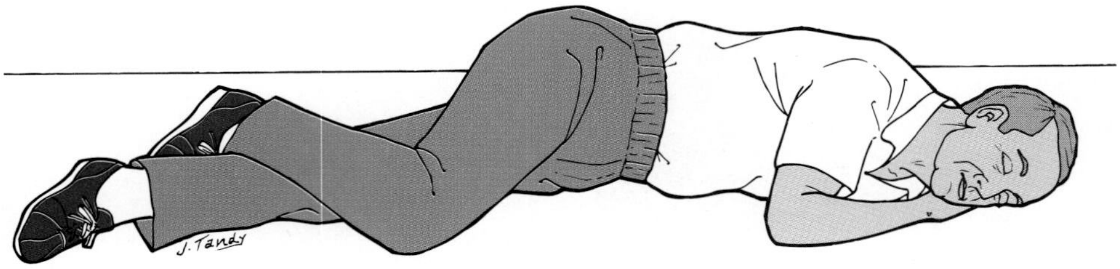

Fig. 31-17 Recovery position.

Recovery Position

The recovery position is a side-lying position (Fig. 31-17). It is used when the person is breathing and has a pulse. Logroll the person into the recovery position, keeping the head, neck, and spine straight. Then keep the person in good alignment. An arm supports the head. This position keeps the airway open and prevents aspiration. Do not use this position if the person might have a neck injury or other trauma.

Self-Administered Heimlich Maneuver

You yourself may choke. You can perform the Heimlich maneuver to relieve the obstructed airway. To do so:

- Make a fist with one hand.
- Place the thumb side of the fist above your navel and below the lower end of the sternum.
- Grasp your fist with your other hand.
- Press inward and upward quickly.
- Press the upper abdomen against a hard surface if the thrust did not relieve the obstruction. Use the back of a chair, a table, or a railing.
- Use as many thrusts as needed.

HEMORRHAGE

Life and body functions require an adequate blood supply. Blood must circulate through the body. If a blood vessel is torn or cut, bleeding occurs. The larger the blood vessel, the greater the bleeding and blood loss. **Hemorrhage** is the excessive loss of blood in a short time. If bleeding is not stopped, death will result.

Hemorrhage may be internal or external. You cannot see internal hemorrhage. Bleeding occurs inside the body into tissues and body cavities. Pain, shock (p. 675), vomiting blood, coughing up blood, and loss of consciousness are signs of internal hemorrhage. There is little you can do for internal bleeding. Activate the EMS system. Then keep the person warm, flat, and quiet until medical help arrives. Fluids are not given. Follow Standard Precautions and the Bloodborne Pathogen Standard in case the person vomits or coughs up blood.

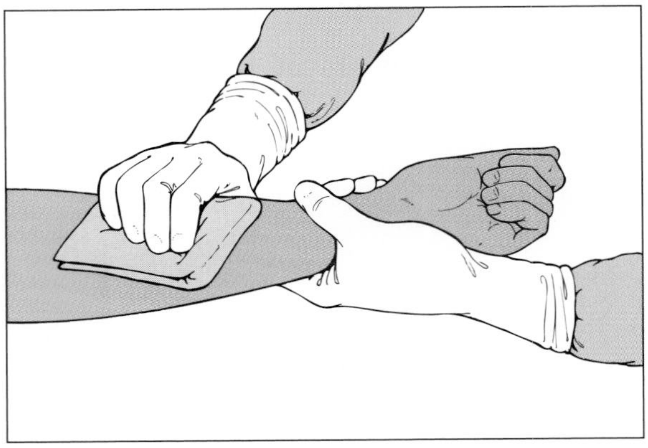

Fig. 31-18 Direct pressure is applied to the wound to stop bleeding. The hand is placed over the wound. *(From Parcel GS, Rinear CE:* Basic emergency care of the sick and injured, *ed 4, St Louis, 1990, McGraw-Hill.)*

External bleeding usually is seen. However, clothing may hide it. Bleeding may be from an injured artery or a vein. Bleeding from an artery is bright red and occurs in spurts. There is a steady flow of blood from a vein. External bleeding must be stopped. You can do the following to control external bleeding:

- Call for help. Have someone activate the EMS system if possible.
- Use Standard Precautions, and follow the Bloodborne Pathogen Standard. Wear gloves if possible.
- Place a sterile dressing directly over the wound. Any clean material (handkerchief, towel, cloth, or sanitary napkin) can be used if there is no sterile dressing.
- Apply pressure with your hand directly over the bleeding site (Fig. 31-18). Do not release the pressure until the bleeding is controlled.
- If direct pressure does control bleeding, apply pressure over the artery above the bleeding site (Fig. 31-19). Use your first three fingers. For example, if bleeding is from the lower arm, apply pressure over the brachial artery. The brachial artery supplies blood to the lower arm.

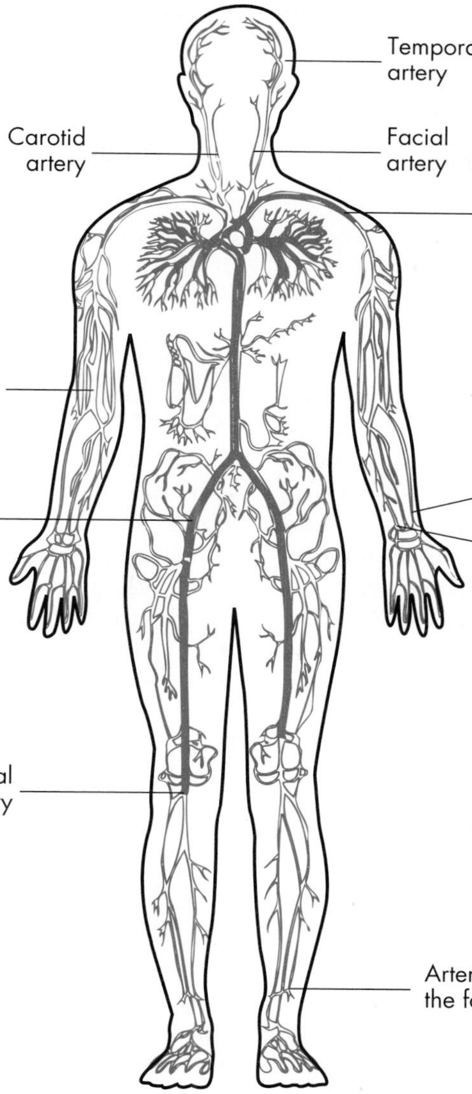

Fig. 31-19 Pressure points to control bleeding. *(From Kidd PS, Sturt P:* Mosby's emergency nursing reference, *St Louis, 1996, Mosby.)*

SHOCK

Shock results when there is not enough blood supply to organs and tissues. Blood loss, heart attack (myocardial infarction), burns, and severe infection can cause shock. Signs and symptoms include:

- Low or falling blood pressure
- Rapid and weak pulse
- Rapid respirations
- Cold, moist, and pale skin
- Thirst
- Restlessness
- Confusion and loss of consciousness as shock worsens

Shock is possible in any person who is acutely ill or injured. Do the following to prevent or to treat shock:

- Keep the person lying down.
- Maintain an open airway.
- Control hemorrhage.
- Keep the person warm. Place blankets over and under the person if possible.
- Reassure the person.
- Activate the EMS system.

SEIZURES

Seizures (convulsions) are violent, sudden, involuntary contractions or tremors of muscles. Seizures are caused by an abnormality in the brain. Causes include head injury during birth or from trauma, high fever, brain tumor, poisoning, seizure disorder, or central nervous system infection. Lack of blood flow to the brain also can cause seizures.

The terms *attack* and *fits* have been used by people outside the health profession in referring to seizures. Do not use these terms. They have unpleasant and disturbing meanings.

The major types of seizures are *partial seizures* and *generalized seizures.* Only a part of the brain is involved with a partial seizure. A body part may jerk. Or the person has hearing or vision problems or stomach discomfort. The person does not lose consciousness.

With generalized seizures the whole brain is involved. The *generalized tonic-clonic seizure (grand mal seizure)* has two phases. The tonic phase is first. The person loses consciousness. If standing or sitting, the person falls to the floor. The body is rigid because all muscles contract at once. The clonic phase is next. Muscle groups contract and relax. This causes jerking and twitching movements of the body. Urinary and fecal incontinence may occur. After the seizure the person usually falls into a deep sleep. The person may experience confusion and headache on awakening.

The *generalized absence (petit mal) seizure* usually lasts a few seconds. There is loss of consciousness, twitching of the eyelids, and staring. No first aid is necessary.

You cannot stop a seizure. However, you can protect the person from injury during a seizure. The following measures are performed:

- Call for help.
- Lower the person to the floor. This protects the person from falling.
- Place a folded bath blanket, towel, cushion, pillow, or other soft item under the resident's head. You may cradle the resident's head in your lap or on a pillow (Fig. 31-20). This prevents the resident's head from striking the floor.
- Turn the person onto his or her side. Make sure the head is turned to the side.
- Loosen tight clothing around the resident's neck (ties, scarves, or collars). Also loosen tight jewelry.
- Move furniture, equipment, and sharp objects away from the person. The person may strike these objects during the uncontrolled body movements.
- Do not try to restrain body movements during the seizure.
- Summon medical help. Do not leave the resident during the seizure.
- Do not put your fingers between the resident's teeth. The person can bite down on your fingers during the seizure.

BURNS

Burns can severely disable a person (Fig. 31-21). They can also cause death. Most burn injuries occur in the home. Infants and children are at risk. So are older persons. Common causes of burns and fires are:

- Scalds from hot liquids
- Playing with matches and lighters
- Electrical injuries (Fig. 31-22)
- Cooking accidents (barbecues, microwaves, stoves, ovens)
- Falling asleep while smoking
- Fireplaces
- Space heaters
- No smoke detectors or nonfunctioning smoke detectors
- Sunburns
- Chemicals

The skin has two layers: the dermis and the epidermis. Burns are described as partial thickness or full thickness. *Partial-thickness burns* involve the dermis and part of the epidermis. These burns are very painful. Nerve endings are exposed. *Full-thickness burns* involve the dermis and the entire epidermis. The fat layer, muscle, and bone may be injured or destroyed. Full-thickness burns are not painful. Nerve endings are destroyed.

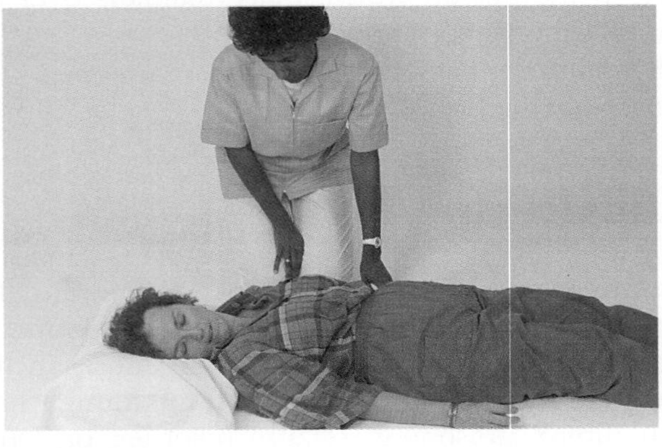

Fig. 31-20 Protect the head during a seizure.

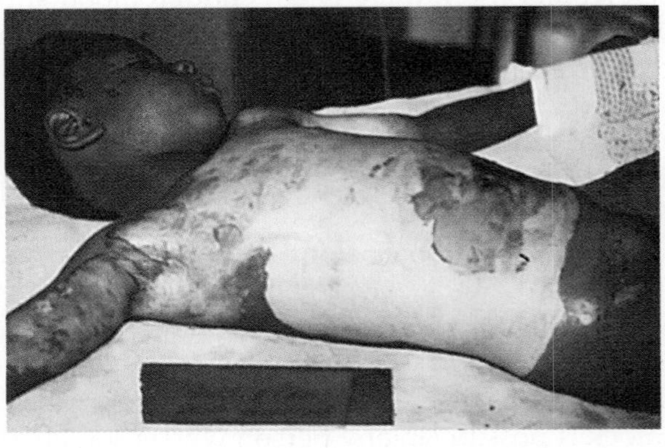

Fig. 31-21 Full-thickness burn from flames. *(Courtesy St. John's Mercy Hospital, St. Louis.)*

A

B

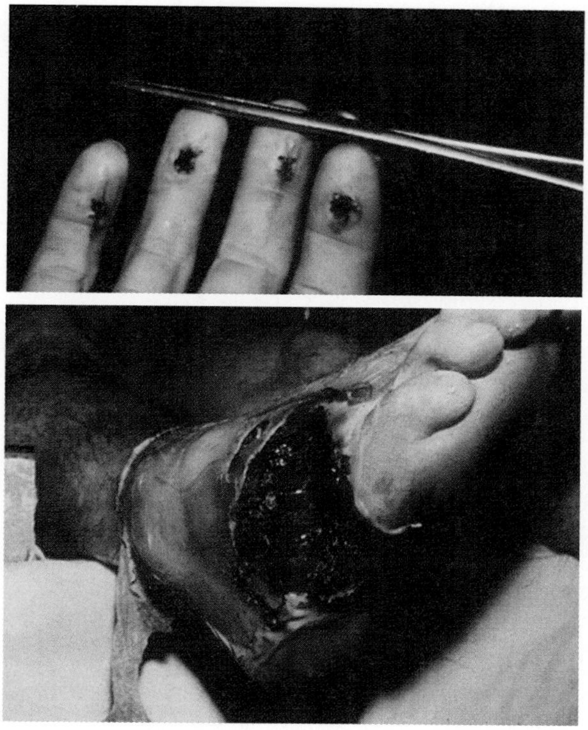

Fig. 31-22 An electrical burn. **A,** The electrical current enters through the hand. **B,** The electrical current exits through the foot. *(From Saunders MJ, Mosby's Paramedic Textbook, 1994, Mosby.)*

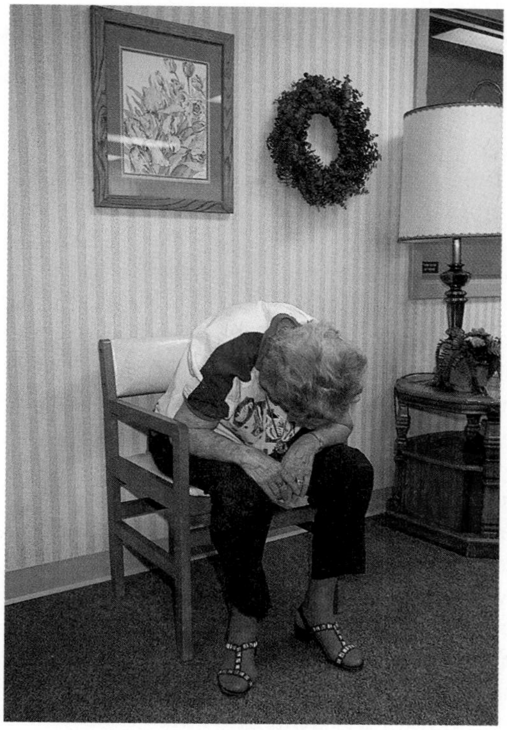

Fig. 31-23 The person bends forward and places the head between the knees to prevent fainting.

Burns vary in seriousness. Burn size and depth, the body part involved, and the person's age affect the severity of the burn. Burns to the face, eyes, ears, hands, and feet are more serious than burns to an arm or leg. Infants, young children, and older persons have a greater risk of dying than do persons of other ages.

Activate the EMS system as soon as possible. Emergency care of burns includes the following:

- Do not touch the person if he or she is in contact with an electrical source. Have the power source turned off or remove the electrical source first. Use an object that does not conduct electricity (rope or wood) to remove the electrical source.
- Remove the person from the fire or burn source.
- Stop the burning process. Extinguish flames with water, or roll the person in a blanket. Or use a coat, sheet, or towel.
- Remove hot clothing that is not sticking to the skin. Also, remove jewelry and any tight clothing. If you cannot remove hot clothing, cool the clothing with water.
- Provide basic life support as needed. This includes activating the EMS system.
- Cover the burn wounds with a clean, moist covering. You can use towels, sheets, or any other clean cloth. Keep the covering wet.
- Do not put oil, butter, salve, or ointments on the burns.
- Cover the person with a blanket or coat to prevent heat loss.

FAINTING

Fainting is the sudden loss of consciousness as a result of an inadequate blood supply to the brain. Hunger, fatigue, fear, and pain are common causes. Some people faint at the sight of blood or injury. Fainting also can be caused by standing in one position for a long time or being in a warm, crowded room. Dizziness, perspiration, and blackness before the eyes are warning signals. The person looks pale. The pulse is weak. Respirations are shallow if the person loses consciousness. Emergency care for fainting includes the following:

- Have the person sit or lie down before fainting occurs.
- If sitting, the person bends forward and places the head between the knees (Fig. 31-23).
- If the person is lying down, elevate his or her legs.
- Loosen tight clothing.
- Keep the person lying down if fainting has occurred.
- Do not let the person get up until symptoms have subsided for about 5 minutes.
- Help the person to a sitting position after recovery from fainting. Observe for symptoms of fainting.

STROKE

Stroke (cerebrovascular accident, brain attack) is described in Chapter 26. A stroke occurs when the brain is suddenly deprived of its blood supply. Usually only part of the brain is affected. A stroke may be caused by a thrombus, an embolus, or cerebral hemorrhage. Cerebral hemorrhage is caused by the rupture of a blood vessel in the brain.

The signs of stroke vary. They depend on the size and location of brain injury. Loss of consciousness or semiconsciousness, rapid pulse, labored respirations, elevated blood pressure, vomiting, and hemiplegia are signs of stroke. The person may have aphasia (the inability to speak). Seizures may occur.

Emergency care includes the following:

- Turn the person onto the affected side. The affected side is limp, and the cheek appears puffy.
- Elevate the head without flexing the neck.
- Loosen tight clothing.
- Keep the person quiet and warm.
- Reassure the person.
- Activate the EMS system

QUALITY OF LIFE

Quality of life must be protected in emergency situations. The person is treated with dignity and respect.

The right to privacy and confidentiality is protected. The person is not exposed unnecessarily. You may be in a place where you cannot close doors, shades, and curtains. The person may be in a lounge, dining area, or public place. Do what you can to protect the person's privacy.

Onlookers are major threats to privacy and confidentiality. If you are giving emergency care, your main concern is the person's illness or injuries. It is hard to give care and manage onlookers at the same time. You can ask someone else to deal with the onlookers. If someone else is giving care, you can help by keeping onlookers away from the person.

People are naturally curious. They want to know what happened, the extent of injuries or illness, and if the person will be okay. You must be careful not to discuss the situation. Information about the person's care, treatment, and condition is confidential. Remember that only doctors can make diagnoses. You can make observations about signs and symptoms. Only the doctor can determine what is wrong with the person.

The right to personal choice also is protected. It is often hard to give the choices in emergencies. However, they are given when possible. Hospital care may be required. The person has the right to choose which hospital to be taken to.

Personal possessions are protected from loss and damage. Dentures and eyeglasses often are lost or broken in an emergency. Watches and other jewelry are easily lost. Clothing may be torn or cut. You must be very careful to protect the person's property. In public places the person's personal items are given to family members, police, or EMS personnel.

The resident has a right to a safe environment. Physical and psychological safety are important. The person is protected from further injury. For example, the person is protected from falls after a stroke. The person having a seizure is protected from head injuries. The person needs to feel safe and secure. Reassurance, explanations about care, and a calm approach are important. They help the person feel safe and secure.

REVIEW QUESTIONS

Circle the BEST answer.

1 The goals of first aid are to
- A Call for help and keep the person warm
- B Prevent death and prevent injuries from becoming worse
- C Stay calm and perform emergency measures
- D Reassure the person and keep bystanders away

2 When giving first aid you should
- A Be aware of your own limitations
- B Move the person
- C Give the person fluids
- D Perform any necessary emergency measures

3 Cardiac arrest is
- A The same as stroke
- B The sudden stopping of heart action and breathing
- C The sudden loss of consciousness
- D The condition that results when there is inadequate blood supply to the organs and tissues of the body

4 Which is *not* a sign of cardiac arrest?
- A No pulse
- B No breathing
- C A sudden drop in blood pressure
- D Unconsciousness

5 You are going to give rescue breathing. You should do the following *except*
- A Pinch the person's nostrils shut
- B Place your mouth tightly over the person's mouth
- C Blow air into the person's mouth as you exhale
- D Cover the person's nose and mouth

6 External chest compressions are performed. The chest is compressed
- A ½ to 1 inch with the index finger and middle finger
- B 1 to 1½ inches with the heel of one hand
- C 1½ to 2 inches with two hands
- D 2 to 2½ inches with one hand in the middle of the sternum

7 Which does *not* determine breathlessness?
- A Looking to see if the chest rises and falls
- B Counting respirations for 30 seconds
- C Listening for the escape of air
- D Feeling for the flow of air

8 Which is used to feel for a pulse during CPR?
- A The apical pulse
- B The brachial pulse
- C The carotid pulse
- D The dorsalis pedis pulse

9 How many breaths are given at the beginning of CPR?
- A 1
- B 2
- C 3
- D 4

10 You are performing adult CPR alone. You should do all of the following *except*
- A Give 2 breaths after every 15 compressions
- B Check for a pulse after 1 minute
- C Give 1 breath after every fifth compression
- D Count out loud

11 CPR is being given by two persons. Breaths are given
- A After every fifth compression
- B After every fifteenth compression
- C After every compression
- D Only when positions are changed

12 The most common cause of obstructed airway in adults is
- A A loose denture
- B Meat
- C Marbles
- D Candy

13 If airway obstruction occurs, the person usually will
- A Clutch at the throat
- B Be able to speak, cough, and breathe
- C Be calm
- D Have a seizure

14 The Heimlich maneuver is used to relieve an obstructed airway. Which statement is *false?*
A The person can be standing, sitting, or lying down.
B A fist is made with one hand.
C The thrusts are given inward and upward at the lower end of the sternum.
D The hands are positioned in the person's midsection, between the waist and lower end of the sternum.

15 A person has an obstructed airway. You should use poking motions to sweep the person's mouth out with your index finger.
A True
B False

16 Arterial bleeding is suspected. Arterial bleeding
A Cannot be seen
B Occurs in spurts
C Is dark red
D Oozes from the wound

17 A resident is hemorrhaging from the left forearm. The first action should be to
A Lower the body part
B Apply pressure to the brachial artery
C Apply direct pressure to the wound
D Cover the person

18 The following statements relate to tonic-clonic seizures. Which statement is *false?*
A There is contraction of all muscles at once.
B Incontinence may occur.
C The seizure usually lasts a few seconds.
D There is loss of consciousness during the seizure.

19 A person is in shock. The signs of shock are
A Rising blood pressure, rapid pulse, and slow respirations
B Rapid pulse, rapid respirations, and warm skin
C Falling blood pressure, rapid pulse and respirations, and skin that is cold, moist, and pale
D Falling blood pressure, slow pulse and respirations, thirst, restlessness, and warm, flushed skin

20 A person is in shock. You should
A Open the airway
B Remove the person's clothing
C Keep the person lying down
D Elevate the person's head

21 A person is about to faint. You should *not*
A Take the person outside for some fresh air
B Have the person sit or lie down
C Loosen tight clothing
D Elevate the legs if the person is lying down

22 A person is having a stroke. Emergency care includes all of the following *except*
A Positioning the person on the affected side
B Giving the person sips of water
C Loosening tight clothing
D Keeping the person quiet and warm

23 A resident was burned. There are no complaints or signs of pain. You know that
A The burn is minor
B The burn is partial thickness
C The burn is full thickness
D The dermis was destroyed

24 Burns are covered with
A A clean, moist cloth or dressing
B Butter, oil, or salve
C Water
D Nothing

25 You can promote quality of life in emergency situations by
A Providing privacy
B Protecting personal possessions from loss or breakage
C Protecting the person from further injury
D All of the above

Answers to these questions are on pp. 700-701.

32 The Dying Person

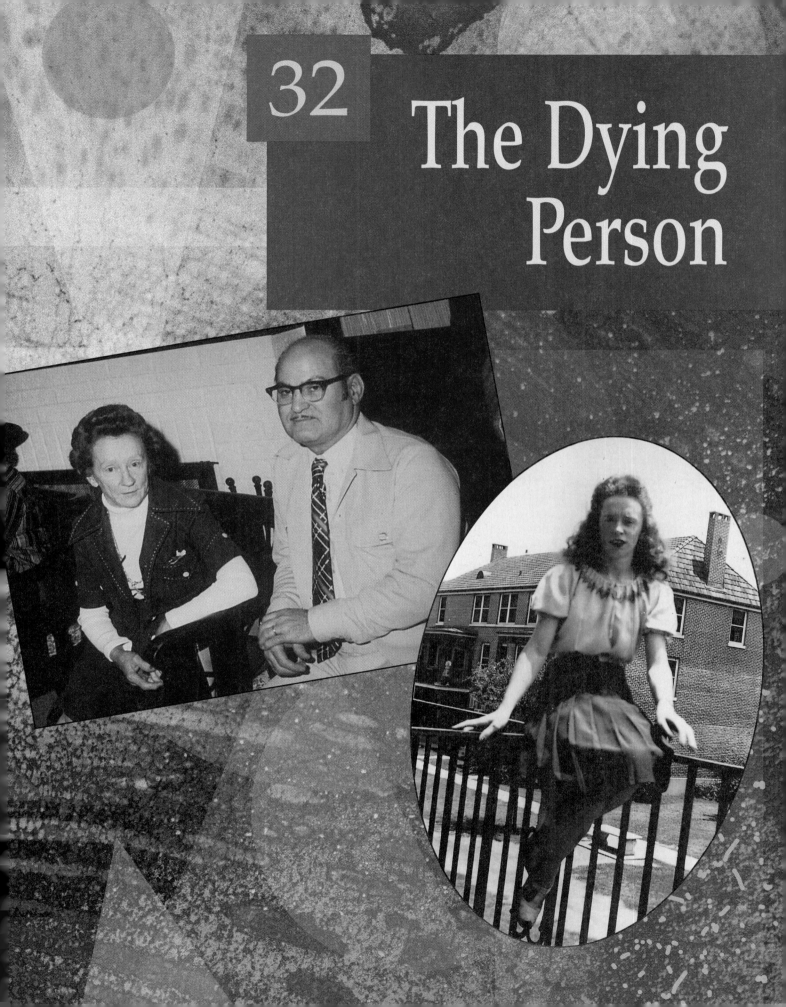

What You Will Learn

- The definition of the key terms listed in this chapter
- How to describe terminal illness
- Two psychological forces that affect living and dying
- How religion and culture affect attitudes about death
- Beliefs about death held by different age-groups
- The five stages of dying
- How to meet the dying resident's psychological, social, and spiritual needs
- How to meet the physical needs of the dying resident
- The needs of the family during the dying process
- The goals of hospice care
- The importance of the Patient Self-Determination Act
- What is meant by a *do not resuscitate* order
- How to promote quality of life for the dying resident
- The signs of approaching death
- The signs of death
- How to assist in giving postmortem care
- The procedure described in this chapter

Key Terms

advance directive A written document stating a person's wishes about health care when that person can no longer make his or her own decisions

postmortem After *(post)* death *(mortem)*

reincarnation The belief that the spirit or soul is reborn in another human body or in another form of life

rigor mortis The stiffness or rigidity *(rigor)* of skeletal muscles that occurs after death *(mortis)*

terminal illness An illness or injury for which there is no reasonable expectation of recovery

Dying residents often are cared for in nursing centers. Some are in hospice programs (p. 686). Death may be sudden and without warning. Often it is expected.

Health care workers see death often. Many are unsure of their feelings about death. They are uncomfortable with dying persons and the subject of death. Dying persons represent helplessness and the failure to cure. They also remind us of our own eventual death or the death of a loved one.

You must examine your own feelings about death. Your attitude about death and dying affects the care you give. Your role is to help meet the resident's physical, psychological, social, and spiritual needs. To do so, you need to understand the dying process. Then you can approach the dying resident with caring, kindness, and respect.

TERMINAL ILLNESS

Many illnesses and diseases can be cured or controlled. Others have no cure. Many injuries can be repaired. Others are so serious that the body cannot continue to function. Recovery is not expected. The disease or injury ends in death. An illness or injury for which there is no reasonable expectation of recovery is a **terminal illness.**

Doctors cannot predict the exact time of death. A person may be given days, months, weeks, or years to live. Predictions can be wrong. Persons who were expected to live for only a short time have lived for years. Others who were expected to live for a longer time died sooner than expected.

Modern medicine has brought cures or has prolonged life in many cases. Future research is likely to bring new cures. Two very powerful psychological forces influence living and dying. They are *hope* and the *will to live*. Persons have died sooner than expected or for no apparent reason when they have given up hope or lost the will to live.

ATTITUDES ABOUT DEATH

Experiences, culture, religion, and age influence a person's attitude about death. Many people fear death. Others refuse to believe they will die. Some look forward to and accept death. Attitudes and beliefs about death often change as a person grows older. They also are affected by changing circumstances.

Dying persons often are cared for in a health care center. The family is often involved in the resident's care. As death nears, the family may gather at the bedside to comfort the dying resident and each other. When death occurs, the funeral director is called. The funeral director takes the body from the center and prepares it for funeral practices.

Many adults and children have never had contact with a dying person. Nor have they been present when death occurred. Some have never attended a visitation or funeral. They have not seen the process of dying and death. Therefore it is frightening, morbid, and a mystery.

Culture and Religion

American practices and attitudes are different from those of other cultures *(see Caring About Culture)*. In some cultures, dying people are cared for at home by the family. Some families care for the body after death and prepare it for burial.

Attitudes about death are closely related to culture and religion. Some believe that life after death is free of suffering and hardship. They also believe there will be reunion with family and loved ones. Many believe there is punishment and suffering in the afterlife for sins and misdeeds. Others do not believe in an afterlife. They believe that death is the end of life. There also are religious beliefs about the form of the human body after death. Some believe that the body keeps its physical form. Others believe that only the spirit or soul is present in the afterlife. **Reincarnation** is the belief that the spirit or soul is reborn in another human body or in another form of life. Many people strengthen their religious beliefs when dying. Religion often provides comfort for the dying person and the family.

Age and Beliefs About Death

Ideas about death change as people grow older. Infants and toddlers have no concept of death. Children between the ages of 3 and 5 start to be curious and have ideas about death. They recognize death of family members or pets and notice dead birds or bugs. They think death is temporary. Children often blame themselves when someone or something dies. They see death as punishment for being bad. When children

CARING ABOUT CULTURE

Death Rites

In Vietnam, quality of life is more important than length of life because of beliefs in reincarnation. There is also the expectation of less suffering in the next life. Therefore the dying are helped to recall their past good deeds and to achieve a fitting mental state. Death at home is preferred over death in the hospital. Upon death, the body is washed and wrapped in clean white sheets. In some areas a coin or jewels (a wealthier family) and rice (a poorer family) are put in the dead person's mouth. This is from the belief that they will help the soul go through the encounters with gods and devils and the soul will be born rich in the next life. Relatives sew small pillows to place under the neck, feet, and wrists of the body. The body is placed in a coffin, and burial is in the ground.

The Chinese have an aversion to death and to anything concerning death. Autopsy and disposal of the body are individual preferences and are not prescribed by religion. Euthanasia is allowed. Donation of body parts is encouraged. The eldest son is responsible for all arrangements for the deceased. The deceased is initially buried in a coffin. After 7 years the body is exhumed and cremated. The urn is reburied in the tomb. White clothing is worn for mourning.

In India, Hindu persons may make indirect references to their own deaths, often accepting God's will. The person's desire to be clear-headed as death approaches must be assessed in planning medical treatment. Providing a time and place for prayer is essential for the family and the person. Prayer helps them deal with anxiety and conflict. The Hindu priest or anyone present may read from the Holy Sanskrit books. Some priests tie strings (signifying a blessing) around the neck or wrist. After death the priest pours water into the mouth of the deceased. Families may prefer that only Hindus touch the body and may wash the body themselves. Blood transfusions, organ transplants, and autopsies are allowed. Cremation is preferred. Reincarnation is a Hindu belief.

Modified from Geissler EM: *Pocket guide to cultural assessment*, ed 2, St Louis, 1998, Mosby.

ask questions about death, adults often give answers that cause fear and confusion. Children who are told "He is sleeping" may be afraid to go to sleep.

Children between the ages of 5 and 7 years know death is final. They do not think that they will die. Death happens to other people. They also think death can be avoided. Children associate death with punishment and body mutilation. It also is associated with witches, ghosts, goblins, and monsters. These ideas come from fairy tales, cartoons, movies, video games, and television.

Adults have more fears about death than children do. They fear pain and suffering, dying alone, and the invasion of privacy. They also fear loneliness and separation from family and loved ones. They worry about who will care for and support those left behind. Adults often resent death. This is particularly true when it interferes with plans, hopes, dreams, and ambitions.

Older persons usually have fewer fears about death than younger adults do. They accept that death will occur. They have had more experiences with dying and death. Many have lost family members and friends. Some welcome death as freedom from pain, suffering, and disability. Death also means reunion with those who have died first. Like younger adults, older persons often fear dying alone.

THE STAGES OF DYING

Dr. Elisabeth Kübler-Ross identified five stages of dying. They are denial, anger, bargaining, depression, and acceptance:

- *Denial* is the first stage. Persons refuse to believe they are dying. "No, not me" is a common response. The person believes a mistake was made. Information about the illness or injury is not heard. The person cannot deal with any problem or decision about the illness or injury. This stage can last for a few hours, days, or much longer. Some people are still in denial when they die.
- *Anger* is the second stage of dying. The person thinks, "Why me?" People in this stage feel anger and rage. They envy and resent those who have life and health. Family, friends, and the health care team are usually targets of their anger. They blame others. Fault is found with those who are loved and needed the most. The health care team and family may have a hard time dealing with residents during this stage. Remember that anger is a normal and healthy reaction. Do not take the resident's anger personally. You must control any urge to attack back or to avoid the resident.
- *Bargaining* is the third stage. Anger has passed. The person now says, "Yes, me, but...." Often there is bargaining with God for more time. Promises are made in exchange for more time. The resident may want to see a child marry, see a grandchild, have one more Christmas, or live for some important event. Usually more promises are made as the resident makes "just one more" request. This stage may not be obvious to you. Bargaining usually is done privately and on a spiritual level.
- *Depression* is the fourth stage. The person thinks, "Yes, me" and is very sad. There is mourning over things that were lost and future loss of life. The resident may cry or say little. Sometimes the resident talks about people and things that will be left behind.
- *Acceptance* is the fifth and final stage of dying. The person is calm and at peace. The person has said what needs to be said. Unfinished business is completed. The resident is ready to accept death. A resident may be in this stage for many months or years. Reaching the acceptance stage does not mean that death is near.

Dying persons do not always go through all five stages. A person may never get beyond a certain stage. Some move back and forth between stages. For example, a person who reached acceptance may move back to bargaining. Then the person may move forward to acceptance. Some people are in one stage until death.

PSYCHOLOGICAL, SOCIAL, AND SPIRITUAL NEEDS

Dying residents continue to have psychological, social, and spiritual needs. They may want family and friends present. They may want to talk about the fears, worries, and anxieties of dying. Some want to be alone. Often they want to talk to a member of the health care team. Residents often need to talk at night. Things are quiet. There are few distractions, and there is more time to think.

There are two very important aspects of communication in dealing with the dying resident. These are *listening* and *touch*:

- *Listening*. The resident needs to talk, express feelings, and share worries and concerns. Let the resident express feelings and emotions in his or her own way. Just being there and listening help meet the resident's psychological and social needs. Do not worry about saying the wrong thing. Do not worry about finding the right words to comfort the resident. Nothing really must be said. Being there for the resident is what counts.

- *Touch.* Touch conveys caring and concern when words cannot. Sometimes the resident does not want to talk but needs to have you nearby. Do not feel that you need to talk. Silence, along with touch, is a powerful and meaningful way to communicate.

Spiritual needs are important. The resident may wish to see a priest, rabbi, minister, or other spiritual leader. The resident also may want to take part in religious practices. Privacy is provided during spiritual moments. Courtesy is given to the spiritual leader. The resident has the right to have religious objects nearby (medals, pictures, statues, or religious books and other spiritual readings). Handle these items like any other valuable.

PHYSICAL NEEDS

Dying may take a few minutes, hours, days, or weeks. There is a general slowing of body processes, weakness, and changes in the level of consciousness. The resident is allowed to be as independent as possible. As the resident weakens, the health care team helps meet basic needs. The resident may totally depend on others for basic needs and activities of daily living. Every effort is made to promote the resident's physical and psychological comfort. The resident is allowed to die in peace and with dignity.

Vision, Hearing, and Speech

Vision blurs and gradually fails during the dying process. The person naturally turns toward light. A darkened room may frighten the person. The eyes may be half open. Secretions may collect in the corners of the eyes. Because of failing vision, you need to explain what is being done to the resident or in the room. The room should be well lit. However, bright lights and glares are avoided. Good eye care is essential (see Chapter 13). If the eyes stay open, a nurse may apply a protective ointment. Then the eyes are covered with moistened pads to prevent injury.

Hearing is one of the last functions lost. Many people hear until the moment of death. Even if unconscious, the resident may hear. Always assume that the dying resident, or any unconscious resident, can hear. Speak in a normal voice, and provide reassurance and explanations about care. Offer words of comfort. Avoid topics that could upset the resident.

Speech becomes difficult. It may be hard to understand the resident. Sometimes the resident cannot speak. The health care team must anticipate the resident's needs. You should not ask questions that need long answers. "Yes" or "no" questions are asked. These are kept to a minimum. Although speech may be difficult or impossible, you must still talk to the resident.

Mouth, Nose, and Skin

Oral hygiene is very important for comfort. Routine mouth care usually is enough if the resident can eat and drink. Frequent oral care is given as death nears and when the resident has difficulty taking oral fluids. Oral hygiene is also important if mucus collects in the mouth and the resident cannot swallow.

Crusting and irritation of the nostrils can occur. Common causes are increased nasal secretions, an oxygen cannula, or a nasogastric (NG) tube. Careful cleansing of the nose is important. The nurse may have you apply a lubricant to the nostrils.

Circulation fails and body temperature rises as death approaches. Although body temperature rises, the skin is cool, pale, and mottled (blotchy). Perspiration increases. Good skin care, bathing, and the prevention of pressure ulcers are necessary. Linens and gowns are changed whenever needed because of perspiration. Although the skin feels cool, only light bed coverings are needed. Blankets may make the resident feel warm and cause restlessness.

Elimination

Dying residents may have urinary and anal incontinence. Incontinence briefs or bed protectors are used. Perineal care is given as necessary. Some residents are constipated and have urinary retention. The doctor may order an enema and Foley catheter. You may be asked to give enemas and perform catheter care (see Chapters 16 and 17).

Comfort and Positioning

Measures are taken to promote comfort. Good skin care, personal hygiene, back massages, proper body alignment, and oral hygiene help to increase comfort. Some residents have severe pain. The nurse gives pain medications ordered by the doctor. Frequent position changes promote comfort. Good body alignment and supportive devices also promote comfort. Care is taken when turning the resident. You may need help to turn the resident slowly and gently. Residents with breathing difficulties usually prefer the semi-Fowler's position.

The Resident's Room

The resident's room should be as pleasant as possible. It should be well lit and well ventilated. Unnecessary equipment is removed. Some equipment is upsetting to look at (suction machines, drainage containers). If possible, this equipment is kept out of the resident's sight.

Mementos, pictures, cards, flowers, religious items, and other significant items comfort and reassure the resident. Arranging them within the resident's view is appreciated. The resident and family are allowed to arrange the room as they wish. This helps meet the needs of love, belonging, and self-esteem. The room should be comfortable and pleasant and reflect the resident's choices. This promotes physical and psychological comfort.

THE RESIDENT'S FAMILY

The family is going through a hard time. It may be very hard to find words to comfort them. You can show your feelings to the family by being available, courteous, and considerate. Use touch to show your concern.

The family usually is allowed to spend a lot of time with their loved one. Sometimes family members stay during the night. The health care team helps to make the family as comfortable as possible. You must respect the resident's and family's right to privacy. They need as much time together as possible. However, the resident's care cannot be neglected just because the family is present. Most centers let family members help give care if they wish. If they do not want to help, you can suggest that they take a break for a beverage or meal.

The family may be very tired, sad, and tearful. They need support and understanding. Watching a loved one die is very painful. So is dealing with the eventual loss of that person. In their grief the family goes through stages like the dying person. Treat the family with courtesy and respect. Visiting with a member of the clergy may be comforting to the family. You need to communicate this request to the nurse immediately.

HOSPICE CARE

Many residents seek hospice care when they are dying (see Chapter 1). Hospices focus on the physical, emotional, social, and spiritual needs of dying residents and their families. Hospice care does not focus on cure or life-saving procedures. Pain relief and comfort measures are stressed. The goal of hospice care is to improve the dying person's quality of life.

A hospice may be part of a health care center or a separate facility. Some centers provide hospice training for staff. Many hospices offer home care. Follow-up care and support groups for survivors are part of hospice services. The hospice also provides support for nursing center staff to help them deal with the death of a resident.

LEGAL ISSUES

Much attention is given to the right to die. Many people do not want to be kept alive by machines or other measures. Consent must be given for any treatment. Residents make their own decisions when they are able. Some make their wishes known about prolonging death before the time comes.

The Patient Self-Determination Act

The Patient Self-Determination Act and OBRA give persons the right to accept or refuse medical treatment. They also have the right to make advance directives. An **advance directive** is a written document stating a person's wishes about health care when that person is no longer able to make his or her own decisions. Advance directives usually prohibit certain types of care if there is no hope of recovery. Living wills and durable power of attorney are common advance directives. OBRA

All health care centers must inform all persons of the right to advance directives on admission. This information must be in writing. The resident's medical record must document whether the resident has made advance directives. The law also protects the resident's quality of care. Quality of care cannot be less because the resident has made advance directives.

Living wills. A living will is a person's written statement about the use of life-sustaining measures. Life-sustaining measures are those that support or maintain life. Tube feedings, mechanical ventilators, and cardiopulmonary resuscitation are some examples. These measures and other machines keep the person alive when death is likely. A living will instructs doctors:

- Not to start measures that prolong dying
- To remove measures that prolong dying

Durable power of attorney. Durable power of attorney for health care is another type of advance directive. The power to make decisions about health care is given to another person. Usually this is a family member or friend. Sometimes it is a lawyer. A person may no longer be able to make decisions about his or her own health care. Then the person with the durable power of attorney has the legal authority to do so.

"Do Not Resuscitate" Orders

When death is sudden and unexpected, every effort is made to save the resident's life. CPR is started (see Chapter 31), and an emergency *code* is called. Nurses, doctors, and other emergency staff members rush to the resident's bedside. They bring emergency and life-saving equipment with them. CPR and other life-support measures are continued until the resident is resuscitated or until the doctor declares the resident dead.

Doctors often write *do not resuscitate (DNR)* or *no code* orders for terminally ill residents. This means that no attempts will be made to resuscitate the resident. The resident is allowed to die in peace and with dignity. The orders are written after consulting with the resident and family. The family and doctor make the decision if the resident is not mentally able. Some residents have advance directives that address resuscitation.

You may not agree with decisions made about treatment and resuscitation. However, you must follow the resident's or family's wishes and the doctor's orders. These may be against your personal, religious, and cultural values. If so, discuss the situation with the nurse. It may be necessary to change your assignments.

SIGNS OF DEATH

There are signs of approaching death. The following signs may occur rapidly or slowly:

- Movement, muscle tone, and sensation are lost. This usually begins in the feet and legs. It eventually spreads to the rest of the body. When the mouth muscles relax, the jaw drops. The mouth may stay open. There is often a peaceful facial expression.
- Peristalsis and other gastrointestinal functions slow down. There may be abdominal distention, fecal incontinence, fecal impaction, nausea, and vomiting.
- Circulation fails, and body temperature rises. The resident feels cool or cold, looks pale, and perspires heavily. The pulse is fast, weak, and irregular. Blood pressure begins to fall.
- The respiratory system fails. Cheyne-Stokes, slow, or rapid and shallow respirations may be observed. Mucus collects in the respiratory tract. This causes the *death rattle* that is heard.
- Pain decreases as the resident loses consciousness. However, some residents are conscious until the moment of death.

The signs of death include no pulse, respirations, or blood pressure. The pupils are fixed and dilated. A doctor determines that death has occurred and pronounces the resident dead.

◈ CARE OF THE BODY AFTER DEATH

Care of the body after *(post)* death *(mortem)* is called **postmortem** care. A nurse is responsible for postmortem care. You may be asked to assist. Postmortem care begins as soon as the doctor pronounces the resident dead. Standard Precautions and the Bloodborne Pathogen Standard are followed. You may have contact with infected blood, body fluids, secretions, or excretions.

Postmortem care is done to maintain good appearance of the body. Discoloration and skin damage are prevented. Postmortem care also includes gathering valuables and personal items for the family. The right to privacy and the right to be treated with dignity and respect apply after death.

Within 2 to 4 hours after death, rigor mortis develops. **Rigor mortis** is the stiffness or rigidity *(rigor)* of skeletal muscles that occurs after death *(mortis)*. Postmortem care involves positioning the body in normal alignment before rigor mortis sets in. The family may wish to see the body before it is taken to the funeral home. The body should appear in a comfortable and natural position for viewing by the family.

In some centers the body is prepared only for viewing. Postmortem care is completed later by the funeral director.

Repositioning of the body is often required during postmortem care. The repositioning is done to bathe soiled areas and to put the body in good alignment. Movement of the body can cause remaining air in the lungs, stomach, and intestines to be expelled. When air is expelled, the body produces sounds. Do not be alarmed or frightened by these sounds. They are normal and expected.

Assisting With Postmortem Care

Pre-Procedure

1. Wash your hands.
2. Collect the following:
   - Postmortem kit if used in your center (shroud, gown, two tags, gauze squares, and safety pins)
   - Valuables list
   - Waterproof bed protectors
   - Wash basin
   - Bath towels
   - Washcloth
   - Tape
   - Dressing
   - Gloves
   - Cotton balls
3. Provide for privacy.
4. Raise the bed to the best level for good body mechanics.

Procedure

5. Make sure the bed is flat.
6. Put on gloves.
7. Position the body supine. Arms and legs are straight. Place a pillow under the head and shoulders (Fig. 32-1).
8. Close the eyes. Gently pull the eyelids over the eyes. Apply moistened cotton balls gently over the eyelids if the eyes will not stay closed.
9. Insert dentures if it is center policy. If not, put them in a labeled denture container.
10. Close the mouth. Place a rolled towel under the chin to support the mouth in the closed position if necessary.
11. Follow center policy about jewelry. Remove all jewelry except for wedding rings if this is center policy. List the jewelry that was removed. Place the jewelry and the list in an envelope for the family.
12. Place a cotton ball over the wedding ring, and secure it in place with tape.
13. Remove drainage bottles, bags, and containers. Leave tubes and catheters in place if an autopsy is to be performed. Ask the nurse about the removal of tubes.
14. Bathe soiled areas with plain water. Dry thoroughly.
15. Place a bed protector under the buttocks.
16. Remove soiled dressings, and replace them with clean ones.
17. Put a clean gown on the body. Make sure the body is positioned as in step 7.
18. Brush and comb the hair if necessary.
19. Fill out the ID tags. Tie one to an ankle or to the right big toe.
20. Cover the body to the shoulders with a sheet if the family will view the body.
21. Collect the resident's belongings. Put them in a bag labeled with the resident's name.
22. Remove all used supplies, equipment, and linens except the shroud and the other ID tag. Make sure the room is neat. Adjust the lighting so it is soft.
23. Remove the gloves, and wash your hands.
24. Let the family view the body. Provide for privacy. Ask the nurse to give the resident's belongings to the family.
25. Put on another pair of gloves.

Assisting With Postmortem Care—cont'd

Procedure—cont'd

26 Place the body on the shroud or cover the body with a sheet after the family has left the room. Apply the shroud (Fig. 32-2, p. 690):
   a Bring the top down over the head.
   b Fold the bottom up over the feet.
   c Fold the sides over the body.

27 Secure the shroud in place with safety pins or tape.

28 Attach the second ID tag to the shroud.

29 Leave the body on the bed for the funeral director. Leave the denture cup with the body.

30 Pull the privacy curtain around the bed, or close the door.

31 Remove the gloves, and wash your hands.

Post-Procedure

32 Put on gloves.

33 Strip the resident's unit after the body was removed.

34 Remove the gloves, and wash your hands.

35 Report the following to the nurse:
   a The time the body was taken by the funeral director
   b What was done with jewelry and personal belongings
   c What was done with dentures

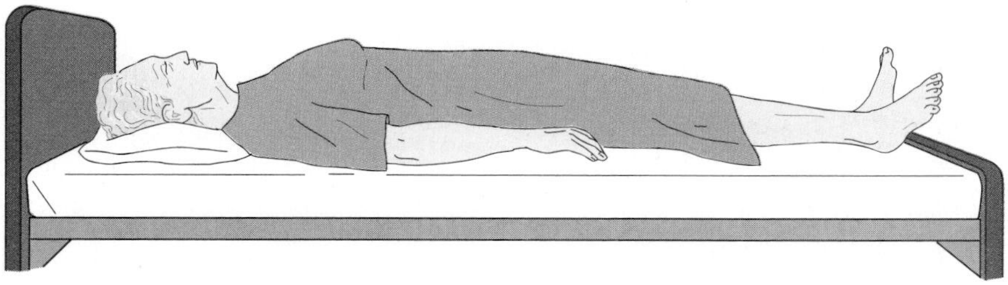

Fig. 32-1 The body is in the dorsal recumbent position. Arms are straight at the sides. There is a pillow under the head and shoulders.

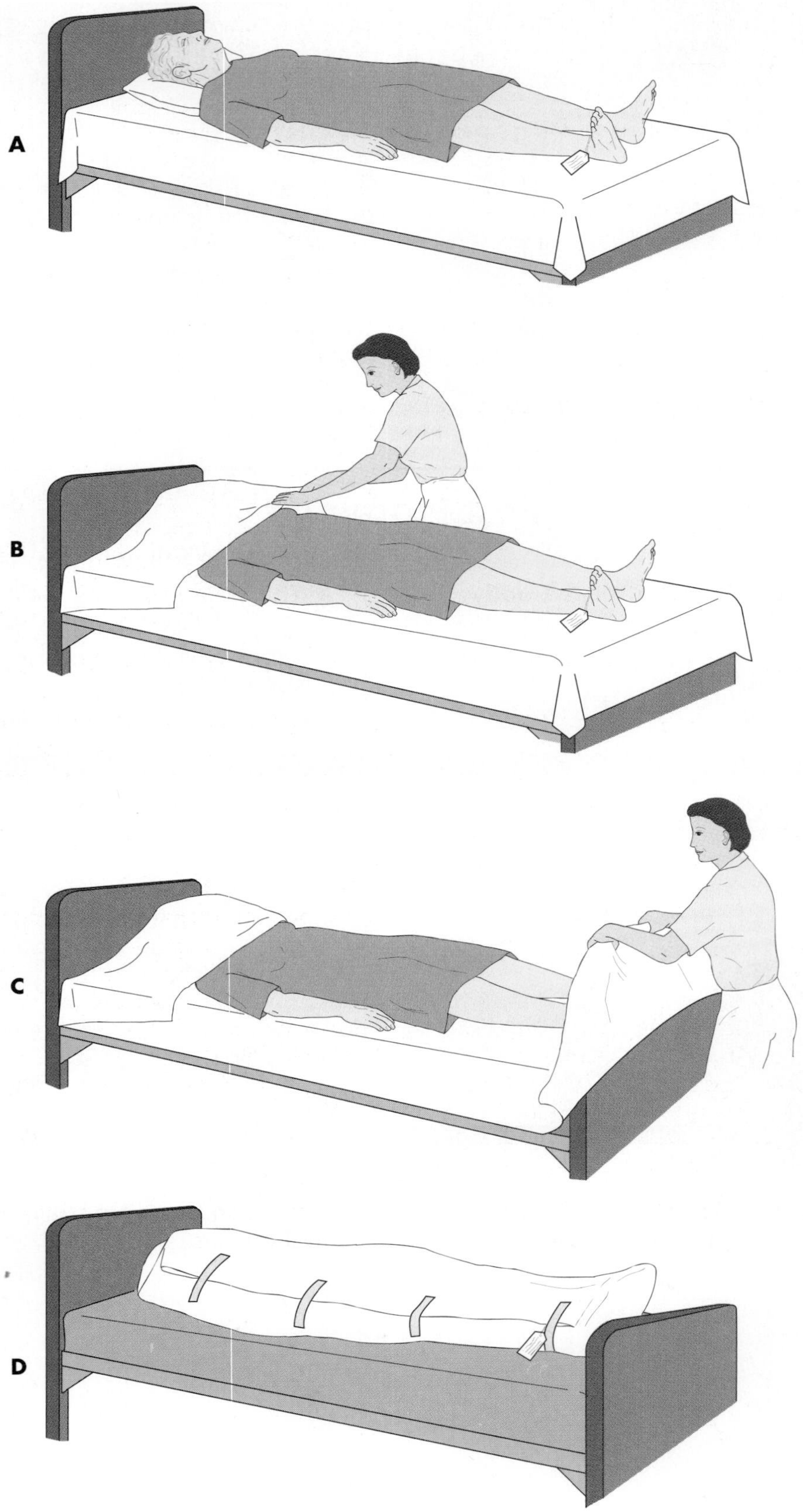

Fig. 32-2 Applying a shroud. **A,** Place the body on the shroud. **B,** Bring the top of the shroud down over the head. **C,** Fold the bottom over the feet. **D,** Fold the sides over the body, tape or pin the sides together, and attach the ID tag.

Quality of Life

Quality of life is important to residents and their families. A resident has the right to die in peace and with dignity. See Box 32-1 on p. 692 for the Dying Person's Bill of Rights. The dying resident also has rights under OBRA.

You must protect the resident's right to privacy and confidentiality. Remember that the resident is not exposed unnecessarily. The resident has the right not to have his or her body seen by others. Proper draping and screening procedures are important.

The resident and family or other visitors have the right to visit in private. The dying resident is likely to be too weak to leave the bed or room. Therefore the roommate may have to leave the room. The nurse and social worker will try to work out an arrangement that is satisfactory to both roommates. The dying resident may be moved to a private room. This gives the resident and family privacy. The family also can stay as long as they like. In addition, a roommate's right to privacy is protected.

The right to confidentiality is important. This right is protected before and after death. The resident's condition and diagnoses are shared only with those involved with the resident's care. The resident's final moments and cause of death also are kept confidential. So are statements, conversations, and reactions of the family.

The dying resident has the right to be free from abuse, mistreatment, and neglect. Some health care workers avoid the dying resident. They are uncomfortable with death and dying. Others have superstitions or religious beliefs about being near dying people. Neglect is possible. Abuse and mistreatment may occur. Family members or health care workers may be the sources of such actions. The dying resident may be too weak to report the abuse or mistreatment. Or the resident may feel that punishment is deserved for needing so much care. The resident has the right to receive kind and respectful care before and after death. You must always report signs of abuse, mistreatment, or neglect to the nurse immediately.

Freedom from restraint applies to the dying resident. Restraints are used only if determined necessary by the health care team and ordered by the doctor. Dying residents often are too weak to be dangerous to themselves or others.

You must protect the resident's personal possessions. The resident may want certain photos and religious items nearby. Religious items may include medals, a rosary, religious books or readings, a crucifix, and candles. It is important to provide such items if possible. The resident's property is protected from loss or damage before and after death. The resident's personal possessions may be passed on as family treasures or mementos.

The resident has a right to a safe and homelike environment. Dying residents usually depend on others for safety. All health care workers are responsible for keeping the environment safe and homelike. Remember that the center is the resident's home. Try to keep equipment and supplies out of view. The room should also be free of unpleasant odors and noises. Do your best to keep the room neat and clean.

The right to personal choice is especially important. Remember that the resident has the right to be involved in treatment and care. The dying resident may refuse treatment. The resident also may have a living will. Some residents are not mentally able to be involved in treatment decisions. The family or legal representative acts on the resident's behalf. The decision may be to allow the resident to die with peace and dignity. Choices to refuse treatment or not to prolong life need to be respected by the health care team.

Box 32-1 The Dying Person's Bill of Rights

- I have the right to be treated as a living human being until I die.
- I have the right to maintain a sense of hopefulness, however changing its focus may be.
- I have the right to be cared for by those who can maintain a sense of hopefulness, however changing this might be.
- I have the right to express my feelings and emotions about my approaching death, in my own way.
- I have the right to participate in decisions concerning my care.
- I have the right to expect continuing medical and nursing attention even though "cure" goals must be changed to "comfort" goals.
- I have the right not to die alone.
- I have the right to be free from pain.
- I have the right to have my questions answered honestly.
- I have the right not to be deceived.
- I have the right to have help from and for my family accepting my death.
- I have the right to die in peace and dignity.
- I have the right to retain my individuality and not be judged for my decisions, which may be contrary to the beliefs of others.
- I have the right to discuss and enlarge my religious and/or spiritual experiences, regardless of what they may mean to others.
- I have the right to expect that the sanctity of the human body will be respected after death.
- I have the right to be cared for by caring, sensitive, knowledgeable people who will attempt to understand my needs and will be able to gain some satisfaction in helping me face my death.

Modified from Barbus AJ: *Am J Nurs* 75(1):99, 1975.

Review Questions

Circle the BEST answer.

1 Which is *true?*
- A Death from terminal illness is sudden and unexpected.
- B Doctors know when death will occur.
- C An illness is terminal when there is no reasonable hope of recovery.
- D All severe injuries result in death.

2 Which two psychological forces influence living and dying?
- A Hope and the will to live
- B Reincarnation and belief in the afterlife
- C Denial and anger
- D Bargaining and depression

3 These statements relate to attitudes about death. Which is *false?*
- A Dying people often are cared for in health care centers.
- B Attitudes about death are influenced by religion.
- C Infants and toddlers understand death.
- D Families often gather around the bed of the dying person.

4 Reincarnation is the belief that
- A There is no afterlife
- B The spirit or soul is reborn into another human body or another form of life
- C The body keeps its physical form in the afterlife
- D Only the spirit or soul is present in the afterlife

5 Children between the ages of 5 and 7 view death as
- A Temporary
- B Final
- C Adults do
- D Going to sleep

6 Adults and older persons usually fear
- A Dying alone
- B Reincarnation
- C The five stages of dying
- D All of the above

7 Persons in the stage of denial
- A Are angry
- B Make "deals" with God
- C Are sad and quiet
- D Refuse to believe they are dying

8 The dying person tries to gain more time during
- A Anger
- B Bargaining
- C Depression
- D Acceptance

9 When caring for the dying resident, you should
- A Use touch and listening
- B Do most of the talking
- C Keep the room darkened
- D Speak in a loud voice

10 As death approaches, the last sense to be lost is
- A Sight
- B Taste
- C Smell
- D Hearing

11 Care of the dying resident includes the following *except*
- A Eye care
- B Mouth care
- C Active range-of-motion exercises
- D Position changes

12 The dying resident is positioned in
- A The supine position
- B Fowler's position
- C Good body alignment
- D The dorsal recumbent position

13 A "do not resuscitate" order was written for a resident. This means that
- A CPR will not be done
- B The resident has a living will
- C Life-prolonging measures will be carried out
- D The resident will be kept alive as long as possible

14 Which are *not* signs of approaching death?
A Increased body temperature and rapid pulse
B Loss of movement and muscle tone
C Increased pain and blood pressure
D Cheyne-Stokes respirations and the death rattle

15 The signs of death are
A Convulsions and incontinence
B No pulse, respirations, or blood pressure
C Loss of consciousness and convulsions
D The eyes stay open, there are no muscle movements, and the body is rigid

16 Postmortem care is done
A After rigor mortis sets in
B After the doctor pronounces the person dead
C When the funeral director arrives for the body
D After the family has viewed the body

Answers to these questions are on p. 701.

ANSWERS

Chapter 1: Introduction to Long-Term Care

1 C
2 B
3 C
4 A
5 B
6 C
7 C
8 A
9 C
10 False
11 True
12 False
13 True
14 False
15 True
16 True
17 True
18 False

Chapter 2: The Nursing Assistant in Long-Term Care

1 False
2 False
3 False
4 True
5 False
6 False
7 True
8 True
9 True
10 True
11 False
12 True
13 False
14 True
15 True
16 True
17 True
18 False
19 True
20 False
21 False
22 False
23 False
24 C
25 A
26 B
27 A
28 A
29 B
30 A
31 C
32 B
33 A
34 A
35 C
36 B
37 A
38 C

Chapter 3: Work Ethics

1 True
2 True
3 False
4 True
5 True
6 True
7 False
8 False
9 True
10 False
11 C
12 D
13 C
14 D
15 B
16 D
17 D
18 B
19 C
20 D
21 C
22 B
23 A
24 A
25 B
26 C
27 D
28 D

Chapter 4: Communicating With the Health Team

1 True
2 False
3 False
4 False
5 True
6 False
7 False
8 False
9 True

10 A
11 D
12 C
13 B
14 C
15 C
16 B
17 C
18 D
19 D
20 B
21 C
22 D
23 B

Chapter 5: Communicating With the Resident

1 C
2 D
3 C
4 B
5 A
6 C
7 B
8 D
9 C
10 A
11 C
12 A
13 A
14 B

Chapter 6: Body Structure and Function

1 A
2 B
3 D
4 C
5 C
6 A
7 B
8 C
9 D
10 D
11 B
12 A
13 B
14 B
15 B
16 C
17 D
18 A
19 D
20 A
21 B

Chapter 7: The Older Person

1 B
2 C
3 A
4 D
5 C
6 D
7 C
8 A
9 B
10 C
11 B
12 D
13 D
14 D
15 C
16 A
17 D
18 B
19 B
20 D
21 A
22 D

Chapter 8: Safety

1 True
2 True
3 True
4 True
5 True
6 False
7 False
8 True
9 True
10 True
11 False
12 True
13 True
14 True
15 False
16 True
17 False
18 True
19 True
20 False
21 False
22 True
23 True
24 False
25 False
26 False
27 D
28 A
29 A
30 D
31 D
32 B
33 C
34 A
35 C

36 D
37 D
38 B
39 B
40 C

Chapter 9: Infection Control

1 False
2 True
3 True
4 False
5 False
6 True
7 True
8 False
9 False
10 True
11 True
12 B
13 D
14 D
15 B
16 D
17 C
18 A
19 D
20 C
21 A
22 D
23 B
24 D
25 C
26 B

Chapter 10: Body Mechanics

1 False
2 True
3 True
4 False
5 False
6 False
7 False
8 True
9 True
10 True
11 True
12 True
13 True
14 True
15 True
16 False
17 False
18 False
19 False
20 True
21 False
22 True

Chapter 11: The Resident's Unit

1 B
2 D
3 A
4 D
5 C
6 True
7 False
8 True
9 False
10 True
11 False

Chapter 12: Bedmaking

1 True
2 True
3 False
4 False
5 False
6 True
7 True
8 False
9 True
10 True
11 True
12 True
13 True
14 False
15 False
16 True

Chapter 13: Hygiene

1 True
2 False
3 False
4 False
5 False
6 False
7 False
8 True
9 False
10 False
11 False
12 True
13 True
14 True
15 True
16 D
17 D
18 B
19 B
20 C
21 C
22 D

Chapter 14: Skin and Nail Care

1 True
2 True
3 True
4 True
5 True
6 False
7 C
8 C
9 C
10 C
11 B
12 A
13 D
14 D
15 B
16 A
17 A
18 A
19 B
20 D

Chapter 15: Grooming

1 D
2 B
3 C
4 A
5 D
6 C
7 B
8 B
9 A
10 A

Chapter 16: Urinary Elimination

1 B
2 D
3 A
4 B
5 B
6 A
7 A
8 D
9 C
10 C
11 D
12 B
13 A
14 B
15 D
16 D
17 A

Chapter 17: Bowel Elimination

1 A
2 B
3 D
4 A
5 C
6 D
7 C
8 C
9 B
10 D
11 D
12 A

Chapter 18: Nutrition

1 False
2 True
3 False
4 False
5 B
6 A
7 A
8 D
9 D
10 C
11 A
12 C
13 A
14 C
15 B
16 D
17 C
18 C
19 C
20 B
21 B
22 A
23 C
24 D
25 D
26 B
27 C
28 B

Chapter 19: Exercise and Activity

1 A
2 B
3 C
4 B
5 D
6 B
7 C
8 A
9 B
10 C
11 B
12 False
13 False
14 True
15 False
16 True

Chapter 20: Comfort, Rest, and Sleep

1 A
2 C
3 D
4 C
5 A
6 B
7 C
8 D
9 B
10 C
11 D
12 A
13 B
14 B
15 True
16 False
17 True

Chapter 21: Measuring Vital Signs

1 C
2 B
3 B
4 B
5 C
6 A
7 B
8 D
9 B
10 C
11 A
12 B

Chapter 22: Admitting, Transferring, and Discharging Residents

1 False
2 True
3 True
4 True
5 False
6 False
7 True
8 False
9 False
10 True
11 True
12 True
13 False
14 True
15 True
16 A
17 C
18 B

Chapter 23: Assisting With the Physical Examination

1 B
2 D
3 C
4 B
5 C
6 B
7 D

Chapter 24: Heat and Cold Applications

1 D
2 B
3 D
4 B
5 C
6 B
7 D
8 A
9 D
10 C
11 A
12 B

Chapter 25: Oxygen Needs

1 A
2 C
3 C
4 B
5 D
6 C
7 D
8 A
9 B
10 A
11 B
12 D
13 B
14 D
15 C
16 A
17 C
18 D
19 B
20 D

Chapter 26: Common Health Problems

1 A
2 C
3 A
4 D
5 C
6 D
7 A
8 A

9 D
10 C
11 B
12 A
13 A
14 B
15 B
16 C
17 A
18 A
19 C
20 B
21 B
22 A
23 D
24 B
25 C
26 D
27 A
28 D
29 B
30 B
31 C
32 A
33 C
34 A
35 D
36 C
37 B
38 D
39 C
40 B
41 D
42 D

Chapter 27: Confusion and Dementia

1 B
2 B
3 C
4 B
5 D
6 D
7 B
8 A
9 D
10 C
11 A
12 D

Chapter 28: Developmental Disabilities

1 D
2 B
3 D
4 B
5 A
6 D
7 C
8 C
9 D
10 B
11 A
12 C
13 A
14 D
15 C

Chapter 29: Rehabilitation and Restorative Care

1 C
2 B
3 A
4 D
5 C
6 A
7 C
8 A
9 C
10 True
11 True
12 True
13 False
14 True
15 False

Chapter 30: Sexuality

1 A
2 D
3 C
4 A
5 B
6 B
7 D
8 B
9 B
10 B

Chapter 31: Basic Emergency Care

1 B
2 A
3 B
4 C
5 D
6 C
7 B
8 C
9 B
10 C
11 A
12 B
13 A
14 C
15 B
16 B
17 C

18 C
19 C
20 C
21 A
22 B
23 C
24 A
25 D

Chapter 32: The Dying Person

1 C
2 A
3 C
4 B
5 B
6 A
7 D
8 B
9 A
10 D
11 C
12 C
13 A
14 C
15 B
16 B

Glossary

abbreviation A shortened form of a word or phrase

abduction Moving a body part away from the midline of the body

abrasion A partial-thickness wound caused by the scraping away or rubbing of the skin

accountable Being responsible for one's actions and the actions of others who perform delegated tasks; answering questions about and explaining one's actions and the actions of others

acetone Ketone bodies that appear in the urine because of the rapid breakdown of fat for energy

active physical restraint A restraint attached to the person's body and to a stationary (non-movable) object; movement and access to one's body are restricted

activities of daily living (ADL) Those self-care activities a person performs daily to remain independent and to function in society

acute illness A sudden illness from which the person is expected to recover

acute pain Pain that is felt suddenly from injury, disease, trauma, or surgery; it generally lasts less than 6 months

adduction Moving a body part toward the midline of the body

admission Official entry of a person into a nursing center or nursing unit

advance directive Written document stating a person's wishes about health care when that person can no longer make his or her own decisions

affect Feelings and emotions

allergy A sensitivity to a substance that causes the body to react with signs and symptoms

alopecia Hair loss

Alzheimer's disease A disease that affects brain tissue; persons suffer increasing memory loss and confusion until they cannot meet their simplest personal needs

ambulation The act of walking

AM care Routine care performed before breakfast; early morning care

amputation The removal of all or part of an extremity

anorexia The loss of appetite

anticoagulant A drug that thins the blood and slows down clotting time; it is given to prevent blood clotting

anxiety A vague, uneasy feeling that occurs in response to stress

aphasia The inability *(a)* to speak *(phasia)*

apical-radial pulse Taking the apical and radial pulses at the same time

apnea The lack or absence *(a)* of breathing *(pnea)*

arterial ulcer An open wound on the lower legs and feet caused by decreased blood flow through the arteries

artery A blood vessel that carries blood away from the heart

arthritis Joint *(arthr)* inflammation *(itis)*

arthroplasty The surgical replacement *(plasty)* of a joint *(arthro)*

asepsis Being free of disease-producing microbes

aspiration Breathing fluid or an object into the lungs

assault Intentionally attempting or threatening to touch a person's body without the person's consent

assessment Collecting information about the resident

assisted living facility A board and care facility or residential care facility

atrophy A decrease in size or a wasting away of tissue

autoclave A pressure steam sterilizer

base of support The area on which an object rests

battery Unauthorized touching of a person's body without the person's consent

benign tumor A tumor that grows slowly and within a localized area

biohazardous waste Items contaminated with blood, body fluids, secretions, or excretions and that may be harmful to others; *bio* means life, and *hazardous* means dangerous or harmful

Biot's respirations Irregular breathing with periods of apnea; respirations may be slow and deep or rapid and shallow

bisexual A person attracted to both sexes

bloodborne pathogens Pathogenic microorganisms present in human blood that can cause disease in humans

blood pressure The amount of force exerted against the walls of an artery by the blood

board and care facility A facility that provides custodial care to a few independent residents, often in a home setting; no licensed nurse is required; also called an *assisted living facility* or *residential care facility*

body alignment The way in which body parts are aligned with one another; posture

body language Facial expressions, gestures, posture, and body movements that send messages to others

body mechanics Using the body in an efficient and careful way

body temperature The amount of heat in the body that is a balance between the amount of heat produced and the amount lost by the body

bowel movement (BM) Defecation

bradycardia A slow *(brady)* heart rate *(cardia)*; the rate is less than 60 beats per minute

bradypnea Slow *(brady)* breathing *(pnea)*; respirations are fewer than 10 per minute

braille A method of writing that uses raised dots; raised dots are arranged to represent each letter of the alphabet; the first ten letters represent the numbers 0 through 9

calorie The amount of energy produced from the burning of food by the body

cancer Malignant tumor

capillary A tiny blood vessel; food, oxygen, and other substances pass from the capillaries to the cells

cardiac arrest The sudden stoppage of breathing and heart action

carrier A human or animal that is a reservoir for pathogens but does not have signs and symptoms of infection

case management A method of organizing nursing care; a case manager (an RN) coordinates resident care from admission through discharge and into the home setting

caster A small wheel made of rubber or plastic

catheter A tube used to drain or inject fluid through a body opening

catheterization The process of inserting a catheter

cell The basic unit of body structure

cerebral palsy (CP) A term applied to a group of disorders characterized by paralysis *(palsy)* that is caused by a defect in the motor region of the brain *(cerebral)*

chart Another term for the medical record

charting Recording

Cheyne-Stokes Respirations gradually increase in rate and depth and then become shallow and slow; breathing may stop (*apnea*) for 10 to 20 seconds

chronic illness An illness, slow or gradual in onset, for which there is no known cure; the illness can be controlled and complications prevented

chronic pain Pain lasting longer than 6 months; it may be constant or occur off and on

chronic wound A wound that does not heal easily

chyme Partially digested food and fluids

circadian rhythm Daily rhythm based on a 24-hour cycle; the day-night cycle or body rhythm

circulatory ulcer An open wound on lower legs and feet caused by a decrease in blood flow through arteries and veins; vascular wound

civil law Laws concerned with relationships between people; private law

clean-contaminated wound A wound occurring from the surgical entry of the urinary, reproductive, respiratory, or gastrointestinal system

clean technique Medical asepsis

clean wound A wound that is not infected; microbes have not entered the wound

closed fracture The bone is broken but the skin is intact; simple fracture

closed wound A wound in which tissues are injured but the skin is not broken

colostomy An artificial opening *(stomy)* between the colon *(colo)* and abdominal wall

coma A state of being unaware of one's surroundings and being unable to react or respond to people, places, or things

comatose The inability to respond to verbal stimuli

comfort A state of well-being; the person has no physical or emotional pain and is calm and at peace

communicable disease A disease caused by pathogens that spread easily; a contagious disease

communication The exchange of information; a message sent is received and interpreted by the intended person

compound fracture The bone is broken and has come through the skin; open fracture

comprehensive care plan A written guide giving direction about the nursing care a resident should receive

compulsion The uncontrolled performance of an act

confidentiality To trust others with personal and private information

conflict A clash between opposing interests and ideas

constipation The passage of a hard, dry stool

constrict To narrow

contagious disease Communicable disease

contaminated wound A wound with a high risk of infection

contamination The process of becoming unclean

contracture The lack of joint mobility caused by abnormal shortening of a muscle

contusion A closed wound caused by a blow to the body

convulsion A seizure; violent and sudden contractions or tremors of muscles

courtesy A polite, considerate, or helpful comment or act

crime An act that violates a criminal law

criminal law Laws concerned with offenses against the public and society in general; public law

culture The values, beliefs, habits, likes, dislikes, customs, and characteristics of a group of people that are passed from one generation to the next

cyanosis Bluish discoloration of the skin

Daily Reference Values (DRVs) The maximum daily intake values for total fat, saturated fat, cholesterol, sodium, carbohydrate, and dietary fiber

Daily Value (DV) How a serving fits into the daily diet; it is expressed in a percentage based on a daily diet of 2000 calories

dandruff The excessive amount of dry, white flakes from the scalp

deconditioning The process of becoming weak from illness or lack of exercise; the loss of muscle strength as a result of inactivity

defamation Injuring a person's name and reputation by making false statements to a third person

defecation The process of excreting feces from the rectum through the anus; a bowel movement

defense mechanism An unconscious reaction that blocks unpleasant or threatening feelings

dehiscence The separation of wound layers

dehydration The excessive loss of water from tissues

delegate Authorizing another person to perform a task

delirium A state of temporary but acute mental confusion that comes on suddenly

delusion A false belief

delusion of grandeur An exaggerated belief about one's own importance, wealth, power, or talents

delusion of persecution A false belief that one is being mistreated, abused, or harassed

dementia A set of chronic signs and symptoms in which a person loses memory and the ability to think and reason; the term used to describe the loss of cognitive function (thinking, remembering, and reasoning) caused by changes in the brain

developmental disability A severe, permanent, physical or mental disability that occurs before 22 years of age

dialysis An artificial way to remove waste and excess fluid from the blood

diarrhea The frequent passage of liquid stools

diastole The period of heart muscle relaxation

diastolic pressure The pressure in the arteries when the heart is at rest

digestion The process of physically and chemically breaking down food so that it can be absorbed for use by the cells

dilate To expand or open wider

diplegia Similar body parts are affected on both sides of the body; paralysis of both arms or both legs

dirty wound An infected wound

disability Any lost, absent, or impaired physical or mental function

disaster A sudden, catastrophic event in which many people are injured and killed and property is destroyed

discharge The official departure of a person from a nursing center or nursing unit

discomfort To ache, hurt, or be sore; pain

disinfection The process of destroying pathogens

distraction To change a person's center of attention

dorsal recumbent position The back-lying or supine position; the legs are together

dorsiflexion A toe-up motion of the foot at the ankle

drawsheet A small sheet placed over the middle of the bottom sheet; it helps keep the mattress and bottom linens clean and dry; can be used to turn and move the person in bed; the cotton drawsheet

dysphagia Difficulty *(dys)* swallowing *(phagia)*

dyspnea Difficult, labored, or painful *(dys)* breathing *(pnea)*

dysuria Painful or difficult *(dys)* urination *(uria)*

early morning care AM care

edema Swelling caused by fluid collecting in tissues

embolus A blood clot that travels through the vascular system until it lodges in a distant vessel

emotional illness Mental illness, mental disorder, psychiatric disorder

enema The introduction of fluid into the rectum and lower colon

enteral nutrition Giving nutrients through the gastrointestinal tract *(enteral)*

enuresis Urinary incontinence in bed at night

epilepsy A condition that produces brief disturbances in the brain's normal electrical functions

ethics Knowledge of what is right conduct and wrong conduct

evaluation Measuring if the goals in the planning step of the nursing process were met

evisceration The separation of the wound along with the protrusion of abdominal organs

expressive aphasia Difficulty expressing or sending out thoughts

expressive-receptive aphasia Difficulty expressing or sending out thoughts and difficulty receiving information

extension Straightening of a body part

external rotation Turning the joint outward

fainting The sudden loss of consciousness as a result of an inadequate blood supply to the brain

false imprisonment Unlawful restraint or restriction of a person's movement

fecal (anal) incontinence The inability to control the passage of feces and gas through the anus

fecal impaction The prolonged retention and accumulation of feces in the rectum

feces The semisolid mass of waste products in the colon

first aid Emergency care given to an ill or injured person before medical help arrives

flatulence The excessive formation of gas or air in the stomach and intestines

flatus Gas or air in the stomach or intestines passed through the anus

flexion Bending a body part

footdrop The foot falls down at the ankle (permanent plantar flexion)

Fowler's position A semi-sitting position; the head of the bed is elevated 45 to 60 degrees

fracture A broken bone

fraud Saying or doing something to trick, fool, or deceive another person

friction The rubbing of one surface against another

full-thickness wound The dermis, epidermis, and subcutaneous tissue are penetrated; muscle and bone may be involved

full visual privacy The resident has the means to be completely free from public view while occupying a bed

functional incontinence The involuntary, unpredicted loss of urine from the bladder

functional nursing A method of organizing nursing care; nursing staff perform specific tasks for all assigned residents

gait belt A transfer belt

gangrene A condition in which there is death of tissue; tissues become black, cold, and shriveled

gastrostomy An opening *(stomy)* in the stomach *(gastro)*

gavage Tube feeding

geriatrics The care of aging people

germicide A disinfectant applied to skin, tissues, or nonliving objects

gerontology The study of the aging process

glucosuria Sugar *(glucose)* in the urine *(uria)*; glycosuria

glycosuria Sugar *(glycos)* in the urine *(uria)*; glucosuria

goal That which is desired in or by the resident as a result of nursing care

gossip To spread rumors or talk about the private matters of others

graduate A calibrated container used to measure fluid

ground That which carries leaking electricity to the earth and away from an electrical appliance

group insurance plan An insurance plan bought by a group for individuals

guided imagery Creating and focusing on an image

hallucination Seeing, hearing, or feeling something that is not real

harassment Troubling, tormenting, offending, or worrying a person by one's behavior or comments

hazardous substance Any chemical that presents a physical hazard or a health hazard in the workplace

hematuria Blood *(hemat)* in the urine *(uria)*

hemiplegia Paralysis *(plegia)* on one side *(hemi)* of the body

hemodialysis Removes waste and fluid from the body (*hemo*) by filtering the blood through an artificial kidney called a *dialyzer*

hemoglobin The substance in red blood cells that carries oxygen and gives blood *(hemo)* its color

hemoptysis Bloody *(hemo)* sputum (*ptysis* meaning "to spit")

hemorrhage The excessive loss *(rrhage)* of blood *(hemo)* from a blood vessel

hemothorax The collection of blood *(hemo)* in the pleural space *(thorax)*

heterosexual A person who is attracted to people of the other sex

hirsutism Excessive body hair in women and children

homosexual A person who is attracted to members of the same sex

horizontal recumbent position The dorsal recumbent position

hormone A chemical substance secreted by the glands into the bloodstream

hospice A health care facility or program for persons dying from a terminal illness

HS care Care given in the evening at bedtime; evening care or PM care

hyperextension Excessive straightening of a body part

hyperglycemia High *(hyper)* sugar *(glyc)* in the blood *(emia)*

hypertension Persistent blood pressure measurements above *(hyper)* the normal systolic (140 mm Hg) or diastolic (90 mm Hg) pressures

hyperthermia A body temperature *(thermia)* that is much higher *(hyper)* than the person's normal range

hyperventilation Respirations that are rapid *(hyper)* and deeper than normal

hypoglycemia Low *(hypo)* sugar *(glyc)* in the blood *(emia)*

hypotension A condition in which the systolic blood pressure is below *(hypo)* 90 mm Hg and the diastolic pressure is below 60 mm Hg

hypothermia A very low (*hypo*) body temperature (*thermia*); body temperature is below 95° F (35° C)

hypoventilation Respirations that are slow *(hypo)*, shallow, and sometimes irregular

hypoxemia A reduced amount *(hypo)* of oxygen *(ox)* in the blood *(emia)*

hypoxia A deficiency *(hypo)* of oxygen *(oxia)* in the cells

ileostomy An artificial opening *(stomy)* between the ileum (small intestine; *ileo*) and the abdominal wall

immunity Protection against a certain disease

implementation Performing or carrying out nursing measures in the care plan

impotence The inability of the male to have an erection

incision An open wound with clean, straight edges; usually intentionally produced with a sharp instrument

infected wound A wound that contains large amounts of bacteria and that shows signs of infection; a dirty wound

infection A disease state resulting from the invasion and growth of microorganisms in the body

insomnia A chronic condition in which the person cannot sleep or stay asleep throughout the night

intentional wound A wound created for therapy

interdisciplinary health care team A variety of health workers who work together to provide health care for residents

interdisciplinary progress note A written description of the care given and the resident's response and progress

internal rotation Turning the joint inward

intravenous therapy Fluid administered through a needle inserted into a vein (IV or IV infusion)

intubation The process of inserting an artificial airway

invasion of privacy Violating a person's right not to have his or her name, photograph, or private affairs exposed or made public without giving consent

jejunostomy An opening *(stomy)* into the middle part of the small intestine *(jejunum)*

job description A listing of the responsibilities and functions the agency expects you to perform

Kardex A type of card file that summarizes information found in the medical record—medications, treatments, diagnosis, routine care measures, special equipment used, and special needs

ketone body Acetone

knee-chest position The person kneels and rests the body on the knees and chest; the head is turned to one side, the arms are above the head or flexed at the elbows, the back is straight, and the body is flexed about 90 degrees at the hips

Kussmaul's respirations Very deep and rapid respirations; a sign of diabetic coma

laceration An open wound with torn tissues and jagged edges

laryngeal mirror An instrument used to examine the mouth, teeth, and throat

lateral position The side-lying position

law A rule of conduct made by a government body

libel Defamation through written statements

licensed practical nurse (LPN) An individual who has completed a 1-year nursing program and who has passed the licensing examination for practical nurses; called *licensed vocational nurse (LVN)* in some states

lithotomy position The person is in a back-lying position, the hips are brought down to the edge of the examination table, the knees are flexed, the hips are externally rotated, and the feet are supported in stirrups

logrolling Turning the resident as a unit in alignment with one motion

malignant tumor A tumor that grows rapidly and invades other tissues; cancer

malpractice Negligence by a professional person

mechanical ventilation Using a machine to move air into and out of the lungs

Medicaid A health insurance program sponsored by state and federal governments

medical asepsis The practices used to remove or destroy pathogens and to prevent their spread from one person or place to another person or place; clean technique

medical diagnosis The identification of a disease or condition by a doctor

medical record A written account of a resident's illness and response to treatment and care given by the health team; chart

Medicare A health insurance plan administered by the Social Security Administration of the federal government

melena A black, tarry stool

menopause The cessation of the menstrual cycle; the time when menstruation stops; it marks the end of the woman's reproductive years

menstruation The process in which the lining of the uterus breaks up and is discharged from the body through the vagina

mental Relating to the mind; something that exists in the mind or is performed by the mind

mental disorder Mental illness, emotional illness, psychiatric disorder

mental health A state of mind in which the person copes with and adjusts to the stresses of everyday living in ways acceptable to society

mental illness A disturbance in the person's ability to cope or adjust to stress; behavior and functioning are impaired; mental disorder, emotional illness, psychiatric disorder

metabolism The burning of food for heat and energy by the cells

metastasis The spread of cancer to other parts of the body

microbe A microorganism

microorganism A small (*micro*) living plant or animal (*organism*) seen only with a microscope; a microbe

micturition The process of emptying urine from the bladder; urination or voiding

mitered corner A way of tucking linens under the mattress to help keep them straight and smooth

mixed incontinence A combination of urge and stress incontinence

morning care Care given after breakfast; cleanliness and skin care measures are more thorough at this time

nasal speculum An instrument used to examine the inside of the nose

nasogastric (NG) tube A tube inserted through the nose *(naso)* into the stomach *(gastro)*

nasointestinal tube A tube inserted through the nose into the duodenum or jejunum of the small intestine

need That which is necessary or desirable for maintaining life and mental well-being

negligence An unintentional wrong in which a person fails to act in a reasonable and careful manner and causes harm to a person or to the person's property

nocturia Frequent urination *(uria)* at night *(noct)*

nonpathogen A microbe that usually does not cause an infection

nonverbal communication Communication that does not involve words

normal flora Microbes that usually live and grow in a certain location

nosocomial infection An infection acquired during a stay at a health care agency

NREM sleep The stage of sleep when there is no rapid eye movement; non-REM sleep

nurse practitioner (NP) A registered nurse with advanced training in physical examination and assessment; some states allow NPs to diagnose and prescribe under a doctor's supervision

nursing assistant An individual who gives basic nursing care under the supervision of a registered nurse or an LPN/LVN; also called *nurse's aide*, *nursing attendant*, and *health care assistant*

nursing center A facility that provides health care services to residents who require regular or continuous care; licensed nursing staff is required; commonly called a *nursing home* or *nursing facility*

nursing diagnosis A statement describing a health problem that can be treated by nursing measures

nursing facility (NF) Nursing center or nursing home

nursing home Nursing facility or nursing center

nursing intervention An action or measure taken by the nursing team to help the resident reach a goal

nursing process The method used by RNs to plan and deliver nursing care; its five steps are assessment, nursing diagnosis, planning, implementation, and evaluation

nursing team The individuals involved in providing nursing care: RNs, LPNs/LVNs, and nursing assistants

nutrient A substance that is ingested, digested, absorbed, and used by the body

nutrition The many processes involved in the ingestion, digestion, absorption, and use of foods and fluids by the body

objective data Information that can be seen, heard, felt, or smelled by another person; signs

observation Using the senses of sight, hearing, touch, and smell to collect information about a resident

obsession A persistent thought or idea

old Those persons between the ages of 65 and 85

old-old Those persons over the age of 85

oliguria Scant amount *(olig)* of urine *(uria)*; usually less than 500 ml in 24 hours

Omnibus Budget Reconciliation Act of 1987 (OBRA) A federal law concerned with the quality of life, health, and safety of residents

open fracture Compound fracture

open wound The skin or mucous membrane is broken

ophthalmoscope A lighted instrument used to examine the internal structures of the eye

optimal level of function A person's highest potential for mental and physical performance

oral hygiene Measures performed to keep the mouth and teeth clean; mouth care

organ Groups of tissues with the same function

orthopnea Being able to breathe *(pnea)* deeply and comfortably only while sitting or standing *(ortho)*

orthopneic position Sitting up in bed *(ortho)* and leaning forward over the bedside table

orthostatic hypotension A drop in *(hypo)* blood pressure when the person stands *(ortho* and *static)*; postural hypotension

ostomy Surgical creation of an artificial opening

otoscope A lighted instrument used to examine the external ear and the eardrum (tympanic membrane)

overflow incontinence The loss of urine when the bladder is too full

oxygen concentration The amount of hemoglobin that contains oxygen (O_2)

pain Discomfort

panic An intense and sudden feeling of fear, anxiety, terror, or dread

paranoia A disorder *(para)* of the mind *(noia)*; false beliefs (delusions) and suspicion about a person or situation

paraphrasing Restating the person's message in your own words

paraplegia Paralysis from the waist down

partial-thickness wound A wound in which the dermis and epidermis of the skin are broken

passive physical restraint A restraint near but not directly attached to the person's body; it does not totally restrict freedom of movement and allows access to certain body parts

pathogen A microbe that is harmful and can cause an infection

pediculosis capitis The infestation of the scalp (*capitis*) with lice

pediculosis corporis The infestation of the body (*corporis*) with lice

pediculosis (lice) The infestation with lice

pediculosis pubis The infestation of the pubic (*pubis*) hair with lice

penetrating wound An open wound in which the skin and underlying tissues are pierced

percussion hammer An instrument used to tap body parts to test reflexes

percutaneous endoscopic gastrostomy (PEG) tube A tube inserted into the stomach *(gastro)* through a stab or puncture wound *(stomy)* made through *(per)* the skin *(cutaneous)*; a lighted instrument *(scope)* allows the doctor to see inside a body cavity or organ *(endo)*

perineal care Cleansing the genital and anal areas

peristalsis Involuntary muscle contractions in the digestive system that move food through the alimentary canal

peritoneal dialysis A process that uses the lining of the abdominal cavity (the *peritoneal membrane*) to remove waste from the body

personal protective equipment Specialized clothing or equipment (e.g., gloves, goggles, gowns) worn for protection against a hazard

phantom pain Pain felt in a body part that is no longer there

phlebitis Inflammation (*itis*) of the vein (*phleb*)

phobia Fear, panic, or dread

plantar flexion The foot *(plantar)* is bent *(flexion)* down at the ankle

plaque A thin film that sticks to the teeth; it contains saliva, microorganisms, and other substances

plastic drawsheet A drawsheet placed between the bottom sheet and the cotton drawsheet to keep the mattress and bottom linens clean and dry

pleural effusion The escape and collection of fluid *(effusion)* in the pleural space *(thorax)*

PM care HS care or evening care

pneumothorax The collection of air *(pneumo)* in the pleural space *(thorax)*

podiatrist A foot (*pod*) doctor

pollutant A harmful chemical or substance in the air or water

polyuria The production of abnormally large amounts *(poly)* of urine *(uria)*

postmortem After *(post)* death *(mortem)*

postural hypotension Orthostatic hypotension

posture The way in which body parts are aligned with one another; body alignment

preceptor A staff member who guides

prefix A word element placed at the beginning of a word to change the meaning of the word

presbyopia Age-related farsightedness

pressure sore A bed sore, decubitus ulcer, or pressure ulcer

pressure ulcer Any injury caused by unrelieved pressure; a decubitus ulcer, bedsore, or pressure sore

primary nursing A method of organizing nursing care; a nurse is responsible for the total care of specific residents on a 24-hour basis

private insurance plan An insurance plan bought by an individual

pronation Turning downward

prone position Lying on the abdomen with the head turned to one side

prosthesis An artificial replacement for a missing body part

pseudodementia False *(pseudo)* disorder of the mind *(dementia)*

psychiatric disorder Mental illness, mental disorder, emotional illness

psychosis A serious mental disorder; the person does not view or interpret reality correctly

pulse The beat of the heart felt at an artery as a wave of blood passes through the artery

pulse deficit The difference between the apical and radial pulse rates

pulse rate The number of heartbeats or pulses felt in 1 minute

puncture wound An open wound made by a sharp object; entry of the skin and underlying tissues; may be intentional or unintentional

purulent drainage Thick green, yellow, or brown drainage

quadriplegia Paralysis from the neck down; paralysis of the arms, legs, and trunk

radiating pain Pain felt at the site of tissue damage and in nearby areas

range of motion (ROM) The movement of a joint to the extent possible without causing pain

receptive aphasia Difficulty receiving information

recording Writing or charting resident care and observations

reflex incontinence The loss of urine at predictable intervals; unconscious incontinence

registered nurse (RN) An individual who has studied nursing for 2, 3, or 4 years and who has passed a licensing examination

regurgitation The backward flow of food from the stomach into the mouth

rehabilitation The process of restoring the disabled person to the highest possible level of physical, psychological, social, and economic functioning

reincarnation The belief that the spirit or soul is reborn in another human body or in another form of life

relaxation To be free from mental or physical stress

religion Spiritual beliefs, needs, and practices

REM sleep The stage of sleep when there is rapid eye movement

reporting A verbal account of resident care and observations

reservoir The environment in which microbes live and grow; host

residential care facility A board and care facility or an assisted living facility

resident unit The personal space, furniture, and equipment provided for the individual by the nursing center

respiration The act of breathing air into (inhalation) and out of (exhalation) the lungs

respiratory arrest Breathing stops but the heart continues to pump for several minutes

respiratory depression Slow, weak respirations that occur at a rate of fewer than 12 per minute; respirations are not deep enough to bring enough air into the lungs

responsibility The duty or obligation to perform some act or function

rest To be calm, at ease, and relaxed; to be free of anxiety and stress

restorative aide A nursing assistant with special training in rehabilitation skills

restraint Any item, object, device, garment, material, or chemical that restricts a person's freedom of movement or access to one's body

reverse Trendelenburg's position The head of the bed is raised, and the foot of the bed is lowered

rigor mortis The stiffness or rigidity *(rigor)* of skeletal muscles that occurs after death *(mortis)*

root A word element containing the basic meaning of the word

rotation Turning the joint

sanguineous drainage Bloody drainage *(sanguis)*

schizophrenia Split (*schizo*) mind (*phrenia*)

seizure The violent and sudden contractions or tremors of muscles; convulsion

self-actualization Experiencing one's potential

self-esteem Thinking well of oneself, seeing oneself as useful, and being well thought of by others

semi-Fowler's position The head of the bed is raised 45 degrees, and the knee portion is raised 15 degrees; or the head of the bed is raised 30 degrees, and the knee portion is not raised

serosanguineous drainage Thin, watery drainage *(sero)* that is blood-tinged *(sanguineous)*

serous drainage Clear, watery fluid (serum)

sex The physical activities involving the organs of reproduction; the activities are done for pleasure or to produce children

sexuality The physical, psychological, social, cultural, and spiritual factors that affect a person's feelings and attitudes about his or her sex

shearing When skin sticks to a surface and muscles slide in the direction the body is moving

shock A condition that results when there is an inadequate blood supply to organs and tissues

side-lying position The lateral position

signs Objective data

simple fracture Closed fracture

Sims' position A left side-lying position in which the upper leg is sharply flexed so that it is not on the lower leg and the lower arm is behind the person

skilled nursing facility (SNF) A facility that provides nursing care for residents who need complex care but do not need hospital services; may be part of a nursing center or a hospital

skin tear A break or rip in the skin that separates the epidermis from underlying tissue

slander Defamation through oral statements

sleep A state of unconsciousness, reduced voluntary muscle activity, and lowered metabolism

spastic Uncontrolled contractions of skeletal muscles

sphygmomanometer The instrument used to measure blood pressure

spore A bacterium protected by a hard shell that forms around the microbe

sputum Expectorated (expelled) mucus

stasis ulcer An open wound on the lower leg and foot caused by poor blood return through the veins; venous ulcer

sterile The absence of all microbes

sterile field A work area free of all pathogens and nonpathogens (including spores)

sterile technique Surgical asepsis

sterilization The process of destroying all microbes

stethoscope An instrument used to listen to the sounds produced by the heart, lungs, and other body organs

stoma An artificial opening to the outside of the body

stomatitis Inflammation *(itis)* of the mouth *(stomat)*

stool Excreted feces

stress The response or change in the body caused by any emotional, physical, social, or economic factor

stress incontinence The loss of small amounts of urine with exercise and certain movements

stressor Any emotional, physical, social, or economic factor that causes stress

subacute care Complex medical care or rehabilitation

subjective data That which is reported by a person and cannot be observed by using the senses; symptoms

suction The process of withdrawing or sucking up fluid (secretions)

suffix A word element placed at the end of a root to change the meaning of the word

suffocation When breathing stops from the lack of oxygen

sundowning Increased signs, symptoms, and behaviors of Alzheimer's disease during hours of darkness

supination Turning upward

supine position The back-lying or dorsal recumbent position

supportive care Care provided on a 24-hour basis that meets a person's basic physical needs

suppository A cone-shaped, solid medication that is inserted into a body opening; it melts at body temperature

surgical asepsis The practices that keep equipment and supplies free of all microbes; sterile technique

symptoms Subjective data

syncope A brief loss of consciousness; fainting

system Organs that work together to perform special functions

systole The period of heart muscle contraction

systolic pressure The amount of force it takes to pump blood out of the heart into the arterial circulation

tachycardia A rapid *(tachy)* heart rate *(cardia)*; the heart rate is over 100 beats per minute

tachypnea Rapid *(tachy)* breathing *(pnea)*; respirations are usually more than 24 per minute

tartar Hardened plaque on teeth

task A function, procedure, activity, or work that does not require an RN's professional knowledge or judgment

team nursing A method of organizing nursing care; a nurse serves as a team leader; the team leader assigns other nurses and nursing assistants to care for certain residents

terminal illness An illness or injury for which there is no reasonable expectation of recovery

thrombus A blood clot

tinnitus Ringing in the ears

tissue A group of cells with similar functions

tort A wrong committed against a person or the person's property

transfer Moving a resident from one room, nursing unit, or nursing center to another

transfer belt A belt used to hold onto a resident during a transfer or when walking with the resident; a gait belt

transsexual A person who believes that he or she is really a member of the other sex

transvestite A person who becomes sexually excited by dressing in the clothes of the other sex

trauma An accident or violent act that injures the skin, mucous membranes, bones, and internal organs

Trendelenburg's position The head of the bed is lowered, and the foot of the bed is raised

triggers Clues for the resident assessment protocols

tumor A new growth of abnormal cells; tumors are benign or malignant

tuning fork An instrument used to test hearing

unconscious incontinence Reflex incontinence

unintentional wound A wound resulting from trauma

ureterostomy An artificial opening (*stomy*) between the ureter (*uretero*) and abdomen

urge incontinence The involuntary loss of urine after feeling a strong need to void

urinary frequency Voiding at frequent intervals

urinary incontinence The inability to control the loss of urine from the bladder

urinary urgency The need to void immediately

urination The process of emptying urine from the bladder; micturition or voiding

vaccine A preparation containing microbes

vaginal speculum An instrument used to open the vagina so that it and the cervix can be examined

vascular wound A circulatory ulcer

vein A blood vessel that carries blood back to the heart

venous ulcer A stasis ulcer

verbal communication Communication that uses the written or spoken word

vertigo Dizziness

vital signs Temperature, pulse, respirations, and blood pressure

voiding Urination or micturition

will A legal statement of how a person wishes to have property distributed after death

word element A part of a word

work ethics Behavior in the workplace

wound A break in the skin or mucous membrane

young-old Those persons between the ages of 55 and 65

APPENDIX A

Minimum Data Set Including Resident Assessment Protocol Summary

*Reprinted with permission of Briggs Corporation, Des Moines, Iowa.

Numeric Identifier_____

MINIMUM DATA SET (MDS) — *VERSION 2.0*
FOR NURSING HOME RESIDENT ASSESSMENT AND CARE SCREENING
BASIC ASSESSMENT TRACKING FORM

SECTION AA. IDENTIFICATION INFORMATION

1.	**RESIDENT NAME** ⊛	a. (First) b. (Middle Initial) c. (Last) d. (Jr./Sr.)
2.	**GENDER** ⊛	1. Male 2. Female
3.	**BIRTHDATE** ⊛	☐☐ — ☐☐ — ☐☐☐☐ Month Day Year
4.	**RACE/ ⊛ ETHNICITY**	1. American Indian/Alaskan Native 4. Hispanic 2. Asian/Pacific Islander 5. White, not of 3. Black, not of Hispanic origin Hispanic origin
5.	**SOCIAL ⊛ SECURITY AND ⊛ MEDICARE NUMBERS** [C in 1st box if non Med. no.]	a. Social Security Number ☐☐☐ — ☐☐ — ☐☐☐☐ b. Medicare number (or comparable railroad insurance number)
6.	**FACILITY PROVIDER NO.** ⊛	a. State No. b. Federal No.
7.	**MEDICAID NO.** ["+" if pending, "N" if not a Medicaid ⊛ recipient]	
8.	**REASONS FOR ASSESS-MENT**	[Note—Other codes do not apply to this form] a. Primary reason for assessment 1. Admission assessment (required by day 14) 2. Annual assessment 3. Significant change in status assessment 4. Significant correction of prior full assessment 5. Quarterly review assessment 10. Significant correction of prior quarterly assessment 0. *NONE OF ABOVE* b. *Codes for assessments required for Medicare PPS or the State* *1. Medicare 5 day assessment* *2. Medicare 30 day assessment* *3. Medicare 60 day assessment* *4. Medicare 90 day assessment* *5. Medicare readmission/return assessment* *6. Other state required assessment* *7. Medicare 14 day assessment* *8. Other Medicare required assessment*
9.	**SIGNATURES OF PERSONS COMPLETING THESE ITEMS:**	

GENERAL INSTRUCTIONS

Complete this information for submission with all full and quarterly assessments (Admission, Annual, Significant Change, State or Medicare required assessments, or Quarterly Reviews, etc.).

a. Signatures Title Date

b. Date

⊛ = Key items for computerized resident tracking

☐ = When box blank, must enter number or letter

☐a. = When letter in box, check if condition applies

Code "—" if information unavailable or unknown

TRIGGER LEGEND

1 - Delirium	10A - Activities (Revise)
2 - Cognitive Loss/Dementia	10B - Activities (Review)
3 - Visual Function	11 - Falls
4 - Communication	12 - Nutritional Status
5A - ADL-Rehabilitation	13 - Feeding Tubes
5B - ADL-Maintenance	14 - Dehydration/Fluid Maintenance
6 - Urinary Incontinence and Indwelling Catheter	15 - Dental Care
7 - Psychosocial Well-Being	16 - Pressure Ulcers
8 - Mood State	17 - Psychotropic Drug Use
9 - Behavioral Symptoms	17* - For this to trigger, O4a, b, or c must = 1-7
	18 - Physical Restraints

Form 1728RHH
R398
© 1997 Briggs Corporation, Des Moines, IA 50306 (800) 247-2343 PRINTED IN U.S.A.
Copyright limited to addition of trigger system.

Resident ______________________ Numeric Identifier ______________________

MINIMUM DATA SET (MDS) — *VERSION 2.0*
FOR NURSING HOME RESIDENT ASSESSMENT AND CARE SCREENING
BACKGROUND (FACE SHEET) INFORMATION AT ADMISSION

SECTION AB. DEMOGRAPHIC INFORMATION

1.	DATE OF ENTRY	*Date the stay began. Note — Does not include readmission if record was closed at time of temporary discharge to hospital, etc. In such cases, use prior admission date.* Month — Day — Year
2.	ADMITTED FROM (AT ENTRY)	1. Private home/apt. with no home health services 2. Private home/apt. with home health services 3. Board and care/assisted living/group home 4. Nursing home 5. Acute care hospital 6. Psychiatric hospital, MR/DD facility 7. Rehabilitation hospital 8. Other
3.	LIVED ALONE (PRIOR TO ENTRY)	0. No 1. Yes 2. In other facility
4.	ZIP CODE OF PRIOR PRIMARY RESIDENCE	
5.	RESIDENTIAL HISTORY 5 YEARS PRIOR TO ENTRY	*(**Check all settings** resident **lived in** during 5 years prior to date of entry given in item AB1 above.)* Prior stay at this nursing home a. Stay in other nursing home b. Other residential facility — board and care home, assisted living, group home c. MH/psychiatric setting d. MR/DD setting e. *NONE OF ABOVE* f.
6.	LIFETIME OCCUPATION(S) (Put "/" between two occupations)	
7.	EDUCATION (*Highest level completed*)	1. No schooling 2. 8th grade/less 3. 9-11 grades 4. High school 5. Technical or trade school 6. Some college 7. Bachelor's degree 8. Graduate degree
8.	LANGUAGE	*(Code for correct response)* a. Primary Language 0. English 1. Spanish 2. French 3. Other **b. If other, specify**
9.	MENTAL HEALTH HISTORY	Does resident's RECORD indicate any history of mental retardation, mental illness, or developmental disability problem? 0. No 1. Yes
10.	CONDITIONS RELATED TO MR/DD STATUS	*(**Check all conditions** that are related to MR/DD status that were manifested before age 22, and are likely to continue indefinitely)* Not applicable — no MR/DD (Skip to AB11) a. MR/DD with organic condition Down's syndrome b. Autism c. Epilepsy d. Other organic condition related to MR/DD e. MR/DD with no organic condition f.
11.	DATE BACKGROUND INFORMATION COMPLETED	Month — Day — Year

[ ] = When box blank, must enter number or letter

[a.] = When letter in box, check if condition applies

Code "—" if information unavailable or unknown

SECTION AC. CUSTOMARY ROUTINE

1. CUSTOMARY ROUTINE *(In year prior to DATE OF ENTRY to this nursing home, or year last in community if now being admitted from another nursing home)*

***(Check all that apply.** If all information UNKNOWN, check last box only.)*

CYCLE OF DAILY EVENTS	
Stays up late at night (e.g., after 9 pm)	a.
Naps regularly during day (at least 1 hour)	b.
Goes out 1+ days a week	c.
Stays busy with hobbies, reading, or fixed daily routine	d.
Spends most of time alone or watching TV	e.
Moves independently indoors (with appliances, if used)	f.
Use of tobacco products at least daily	g.
NONE OF ABOVE	h.
EATING PATTERNS	
Distinct food preferences	i.
Eats between meals all or most days	j.
Use of alcoholic beverage(s) at least weekly	k.
NONE OF ABOVE	l.
ADL PATTERNS	
In bedclothes much of day	m.
Wakens to toilet all or most nights	n.
Has irregular bowel movement pattern	o.
Showers for bathing	p.
Bathing in PM	q.
NONE OF ABOVE	r.
INVOLVEMENT PATTERNS	
Daily contact with relatives/close friends	s.
Usually attends church, temple, synagogue (etc.)	t.
Finds strength in faith	u.
Daily animal companion/presence	v.
Involved in group activities	w.
NONE OF ABOVE	x.
UNKNOWN — Resident/family unable to provide information	y.

END

SECTION AD. FACE SHEET SIGNATURES

SIGNATURES OF PERSONS COMPLETING FACE SHEET:

a. Signature of RN Assessment Coordinator — Date

b. Signatures — Title — Sections — Date

c. — Date

d. — Date

e. — Date

f. — Date

g. — Date

NOTE: Normally, the MDS Face Sheet is completed once, when an individual first enters the facility. However, the face sheet is also required if the person is reentering this facility after a discharge where return had not previously been expected. It is not completed following temporary discharges to hospitals or after therapeutic leaves/home visits.

Form 1728RHH

Resident ______ Numeric Identifier ______

MINIMUM DATA SET (MDS) — *VERSION 2.0*
FOR NURSING HOME RESIDENT ASSESSMENT AND CARE SCREENING
FULL ASSESSMENT FORM
(Status in last 7 days, unless other time frame indicated)

SECTION A. IDENTIFICATION AND BACKGROUND INFORMATION

1.	RESIDENT NAME	a. (First) b. (Middle Initial) c. (Last) d. (Jr./Sr.)
2.	ROOM NUMBER	
3.	ASSESS-MENT REFERENCE DATE	a. *Last day of MDS observation period* Month — Day — Year b. Original (0) or corrected copy of form (enter number of correction)
4a.	DATE OF REENTRY	Date of reentry from most recent temporary discharge to a hospital in last 90 days (or since last assessment or admission if less than 90 days) Month — Day — Year
5.	MARITAL STATUS	1. Never married 2. Married 3. Widowed 4. Separated 5. Divorced
6.	MEDICAL RECORD NO.	
7.	CURRENT PAYMENT SOURCES FOR N.H. STAY	(*Billing Office to indicate;* **check all that apply in last 30 days**) Medicaid per diem a. Medicare per diem b. Medicare ancillary part A c. Medicare ancillary part B d. CHAMPUS per diem e. VA per diem f. Self or family pays for full per diem g. Medicaid resident liability or Medicare co-payment h. Private insurance per diem (including co-payment) i. Other per diem j.
8.	REASONS FOR ASSESS-MENT [*Note—If this is a discharge or reentry assessment, only a limited subset of MDS items need be completed*]	a. Primary reason for assessment 1. Admission assessment (required by day 14) 2. Annual assessment 3. Significant change in status assessment 4. Significant correction of prior full assessment 5. Quarterly review assessment 6. Discharged—return not anticipated 7. Discharged—return anticipated 8. Discharged prior to completing initial assessment 9. Reentry 10. Significant correction of prior quarterly assessment 0. NONE OF ABOVE **b. *Codes for assessments required for Medicare PPS or the State*** 1. Medicare 5 day assessment 2. Medicare 30 day assessment 3. Medicare 60 day assessment 4. Medicare 90 day assessment 5. Medicare readmission/return assessment 6. Other state required assessment 7. Medicare 14 day assessment 8. Other Medicare required assessment
9.	RESPONSI-BILITY/ LEGAL GUARDIAN	(***Check all that apply***) Legal guardian a. Other legal oversight b. Durable power of attorney/health care c. Durable power of attorney/financial d. Family member responsible e. Patient responsible for self f. *NONE OF ABOVE* g.
10.	ADVANCED DIRECTIVES	(*For those items with supporting documentation in the medical record,* ***check all that apply***) Living will a. Do not resuscitate b. Do not hospitalize c. Organ donation d. Autopsy request e. Feeding restrictions f. Medication restrictions g. Other treatment restrictions h. *NONE OF ABOVE* i.

SECTION B. COGNITIVE PATTERNS

1.	COMATOSE	(*Persistent vegetative state/no discernible consciousness*) 0. No 1. Yes ***(If yes, skip to Section G)***
2.	MEMORY	(*Recall of what was learned or known*) a. Short-term memory OK—seems/appears to recall after 5 minutes 0. Memory OK 1. Memory problem **2** b. Long-term memory OK—seems/appears to recall long past 0. Memory OK 1. Memory problem **2**
3.	MEMORY/ RECALL ABILITY	(***Check all*** *that resident was* ***normally able to recall during last 7 days***) Current season a. Location of own room b. Staff names/faces c. That he/she is in a nursing home d. *NONE OF ABOVE are recalled* e.
4.	COGNITIVE SKILLS FOR DAILY DECISION-MAKING	(*Made decisions regarding tasks of daily life*) 0. *INDEPENDENT*—decisions consistent/reasonable 1. *MODIFIED INDEPENDENCE*—some difficulty in new situations only **2** 2. *MODERATELY IMPAIRED*—decisions poor; cues/ supervision required **2** 3. *SEVERELY IMPAIRED*—never/rarely made decisions **2, 5B**
5.	INDICATORS OF DELIRIUM— PERIODIC DISOR-DERED THINKING/ AWARENESS	(*Code for behavior in the* ***last 7 days.***) [***Note: Accurate assessment requires conversations with staff and family who have direct knowledge of resident's behavior over this time.***] 0. Behavior not present 1. Behavior present, not of recent onset 2. Behavior present, over last 7 days appears different from resident's usual functioning (e.g., new onset or worsening) a. EASILY DISTRACTED—(e.g., difficulty paying attention; gets sidetracked) 2 = **1, 17*** b. PERIODS OF ALTERED PERCEPTION OR AWARENESS OF SURROUNDINGS—(e.g., moves lips or talks to someone not present; believes he/she is somewhere else; confuses night and day) 2 = **1, 17*** c. EPISODES OF DISORGANIZED SPEECH—(e.g., speech is incoherent, nonsensical, irrelevant, or rambling from subject to subject; loses train of thought) 2 = **1, 17*** d. PERIODS OF RESTLESSNESS—(e.g., fidgeting or picking at skin, clothing, napkins, etc.; frequent position changes; repetitive physical movements or calling out) 2 = **1, 17*** e. PERIODS OF LETHARGY—(e.g., sluggishness; staring into space; difficult to arouse; little body movement) 2 = **1, 17*** f. MENTAL FUNCTION VARIES OVER THE COURSE OF THE DAY—(e.g., sometimes better, sometimes worse; behaviors sometimes present, sometimes not) 2 = **1, 17***
6.	CHANGE IN COGNITIVE STATUS	Resident's cognitive status, skills, or abilities have changed as compared to status of **90 days ago** (or since assessment if less than 90 days) 0. No change 1. Improved 2. Deteriorated **1, 17***

SECTION C. COMMUNICATION/HEARING PATTERNS

1.	HEARING	(*With hearing appliance, if used*) 0. *HEARS ADEQUATELY*—normal talk, TV, phone 1. *MINIMAL DIFFICULTY* when not in quiet setting **4** 2. *HEARS IN SPECIAL SITUATIONS ONLY*—speaker has to adjust tonal quality and speak distinctly **4** 3. *HIGHLY IMPAIRED/*absence of useful hearing **4**
2.	COMMUNI-CATION DEVICES/ TECH-NIQUES	(***Check all that apply*** *during last 7 days*) Hearing aid, present and used a. Hearing aid, present and not used regularly b. Other receptive comm. techniques used (e.g., lip reading) c. *NONE OF ABOVE* d.
3.	MODES OF EXPRESSION	(***Check all used by*** *resident to make needs known*) Speech a. Writing messages to express or clarify needs b. American sign language or Braille c. Signs/gestures/sounds d. Communication board e. Other f. *NONE OF ABOVE* g.
4.	MAKING SELF UNDER-STOOD	(*Expressing information content—however able*) 0. *UNDERSTOOD* 1. *USUALLY UNDERSTOOD*—difficulty finding words or finishing thoughts **4** 2. *SOMETIMES UNDERSTOOD*—ability is limited to making concrete requests **4** 3. *RARELY/NEVER UNDERSTOOD* **4**
5.	SPEECH CLARITY	(*Code for speech in the* ***last 7 days)*** 0. *CLEAR SPEECH*—distinct, intelligible words 1. *UNCLEAR SPEECH*—slurred, mumbled words 2. *NO SPEECH*—absence of spoken words
6.	ABILITY TO UNDER-STAND OTHERS	(*Understanding verbal information content—however able*) 0. *UNDERSTANDS* 1. *USUALLY UNDERSTANDS*—may miss some part/ intent of message **2, 4** 2. *SOMETIMES UNDERSTANDS*—responds adequately to simple, direct communication **2, 4** 3. *RARELY/NEVER UNDERSTANDS* **2, 4**
7.	CHANGE IN COMMUNI-CATION/ HEARING	Resident's ability to express, understand, or hear information has changed as compared to status of ***90 days ago*** (*or since last assessment if less than 90 days*) 0. No change 1. Improved 2. Deteriorated **17***

TRIGGER LEGEND
1 - Delirium
2 - Cognitive Loss/Dementia
4 - Communication
5B - ADL Maintenance
17* - Psychotropic Drugs
(For this to trigger, O4a, b, or c must = 1-7)

☐ = When box blank, must enter number or letter.

a. = When letter in box, check if condition applies

Code "—" if information unavailable or unknown

Form 1728RHH

MDS 2.0 1/30/98

Resident ______________________

SECTION D. VISION PATTERNS

1.	VISION	*(Ability to see in adequate light and with glasses if used)* 0. *ADEQUATE*—sees fine detail, including regular print in newspapers/books 1. *IMPAIRED*—sees large print, but not regular print in newspapers/books **3** 2. *MODERATELY IMPAIRED*—limited vision; not able to see newspaper headlines, but can identify objects **3** 3. *HIGHLY IMPAIRED*—object identification in question, but eyes appear to follow objects **3** 4. *SEVERELY IMPAIRED*—no vision or sees only light, colors, or shapes; eyes do not appear to follow objects	
2.	VISUAL LIMITATIONS/ DIFFICULTIES	Side vision problems—decreased peripheral vision (e.g., leaves food on one side of tray, difficulty traveling, bumps into people and objects, misjudges placement of chair when seating self) **3**	a.
		Experiences any of following: sees halos or rings around lights; sees flashes of light; sees "curtains" over eyes	b.
		NONE OF ABOVE	c.
3.	VISUAL APPLIANCES	Glasses; contact lenses; magnifying glass 0. No 1. Yes	

SECTION E. MOOD AND BEHAVIOR PATTERNS

1. INDICATORS OF DEPRESSION, ANXIETY, SAD MOOD

(Code for indicators observed in last 30 days, irrespective of the assumed cause)
0. Indicator not exhibited in last 30 days
1. Indicator of this type exhibited up to five days a week
2. Indicator of this type exhibited daily or almost daily (6, 7 days a week)

VERBAL EXPRESSIONS OF DISTRESS

a. Resident made negative statements—e.g., *"Nothing matters; Would rather be dead; What's the use; Regrets having lived so long; Let me die"* 1 or 2 = **8**

b. Repetitive questions—e.g., *"Where do I go; What do I do?"* 1 or 2 = **8**

c. Repetitive verbalizations—e.g., calling out for help *("God help me")* **1 or 2 = 8**

d. Persistent anger with self or others—e.g., easily annoyed, anger at placement in nursing home; anger at care received 1 or 2 = **8**

e. Self deprecation—e.g., *"I am nothing; I am of no use to anyone"* 1 or 2 = **8**

f. Expressions of what appear to be unrealistic fears—e.g., fear of being abandoned, left alone, being with others 1 or 2 = **8**

g. Recurrent statements that something terrible is about to happen—e.g., believes he or she is about to die, have a heart attack 1 or 2 = **8**

h. Repetitive health complaints—e.g., persistently seeks medical attention, obsessive concern with body functions 1 or 2 = **8**

i. Repetitive anxious complaints/concerns (non-health related) e.g., persistently seeks attention/reassurance regarding schedules, meals, laundry/clothing, relationship issues 1 or 2 = **8**

SLEEP-CYCLE ISSUES

j. Unpleasant mood in morning 1 or 2 = **8**

k. Insomnia/change in usual sleep pattern 1 or 2 = **8**

SAD, APATHETIC, ANXIOUS APPEARANCE

l. Sad, pained, worried facial expressions—e.g., furrowed brows 1 or 2 = **8**

m. Crying, tearfulness 1 or 2 = **8**

n. Repetitive physical movements—e.g., pacing, hand wringing, restlessness, fidgeting, picking 1 or 2 = **8, 17***

LOSS OF INTEREST

o. Withdrawal from activities of interest—e.g., no interest in longstanding activities or being with family/friends 1 or 2 = **7, 8**

p. Reduced social interaction 1 or 2 = **8**

2. MOOD PERSISTENCE — **One or more indicators of depressed, sad or anxious mood were not easily altered by attempts to "cheer up", console, or reassure the resident over last 7 days**
0. No mood indicators 1. Indicators present, easily altered **8** 2. Indicators present, not easily altered **8**

3. CHANGE IN MOOD — Resident's mood status has changed as compared to status of **90 days ago** (or since last assessment if **less than 90 days**)
0. No change 1. Improved 2. Deteriorated **1, 17***

4. BEHAVIORAL SYMPTOMS

*(A) **Behavioral** symptom **frequency in last 7 days***
0. Behavior not exhibited in last 7 days
1. Behavior of this type occurred 1 to 3 days in last 7 days
2. Behavior of this type occurred 4 to 6 days, but less than daily
3. Behavior of this type occurred daily

*(B) **Behavioral** symptom **alterability in last 7 days***
0. Behavior not present OR behavior was easily altered
1. Behavior was not easily altered

	(A)	(B)
a. WANDERING (moved with no rational purpose, seemingly oblivious to needs or safety) A = 1, 2, or 3 = **9, 11**		
b. VERBALLY ABUSIVE BEHAVIORAL SYMPTOMS (others were threatened, screamed at, cursed at) A = 1, 2, or 3 = **9**		
c. PHYSICALLY ABUSIVE BEHAVIORAL SYMPTOMS (others were hit, shoved, scratched, sexually abused) A = 1, 2, or 3 = **9**		
d. SOCIALLY INAPPROPRIATE/DISRUPTIVE BEHAVIORAL SYMPTOMS (made disruptive sounds, noisiness, screaming, self-abusive acts, sexual behavior or disrobing in public, smeared/threw food/feces, hoarding, rummaged through others' belongings) A = 1, 2, or 3 = **9**		
e. RESISTS CARE (resisted taking medications/injections, ADL assistance, or eating) A = 1, 2, or 3 = **9**		

Numeric Identifier ______________________

5. CHANGE IN BEHAVIORAL SYMPTOMS — Resident's behavior status has changed as compared to **status of 90 days ago** (or since last assessment if less than 90 days)
0. No change 1. Improved **9** 2. Deteriorated **1, 17***

SECTION F. PSYCHOSOCIAL WELL-BEING

1.	SENSE OF INITIATIVE/ INVOLVEMENT	At ease interacting with others	a.
		At ease doing planned or structured activities	b.
		At ease doing self-initiated activities	c.
		Establishes own goals **7**	d.
		Pursues involvement in life of facility (e.g., makes/keeps friends; involved in group activities; responds positively to new activities; assists at religious services)	e.
		Accepts invitations into most group activities	f.
		NONE OF ABOVE	g.
2.	UNSETTLED RELATIONSHIPS	Covert/open conflict with or repeated criticism of staff **7**	a.
		Unhappy with roommate **7**	b.
		Unhappy with residents other than roommate **7**	c.
		Openly expresses conflict/anger with family/friends **7**	d.
		Absence of personal contact with family/friends	e.
		Recent loss of close family member/friend	f.
		Does not adjust easily to change in routines	g.
		NONE OF ABOVE	h.
3.	PAST ROLES	Strong identification with past roles and life status **7**	a.
		Expresses sadness/anger/empty feeling over lost roles/status **7**	b.
		Resident perceives that daily routine (customary routine, activities) is very different from prior pattern in the community **7**	c.
		NONE OF ABOVE	d.

SECTION G. PHYSICAL FUNCTIONING AND STRUCTURAL PROBLEMS

1. (A) ADL SELF-PERFORMANCE—***(Code for resident's PERFORMANCE OVER ALL SHIFTS during last 7 days—****Not including setup)*
0. *INDEPENDENT*—No help or oversight—OR—Help/oversight provided only 1 or 2 times during last 7 days
1. *SUPERVISION*—Oversight, encouragement or cueing provided 3 or more times during last 7 days—OR—Supervision (3 or more times) plus physical assistance provided only 1 or 2 times during last 7 days
2. *LIMITED ASSISTANCE*—Resident highly involved in activity; received physical help in guided maneuvering of limbs or other nonweight bearing assistance 3 or more times—OR—More help provided only 1 or 2 times during last 7 days
3. *EXTENSIVE ASSISTANCE*—While resident performed part of activity, over last 7-day period, help of following type(s) provided 3 or more times:
—Weight-bearing support
—Full staff performance during part (but not all) of last 7 days
4. *TOTAL DEPENDENCE*—Full staff performance of activity during entire 7 days
8. *ACTIVITY DID NOT OCCUR* during entire 7 days

(B) ADL SUPPORT PROVIDED—***(Code for MOST SUPPORT PROVIDED OVER ALL SHIFTS during last 7 days; code regardless of*** *resident's self-performance classification)*
0. No setup or physical help from staff
1. Setup help only
2. One person physical assist
3. Two+ persons physical assist
8. ADL activity itself did not occur during entire 7 days

			(A) SELF-PERF	(B) SUPPORT
a.	BED MOBILITY	How resident moves to and from lying position, turns side to side, and positions body while in bed A = 1 = **5A**; A = 2, 3, or 4 = **5A, 16**; A = 8 = **16**		
b.	TRANSFER	How resident moves between surfaces—to/from: bed, chair, wheelchair, standing position (EXCLUDE to/from bath/toilet) A = 1, 2, 3, or 4 = **5A**		
c.	WALK IN ROOM	How resident walks between locations in his/her room A = 1, 2, 3, or 4 = **5A**		
d.	WALK IN CORRIDOR	How resident walks in corridor on unit A = 1, 2, 3, or 4 = **5A**		
e.	LOCOMOTION ON UNIT	How resident moves between locations in his/her room and adjacent corridor on same floor. If in wheelchair, self-sufficiency once in chair A = 1, 2, 3, or 4 = **5A**		
f.	LOCOMOTION OFF UNIT	How resident moves to and returns from off unit locations (e.g., areas set aside for dining, activities, or treatments). **If facility has only one floor**, how resident moves to and from distant areas on the floor. If in wheelchair, self-sufficiency once in chair A = 1, 2, 3, or 4 = **5A**		
g.	DRESSING	How resident puts on, fastens, and takes off all items of **street clothing**, including donning/removing prosthesis A = 1, 2, 3, or 4 = **5A**		
h.	EATING	How resident eats and drinks (regardless of skill). Includes intake of nourishment by other means (e.g., tube feeding, total parenteral nutrition) A = 1, 2, 3, or 4 = **5A**		
i.	TOILET USE	How resident uses the toilet room (or commode, bedpan, urinal); transfers on/off toilet, cleanses, changes pad, manages ostomy or catheter, adjusts clothes A = 1, 2, 3, or 4 = **5A**		
j.	PERSONAL HYGIENE	How resident maintains personal hygiene, including combing hair, brushing teeth, shaving, applying makeup, washing/drying face, hands, and perineum (EXCLUDE baths and showers) A = 1, 2, 3, or 4 = **5A**		

TRIGGER LEGEND
1 - Delirium
3 - Visual Function
5A - ADL Rehabilitation
7 - Psychosocial Well-Being
8 - Mood State
9 - Behavior Symptoms
11 - Falls
17* - Psychotropic Drugs (*For this to trigger, O4a, b, or c must = 1-7)

Resident ______________________ Numeric Identifier ______________________

2.	**BATHING**	How resident takes full-body bath/shower, sponge bath, and transfers in/out of tub/shower (EXCLUDE washing of back and hair). ***Code for most dependent** in self-performance and support.* A = 1, 2, 3 or 4 =**5A** (A) BATHING SELF-PERFORMANCE codes appear below. (A) (B) **0.** Independent—No help provided **1.** Supervision—Oversight help only **2.** Physical help limited to transfer only **3.** Physical help in part of bathing activity **4.** Total dependence **8.** Activity itself did not occur during entire 7 days *(Bathing support codes are as defined in **Item 1, code B above**)*
3.	**TEST FOR BALANCE** (See training manual)	*(Code for ability during test in the **last 7 days**)* **0.** Maintained position as required in test **1.** Unsteady, but able to rebalance self without physical support **2.** Partial physical support during test; or stands (sits) but does not follow directions for test **3.** Not able to attempt test without physical help a. Balance while standing b. Balance while sitting—position, trunk control 1, 2, or 3 = **17***
4.	**FUNCTIONAL LIMITATION IN RANGE OF MOTION** (see training manual)	*(Code for limitations during **last 7 days** that interfered with daily functions or placed resident at risk of injury)* *(A) RANGE OF MOTION*: **0.** No limitation; **1.** Limitation on one side; **2.** Limitation on both sides *(B) VOLUNTARY MOVEMENT*: **0.** No loss; **1.** Partial loss; **2.** Full loss (A) (B) **a.** Neck **b.** Arm—Including shoulder or elbow **c.** Hand—Including wrist or fingers **d.** Leg—Including hip or knee **e.** Foot—Including ankle or toes **f.** Other limitation or loss
5.	**MODES OF LOCOMOTION**	***(Check all that apply** during **last 7 days**)* Cane/walker/crutch a. Wheeled self b. Other person wheeled c. Wheelchair primary mode of locomotion d. *NONE OF ABOVE* e.
6.	**MODES OF TRANSFER**	***(Check all that apply** during **last 7 days**)* Bedfast all or most of time **16** a. Bed rails used for bed mobility or transfer b. Lifted manually c. Lifted mechanically d. Transfer aid (e.g., slide board, trapeze, cane, walker, brace) e. *NONE OF ABOVE* f.
7.	**TASK SEGMENTATION**	Some or all of ADL activities were broken into subtasks during **last 7 days** so that resident could perform them **0.** No **1.** Yes
8.	**ADL FUNCTIONAL REHABILITATION POTENTIAL**	Resident believes he/she is capable of increased independence in at least some ADLs **5A** a. Direct care staff believe resident is capable of increased independence in at least some ADLs **5A** b. Resident able to perform tasks/activity but is very slow c. Difference in ADL Self-Performance or ADL Support, comparing mornings to evenings d. *NONE OF ABOVE* e.
9.	**CHANGE IN ADL FUNCTION**	Resident's ADL self-performance status has changed as compared to status of **90 days ago** (or since last assessment if less than 90 days) **0.** No change **1.** Improved **2.** Deteriorated

SECTION H. CONTINENCE IN LAST 14 DAYS

1.	CONTINENCE SELF-CONTROL CATEGORIES ***(Code for resident's PERFORMANCE OVER ALL SHIFTS)***	**0.** *CONTINENT*—Complete control *(includes use of indwelling urinary catheter or ostomy device that does not leak urine or stool)* **1.** *USUALLY CONTINENT*—BLADDER, incontinent episodes once a week or less; BOWEL, less than weekly **2.** *OCCASIONALLY INCONTINENT*—BLADDER, 2 or more times a week but not daily; BOWEL, once a week **3.** *FREQUENTLY INCONTINENT*—BLADDER, tended to be incontinent daily, but some control present (e.g., on day shift); BOWEL, 2-3 times a week **4.** *INCONTINENT*—Had inadequate control. BLADDER, multiple daily episodes; BOWEL, all (or almost all) of the time
a.	**BOWEL CONTINENCE**	Control of bowel movement, with appliance or bowel continence programs, if employed 1, 2, 3 or 4 = **16**
b.	**BLADDER CONTINENCE**	Control of urinary bladder function (if dribbles, volume insufficient to soak through underpants), with appliances (e.g., foley) or continence programs, if employed 2, 3 or 4 = **6**
2.	**BOWEL ELIMINATION PATTERN**	Bowel elimination pattern regular—at least one movement every three days a. Constipation **17*** b. Diarrhea c. Fecal impaction **17*** d. *NONE OF ABOVE* e.
3.	**APPLIANCES AND PROGRAMS**	Any scheduled toileting plan a. Bladder retraining program b. External (condom) catheter **6** c. Indwelling catheter **6** d. Intermittent catheter **6** e. Did not use toilet room/commode/urinal f. Pads/briefs used **6** g. Enemas/irrigation h. Ostomy present i. *NONE OF ABOVE* j.
4.	**CHANGE IN URINARY CONTINENCE**	Resident's urinary continence has changed as compared to status of **90 days ago** (or since last assessment if less than 90 days) **0.** No change **1.** Improved **2.** Deteriorated

SECTION I. DISEASE DIAGNOSES

Check only **those diseases that have a relationship** to current ADL status, cognitive status, mood and behavior status, medical treatments, nursing monitoring, or risk of death. (Do not list inactive diagnoses)

1. DISEASES ***(If none apply, CHECK the NONE OF ABOVE box)***

ENDOCRINE/METABOLIC/NUTRITIONAL		Hemiplegia/Hemiparesis	v.
Diabetes mellitus	a.	Multiple sclerosis	w.
Hyperthyroidism	b.	Paraplegia	x.
Hypothyroidism	c.	Parkinson's disease	y.
HEART/CIRCULATION		Quadriplegia	z.
Arteriosclerotic heart disease (ASHD)	d.	Seizure disorder	aa.
Cardiac dysrhythmias	e.	Transient ischemic attack (TIA)	bb.
Congestive heart failure	f.	Traumatic brain injury	cc.
Deep vein thrombosis	g.	**PSYCHIATRIC/MOOD**	
Hypertension	h.	Anxiety disorder	dd.
Hypotension **17***	i.	Depression **17***	ee.
Peripheral vascular disease **16**	j.	Manic depression (bipolar disease)	ff.
Other cardiovascular disease	k.	Schizophrenia	gg.
MUSCULOSKELETAL		**PULMONARY**	
Arthritis	l.	Asthma	hh.
Hip fracture	m.	Emphysema/COPD	ii.
Missing limb (e.g., amputation)	n.	**SENSORY**	
Osteoporosis	o.	Cataracts **3**	jj.
Pathological bone fracture	p.	Diabetic retinopathy	kk.
NEUROLOGICAL		Glaucoma **3**	ll.
Alzheimer's disease	q.	Macular degeneration	mm.
Aphasia	r.	**OTHER**	
Cerebral palsy	s.	Allergies	nn.
Cerebrovascular accident (stroke)	t.	Anemia	oo.
Dementia other than Alzheimer's disease	u.	Cancer	pp.
		Renal failure	qq.
		NONE OF ABOVE	rr.

2. INFECTIONS ***(If none apply, CHECK the NONE OF ABOVE box)***

Antibiotic resistant infection (e.g., Methicillin resistant staph)	a.	Septicemia	g.
Clostridium difficile (c. diff.)	b.	Sexually transmitted diseases	h.
Conjunctivitis	c.	Tuberculosis	i.
HIV infection	d.	Urinary tract infection **in last 30 days 14**	j.
Pneumonia	e.	Viral hepatitis	k.
Respiratory infection	f.	Wound infection	l.
		NONE OF ABOVE	m.

3. OTHER CURRENT OR MORE DETAILED DIAGNOSES AND ICD-9 CODES

Dehydration 276.5 = **14**

a. ______________________ •
b. ______________________ •
c. ______________________ •
d. ______________________ •
e. ______________________ •

SECTION J. HEALTH CONDITIONS

1. PROBLEM CONDITIONS ***(Check all problems present in last 7 days** unless other time frame is indicated)*

INDICATORS OF FLUID STATUS		Dizziness/Vertigo **11, 17***	f.
Weight gain or loss of 3 or more pounds within a 7 day period **14**	a.	Edema	g.
Inability to lie flat due to shortness of breath	b.	Fever **14**	h.
Dehydrated; output exceeds input **14**	c.	Hallucinations **17***	i.
Insufficient fluid; did **NOT** consume all/almost all liquids provided during **last 3 days 14**	d.	Internal bleeding **14**	j.
OTHER		Recurrent lung aspirations in **last 90 days 17***	k.
Delusions	e.	Shortness of breath	l.
		Syncope (fainting) **17***	m.
		Unsteady gait **17***	n.
		Vomiting	o.
		NONE OF ABOVE	p.

TRIGGER LEGEND
3 - Visual Function
5A - ADL Rehabilitation
6 - Urinary Incontinence/Indwelling Catheter
11 - Falls
14 - Dehydration/Fluid Maintenance
16 - Pressure Ulcers
17* - Psychotropic Drugs
(*For this to trigger, O4a, b, or c must = 1-7)

Resident _____ Numeric Identifier _____

2.	PAIN SYMPTOMS	(Code the **highest level of pain** present in **the last 7 days**)	
		a. FREQUENCY with which resident complains or shows evidence of pain	b. INTENSITY of pain
		0. No pain **(skip to J4)**	1. Mild pain
		1. Pain less than daily	2. Moderate pain
		2. Pain daily	3. Times when pain is horrible or excruciating

3.	PAIN SITE	(If pain present, **check all sites** that apply in last 7 days)			
		Back pain	a.	Incisional pain	f.
		Bone pain	b.	Joint pain (other than hip)	g.
		Chest pain while doing usual activities	c.	Soft tissue pain (e.g., lesion, muscle)	h.
		Headache	d.	Stomach pain	i.
		Hip pain	e.	Other	j.

4.	ACCIDENTS	(Check all that apply)		Hip fracture in last 180 days **17***	c.
		Fell in past 30 days **11, 17***	a.	Other fracture in last 180 days	d.
		Fell in past 31-180 days **11, 17***	b.	NONE OF ABOVE	e.

5.	STABILITY OF CONDITIONS	Conditions/diseases make resident's cognitive, ADL, mood or behavior patterns unstable—(fluctuating, precarious, or deteriorating)	a.
		Resident experiencing an acute episode or a flare-up of a recurrent or chronic problem	b.
		End-stage disease, 6 or fewer months to live	c.
		NONE OF ABOVE	d.

SECTION K. ORAL/NUTRITIONAL STATUS

1.	ORAL PROBLEMS	Chewing problem	a.
		Swallowing problem **17***	b.
		Mouth pain **15**	c.
		NONE OF ABOVE	d.

2.	HEIGHT AND WEIGHT	Record **(a.)** height in inches and **(b.)** weight in pounds. Base weight on most recent measure in **last 30 days**; measure weight consistently in accord with standard facility practice—e.g., in a.m. after voiding, before meal, with shoes off, and in nightclothes.		
		a. HT (in.)	b. WT (lb.)	

3.	WEIGHT CHANGE	a. Weight loss—5% or more in **last 30 days**; or 10% or more in **last 180 days** 0. No 1. Yes **12**	
		b. Weight gain—5% or more in **last 30 days**; or 10% or more in **last 180 days** 0. No 1. Yes	

4.	NUTRI- TIONAL PROBLEMS	Complains about the taste of many foods **12**	a.	Leaves 25% or more of food uneaten at most meals **12**	c.
		Regular or repetitive complaints of hunger	b.	NONE OF ABOVE	d.

5.	NUTRI- TIONAL APPROACH- ES	(Check all that apply in last 7 days)		Dietary supplement between meals	f.
		Parenteral/IV **12, 14**	a.	Plate guard, stabilized built-up utensil, etc.	g.
		Feeding tube **13, 14**	b.	On a planned weight change program	h.
		Mechanically altered diet **12**	c.	NONE OF ABOVE	i.
		Syringe (oral feeding) **12**	d.		
		Therapeutic diet **12**	e.		

6.	PARENTERAL OR ENTERAL INTAKE	**(Skip to Section L if neither 5a nor 5b is checked)** a. Code the proportion of **total calories** the resident received through parenteral or tube feedings in the **last 7 days**	
		0. None 3. 51% to 75% 1. 1% to 25% 4. 76% to 100% 2. 26% to 50%	
		b. Code the average **fluid intake** per day by IV or tube in **last 7 days** 0. None 3. 1001 to 1500 cc/day 1. 1 to 500 cc/day 4. 1501 to 2000 cc/day 2. 501 to 1000 cc/day 5. 2001 or more cc/day	

SECTION L. ORAL/DENTAL STATUS

1.	ORAL STATUS AND DISEASE PREVEN- TION	Debris (soft, easily movable substances) present in mouth prior to going to bed at night **15**	a.
		Has dentures or removable bridge	b.
		Some/all natural teeth lost—does not have or does not use dentures (or partial plates) **15**	c.
		Broken, loose, or carious teeth **15**	d.
		Inflamed gums (gingiva); swollen or bleeding gums; oral abscesses; ulcers or rashes **15**	e.
		Daily cleaning of teeth/dentures or daily mouth care—by resident or staff Not ✓ = **15**	f.
		NONE OF ABOVE	g.

SECTION M. SKIN CONDITION

1.	ULCERS (Due to any cause)	(Record the number of ulcers at each ulcer stage—regardless of cause. If none present at a stage, record "0" (zero). Code all that apply during **last 7 days**. Code 9 = 9 or more.) **[Requires full body exam.]**	Number at Stage
		a. Stage 1. A persistent area of skin redness (without a break in the skin) that does not disappear when pressure is relieved.	
		b. Stage 2. A partial thickness loss of skin layers that presents clinically as an abrasion, blister, or shallow crater.	
		c. Stage 3. A full thickness of skin is lost, exposing the sub-cutaneous tissues—presents as a deep crater with or without undermining adjacent tissue.	
		d. Stage 4. A full thickness of skin and subcutaneous tissue is lost, exposing muscle or bone.	

2.	TYPE OF ULCER	(For each type of ulcer, **code for the highest stage in the last 7 days** using scale in item M1—i.e., 0=none; stages 1, 2, 3, 4)	
		a. Pressure ulcer—any lesion caused by pressure resulting in damage of underlying tissue 1 = **16**; 2, 3, or 4 = **12, 16**	
		b. Stasis ulcer—open lesion caused by poor circulation in the lower extremities	

3.	HISTORY OF RESOLVED ULCERS	Resident had an ulcer that was resolved or cured in **LAST 90 DAYS** 0. No 1. Yes **16**	

4.	OTHER SKIN PROBLEMS OR LESIONS PRESENT	(Check all that apply during **last 7 days**)	
		Abrasions, bruises	a.
		Burns (second or third degree)	b.
		Open lesions other than ulcers, rashes, cuts (e.g., cancer lesions)	c.
		Rashes—e.g., intertrigo, eczema, drug rash, heat rash, herpes zoster	d.
		Skin desensitized to pain or pressure **16**	e.
		Skin tears or cuts (other than surgery)	f.
		Surgical wounds	g.
		NONE OF ABOVE	h.

5.	SKIN TREAT- MENTS	(Check all that apply during **last 7 days**)	
		Pressure relieving device(s) for chair	a.
		Pressure relieving device(s) for bed	b.
		Turning/repositioning program	c.
		Nutrition or hydration intervention to manage skin problems	d.
		Ulcer care	e.
		Surgical wound care	f.
		Application of dressings (with or without topical medications) other than to feet	g.
		Application of ointments/medications (other than to feet)	h.
		Other preventative or protective skin care (other than to feet)	i.
		NONE OF ABOVE	j.

6.	FOOT PROBLEMS AND CARE	(Check all that apply during **last 7 days**)	
		Resident has one or more foot problems—e.g., corns, calluses, bunions, hammer toes, overlapping toes, pain, structural problems	a.
		Infection of the foot—e.g., cellulitis, purulent drainage	b.
		Open lesions on the foot	c.
		Nails/calluses trimmed during **last 90 days**	d.
		Received preventative or protective foot care (e.g., used special shoes, inserts, pads, toe separators)	e.
		Application of dressings (with or without topical medications)	f.
		NONE OF ABOVE	g.

SECTION N. ACTIVITY PURSUIT PATTERNS

1.	TIME AWAKE	(Check appropriate time periods over last 7 days) Resident awake all or most of time (i.e., naps no more than one hour per time period) in the:			
	10B only if BOTH N1a = ✓ and N2 = 0	Morning **10B**	a.	Evening	c.
		Afternoon	b.	NONE OF ABOVE	d.

(IF RESIDENT IS COMATOSE, SKIP TO SECTION O)

2.	AVERAGE TIME INVOLVED IN ACTIVITIES	(When awake and not receiving treatments or ADL care) 0. Most—more than 2/3 of time **10B** 1. Some—from 1/3 to 2/3 of time	2. Little—less than 1/3 of time **10A** 3. None **10A**

3.	PREFERRED ACTIVITY SETTINGS	(Check all settings in which activities are **preferred**)			
		Own room	a.		
		Day/activity room	b.	Outside facility	d.
		Inside NH/off unit	c.	NONE OF ABOVE	e.

4.	GENERAL ACTIVITY PREFER- ENCES (Adapted to resident's current abilities)	(Check all PREFERENCES whether or not activity is currently available to resident)			
		Cards/other games	a.	Trips/shopping	g.
		Crafts/arts	b.	Walking/wheeling outdoors	h.
		Exercise/sports	c.	Watching TV	i.
		Music	d.	Gardening or plants	j.
		Reading/writing	e.	Talking or conversing	k.
		Spiritual/religious activities	f.	Helping others	l.
				NONE OF ABOVE	m.

TRIGGER LEGEND

10A - Activities (Revise)	**13** - Feeding Tubes	**17*** - Psychotropic Drugs
10B - Activities (Review)	**14** - Dehydration/Fluid Maintenance	(*For this to trigger, O4a, b, or c must = 1-7)
11 - Falls	**15** - Dental Care	
12 - Nutritional Status	**16** - Pressure Ulcers	

Form 1728RHH © 1997 Briggs Corporation, Des Moines, IA 50306 (800) 247-2343 PRINTED IN U.S.A. Copyright limited to addition of trigger system.

Resident ______ Numeric Identifier ______

5.	PREFERS CHANGE IN DAILY ROUTINE	*Code for resident preferences in daily routines* 0. No change 1. Slight change 2. Major change a. Type of activities in which resident is currently involved 1 or 2 = **10A** b. Extent of resident involvement in activities 1 or 2 = **10A**

SECTION O. MEDICATIONS

1.	NUMBER OF MEDICATIONS	***(Record the number of different** medications used in the **last 7 days**; enter "0" if none used)*
2.	NEW MEDICATIONS	*(Resident currently receiving medications that were initiated during the **last 90 days**)* 0. No 1. Yes
3.	INJECTIONS	***(Record the number of DAYS** injections of any type received during the **last 7 days**; enter "0" if none used)*
4.	DAYS RECEIVED THE FOLLOWING MEDICATION	***(Record the number of DAYS** during **last 7 days**; enter "0" if not used. Note—enter "1" for long-acting meds used less than weekly)* (**NOTE:** For **17** to actually be triggered, O4a, b, or c MUST = 1-7 AND at least one additional item marked **17*** must be indicated. See sections B, C, E, G, H, I, J, and K.) a. Antipsychotic 1-7 = **17** d. Hypnotic b. Antianxiety 1-7 = **11, 17** e. Diuretic 1-7 = **14** c. Antidepressant 1-7 = **11, 17**

SECTION P. SPECIAL TREATMENTS AND PROCEDURES

1.	SPECIAL TREATMENTS, PROCEDURES, AND PROGRAMS	**a. SPECIAL CARE**—*Check treatments or programs received during the **last 14 days***

TREATMENTS

Chemotherapy	a.
Dialysis	b.
IV medication	c.
Intake/output	d.
Monitoring acute medical condition	e.
Ostomy care	f.
Oxygen therapy	g.
Radiation	h.
Suctioning	i.
Tracheostomy care	j.
Transfusions	k.
Ventilator or respirator	l.

PROGRAMS

Alcohol/drug treatment program	m.
Alzheimer's/dementia special care unit	n.
Hospice care	o.
Pediatric unit	p.
Respite care	q.
Training in skills required to return to the community (e.g., taking medications, house work, shopping, transportation, ADLs)	r.
NONE OF ABOVE	s.

b. THERAPIES—*Record the number of days and total minutes each of the following therapies was administered (for at least 15 minutes a day) in the **last 7 calendar days** (Enter 0 if none or less than 15 min. daily)* **[Note—count only post admission therapies]**

(A) = # of days administered for **15 minutes or more**
(B) = **total # of minutes** provided in **last 7 days**

	DAYS (A)	MIN (B)
a. Speech-language pathology and audiology services		
b. Occupational therapy		
c. Physical therapy		
d. Respiratory therapy		
e. Psychological therapy (by any licensed mental health professional)		

2.	INTERVENTION PROGRAMS FOR MOOD, BEHAVIOR, COGNITIVE LOSS	(Check all interventions or strategies used in **last 7 days**—no matter where received)	
		Special behavior symptom evaluation program	a.
		Evaluation by a licensed mental health specialist in **last 90 days**	b.
		Group therapy	c.
		Resident-specific deliberate changes in the environment to address mood/behavior patterns—e.g., providing bureau in which to rummage	d.
		Reorientation—e.g., cueing	e.
		NONE OF ABOVE	f.
3.	NURSING REHABILITATION/ RESTORATIVE CARE	*Record the NUMBER OF DAYS each of the following rehabilitation or restorative techniques or practices was **provided to the resident for more than or equal to 15 minutes** per day in the **last 7 days** (Enter 0 if none or less than 15 min. daily.)*	

a. Range of motion (passive)	f. Walking
b. Range of motion (active)	g. Dressing or grooming
c. Splint or brace assistance	h. Eating or swallowing
TRAINING AND SKILL PRACTICE IN:	i. Amputation/ prosthesis care
d. Bed mobility	j. Communication
e. Transfer	k. Other

4.	DEVICES AND RESTRAINTS	*(Use the following codes for **last 7 days**:)* 0. Not used 1. Used less than daily 2. Used daily Bed rails a. —Full bed rails on all open sides of bed b. —Other types of side rails used (e.g., half rail, one side) c. Trunk restraint 1 = **11, 18**; 2 = **11, 16, 18** d. Limb restraint 1 or 2 = **18** e. Chair prevents rising 1 or 2 = **18**
5.	HOSPITAL STAY(S)	Record number of times resident was admitted to hospital with an overnight stay in **last 90 days** (or since last assessment if less than 90 days). *(Enter 0 if no hospital admissions)*
6.	EMERGENCY ROOM (ER) VISIT(S)	Record number of times resident visited ER without an overnight stay in **last 90 days** (or since last assessment if less than 90 days). *(Enter 0 if no ER visits)*
7.	PHYSICIAN VISITS	In the **LAST 14 DAYS** (or since admission if less than 14 days in facility) how many days has the physician (or authorized assistant or practitioner) examined the resident? *(Enter 0 if none)*
8.	PHYSICIAN ORDERS	In the **LAST 14 DAYS** (or since admission if less than 14 days in facility) how many days has the physician (or authorized assistant or practitioner) changed the resident's orders? *Do not include order renewals without change. (Enter 0 if none)*
9.	ABNORMAL LAB VALUES	Has the resident had any abnormal lab values during the **last 90 days** (or since admission)? 0. No 1. Yes

SECTION Q. DISCHARGE POTENTIAL AND OVERALL STATUS

1.	DISCHARGE POTENTIAL	a. Resident expresses/indicates preference to return to the community 0. No 1. Yes b. Resident has a support person who is positive toward discharge 0. No 1. Yes c. Stay projected to be of a short duration—discharge projected **within 90 days** (do not include expected discharge due to death) 0. No 1. Within 30 days 2. Within 31-90 days 3. Discharge status uncertain
2.	OVERALL CHANGE IN CARE NEEDS	Resident's overall self sufficiency has changed significantly as compared to status of **90 days ago** (or since last assessment if less than 90 days) 0. No change 1. Improved—receives fewer supports, needs less restrictive level of care 2. Deteriorated—receives more support

SECTION R. ASSESSMENT INFORMATION

1.	PARTICIPATION IN ASSESSMENT	a. Resident:	0. No	1. Yes	
		b. Family:	0. No	1. Yes	2. No family
		c. Significant other:	0. No	1. Yes	2. None

2. **SIGNATURES OF PERSONS COMPLETING THE ASSESSMENT:**

a. Signature of RN Assessment Coordinator (sign on above line)
b. Date RN Assessment Coordinator signed as complete ☐☐ – ☐☐ – ☐☐☐☐ (Month, Day, Year)

c. Other Signatures	Title	Sections	Date
d.			Date
e.			Date
f.			Date
g.			Date
h.			Date

TRIGGER LEGEND
10A - Activities (Revise)
11 - Falls
14 - Dehydration/Fluid Maintenance
16 - Pressure Ulcers
17 - Psychotropic Drugs
17* - For this to trigger, O4a, b, or c must = 1-7
18 - Physical Restraints

Form 1728RHH

MDS 2.0 1/30/98

Resident ______________________ Numeric Identifier ______________________

SECTION T. THERAPY SUPPLEMENT FOR MEDICARE PPS

1. SPECIAL TREATMENTS AND PROCEDURES

a. **RECREATION THERAPY**—*Enter number of days and total minutes of recreation therapy administered* ***(for at least 15 minutes a day)*** *in the* ***last 7 days*** *(Enter 0 if none)*

(A) = # **of days** administered for 15 minutes or more
(B) = **total # of minutes** provided in last 7 days

DAYS (A)	MIN (B)

Skip unless this is a Medicare 5 day or Medicare readmission/return assessment.

b. **ORDERED THERAPIES**—*Has physician ordered any of following therapies to begin in FIRST 14 days of stay—physical therapy, occupational therapy, or speech pathology service?*

0. No 1. Yes

If not ordered, skip to item 2

c. Through day 15, provide an estimate of the number of days when at least 1 therapy service can be expected to have been delivered.

d. Through day 15, provide an estimate of the number of therapy minutes (across the therapies) than can be expected to be delivered.

2. WALKING WHEN MOST SELF SUFFICIENT

Complete item 2 if ADL self-performance score for TRANSFER (G.1.b.A) is 0, 1, 2, or 3 AND at least one of the following are present:

- Resident received physical therapy involving gait training (**P.1.b.c**)
- Physical therapy was ordered for the resident involving gait training (**T.1.b**)
- Resident received nursing rehabilitation for walking (**P.3.f**)
- Physical therapy involving walking has been discontinued within the past 180 days

Skip to item 3 if resident did not walk in last 7 days

FOR FOLLOWING FIVE ITEMS, BASE CODING ON THE EPISODE WHEN THE RESIDENT WALKED THE FARTHEST WITHOUT SITTING DOWN. INCLUDE WALKING DURING REHABILITATION SESSIONS.)

a. **Furthest distance walked** without sitting down during this episode.

0. 150+ feet
1. 51-149 feet
2. 26-50 feet
3. 10-25 feet
4. Less than 10 feet

b. **Time walked** without sitting down during this episode.

0. 1-2 minutes
1. 3-4 minutes
2. 5-10 minutes
3. 11-15 minutes
4. 16-30 minutes
5. 31+ minutes

c. **Self-Performance in walking** during this episode.

0. *INDEPENDENT*—No help or oversight
1. *SUPERVISION*—Oversight, encouragement or cueing provided
2. *LIMITED ASSISTANCE*—Resident highly involved in walking; received physical help in guided maneuvering of limbs or other nonweight bearing assistance
3. *EXTENSIVE ASSISTANCE*—Resident received weight bearing assistance while walking

d. **Walking support provided** associated with this episode (code regardless of resident's self-performance classification).

0. No setup or physical help from staff
1. Setup help only
2. One person physical assist
3. Two+ persons physical assist

e. **Parallel bars** used by resident in association with this episode.

0. No 1. Yes

3. CASE MIX GROUP

Medicare ☐☐☐☐☐ **State** ☐☐☐☐☐

SECTION V. RESIDENT ASSESSMENT PROTOCOL SUMMARY Numeric Identifier______________

Resident's Name:	Medical Record No.:

1. Check if RAP is triggered.
2. For each triggered RAP, use the RAP guidelines to identify areas needing further assessment. Document relevant assessment information regarding the resident's status.
   - Describe:
     —Nature of the condition (may include presence or lack of objective data and subjective complaints).
     —Complications and risk factors that affect your decision to proceed to care planning.
     —Factors that must be considered in developing individualized care plan interventions.
     —Need for referrals/further evaluation by appropriate health professionals.
   - Documentation should support your decision-making regarding whether to proceed with a care plan for a triggered RAP and the type(s) of care plan interventions that are appropriate for a particular resident.
   - Documentation may appear anywhere in the clinical record (e.g., progress notes, consults, flowsheets, etc.).
3. Indicate under the Location of RAP Assessment Documentation column where information related to the RAP assessment can be found.
4. For each triggered RAP, indicate whether a new care plan, care plan revision, or continuation of current care plan is necessary to address the problem(s) identified in your assessment. The Care Planning Decision column must be completed within 7 days of completing the RAI (MDS and RAPs).

A. RAP Problem Area	(a) Check if Triggered	Location and Date of RAP Assessment Documentation	(b) Care Planning Decision—check if addressed in care plan
1. DELIRIUM			
2. COGNITIVE LOSS			
3. VISUAL FUNCTION			
4. COMMUNICATION			
5. ADL FUNCTIONAL/ REHABILITATION POTENTIAL			
6. URINARY INCONTINENCE AND INDWELLING CATHETER			
7. PSYCHOSOCIAL WELL-BEING			
8. MOOD STATE			
9. BEHAVIORAL SYMPTOMS			
10. ACTIVITIES			
11. FALLS			
12. NUTRITIONAL STATUS			
13. FEEDING TUBES			
14. DEHYDRATION/FLUID MAINTENANCE			
15. ORAL/DENTAL CARE			
16. PRESSURE ULCERS			
17. PSYCHOTROPIC DRUG USE			
18. PHYSICAL RESTRAINTS			

B. ______________________________________ 2. ☐☐ – ☐☐ – ☐☐☐☐

1. Signature of RN Coordinator for RAP Assessment Process — Month Day Year

______________________________________ 4. ☐☐ – ☐☐ – ☐☐☐☐

3. Signature of Person Completing Care Planning Decision — Month Day Year

Form 1728RHH

MDS 2.0 1/30/98

APPENDIX B

NNAAP™ SKILL

National Nurse Aide Assessment Program (NNAAP™) Written Examination Content Outline

The NNAAP Written Examination is comprised of seventy (70) multiple choice questions. Ten (10) of these questions are pre-test (non-scored) questions on which statistical information will be collected.

I. Physical Care Skills

A. Activities of Daily Living .... *12% of exam*
1. Hygiene
2. Dressing and Grooming
3. Nutrition and Hydration
4. Elimination
5. Rest/Sleep/Comfort

B. Basic Nursing Skills .... *29% of exam*
1. Infection Control
2. Safety/Emergency
3. Therapeutic/Technical Procedures
4. Data Collection and Reporting

C. Restorative Skills .... *6% of exam*
1. Prevention
2. Self Care/Independence

II. Psychosocial Care Skills

A. Emotional and Mental Health Needs .... *20% of exam*
B. Spiritual and Cultural Needs .. *2% of exam*

III. Role of the Nurse Aide

A. Communication .... *6% of exam*
B. Client Rights .... *14% of exam*
C. Legal and Ethical Behavior .... *3% of exam*
D. Member of the Health Care Team .... *8% of exam*

National Nurse Aide Assessment Program (NNAAP™) Skills Examination*

LIST OF SKILLS

1. Washes hands
2. Measures and records weight of ambulatory client
3. Provides mouth care
4. Dresses client with affected right arm
5. Transfers client from bed to wheelchair
6. Assists client to ambulate
7. Cleans and stores dentures
8. Performs passive range of motion on one shoulder
9. Performs passive range of motion on one knee and one ankle
10. Measures and records urinary output
11. Assists client with use of bedpan
12. Provides perineal care for incontinent client
13. Provides catheter care
14. Takes and records oral temperature
15. Takes and records radial pulse and counts and records respirations

16a. Takes and records client's blood pressure (one-step procedure)

16b. Takes and records client's blood pressure (two-step procedure)

17. Puts one knee-high elastic stocking on client
18. Makes an occupied bed
19. Provides foot care
20. Provides fingernail care
21. Feeds client who cannot feed self
22. Positions client on side
23. Gives modified bed bath (face, and one arm, hand, and underarm)
24. Shampoos client's hair in bed

Courtesy of the National Council of State Boards of Nursing, Chicago, Illinois.

Prepared by ASI for the National Nurse Aide Assessment Program (NNAAP™) © 1998 by ASI Suite 300, Three Bala Plaza West • Bala Cynwyd, PA 19004-3481 • (610) 617-9300

***All states do not participate in the program. Such states have other arrangements for nurse aide competency and evaluation program.**

Index

B

C

D

O

U

KEY TERMS—cont'd

Omnibus Budget Reconciliation Act of 1987 (OBRA) A federal law concerned with the quality of life, health, and safety of residents

primary nursing A method of organizing nursing care; a nurse is responsible for the total care of specific residents on a 24-hour basis

private insurance plan An insurance plan bought by an individual

registered nurse (RN) An individual who has studied nursing for 2, 3, or 4 years and who has passed a licensing examination

residential care facility A board and care facility or an assisted living facility

restorative aide A nursing assistant with special training in rehabilitation skills

skilled nursing facility (SNF) A facility that provides nursing care for residents who need complex care but do not need hospital services; may be part of a nursing center or a hospital

subacute care Complex medical care or rehabilitation

supportive care Care provided on a 24-hour basis that meets a person's basic physical needs

team nursing A method of organizing nursing care; a nurse serves as a team leader; the team leader assigns other nurses and nursing assistants to care for certain residents

This chapter describes the purposes, goals, and services of long-term care. Emphasis is given to nursing centers that employ nursing assistants. The chapter also describes the organization of nursing centers, the nursing team, private and government insurance programs, and some of the federal laws regarding resident care.

LONG-TERM CARE CENTERS

Long-term care centers provide health care services to persons unable to care for themselves at home but who do not need hospital care. Services range from supportive care to very complex care. Medical, nursing, dietary, recreational, rehabilitative, and social services are provided.

Persons living in long-term care centers are called *residents,* not patients. The center is their permanent or temporary home. Long-term care centers are designed and constructed to meet the special needs of elderly or disabled residents. Some residents return home when well enough. Others require nursing care until death occurs.

Board and Care Facilities

A **board and care facility** (**assisted living facility** or **residential care facility**) often is in a home setting. It also may be a separate wing or building of a nursing center. Supportive care is provided. **Supportive care** is care that is provided on a 24-hour basis and that meets the person's basic physical needs. A safe environment is provided for persons who need supervision but not 24-hour nursing care. Services include three meals a day, housekeeping, laundry services, transportation, a 24-hour caregiver, an emergency call system, personal care, and medication reminders. Residents need very little assistance with personal care. They usually can dress and tend to grooming and bathroom needs with little assistance. The caregiver may be a nursing assistant. In many states, board and care facilities are regulated and require a license.

Nursing Centers

A **nursing center** provides heath care services to residents who require regular or continuous care. **Nursing facility (NF)** and **nursing home** are other names. A licensed nursing staff is required. Residents usually have more severe health problems than do persons in board and care facilities. Services range from supportive care to more complex care. Medical, nursing, dietary, recreational, rehabilitative, and social services usually are provided. Licensed nurses, nursing assistants, physical therapists, dietary personnel, and other health care workers are needed to provide such services (p. 5). These employees have specific skills and knowledge. The focus of their care is always on the residents.

Some nursing centers also provide more complex care. They are called **skilled nursing facilities (SNFs).** A part of the center (skilled nursing unit) is reserved for residents with more severe health problems. These residents have many health problems but do not require hospital services. Many residents are admitted to SNFs directly from a hospital. They stay for a short time to recover from an illness or surgery or to be rehabilitated. Others do not recover enough to return home. These residents transfer to other types of centers or become permanent residents of the nursing center. *(See Subacute Care, p. 4.)*

Subacute Care

Some long-term care centers provide **subacute care**—complex medical care or rehabilitation for persons who no longer need hospital care. Subacute care is provided on special units. Persons on these units may be called *patients.* The length of stay on a subacute unit is usually short. Many patients get well and go home. Some may need long-term care until death.

SNFs and subacute units may also be in hospitals. Persons in a hospital-based SNF or subacute unit are called patients because they stay for a short time. They usually transfer to another SNF or nursing center after a few weeks.

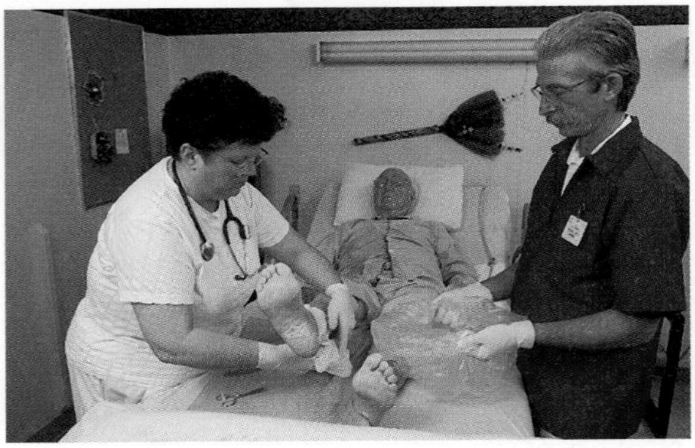

Fig. 1-1 A nursing assistant helping an RN give care to a resident.

Purposes and goals of nursing centers

Nursing centers have several purposes. Most residents suffer from one or more chronic illnesses. One goal is to *promote good physical and mental health.* Residents are helped to accept the limits of their chronic diseases and to function within those limits. Residents are helped to change habits that can make their illnesses worse. They are encouraged to eat proper diets and to get the proper amount and type of exercise. They also are encouraged to focus on their abilities rather than their disabilities and to do as much for themselves as possible.

Families need to accept the physical and mental changes that they see in their loved ones. They are helped to understand the reasons for these physical and mental changes. They are taught how to assist their loved ones to maintain the highest possible level of functioning and to accept the limits of the chronic illnesses.

Preventing communicable disease is another goal. A communicable disease can be spread from one person to another (see Chapter 9). Communicable diseases—(for example, colds and influenza (flu)—can create major health problems for older and disabled persons. You are involved in resident care. You may be the first person to detect the signs and symptoms of a communicable disease.

Treating chronic illness is another major goal. A **chronic illness** is slow or gradual in onset. There is no known cure. The illness can be controlled and complications can be prevented with proper treatment. Chronic illness is different from acute illness. An **acute illness** begins suddenly. The person is expected to recover. Persons with acute illnesses may need hospital care.

Nurses observe residents for changes in health status. Nurses are involved in the treatment of illness by giving care and carrying out therapeutic measures ordered by doctors. You assist nurses. Therefore you are involved in observing and caring for residents (Fig. 1-1).

Rehabilitation or *restorative care* is aimed at helping residents return to their highest possible level of physical and mental functioning. In the past, rehabilitation focused primarily on persons who could return home. Now all residents are helped to become or remain as independent as possible. This includes those residents who will be in nursing centers for the rest of their life.

Restorative care begins when a person is admitted to the center. Often residents are deconditioned after an acute illness. **Deconditioning** is the process of becoming weak from illness or the lack of exercise. Disabilities can result from strokes, fractures, or surgery. Many health care workers are involved in helping the person become as independent as possible. These include physical therapists, occupational therapists, speech/language therapists, and restorative aides. **Restorative aides** are nursing assistants with special rehabilitation training. They assist other health care workers in the restorative program. The entire staff follows the rehabilitation program. They help residents reach and maintain their highest level of functioning.

Other services. Some nursing centers provide educational experiences for students. The students may be studying to become nurses, nursing assistants, nurse practitioners, or other health team members. Medical students also study in nursing centers. All students are concerned with the center's purposes and goals. They assist in promoting health, treating illness, and preventing communicable disease. They also assist with restorative care.

Nursing centers provide dietary, respiratory therapy, recreational therapy, and social services. Some also provide laboratory and portable x-ray services. Many centers have special units for different types of care. These include hospice and Alzheimer's disease units.

- *Hospice units*—A **hospice** is a health care agency or program for persons who are dying. The physical, emotional, social, and spiritual needs of the person and family are provided for in a setting that allows much freedom. Children and pets usually can visit at any time. Family and friends can take part in giving care. Hospice care is provided by hospitals, long-term care centers, and home care agencies.
- *Alzheimer's units (dementia care units)*—An Alzheimer's unit is designed for residents with **Alzheimer's disease** and other types of dementia (see Chapter 27). Alzheimer's disease affects brain tissue. Affected persons suffer increasing memory loss and confusion until they cannot take care of their own simplest personal needs. Eventually, they may forget their own name. They often wander about and may become agitated or even combative. The Alzheimer's unit usually is closed off from the rest of the center. Keeping the unit closed provides a safer environment for these special residents to wander freely. Alzheimer's disease is progressive. Because they no longer wander during the middle and end stages of the disease, residents may no longer need a closed unit. They are cared for on other units in the nursing center. Special programming is required to meet the needs of residents with Alzheimer's disease (see Chapter 27).

Nursing Center Organization

Nursing centers usually are owned by an individual or by a corporation. The owner is responsible for making sure that the center provides adequate and safe care at the lowest possible cost. The owner must make sure that local, state, and federal regulations are followed. The owner makes center policies and hires others to manage the center. Corporate-owned centers usually have a regional manager. The regional manager hires an administrator for the center. If the center is privately owned, the owner also may be the center's administrator.

In larger centers, department directors report to the administrator (Fig. 1-2, p. 6). A finance director is responsible for resident billing. Housekeeping, maintenance, and laundry supervisors are common positions. A social services director focuses on the social needs of residents and their families. Activity directors or recreational therapists plan and organize resident activities. A director of staff development is responsible for staff training and in-service programs. Federal law requires that all nursing centers have a medical director. The medical director is a doctor who is a consultant to the staff for all medical problems not handled by a resident's personal doctor. The medical director also helps guide resident care policies and programs. The director of nursing is in charge of the entire nursing staff and the activities involved in providing safe nursing care to residents. The nursing service department is discussed later in this chapter.

The Interdisciplinary Health Care Team

The **interdisciplinary health care team** involves a variety of workers whose skills and knowledge are directed to the total care of the resident (Table 1-1, pp. 7-8). Team members provide supportive services for the overall goal of quality resident care. They work together to meet each resident's needs. Because many health care workers are involved in the care of each resident, coordination of care is needed. The nursing staff usually is responsible for coordinating care. An RN serves in the key leadership position. Figure 1-3 on p. 9 shows the members of the interdisciplinary health care team, with the resident as the focus of all health care workers.

Nursing Service

Nursing service is a major department in nursing centers. The director of nursing (DON) is responsible for the entire nursing staff. This includes the activities involved in giving safe resident care. Nurse managers (usually RNs) assist the DON in managing and carrying out the nursing department functions. Nurse managers may be responsible for a shift worked or a specific nursing department function. A nursing function may be staff development, restorative nursing, infection control, or continuous quality improvement. There may be shift supervisors. They coordinate resident care for each shift. Each unit usually has a nurse in charge. The nurse in charge usually is an RN but may be an LPN/LVN in some states. The nurse in charge is responsible for all resident care and the actions of nursing staff on a unit. Staff RNs report to the nurse in charge. LPNs/LVNs report to staff RNs or to the nurse in charge. You report to the RN or LPN/LVN supervising your work.

Nursing education or staff development personnel plan and present educational programs to the nursing team. They provide new and changing information so that current and safe care is given. They also provide information on new equipment. This staff also may educate and train nursing assistants. They also conduct new employee orientation programs.

THE NURSING TEAM

The **nursing team** involves RNs, LPNs/LVNs, and nursing assistants. Each has a different role and responsibilities. All are concerned with the physical, social, emotional, and spiritual needs of residents and families.

Text continued on p. 9

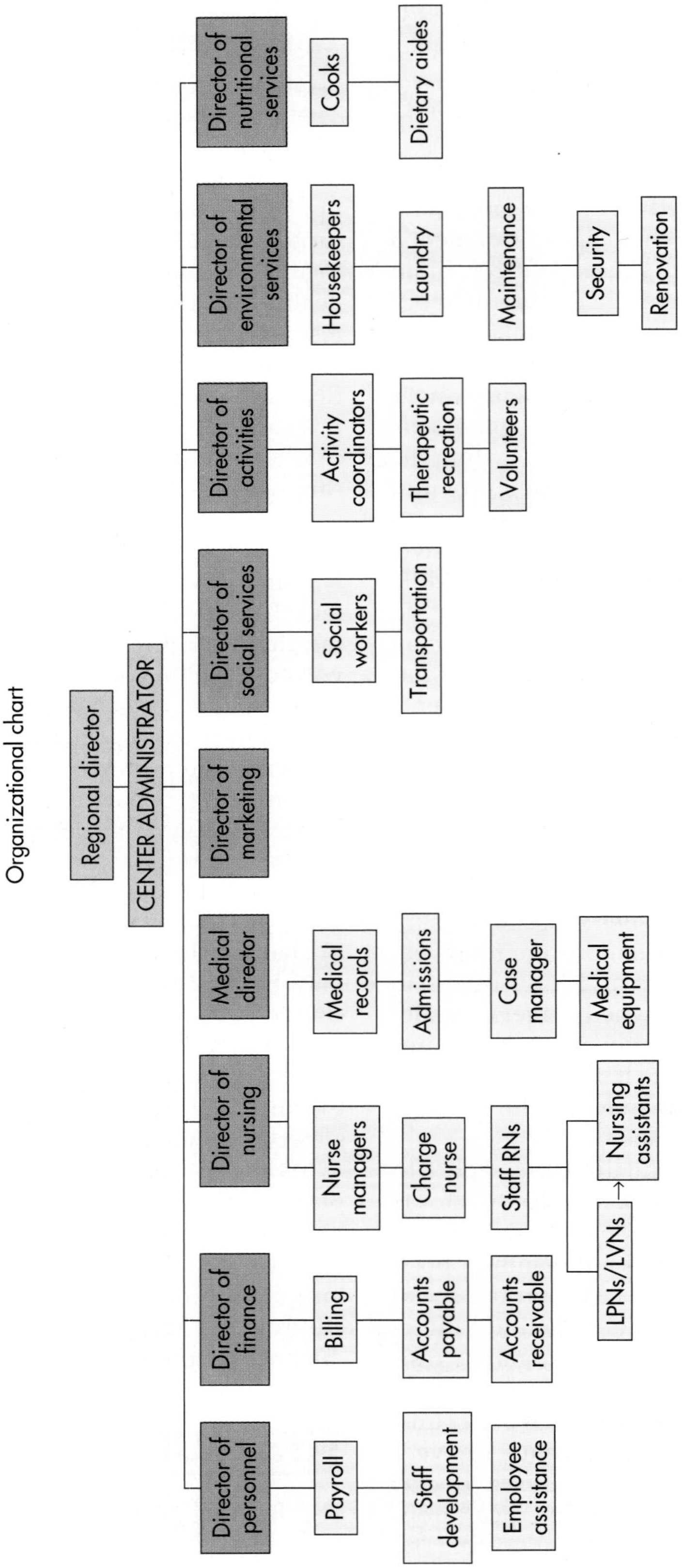

Fig. 1-2 Organization of a nursing center.

Table 1-1 Members of the Interdisciplinary Health Care Team

Title	Description	Credentials
Activities Director	Works in nursing centers; assesses, plans, and implements recreational needs of residents	Required training varies with state and/or center policies; ranges from no required training to bachelor's degree
Audiologist	Tests hearing; prescribes hearing aids; and works with hearing impaired persons	Master's degree in audiology, 1 year of supervised employment, and a national examination
Chaplain	Works in all types of health care settings to assist patients and residents with their spiritual needs	Priest, minister, rabbi, sister, deacon, or other pastoral training
Dental Hygienist	Focuses on prevention of dental disorders; works under direction of a licensed dentist	Graduation from accredited dental hygiene program and state licensure
Dentist	Prevents and treats disorders and diseases of the teeth, gums, and oral structures	Doctor of Dental Science (DDS) and state licensure
Dietitian	Assesses and plans for nutritional needs of patients and residents; teaches individuals and families about good nutrition, food selection, and preparation	Bachelor's degree; Registered Dietitians (RD) must pass national registration examination; some states require licensure
Licensed Practical/ Vocational Nurse (LPN/LVN)	Provides direct patient/resident care, including adminstering medications, under the direction of an RN	Graduate of a state-approved program (usually 1 year in length) and state licensure
Medical Laboratory Technician	Collects samples and performs laboratory tests on blood, urine, and other body fluids	Graduate of a 2-year program and national certifying examination; state licensure may be required
Medical Records Technician	Maintains medical records for legal and insurance purposes; transcribes medical reports, files records, and completes required reports	Graduates of two-year programs take the national Accredited Record Technician (ART) examination
Nursing Assistant	Assists RNs and LPNs/LVNs; gives direct bedside patient/resident care; must be supervised by a licensed nurse	Completion of state-approved training program (federal law requires at least 75 hours of training); successful completion of competency evaluation (written and skills test)
Occupational Therapist	Assists individuals to learn or regain the skills needed to perform activities of daily living; designs adaptive equipment for activities of daily living	Bachelor of Science degree in occupational therapy and national certification; state licensure may be required
Occupational Therapy Assistant	Performs tasks and services under supervision of occupational therapist	Graduation from accredited program (usually 2 years in length) and national certification; state licensure may be required

Continued

CONT'D TABLE 1-1 MEMBERS OF THE INTERDISCIPLINARY HEALTH CARE TEAM

Title	Description	Credentials
Pharmacist	Fills medication and prescription orders written by physician; monitors and evaluates drug interactions; consults with physicians and nurses regarding drug actions and interactions	Bachelor of Science in Pharmacy and state licensure
Physical Therapist	Assists persons with musculoskeletal problems; focuses on restoring function and preventing disability from illness or injury	Bachelor of Science in physical therapy and state licensure
Physical Therapy Assistant	Performs selected physical therapy tasks and functions under direction of physical therapist	Associate degree from accredited program; national certification required in many states
Physician (Doctor)	Diagnoses and treats diseases and injuries	Medical school graduation, residency, and National Board Examination; state licensure
Physician's Assistant	Assists physician in diagnosis and treatment of ill and injured persons; able to perform many medical tasks under direction of physician	Completion of required training program and national certification; state licensure may be required
Podiatrist	Prevents, diagnoses, and treats foot disorders	Doctor of Podiatric Medicine (DPM) and state and/or national board examination
Radiographer/ Radiologic Technologist	Takes x-rays ordered by physician and processes film for viewing	Graduation from accredited program and National Registry Examination
Registered Nurse (RN)	Assesses, makes nursing diagnoses, plans, implements, and evaluates nursing care; supervises LPNs and nursing assistants	Graduate of state-approved nursing program with associate degree, diploma, or bachelor's degree; state licensure
Respiratory Therapist	Assists in treatment of lung and heart disorders; gives respiratory treatments and therapies ordered by physician	Graduation from a 1- or 2-year program and certification by National Board of Respiratory Therapy
Social Worker	Helps residents and families deal with social, emotional, and environmental issues affecting illness and recovery; coordinates community agencies to assist patient and family	Bachelor of Social Work (BSW) or Master of Social Work (MSW)
Speech-Language Pathologist	Evaluates speech and language and treats persons with speech, voice, hearing, and communication disorders	Master's degree in speech/ language pathology, 1 year supervised work experience, and national examination